W9-BMS-949

Ultrasound THE REQUISITES

SERIES EDITOR

James H. Thrall, MD
Radiologist-in-Chief
Department of Radiology
Massachusetts General Hospital
Boston, Massachusetts

OTHER VOLUMES IN THE REQUISITES™ SERIES

Gastrointestinal Radiology

Pediatric Radiology

Neuroradiology

Nuclear Medicine

Cardiac Radiology

Genitourinary Radiology

Musculoskeletal Imaging

Mammography

Vascular and Interventional Radiology

Thoracic Imaging

Ultrasound

THE REQUISITES

Second Edition

William D. Middleton, MD, FACR
Professor of Radiology
Mallinckrodt Institute of Radiology
Washington University School of Medicine
St. Louis, Missouri

Alfred B. Kurtz, MD, FACR
Professor of Radiology
Jefferson Medical College
Thomas Jefferson University
Philadelphia, Pennsylvania

Barbara S. Hertzberg, MD, FACR
Professor of Radiology
Associate Professor of Obstetrics and Gynecology
Co-Director, Fetal Diagnostic Center
Duke University Medical Center
Durham, North Carolina

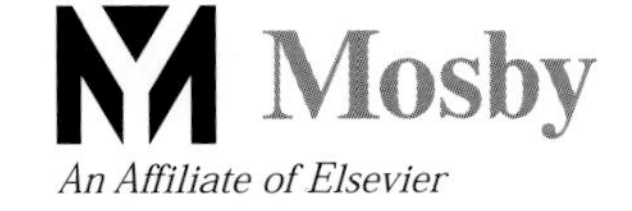

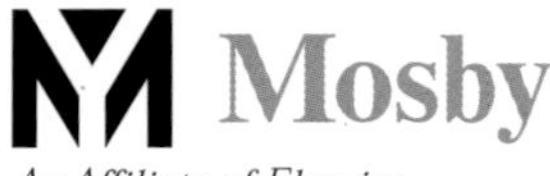

An Affiliate of Elsevier

11830 Westline Industrial Drive
St. Louis, Missouri 63146

THE REQUISITES™
THE REQUISITES
THE REQUISITES
THE REQUISITES
THE REQUISITES

Publishing Director, Surgery: Richard Lampert
Developmental Editor: Christy Bracken
Acquisitions Editor: Hilarie Surrena
Project Manager: Norman Stellander
Book Designer: Ellen Zanolle
CE/HYP

ULTRASOUND: THE REQUISITES ISBN 0-323-01702-9

Notice

Radiology is an ever-changing field. Standard safety precautions must be followed, but as new research and clinical experience broaden our knowledge, changes in treatment and drug therapy may become necessary or appropriate. Readers are advised to check the most current product information provided by the manufacturer of each drug to be administered to verify the recommended dose, the method and duration of administration, and contraindications. It is the responsibility of the treating physician, relying on experience and knowledge of the patient, to determine dosages and the best treatment for each individual patient. Neither the publisher nor the editor assumes any liability for any injury and/or damage to persons or property arising from this publication.

The Publisher

Library of Congress Cataloging-in-Publication Data

Middleton, William D.
Ultrasound : the requisites / William D. Middleton, Albert B. Kurtz, Barbara S. Hertzberg.
p. cm.
Includes index.
ISBN 0-323-01702-9
1. Diagnosis, Ultrasonic. I. Kurtz, Alfred B. II. Hertzberg, Barbara S. III. Title.

RC78.7.U4M533 2004
616.07'543–dc22

2003065106

Printed in China

Last digit is the print number: 9 8 7 6 5 4 3 2

To our families:

Our parents, Bill and Joyce, Lenard and Esther, and Julius and Sunny, who tirelessly fostered our growth and blessed our lives with constant love, support, and encouragement.

Our spouses, Mary, Barbara, and Mike, who recognized our love of teaching and accepted the time commitment required to complete a project of this magnitude.

Our children, B.I. and Dana; Amy, Liza, and Dana; and Brian, Jeffrey, and Andrew; who will see this book and perhaps understand that from effort and dedication comes knowledge and satisfaction.

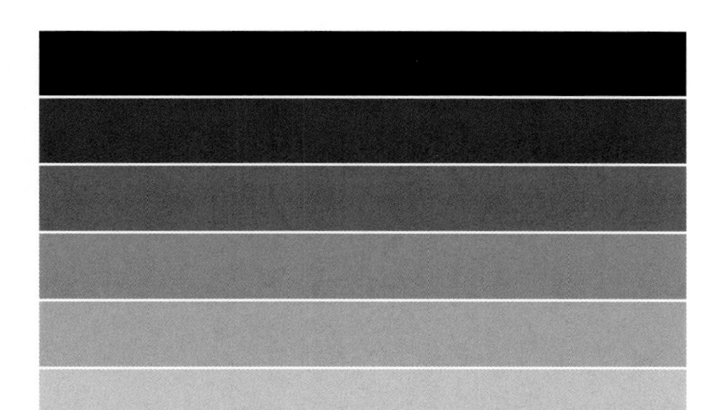

Foreword

The first edition of *Ultrasound: The Requisites* was extremely well received in the entire radiology community for its high quality and thoughtful selection of material presented. The second edition promises to be even better while maintaining the goal of concentrating on the most important core material in the major clinical applications of ultrasound. By the same token, the field of ultrasound has evolved and expanded enormously since the first edition. Drs. Kurtz and Middleton have invited Dr. Barbara S. Hertzberg to join them to take advantage of her substantial knowledge and experience and to help with the formidable task of ensuring that all material in their book is up-to-date and in keeping with current practice.

One of the ongoing challenges in structuring any textbook devoted to ultrasound is the diversity between departments of radiology in how diagnostic ultrasound is both practiced and taught. While it is the case that some institutions approach ultrasound as a modality embracing all applications and other departments incorporate ultrasound into an organ system approach to specialization, the knowledge base is the same. Mindful of this the authors of the second edition of *Ultrasound: The Requisites* maintain the excellent approach adopted in the original book of making each chapter a self-contained unit that covers the relevant clinical applications by organ system and related technical considerations.

The chapter outline of the current edition of *Ultrasound: The Requisites* has changed significantly from that of the first edition to reflect changes in clinical applications but also to address the increasing importance of understanding the physical principles contributing to ultrasound images. Thus, the first chapter is now devoted to "Practical Physics" and is a welcome addition for anyone performing ultrasound on a regular basis. What has not changed is the author's dedication to providing the best illustrative material available, and the second edition is again richly endowed with high-quality images. Material in the text is again reinforced in tables and boxes, allowing the reader to quickly review differential diagnoses and alternative etiologies of sonographic findings.

With the extensive restructuring, the addition of new chapters, and the replacement of many original images with fresh new examples, one could argue that the second edition of *Ultrasound: The Requisites* is really a brand new book. However, what is even more important is the continued unique ability of the authors to connect with the reader and to present very sophisticated and often difficult material in an accessible "reader friendly" manner.

I believe that residents in radiology will find the second edition of *Ultrasound: The Requisites* to again be an excellent vehicle for introducing themselves to the subject. The text continues to provide both basic and state-of-the-art information in all chapters. As noted, this book exemplifies the philosophy of the entire Requisites series. That is, the book can be read and reread during successive ultrasound rotations during a residency program so that material becomes familiar. Physicians in practice and in fellowship programs should also continue to find *Ultrasound: The Requisites* attractive for the same reasons—it is a concise way to expand or refresh their knowledge in this subspecialty area.

The Requisites series has been out for over a decade. The philosophy of the series is that when well done "less can be more" has proven to be robust and well received by residents, fellows, and practicing radiologists alike. The key has indeed been the selectivity of material and quality of presentation rather than more pages of text. Each book represents the respective authors' best assessment of what is truly important in their respective areas of expertise.

The books in the series have never been intended to be exhaustive but instead provide the basic conceptional, factual, and interpretive material required for clinical practice.

I congratulate Drs. Middleton, Kurtz, and Hertzberg for their outstanding new contribution to the Requisites in Radiology series. It is truly a tour de force that will benefit its readers and their patients.

James H. Thrall, MD

Radiologist-in-Chief
Massachusetts General Hospital
Professor of Radiology
Harvard Medical School

Preface

The first edition of *Ultrasound: The Requisites* started with the concept of presenting complex material in an uncomplicated way. Rather than a large, all-encompassing tome, we had hoped that our final product would be a book that each resident could read during a short time on an ultrasound rotation. We had further hoped that every time the resident returned to the book, further insight into ultrasound could be obtained. We were most gratified by the feedback of residents and felt that our efforts in writing the first edition of the book had been well worth the time and effort.

As ultrasound has expanded, so has the need for a second edition. We had anticipated that advances in technology and new and revised understanding of clinical matters would necessitate a revision within 6 to 8 years. That turned out to be correct, and approximately 5 years after the first edition was published, we began work on the second edition. The most important initial decision was to include Dr. Barbara Hertzberg as an additional author. We believe that our unique and shared experience, talents, and knowledge have combined to allow for a more thorough review of the field of ultrasonography.

We had been told that to qualify as a new edition, we would need to change 30% of the original book. But the three of us felt that even more was needed to keep the book on pace with the advances in sonography. We have therefore added new chapters and have reorganized older chapters to allow for additional material and a better flow of information. A new physics chapter has been added to explain the practical aspects of ultrasound physics and common artifacts. We have included a new chapter on general abdominal conditions that covers abnormalities that did not fit into any of the organ-specific chapters of the first edition. We have added new material on the lower genitourinary tract and the chest and have significantly expanded musculoskeletal sonography. The chapters covering first trimester pregnancy and ectopic pregnancy have been integrated, and the material on ectopic pregnancy has been expanded. New material has also been added on a variety of fetal abnormalities.

Since images are everything (or at least are very important), we have replaced most of the images from the first edition with new and more current examples and we have dramatically increased the total number of images. We have also altered our approach to the figures. Whenever possible, we have tried to combine, in one figure, as many images as necessary to illustrate the full spectrum of a particular condition. We believe that this makes it easier for the reader to quickly grasp the important sonographic characteristics of commonly seen abnormalities and allows the reader to appreciate when there is overlap in the appearance of different lesions. We also believe that these figures will provide an easy visual reference when the practicing radiologist encounters an abnormality in real life and is attempting to develop a differential diagnosis.

All told, this second edition of *Ultrasound: The Requisites* is a very different book from the first edition. Yet with all of these changes, we have tried to maintain the essential qualities of the first edition that made it so popular, adhering to the principle that it is better to master a simplified version of a field than to misunderstand or forget a complicated version. We sincerely hope that the innovations introduced in this new edition lead to a continued improvement, understanding, and appreciation of the art and practice of ultrasonography.

William D. Middleton
Alfred B. Kurtz
Barbara S. Hertzberg

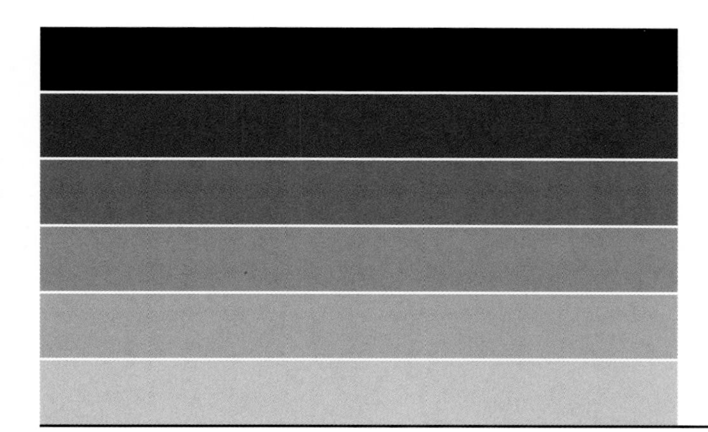

Acknowledgments

Many people contributed to the production of this book. We would like to thank all of our colleagues who have performed the much-needed clinical work while we worked on this project. We are indebted to the hard work and skill of the sonographers we work with. Their dedication and commitment led to the creation of many of these wonderful images. We acknowledge our secretaries who assisted in ways that are too numerous to list but without whose efforts this book would not have been possible. Most importantly, we recognize the intense desire to learn ultrasound shown by the radiology residents at the Mallinckrodt Institute of Radiology, Thomas Jefferson University, and Duke University. Their devotion has inspired us to try to produce a text worthy of their efforts, as well as the efforts of residents and practicing physicians throughout this country and abroad.

Contents

General and Vascular

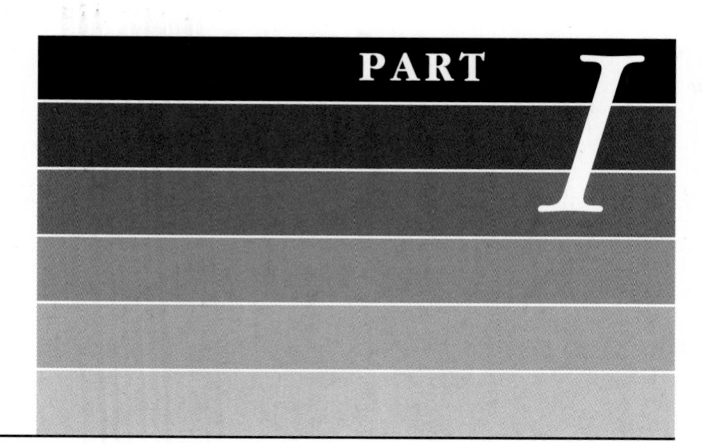

CHAPTER 1

Practical Physics

For Key Features summary see p. 26

Sonography has been a valuable method of imaging the body for many years. One of the most important of the many reasons sonography is an especially attractive technique is its lack of ionizing radiation. Sonography can provide clinically useful information without clinically significant biologic effects on the patient. This is especially critical in obstetrics and is also very important in the pediatric patient population. A second unique aspect of sonography is the real-time nature of the examination. This makes it possible to evaluate rapidly moving structures such as the heart and easier to examine the fetus and patients who cannot suspend respiration or cannot cooperate. A third advantage of sonography is its multiplanar imaging capability. Real-time equipment and three-dimensional capabilities make possible great flexibility in the selection of imaging planes and the ease of altering these planes, which allows for rapid determination of the origin of pathologic masses and analysis of spatial relationships of various structures. The portable nature of the equipment is another advantage that sonography has over other cross-sectional modalities such as computed tomography (CT) and magnetic resonance imaging (MRI). Another advantage of sonography is its excellent resolution of superficial structures. Doppler techniques add the advantage of qualitative and quantitative evaluation of blood flow. Finally, in the era of medical cost containment, sonography is an attractive imaging study for many clinical problems, especially in situations in which multiple sequential examinations are necessary or when screening of large patient populations is desired. All of these factors make sonography an extremely valuable tool in the investigation of a vast array of disorders.

Any radiologist who performs diagnostic sonography must have an understanding of the physical principles of this technique and the instrumentation available for detecting and displaying the acoustic information. In this chapter the discussion is limited to the practical physical principles that are most relevant to the practice of diagnostic ultrasound evaluation.

ACOUSTICS

Sound is the result of mechanical energy that produces alternating compression and rarefaction of the conducting medium as it travels in the form of a wave. Human hearing encompasses a range from 20 hertz (Hz) to 20 kilohertz (kHz). Ultrasound differs from audible sound only in its higher frequency, hence the name "ultrasound" (i.e., >20 kHz). Diagnostic sonography generally operates at frequencies of 1 to 20 megahertz (MHz).

Ultrasound uses short sound pulses that are transmitted into the body. The velocity of propagation is constant for a given tissue and is not affected by the frequency or wavelength of the pulse. The more closely packed the molecules, the faster the speed of sound. So in biologic tissues, the speed of sound is lowest in gases, faster in fluid, faster yet in soft tissue, and fastest in bones. In soft tissues, the assumed average propagation velocity is 1540 m/sec.

Sound pulses transmitted into the body can be reflected, scattered, refracted, or absorbed. Reflection or backscatter occurs whenever the pulse encounters an interface between tissues that have different acoustic impedances. Acoustic impedance is the product of the speed of sound and the tissue density. The strength of reflection depends on the difference in acoustic impedance between the tissues as well as the size of the interface, its surface characteristics, and its orientation with respect to the transmitted sound pulse. The greater the acoustic impedance mismatch, the greater the backscatter or reflection. Large interfaces that are smooth are referred to as specular reflectors. If specular reflectors are oriented perpendicular to the direction of the transmitted pulse, they will reflect the sound directly back to the active crystal elements in the transducer and produce a strong signal. Specular reflectors not oriented perpendicular to the sound will produce a weaker signal. Scattering refers to the redirection of sound in multiple directions. Scattering produces a weak signal and occurs when the pulse encounters a small acoustic interface or large interface that is rough. The results of these interactions are illustrated in Figure 1-1.

Refraction refers to a change in the direction of the sound and occurs when sound encounters an interface between two tissues that transmit sound at different speeds. Because the sound frequency remains constant, the wavelength changes to accommodate the difference in the speed of sound in the two tissues. The result of this change in wavelength is a redirection of the sound pulse as it passes through the interface (Fig. 1-2). Refraction is important because it is one of the causes of mislocalization of a structure on an ultrasound image. Refraction is discussed in more detail later in this chapter in the section on artifacts.

Absorption refers to the loss of sound energy secondary to its conversion to thermal energy. Absorption is greater in soft tissues than in fluid, and it is greater in bone than in soft tissues. Sound absorption is a major cause of acoustic shadowing. The combined effects of reflection, scattering, and absorption result in attenuation in the intensity of the sound pulse as it travels through matter.

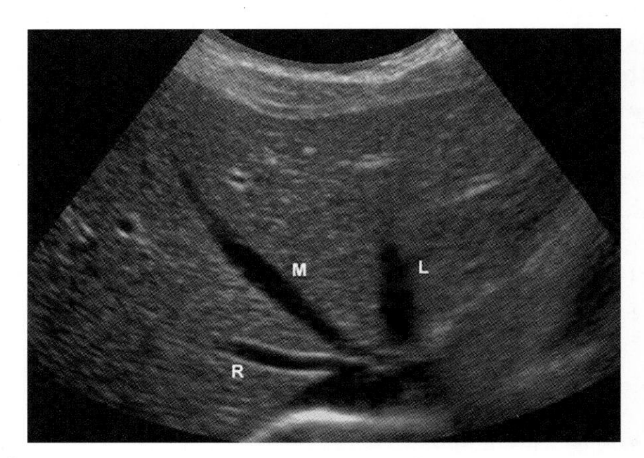

Figure 1-1 Interactions of sound with anatomic structures. Transverse view of the liver demonstrates the right (R), middle (M), and left (L) hepatic veins. They appear anechoic (black) because the intraluminal blood contains very weak reflectors. The walls of the hepatic veins are specular reflectors, and their appearance will depend on their orientation to the sound beam. Because the right hepatic vein is oriented perpendicular to the direction of sound, its walls appear echogenic. The left and middle hepatic veins are not oriented perpendicular to the sound beam so their walls are hypoechoic. The liver parenchyma appears intermediate in echogenicity because it contains multiple small tissue interfaces that scatter the sound.

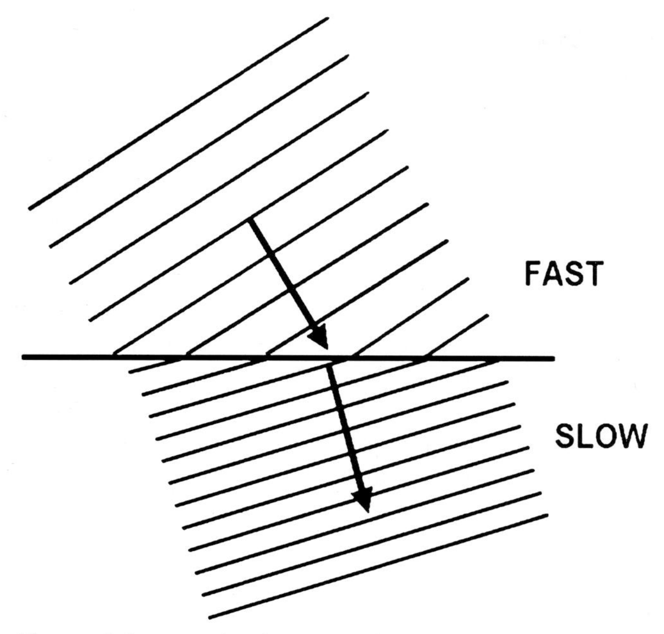

Figure 1-2 Sound refraction. When sound travels obliquely through an interface between substances that transmit sound at different speeds, the wavelength changes. The result is a redirection or bending of the sound that is called *refraction.*

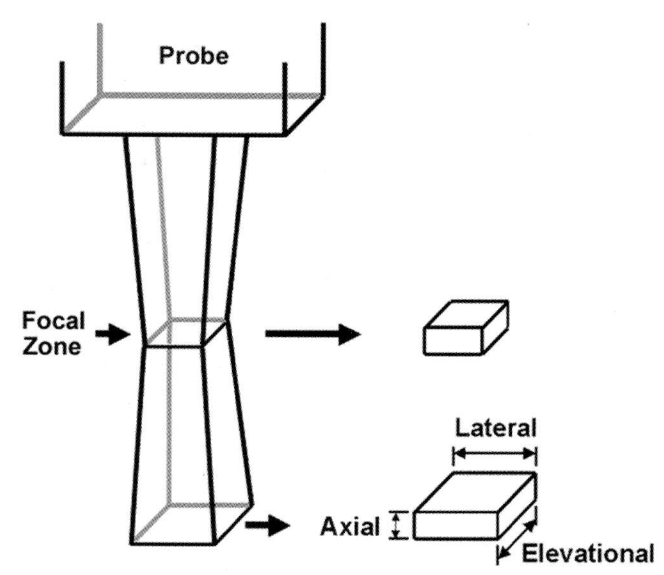

Figure 1-3 Ultrasound resolution. This schematic shows a sound beam being produced by an ultrasound probe. The ultrasound beam is narrowest at the level of the focal zone, resulting in the best lateral resolution at this level. The focal zone can be adjusted up and down by the operator. The elevational resolution, which is equivalent to the slice thickness, is dependent on the shape of the transducer's crystal elements and is not variable. In this diagram the elevational focal zone and the lateral focal zone are at the same level, but that is not always the case. The axial resolution is dependent on the transmit frequency and improves with higher-frequency transducers.

INSTRUMENTATION

Piezoelectric Crystals

Ceramic crystals that deform and vibrate when they are electronically stimulated generate the sound pulses used for diagnostic sonography. Each pulse consists of a band of frequencies referred to as the bandwidth. The center frequency produced by a transducer is the resonant frequency of the crystal element and depends on the thickness of the crystal. Echoes that return to the transducer distort the crystal elements and generate an electric pulse that is processed into an image. High-amplitude echoes produce greater crystal deformation and generate a larger electronic voltage. They are then displayed on the image as brighter pixels than low-amplitude echoes. Because of this, standard two-dimensional gray-scale images are often referred to as B-mode, or brightness mode, images.

The size and configuration of the transmitted sound pulse determines the resolution of the image. Resolution must be considered in three dimensions, as illustrated in Figure 1-3. *Axial resolution* refers to the ability to resolve objects within the imaging plane that are located at different depths along the direction of the sound pulse. This depends on the length of the generated sound pulse, which in turn depends on the wavelength. Because wavelength is inversely proportional to the frequency, higher-frequency probes produce shorter pulses and better axial resolution. Unfortunately, high-frequency sound does not penetrate as deeply into tissues, so high-frequency probes are only useful for superficial structures. *Lateral resolution* refers to the ability to resolve objects within the imaging plane that are located side by side at the same depth from the transducer. This depends on the in-plane diameter of the pulse and can be varied within limits by adjusting the focal zone. *Elevation resolution* (azimuth resolution) refers to the ability to resolve objects that are the same distance from the transducer but are located perpendicular to the plane of imaging. This depends on the out-of-plane diameter of the pulse, which is equivalent to the thickness of the tomographic slice. Slice thickness is generally determined by the shape of the crystal elements or the characteristics of fixed acoustic lenses and is not adjustable by the user.

Static B-Mode Systems

The early two-dimensional units attached a B-mode transducer to an articulated arm that was capable of determining the exact location and orientation of the transducer in space. The distance of the reflector from the transducer was obtained by converting the time taken for the echo to return to the transducer based on the speed of sound in soft tissues (1540 m/sec). This allowed the origin of the returning echoes to be localized in two dimensions. Then, by moving the transducer across the patient's body, a series of B-mode lines of information could be added together to produce a two-dimensional image. With static B-mode imaging it became possible to view large organs, such as the liver, in one cross-sectional image. The major disadvantage of static B-mode imaging was its lack of real-time capabilities. Because of this limitation, static articulated-arm B-mode devices have now been replaced by real-time units.

Real-Time Transducers

Mechanical Transducers

Real-time images can be generated with a variety of transducers. The simplest design is the mechanical sector transducer, which uses a single large piezoelectric element to generate and receive the ultrasound pulses. Beam steering is accomplished by an oscillating or rotating motion of the crystal element itself or by reflection of the sound pulse off an oscillating acoustic mirror. Beam focusing is done by using different-shaped crystal elements or by attaching an acoustic lens to the transducer. Although the mechanical movement is fast enough to produce gray-scale images in real time, it is not fast enough to produce real-time color Doppler images. Another disadvantage of the mechanical sector transducer is the fixed focal zone. This forces the operator to switch to a completely different transducer to vary the focus distance.

Multi-element Array Transducers

Because of their lack of flexibility, mechanical sector transducers have been largely replaced by multi-element transducers, commonly called arrays. The array transducers contain groups of small crystal elements arranged in a sequential fashion. Transmitted sound pulses are created by the summation of multiple pulses from many different elements. By altering the timing and sequence of activation of the different elements, the transmitted pulse can be steered in different directions and focused at different depths. In fact, the multi-element arrays can scan in real time while focusing at multiple levels.

The image created by array transducers consists of multiple scan lines arranged side by side. The length of the scan line multiplied by the speed of sound determines how much time it takes to generate each line. This time must be doubled because sound travels the length of the scan line and then back to the transducer. This travel time can then be multiplied by the total number of lines in the image to determine the time required to generate an entire frame of the real-time image. Because the speed of sound is essentially constant, the frame rate of the image can be adjusted by changing the depth of the image (length of the scan line), the width of the image (number of scan lines), or the line density (number of lines per centimeter).

Phased-Array Transducer

With the phased-array transducer, every element in the array participates in the formation of each transmitted pulse. Because the sound beams are steered at varying angles from one side of the transducer to the other, a sector image format is produced (Fig. 1-4A). Compared with the other electronic array transducers (discussed later), the phased-array probe is smaller and therefore capable of scanning in areas where acoustic access is limited, such as between ribs. However, phased arrays have a small superficial field of view and poor near-field focusing capabilities. The focusing capabilities in the periphery of the image are also limited. Phased arrays are good for performance of deep Doppler imaging but poor for superficial Doppler imaging.

Linear-Array or Linear-Sequenced-Array Transducers

Unlike phased arrays in which all crystal elements are used to generate each transmitted sound pulse, linear arrays activate a limited group of adjacent elements to generate each pulse. Typically, each sound pulse travels in the same direction (parallel) and is oriented perpendicular to the transducer surface, resulting in a rectangular image (see Fig. 1-4C). However, it is also possible to steer the pulses so that the image is trapezoidal. The major advantages of linear-array transducers are high resolution in the near field and a large superficial field of view. Focusing is uniform in the center and periphery of the image when there is no beam steering. Some loss of focusing and resolution occurs when the format is changed to a trapezoid. The major disadvantages of linear arrays are their large size, which limits their use in areas where access is limited, and their limited deep field of view.

Curved-Array Transducers

If the surface of a linear array is re-formed into a curved convex shape, a sector-shaped image with a convex apex is produced (see Fig. 1-4B). Compared with a standard linear array, this results in a wider far field of view but reduces the resolution of the probe. Curved arrays can be formed in different sizes and shapes. Probes with a short radius of curvature can be used for endoluminal scanning, and probes with a larger radius of curvature can be used for general abdomen and obstetric scanning. Other names for curved arrays are curved linear, convex linear, and curvilinear. The advantages of the commonly used transducers are listed in Table 1-1.

Annular-Array Transducers

All of the transducers just described allow for electronically controlled focusing of the sound beam in the plane of the image but not in the elevational plane. Focusing the beam in the elevation plane affects the out-of-plane resolution, which is identical to the slice thickness. Annular-array transducers allow concentric beam

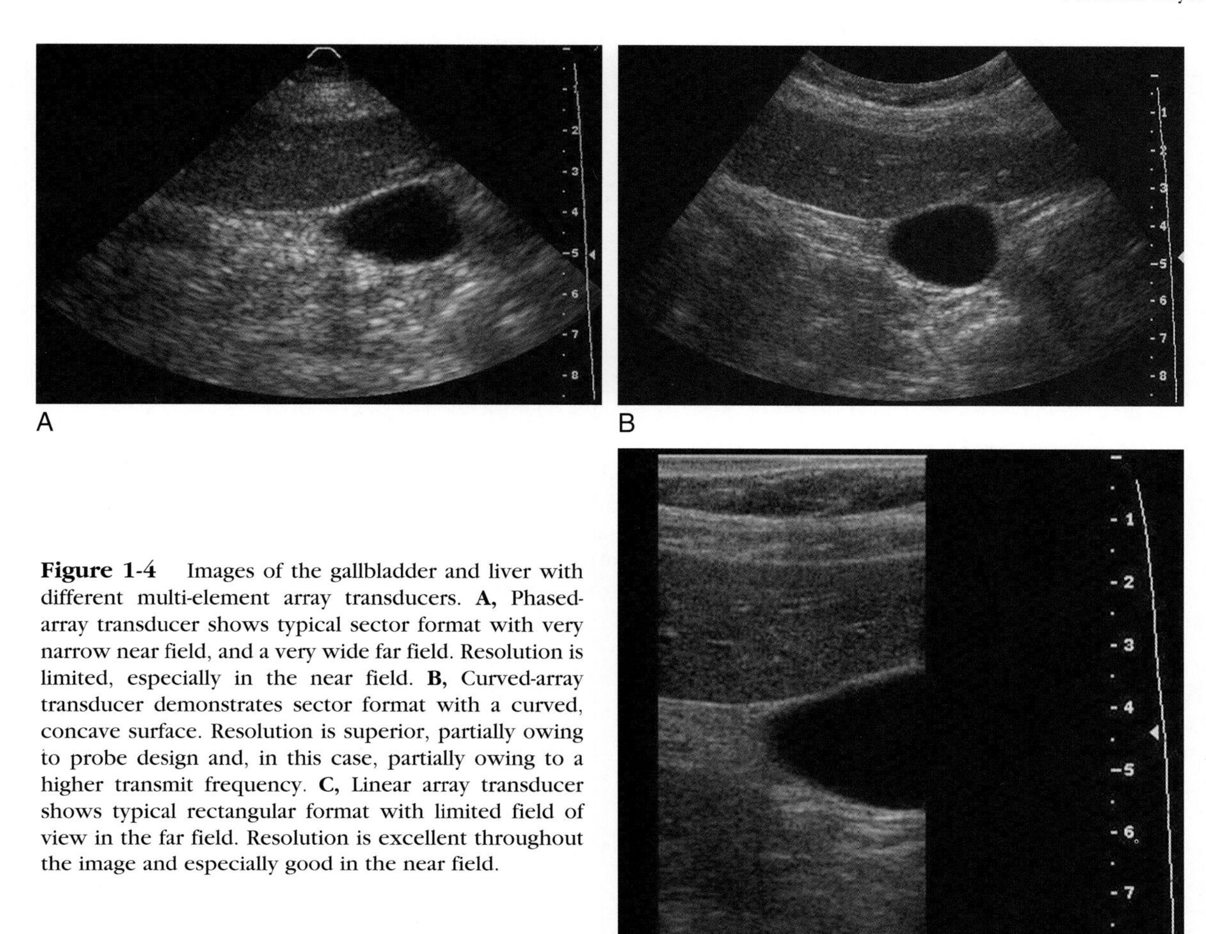

Figure 1-4 Images of the gallbladder and liver with different multi-element array transducers. **A,** Phased-array transducer shows typical sector format with very narrow near field, and a very wide far field. Resolution is limited, especially in the near field. **B,** Curved-array transducer demonstrates sector format with a curved, concave surface. Resolution is superior, partially owing to probe design and, in this case, partially owing to a higher transmit frequency. **C,** Linear array transducer shows typical rectangular format with limited field of view in the far field. Resolution is excellent throughout the image and especially good in the near field.

focusing in the imaging plane as well as the elevation plane, thereby permitting variations in slice thickness. These transducers contain multiple ring-shaped concentrically arranged elements, which nestle within one another like a target. The ring arrangement produces a cone-shaped beam that reduces section thickness, thereby theoretically allowing for the detection and characterization of smaller structures. The major disadvantage of the annular arrays is that they cannot steer electronically. Because mechanical steering is much slower than electronic steering, time-consuming imaging techniques such as color Doppler sonography are not practical with the annular-array transducers.

Table 1-1 Advantages of Different Transducers

Phased array	Easy to use where access is limited
	Large deep field of view
Linear array	Excellent resolution
	Large superficial field of view
Curved array	Good resolution
	Large deep and superficial field of view

Two-Dimensional Arrays

Another solution to variable focusing in the elevation plane is the two-dimensional array. These probes have crystal elements that are stacked in columns as well as rows. They allow for variable slice thickness while maintaining the other advantages of electronically controlled arrays, such as the ability to perform color Doppler.

Intraluminal Probes

Small transducers that can be placed within various body lumens are now widely available. These transducers can be positioned close to the organ of interest; thus, higher frequencies can be used and higher-resolution images can be obtained. In addition, the ability to image organs without having to transmit the sound beam through the abdominal wall helps to minimize the image-degrading properties of adipose tissue. The overall result is that the images are of much higher quality than those obtained with a standard transabdominal approach. The disadvantage is the limited imaging depth. Endovaginal and endorectal transducers are used most commonly (Fig. 1-5). Very small transducers have been added to flexible endoscopes to evaluate pathologic

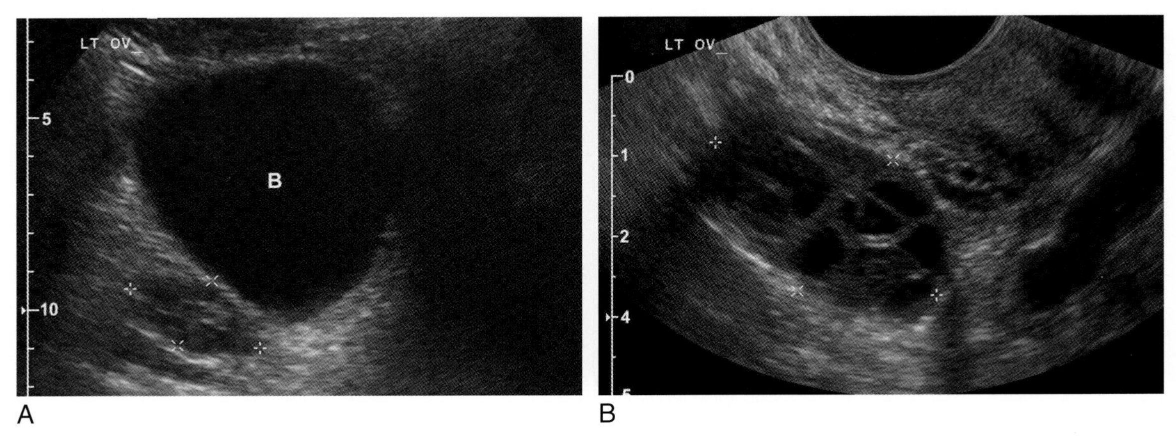

Figure 1-5 Endoluminal probe. **A,** Transabdominal view using a 3.5-MHz transducer demonstrates the left ovary *(cursors)* posterior to the urinary bladder (B). Ovarian follicles are difficult to see well. **B,** Transvaginal view with a 5.5-MHz transducer demonstrates the left ovary *(cursors).* Ovarian follicles are seen much more clearly than on the transabdominal view. The ovary appears much larger because the field of view for transvaginal scanning is much smaller than for transabdominal scanning.

processes in both the upper and lower gastrointestinal tract. Intra-arterial probes that fit on the end of catheters are the most recent addition to the group of intraluminal sonographic devices.

HARMONIC IMAGING

In conventional scanning, the sound frequency of the echoes used to create the image is the same frequency as the transmitted sound pulses. Conventional sound pulses and their returning echoes progressively decrease in intensity as they travel through the body. Harmonic frequencies are higher-integer multiples of the fundamental transmitted frequency. They are produced as the sound wave travels through tissues and progressively increase in intensity before eventually decreasing because of attenuation. With harmonic imaging, a filter is used to remove the fundamental echoes so that only the high-frequency harmonic signal is processed to produce an image. Although many harmonic frequencies are generated with propagation of the initial pulse, the current technology uses only the second harmonic, which is twice the transmitted frequency.

Harmonic beams are narrower than the transmitted beam and have fewer side lobes (side lobes are discussed in more detail in the section on artifacts). The reduced width of the beam improves lateral resolution, and the reduction in side lobes improves the signal-to-noise ratio. Furthermore, harmonic signals are produced after the beam enters the tissues of the body so that the degrading effect of body wall fat is minimized (Fig. 1-6).

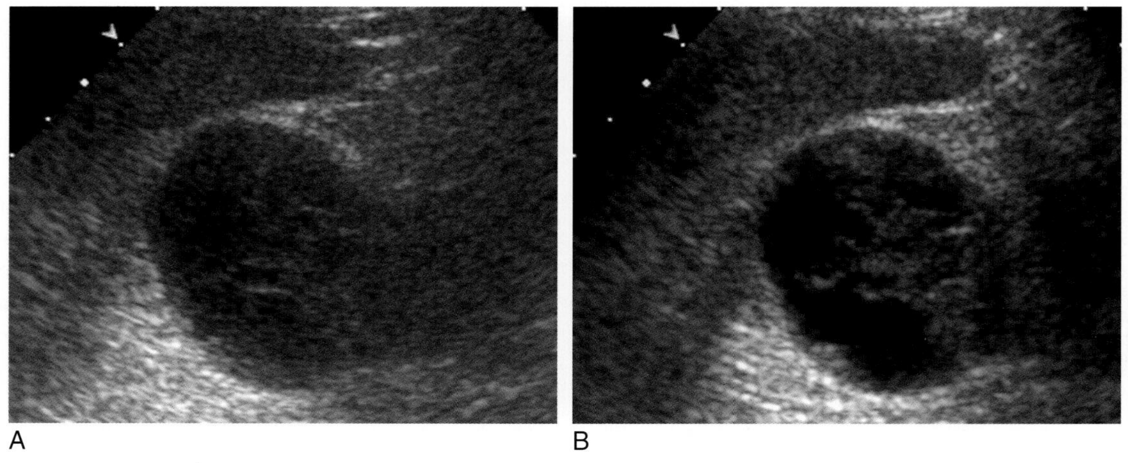

Figure 1-6 Tissue harmonic imaging. **A,** Conventional fundamental frequency scan of a renal cyst demonstrates amorphous internal echoes. **B,** Harmonic imaging demonstrates well-defined solid material within this renal cyst secondary to internal hemorrhage.

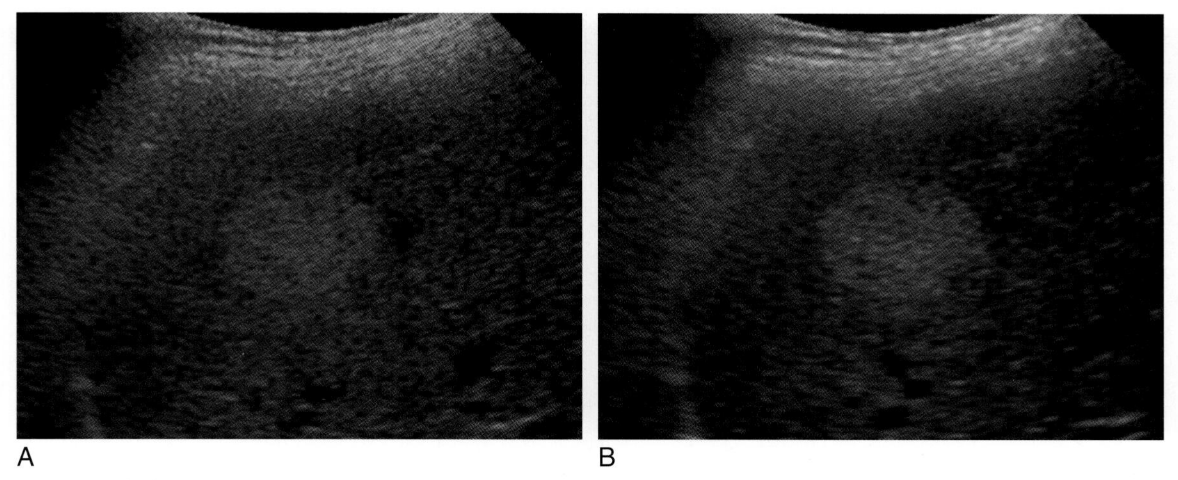

Figure 1-7 Real-time compound imaging. **A,** Conventional image of the liver demonstrates a hemangioma with poorly defined margins. **B,** Similar image obtained with real-time compounding demonstrates better demarcation of the hemangioma from the adjacent liver parenchyma.

For this reason, harmonic imaging is theoretically even more valuable in obese patients.

REAL-TIME COMPOUNDING

With conventional linear-array and curved-array imaging, the sound beams are directed perpendicular to the surface of the probe. With real-time compounding, the sound is steered at multiple angles, as well as perpendicular. By averaging signals originating from the different sound angles, the theoretical result is to accentuate high-level reflectors and de-emphasize weak reflectors and noise. The net result is an improvement in signal-to-noise ratio and tissue contrast (Fig. 1-7).

EXTENDED-FIELD-OF-VIEW IMAGING

One disadvantage of real-time ultrasound is its limited field of view. This is especially true with high-resolution linear-array transducers because of their rectangular image format. Thus, spatial relationships and sizes often must be mentally synthesized from multiple real-time images that display only portions of the relevant anatomy. In addition, it is often difficult to display pertinent findings and relevant anatomy to someone who was not involved with the real-time scanning.

With the use of new computer algorithms, an image-registration-based position-sensing technique now allows for generation of panoramic images in real time with no loss in resolution and without an external position sensor. The technique uses an echo-tracking-based process for estimating probe motion that is applicable to all conventional real-time transducers and is becoming available on most modern systems (Fig. 1-8).

THREE-DIMENSIONAL ULTRASOUND IMAGING

Three-dimensional (3D) sonography has undergone continued refinement for many years. Data for 3D sonography are acquired as a stack of parallel cross-sections with the use of a 2D scanner or as a volume with the use of a mechanical or an electronic array probe. The resultant 3D images can be displayed with a variety of formats, including multiplanar reformatting (Fig. 1-9A), surface rendering (see Fig. 1-9B), volume rendering, and virtual endoscopy. 3D imaging is also possible in the color Doppler mode (see Fig. 1-9C). Clinical applications

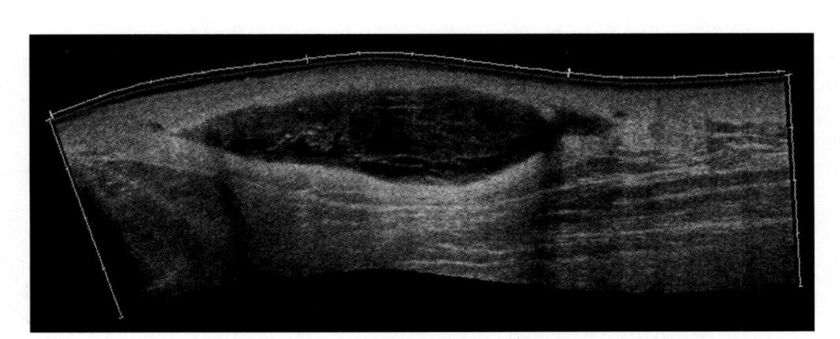

Figure 1-8 Extended-field-of-view imaging. Longitudinal view of the leg demonstrates a hematoma measuring approximately 8 cm in length. This is too large to be visualized with standard transducers but is well demonstrated with extended field of view scanning.

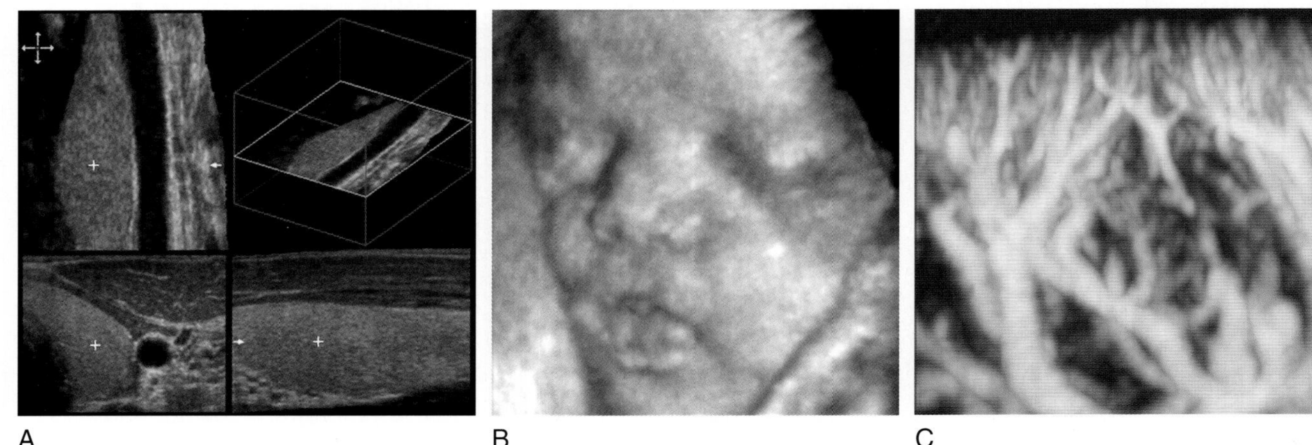

Figure 1-9 Three-dimensional imaging. **A,** Multiplanar reformatting of the thyroid and carotid in the sagittal and coronal plane obtained from source images in the axial plane. **B,** Surface rendering of a fetal face. (This image was provided by Dr. George Bega, Philadelphia, PA.) **C,** Three-dimensional volume-rendered image of renal cortical blood flow obtained with power Doppler imaging.

are expanding, but the biggest impact is currently in the evaluation of fetal anatomy.

GRAY-SCALE IMAGE OPTIMIZATION

Transducer

The transducer used should be matched to the application. Superficial structures should be scanned with high-frequency probes to allow for the best possible resolution. Typically, transmit frequencies vary from 7 to 15 MHz for thyroid, scrotal, and musculoskeletal scans. Because of limited penetration, high-frequency probes cannot be used for deep structures. Therefore, lower frequencies ranging from 2 to 5 MHz are typically used for abdominal, pelvic, and obstetric scans. With some probes it is possible to select different frequencies on the same probe. With others, a new probe must be selected to change frequency. The probe used is indicated on the image using the letters P, L, and C to indicate phased, linear, and curved. The numbers following these letters indicate the frequency or range of frequencies of the probe. Other numbers associated with probe designation may indicate the size of the probe (for linear arrays) or the radius of curvature (for curved arrays).

Power Output

The power output determines the strength of the pulse that is transmitted. When the transmitted pulse is stronger, the returning echoes are stronger and the resulting image is brighter. Power output is typically displayed as either a percent of maximum or as a decibel (dB). The decibel is a logarithmic scale in which a difference of 1 dB equates to a 10-time difference in power. In addition, indices are now used to give the operator an idea about the likelihood of biologic effects. The thermal index (TI), which is usually displayed during Doppler examinations, is a number that estimates the temperature increase in degrees Centigrade assuming worst-case conditions. It can be calibrated for soft tissues, bone, and the cranium. The mechanical index (MI) predicts cavitation and is usually displayed during gray-scale imaging. If an index can reach 1.0 for a given mode of operation, then it must be displayed. Power output should be increased when attenuation of sound limits penetration and diagnostic information cannot be obtained even after proper adjustment of gain and transducer frequency (Fig. 1-10). Otherwise, preprogrammed power levels should be employed. In all situations it is prudent to limit the power used and the time of examinations as much as possible, especially during pulsed Doppler examinations.

Gain

Because of sound attenuation, an interface in the deep tissues will produce a weaker reflection and less distortion of the probes crystal elements than a similar interface in the near tissues. To compensate for this, signals from deeper tissues are electronically amplified after they return to the transducer. Because the depth of the interface is determined by the amount of time it takes for the transmitted sound pulse to return to the transducer, this variable amplification is referred to as the time gain compensation (TGC). The amount of gain

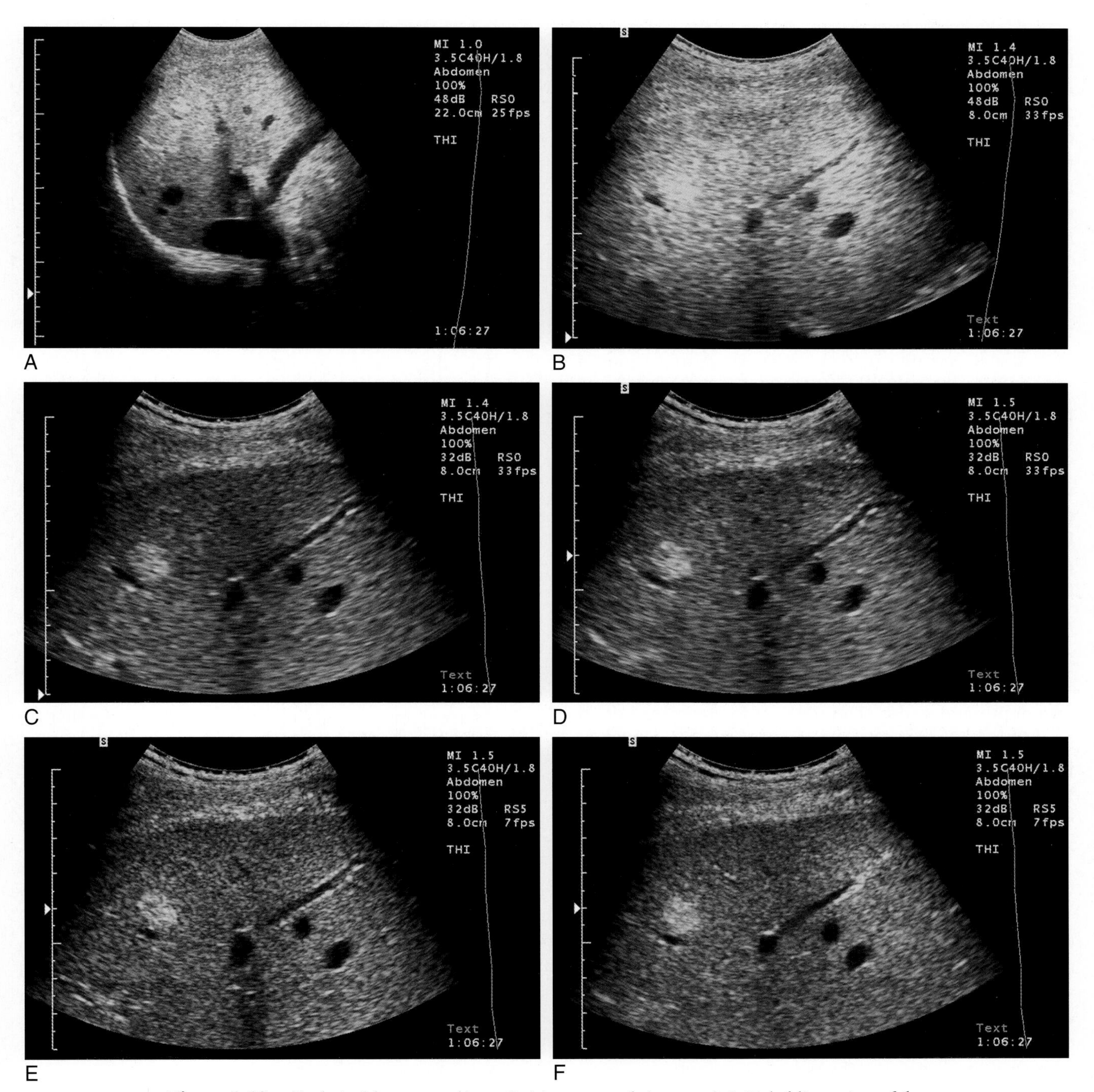

Figure 1-10 Technical factors used in optimizing gray-scale images. **A,** Initial oblique view of the liver before any image optimization. **B,** Decreasing the field of view from a depth of 22 cm to a depth of 8 cm focuses attention on the superficial aspect of the liver where an abnormality was suspected. **C,** Adjusting the time gain compensation curve normalizes echogenicity throughout the liver and makes it easier to identify an echogenic hemangioma. **D,** Adjusting the focal zone to the level of the hemangioma improves resolution at this level. **E,** Increasing the line density decreases pixel size and further improves resolution. **F,** Increasing image persistence results in reduction in noise and an overall smoothing effect on the image.

is shown to the side of the image in the form of a line or curve. The TGC curve is moved a variable amount to the right (indicating increased gain) in the deeper aspects of the image. Because different tissues attenuate sound to a different degree, the TGC curve requires frequent readjustments as different structures are scanned (see Fig. 1-10).

In addition to the TGC curve, the overall gain, which affects the brightness of the entire image, can also be adjusted. Similar to the power output, the overall gain is usually displayed as a percent of maximum or as a decibel level. In fact, in many ways, gain has an effect on the image that is similar to power. However, because gain amplifies the electronic signal produced by the returning echo, it does not affect the strength of the pulse transmitted into the patient. As mentioned earlier, it is best to try to equilibrate and optimize image brightness using gain controls first and increase power only if gain modification is unsuccessful.

Focal Zone

As mentioned earlier, with the electronic array transducers it is possible to focus the transmitted sound at different depths. This control is also referred to as the transmit zone and is usually indicated at the side of the image as an arrowhead. When scanning a particular structure, the focal zone should be placed at the level of interest (see Fig. 1-10). When necessary, it is possible to create separate image parts using focal zones at multiple levels and "pasting" these parts together to create a complete image (see Fig. 1-10). The tradeoff for multilevel focusing is a decrease in the frame rate.

Field of View

The field of view of a real-time image can be divided into depth and width. The tradeoff for increased depth or width is reduced frame rate. Depth is usually displayed on the image as centimeters or as a scale on the side of the image (see Fig. 1-10). Width is usually adjusted using submenus.

Line Density

As described earlier, each image is composed of multiple adjacent scan lines. The density of scan lines can be adjusted for linear arrays (scan lines per centimeter) as well as phased arrays and curved arrays (scan lines per degree). Increasing the line density will decrease the size of the pixels and improve resolution. The tradeoff for increased line density is decreased frame rate.

Gray-Scale Curves

Each pixel in an ultrasound image has a designated echo-amplitude depending on the strength of the reflections from that pixel. The exact way that gray-scale values are matched with echo-amplitudes can be varied by changing the gray-scale curves. Analogous to CT, where changing the center and window settings causes different structures to be emphasized, changing the gray-scale curves can emphasize different aspects of the ultrasound image. For instance, all of the low-amplitude echoes can be assigned a value of black and the rest of the range of gray-scale values can be spread out among the high echo-amplitudes. This will make it easier to visualize differences between the bright reflectors. On the other hand, all of the high echo-amplitudes can be assigned a value of white and the rest of the range of gray-scale values can be spread out among the low echo-amplitudes to emphasize differences in the weak reflectors. There are usually 5 to 10 curves to choose from. The gray-scale curve used is often displayed on the image by the letter "C" followed by the curve number.

Dynamic Range

The dynamic range refers to the range of signal strengths that can be effectively handled by the scanner. Because the range is greater for the amplifier than the display monitor, the received signals must be compressed before they are displayed. Less compression (i.e., a higher dynamic range) allows for distinction of subtle differences in echo-amplitude and produces an image that appears smoother. More compression (i.e., a lower dynamic range) limits the range of distinguishable echo-amplitudes and produces images that have higher apparent contrast.

Persistence

By averaging several frames of a real-time scan that are temporally contiguous, background noise can be reduced and image quality improves. For instance, the actual frame number 1, 2, and 3 could be averaged together to create the first frame that is displayed. Then the actual frames 2, 3, and 4 could be averaged to create the second frame that is displayed, and so on. This process is referred to as persistence, and it assumes that structures are either motionless or move very slowly. The disadvantage of high persistence is that blurring occurs when internal structures are moving, or when the transducer is moving. For instance, high levels of persistence can mask fetal heart motion.

A review of the effects of the various technical parameters is shown in Table 1-2.

DOPPLER SONOGRAPHY

Real-time gray-scale images use only the amplitude of the returning echoes to generate gray-scale information. An analysis of the frequency of the returning echo can also yield important information. Because of the Doppler effect, sound that reflects off a moving object undergoes a change in frequency. Objects moving toward the transducer reflect sound at a higher frequency than that of the incident pulse, and objects

Table 1-2 Gray-Scale Technical Parameters

Parameter	Effect on Image
Transmit frequency	Varies resolution Varies penetration
Power output	Varies power of transmitted pulse Changes image brightness Contributes to artifact generation Determines patient exposure
Gain	Varies amplification of returning signals Changes image brightness Compensates for sound attenuation
Focal zone	Varies depth of maximum beam focusing Determines lateral resolution Alters frame rate when multi-zone focusing
Field of view	Varies image size Alters frame rate
Gray-scale curves	Translates echo-amplitudes to gray-scale values Changes image contrast
Line density	Determines scan lines per centimeter or degree Alters frame rate Alters resolution and pixel size
Dynamic range	Varies the range of displayed gray scale values Changes image contrast
Persistence	Averages sequential real-time frames Improves signal-to-noise-of stationary objects Blurs moving objects

moving away reflect sound at a lower frequency. The difference between the transmitted and received frequency is called the Doppler frequency shift. The magnitude of the Doppler frequency shift is determined by the equation:

$$Fd = Ft - Fr = 2 \times Ft \times \left(\frac{V}{c}\right) \times \cos\theta$$

where Fd = the Doppler frequency shift, Ft = the transmitted frequency, Fr = the received frequency, V = the speed of moving target (blood flow velocity), c = the speed of sound in soft tissue, and θ = the angle between the direction of blood flow and the direction of the transmitted sound pulse (Fig. 1-11).

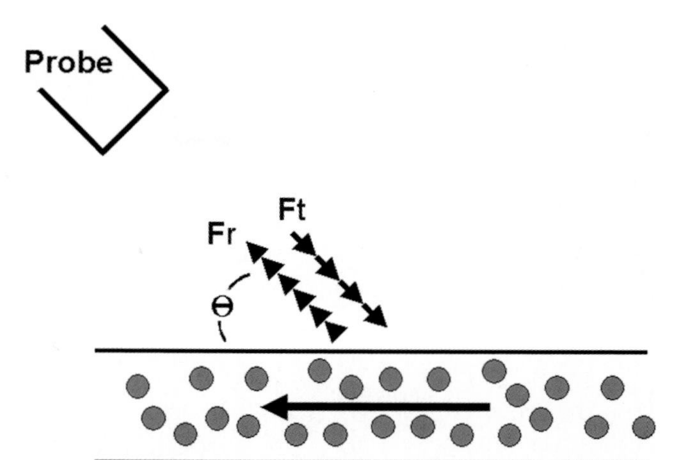

Figure 1-11 Doppler effect. When sound reflects off of moving targets such as red blood cells in a vessel, the sound frequency is changed. The difference in the transmitted frequency (Ft) and the received frequency (Fr) is referred to as the Doppler frequency shift. The angle between the direction of sound and the direction of motion of the target θ is referred to as the Doppler angle.

Pulsed Doppler

As with gray-scale imaging, pulsed Doppler devices transmit short pulses of sound and then wait for the returning echo. By varying the delay time between the transmission and reception of the sound wave, it is possible to determine the location (i.e., depth) from which the Doppler signal arises. This location is referred to as the sample volume or Doppler gate. The size of the sample volume can be varied by changing the duration of the time that the probe receives returning signals. By using a standard gray-scale image to visualize the vessels of interest, the position of the Doppler sample volume can be adjusted so that signals are obtained from specific vessels. This combination of gray-scale sonography with pulsed Doppler sonography is called duplex Doppler sonography (Fig. 1-12). The waveform that displays the Doppler information has the Doppler frequency shift on the vertical axis and time on the horizontal axis. The Doppler shift from objects moving toward the transducer is positive and is typically displayed above the baseline, and the shift from objects moving away from the transducer is negative and typically displayed below the line.

As indicated in the Doppler equation, the frequency shift is proportional to the velocity. So when analyzing blood flow, the size of the waveform varies with the flow velocity. The frequency shift is also proportional to the $\cos\theta$. At a Doppler angle of 90 degrees (blood flow perpendicular to direction of sound), the $\cos\theta = 0$ and no Doppler frequency shift will be detected. On the other hand, at a Doppler angle of 0 degrees (blood flow and sound direction are parallel), the $\cos\theta = 1$. Because this is the maximum possible value for the $\cos\theta$, the Doppler frequency shift is maximized at an angle of 0 degrees. Therefore, orienting the transmitted Doppler pulse with respect to the blood vessel so that the Doppler angle is as close to 0 degrees as possible will obtain the largest Doppler signal (see Fig. 1-12B).

In many situations, it is important to calculate the exact blood flow velocity. This can be done by rearranging

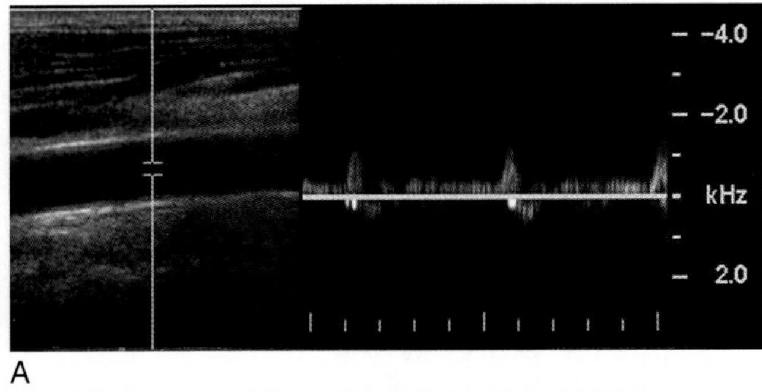

A

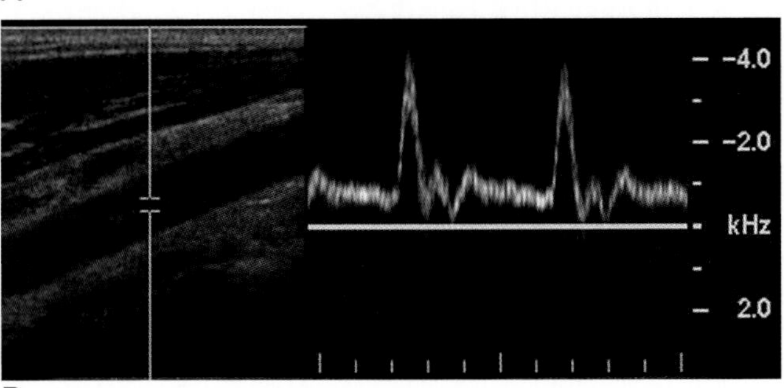

B

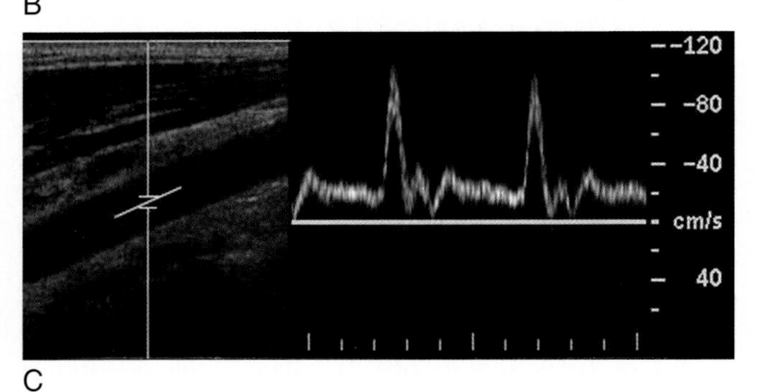

C

Figure 1-12 Duplex Doppler. **A,** Gray-scale image of the common carotid artery provides the map on which a Doppler sample volume can be positioned. The resulting waveform represents the Doppler frequency shift (kHz) along the vertical axis and time along the horizontal axis. In this image, the waveform is weak and small because the Doppler angle between the direction of the sound pulse and the direction of the vessel is close to 90 degrees. **B,** To improve the Doppler waveform, the transducer has been angled so that the Doppler angle is now closer to 60 degrees. This results in a higher Doppler frequency shift and a stronger signal. **C,** By adding an angle indicator line to the image and rotating it so it is parallel to the long axis of the vessel, the frequency shift information displayed on the vertical axis can be converted to velocity (cm/sec).

the Doppler equation to solve for velocity:

$$V = Fd \times \frac{1}{Ft} \times C \times \frac{1}{\cos\theta} \times \frac{1}{2}$$

The transmit frequency and speed of sound are both known. The frequency shift is determined by the waveform. The only other variable required to determine the velocity is the Doppler angle. This is determined by aligning an angle indicator line parallel to the vessel and then measuring the angle between this line and the Doppler beam. When this is done, the Doppler scale can be recalibrated for velocity rather than frequency (see Fig. 1-12C). It is important to realize that the image allows for estimation of the direction of blood flow only within several degrees. Unfortunately there is always some degree of unavoidable error in the value used for θ, and, thus, there is some degree of error in the calculation of velocity. The Doppler equation shows that velocity is directly proportional to 1/cosθ. Figure 1-13 is a graph plotting 1/cosθ with respect to θ. At Doppler angles less than 60 degrees, there is little change in 1/cosθ for small differences in θ. However, above 60 degrees, small differences in the angle θ produce large differences in the value of 1/cosθ. Therefore, to avoid significant errors in calculating velocities, it is important to maintain a Doppler angle of 60 degrees or less.

A number of measurements are used to analyze arterial waveforms. The most common is the *resistive index:*

$$RI = 1 - \left(\frac{D}{S}\right) = \frac{(S - D)}{S}$$

where S is the peak systolic velocity (or frequency shift) and D is the end-diastolic velocity (or frequency shift). The resistive index goes up when resistance to flow goes up. When there is no diastolic flow, the resistive index is 1. Because the calculation depends only on the ratio of

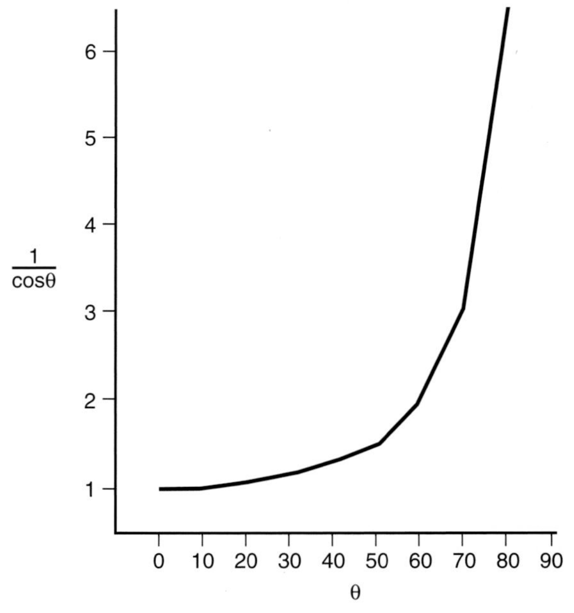

Figure 1-13 Explanation for performing velocity calculations at a Doppler angle less than 60 degrees. Velocity is proportional to the inverse of cosθ. Between 0 degrees and 60 degrees, small differences in θ correlate with small differences in the inverse of cosθ. Above 60 degrees, small differences in θ result in large differences in the inverse of cosθ.

systolic to diastolic flow, it is independent of the Doppler angle. Parenchymal organs should normally have a resistive index of between 0.5 and 0.7.

Another common measurement is the *pulsatility index:*

$$PI = \frac{(S - D)}{m}$$

where m is the mean flow velocity throughout the cardiac cycle. The pulsatility index is probably a truer indication of vascular resistance than the resistive index, but because it is harder to measure, it has not gained widespread use. Like the resistive index, the pulsatility index is independent of Doppler angle.

In addition to these measurements of vascular resistance, measurements of systolic acceleration are also becoming more widely used as a means of detecting proximal arterial stenosis. Acceleration is obtained by measuring the slope (change in velocity/change in time) of the early systolic upstroke. Unlike the resistive index and pulsatility index, systolic acceleration requires determination of an absolute difference in velocities and thus must be calculated from an angle-corrected velocity waveform.

Color Doppler

Color Doppler sonography is sensitive to Doppler signals throughout an adjustable portion of the field of view. It provides a real-time image, displaying tissue morphology in gray scale and blood flow in color. Color Doppler sonography analyzes the phase information, frequency, and amplitude of the returning echoes. Signals from moving red blood cells are assigned a color (red versus blue) based on the direction of the phase shift (i.e., the direction of blood flow toward or away from the transducer). The color shade for each pixel is based on the mean frequency shift arising from that pixel. High-frequency shifts are assigned a lighter color, and lower-frequency shifts are assigned a darker color (Fig. 1-14A). Stationary objects produce no phase shift and are assigned a gray-scale value, as in conventional gray-scale imaging.

Because color Doppler studies visualize flow throughout the vessel, areas of abnormal flow can be visualized rapidly, thus avoiding the time-consuming point by point interrogation required with pulsed duplex Doppler analysis. In addition, pulsed duplex Doppler analysis relies on the gray-scale image to identify a vessel for interrogation. Therefore, analysis of small vessels, such as in the testis, can be extremely difficult because the vessels are too small to be resolved with gray-scale imaging. Color Doppler sonography is capable of showing these small vessels. In practice, it is often used to identify vessels, or to identify focal areas of flow disturbance, and then waveforms from these areas are obtained with pulsed Doppler analysis.

Power Doppler

Power Doppler imaging estimates the power or strength of the Doppler signal rather than the mean frequency shift. The Doppler detection sequence used in power Doppler imaging is identical to that employed in frequency-based color Doppler imaging. However, once the Doppler shift has been detected, the frequency components are ignored in lieu of the total energy of the Doppler signal. The color and hue relate to the moving blood volume rather than the direction or the velocity of flow (see Fig. 1-14B).

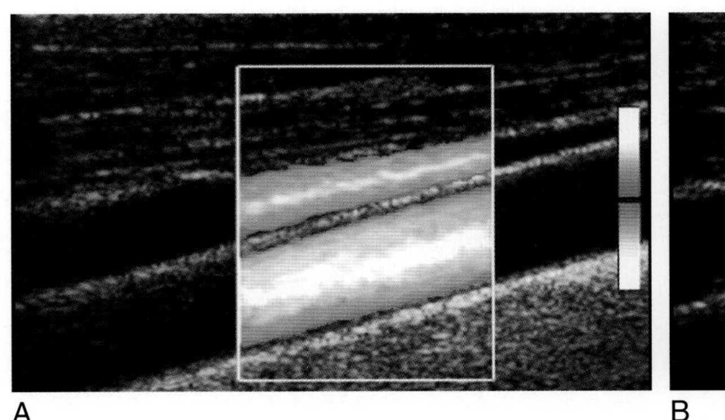

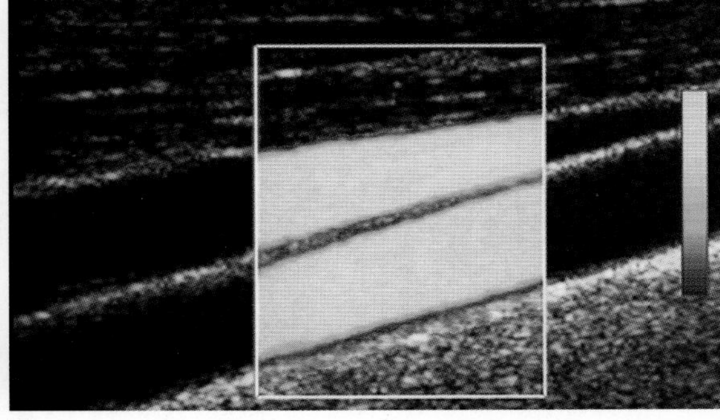

Figure 1-14 Color and power Doppler. **A,** Color Doppler image of the common carotid artery and internal jugular vein. Blood flow oriented away from the sound pulse is displayed in red, and flow toward the sound pulse is displayed in blue. Because the velocity is highest in the center of the vessels, the frequency shifts are also highest in these regions and the color assignment shifts toward lighter shades of blue in the jugular vein and lighter shades of red in the carotid artery. **B,** Power Doppler view of a similar area demonstrates flow in both vessels. Information concerning direction of flow and velocity is not displayed on power Doppler scans.

Power Doppler imaging has several theoretical advantages over color Doppler imaging. In conventional color Doppler imaging, noise appears over the entire Doppler frequency shift, which means that gain settings must be limited to reduce excessive noise. If the gain is too high, a background of random noise obscures true signal. In the power Doppler display, low-level noise is assigned as a homogeneous color background, even when the gain is increased greatly. This allows for the use of higher gain settings and a minimal increase in the sensitivity to blood flow. In addition, the power of the signal is not affected by the Doppler angle, so flow can be seen in vessels that travel close to a right angle to the ultrasound beam.

Unfortunately, power Doppler sonography has significant limitations. Perhaps the most significant is that it gives no information about direction or velocity of blood flow. It is also very susceptible to flash artifact, which are zones of intense color that result from motion of soft tissues and motion of the transducer. Because of these limitations and only marginal and often imperceptible increases in flow sensitivity, power Doppler sonography has remained an ancillary mode with color Doppler analysis being the primary flow imaging technique. Box 1-1 compares the advantages of color Doppler and power Doppler imaging.

Box 1-1 Advantages of Color Doppler and Power Doppler

COLOR DOPPLER	POWER DOPPLER
Determines flow direction	Slightly more sensitive
Determines relative flow velocity	Less affected by Doppler angle
Less affected by tissue motion	
Less affected by probe motion	

DOPPLER OPTIMIZATION

Transducer Frequency

Because the Doppler frequency shift is proportional to the transmitted frequency, higher-frequency transducers cause a higher Doppler frequency shift that is easier to detect. Additionally, the strength of the reflection from small objects such as red blood cells is proportional to the fourth power of the transmitted frequency. Therefore, higher-frequency probes result in a stronger reflection from red blood cells. These effects improve the sensitivity of higher-frequency probes. They are unfortunately counterbalanced by decreased penetration of higher-frequency sound. Whenever it becomes difficult to detect flow in a given vessel, it is a good idea to use a variety of different probes operating at different frequencies. For deep applications, it is often advantageous to switch to a lower-frequency probe, whereas higher-frequency probes are often better for superficial structures (Fig. 1-15).

Gain

Doppler gain is a receiver end amplification of the Doppler signal that can be applied to either the Doppler

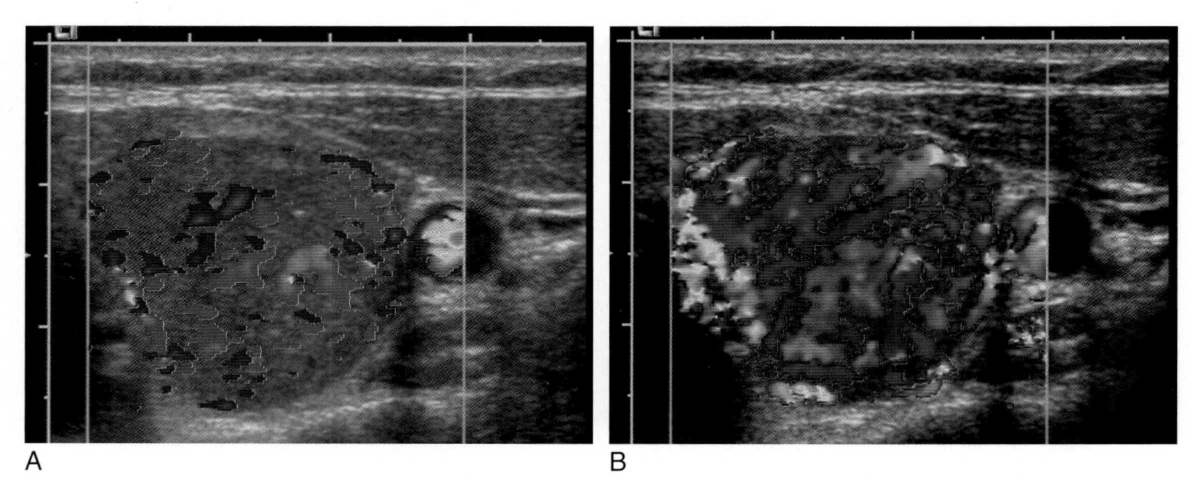

Figure 1-15 Effect of transmit frequency on Doppler signal strength. **A,** Transverse view of the thyroid with transmit frequency of 4 MHz shows a nodule with scattered internal vessels. **B,** Similar view with transmit frequency of 7 MHz shows improved sensitivity and more extensive internal vascularity.

waveform or to the color Doppler image. In most situations, the gain should be increased to a maximum value just before the point where random noise begins to obscure the pulsed Doppler waveform, or with color Doppler to the point where color starts to appear in nonvascular spaces of the color image (Fig. 1-16). The Doppler gain affects only the Doppler portion of the image and does not affect the gray-scale background.

Power

As with gray-scale imaging, power output refers to the strength of the transmitted ultrasound pulse. Stronger or more powerful sound pulses will produce stronger reflections that are more easily detected. Power output affects both the gray-scale and Doppler images. In general, increasing the power output improves

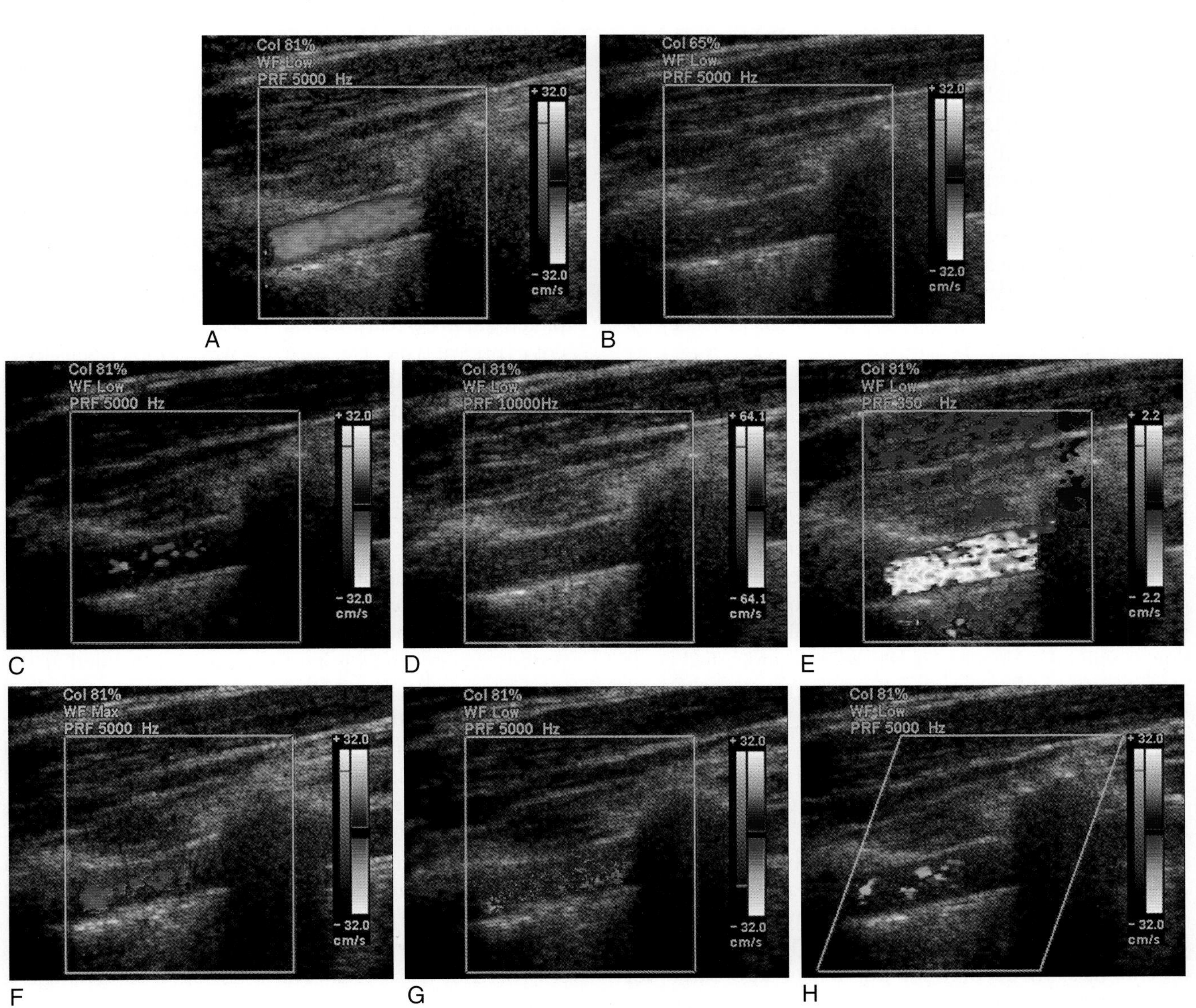

Figure 1-16 Effect of technical parameters on Doppler sensitivity. **A,** Longitudinal view of the vertebral artery with the technical parameters optimized. **B,** In this image the Doppler gain (65%) is too low and vertebral flow is difficult to detect. **C,** The power output is too low and vertebral flow is difficult to detect. Because power also affects the gray scale echoes, the entire image is dark. **D,** The pulse repetition frequency (PRF) (10,000 Hz) is too high. This also causes the Doppler scale to increase to ±64.1 cm/sec. **E,** The PRF is too low (350 Hz) and artifactual color is seen in the soft tissues around the vertebral flow. The Doppler scale is ±2.2 cm/sec. **F,** The wall filter (WF Max) is too high. **G,** The color priority (seen as a green line in the gray-scale bar next to the color Doppler scale) is too low. **H,** The Doppler color box has been steered to the left. Although this has resulted in a more optimal Doppler angle and a higher Doppler frequency shift, the weaker signal strength has resulted is poorer sensitivity.

Doppler sensitivity (see Fig. 1-16). This can be very important in deep abdominal applications where tissue attenuation significantly weakens the Doppler signal. However, increasing the power output also causes increased patient exposure and can lead to a number of artifacts. Therefore, power levels should be kept as low as is reasonably achievable to obtain the desired information.

Pulse Repetition Frequency (Doppler Scale)

The pulse repetition frequency (PRF) refers to the number of sound pulses transmitted per second. High PRFs result in a high Doppler scale whereas lower PRFs result in a lower Doppler scale. On most units, there is a control labeled Doppler scale, but one should realize that adjusting the Doppler scale is really changing the PRF. The advantage of a high PRF or high Doppler scale is display of high velocity flow without aliasing. The advantage of a low PRF or low Doppler scale is improved sensitivity to low velocity blood flow (see Fig. 1-16).

Ensemble Length

An uncommonly used means of improving the Doppler sensitivity is to increase the number of sound pulses used to generate each individual line of color Doppler information. This control has been referred to as the dwell time, the ensemble length, or the color sensitivity. When more pulses are used it is easier to detect frequency shifts at a given location so the sensitivity improves. Realize that when more pulses are used per line, it will take longer to generate each individual color Doppler frame and the tradeoff is a lowered frame rate.

Wall Filter

In many situations it is important to eliminate artifactual or unwanted signals, such as frequency shifts arising from pulsating vessel walls or moving soft tissues. The wall filter is a high-pass filter that allows frequency shifts above a certain level to be displayed while lower-frequency shifts are not displayed. This can reduce or eliminate tissue motion, but it can also filter out true low-velocity flow if it is adjusted improperly (see Fig. 1-16).

Color Priority

Another way to eliminate unwanted color information is to establish a gray-scale value above which color information is suppressed. This is based on the assumption that blood flow should only be demonstrated in blood vessels and that blood vessels should appear anechoic or very hypoechoic. Therefore, any color assignment arising from a pixel that is not anechoic or very hypoechoic must be artifactual. When dealing with large superficial vessels such as the carotids, these assumptions more or less apply and the color priority can be adjusted to prevent color assignment from overwriting the gray-scale information arising from the pulsating vessel wall. However, when dealing with small vessels that are not resolvable on gray-scale imaging, it is possible to completely suppress real color information by misadjusting the color priority (see Fig. 1-16). When Doppler sensitivity is inadequate to detect flow, the color priority should be increased to its maximum value so that no color information is being suppressed.

Box 1-2 How to Improve Doppler Sensitivity

BASIC CONTROLS	ADVANCED CONTROLS
Increase Doppler gain	Decrease wall filter
Increase power output	Increase pulses per line
Decrease Doppler scale	Increase color priority
Decrease Doppler angle	Decrease Doppler steering
Adjust transmit frequency	

Beam Steering

Whenever the Doppler pulse is directed at an angle other than perpendicular to the transducer surface, it is being steered. Steering is an option on linear-array transducers, and it occurs automatically with phased-array probes whenever Doppler imaging is performed at the edge of the sector image. Steered pulses are less focused and lose a greater percentage of their energy to side lobes. In addition, the echoes returning from a steered pulse strike the surface of the transducer at an angle and produce less of an effect on the crystals and a weaker electronic impulse than nonsteered echoes (analogous to the different force exerted on a billiard table cushion when a ball strikes the cushion at an angle versus head on). Thus, for a variety of reasons, signal strength of returning echoes is less when the Doppler beam is steered. This may occur even when the Doppler angle is more optimal with a steered beam (see Fig. 1-16). The various ways that Doppler sensitivity can be improved are listed in Box 1-2.

ARTIFACTS

Ultrasound images are generated based on a number of assumptions. The most basic is that sound travels in a straight line and at a constant speed. Therefore, if the direction of a sound pulse transmitted into the body is controlled, the origin of a returning echo can be determined by analysis of timing. Other assumptions are that the only source of sound is the transducer, that sound is attenuated uniformly throughout the scan plane, and that each reflector in the body will only produce one echo. Finally, as with any cross-sectional imaging method, thickness of the slice is assumed to be infinitely thin. Deviations from these assumptions produce artifacts that result in inaccurate reproduction of internal structures.

Shadowing

Acoustic shadowing is so common in ultrasound images that it is often not even considered to be an artifact. It occurs when the energy of transmitted sound is decreased by reflection and/or absorption. The shadowing that occurs behind gas is due to the high degree of reflection at gas/tissue interfaces. Because the energy of a sound pulse reflected off of gas is essentially the same as the transmitted pulse, the reflected pulse will interact with the interfaces in front of the gas and produce secondary reflections that travel back to the gas surface and then reflect from this surface back to the transducer. These secondary reflections produce low-level echoes in the shadow deep to the gas, accounting for the "dirty" appearance. The shadowing that occurs behind stones, calcifications, and bones is caused primarily by sound attenuation by these structures. Because most of the sound is absorbed by these structures, much less energy is available for the generation of secondary reflections and the associated shadow tends to be more anechoic and "clean" appearing (Fig. 1-17). Unfortunately, there are many exceptions to the rule that gas produces dirty shadowing and stones produce clean shadowing; therefore, it is hard to rely too heavily on these characteristics.

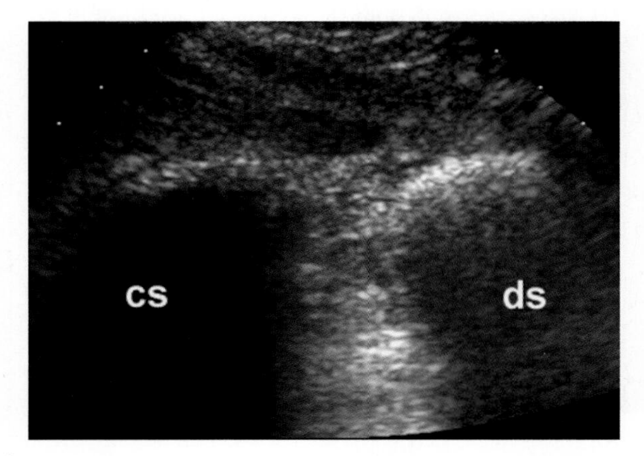

Figure 1-17 Clean vs. dirty shadowing. A gallbladder filled with stones demonstrates a classic clean shadow (cs). A gas-filled loop of bowel demonstrates classic dirty shadowing (ds).

Partial shadowing can occasionally occur behind highly attenuating soft tissues. This occurs most often behind fat-containing structures when they are surrounded by other soft tissues (Fig. 1-18A and B). Partial shadowing may also occur behind calcifications and stones if the cross section of the ultrasound beam (at the depth of the stone) is greater than the diameter of the stone. Therefore, the focal zone of the transducer should be adjusted so the tightest focusing occurs at the level of the stone (see Fig. 1-18C and D). Because higher-frequency probes can be focused more drastically and because high-frequency sound is less penetrating, it is usually easier to show shadowing with high-frequency probes.

Posterior Enhancement

As sound passes through solid tissues it is gradually attenuated. Fluid-containing structures attenuate the sound much less than solid structures so that the strength of the sound pulse is greater after passing through fluid than through an equivalent amount of solid tissue. Therefore, interfaces deep to cystic structures will produce stronger reflections and appear brighter than identical interfaces deep to solid tissues. This artifact produced by increased through transmission is quite helpful in distinguishing cystic from solid lesions (Fig. 1-19A), particularly when their gray scale appearance is nonspecific. However, it is important to realize that solid masses that attenuate sound less than adjacent soft tissues may also be associated with increased through transmission (see Fig. 1-19B).

Mirror Images

Acoustic mirrors can be compared with optical mirrors. With optical mirrors, a smooth flat surface that reflects a large amount of light will cause a visual duplication of structures. Surfaces that reflect more light (like a silvered piece of glass) act as better mirrors than surfaces that reflect less light (like a clear piece of glass). Flat surfaces will produce a mirror image that is identical in size and shape to the original object, but curved surfaces (like mirrors at the carnival) will produce a distorted mirror image. Because gas reflects almost 100% of the sound that hits it, gas is the best acoustic mirror in the body. This is particularly true where there are large, smooth gas interfaces—such as the lung (Fig. 1-20A). Therefore, mirror images are very common on sonograms that include the interface between lung and adjacent soft tissues.

The base of the right lung serves as a mirror on right upper quadrant scans and is capable of duplicating the

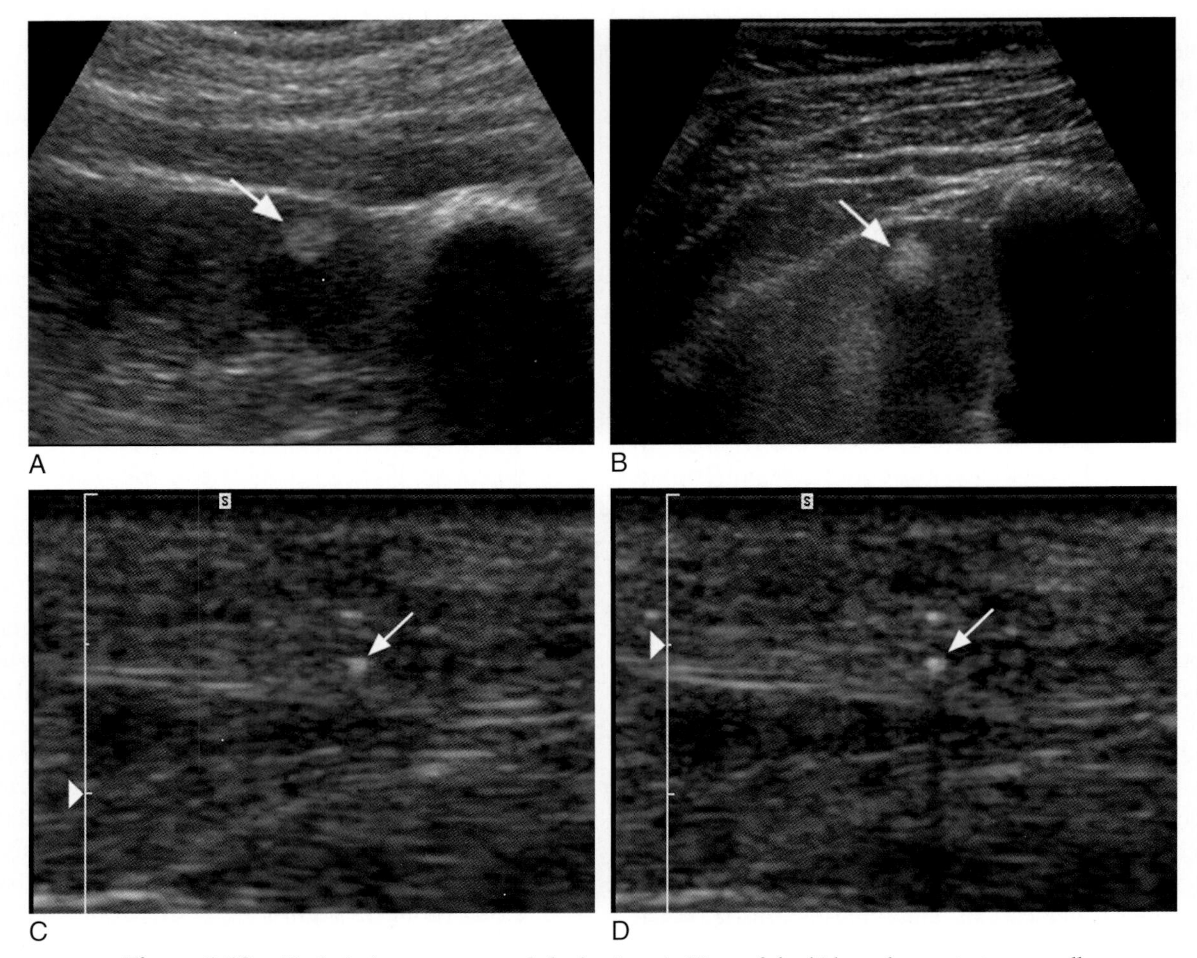

Figure 1-18 Technical parameters and shadowing. **A,** View of the kidney demonstrates a small echogenic mass *(arrow)*. **B,** Similar view using a higher frequency transducer demonstrates mild shadowing deep to the mass *(arrow)*. The presence of shadowing increases diagnostic confidence that this represents a fat-containing angiomyolipoma. **C,** View of the hand in a patient with a foreign body *(arrow)* shows a small bright reflector in the soft tissues but no posterior shadowing. **D,** Similar view with the focal zone readjusted to the level of the foreign body shows definite posterior shadowing *(arrow)*.

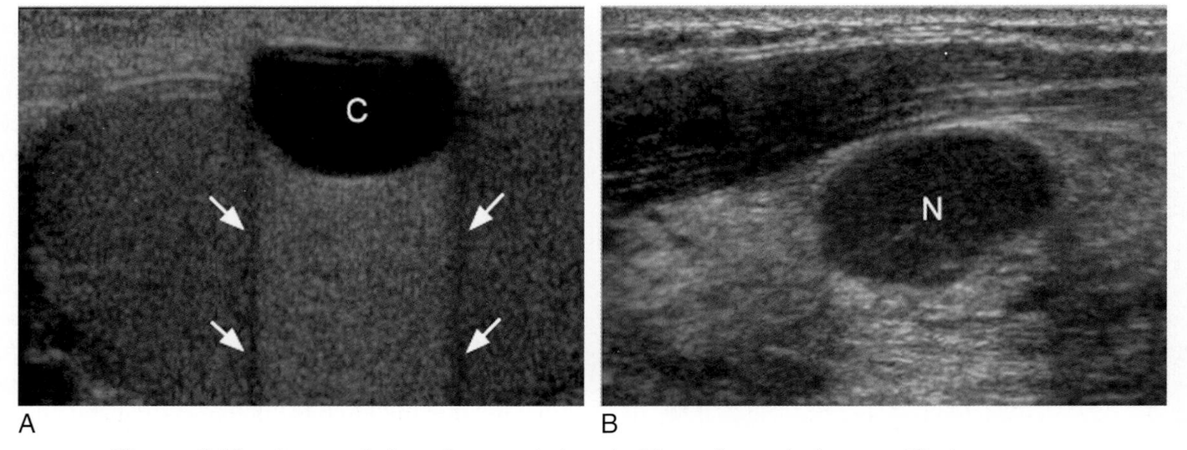

Figure 1-19 Increased through transmission. **A,** View of a testicular cyst (C) demonstrates classic posterior enhancement in the testicular parenchyma deep to the cyst. Also note the refractive shadowing *(arrows)* arising from each edge of the cyst. **B,** View of the neck demonstrates a lymph node (N) that is entirely solid but also shows clear posterior enhancement.

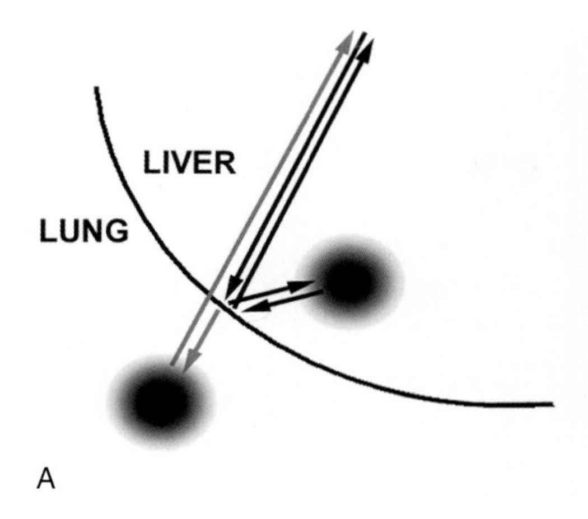

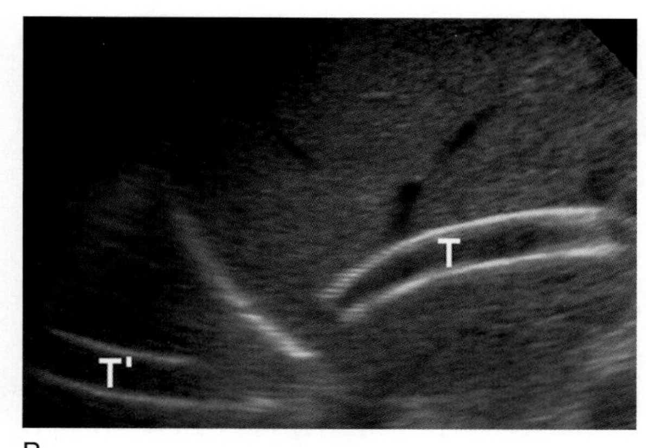

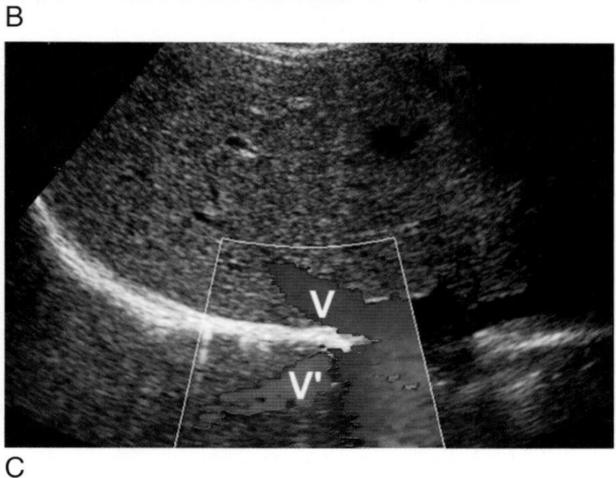

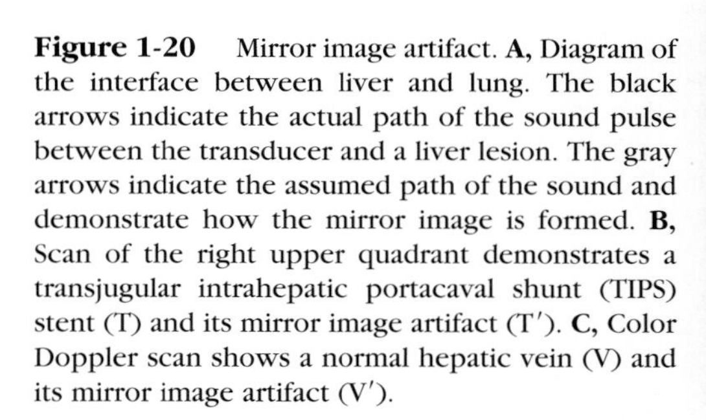
Figure 1-20 Mirror image artifact. **A,** Diagram of the interface between liver and lung. The black arrows indicate the actual path of the sound pulse between the transducer and a liver lesion. The gray arrows indicate the assumed path of the sound and demonstrate how the mirror image is formed. **B,** Scan of the right upper quadrant demonstrates a transjugular intrahepatic portacaval shunt (TIPS) stent (T) and its mirror image artifact (T′). **C,** Color Doppler scan shows a normal hepatic vein (V) and its mirror image artifact (V′).

liver itself, liver lesions, and the diaphragm (see Fig. 1-20B). The trachea is another structure with a large smooth gas interface. It is therefore capable of acting as a mirror on scans of the neck.

Because color Doppler scanning creates images with marked contrast between vascular structures and soft tissues (i.e., color vs. gray scale), mirror image artifacts are particularly common on color Doppler scans. As with gray-scale imaging, color Doppler mirror images occur most frequently around the lung (see Fig. 1-20C). However, the increased contrast also allows weaker acoustic interfaces, such as bone or even the back wall of the carotid, to act as mirrors for color Doppler imaging.

Refraction

Sound is refracted when it passes obliquely through an interface between two substances that transmit sound at different speeds (see Fig. 1-2). This is analogous to redirection of light by an optical lens. Because the speed of sound is least in fat (approximately 1450 m/sec) and greatest in soft tissues (approximately 1540 m/sec), refraction artifacts are most prominent at fat/soft tissue interfaces. The most widely recognized refraction artifact occurs at the junction of the rectus abdominis muscle and abdominal wall fat. The end result is a duplication of deep abdominal and pelvic structures seen when scanning through the abdominal midline (Fig. 1-21). Duplication artifacts can also arise when scanning the kidneys, owing to refraction of sound at the interface between the spleen (or liver) and adjacent fat.

Soft tissue and fluid interfaces can also produce refraction artifacts because the speed of sound in body fluids (1480 m/sec) is slower than in soft tissues. This can produce duplication of structures deep to the refracting interface just as with soft tissue/fat interfaces. Because refraction is also accompanied by defocusing and loss of beam energy, shadowing may also occur at the edge of cystic structures (see Fig. 1-19A).

Reverberation

When sound reflects off of strong acoustic interfaces in the near field, the returning pulse may be strong enough to reflect off of the transducer itself and back into the body so that it can interact with the same near-field interfaces a second time or multiple times. This produces an additional set of echoes that are interpreted as arising deep to the original reflector. In many cases these reverberation echoes are lost in the gray scale background of soft tissues. However, when they occur

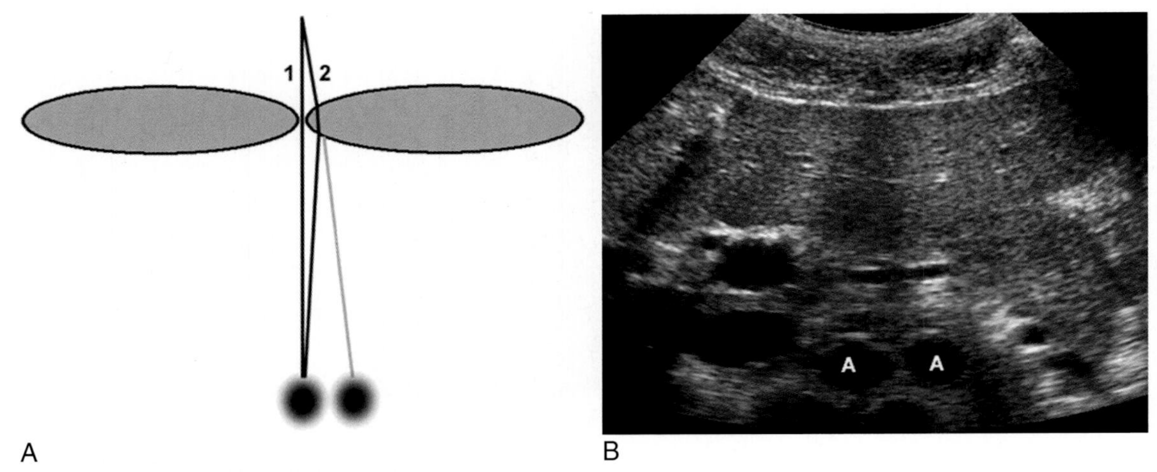

Figure 1-21 Refraction artifact. **A,** Diagram showing how sound beam refraction results in a duplication artifact. When sound pulse No. 1 goes between the rectus muscles, it travels in a straight line and the structure positioned in the midline is localized correctly. When sound pulse No. 2 travels through the medial edge of the rectus muscle, it is refracted as it enters the muscle and as it exits the muscle so that it is redirected toward the midline structure. The gray line indicates the assumed path of sound pulse No. 2 and illustrates how midline structures can be duplicated. **B,** Transverse midline view of the upper abdomen shows duplication of the aorta (A) secondary to rectus muscle refraction.

in cystic structures, the anechoic background of the fluid allows the reverberations to be seen. They may appear as bright bands or as diffuse low-level echoes in the superficial aspect of cystic spaces (Fig. 1-22A). They can be decreased or eliminated by decreasing power output and gain. When possible, they can also be minimized by positioning the transducer so that the cystic structure is no longer in the near field (see Fig. 1-22B). Occasionally, reverberation artifacts will be seen in soft tissues and these may be more difficult to recognize. Nevertheless, if they are suspected, the original interface can usually be identified and confirmed to be halfway between the transducer and the reverberation artifact.

Ring Down

Ring down occurs most frequently due to gas, and it has been shown that multiple bubbles of gas are required to produce this artifact. When the sound pulse reaches the gas bubbles, it excites the fluid that is trapped between the bubbles and causes the fluid to resonate. This results in a continuous sound wave following the original echo back to the transducer. This sound is interpreted as having originated from reflectors deep to the gas so a series of bright echoes is produced deep to the gas (Fig. 1-23A). Metal is also capable of producing a ring-down artifact (Fig. 1-23B).

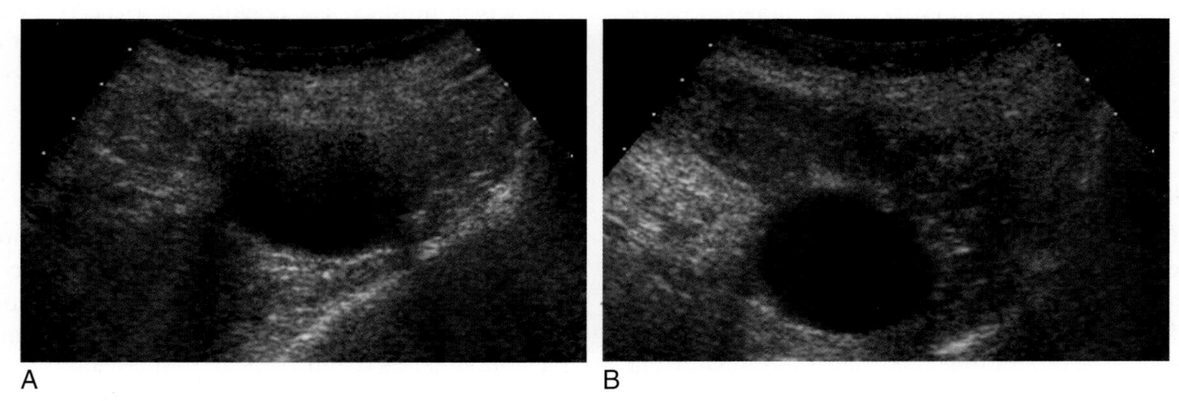

Figure 1-22 Reverberation artifact. **A,** View of the left pelvis demonstrates an ovarian cyst. Diffuse low-level echoes are seen in the superficial aspect of the cyst secondary to near-field reverberations. **B,** With the transducer repositioned so that the cyst is located in the deeper aspect of the field of view, the near-field reverberations are no longer seen within the cyst.

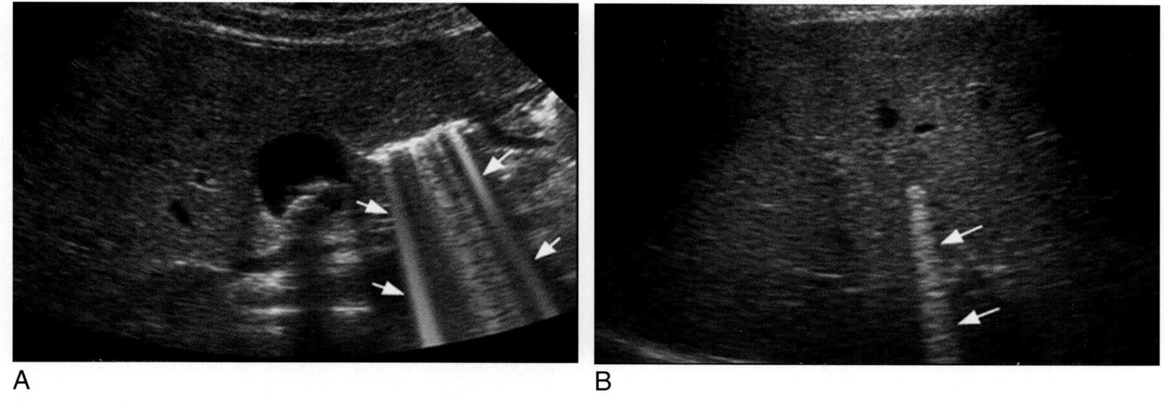

Figure 1-23 Ring-down artifact. **A,** View of the right upper quadrant shows multiple ring-down artifacts *(arrows)* arising from a gas-filled loop of bowel in the right upper quadrant. **B,** View of the liver shows a ring-down artifact *(arrows)* arising from a shotgun pellet embedded within the liver.

Side Lobe

The majority of the sound energy transmitted by the ultrasound transducer is concentrated in the center beam. However, weak side lobes radiate outward from the center beam. Because these side lobes are weak, they generally do not result in significant artifacts. Artifacts are occasionally produced when a side lobe reflects off of a strong reflector and produces an echo that is strong enough to be detected. Because the side-lobe reflection is assumed to have arisen from the center beam, an artifactual low-level echo is created on the image. Side-lobe artifacts are usually obscured when they occur over soft tissues but become visible when displayed on the anechoic background of cystic structures (Fig. 1-24).

Slice Thickness

The thickness of the ultrasound beam can be separated into a component in the plane of imaging and a component out of the plane of imaging. Although each of these components of thickness can be minimized by a combination of electronic and mechanical focusing, the beam always has a finite thickness. When part of the ultrasound beam interacts with a fluid-filled structure and part interacts with solid tissue there is artifactual generation of low-level echoes within the cystic space.

Aliasing

Aliasing is a well-known artifact that occurs when the Doppler sampling rate (i.e., the PRF) is less than twice the Doppler frequency shift. A similar effect is seen when the frame rate of a movie (analogous to the PRF) is too slow to reproduce the rotation of a wheel and the wheel appears to rotate backward. On Doppler waveforms, aliasing causes the high-frequency components to wrap around from the positive extreme of the scale to the negative extreme or vice versa (Fig. 1-25). When aliasing occurs on color Doppler images, the wraparound effect causes the color representing the highest positive frequency shift to change to the color representing the highest negative frequency shift, or vice versa. This change in color assignment can be distinguished from true flow reversal because the change is between light color shades rather than dark color shades (Fig. 1-26). When aliasing is severe, there can be multiple wraparounds of the Doppler waveform or the color assignment and this can produce an appearance of random frequency shifts that simulates noise or severe flow turbulence. Although aliasing is artifactual, when properly recognized it can be useful because it dramatically identifies areas of high flow velocity. Aliasing can be diminished or eliminated by increasing the PRF. In most instances, the maximum PRF is limited by the depth of the vessel, because it takes a finite amount of time to deliver the Doppler pulse to the vessel and wait for the echo to return to the transducer before the next pulse is transmitted. Another means of decreasing or eliminating aliasing is to decrease the observed frequency shift. This can be done by manipulating the transducer so that the vessel is scanned at a Doppler angle closer to 90 degrees or by switching to a lower-frequency transducer.

Tissue Vibration

Tissue vibration is another artifact that is occasionally encountered in areas of turbulent blood flow. Turbulence causes pressure fluctuations in the lumen of the vessel that can produce vibration of the vessel wall and

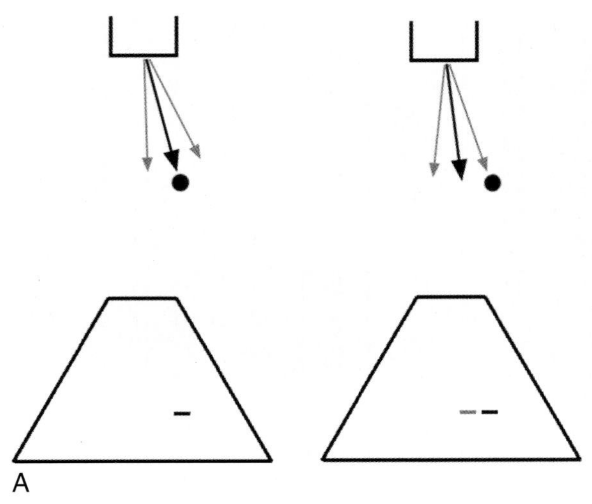

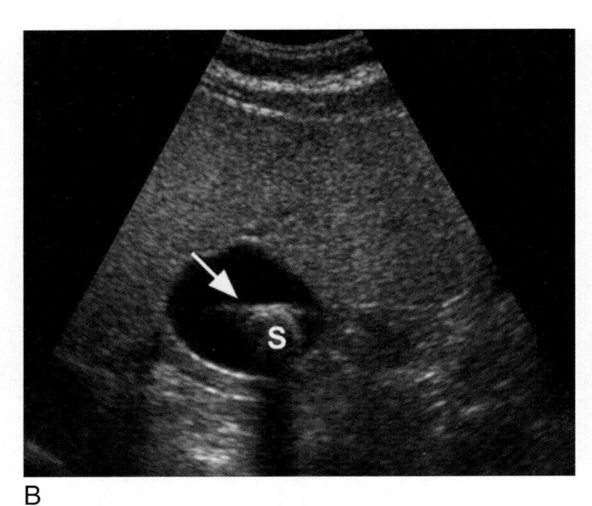

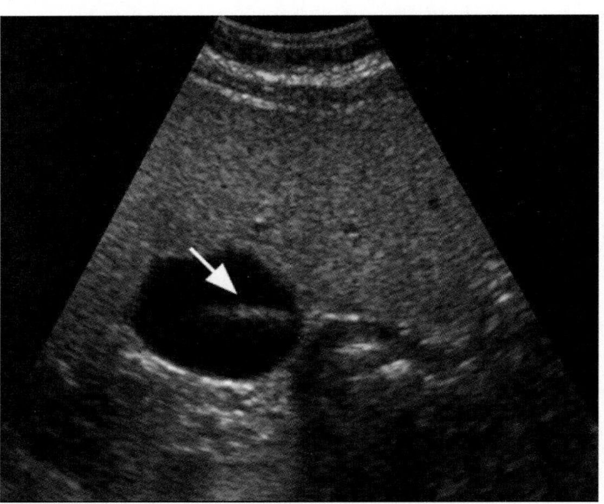

Figure 1-24 Side lobe artifact. **A,** Diagram showing how side lobe artifacts are generated. When the main sound beam *(black arrow)* is directed toward a strong reflector *(black circle),* the image (shown below) displays a single echo *(short black line).* The side lobes *(gray arrows)* do not reflect off of anything and no artifact is generated. When the main sound beam shifts to the left, one of the side lobes is directed toward the strong reflector. The reflection from the side lobe is weaker than the reflection from the main beam, but is sufficient to produce an echo *(short gray line)* on the image. The artifactual echo is located immediately adjacent to the real echo. **B,** Scan of the gallbladder shows a shadowing stone (S). Side lobe artifacts *(arrow)* are seen adjacent to the anterior aspect of the gallstone. **C,** Scan of the gallbladder immediately next to the gallstone still shows the side lobe artifact *(arrow).* This occurs because the side lobes extend around the main beam for 360 degrees and can reflect off of structures that are not in the plane of imaging.

of the perivascular soft tissues. When the tissue interfaces vibrate, they may produce a detectable Doppler frequency shift and this will be assigned a color. Because the vibrational motion is both toward and away from the transducer, the color assignment is a mixture of red and blue (Fig. 1-27A). Although this artifact can obscure underlying vessel anatomy, it can also be a valuable marker of vascular pathology. In fact, it is often the most dramatic finding in situations that promote turbulent blood flow such as arteriovenous fistulas or deep abdominal arterial stenoses. This artifact is also visible on pulsed Doppler waveforms as a small but strong signal that is most prominent during systole and is symmetric above and below the baseline (see Fig. 1-27B).

CONTRAST AGENTS

Microbubble-based intravenous contrast agents are being developed and refined by a number of pharmaceutical companies. Different gases and encapsulating agents are utilized to vary the durability, size, and metabolism of the bubbles. In general, they all share the properties of being small enough to pass through the pulmonary and systemic circulation and being durable enough to recirculate for several minutes.

One of the primary characteristics of the bubbles is that they increase the strength of the backscattered signal from blood by several orders of magnitude. Thus, the Doppler signal from flowing blood is considerably easier to detect after administration of intravenous contrast agents. This allows for improvement in vascular examinations where vessels may be difficult to see (e.g., the renal arteries), where the flow may be slow (e.g., the portal vein), or where the signal may be attenuated by overlying structures (e.g., transcranial Doppler).

Another characteristic of microbubbles is that they oscillate when they are subjected to ultrasound waves. This generates harmonic signals that are stronger than the harmonic signals generated by soft tissues. Therefore, post-contrast harmonic imaging allows for visualization of blood flow and enhanced soft tissues in the

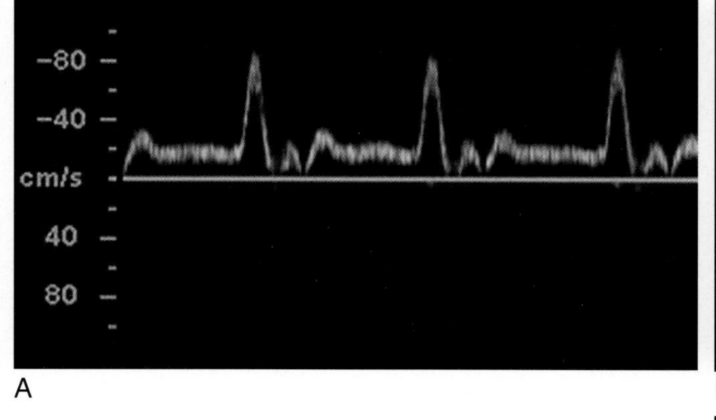

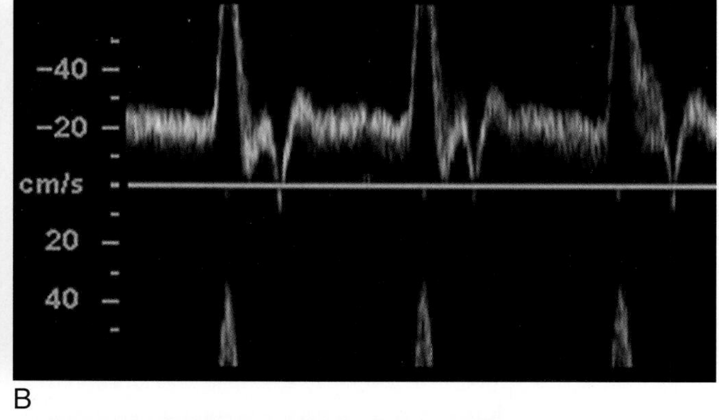

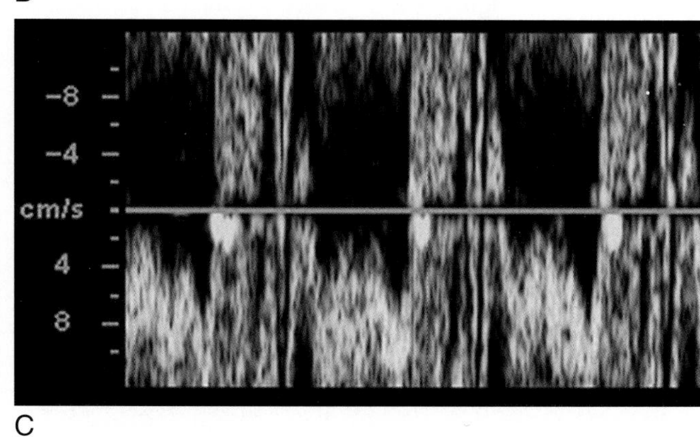

Figure 1-25 Pulsed Doppler aliasing artifact. **A,** Doppler waveform from the common carotid artery using a high Doppler scale (±80 cm/sec) displays the entire waveform without aliasing artifact. **B,** With a smaller Doppler scale (±40 cm/sec), the systolic peaks can no longer be displayed above the baseline and therefore become aliased below the baseline. **C,** With an even smaller Doppler scale (±8 cm/sec), more severe aliasing occurs. Diastolic flow becomes aliased below the baseline, and systolic flow begins to overlap on itself, owing to multiple wraparounds.

gray-scale mode (Fig. 1-28). This has significant advantages to color and power Doppler imaging because the frame rates are higher in gray-scale imaging and the resolution is better. In addition, the blooming artifacts that occur with post-contrast color and power Doppler imaging are not present in gray-scale harmonic imaging.

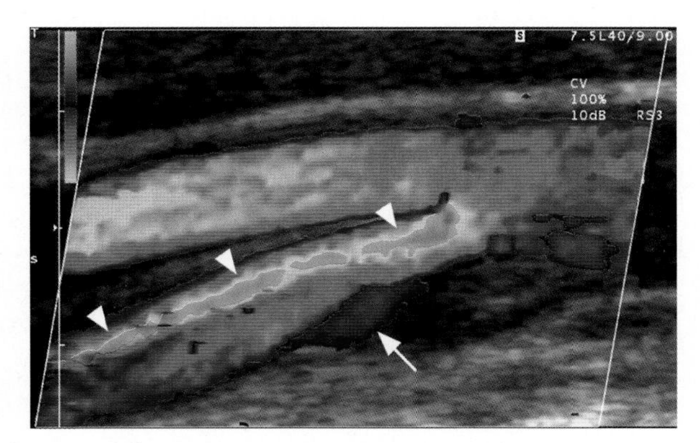

Figure 1-26 Color Doppler aliasing. Longitudinal view of the carotid bifurcation shows aliasing *(arrowheads)* in the flow jet. Note how the transition from one color to the other occurs in the light shades with aliasing and occurs in the darker color shades with reversed flow *(arrow).*

Pulse inversion imaging is another technique that has been developed to take advantage of unique properties of contrast agents. With this technique, a pulse is transmitted and the returning signals are digitally stored. A second pulse that is the inverse of the first is then transmitted, and the returning signal is again digitally stored. The system then sums the two signals together. Because the fundamental soft tissue signals are inverted, they cancel each other out. Because the harmonic signal from the contrast agent is nonlinear, the summation process does not cancel it out, and the image shows contrast to a much greater degree than soft tissue. This maintains the superior resolution attained with gray-scale imaging, reduces clutter from background tissues, and further enhances signals from contrast.

The techniques just described can be utilized in two modes to emphasize different facets of contrast distribution. Continuous imaging at low output powers will display flowing contrast medium in larger vessels. However, if the scanning is stopped for a period of time, contrast medium will accumulate in the microvasculature. After a delay, resumption of scanning at high output levels will cause bubble destruction (that proceeds from the near field to the far field) and an even stronger signal from the contrast agent. The resulting image gives additional information about the vascular volume of normal and abnormal tissues.

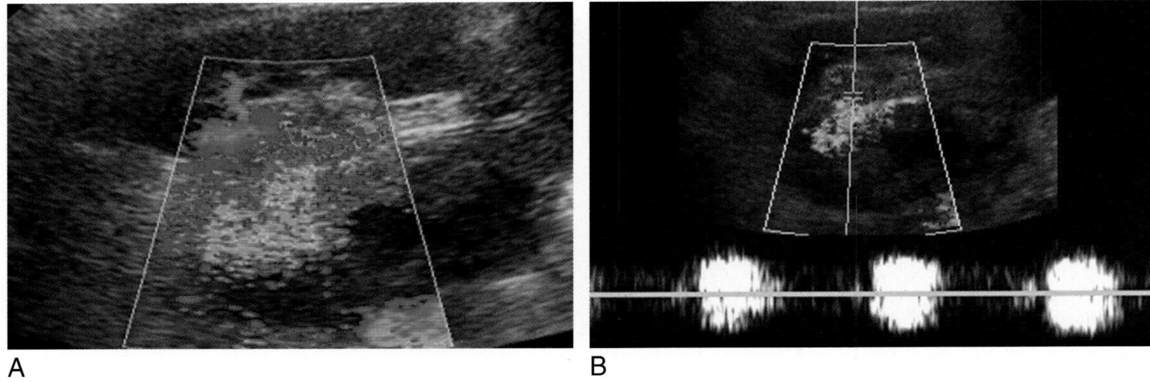

Figure 1-27 Tissue vibration artifact. **A,** Transverse view of a renal transplant with renal artery stenosis demonstrates random red and blue color assignment outside the expected confines of the vessels in the region of the renal hilum. This reflects vibrating soft tissue interfaces. **B,** Pulsed Doppler waveform from this region demonstrates a strong signal during systole that shows symmetric components above and below the baseline. This also reflects the presence of underlying soft tissue vibration.

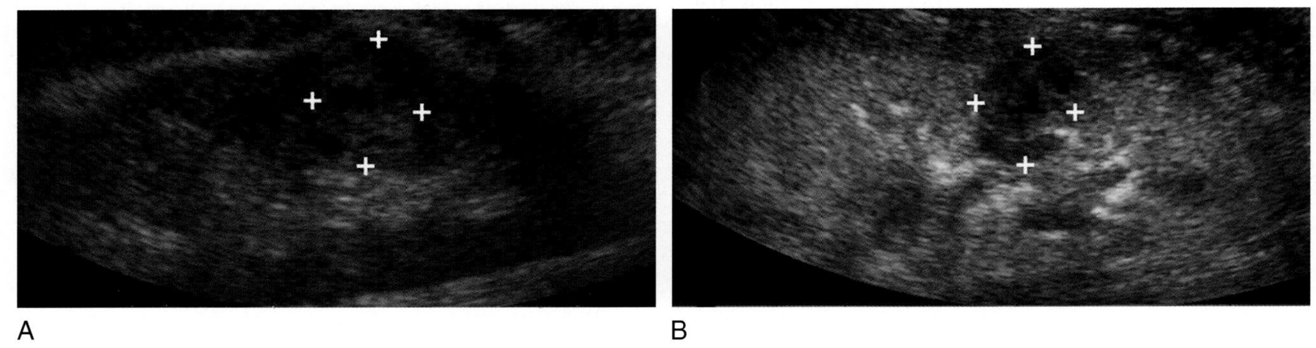

Figure 1-28 Microbubble contrast agent enhancement. **A,** Longitudinal view of the kidney before administration of contrast agent shows a renal mass *(cursors)* that is difficult to distinguish from the normal renal parenchyma. **B,** Similar view during intravenous injection of contrast agent shows intense enhancement of the renal parenchyma and allows for easy visualization of the mass *(cursors).* This proved to be a renal cell cancer.

Key Features

Sound can be reflected, scattered, refracted, and absorbed.
The speed of sound in soft tissues is 1540 m/sec. Sound is slower in fat and fluids.
Large, smooth interfaces are called specular reflectors.
The higher the transmit frequency, the better the resolution.
The lower the transmit frequency, the better the penetration.
Sound pulses are produced, and the returning echoes are received by piezoelectric crystals housed in the transducer.
Resolution is divided into axial, lateral, and elevational.
Harmonic imaging extracts information from the harmonic signals generated by the interaction of the fundamental sound pulse and body tissue.
Real-time compounding adds signals generated by pulses traveling in different directions.
Doppler frequency shift is directly proportional to the blood flow velocity and the cosine of the Doppler angle.
Velocity should only be estimated at Doppler angles of 60 degrees or less.
The resistive index (RI) and pulsatility index (PI) are unitless indices independent of the Doppler angle that increase as the vascular resistance increases.
Differential attenuation of sound causes shadowing and posterior enhancement.
Large smooth interfaces that reflect a large amount of sound can produce mirror image artifacts.
Sound refraction can cause duplication artifacts.
Reverberation artifacts commonly occur in the near field.
Ring-down artifacts usually indicate gas bubbles.
Doppler aliasing occurs when the frequency shift exceeds the Doppler scale.
Turbulent blood flow can cause vibration in perivascular tissues and lead to extravascular Doppler signals.

SUGGESTED READINGS

Avruch L, Cooperberg PL: The ring-down artifact. J Ultrasound Med 4:21-28, 1985.

Balen FG, Allen CM, Lees WR: Ultrasound contrast agents. Clin Radiol 49:77-82, 1994.

Bude RO, Rubin JM: Power Doppler sonography. Radiology 200:21-23, 1996.

Bude RO, Rubin JM: Relationship between the resistive index and vascular compliance and resistance. Radiology 211: 411-417, 1999.

Burns PN: Contrast agents for ultrasound imaging and Doppler. In Rumack CM, Wilson ST, Charboneau JW (eds): Diagnostic Ultrasound. St. Louis, Mosby, 1998, pp 57-84.

Choudhry S, Gorman B, Charboneau JW, et al: Comparison of tissue harmonic imaging with conventional US in abdominal disease. Radiographics 20:1127-1135, 2000.

Desser TS, Jedrzejewicz T, Haller MI: Color and power Doppler sonography: Techniques, clinical applications, and trade-offs for image optimization. Ultrasound Q 14(3): 128-149, 1998.

Downey DB, Fenster A, Williams JC: Clinical utility of three-dimensional US. Radiographics 20:559-571, 2000.

Fiske CE, Filly RA: Pseudo-sludge: A spurious ultrasound appearance within the gallbladder. Radiology 144:631-632, 1982.

Goldberg BB, Liu J-B, Forsberg F: Ultrasound contrast agents: A review. Ultrasound Med Biol 20:319-333, 1994.

Goldstein A, Madrazo BL: Slice-thickness artifacts in gray-scale ultrasound. J Clin Ultrasound 9:365-375, 1981.

Goldstein A: AAPM Tutorials: Overview of the physics of US. Radiographics 13:701-704, 1993.

Keogh CF, Cooperberg PL: Is it real or is it an artifact. Ultrasound Q 17:201-210, 2001.

Kremkau FW: AAPM Tutorial: Multiple-element transducers. Radiographics 13:1163-1176, 1993.

Kremkau FW, Taylor KJW: Artifacts in ultrasound imaging. J Ultrasound Med 5:227-237, 1986.

Laing FC: Commonly encountered artifacts in clinical ultrasound. Semin Ultrasound 4:27-43, 1983.

Laing FC, Kurtz AB: The importance of ultrasonic side-lobe artifacts. Radiology 145:763-768, 1982.

Mayo J, Cooperberg PL: Displacement of the diaphragmatic echo by hepatic cysts: A new explanation with computer simulation. J Ultrasound Med 3:337-340, 1984.

Middleton WD: Color Doppler: Image interpretation and optimization. Ultrasound Q 14:194-208, 1998.

Middleton WD, Melson GL: Diaphragmatic discontinuity associated with perihepatic ascites: A sonographic refractive artifact. AJR Am J Roentgenol 151:709-711, 1988.

Middleton WD, Melson GL: Renal duplication artifact in US imaging. Radiology 173:427-429, 1989.

Middleton WD, Melson GL: The carotid ghost. A color Doppler ultrasound duplication artifact. J Ultrasound Med 9:487-493, 1990.

Muller N, Cooperberg PL, Rowley VA, et al: Ultrasonic refraction by the rectus abdominis muscles: The double image artifact. J Ultrasound Med 3:515-519, 1984.

Nelson TR, Pretorius DH: Three-dimensional ultrasound imaging. Ultrasound Med Biol 24:1243-1270, 1998.

Reading CC, Charboneau JW, Allison JW, Cooperberg PL: Color and spectral Doppler mirror image artifact of the subclavian artery. Radiology 174:41-42, 1009.

Robinson DE, Wilson LS, Kossoff G: Shadowing and enhancement in ultrasonic echograms by reflection and refraction. J Clin Ultrasound 9:181-188, 1981.

Rubin JM: AAPM Tutorial: Spectral Doppler US. Radiographics 14:139-150, 1994.

Rubin JM, Adler RS, Bude RO, et al: Clean and dirty shadowing at US: A reappraisal. Radiology 181:231-236, 1991.

Sauerbrei EE: The split image artifact in pelvic ultrasonography: The anatomy and physics. J Ultrasound Med 4:29-34, 1985.

Shapiro RS, Winsberg F: Comet-tail artifact from cholesterol crystals: Observations in the postlithotripsy gallbladder and an in vitro model. Radiology 177:153-156, 1990.

Sommer FG, Taylor KJW: Differentiation of acoustic shadowing due to calculi and gas collections. Radiology 135:399-403, 1980.

Weng L, Tirumalai AP, Lowery, CM, et al: US Extended-field-of-view imaging technology. Radiology 203:877, 1997.

Wilson SR, Burns PN, Wilkinson LM, et al: Gas at abdominal US: Appearance, relevance, and analysis of artifacts. Radiology 210:113-123, 1999.

Ziskin MC: Fundamental physics of ultrasound and its propagation in tissue. Radiographics 13:705-709, 1993.

CHAPTER 2 Gallbladder

For Key Features summary see p. 46

ANATOMY

The gallbladder is a long oval organ that is positioned beneath the liver immediately adjacent to the interlobar fissure (Fig. 2-1). The fissure can be a useful landmark for locating small contracted gallbladders or gallbladders that are completely filled with stones. Likewise, the gallbladder can be used as a landmark for identifying the junction between the left and right lobes of the liver. The upper limit of normal for the transverse dimension of the gallbladder is 4 cm. The length of the gallbladder is more variable but generally does not exceed 10 cm. The normal upper limit for the gallbladder wall thickness is 3 mm. When the gallbladder contracts, the echogenic mucosa and the hypoechoic muscularis become apparent and the wall may appear thickened (Fig. 2-2). However, even with gallbladder contraction, the wall usually remains less than 3 mm thick. See Table 2-1 for the characteristics of a normal gallbladder.

Variations in shape of the gallbladder are common. There are frequently one or more junctional folds in the gallbladder neck, and occasionally there are folds throughout the gallbladder (Fig. 2-3A and B). When the gallbladder fundus folds on itself, it is referred to as a phrygian cap (see Fig. 2-3C). Gallbladder folds may mimic septations, but it should be possible to demonstrate a change in the outer contour of the gallbladder. Septations are rare and generally appear thinner than folds. They separate the gallbladder into segments that communicate through a small pore (Fig. 2-4).

Variations in the location of the gallbladder are also rare; intrahepatic gallbladders are probably the most frequently recognized. Most intrahepatic gallbladders are located immediately above the interlobar fissure (Fig. 2-5). Gallbladder duplication is another rare congenital anomaly that may be complete (Fig. 2-6A) or partial (see Fig. 2-6B). Agenesis of the gallbladder has also been reported.

TECHNIQUE

Ideally, patients should fast 8 hours after midnight before a gallbladder sonogram to ensure adequate gallbladder distention and to reduce upper abdominal bowel gas. A recent meal makes the examination harder to perform and interpret and decreases diagnostic sensitivity. However, in most cases diagnostic information can be obtained even in non-fasting patients, so a recent meal is not an absolute contraindication to performing a gallbladder sonogram.

Most gallbladder examinations start with the patient in the supine position using a 3- to 5-MHz sector transducer. The gallbladder should be scanned from both a subcostal and intercostal approach whenever possible. Often one approach will display a pathologic process and/or diminish artifacts better. When scanning from a subcostal view, a deep inspiration will usually allow better visualization. Frequently there are artifactual low-level echoes in the gallbladder lumen resulting from reverberations. They can often be eliminated by scanning from a more lateral and superior approach (often

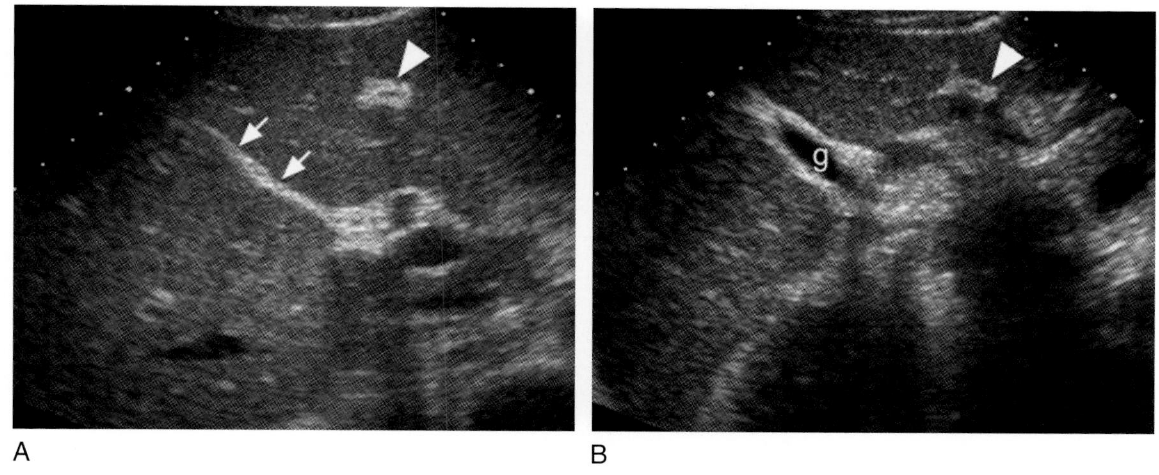

Figure 2-1 Relationship of gallbladder to interlobar fissure. **A,** Transverse view shows the ligamentum teres *(arrowhead)* and the interlobar fissure *(arrows)*. **B,** Transverse view slightly inferior to part A shows a contracted gallbladder (g) located immediately inferior to the interlobar fissure.

from an intercostal space) and using more of the liver as a window. Scans should routinely be obtained with the patient in a variety of positions (left posterior oblique, left lateral decubitus, prone, upright) to document mobility of intraluminal structures, such as stones and sludge, and nonmobility of polyps and tumors. In some patients the gallbladder may be hard to see in the prone position. Nevertheless, stones that fall into the fundus when the patient is prone can be seen on real-time imaging, falling back into the neck as the patient rolls from a prone to a supine position. Upright views can be obtained in the sitting position, although it is usually easier to scan with the patient standing. Although it is important to visualize the entire gallbladder, seeing the gallbladder neck is especially important, because stones can be missed if the entire neck is not visualized, if a stone is positioned behind a junctional fold, or if the stone is impacted in the neck of the organ (Fig. 2-7). It is also important to ensure that abnormalities in the fundus are not obscured by bowel gas.

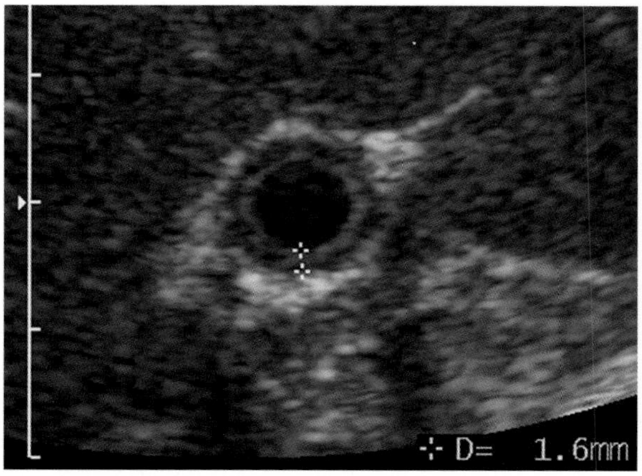

Figure 2-2 Contracted gallbladder. Transverse view shows the echogenic mucosal layer and the hypoechoic muscular layer. Despite apparent thickening, the wall measures only 1.6 mm thick *(cursors)*.

GALLSTONES

Gallstones are present in up to 10% of the population. In North America, 75% are cholesterol and 25% are pigment. The majority of gallstones are asymptomatic (silent). Surgery is seldom performed on silent stones because they become symptomatic at a rate of only 2% per year. Symptoms rarely develop after an asymptomatic period of 10 to 15 years.

The most common symptom of gallstones is biliary colic, which manifests as acute right upper quadrant or epigastric pain lasting for up to 6 hours and ending when the stone disimpacts from the gallbladder neck or passes completely through the cystic duct. Gallstones may also cause nonspecific dyspeptic symptoms.

Table 2-1 Characteristics of the Normal Gallbladder

Characteristic	Appearance
Location	Inferior to interlobar fissure Between left and right lobe
Size	<4 cm transverse <10 cm longitudinal
Wall thickness	<3 mm
Lumen	Anechoic

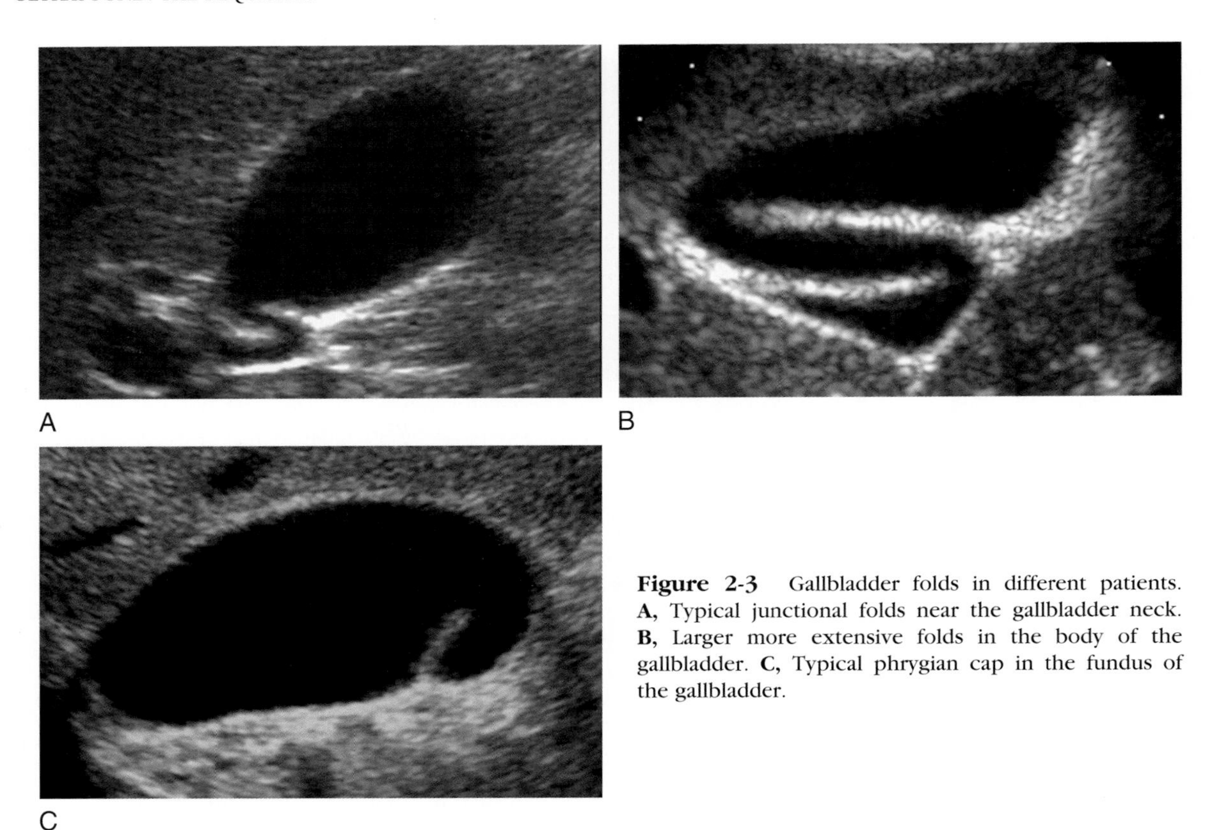

Figure 2-3 Gallbladder folds in different patients. **A,** Typical junctional folds near the gallbladder neck. **B,** Larger more extensive folds in the body of the gallbladder. **C,** Typical phrygian cap in the fundus of the gallbladder.

Sonography has assumed an important role in evaluating the gallbladder because it is the most sensitive means of detecting gallstones. Multiple studies have documented sensitivities of greater than 95% and positive and negative predictive values that are close to 100%. Even in obese patients, sonography is the best way to detect stones.

Gallstones appear as mobile, echogenic, intraluminal structures that cast acoustic shadows (Fig. 2-8). Shadowing occurs because of sound beam absorption by the stone. Demonstration of shadowing is important in distinguishing stones from other intraluminal abnormalities. Shadowing primarily depends on the size of the stone. Stones smaller than 3 mm may not cast a

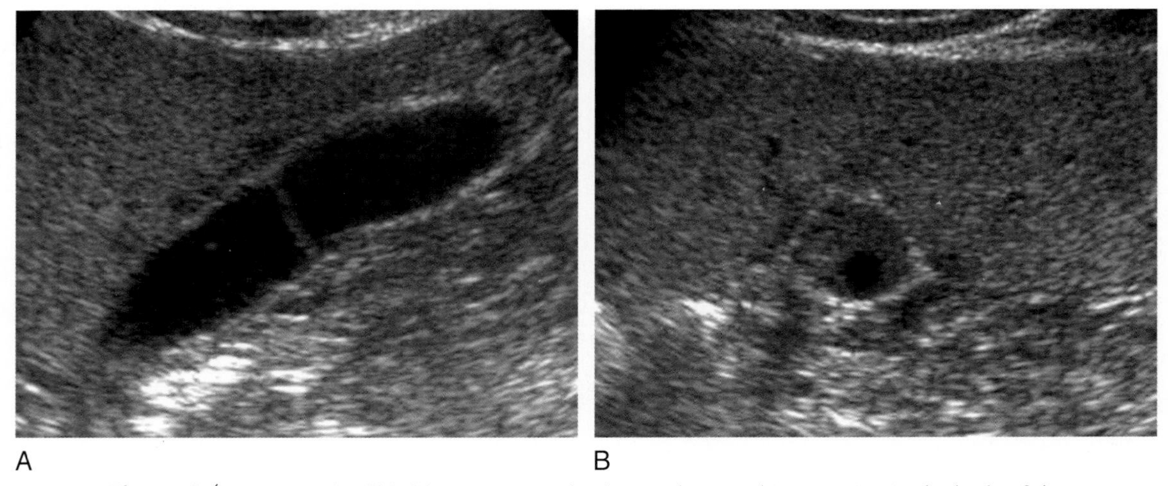

Figure 2-4 Septated gallbladder. **A,** Longitudinal view shows a thin septation in the body of the gallbladder with little deformation of the outer gallbladder contour. **B,** Transverse view through the septation shows a small, round defect in the periphery of the septation that allows for communication between the two segments of the gallbladder.

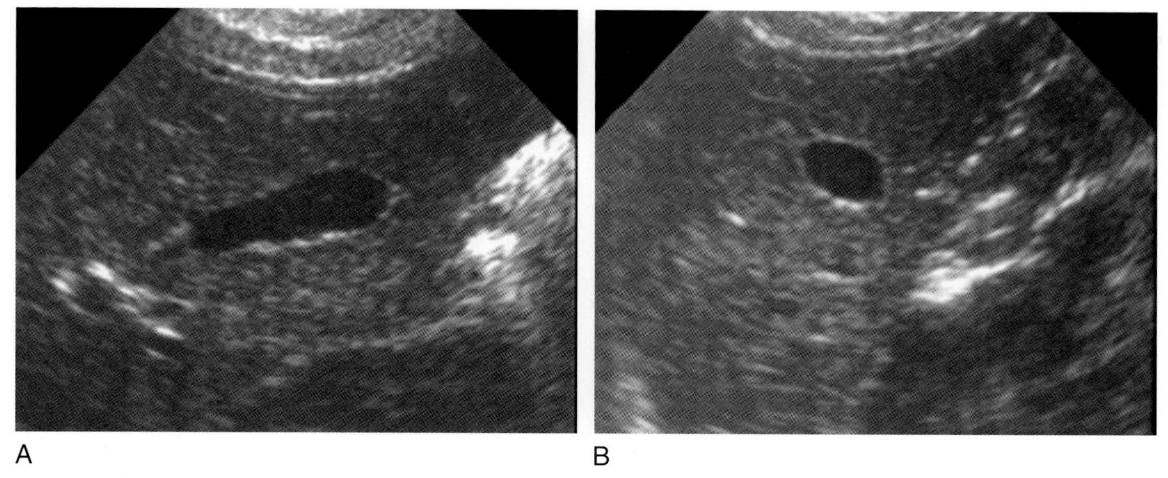

Figure 2-5 Intrahepatic gallbladder. **A,** Longitudinal view of the liver shows a gallbladder completely surrounded by hepatic parenchyma. **B,** Transverse view of the gallbladder shows similar findings.

detectable shadow. In contrast, shadowing is largely independent of stone composition. In particular, calcification is not necessary for shadow production. To a large degree, all stones appear similar on sonography.

Technical factors need to be optimized to demonstrate shadowing from small stones. Because sound absorption increases at higher frequencies, non-shadowing stones may be converted into shadowing stones by switching to a higher-frequency transducer (Fig. 2-9A and B). Another important factor is the focal zone. Because the beam profile is narrowest at the focal zone, it should be set at the depth of the stone so that the stone will absorb a greater percentage of the sound beam (see Fig. 2-9C and D). If there are multiple small stones, shadowing may be best demonstrated by positioning the patient so that the stones are clumped together (see Fig. 2-9E and F).

The major differential considerations are gallbladder polyps and sludge balls (Table 2-2). Polyps are small soft tissue structures that are adherent to the gallbladder wall. They do not move or shadow. Sludge balls (tumefactive sludge) are almost always mobile but do not produce a shadow. In addition, sludge balls are usually quite a bit larger than non-shadowing stones.

A gallbladder completely filled with stones is harder to recognize than when it is filled with bile. All that is apparent is an echogenic shadowing structure in the right upper quadrant that could potentially be confused with a gas-filled loop of bowel. If an identifiable gallbladder is seen elsewhere, then the problem is solved.

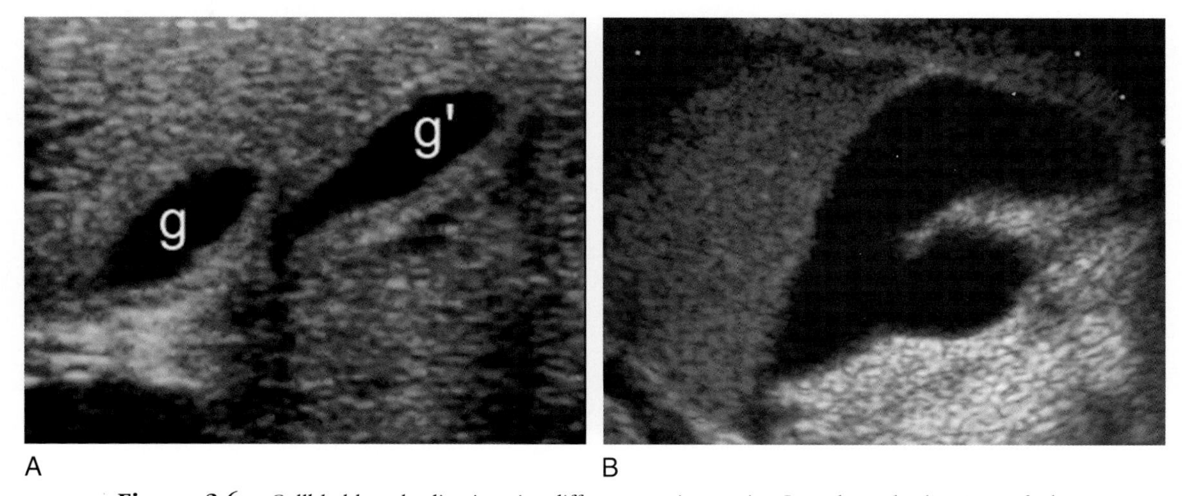

Figure 2-6 Gallbladder duplication in different patients. **A,** Complete duplication of the gallbladder into two separate structures (g, g′). **B,** Partial duplication of the gallbladder into two separate fundal segments.

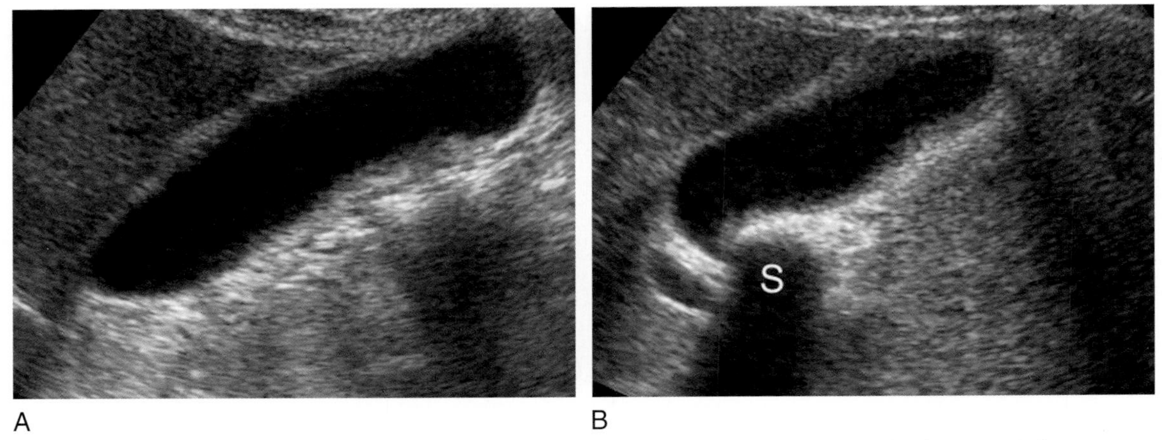

Figure 2-7 Importance of visualizing entire gallbladder neck. **A,** Longitudinal view of the gallbladder shows an apparently stone-free lumen. **B,** Longitudinal view showing more of the gallbladder neck demonstrates a shadowing stone (S) within a folded segment of the gallbladder neck.

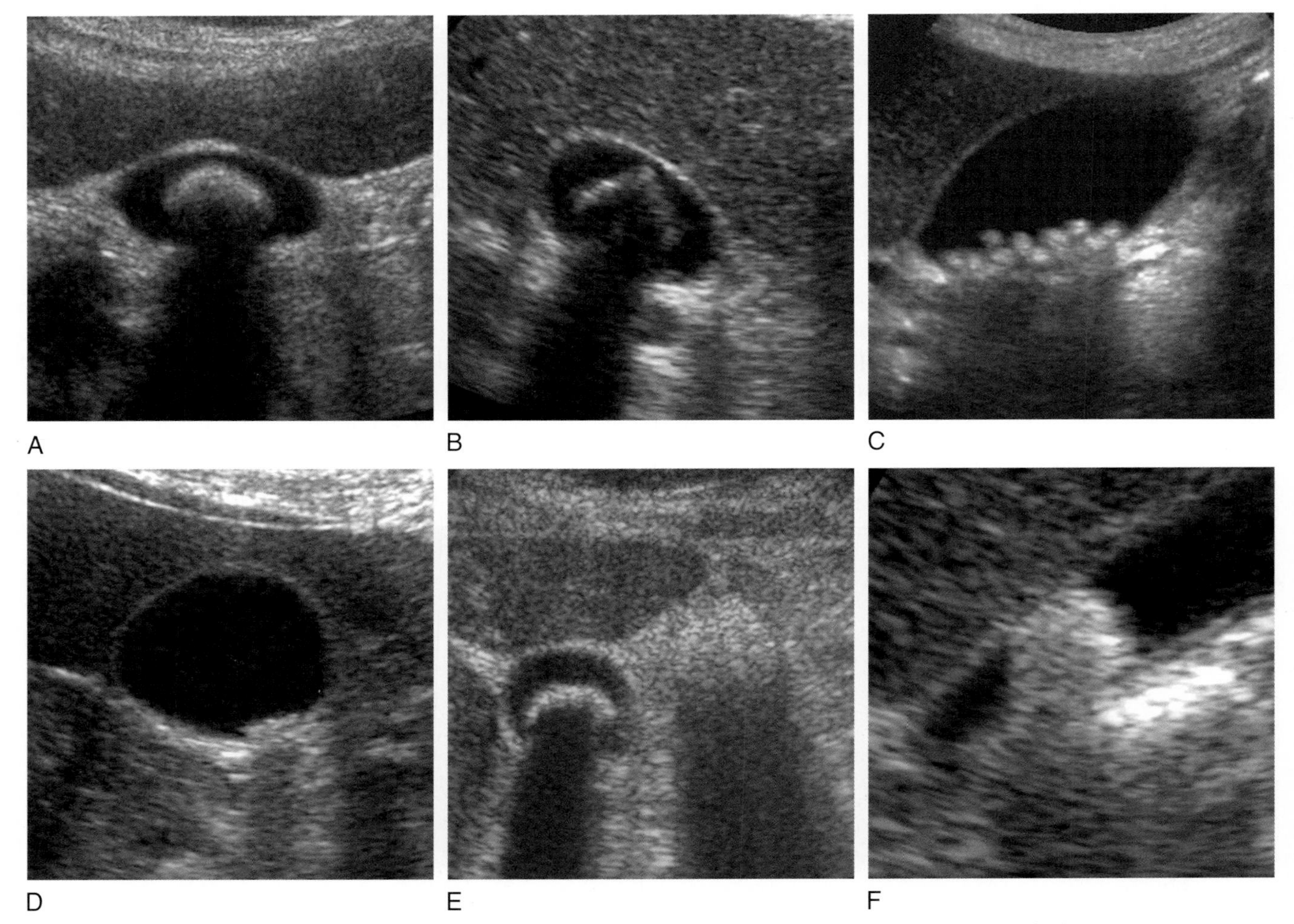

Figure 2-8 Gallstones in different patients. **A,** Typical stone with distinct clean acoustic shadow. **B,** Faceted stone. **C,** Multiple small stones layering in the dependent portion of the gallbladder. **D,** Very small stones with a faint acoustic shadow layering in the dependent portion of the gallbladder. **E,** Gallstone with a clean acoustic shadow immediately adjacent to a gas-filled loop of bowel with a dirty acoustic shadow. **F,** Unusual gallstone with a dirty acoustic shadow.

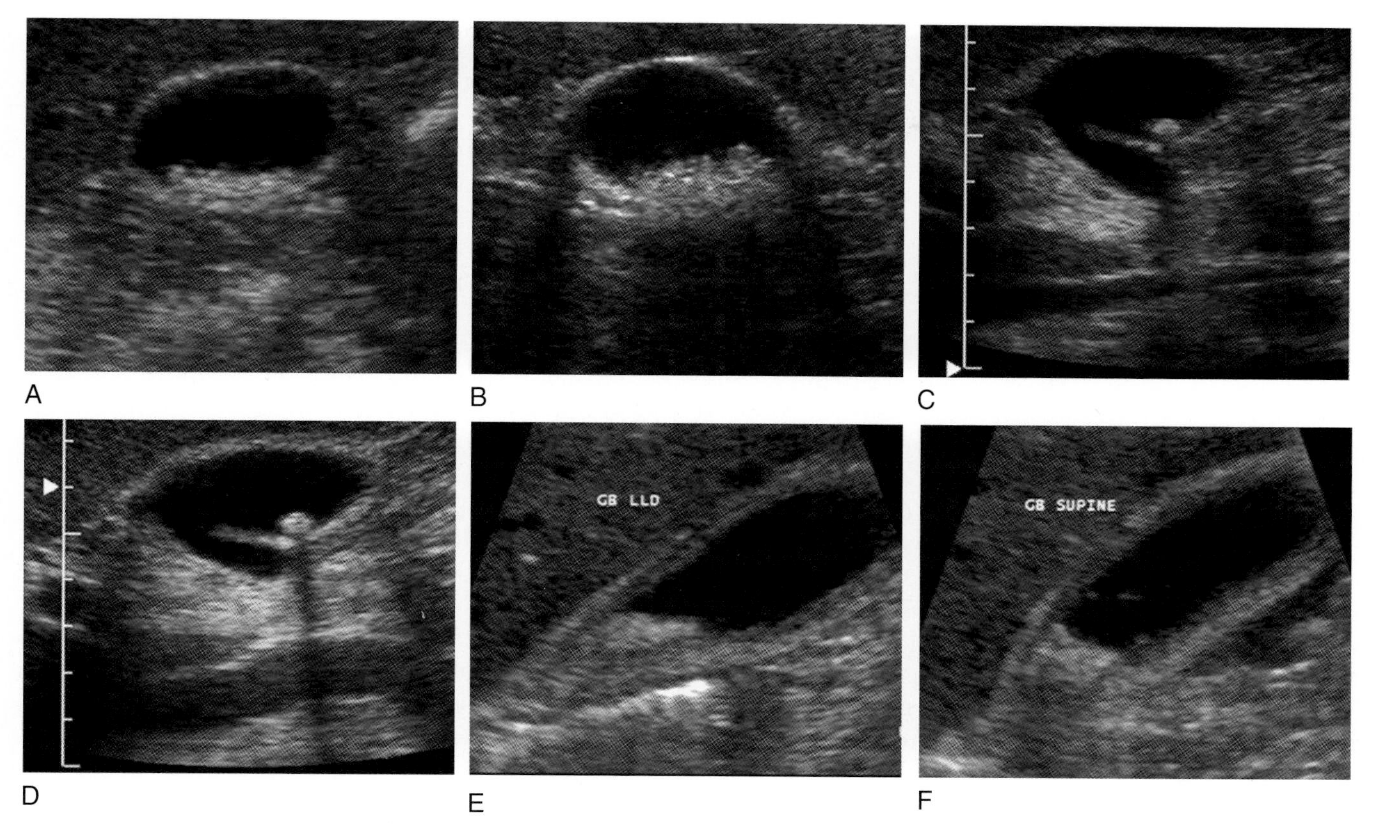

Figure 2-9 Importance of technical parameters in demonstrating gallstone shadowing in different patients. **A,** Transverse view of the gallbladder obtained at 3.6 MHz shows stones but no shadowing. **B,** A similar view obtained at 6.0 MHz shows readily detectable shadowing. **C,** View of the gallbladder with the focal zone placed at the deep aspect of the field of view shows only faint acoustic shadowing from the gallstone. **D,** Another view with the focal zone placed at the level of the gallstone shows distinct acoustic shadowing. **E,** View of the gallbladder with the patient in a left lateral decubitus position shows echogenic material in the neck of the gallbladder but no definite acoustic shadowing. **F,** Similar view but with the patient in the supine position results in consolidation of the material and production of an acoustic shadow confirming that this represents small stones rather than sludge.

If not, the character of the shadow is important. In most cases stones produce a clean shadow and gas produces a dirty shadow (see Fig. 2-8E). Exceptions to this rule occur occasionally (see Fig. 2-8F) and are probably a result of differences in the surface characteristics of gallstones. Another sign that can assist in differentiating a stone-filled gallbladder and gas-filled bowel is the wall-echo-shadow (WES) complex. This consists of three arc-shaped lines followed by a shadow (Fig. 2-10). The first line is echogenic and represents pericholecystic fat as well as the interface between the gallbladder wall and the liver. The second line is hypoechoic and represents the gallbladder wall itself. The third is echogenic and arises from the stones. Although a WES complex is a very reliable sign of a stone-filled gallbladder, it is not possible to demonstrate it in every case. Therefore, it is a useful finding when seen but it is not useful when absent.

As mentioned earlier, the vast majority of gallstones fall into the dependent aspect of the gallbladder. When there are multiple small stones arranged in a layer along the dependent gallbladder wall, they might be confused with the wall itself. In such cases, identification of the stones and detection of an acoustic shadow are usually easier on transverse views (see Fig. 2-8D).

When the density of bile is unusually high, stones may float (Fig. 2-11). This occurs when the specific gravity of bile is greater than the specific gravity of the stones and indicates that the floating stones are composed of

Table 2-2 Intraluminal Abnormalities in the Gallbladder

Ultrasound characteristics	Common	Uncommon
Shadowing and mobile	Stones	Nothing else
Non-shadowing and mobile	Sludge	Stones (<3 mm)
Non-shadowing and nonmobile	Polyps	Sludge

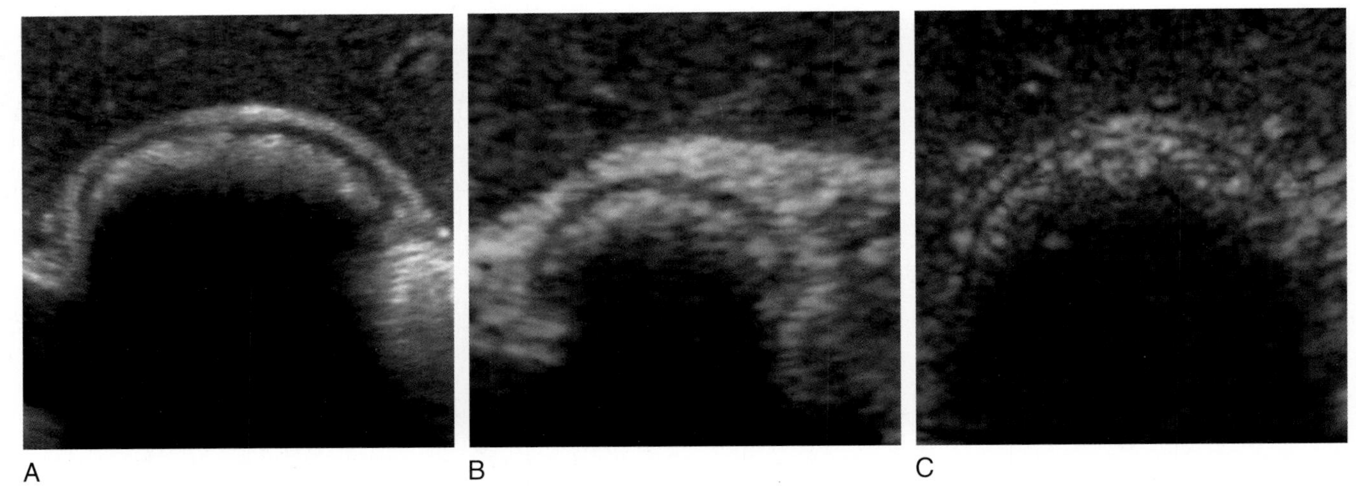

Figure 2-10 Typical examples of the wall-echo-shadow complex in different patients. The complex varies from a very distinct series of arc-shaped lines (**A** and **B**) to less distinct lines (**C**).

cholesterol. One of the most common situations in which the specific gravity of bile increases is when intravenous contrast medium has been injected and there is some degree of vicarious excretion in the gallbladder.

SLUDGE

Sludge consists of calcium bilirubinate granules and cholesterol crystals, often in the setting of thick, viscous bile. It appears as low- to high-level, non-shadowing reflectors in the gallbladder. Typically, sludge localizes in the dependent portion of the gallbladder and forms a bile-sludge level (Fig. 2-12A and B), although it may fill the entire gallbladder lumen (see Fig. 2-12C and D). Sludge may form mass-like aggregates called sludge balls or tumefactive sludge (see Fig. 2-12E). Stones may coexist with sludge, in which case shadowing will be seen (see Fig. 2-12B and D). In some cases the crystalline components of sludge float in the non-dependent portion of the gallbladder lumen (see Fig. 2-12F). This should not be confused with stones. Although typically

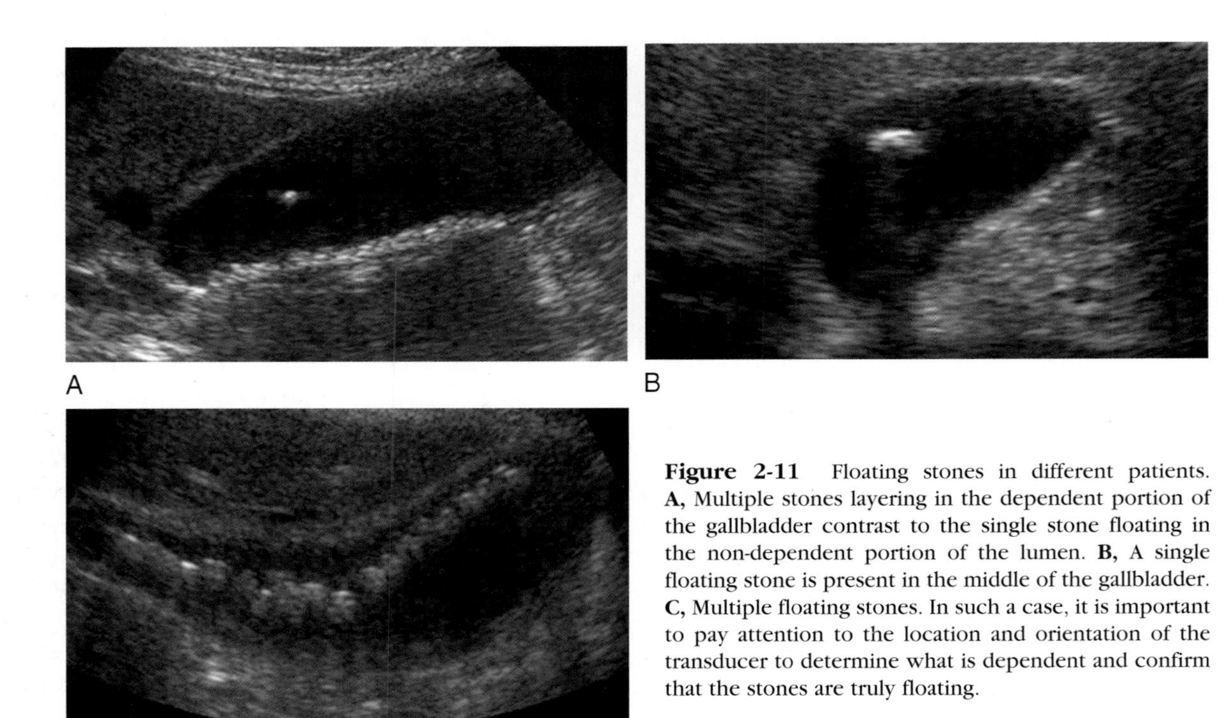

Figure 2-11 Floating stones in different patients. **A,** Multiple stones layering in the dependent portion of the gallbladder contrast to the single stone floating in the non-dependent portion of the lumen. **B,** A single floating stone is present in the middle of the gallbladder. **C,** Multiple floating stones. In such a case, it is important to pay attention to the location and orientation of the transducer to determine what is dependent and confirm that the stones are truly floating.

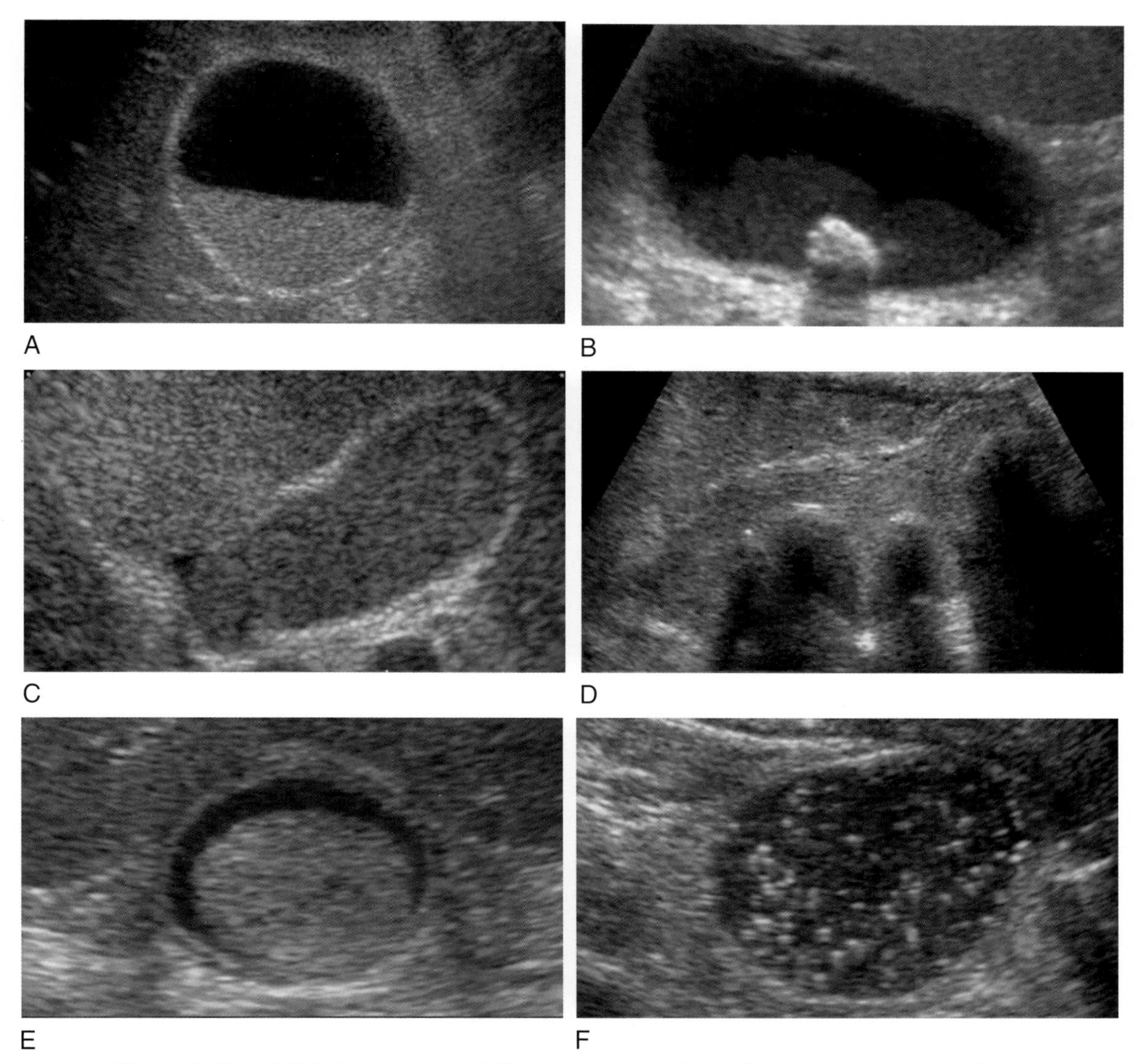

Figure 2-12 Gallbladder sludge in different patients. **A,** Typical echogenic sludge layering in the dependent portion of the gallbladder lumen. **B,** Less echogenic sludge with associated gallstone. **C,** Sludge completely filling the gallbladder lumen. **D,** Sludge completely filling the gallbladder with associated stones. **E,** Sludge ball occupying most of the gallbladder lumen. **F,** Sludge with multiple distinct crystals, many of which demonstrate short comet-tail artifacts.

homogeneous, sludge may have a very inhomogeneous appearance, with prominent hypoechoic regions. It can also form echogenic bands that can be confused with sloughed membranes. The lack of shadowing distinguishes the different forms of sludge from gallstones, and mobility distinguishes sludge from polyps and tumors. In rare cases, it will not be possible to demonstrate mobility of sludge. In such cases a follow-up examination several weeks later is often helpful to demonstrate mobility or a change in appearance and thus excludes gallbladder neoplasm. Color Doppler imaging is also potentially useful in isolated cases because detection of blood flow excludes tumefactive sludge from the differential diagnosis. Lack of detectable flow is not helpful because it can occur in hypovascular tumors in addition to tumefactive sludge. Intraluminal blood and pus can both mimic all of the characteristics of sludge.

The clinical significance of sludge is not entirely clear, but in most patients it can probably be thought of as an asymptomatic dynamic equilibrium between crystal development and elimination. Nonetheless, in a minority of patients it probably represents the early stage of gallstone formation. It is also believed that biliary crystals can cause pancreatitis, and this can make the detection of sludge important in patients with pancreatitis of unknown origin.

ACUTE CHOLECYSTITIS

In the majority of cases, acute cholecystitis occurs from persistent obstruction of the cystic duct or gallbladder neck by an impacted gallstone. If the stone does not spontaneously disimpact or some form of therapy is not initiated, the gallbladder may become necrotic and perforate. Surgery is the treatment of choice and is typically performed at presentation if the duration of symptoms is less than 48 to 72 hours. Otherwise, antibiotics and supportive care can control the inflammatory process and the patient's symptoms so that cholecystectomy can be performed electively.

There are a number of sonographic findings that support the diagnosis of acute cholecystitis and the diagnosis of advanced acute cholecystitis (Boxes 2-1 and 2-2). They include (1) gallstones, (2) gallbladder wall thickening, (3) gallbladder enlargement, (4) pericholecystic fluid, (5) a stone impacted in the gallbladder neck or cystic duct, and (6) focal tenderness directly over the gallbladder. By themselves, none of these findings is pathognomonic for acute cholecystitis, but the combination of several findings in the appropriate clinical setting is highly suggestive. The positive predictive value of gallstones and a positive sonographic Murphy's sign is 92%, whereas the negative predictive value is 95%.

Gallbladder wall thickening greater than or equal to 3 mm occurs in the majority of patients with acute cholecystitis (Fig. 2-13A and B). Unfortunately there are many other causes of wall thickening, and the sonographic appearance of the thickened gallbladder wall is not helpful in distinguishing cholecystitis from other abnormalities. However, irregular, striated sonolucencies in a thickened wall may imply a more advanced case of cholecystitis. Gallbladder enlargement is an important sign of cholecystitis, and the width of the gallbladder is more important than the length (see Fig. 2-13C). As mentioned earlier, gallstones are present in approximately 95% of cases of cholecystitis. In some instances, it is possible to identify the impacted stone that is causing the obstruction in the gallbladder neck or cystic duct (see Fig. 2-13D). However, in many cases non-obstructing stones are seen but the obstructing stone is not. Pericholecystic fluid collections occur in less than 20% of patients with acute cholecystitis. They typically appear as loculated collections in the peritoneal cavity, most frequently near the fundus (see Fig. 2-13E and F). Pericholecystic fluid is important to recognize because it usually indicates more advanced cholecystitis and the need for more urgent intervention. On the other hand, reactive effusions are common and do not have the same implications. Collections between the gallbladder and the liver are also common and probably represent edema in loose areolar tissue rather than pericholecystic fluid.

Box 2-1 Sonographic Signs of Acute Cholecystitis

Gallstones
Wall thickening ($\geq$ 3 mm)
Gallbladder enlargement
Pericholecystic fluid
Impacted stone
Sonographic Murphy's sign

Box 2-2 Sonographic Signs of Advanced Acute Cholecystitis

Pericholecystic fluid
Sloughed mucosal membranes
Irregular striated intramural sonolucencies
Wall disruption
Wall ulceration
Focal wall bulge

In addition to pericholecystic fluid collections and irregular striated thickening of the gallbladder wall, other signs of advanced cholecystitis and wall necrosis include focal ulceration of the mucosa, sloughed mucosal membranes, focal bulges of the gallbladder wall, and intramural abscess (Fig. 2-14). All of these abnormalities are rare; and, as mentioned earlier, membranous sludge can simulate sloughed mucosal membranes.

The sonographic diagnosis of acute cholecystitis remains in doubt in some patients. In these patients, hepatobiliary scintigraphy is extremely valuable as a problem-solving technique to exclude or establish the diagnosis of acute cholecystitis. The American College of Radiology states in its appropriateness criteria that patients with suspected acute cholecystitis can be evaluated first with either ultrasound or scintigraphy. However, ultrasound receives a higher rating. There are several reasons for this.

1. Approximately 70% of patients with clinically suspected acute cholecystitis will have some other problem, and by showing a normal gallbladder, ultrasound can rapidly exclude cholecystitis in the majority of these patients.
2. Ultrasound is much more likely to identify a specific alternative diagnosis than is biliary scintigraphy.
3. Ultrasound is a relatively inexpensive means of obtaining morphologic information about all of the right upper quadrant organs. This is becoming particularly more important in the era of laparoscopic cholecystectomies because the surgeon has less capability of examining these organs during the operation.

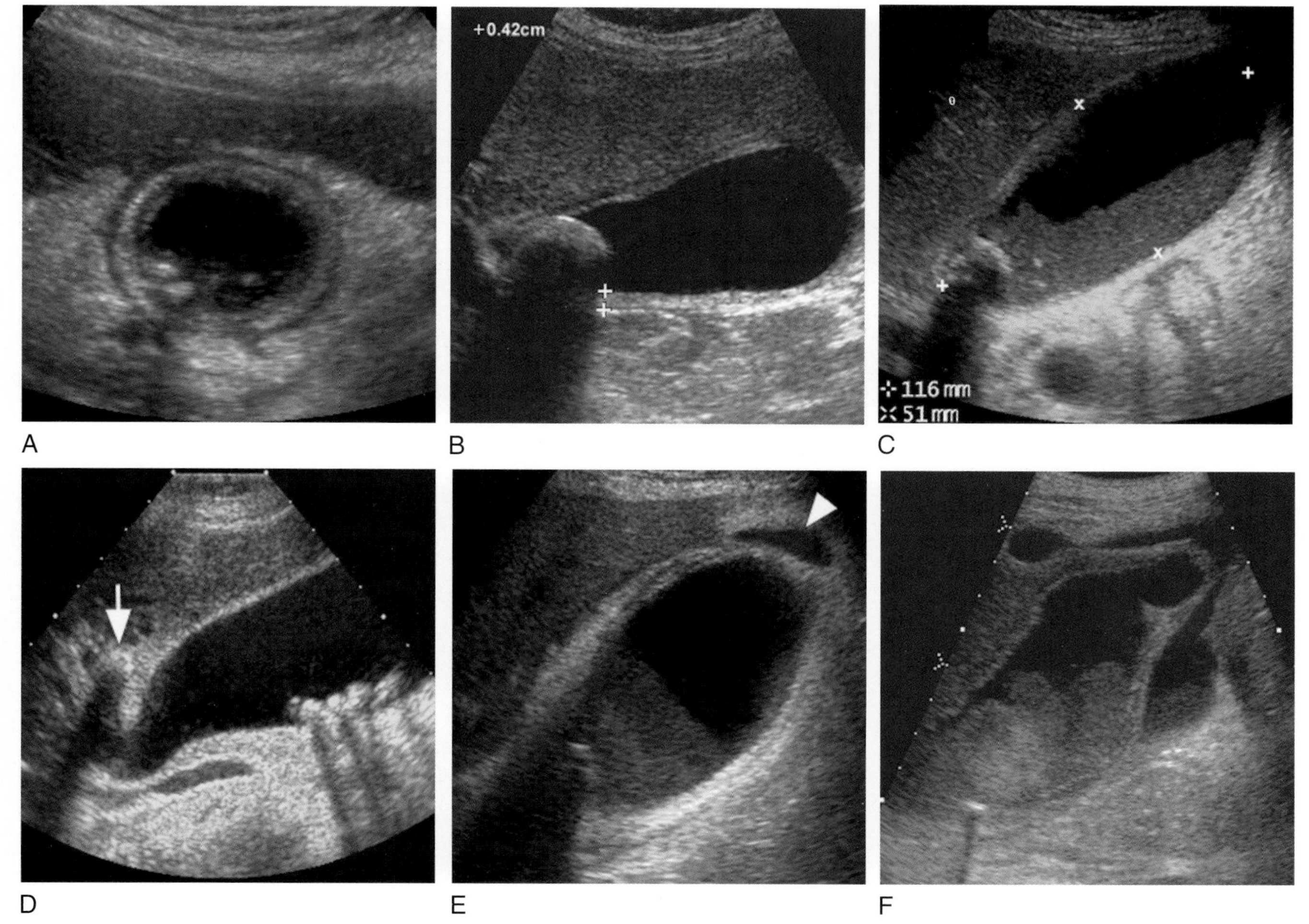

Figure 2-13 Acute cholecystitis in different patients. **A,** Transverse view shows stones, sludge, and gallbladder wall thickening as well as echogenic inflammatory changes in the adjacent fat. **B,** Longitudinal view shows wall thickening (0.42 cm, *cursors*) and a stone in the neck of the gallbladder. **C,** Longitudinal view shows an enlarged gallbladder (116 × 51 mm) with stones and sludge. **D,** Longitudinal view shows a gallstone impacted in the cystic duct *(arrow)* in addition to multiple non-impacted stones in the gallbladder lumen. **E,** Longitudinal view shows wall thickening, sludge, stones, and a small collection of pericholecystic fluid *(arrowhead)* near the gallbladder fundus. **F,** Longitudinal view shows findings similar to that in **E** but more extensive pericholecystic fluid around the gallbladder fundus.

4. The size of the gallbladder, size of the largest stone, status of the gallbladder wall, and presence of biliary dilatation are all important preoperative data that can be obtained with sonography but not with scintigraphy.
5. Most ultrasound examinations that are considered false positive for acute cholecystitis occur in patients with symptomatic gallstones. Because these patients require cholecystectomy anyway, the impact of a preoperative diagnosis of acute cholecystitis is minimal.

Approximately 5% of cases of acute cholecystitis occur in the absence of gallstones and are referred to as acalculous cholecystitis. The etiology is multifactorial and includes ischemia, gallbladder wall infection, chemical toxicity to the gallbladder wall, and cystic duct obstruction. Acalculous cholecystitis occurs predominantly in very sick patients, particularly after major surgery, extensive burns, major trauma, and prolonged total parenteral nutrition. Therefore, the absence of stones is not a reliable means of excluding cholecystitis in this group of patients. Secondary signs must be relied on to make the diagnosis (Fig. 2-15). Unfortunately, most very ill patients have many potential causes of secondary signs, such as gallbladder enlargement and wall thickening. It can also be difficult to assess for tenderness in a semiresponsive patient. Therefore, sonography has significant limitations in the diagnosis of acalculous cholecystitis. Scintigraphy is probably more sensitive than sonography, but it is also prone to false-positive results.

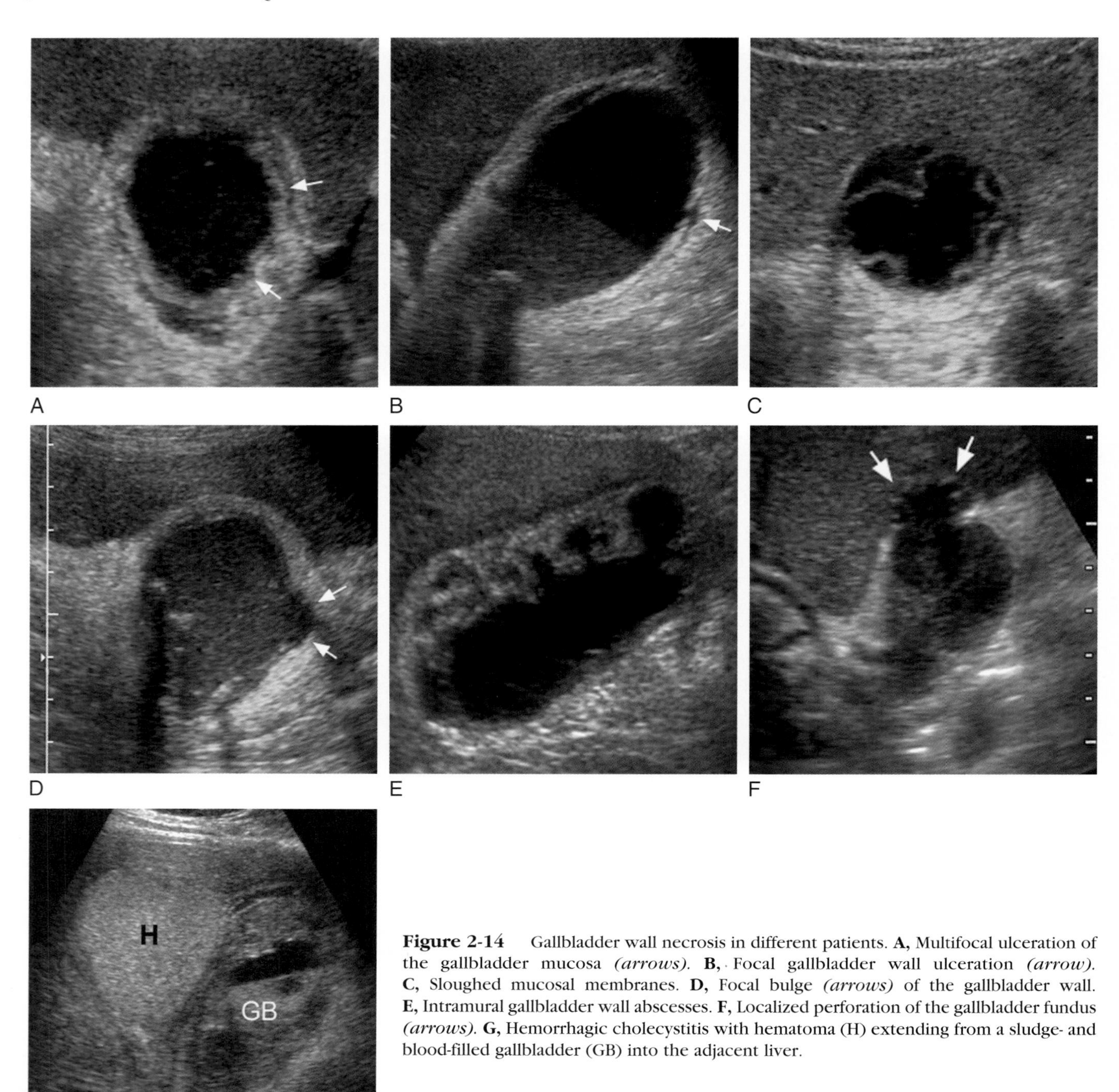

Figure 2-14 Gallbladder wall necrosis in different patients. **A,** Multifocal ulceration of the gallbladder mucosa *(arrows).* **B,** Focal gallbladder wall ulceration *(arrow).* **C,** Sloughed mucosal membranes. **D,** Focal bulge *(arrows)* of the gallbladder wall. **E,** Intramural gallbladder wall abscesses. **F,** Localized perforation of the gallbladder fundus *(arrows).* **G,** Hemorrhagic cholecystitis with hematoma (H) extending from a sludge- and blood-filled gallbladder (GB) into the adjacent liver.

Emphysematous cholecystitis is another unusual form that tends to occur in elderly men. Because it is caused by ischemia, it occurs more often in diabetics and is often not associated with gallstones. The gas that develops results from infection with gas-forming organisms and can occur in the gallbladder wall and/or lumen. Perforation of the gallbladder is five times more likely with emphysematous cholecystitis than with gallstone-induced cholecystitis; thus, the distinction is clinically significant. Sonographically, emphysematous cholecystitis usually manifests as very bright reflections from a non-dependent portion of the gallbladder wall (Fig. 2-16A). The associated acoustic shadow is usually dirty (see Fig. 2-16B) and in many cases has a demonstrable

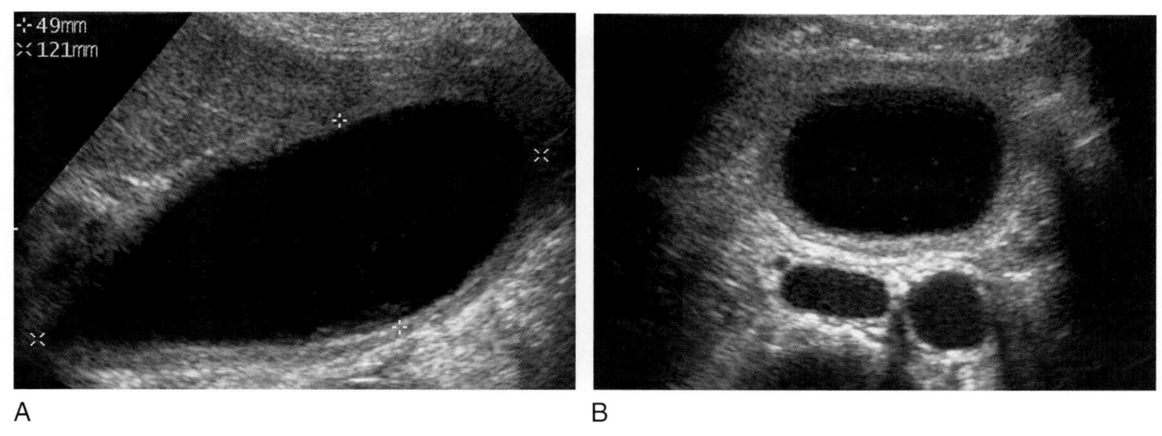

Figure 2-15 Acalculous cholecystitis. Longitudinal (**A**) and transverse (**B**) views show an enlarged gallbladder (49 × 121 mm) with wall thickening but no detectable stones.

ring-down artifact (see Fig. 2-16C) that is a reliable sign of gas.

CARCINOMA

Gallbladder cancer is the fifth most common gastrointestinal malignancy. It probably occurs because of chronic irritation of the gallbladder wall by stones. Therefore, the vast majority of gallbladder cancers are associated with gallstones and develop more commonly in women than in men. The 5-year survival rate for patients with gallbladder cancer is less than 20%, although the prognosis for patients with tumor confined to the gallbladder wall is much better. Unfortunately, up to 80% of these patients have direct tumor invasion of the liver or portal node involvement at the time of diagnosis.

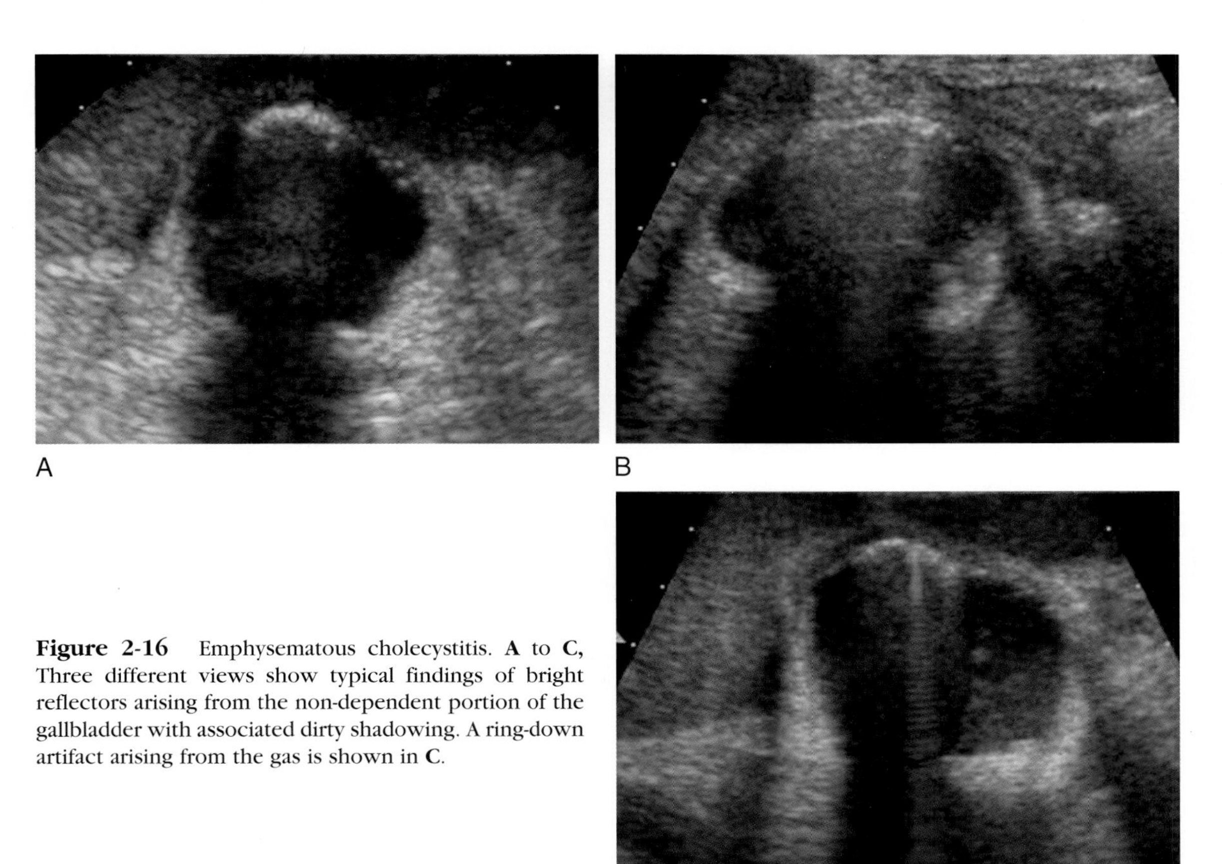

Figure 2-16 Emphysematous cholecystitis. **A** to **C**, Three different views show typical findings of bright reflectors arising from the non-dependent portion of the gallbladder with associated dirty shadowing. A ring-down artifact arising from the gas is shown in **C**.

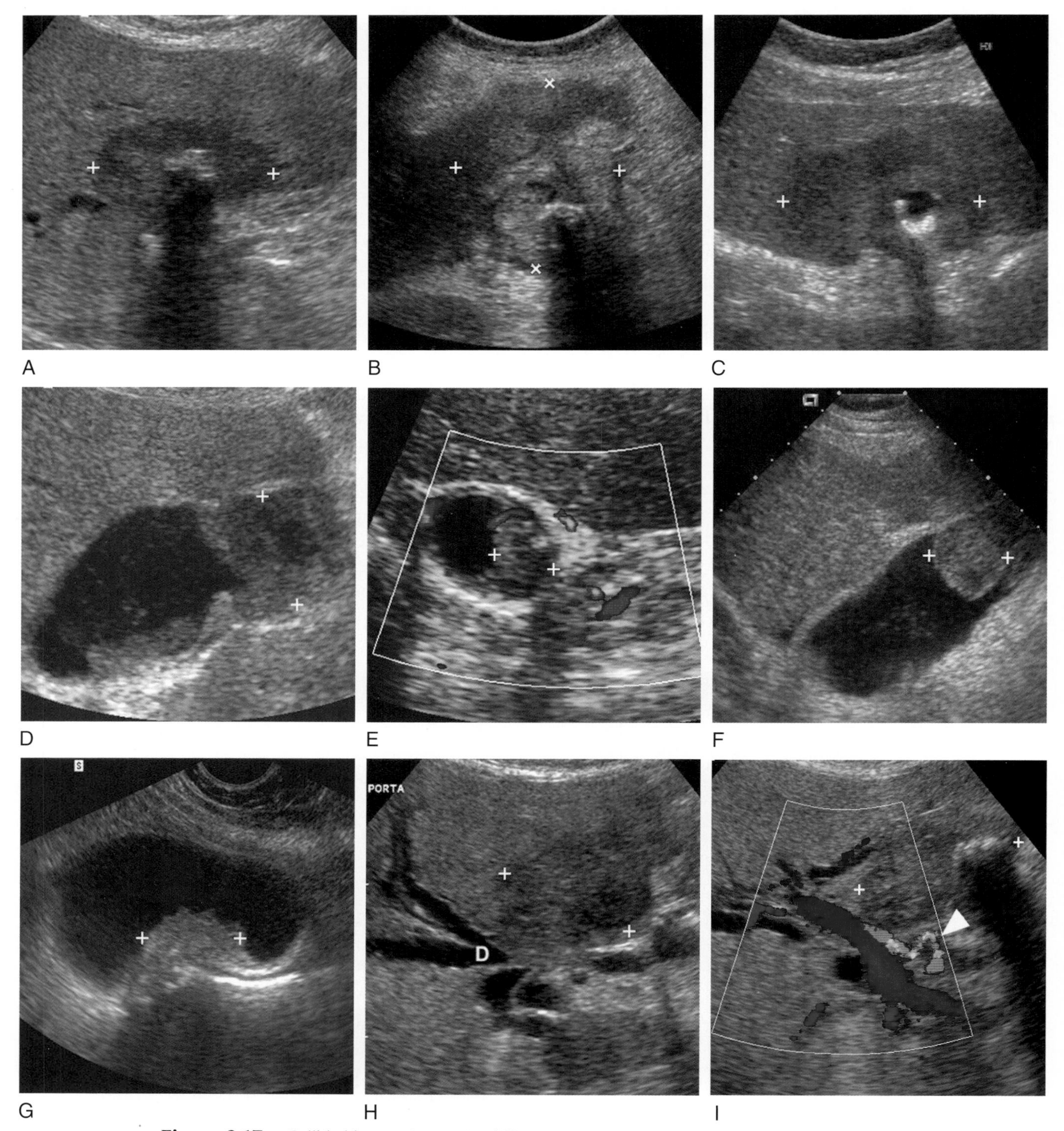

Figure 2-17 Gallbladder carcinoma in different patients. **A,** Homogeneous hypoechoic mass *(cursors)* obliterating the gallbladder lumen and engulfing a gallstone. **B,** Large heterogeneous mass *(cursors)* obliterating the gallbladder lumen and engulfing a gallstone. **C,** Homogeneous mass *(cursors)* partially obliterating the gallbladder lumen. **D,** Focal thickening of the gallbladder wall *(cursors)* in the region of the fundus. **E,** Focal thickening *(cursors)* of the medial aspect of the gallbladder wall. **F,** Large polypoid mass *(cursors)* in the gallbladder fundus. **G,** Smaller sessile polypoid mass *(cursors)* in the body of the gallbladder. **H,** Hypoechoic mass *(cursors)* in the gallbladder fossa invading the porta hepatis and causing bile duct obstruction with dilated intrahepatic bile ducts (D). **I,** Hypoechoic mass *(cursors)* engulfing a gallstone and invading the porta hepatitis and encasing the hepatic artery *(arrowhead).*

Box 2-3 Sonographic Appearance of Gallbladder Cancer

Mass centered on gallbladder fossa with associated stones
Eccentric irregular wall thickening
Bulky intraluminal polypoid mass
Infiltration of adjacent liver or vessels
Periportal and/or peripancreatic lymphadenopathy
Bile duct obstruction

The most common sonographic appearance for gallbladder cancer is a soft tissue mass centered in the gallbladder fossa that completely (Fig. 2-17A and B) or partially obliterates the lumen (see Fig. 2-17C). Identification of gallstones within the mass can help to confirm that the origin of the mass is the gallbladder rather than adjacent organs. Fifteen to 30 percent of gallbladder cancers appear as focal or diffuse gallbladder wall thickening (see Fig. 2-17D and E). In the vast majority of these cases the thickening is irregular, asymmetric, and eccentric. The least common form of gallbladder cancer is a polypoid intraluminal mass (see Fig. 2-17F and G). This form is almost always larger than a centimeter (usually much larger). Size is therefore a good way to distinguish cancer from gallbladder polyps. The sonographic findings in gallbladder cancer are reviewed in Box 2-3.

The differential diagnosis for gallbladder masses includes tumefactive sludge (see Fig. 2-12C), inflammatory wall thickening, polyps (Fig. 2-18), metastases (Fig. 2-19), and focal adenomyomatosis (Fig. 2-20D). The causes of gallbladder masses are reviewed in Box 2-4. When the diagnosis of cancer is in doubt, detection of metastatic disease in the regional lymph nodes or peritoneal cavity, or invasion of adjacent organs, especially the liver, bile ducts, or vessels (Fig. 2-17H and I, can be very useful.

POLYPS

Cholesterolosis is a condition in which triglycerides, cholesterol precursors, and cholesterol esters are deposited within the lamina propria of the gallbladder. Although the cause is unknown, cholesterolosis does not appear to be related to serum lipid level, atherosclerosis, diabetes, cholesterol stones, or hyperconcentration of cholesterol in the bile.

Most cases of cholesterolosis are of the planar variety and produce no detectable changes in the appearance or thickness of the gallbladder wall on ultrasound or other imaging tests. It is sometimes referred to as strawberry gallbladder because the mucosa bears a resemblance to the surface of a strawberry. A minority of cases of cholesterolosis are of the polypoid variety and can be detected by imaging tests such as ultrasound (see Fig. 2-18). Cholesterol polyps are by far the most common type of gallbladder polyp. They are not true neoplasms but rather enlarged papillary fronds filled with lipid-laden macrophages, and they are attached to the wall by means of a slender stalk. The stalk is rarely seen so they typically appear as a mass that is adjacent to the wall but barely attached to the wall. This is referred to as the "ball on the wall" sign. There are usually multiple polyps, although it is not uncommon to detect only the largest one sonographically. Cholesterol polyps are usually 5 mm or less and only rarely get bigger than 10 mm. They can be distinguished from gallbladder stones by their lack of a shadow and nonmobile nature and from sludge balls by their lack of mobility. Their small size and multiplicity help to distinguish them from true neoplasms of the gallbladder wall. Other types of gallbladder polyps occur but are less common than cholesterol polyps. These include adenomas, papillomas, leiomyomas, lipomas, and neuromas. These lesions are true neoplasms and are almost always solitary and are usually larger than cholesterol polyps (see Fig. 2-18E). Larger polyps may have detectable blood flow on color Doppler imaging (see Fig. 2-18F).

Metastatic disease to the gallbladder is very uncommon but can produce multiple polypoid lesions. Melanoma has the greatest tendency to spread to the gallbladder (see Fig. 2-19), and detection of gallbladder polyps should be viewed with a high level of suspicion in patients with a history of melanoma. Generally there will be other evidence of metastatic disease in the liver, lymph nodes, or elsewhere in the abdomen.

It has been well established that polypoid lesions of the gallbladder wall that are 5 mm or less require no further evaluation or therapy. Lesions that are between 5 and 10 mm should be monitored to ensure their stability, realizing that the yield of follow-up studies will be very low. If small polyps are multiple, they are almost certainly cholesterol polyps and can be ignored. Lesions that are larger than 10 mm should probably be removed because of the possibility of cancer and the low risk of cholecystectomy. It should be recognized that most polyps that are just slightly larger than 10 mm will still be benign, but as polyps enlarge, the risk of malignancy increases progressively.

ADENOMYOMATOSIS

Adenomyomatosis is one of two forms of hyperplastic cholecystoses (cholesterolosis is the other). Like cholesterolosis, the etiology is unknown. Pathologically, adenomyomatosis is characterized by mucosal hyperplasia

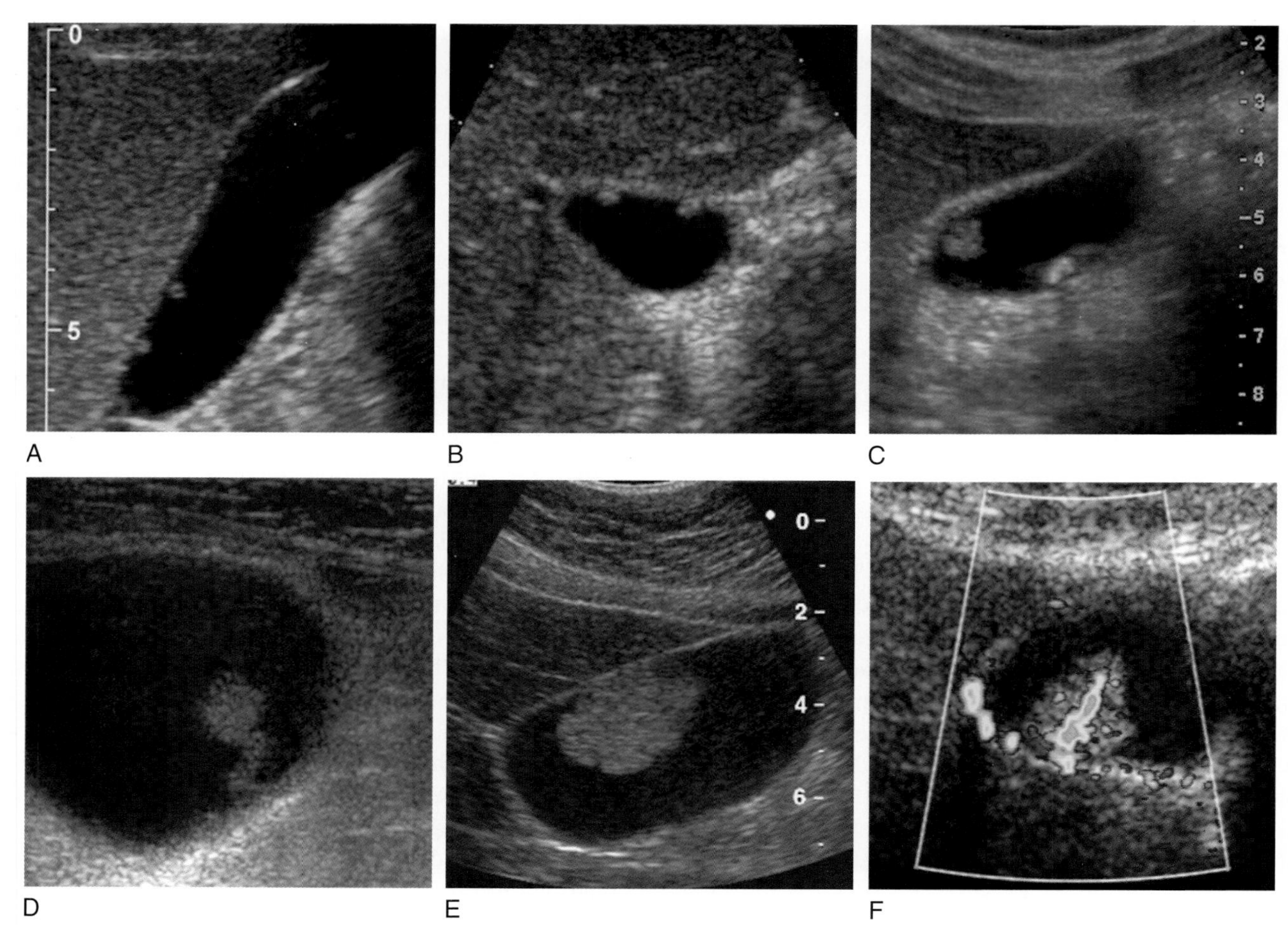

Figure 2-18 Gallbladder polyps in different patients. Longitudinal (**A**) and transverse (**B**) views show two small (<5 mm) non-shadowing polypoid defects along the non-dependent portion of the gallbladder typical of cholesterol polyps. **C,** Oblique view shows a stone in the dependent portion and a non-shadowing polypoid filling defect in the non-dependent portion. This is slightly larger than expected for a typical cholesterol polyp but demonstrates the typical "ball on the wall" sign. **D,** Unusual case showing the stalk of a cholesterol polyp. **E,** Three-centimeter polyp that was pathologically proven to represent an adenoma. **F,** Color Doppler view shows the vascular pedicle of a polyp, which helps to distinguish this from tumefactive sludge.

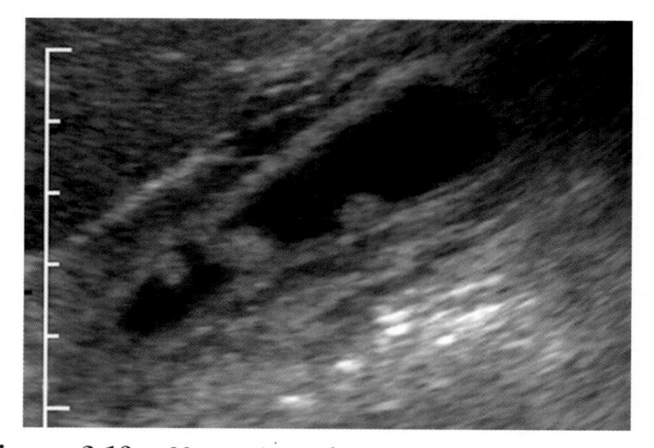

Figure 2-19 Metastatic melanoma. Longitudinal view of the gallbladder shows several polypoid lesions in a patient with widely metastatic melanoma. Gallbladder wall edema is also present owing to portal hypertension caused by diffuse liver metastases.

and thickening of the muscular layer of the gallbladder. Mucosal herniations into the muscular layer are called Rokitansky-Aschoff sinuses, and they frequently contain cholesterol crystals. Adenomyomatosis is unrelated to gallstones and occurs equally in men and women.

Sonographically, the cholesterol crystals deposited in the Rokitansky-Aschoff sinuses result in bright reflections and short comet-tail artifacts arising from the gallbladder wall (see Fig. 2-20A to C). The comet-tail artifact is the most obvious finding in many cases of adenomyomatosis and is almost exclusively seen along the near wall of the gallbladder. This does not reflect focal disease but instead occurs because the artifact is only visible when it is displayed in the anechoic background of intraluminal bile behind the near wall and not visible in the echogenic background of the tissues deep to the back

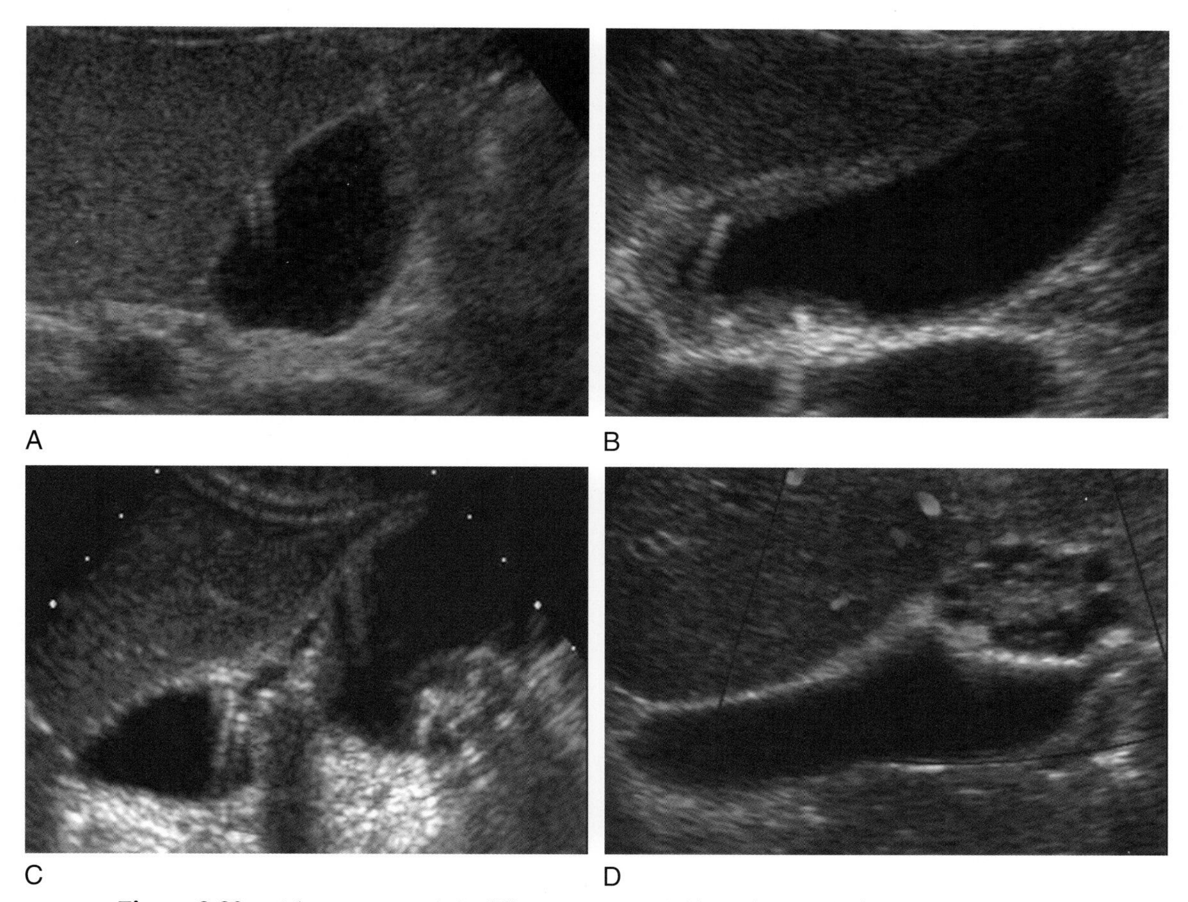

Figure 2-20 Adenomyomatosis in different patients. **A,** Typical example showing comet-tail artifacts from the superficial wall of the gallbladder but no other abnormalities. **B,** Focal thickening of the gallbladder wall near the gallbladder neck with associated comet-tail artifacts. **C,** Focal segmental wall thickening in the midportion of the gallbladder with associated waisting of the gallbladder contour and comet-tail artifacts. Stones are present in the fundal segment. **D,** Focal mass in the fundus of the gallbladder with multiple cystic spaces owing to unusually large Rokitansky-Aschoff sinuses.

wall. Rarely, large Rokitansky-Aschoff sinuses will be resolved as cystic or hypoechoic spaces in the gallbladder wall. Adenomyomatosis may also appear as diffuse wall thickening, focal segmental annular thickening (see Fig. 2-20C), or a localized mass (see Fig. 2-20D). In many cases ultrasound will show such characteristic findings that the diagnosis is unequivocal. However, when the diagnosis of adenomyomatosis is in doubt, an oral cholecystogram can be obtained because it may demonstrate the Rokitansky-Aschoff sinuses and establish the diagnosis more definitively.

Box 2-4 Causes of Gallbladder Masses

COMMON	UNCOMMON
Polyps	Metastases
Adenomyomatosis	Chronic cholecystitis
Gallbladder cancer	
Tumefactive sludge	

GALLBLADDER WALL THICKENING

As mentioned previously, the normal upper limit for the gallbladder wall is 3 mm. A large number of processes can result in a thickened gallbladder wall (Box 2-5). In addition to acute cholecystitis, gallbladder cancer, and adenomyomatosis, other abnormalities related to the biliary tract that can thicken the gallbladder wall are AIDS cholangiopathy and sclerosing cholangitis.

A large number of non-biliary processes can also cause gallbladder wall thickening due to edema (Fig. 2-21).

Box 2-5 Causes of Gallbladder Wall Thickening

BILIARY	NON-BILIARY
Cholecystitis	Hepatitis
Adenomyomatosis	Pancreatitis
Cancer	Heart failure
AIDS cholangiopathy	Hypoproteinemia
Sclerosing cholangitis	Cirrhosis
	Portal hypertension
	Lymphatic obstruction

Interestingly, non-biliary-related edema of the gallbladder wall usually produces more marked thickening than does acute cholecystitis. Hypoproteinemia (from cirrhosis, nephrotic syndrome, etc.), congestive heart failure, venous congestion from portal hypertension, lymphatic obstruction from portal lymph node disease, and adjacent inflammatory processes such as pancreatitis are all potential causes. Hepatitis is another cause of gallbladder wall thickening that is often overlooked, despite the fact that it can cause marked thickening (see Fig. 2-21C). This may be due to the adjacent inflammation of the liver or excretion of the virus in the bile and direct infection of the gallbladder. Hepatitis also frequently causes gallbladder contraction. Gallbladder varices can also occur in patients with portal hypertension and can simulate wall thickening on gray-scale imaging but should be readily distinguishable on color Doppler imaging (Fig. 2-22).

Most non-biliary causes of gallbladder wall thickening produce concentric thickening that may be uniform in echogenicity or may have a regular or irregular layered appearance with both hypoechoic and echogenic components. The actual sonographic appearance of the thickened wall is not helpful in distinguishing acute cholecystitis from non-biliary thickening. However, in most cases the clinical setting and the presence or absence of a sonographic Murphy's sign can help to make the diagnosis. In some instances, associated sonographic signs can be very useful. For instance, heart failure often produces abnormally pulsatile portal venous flow and cirrhosis produces secondary signs of portal hypertension and a nodular liver surface.

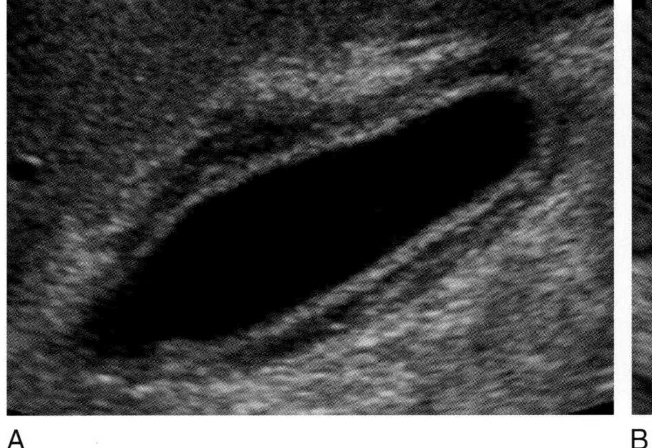

A

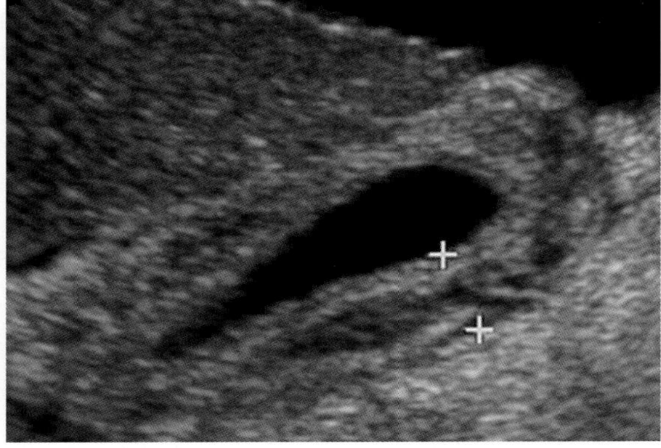

B

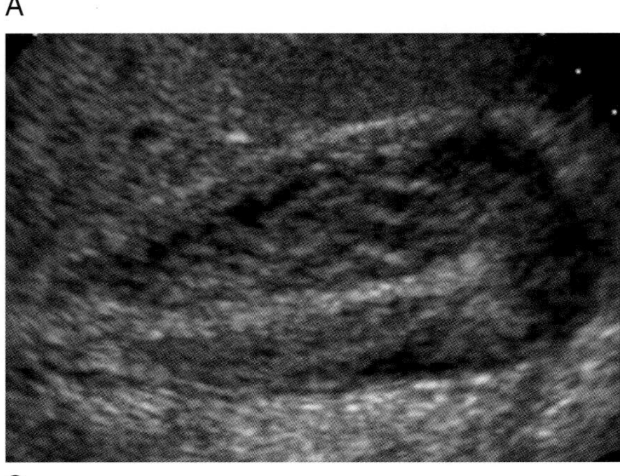

C

Figure 2-21 Gallbladder wall thickening in different patients. Longitudinal views of the gallbladder show diffuse thickening secondary to congestive heart failure (**A**), cirrhosis and portal hypertension (**B**), and hepatitis (**C**). In the case of hepatitis, the gallbladder lumen is completely contracted and the coapted mucosal layers are seen as a thin echogenic line in the center of the gallbladder.

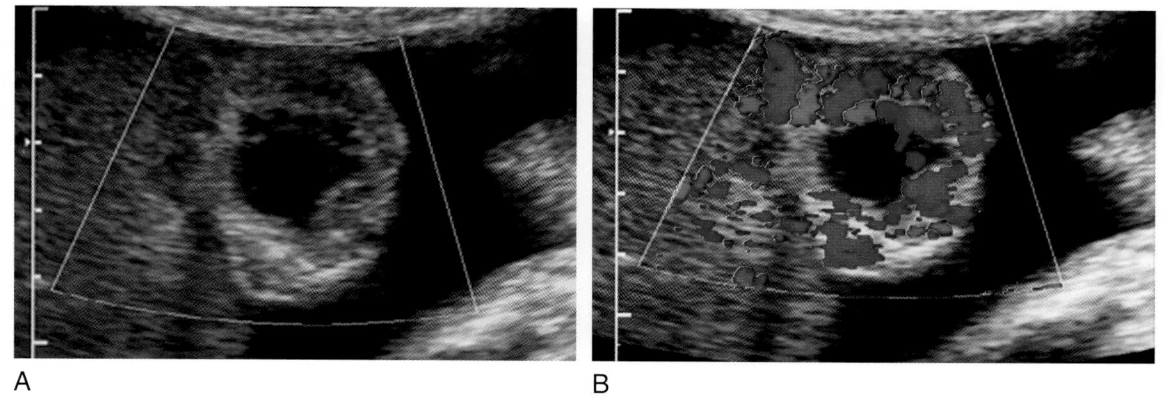

Figure 2-22 Gallbladder wall varices. Transverse gray-scale (**A**) and color Doppler (**B**) views of the gallbladder show wall thickening secondary to diffuse gallbladder wall varices.

PORCELAIN GALLBLADDER

Extensive calcification of the gallbladder produces a brittle bluish wall that has led to the term *porcelain gallbladder*. It is associated with chronic gallbladder inflammation, and 95% of the cases have gallstones. The clinical significance of porcelain gallbladder is the increased risk of gallbladder carcinoma. Estimates of this risk range from 13% to 61%. Because many uncomplicated and occult cases of porcelain gallbladder probably never come to clinical attention, the true incidence of carcinoma in this condition is probably overestimated in the literature. Nonetheless, most authorities would still recommend prophylactic cholecystectomy unless there are medical contraindications to surgery.

When the gallbladder wall is heavily calcified and the wall is diffusely involved, it will appear as an echogenic arc with dense posterior shadowing (Fig. 2-23A). Less extensive calcification will produce only partial shadowing so that the back wall of the gallbladder remains visible (see Fig. 2-23B). In early cases, only segments of the gallbladder wall may be affected. Given the increased risk of gallbladder carcinoma, whenever wall calcification is detected, a careful search should be made for evidence of malignancy (see Fig. 2-23C).

The major differential diagnosis for porcelain gallbladder is an entirely stone-filled gallbladder and

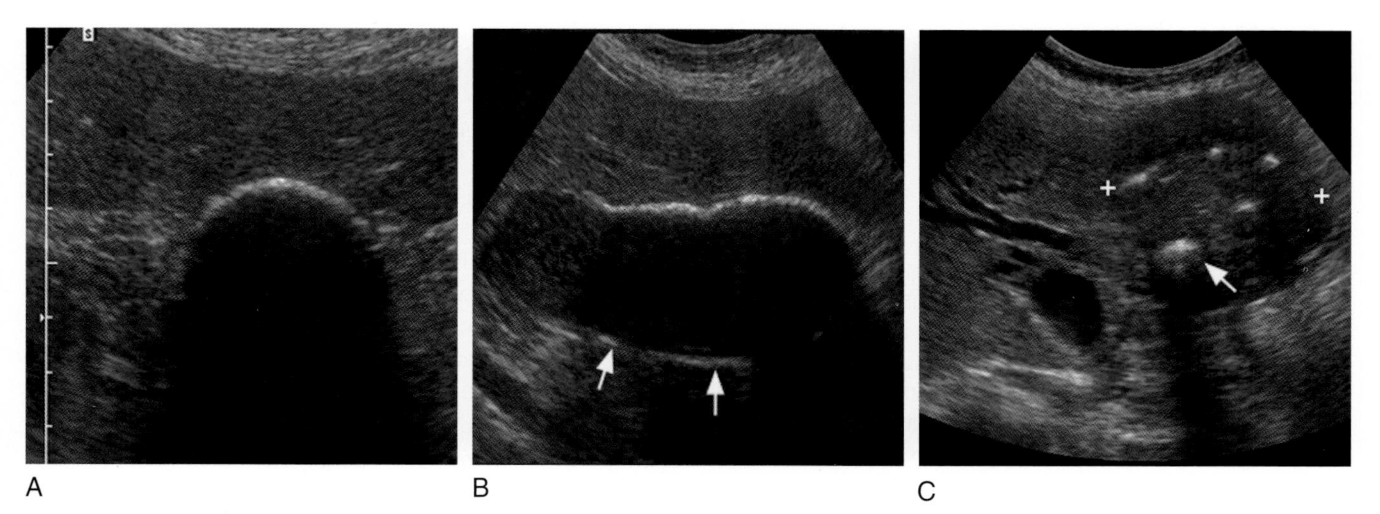

Figure 2-23 Porcelain gallbladder in different patients. **A,** Transverse view shows an echogenic superficial gallbladder wall with complete shadowing of the remainder of the gallbladder lumen and back wall. **B,** Longitudinal view of the gallbladder shows an echogenic superficial wall with shadowing of the deep gallbladder wall in the region of the fundus but sound penetration and visualization of the back wall in the body of the gallbladder *(arrows)*. **C,** Large mass *(cursors)* caused by gallbladder carcinoma that has engulfed displaced areas of echogenic gallbladder wall calcification as well as a gallstone *(arrow)*.

Table 2-3 Causes of Shadowing from Gallbladder Fossa

	Shadow	Wall-Echo-Shadow Complex	Back Wall
Gallbladder full of stones	Usually clean	Often	Not seen
Porcelain gallbladder	Variable	Rare	May be seen
Intramural gas	Usually dirty	Rare	May be seen

emphysematous cholecystitis. If a wall-echo-shadow complex is seen, then it is almost certainly a stone-filled gallbladder. If the back wall of the gallbladder is visible, then a gallbladder filled with stones can be excluded. If ring-down artifact is detected, emphysematous cholecystitis can be diagnosed. In cases where it is not possible to distinguish these three possibilities sonographically, abdominal radiographs and/or CT will be helpful. Table 2-3 summarizes the causes of shadowing from the gallbladder fossa.

Key Features

- Gallstones appear as mobile, dependent, shadowing echogenic structures in the gallbladder lumen. Sonography is the most accurate means of detecting gallstones.
- The wall-echo-shadow complex is a sign of a completely stone-filled gallbladder.
- Sonography is the method of choice in the initial evaluation of patients with suspected acute cholecystitis. Findings include gallstones, wall thickening, gallbladder enlargement, impacted stone, pericholecystic fluid, and a sonographic Murphy sign.
- Gallbladder cancer typically presents late as a mass obliterating the gallbladder and engulfing gallstones. Wall thickening and intraluminal masses are less common findings.
- Cholesterolosis is a benign, usually asymptomatic condition that may produce cholesterol polyps, which are usually small and are the most common polypoid lesion of the gallbladder wall. They appear as a non-mobile, non-shadowing "ball on the wall."
- Adenomyomatosis is a benign, usually asymptomatic condition that may produce focal or diffuse wall thickening. Cholesterol crystals deposited in Rokitansky-Aschoff sinuses are a characteristic finding.
- Gallbladder wall thickening is a nonspecific finding with a lengthy differential diagnosis. Extensive wall thickening is usually due to systemic edema-forming states rather than cholecystitis.
- Calcification of the gallbladder wall places a patient at a significantly increased risk of gallbladder cancer.

SUGGESTED READINGS

Berk RN, Armbuster RG, Saltzstein SL: Carcinoma in the porcelain gallbladder. Radiology 106:29-31, 1973.

Berk RN, van der Vegt JH, Lichtenstein JE: The hyperplastic cholecystoses: Cholesterolosis and adenomyomatosis. Radiology 146:593-601, 1983.

Boland GWL, Slater G, Lu DSK, et al: Prevalence and significance of gallbladder abnormalities seen on sonography in intensive care unit patients. AJR Am J Roentgenol 174:973-977, 2000.

Bortoff GA, Chen MYM, Ott DJ, et al: Gallbladder stones: Imaging and intervention. Radiographics 20:751-766, 2000.

Brandt DJ, et al: Gallbladder disease in patients with primary sclerosing cholangitis. AJR Am J Roentgenol 150:571-574, 1988.

Callen PW, Filly RA: Ultrasonographic localization of the gallbladder. Radiology 133:687-691, 1979.

Carroll BA: Gallbladder wall thickening secondary to focal lymphatic obstruction. J Ultrasound Med 2:89-91, 1983.

Carroll BA: Gallstones: In vitro comparison of physical, radiographic, and ultrasonic characteristics. Am J Roentgenol 131:223-226, 1978.

Collett JA, Allan RB, Chisholm RJ, et al: Gallbladder polyps: Prospective study. J Ultrasound Med 17:207-211, 1998.

Cooperberg PL, Gibney RG: Imaging of the gallbladder. Radiology 163:605-613, 1987.

Costi R, Sarli L, Caruso G, et al: Preoperative ultrasonographic assessment of the number and size of gallbladder stones. J Ultrasound Med 21:971-976, 2002.

Cover KL, Slasky BS, Skolnick ML: Sonography of cholesterol in the biliary system. J Ultrasound Med 4:647-653, 1985.

Eelkema HH, Hodgson JR, Stauffer MH: Fifteen year follow-up of polypoid lesions of the gallbladder diagnosed by cholecystography. Gastroenterology 42:144-147, 1962.

Filly RA, et al: In vitro investigation of the origin of echoes within biliary sludge. J Clin Ultrasound 8:193-200, 1980.

Fiske CE, Laing FC, Brown TW: Ultrasonographic evidence of gallbladder wall thickening in association with hypoalbuminemia. Radiology 135:713-716, 1980.

Grieco RV, Bartone NF, Vasilas A: A study of fixed filling defects in the well opacified gallbladder and their evolution. AJR Am J Roentgenol 90:844-853, 1963.

Harvey RT, Miller WT Jr: Acute biliary disease: Initial CT and follow-up US versus initial US and follow-up CT. Radiology 213:831-836, 1999.

Jeanty P, Amman W, Cooperberg PL: Mobile intraluminal masses of the gallbladder. J Ultrasound Med 2:65-71, 1983.

Jivegord I, Thornell E, Svanvik J: Pathophysiology of acute obstructive cholecystitis: Implications for nonoperative management. Br J Surg 74:1084-1086, 1987.

Jutras JA: Hyperplastic cholecystosis. AJR Am J Roentgenol 83:795-827, 1960.

Juttner HU, et al: Thickening of the gallbladder wall in acute hepatitis: Ultrasound demonstration. Radiology 142:465-466, 1982.

Kane RA, et al: Porcelain gallbladder ultrasound and CT appearance. Radiology 152:137-141, 1984.

Kidney M, Goiney R, Cooperberg PL: Adenomyomatosis of the gallbladder: A pictorial exhibit. J Ultrasound Med 5: 331-333, 1986.

Koga A, et al: Diagnosis and operative indications for polypoid lesions of the gallbladder. Arch Surg 123:26-29, 1988.

Lafortune M, et al: The V-shaped artifact of the gallbladder wall. AJR Am J Roentgenol 147:505-508, 1986.

Laing FC, et al: Ultrasonic evaluation of patients with acute right upper quadrant pain. Radiology 140:449-455, 1981.

Laing FC: Diagnostic evaluation of patients with suspected acute cholecystitis. Radiol Clin North Am 21:477-493, 1983.

Lane J, Buck JL, Zeman RK: Primary carcinoma of the gallbladder: A pictorial essay. Radiographics 9:209-228, 1989.

Lee SP, Maher K, Nicholls JF: Origin and fate of biliary sludge. Gastroenterology 94:170-176, 1988.

Lee SP, Nicholls JF: Nature and composition of biliary sludge. Gastroenterology 90:677-686, 1986.

Levy AD, Murakata LA, Abbott RM, Rohrmann CA Jr: Benign tumors and tumorlike lesions of the gallbladder and extrahepatic bile ducts: Radiologic-pathologic correlation. Radiographics 22:387-413, 2002.

Levy AD, Murkata LA, Rohrmann CA Jr: Gallbladder carcinoma: Radiologic-pathologic correlation. Radiographics 21:295-314, 2001.

Lim JH, Ko YT, Kim SY: Ultrasound changes of the gallbladder wall in cholecystitis: Sonographic-pathologic correlation. Clin Radiol 38:389-393, 1987.

MacDonald FR, Cooperberg PL, Cohen MM: The WES triad—a specific sonographic sign of gallstones in the contracted gallbladder. Gastrointest Radiol 6:39-41, 1981.

Matron KI, Doubilet P: How to study the gallbladder. Ann Intern Med 109:752-754, 1988.

Melson GL, Reiter F, Evens RG: Tumorous conditions of the gallbladder. Semin Roentgenol 11:269-282, 1976.

Mentzer RM, et al: A comparative appraisal of emphysematous cholecystitis. Am J Surg 124:10-15, 1975.

Mirvis SE, et al: The diagnosis of acute acalculous cholecystitis: A comparison of sonography, scintigraphy, and CT. AJR Am J Roentgenol 147:1171-1175, 1986.

Muguruma N, Okamura S, Ichikawa S, et al: Endoscopic sonography in the diagnosis of gallbladder wall lesions in patients with gallstones. J Clin Ultrasound 29:395-400, 2001.

Nemcek AA, et al: The effervescent gallbladder: A sonographic sign of emphysematous cholecystitis. AJR Am J Roentgenol 150:575-577, 1988.

Ochsner SF: Solitary polypoid lesions of the gallbladder. Radiol Clin North Am 4:501-510, 1966.

Parulekar SG: Sonographic findings in acute emphysematous cholecystitis. Radiology 145:117-119, 1982.

Paulson BA, Pozniak MA: Ultrasound case of the day: Gallbladder varices. Radiographics 13:215-217, 1993.

Phillips G, et al: Ultrasound patterns of metastatic tumors in the gallbladder. J Clin Ultrasound 10:379-383, 1982.

Price RJ, et al: Sonography of polypoid cholesterolosis. AJR Am J Roentgenol 139:1197-1198, 1982.

Raghavendra BN, et al: Acute cholecystitis: Sonographicpathologic analysis. AJR Am J Roentgenol 137:327-332, 1981.

Raghavendra BN, et al: Sonography of adenomyomatosis of the gallbladder: Radiologic-pathologic correlation. Radiology 146:747-752, 1983.

Ralls PW, et al: Prospective evaluation of 99mTc-IDA cholescintigraphy and gray-scale ultrasound in the diagnosis of acute cholecystitis. Radiology 144:369-371, 1982.

Ralls PW, et al: Real-time sonography in suspected acute cholecystitis: Prospective evaluation of primary and secondary signs. Radiology 155:767-771, 1985.

Ralls PW, et al: Prospective evaluation of the sonographic Murphy sign in suspected acute cholecystitis. J Clin Ultrasound 10:113-115, 1982.

Rice J, et al: Sonographic appearance of adenomyomatosis of the gallbladder. J Clin Ultrasound 9:336-337, 1981.

Romano AJ, et al: Gallbladder and bile duct abnormalities in AIDS: Sonographic findings in eight patients. AJR Am J Roentgenol 150:123-127, 1988.

Rooholamini SA, Tehrani NS, Razavi MK, et al: Imaging of gallbladder carcinoma. Radiographics 14:291-306, 1994.

Ryubicki FJ: The WES sign. Radiology 214:881-882, 2000.

Sharp KW: Acute cholecystitis. Surg Clin North Am 68: 269-279, 1988.

Shieh CJ, Dunn E, Standard JE: Primary carcinoma of the gallbladder: A review of a 16-year experience at the Waterbury Hospital Health Center. Cancer 47:996-1004, 1981.

Shlaer WJ, Leopold GR, Scheible FW: Sonography of the thickened gallbladder wall: A nonspecific finding. AJR Am J Roentgenol 136:337- 339, 1981.

Shuman WP, et al: Evaluation of acute right upper quadrant pain: Sonography and 99mTc-HIDA cholescintigraphy. AJR Am J Roentgenol 139:61-64, 1982.

Shuman WP, et al: Low sensitivity of sonography and cholescintigraphy in acalculous cholecystitis. AJR Am J Roentgenol 142:531-534, 1984.

Sommer FG, Taylor KJW: Differentiation of acoustic shadowing due to calculi and gas collections. Radiology 135:399-403, 1980.

Sood BP, Kalra N, Gupta S, et al: Role of sonography in the diagnosis of gallbladder perforation. J Clin Ultrasound 30: 270-274, 2002.

Soyer P, Gouhiri M, Boudiaf M, et al: Pictorial essay: Carcinoma of the gallbladder: Imaging features with surgical correlation. AJR Am J Roentgenol 169:781-785, 1997.

Teefey SA, Baron RA, Bigler SA: Sonography of the gallbladder: Significance of striated (layered) thickening of the gallbladder wall. AJR Am J Roentgenol 156:945-947, 1991.

Weiner SN, et al: Sonography and computed tomography in the diagnosis of carcinoma of the gallbladder. AJR Am J Roentgenol 142:735-739, 1984.

Yamada K, Yamada H: Gallbladder wall thickening in mononucleosis syndromes. J Clin Ultrasound 29:322-325, 2001.

Yeh HC, Goodman J, Rabinowitz JG: Floating gallstones in bile without added contrast material. AJR Am J Roentgenol 146: 49-50, 1986.

CHAPTER 3

Liver

For Key Features summary see p. 83

ANATOMY

The liver is the largest solid organ in the normal abdomen, occupying most of the right upper quadrant. The right lobe contains an anterior and posterior segment, and the left lobe contains a medial and lateral segment. The right hepatic vein runs between the right anterior and posterior segments, the left hepatic vein runs between the left medial and lateral segments, and the middle hepatic vein runs between the left medial and the right anterior segment (Fig. 3-1A). The middle and left hepatic veins usually join together just before entering the inferior vena cava (IVC). Smaller, dorsal hepatic veins from the posterior right lobe and the caudate lobe often drain into the vena cava below the level of the three main veins (Fig. 3-2). Whereas the hepatic veins separate the hepatic segments, the portal veins run through the middle of the segments, and each branch is named according to the segment it supplies. The exception is the umbilical segment of the left portal vein, which runs between the left medial and lateral segments (see Fig. 3-1B). The portal veins can be distinguished from the hepatic veins by the periportal fibrofatty tissue, which produces brighter echoes around the portal veins as well as the adjacent hepatic arteries and bile ducts (see Fig. 3-1A).

The ligamentum teres is a useful landmark that travels between the medial and lateral segments of the left lobe (see Fig. 3-1C to F). It contains the fibrous remnant of the umbilical vein and travels from the umbilicus to the anterior aspect of the umbilical segment of the left portal vein. The interlobar fissure is a shallow indentation on the posterior aspect of the liver that separates the right and left lobes (see Fig. 3-1C) and identifies the location of the gallbladder fossa (see Fig 3-1D). The caudate lobe is a small segment of the liver located immediately anterior to the IVC. It is contiguous with the right lobe and separated from the lateral segment of the left lobe by the fissure for the ligamentum venosum (see Fig. 3-1B and E). The fissure for the ligamentum venosum extends to the posterior aspect of the umbilical segment of the left portal vein (see Fig. 3-1B). Table 3-1 reviews these important hepatic landmarks and the segmental anatomy of the liver.

Because surgeons can now resect subsegments of the liver, it is important to expand the classic segmental

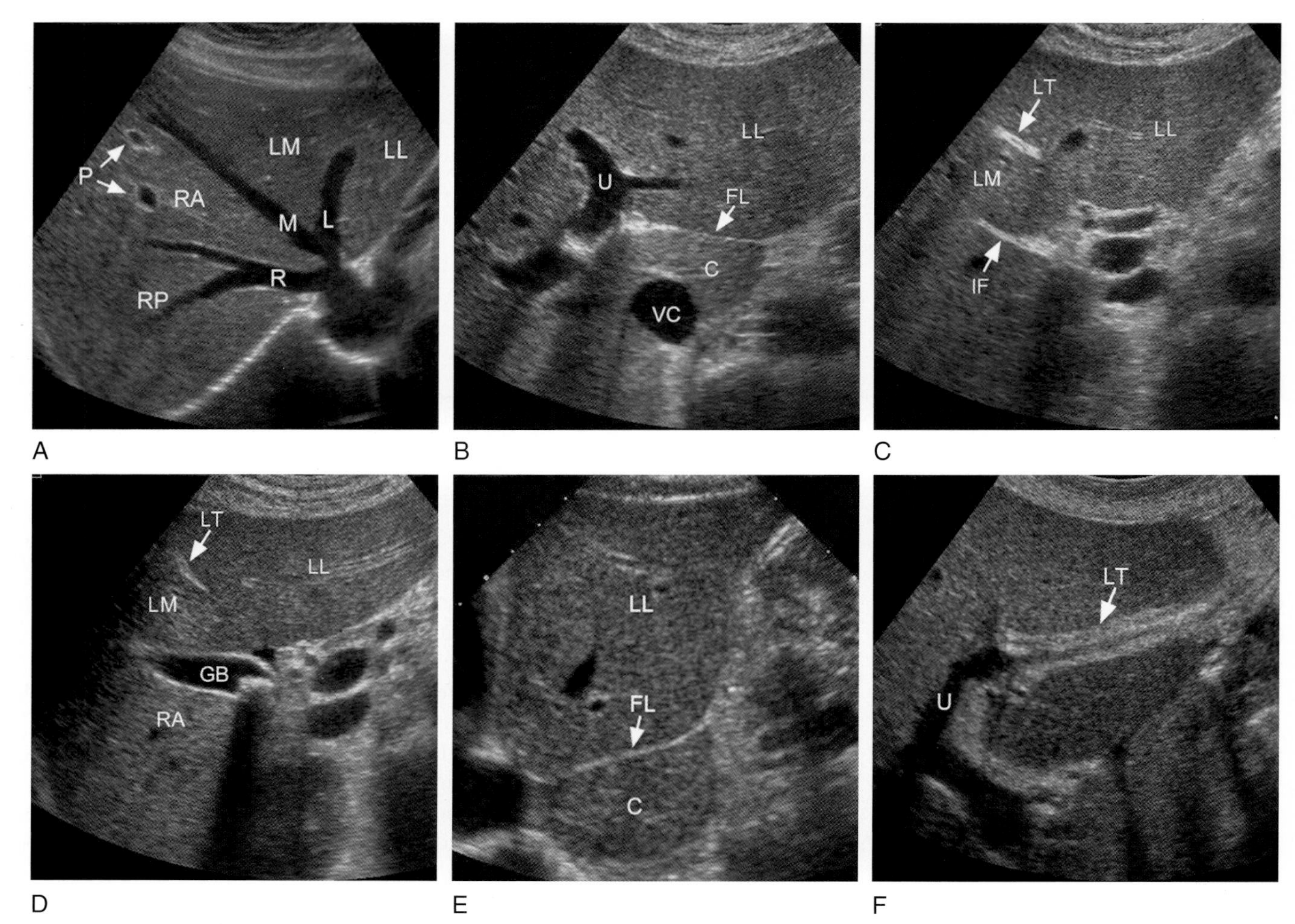

Figure 3-1 Normal liver anatomy. **A,** Transverse view of the hepatic vein confluence shows the right (R), middle (M), and left (L) hepatic veins. The segments of the liver are also shown: left lateral segment (LL), left medial segment (LM), right anterior segment (RA), and right posterior segment (RP). Two portal vein branches (P) in the right anterior segment differ from the hepatic veins by the echogenic fibrofatty tissue surrounding the vessel. **B,** Transverse view at the level of the left portal vein shows the fissure for the ligamentum venosum (FL) separating the caudate lobe (C) and the left lateral segment (LL). The fissure for the ligamentum venosum connects to the umbilical segment of the left portal vein (U). Also seen is the inferior vena cava (VC). **C,** Transverse view just inferior to **B** shows the ligamentum teres (LT) immediately below the anterior aspect of the umbilical segment of the left portal vein. The interlobar fissure (IF) is seen posteriorly. The left lateral segment (LL) and the left medial segment (LM) are separated by the ligamentum teres. **D,** Transverse view just inferior to previous image shows the gallbladder (GB) immediately below the interlobar fissure. The interlobar fissure and the gallbladder fossa separate the left medial segment (LM) from the right anterior segment (RA). The ligamentum teres (LT) and the left lateral segment (LL) are also seen. A gallstone is present in the gallbladder. **E,** Longitudinal view from the midline of the abdomen shows the caudate lobe (C) and the left lateral segment (LL) separated by the fissure for the ligamentum venosum (FL). **F,** Longitudinal view through the left lobe shows the umbilical segment of the left portal vein (U) and the ligamentum teres (LT). Note that the ligamentum teres connects to the anterior most aspect of the umbilical segment of the left portal vein.

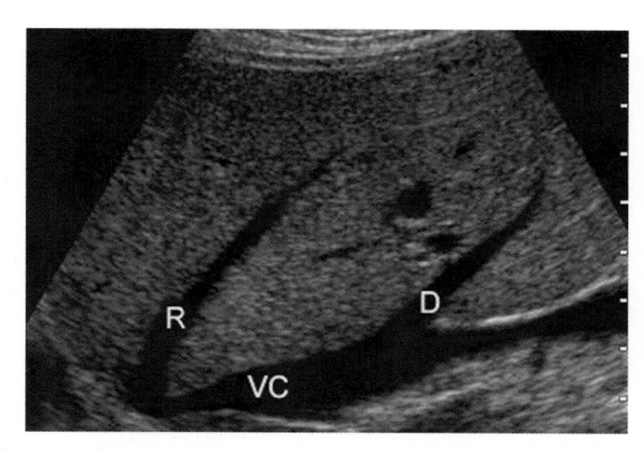

Figure 3-2 Dorsal right hepatic vein. Longitudinal view of the right lobe of the liver shows the right hepatic vein (R) draining into the vena cava (VC) superiorly. A dorsal right hepatic vein (D) is also seen draining into the vena cava inferiorly.

nomenclature. The Couinaud system divides the left lateral, right anterior, and right posterior segments into superior and inferior subsegments and maintains the caudate lobe and the medial left segment as single segments. This results in eight anatomic subsegments numbered as follows: I—caudate, II—left lateral superior, III—left lateral inferior, IV—left medial, V—right anterior inferior, VI—right posterior inferior, VII—right posterior superior, and VIII—right anterior superior. A separate portal venous branch supplies each of these subsegments.

The common hepatic artery normally arises from the celiac axis and passes anterior to the portal vein (Fig. 3-3A and B). The gastroduodenal artery arises from the common hepatic and descends along the anterior aspect of the pancreatic head. Beyond the gastroduodenal artery, the hepatic artery is called the proper hepatic artery. The proper hepatic artery ascends in the gastroduodenal ligament to the porta hepatis. It then divides into the right and left hepatic artery. The right hepatic artery passes posterior to the common bile duct and anterior to the portal vein (see Chapter 4).

Variations in the hepatic arteries are very common. A replaced (i.e., the only existing vessel arises from an anomalous origin) or an accessory (i.e., an additional vessel arises from an anomalous origin) right hepatic artery arising from the superior mesenteric artery is present in approximately 20% of individuals. Replaced or accessory left hepatic arteries arising from the left gastric artery are just as common. They pass into the left lobe of the liver through the fissure for the ligamentum venosum rather than the porta hepatis (see Fig. 3-3C and D). Replaced/accessory right hepatic arteries pass posterior to the portal vein and anterior to the vena cava (see Fig. 3-3E and F).

Table 3-1 Hepatic Segmental Landmarks

Segments	Separating Landmarks
Left lateral/left medial	Ligamentum teres, umbilical segment of left portal vein, left hepatic vein
Left medial/right anterior	Interlobar fissure, gallbladder, middle hepatic vein
Right anterior/right posterior	Right hepatic vein
Caudate lobe/left lobe	Fissure for ligamentum venosum

A common variation that is seen in the periphery of the liver is deep fissures caused by hypertrophied diaphragmatic muscle bundles (Fig. 3-4). In certain imaging planes, these may appear as echogenic lesions on the surface of the liver. However, because they are long bands of muscle, it is possible to rotate the transducer parallel to the long axis of the band and show that the "lesion" is linear and not spherical. True accessory fissures also occur but are not commonly visualized on sonography.

The size of the liver can be difficult to gauge on sonography because its shape and volume distribution between right and left lobe is so variable. Normal upper limits of liver length measured in the midclavicular line range from 13 to 17 cm (15 cm is used most frequently). Indirect signs of hepatomegaly include extension of the right lobe below the lower pole of the kidney (in the absence of a Riedel lobe), rounding of the inferior tip of the liver, and extension of the left lobe into the left upper quadrant above the spleen.

The liver parenchyma is normally homogeneous and is only interrupted by the portal triads and the hepatic veins. Echogenicity of the liver should be slightly greater than or equal to that of the right kidney but less than that of the spleen (Table 3-2). The liver is less echogenic than the spleen and is usually less echogenic than the pancreas, although the liver and pancreas may be isoechoic in younger individuals.

TECHNIQUE

The liver is usually best scanned with a sector or a curved-array transducer, with center frequency ranging from 2 to 5 MHz. Linear-array transducers of even higher frequency are useful for imaging superficial abnormalities, diffuse parenchymal abnormalities (e.g., cirrhosis), and the surface of the liver. The left lobe can be imaged effectively in most patients from an anterior subxiphoid approach. The right lobe should be scanned from both a subcostal and intercostal approach to optimize detection and characterization of focal lesions. Intercostal scans are usually most effective with the patient supine and

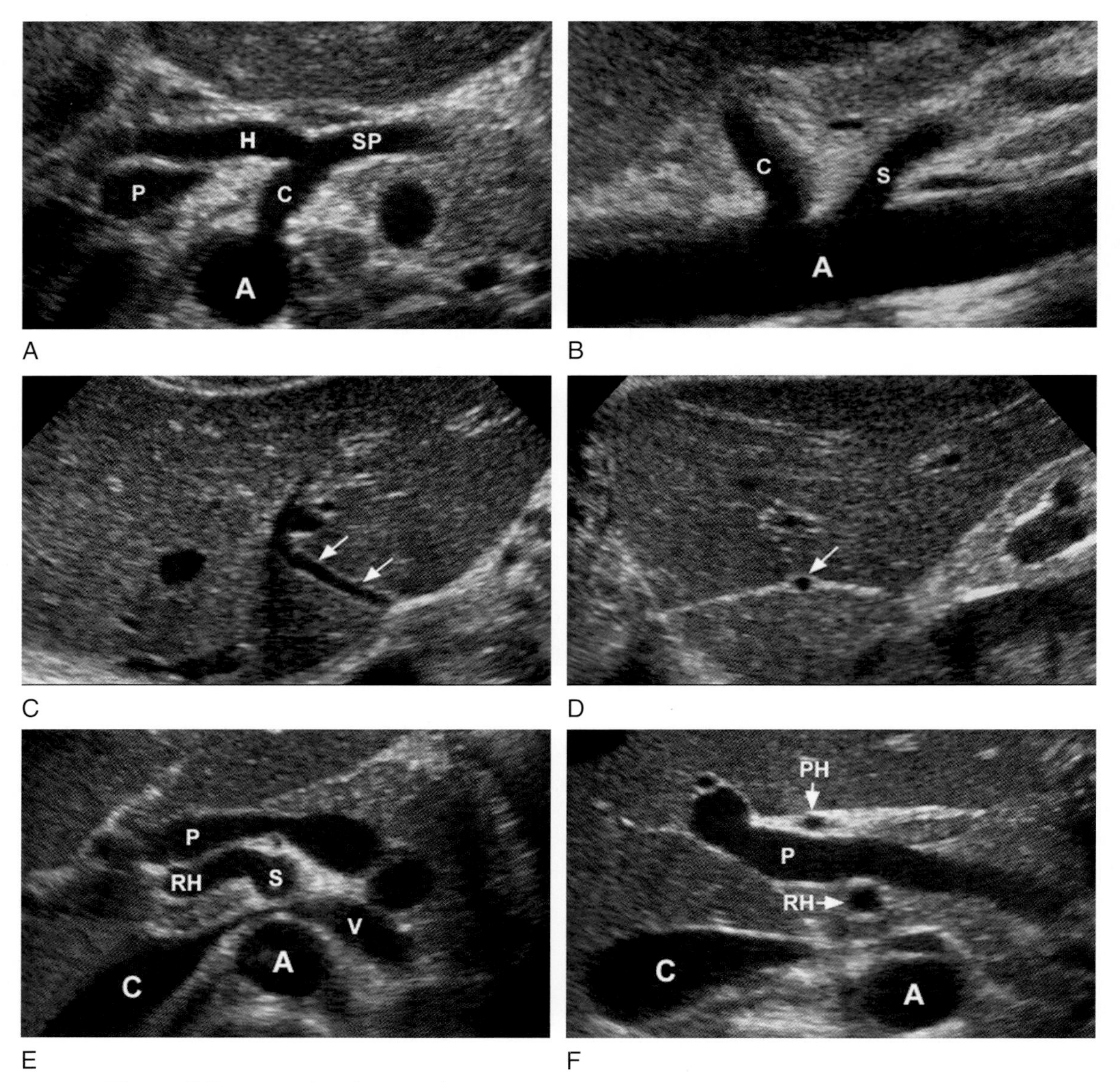

Figure 3-3 Normal and variant hepatic artery anatomy. Transverse (**A**) and longitudinal (**B**) views of the normal celiac axis show the celiac (C) arising from the aorta (A). On the transverse view, the common hepatic artery (H) is seen traveling anterior to the portal vein (P). The splenic artery (SP) is also seen. On the longitudinal view, the superior mesenteric artery (S) is seen inferior to the celiac axis. Transverse (**C**) and longitudinal (**D**) views of a replaced left hepatic artery *(arrows)*. On the longitudinal view, the artery appears as a small round dot within the echogenic linear fissure for the ligamentum venosum. Transverse (**E**) and longitudinal (**F**) views of a replaced right hepatic artery. On the transverse view, the replaced right hepatic artery (RH) is seen arising from the superior mesenteric artery (S). Also seen is the aorta (A), vena cava (C), left renal vein (V), and portal vein (P). The longitudinal view shows the replaced right hepatic artery posterior to the portal vein and the proper hepatic artery (PH) anterior to the portal vein.

are best done during normal respiration so that the right lung base and its associated shadowing are not obscuring the superior aspects of the liver. Rib shadowing can be minimized by imaging in an oblique plane that is parallel to the long axis of the intercostal spaces. Subcostal scanning should be performed with the patient in a left lateral decubitus or left posterior oblique position so that the liver shifts slightly medial and inferior. More inferior displacement of the liver and further enhancement of subcostal and subxiphoid scanning can be achieved by imaging during deep patient inspiration. It is important to angle the transducer superiorly while scanning from a subcostal approach so that the dome of the liver can be visualized.

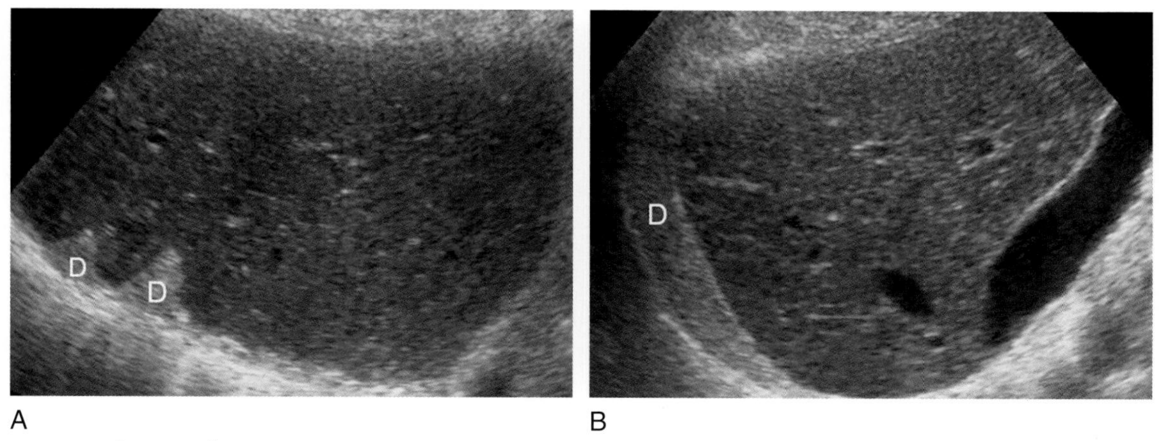

Figure 3-4 Diaphragmatic fissures. **A,** Two adjacent echogenic triangular defects are identified on the surface of the liver. These represent two external fissures caused by the diaphragm (D). **B,** View 90 degrees from that in **A** shows the larger of these two defects as an elongated band of diaphragmatic muscle external to the liver.

CYSTS

Simple hepatic cysts are the most common focal liver lesions. Because the liver is such a homogeneous organ, cysts are usually easy to detect and generally display the three classic sonographic criteria of an anechoic lumen, increased through transmission, and a well-defined back wall (Fig. 3-5A and B). Many hepatic cysts have at least a partial septation or puckering of the wall that disturbs the normally smooth contour of uncomplicated cysts (see Fig. 3-5C). Cysts are referred to as complex if they have internal echoes, a thick wall, septations that are numerous or thick, solid elements, or calcification. Complex cystic lesions include hematomas, abscesses, bilomas, echinococcus, cystic metastases, and hemorrhagic or necrotic tumors. Biliary cystadenomas and cystadenocarcinomas are rare neoplasms that appear as multiseptated cystic masses (Box 3-1). Vascular lesions such as aneurysms, arterioportal fistulas, and portal hepatic vein fistulas can simulate cysts on gray-scale sonography but are easily distinguished with Doppler analysis (Fig. 3-6). Lymphoma is a solid tumor that can rarely simulate a cyst.

The liver is involved in 40% to 50% of cases of autosomal dominant polycystic disease. Despite extensive replacement by cysts, liver function remains normal in the majority of patients unless there is associated hepatic fibrosis. Symptoms may arise from the mass effect of the numerous cysts or result from cyst hemorrhage (Fig. 3-7).

Table 3-2 Characteristics of Normal Liver

Characteristic	Appearance
Size	<15 cm
Echogenicity	≥Right kidney, <pancreas, <spleen
Parenchyma	Homogeneous
Surface	Smooth

BENIGN TUMORS

Hemangiomas

Hemangiomas are the most common benign liver neoplasm, occurring in approximately 7% of adults. They are found more often in women than men. With the exception of cysts, hemangiomas are the most common incidental lesions detected on hepatic sonography. Structurally, they are much like a sponge filled with blood. Multiple, small, blood-filled spaces are separated by fibrous septations and lined by endothelial cells. Approximately 10% are multiple. It is unusual for hemangiomas to bleed or to cause symptoms, although giant hemangiomas may have enough mass effect to be symptomatic. Platelet sequestration and destruction by hemangiomas has been reported as a rare cause of thrombocytopenia (Kasabach-Merritt syndrome).

The typical appearance is a homogeneous, hyperechoic mass that is usually less than 3 cm in size. Sixty to 70 percent of hemangiomas are typical (Fig. 3-8). The margins are usually sharp and smooth, and they may be round or slightly lobulated. Larger lesions are more likely to appear atypical as a result of fibrosis, thrombosis, and necrosis. Calcifications can occur but are rare.

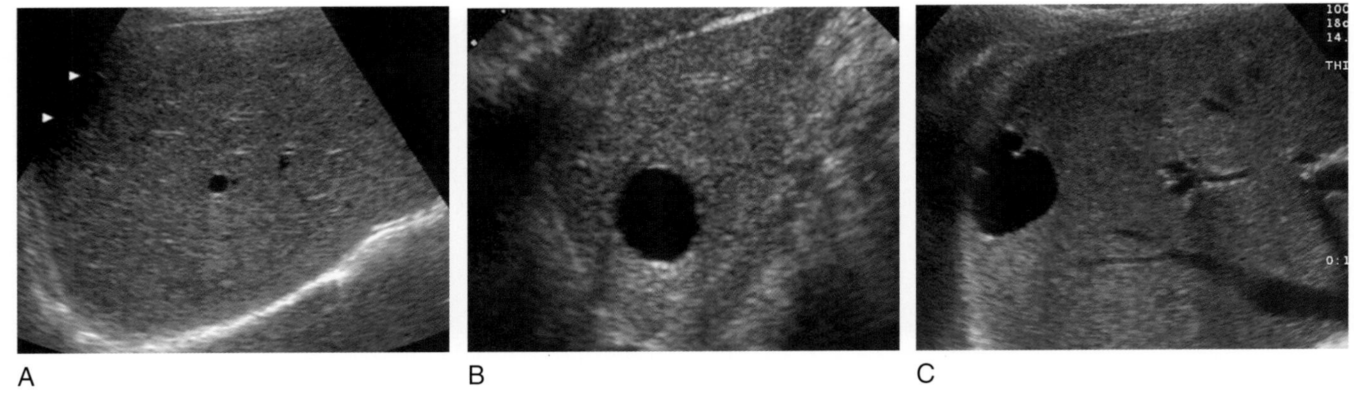

Figure 3-5 Hepatic cysts in different patients. **A,** Small hepatic cyst (<1 cm). Despite the small size, the cyst is anechoic with a well-defined back wall and minimal but detectable increased through transmission. **B,** Larger hepatic cyst shows classic findings and obvious increased through transmission. **C,** Hepatic cyst shows peripheral puckering, which is frequently seen in otherwise simple hepatic cysts.

Box 3-1 Causes of Cystic Lesions in the Liver

COMMON	UNCOMMON	RARE
Cysts	Abscess	Aneurysm
	Hematoma	Arterioportal fistula
	Cystic metastases	Portal-hepatic vein fistula
	Biloma	Hemorrhagic adenoma
	Echinococcus	Biliary cystadenoma (carcinoma)

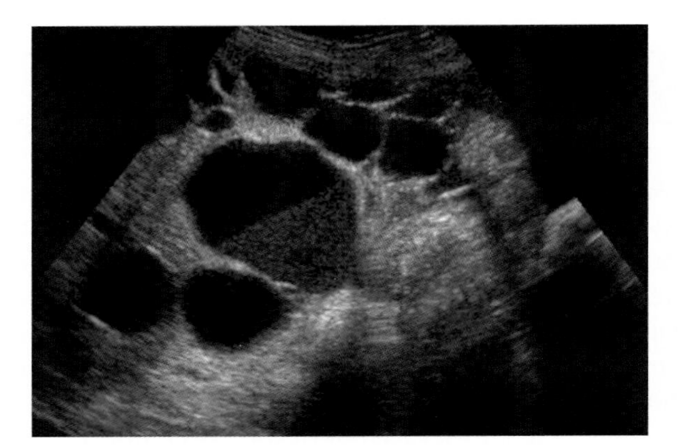

Figure 3-7 Polycystic disease. Transverse view of the liver demonstrates multiple simple hepatic cysts. The largest cyst shows a fluid cellular layer secondary to hemorrhage.

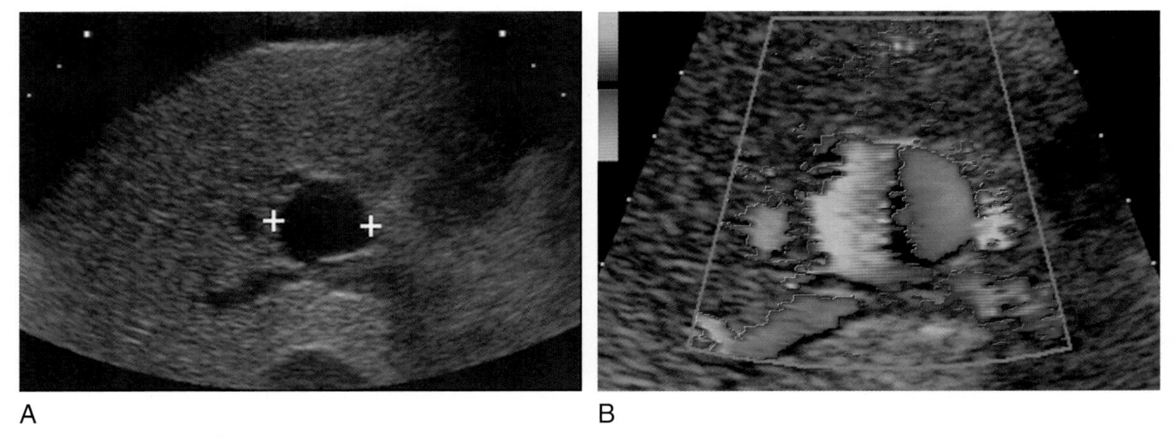

Figure 3-6 Portal vein aneurysm simulating a hepatic cyst. **A,** Gray-scale view of the liver demonstrates an anechoic structure *(cursors)* with a well-defined back wall and increased through transmission. This has a typical appearance of a hepatic cyst. **B,** Doppler analysis demonstrates flow throughout the lesion. Pulsed Doppler analysis showed a venous waveform consistent with a portal vein aneurysm.

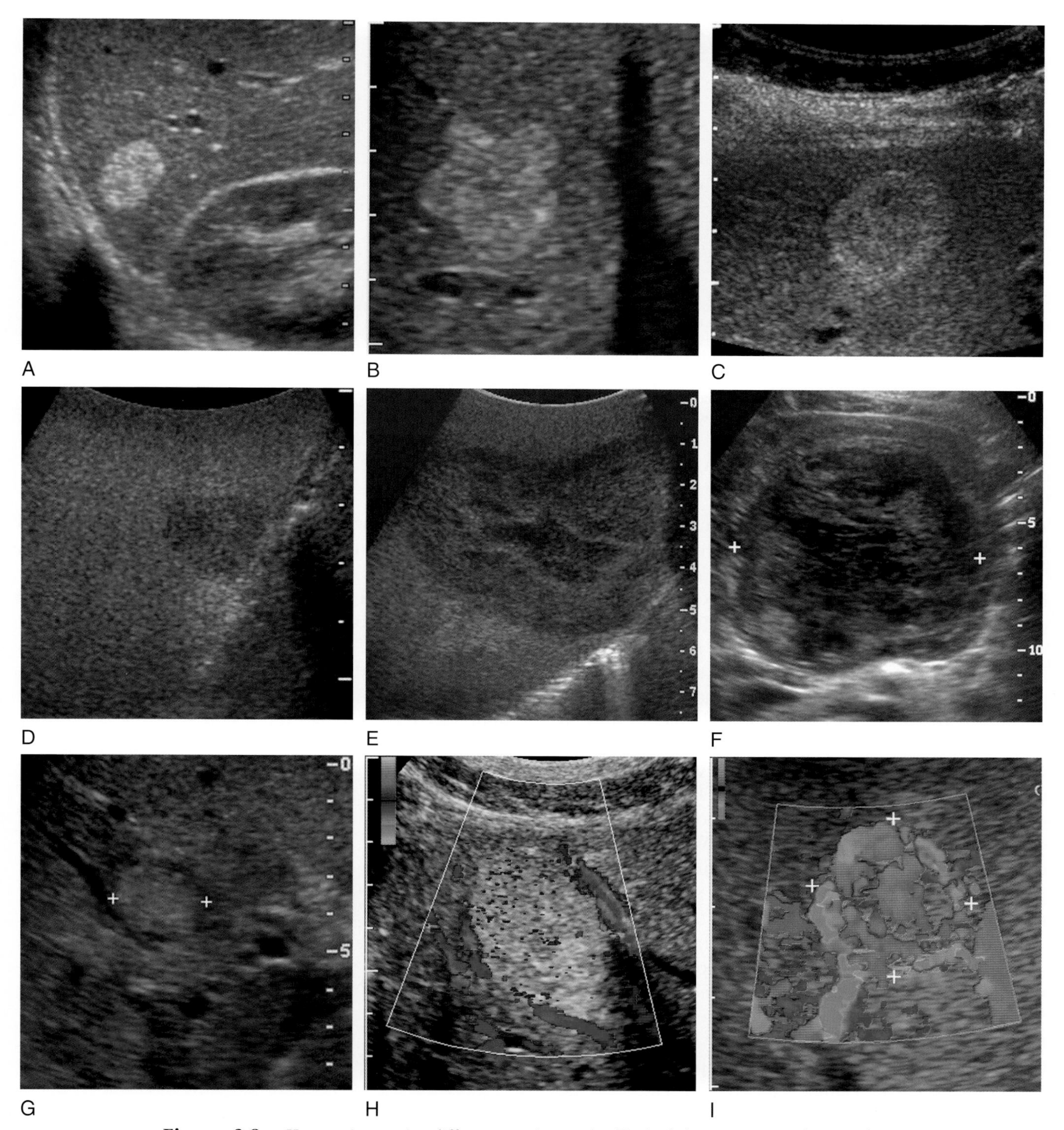

Figure 3-8 Hemangiomas in different patients. **A,** Typical homogeneous hyperechoic well-defined mass. **B,** Homogeneous hyperechoic mass with scalloping of the margin. **C,** Lesion with isoechoic center and a thick peripheral hyperechoic halo. This appearance is sometimes referred to as a reverse target appearance. **D,** Atypical hemangioma appearing as a hypoechoic lesion with slight through transmission. This occurred in the setting of an otherwise fatty infiltrated liver. **E,** Large atypical hemangioma that is predominantly hypoechoic and heterogeneous with a large central region of decreased echogenicity likely caused by fibrosis or thrombosis. **F,** Large atypical hemangioma *(cursors)* that is diffusely heterogeneous. **G,** Small hemangioma *(cursors)* that has a targetoid appearance. This appearance, which closely simulates a malignant lesion, is only rarely seen with hemangiomas. **H,** Color Doppler view of a typical hemangioma showing flow in vessels adjacent to the lesion but no flow within the lesion. **I,** Color Doppler view of an atypical hemangioma with abundant detectable internal flow *(cursors).*

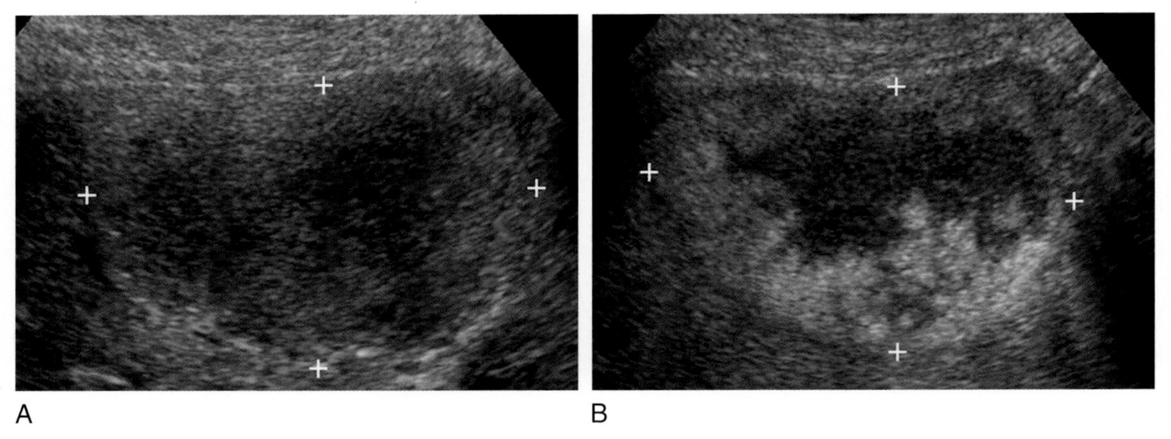

Figure 3-9 Contrast enhancement of hemangioma. **A,** View of a large atypical hemangioma *(cursors)* shows heterogeneous echotexture that is predominantly hypoechoic. **B,** After administration of intravenous contrast material, peripheral contrast enhancement is seen with a typical puddling pattern similar to what is well described on CT.

A significant percentage of atypical hemangiomas have a hyperechoic periphery and a hypoechoic center. This "reverse target" appearance is fairly characteristic of hemangiomas and is only rarely seen in malignant disease. Posterior enhancement is often included in the description of hemangiomas, but it is not a common finding; and because other solid liver tumors can have posterior enhancement, it is not a useful finding. Despite the vascular nature of hemangiomas, blood flow is generally too slow to be detected with Doppler techniques. Therefore, detection of flow within a hepatic mass that otherwise appears like a hemangioma on gray-scale imaging should raise suspicion for metastatic disease or hepatocellular carcinoma. With intravenous ultrasound contrast agents, hemangiomas demonstrate peripheral puddling similar to what is seen on contrast medium–enhanced CT (Fig. 3-9).

As one would expect for a benign lesion, hemangiomas are usually stable over time. However, approximately 10% will undergo a decrease in echogenicity, and 5% will regress partially or completely. Only 2% of hemangiomas enlarge on follow-up scans. Rarely a hemangioma will change its sonographic appearance during the course of a single examination (Fig. 3-10); no other hepatic lesion is known to do this.

The differential diagnosis for hyperechoic masses in the liver primarily includes other neoplasms, especially liver metastases and hepatocellular cancer. Focal fatty infiltration can also produce nodular regions of increased echogenicity. Minimal shadowing is occasionally seen with focal nodular fat but is not a feature of hemangiomas.

The work-up of a homogeneous hyperechoic hepatic mass depends on the patient's risk of malignancy. If the patient has a prior history or current evidence of an extrahepatic malignancy capable of metastasizing to the liver, or a history of chronic liver disease, the suspected diagnosis of hemangioma should be confirmed with another imaging modality. MRI is probably most useful, although CT can also be used for larger lesions. If the lesion is larger than 2 cm and not adjacent to the heart or major hepatic vascular structures, technetium 99m–tagged red blood cell (RBC) scintigraphy can be used. If the patient does not have these risk factors, a homogeneous hyperechoic liver lesion requires no further evaluation.

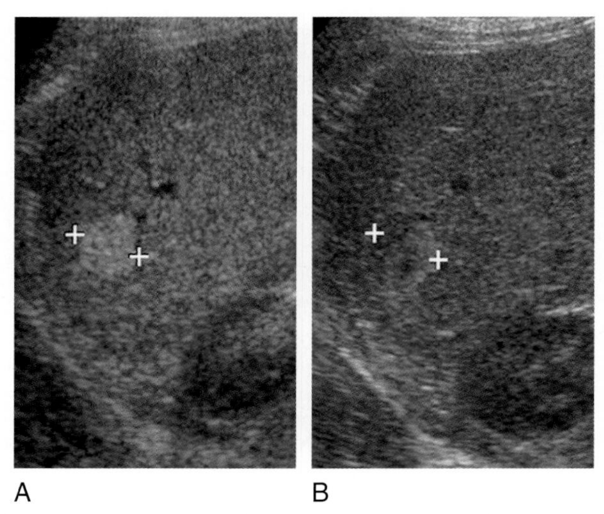

Figure 3-10 A rapid change of hemangioma. **A,** Initial view of hemangioma *(cursors)* shows a typical homogeneous hyperechoic pattern. **B,** Similar view obtained 33 seconds later demonstrates change in the appearance of this lesion to a predominantly hypoechoic pattern. (Case courtesy of Dr. Andy Fisher, Denver, CO.)

Occasionally, noninvasive tests will not establish the diagnosis of hemangioma in a patient at risk for malignancy, and the patient will require a biopsy. Despite the vascular nature of hemangiomas, biopsies can be performed safely. However, the needle should pass through normal parenchyma before entering the hemangioma to achieve some tamponade effect. Core needle biopsies using a 20-gauge or larger needle can obtain sufficient tissue for diagnosis in the majority of cases. Fine-needle aspirations generally obtain only blood and are not sufficient to make the diagnosis.

Focal Nodular Hyperplasia

Focal nodular hyperplasia (FNH) is a benign tumor of the liver that is composed of Kupffer cells, hepatocytes, and biliary structures but lacks the typical normal lobular hepatic features of portal triads and central veins. Although uncommon, it is the second most frequently encountered benign liver tumor after hemangiomas. Interestingly, the two lesions occur together at an increased rate, especially in patients with multifocal FNH. It is hypothesized that FNH develops from a congenital vascular malformation that promotes focal hyperemia and hepatocellular hyperplasia. It is typically unencapsulated and often has a central, stellate scar. Ten to 20 percent are multiple. FNH is supplied by an internal arterial network that is arranged in a spoke-wheel pattern. They are much more common in women (80% to 90%). Unlike hepatic adenomas, they are not related to use of birth control pills, although birth control pills may promote their growth. They seldom bleed or cause any clinical symptoms, although pain may be encountered when the lesions are large.

FNH is usually detected as an incidental mass that enhances brightly and transiently during the arterial phase of CT scans. Sonography is not typically part of the work-up of suspected FNH unless it is used to guide percutaneous biopsy. This may change with the more widespread use of intravenous ultrasound contrast agents. Although the appearance of FNH varies on sonography, most are isoechoic or nearly isoechoic to liver parenchyma (Fig. 3-11). This makes sense because their cellular makeup is similar to that of liver. They may also have a target appearance. Calcification, cystic changes, hemorrhagic areas, and necrosis are very uncommon. The central stellate scar, which is frequently seen on CT and MRI, is uncommonly seen on conventional ultrasound (but should be seen with contrast medium enhancement). However, the spoke-wheel pattern of internal vascularity is better displayed on color or power Doppler imaging than on CT or MRI. This is composed of one or occasionally more than one dominant feeding artery that enters the tumor from the periphery, travels to the center of the lesion, and then divides into multiple branches that radiate back out to the periphery of the lesion (see Fig. 3-11B and E).

The differential diagnosis of FNH includes fibrolamellar carcinoma, hepatic adenoma, hepatocellular carcinoma, hemangioma, and vascular metastases. In most cases the clinical history will point in the right direction. Fibrolamellar cancer most closely simulates FNH because it has a central scar and a spoke-wheel pattern of vascularity. Any features of malignancy (metastases or adenopathy) or lesional calcification or necrosis would suggest fibrolamellar cancer.

When a lesion suspected to represent FNH is initially detected with ultrasound, hepatic scintigraphy with sulfur colloid can be very useful. Because of the concentration of Kupffer cells, approximately 60% of FNH will be either hot (more intense than adjacent liver) or warm (isointense to adjacent liver). The typical features on ultrasound (in particular the spoke-wheel arterial pattern) and these findings on sulfur colloid scans are sufficient to make the diagnosis with a high degree of certainty. If the lesion is cold on sulfur colloid scans, then FNH remains a possibility, but other lesions also need to be considered. MRI with reticuloendothelial contrast agents is also becoming a popular way of confirming suspected FNH.

Hepatic Adenoma

Adenomas are rare benign tumors that contain normal (or occasionally slightly abnormal) hepatocytes but few Kupffer cells and virtually no bile ductules. Tumor capsules are usually absent or incomplete. Adenomas occur most commonly in women taking birth control pills, and their incidence is related to both dose and duration of use of oral contraceptives. They also occur in men taking anabolic steroids. Multiple adenomas may occur in patients with type I glycogen storage disease, and multiplicity defines a condition known as hepatic adenomatosis. Their propensity to bleed makes them surgical lesions despite their benign histology. They also have a low but real risk of malignant degeneration. Their sonographic appearance is varied and nonspecific, and in most cases additional imaging is necessary to confirm the diagnosis. They are usually not suspected in a patient unless the clinical history includes known use of oral contraceptives or previous bleeding episodes.

Simple, small uncomplicated adenomas tend to be homogeneous and are often hypoechoic. Internal hemorrhage or necrosis usually produces a heterogeneous appearance and/or complex cystic components (Fig. 3-12). Intratumoral fat may result in a hyperechoic appearance. Calcifications occur in 10% of cases. Free intraperitoneal fluid may be seen in cases of intraperitoneal rupture.

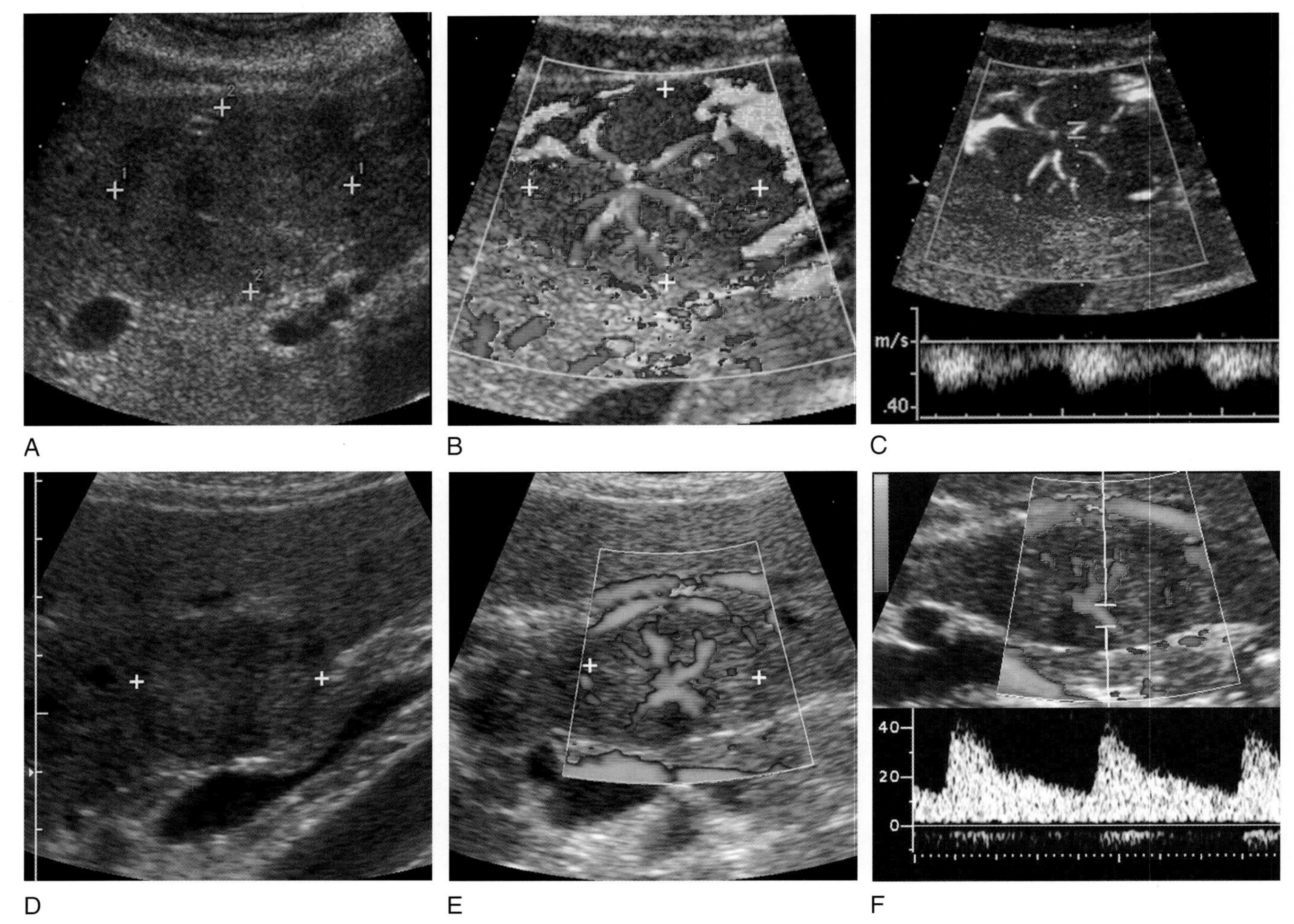

Figure 3-11 Focal nodular hyperplasia in different patients. Gray-scale (**A**), color Doppler (**B**), and pulsed Doppler (**C**) views of a patient with typical focal nodular hyperplasia *(cursors)*. The gray-scale view shows a slightly heterogeneous mass that is predominantly isoechoic to the liver. Color Doppler imaging shows the typical spoke-wheel arrangement of internal vascularity. Pulsed Doppler waveform confirms the arterial nature of the central vascular flow. **D** to **F**, Similar views of another patient with focal nodular hyperplasia *(cursors)*. The gray-scale view shows a target lesion that is slightly hyperechoic centrally but has a hypoechoic halo. Color Doppler view again demonstrates the spoke-wheel pattern, and the pulsed Doppler view confirms arterial flow within the lesion.

MALIGNANT TUMORS

Metastases

The lungs and liver are the most frequent sites of distant metastatic disease, and metastases are the most common malignant liver lesion in North America. Up to 50% of patients dying of cancer have liver metastases. Metastases are multiple in up to 98% of cases, and they usually involve both lobes of the liver. Signs and symptoms of liver disease are absent in approximately one half of patients with liver metastases. Liver function tests are also unreliable in detecting liver metastases. Therefore, imaging plays a critical role in patients with suspected liver metastases.

The majority of metastatic lesions have a target appearance with an echogenic or isoechoic center and a hypoechoic halo (Fig. 3-13). When the halo is thin, it may represent dilated peritumoral sinusoids or compressed liver parenchyma. Thick halos represent proliferating tumor. After metastases, the most common cause of target lesions is hepatocellular carcinoma. Lymphoma can also produce target lesions. Abscesses, adenomas, and FNH may appear as target lesions, but these lesions

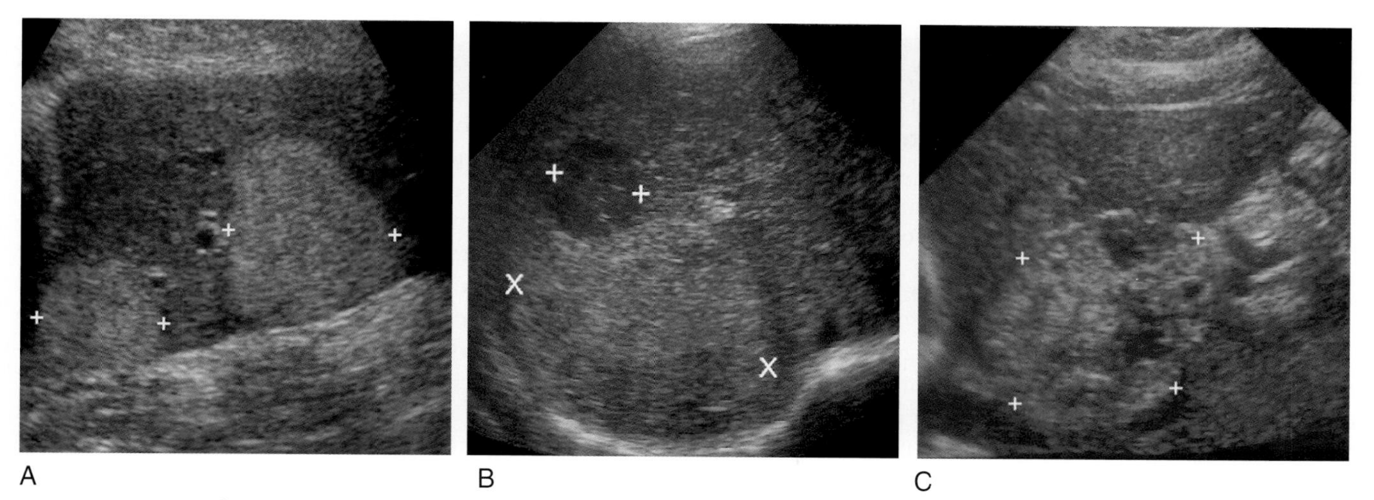

Figure 3-12 Hepatic adenomas in different patients. **A,** Two hepatic adenomas *(cursors)* with homogeneous hyperechoic appearance simulating hemangiomas. **B,** Two adenomas *(cursors)* with variable appearance. The smaller lesion is predominantly hypoechoic. **C,** Heterogeneous lesion *(cursors)* with scattered hypoechoic areas and cystic-appearing areas likely secondary to internal hemorrhage.

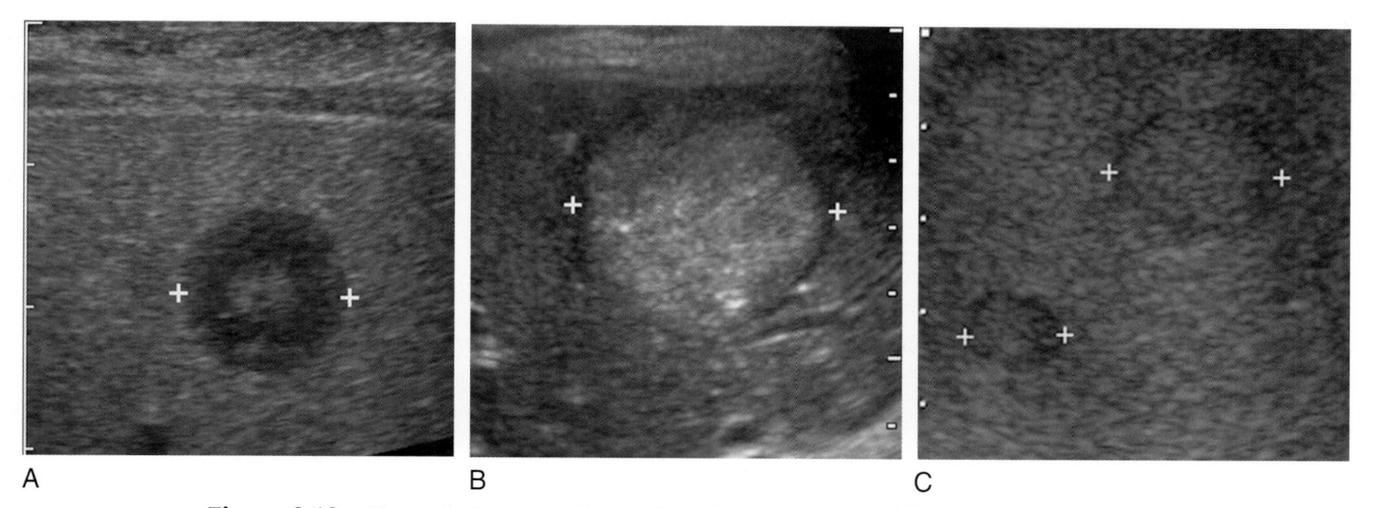

Figure 3-13 Target lesions secondary to hepatic metastases in different patients. **A,** Lesion *(cursors)* with isoechoic center and a thick hypoechoic halo. In this case, the hypoechoic halo almost certainly represents proliferating tumor. **B,** Hyperechoic lesion *(cursors)* with thin peripheral hypoechoic halo. In this case, the halo may represent compressed liver parenchyma or dilated hepatic sinusoids. **C,** Isoechoic lesions *(cursors)* that are visible only due to their thin hypoechoic halo.

Box 3-2 Hepatic Target Lesions

COMMON	UNCOMMON
Metastases	Lymphoma
Hepatocellular cancer	Focal nodular hyperplasia
	Fungal microabscess
	Adenoma

are not nearly as common as the malignant lesions just mentioned. Hemangioma is a very common lesion but only rarely produces a target appearance. It is important to realize that target lesions are much more likely to be malignant than benign (Box 3-2).

In addition to target lesions, metastases can have a variety of sonographic appearances, as illustrated in Figure 3-14. Although it is not possible to predict the primary tumor based on the sonographic appearance of the liver metastases, some trends are useful. Hyperechoic metastases tend to arise from the gastrointestinal tract, most commonly from the colon. Neuroendocrine tumors are another relatively common cause of hyperechoic metastases. The colon is also the most common source for calcified metastases, although mucinous primary tumors of the ovary, breast, and stomach can also calcify (Box 3-3). Cystic hepatic metastases are unusual but do occur. They generally have thick walls, thick septations, or obvious solid components and therefore do not mimic simple hepatic cysts. Cystic

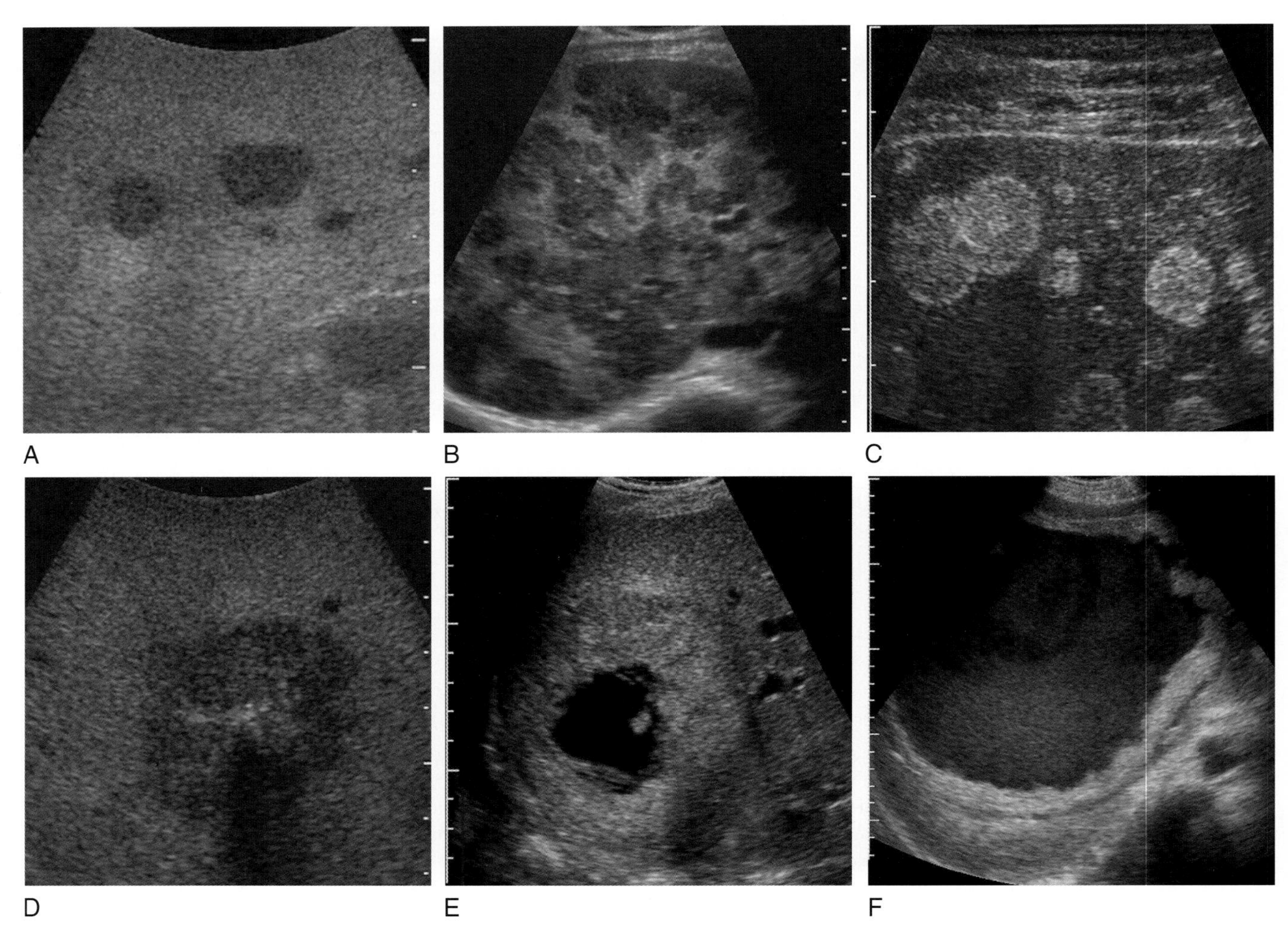

Figure 3-14 Liver metastases with a variety of sonographic appearances in different patients. **A,** Two adjacent metastases from colon carcinoma with homogeneous hypoechoic appearance and slightly increased through transmission. **B,** Multiple lesions that are confluent in areas secondary to breast cancer. All are hypoechoic. **C,** Multiple metastases secondary to osteosarcoma. All are hyperechoic and similar in appearance to hepatic hemangiomas. **D,** Metastasis secondary to colon cancer that is predominantly hypoechoic with a central shadowing echogenic region due to calcification. **E,** Metastasis from squamous cell carcinoma of the head and neck shows a large slightly hyperechoic lesion with peripheral hypoechoic halo and a central area of liquefaction secondary to necrosis. **F,** Metastasis from leiomyosarcoma shows a large cystic mass with low-level internal echoes and a thick hyperechoic wall. This lesion replaces most of the right lobe of the liver.

Box 3-3 Calcified Hepatic Masses

LARGE, WITH OR WITHOUT MASS	SMALL, WITHOUT MASS
Metastases	Granulomas
Fibrolamellar hepatocellular cancer	Pneumocystis
Old hematoma	Biliary stones
Old abscess	Hepatic arteries

Box 3-4 Diffuse Hepatic Inhomogeneity

COMMON	UNCOMMON
Cirrhosis	Hepatocellular cancer
Metastases	Hepatic fibrosis
Fatty infiltration	Lymphoma

spaces in metastases may result from a cystic primary tumor (ovary) or from necrosis, such as squamous cell carcinomas, sarcomas, and large lesions from any primary tumor.

With widespread hepatic metastases the liver may appear diffusely heterogeneous and it may be difficult to identify individual lesions. High-resolution views focused on the superficial aspect of the liver increase the chance of identifying individual lesions (Fig. 3-15). This pattern is particularly typical for breast cancer. The differential diagnosis for this appearance includes cirrhosis, hepatic fibrosis, hepatic lymphoma, fatty infiltration, and diffuse hepatocellular carcinoma (Box 3-4).

In many clinical situations when metastatic disease is suspected, definite tissue confirmation is required before therapy can be initiated. With experience, liver lesions can be sampled with ultrasound guidance with a high degree of success. Even lesions less than 1 cm can be sampled with 90% success rates (Fig. 3-16). Because the course of the needle can be followed in real time, ultrasound-guided biopsies can be performed much more rapidly than CT-guided biopsies. When there is a known extrahepatic primary malignancy, it is usually adequate to perform fine-needle aspirations (using 22- to 25-gauge needles) for cytologic analysis. When there is no known primary tumor, suspected liver metastases should be sampled with core needles (using 18- to 20-gauge needles). This allows immunohistochemical studies to be done so that the primary tumor can be identified with more certainty.

Hepatocellular Carcinoma

Hepatocellular carcinoma (HCC) is the most common primary malignancy of the liver. It is sometimes referred to as hepatoma. Although HCC can occur in normal livers, it is strongly associated with chronic liver disease, especially hepatitis B and C infection and cirrhosis. HCC is a major health problem in Asia and sub-Saharan Africa, owing to the high prevalence of hepatitis and aflatoxin ingestion. In non-Asian populations, alcoholic cirrhosis is the most important condition predisposing to HCC. Other predisposing factors include hemochromatosis, Wilson's disease, and type I glycogen storage disease.

Cirrhotic livers pathologically display a spectrum of nodular lesions. Regenerating nodules form because of

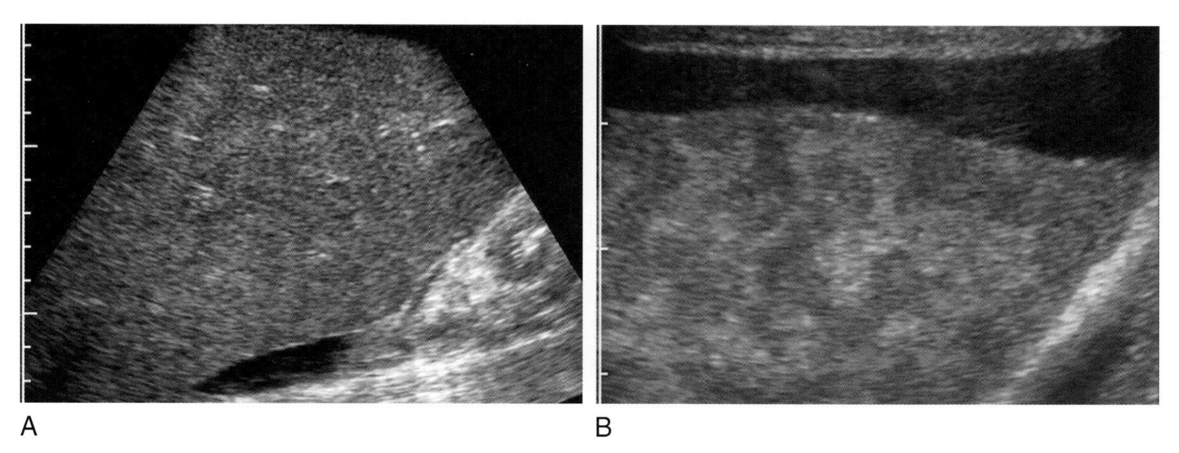

Figure 3-15 Diffuse hepatic metastases. **A,** Standard view of the liver demonstrates mild heterogeneity of the hepatic parenchyma. It is difficult to define individual lesions on this image. **B,** High-resolution view of the superficial aspect of the liver demonstrates multiple discrete hypoechoic lesions less than 1 cm.

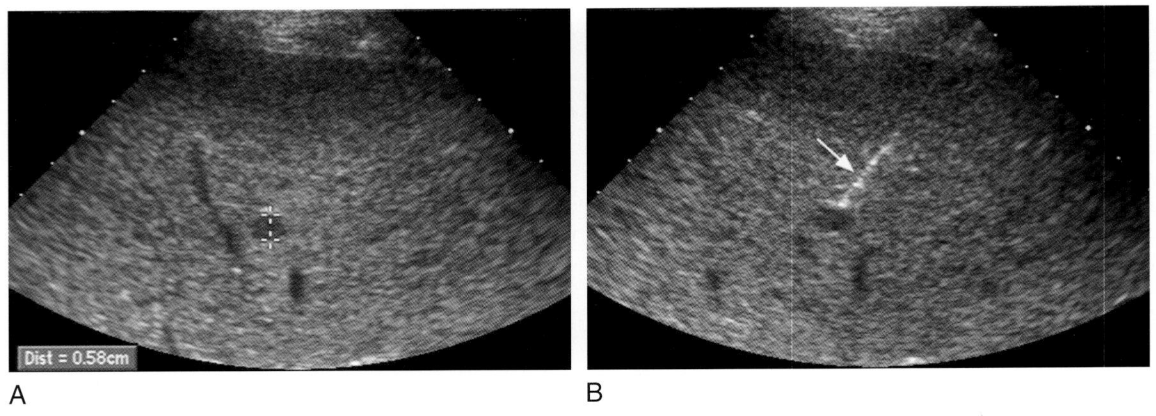

Figure 3-16 Ultrasound-guided liver biopsy. **A,** View of the liver shows a 5.8-mm hypoechoic lesion *(cursors)* in a patient with a history of melanoma. **B,** Fine-needle aspiration performed with a 22-gauge needle *(arrow)*. Cytologic analysis was positive for metastatic melanoma.

replication of hepatocytes and resulting compression and distortion of adjacent stroma and fibrous tissue. Adenomatous hyperplasia (also known as nodular hyperplasia, adenomatous hyperplastic nodules, and microregenerative nodules) is defined as a nodule that is significantly larger than the other regenerative nodules in a cirrhotic liver. They are usually larger than 1 cm and may contain atypical cells or actual malignant foci. In the latter case they are considered early HCC. It is believed that many HCCs develop from the following sequence: regenerative nodule to adenomatous hyperplasia to atypical adenomatous hyperplasia to HCC.

The growth pattern of HCC is quite variable: it may be solitary, multifocal, or diffuse and infiltrating. One pattern that is typical is a large dominant lesion with scattered smaller satellite lesions. Echogenicity is also variable, and in general the sonographic appearance is nonspecific. Figure 3-17 shows a variety of appearances of HCC. Calcification and cystic changes can occur but are very unusual. Most HCCs are hypervascular with chaotic-appearing internal vessels. Post-contrast scans are reported to show enhancement to a greater degree than adjacent liver parenchyma.

HCC has a strong tendency to invade the hepatic vasculature. Estimates of venous invasion range as high as 30% to 60% for the portal veins and 15% for the hepatic veins. These figures tend to apply to extensive tumors that are typically seen in non-screened populations. The incidence of venous invasion is much lower for small tumors that are typically seen in high-risk populations that are being screened for HCC. Regardless of the rate of vascular invasion, detection of intravenous soft tissue in a patient with a hepatic mass or masses strongly suggests HCC. Tumor thrombus tends to expand the lumen of the vein to a greater extent than bland thrombus. In many patients, arterial flow is detectable within tumor thrombus on Doppler analysis. This is a reliable sign that distinguishes tumor thrombus from bland thrombus. Because the tumor thrombus and its arterial supply invades peripheral portal veins and then grows into the more central portal veins, the arterial flow in tumor thrombus is hepatofugal in direction.

Fibrolamellar HCC is an unusual variant that occurs in younger patients without coexistent liver disease and has a much better prognosis than typical HCC. It is usually solitary and is more likely to contain calcification than typical HCC (Fig. 3-18). The central scar that is often present histologically is only occasionally seen sonographically.

Sonography is widely used in Asia to screen patients at risk for HCC, with a reported sensitivity of up to 95%. In North America, sensitivity is lower owing to the larger body habitus of the patient population. Nevertheless, ultrasound is frequently used in North America in the surveillance schemes of patients with hepatitis. In advanced cirrhosis, the diffuse hepatic inhomogeneity and nodularity reduces sensitivity as low as 50%. Interestingly, large tumors that involve liver segments diffusely are often harder to detect with sonography than are smaller tumors. Given this, it is likely that sonographic sensitivity is higher when patients are screened earlier in their disease, before the development of HCC. Any solid mass detected on an initial sonogram in a patient with cirrhosis should be considered malignant until proved otherwise. Even masses that have a typical appearance of hemangioma have a 50% chance of being HCC. In screened high-risk populations, new masses that develop over the course of surveillance have a risk of being HCC approaching 100%, regardless of the appearance.

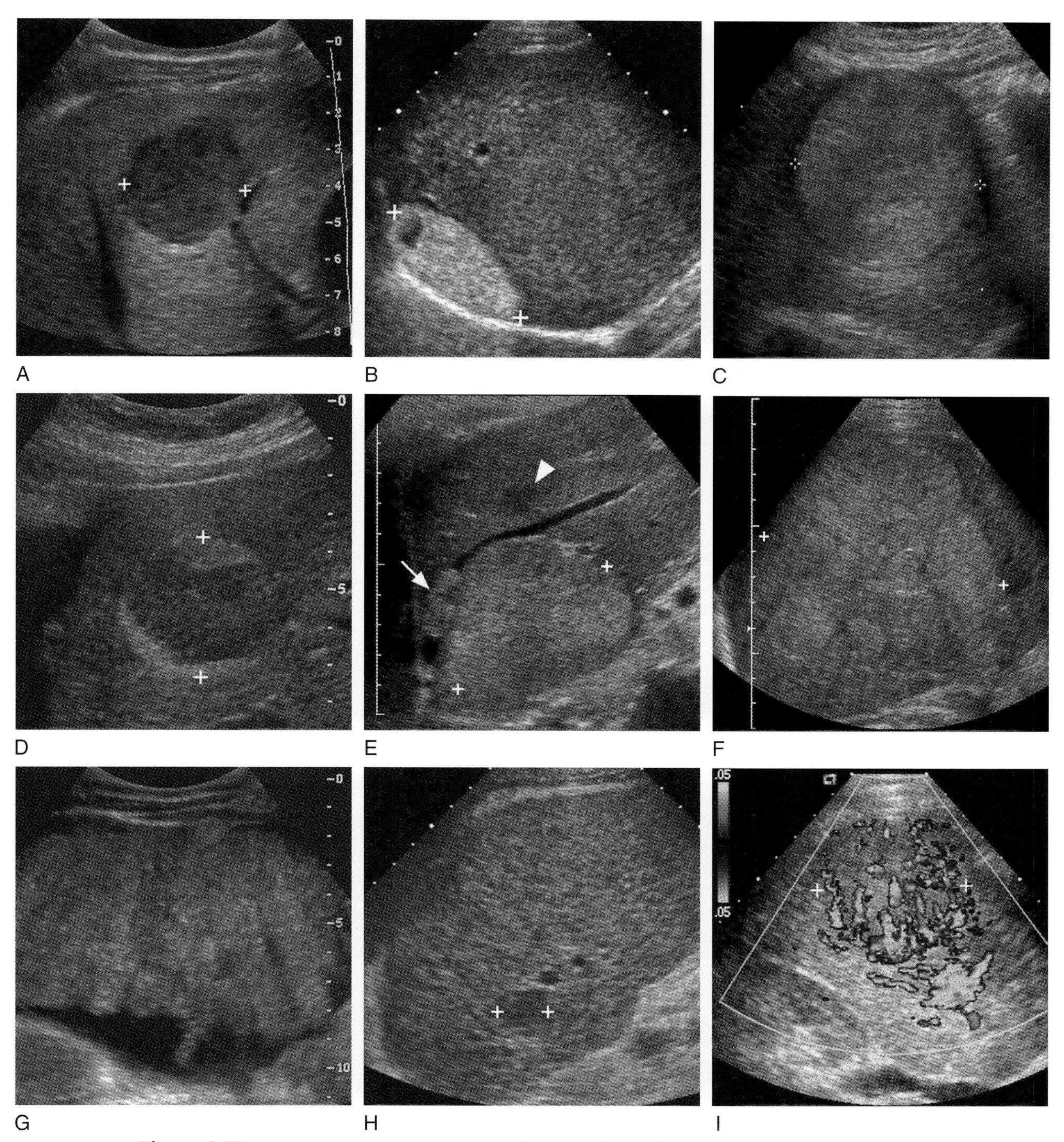

Figure 3-17 Hepatocellular carcinoma in different patients. **A,** Relatively homogeneous hypoechoic lesion *(cursors)* with increased through transmission. **B,** Hyperechoic lesion *(cursors)* with a small central hypoechoic focus. Fatty components were identified on computed tomography, accounting for the hyperechoic appearance. **C,** Target lesion *(cursors)* that is predominantly hyperechoic with a thin hypoechoic halo. **D,** Mixed echogenicity lesion *(cursors)* with a large hypoechoic region centrally and areas of hyperechogenicity peripherally. **E,** Large hyperechoic lesion *(cursors)* with invasion of the adjacent hepatic vein *(arrow)*. A small hypoechoic satellite lesion *(arrowhead)* is seen anteriorly. **F,** Large, slightly hyperechoic lesion *(cursors)* replacing most of the right lobe of the liver. Large lesions such as this one are often difficult to detect sonographically. **G,** Diffusely infiltrating tumor entirely replacing the visualized portion of the liver and resulting in a diffuse heterogeneous multinodular appearance. **H,** Diffusely nodular hepatic parenchyma secondary to advanced cirrhosis with a dominant approximately 2-cm hypoechoic mass *(cursors)* biopsy proven to be hepatocellular cancer. **I,** Color Doppler view showing intense hypervascularity typical of hepatocellular cancer.

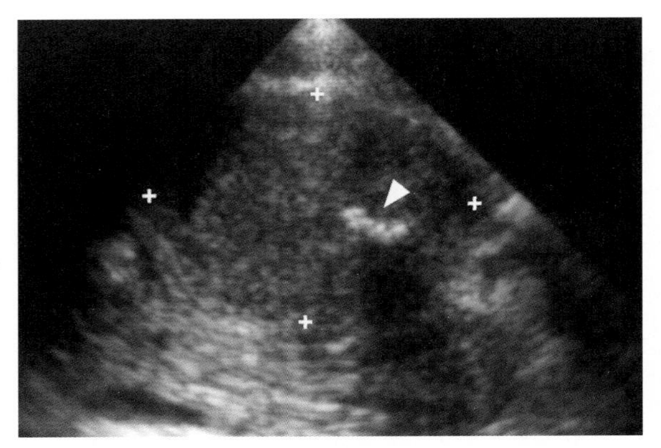

Figure 3-18 Fibrolamellar hepatocellular carcinoma. Transverse view of the left lobe of the liver shows a solid mass *(cursors)* with a focal region of calcification *(arrowhead)*. The patient was a 23-year-old man with no history of previous liver disease.

Lymphoma

Hepatic lymphoma usually presents in the setting of advanced disease elsewhere and is of the non-Hodgkin variety. Primary hepatic lymphoma occurs most often in the setting of an immunocompromised state such as AIDS or post transplantation. On sonography, it usually simulates metastatic disease, typically appearing as target lesions or as homogeneous hypoechoic masses (Fig. 3-19). Unlike metastatic disease, it is very unusual for lymphoma to appear hyperechoic, to contain cystic spaces, or to contain calcification. Because lymphoma is a very homogeneous tumor, it may generate very few internal reflections. This is why it is typically hypoechoic. In rare instances, it can appear anechoic and simulate a cyst. It may also have some detectable posterior enhancement, although this is less than expected for a cyst of similar size.

INFECTIONS

Pyogenic Abscess

Pyogenic liver abscesses are most often a secondary development of seeding from intestinal sources, such as appendicitis or diverticulitis; as a direct extension from cholecystitis or cholangitis; or from endocarditis. Like abscesses elsewhere in the body, hepatic abscesses typically appear as complex fluid collections with a mixed echogenicity (Fig. 3-20). However, it is important to realize that abscesses in the liver may mimic solid hepatic masses. The presence of through transmission will often provide a clue to the liquefied nature of the mass. Contrast medium–enhanced CT usually shows findings characteristic of an abscess even when the ultrasound evaluation shows an apparently solid lesion. Abscesses

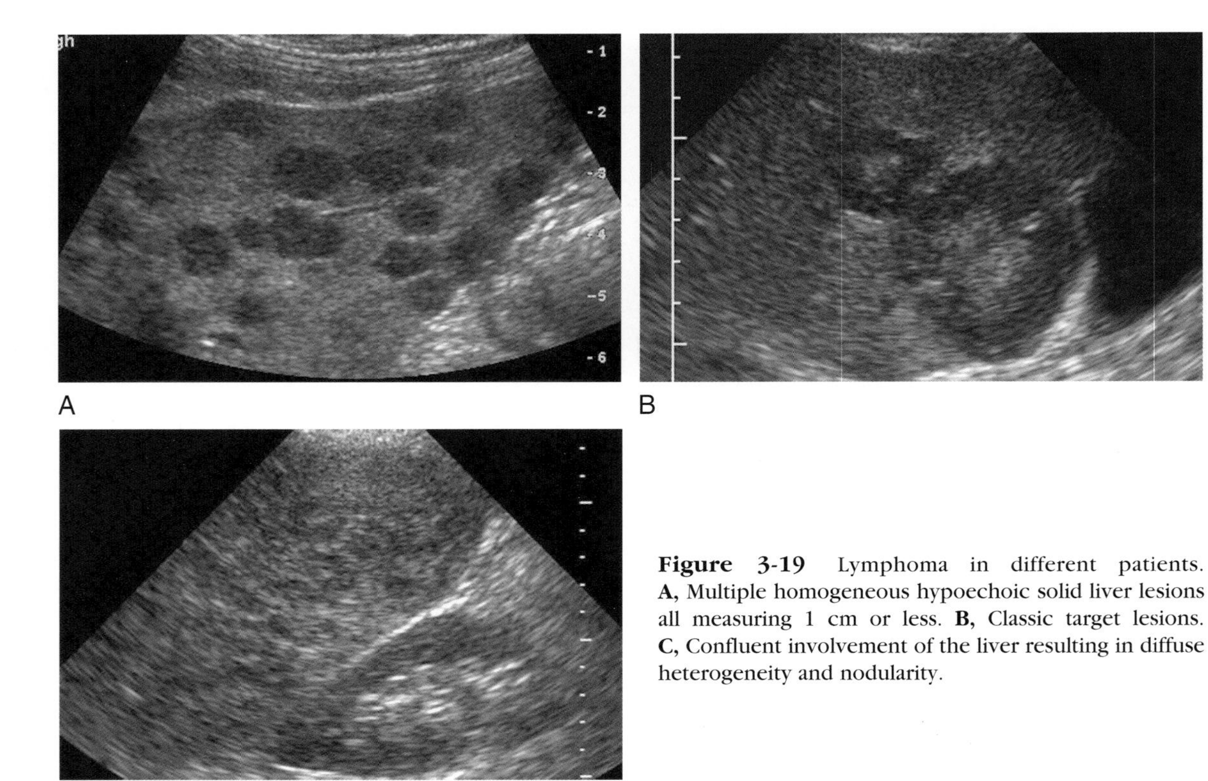

Figure 3-19 Lymphoma in different patients. **A,** Multiple homogeneous hypoechoic solid liver lesions all measuring 1 cm or less. **B,** Classic target lesions. **C,** Confluent involvement of the liver resulting in diffuse heterogeneity and nodularity.

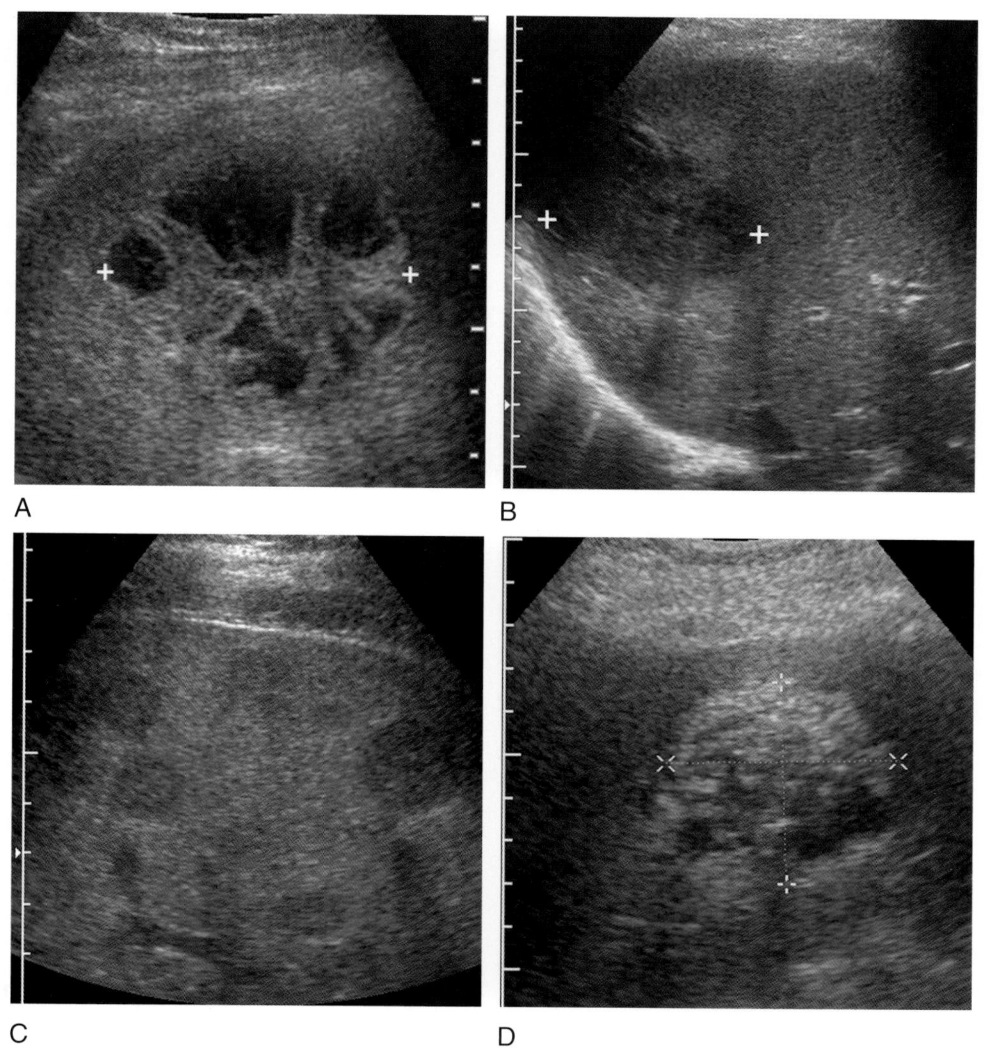

Figure 3-20 Liver abscesses in different patients. **A,** Complex cystic lesion *(cursors)* typical of a hepatic abscess. **B,** Large hypoechoic lesion *(cursors)* with increased through transmission. **C,** Multiple small hypoechoic solid-appearing lesions. **D,** Large heterogeneous, predominantly hyperechoic, lesion *(cursors).*

may also appear as thick-walled cystic lesions or as cysts with fluid-fluid levels. Gas may result in highly reflective regions with shadowing or ring-down artifacts. Abscesses may calcify with healing. The differential diagnosis for these various appearances primarily includes hematoma, hemorrhagic cyst, and necrotic or hemorrhagic tumor.

Fungal Abscess

Fungal infections of the liver usually occur in immunocompromised patients; the most common organism is *Candida.* Although it usually causes very small lesions (referred to as microabscesses), larger lesions occasionally occur (Fig. 3-21). The typical sonographic appearance is a target lesion with a central echogenic region and a peripheral hypoechoic halo. Early lesions may have a hypoechoic focus centrally, caused by necrosis and fungal elements. This appearance has been called a "wheel within a wheel." With healing, candidal abscesses become uniformly hyperechoic and ultimately may calcify.

Granulomatous Disease

Pneumocystis carinii infection of the liver is becoming increasingly common in patients with AIDS. Aerosolized pentamidine controls the infection in the lungs but does not achieve the sufficient systemic concentration necessary to prevent dissemination to other

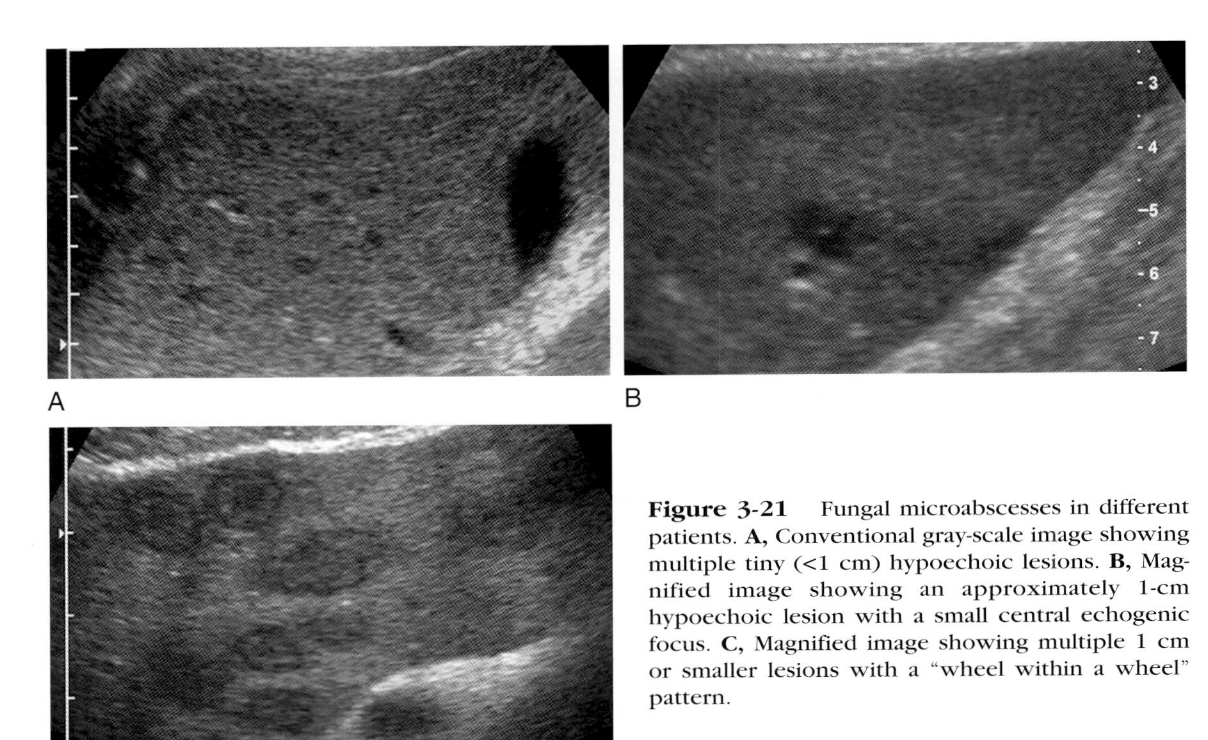

Figure 3-21 Fungal microabscesses in different patients. **A,** Conventional gray-scale image showing multiple tiny (<1 cm) hypoechoic lesions. **B,** Magnified image showing an approximately 1-cm hypoechoic lesion with a small central echogenic focus. **C,** Magnified image showing multiple 1 cm or smaller lesions with a "wheel within a wheel" pattern.

organs, including the liver, spleen, pancreas, and kidneys. Pathologically, the lesions in these various organs are granulomas that may or may not show calcification. Sonographically, the appearance is very characteristic and consists of multiple echogenic foci scattered throughout the liver (Fig. 3-22). The same appearance has been reported in a very limited number of cases of *Mycobacterium avium-intracellulare* and cytomegalovirus infection of the liver. Small punctate calcified granulomas are very common in areas where histoplasmosis is endemic.

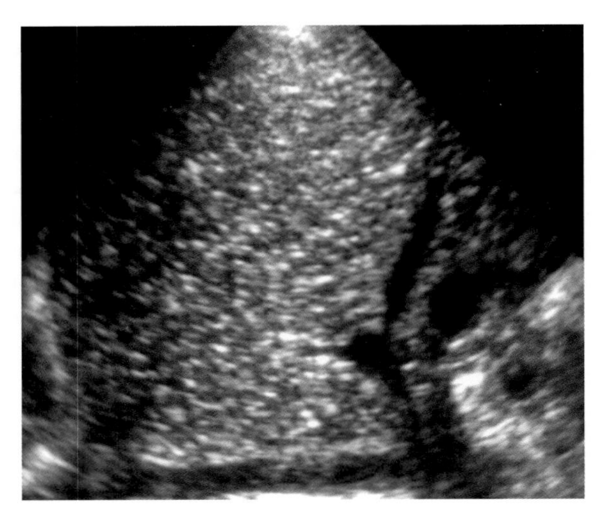

Figure 3-22 *Pneumocystis carinii* infection of the liver. Longitudinal view demonstrates multiple diffuse non-shadowing small hyperechoic foci throughout the liver. Similar foci were seen in the kidneys bilaterally.

Parasitic Infection

Echinococcal disease is usually caused by a tapeworm, *Echinococcus granulosus.* Humans are a secondary host who get infected by ingesting egg-infested vegetables. The liver is the most commonly affected organ, although the lungs, spleen, bones, kidneys, and central nervous system can also be affected. Echinococcal cysts in the liver have an external membrane called the ectocyst and an internal germinal layer called the endocyst. In addition, the host forms a fibrous capsule around the cyst that is called the pericyst. Sonographically, hydatid cysts may appear as relatively simple cysts, cysts with multiple internal daughter cysts, cysts with detached floating endocystic membranes, cysts with internal debris, and cysts with internal or peripheral calcification (Fig. 3-23).

Other parasitic infections of the liver include amebic abscesses and schistosomiasis. Amebic abscesses result from primary colonic involvement with hepatic seeding through the portal vein and are indistinguishable from pyogenic abscesses. Schistosomiasis is rare in the United States but quite common worldwide. Ova reach the

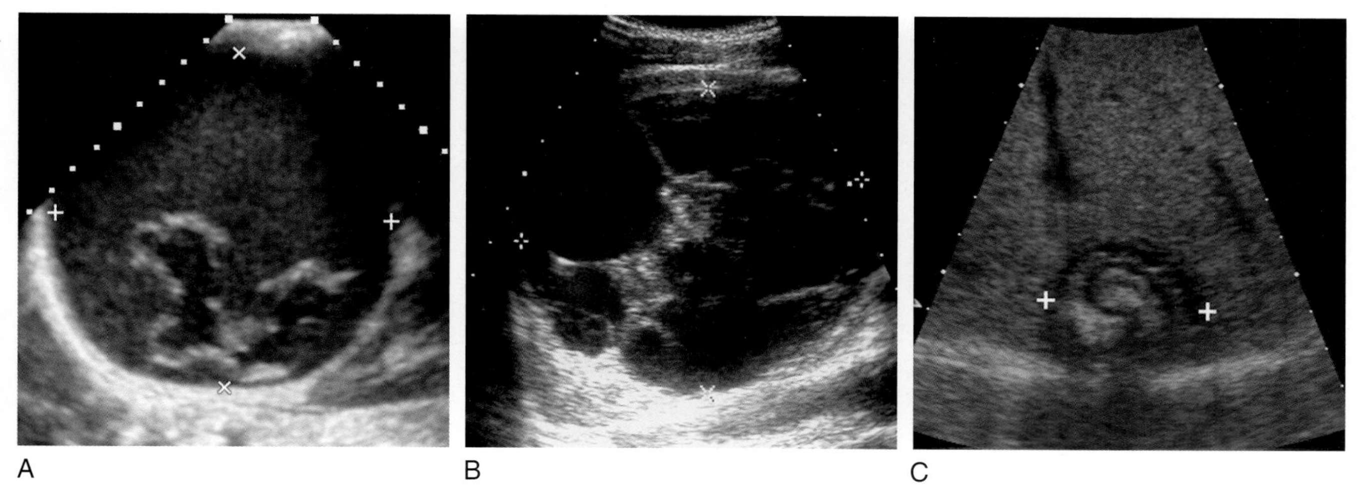

Figure 3-23 Echinococcal cysts in different patients. **A,** Cystic lesion *(cursors)* containing diffuse low-level echoes and a detached endocystic membrane. **B,** Complex cyst *(cursors)* with multiple internal daughter cysts. **C,** Partially calcified lesion *(cursors)* with posterior shadowing and detached endocystic membranes arranged in a spiral fashion.

peripheral portal triads and cause a granulomatous reaction. The resulting periportal fibrosis appears as thickened echogenic portal triads.

TRAUMA

In the setting of blunt abdominal trauma, sonography is now being used to evaluate for potential hemoperitoneum. However, acute hepatic lacerations are difficult to detect with sonography. This is because acute hematomas are often isoechoic to liver parenchyma and produce only subtle alterations in hepatic echogenicity (Fig. 3-24). Like hematomas elsewhere, hepatic hematomas become progressively more liquefied over a matter of days to weeks. Because of this limitation, CT is the modality of choice for detecting and quantifying liver hematoma. Sonography is a useful problem-solving tool when questions concerning the biliary tract or hepatic vasculature arise.

DIFFUSE PARENCHYMAL DISEASE

Hepatitis

Hepatitis usually results in no detectable sonographic abnormality. In a limited number of patients it can cause increased echogenicity of the portal triads, which appear as small bright areas on views of the liver periphery (Fig. 3-25). This appearance has been referred to as

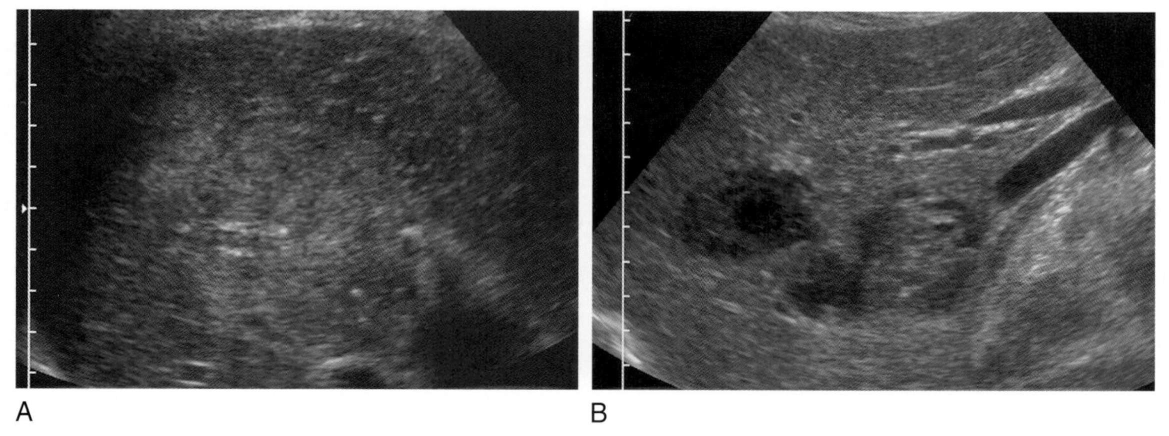

Figure 3-24 Hepatic laceration in different patients. **A,** Oblique view of the liver shows a poorly marginated vague area of increased echogenicity throughout the central aspect of the liver. **B,** Oblique view through the liver demonstrates a subacute laceration with one hematoma containing more echogenic clot and other hematomas that have developed more liquefactive areas.

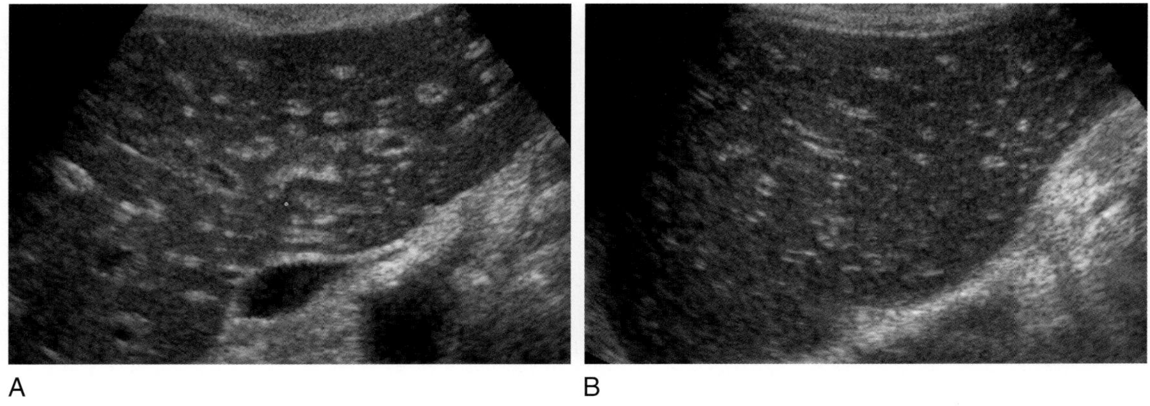

Figure 3-25 Hepatitis in different patients. **A,** Transverse view through the middle aspect of the liver demonstrates multiple portal triads that stand out because of their unusually echogenic borders. **B,** Transverse view through the peripheral aspect of the liver shows echogenic portal triads that are more numerous than typically seen in the periphery of the liver.

the "starry sky" sign. Unfortunately, it can be seen in the absence of hepatitis, and, when present, it is often subtle. Hepatitis can also produce marked thickening of the gallbladder wall, contraction of the gallbladder lumen, and periportal lymphadenopathy.

Fatty Infiltration

Fatty infiltration of the liver is characterized pathologically by intracellular deposition of triglycerides within hepatocytes. It is extremely common in North America and is usually due to obesity. Other common causes include alcohol abuse, cholesterol-lowering medications, and certain chemotherapy agents. In addition, corticosteroids, diabetes, malnutrition, total parenteral nutrition, and toxins (such as carbon tetrachloride) are potential causes.

Fatty infiltration of the liver causes a variety of fairly characteristic abnormalities on sonography. These are illustrated in Figure 3-26. Fatty infiltration most often manifests in a diffuse distribution and results in uniform increased echogenicity of the liver. Because the normal liver is only slightly more echogenic than the kidney, the diagnosis of fatty infiltration is best made by noting a marked discrepancy between the hyperechoic liver and the less echogenic kidney. In addition, because the normal pancreas is more echogenic than the liver, fatty infiltration should be considered whenever the liver appears hyperechoic compared with the pancreas. More advanced fatty infiltration will cause significant sound beam attenuation and will make the hepatic vessels, and in some cases the diaphragm, difficult to visualize. Another characteristic of fatty infiltration is an increased concentration of tiny reflections from the liver parenchyma that result in a finer echotexture than normal liver. With experience, this echotexture can be recognized with reasonable accuracy.

In many cases of otherwise diffuse fatty infiltration, there will be focal areas of spared normal liver parenchyma that appear hypoechoic with respect to the fatty infiltrated parenchyma. If the fatty infiltration is not recognized, the spared areas of normal parenchyma may be mistaken as focal hypoechoic lesions. Fortunately, the spared parenchyma is usually located in front of the right portal vein or portal bifurcation or around the gallbladder. The combination of these typical locations and the fact that focal sparing is usually not spherical generally allows for a confident diagnosis of focal fatty sparring. In fact, when the presence or absence of fatty infiltration in the liver is uncertain, it is often possible to detect the characteristic areas of focal sparing, which allows for a more confident diagnosis of fatty infiltration in the remainder of the liver.

In cases in which fatty infiltration of the liver is patchy, the geographic margins of the abnormally echogenic fatty liver and the lack of mass effect on hepatic vessels serve as clues to the diagnosis. Occasionally, fatty infiltration will be focal and nodular. This frequently occurs in the anterior aspect of the left lobe (especially the medial segment) immediately adjacent to the falciform ligament. Another typical location for focal fatty infiltration is anterior to the portal vein bifurcation, which is exactly where focal fatty sparing also typically occurs. The paradoxical deposition and lack of deposition of fat in this location is not well understood but may be related to relative differences in perfusion to this area. Regardless of the cause, if an elongated hyperechoic lesion is seen in these typical locations in patients with no known primary malignancy, the diagnosis of focal fatty infiltration is almost

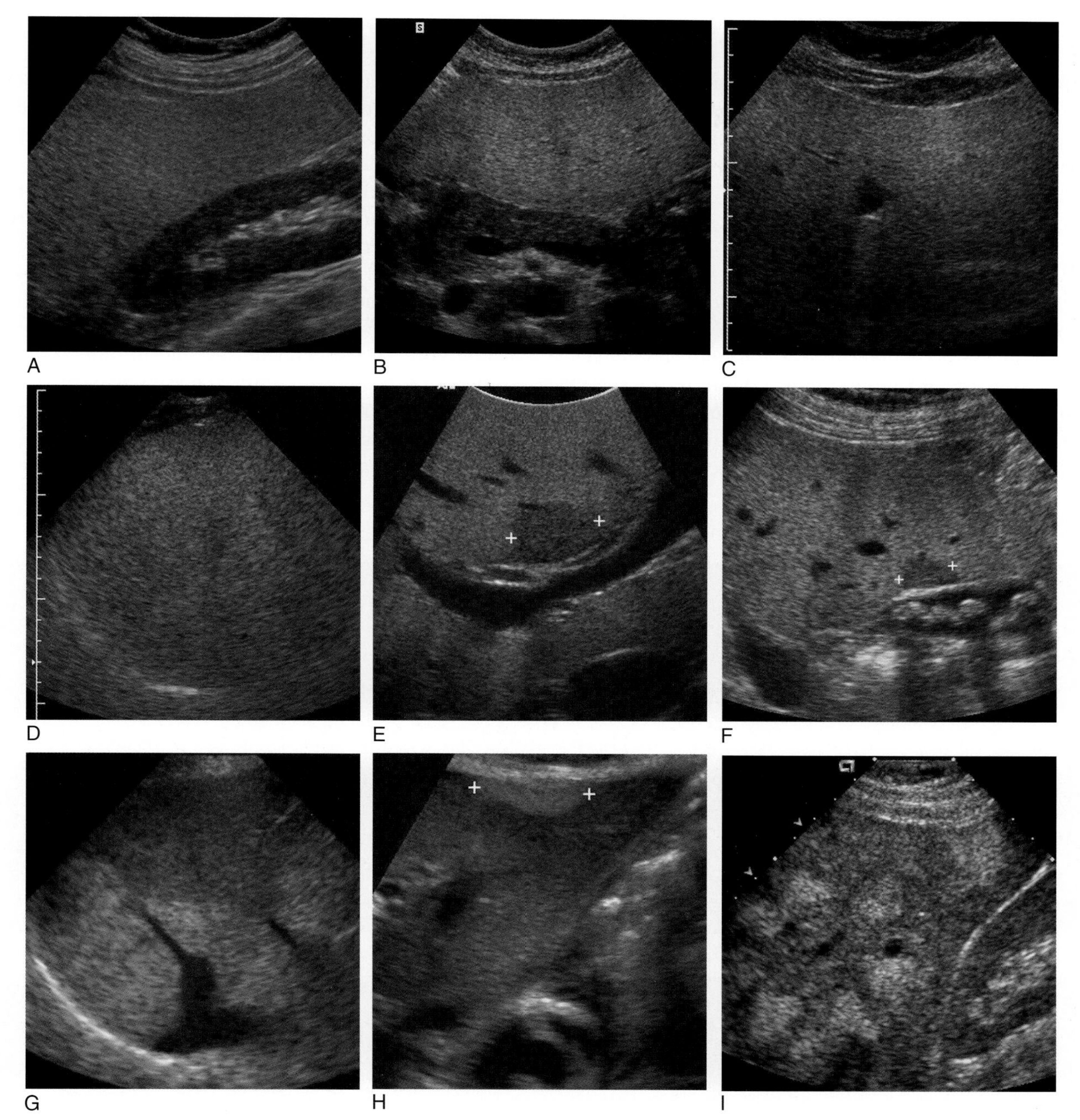

Figure 3-26 Fatty infiltration of the liver in different patients. **A,** Longitudinal view of the liver and right kidney shows marked discrepancy between the hyperechoic liver and the normal right kidney. **B,** Transverse view through the liver shows marked discrepancy between the hyperechoic liver and the normal pancreas. **C,** Transverse view of the liver demonstrates attenuation of the sound beam with progressive decreased echogenicity of the deeper aspects of the liver, indicating more advanced fatty infiltration. **D,** Transverse view shows loss of detectable internal vascular structures in the liver and very poor definition of the diaphragm, indicating very advanced fatty infiltration. **E,** Transverse view through the portal bifurcation demonstrates a focal area of decreased echogenicity *(cursors)* anterior to the portal vein secondary to focal parenchymal sparing. **F,** Longitudinal view showing a gallbladder with stones and a focal area of decreased hepatic parenchymal echogenicity *(cursors)* adjacent to the gallbladder due to focal parenchymal sparing. **G,** Oblique view through the liver shows a non-spherical area of increased echogenicity posteriorly that does not displace the hepatic vein in that area. This is typical of a focal region of fatty infiltration. **H,** Longitudinal view through the left lobe of the liver shows an oval area of increased echogenicity anteriorly *(cursors)* secondary to focal nodular fatty infiltration. This was located immediately adjacent to the ligamentum teres. **I,** Longitudinal view of the liver demonstrating multiple focal nodular areas of increased echogenicity. MRI confirmed this was multifocal fatty infiltration.

certain and no further evaluation is necessary. On the other hand, fatty infiltration may rarely cause focal or multifocal nodular regions of increased echogenicity in atypical locations. This can closely simulate metastatic disease or hemangiomas. In such cases, MRI should be considered to confirm the diagnosis of nodular fatty infiltration.

Cirrhosis

Cirrhosis is caused by hepatocellular death and resulting fibrosis and regeneration. It occurs most commonly from alcohol abuse, which causes micronodular changes (<1 cm). Hepatitis is the next most common cause, and it results in macronodular cirrhosis (nodules between 1 and 5 cm). Surface nodularity can easily be detected sonographically in the presence of ascites and is a reliable sign of cirrhosis (Fig. 3-27). In the absence of ascites, surface nodularity is best detected using a high-resolution linear- or curved-array transducer focused on the liver surface. Nodularity can also be seen where liver interfaces with structures that are anechoic (e.g., anechoic gallbladder or hepatic veins) or echogenic structures (e.g., perihepatic fat). Coarsening and nodularity of the liver parenchyma is another useful sign of cirrhosis that can be seen especially well with the high-resolution probes focused on the superficial liver parenchyma (see Fig. 3-27). Although the liver shrinks in advanced disease, there is frequently an initial redistribution of liver volume toward the caudate lobe and the lateral segment of the left lobe. Ratios comparing the size of the caudate lobe and the right lobe have been used in the past to make the diagnosis of cirrhosis. This technique has now been replaced by more direct analysis of the liver

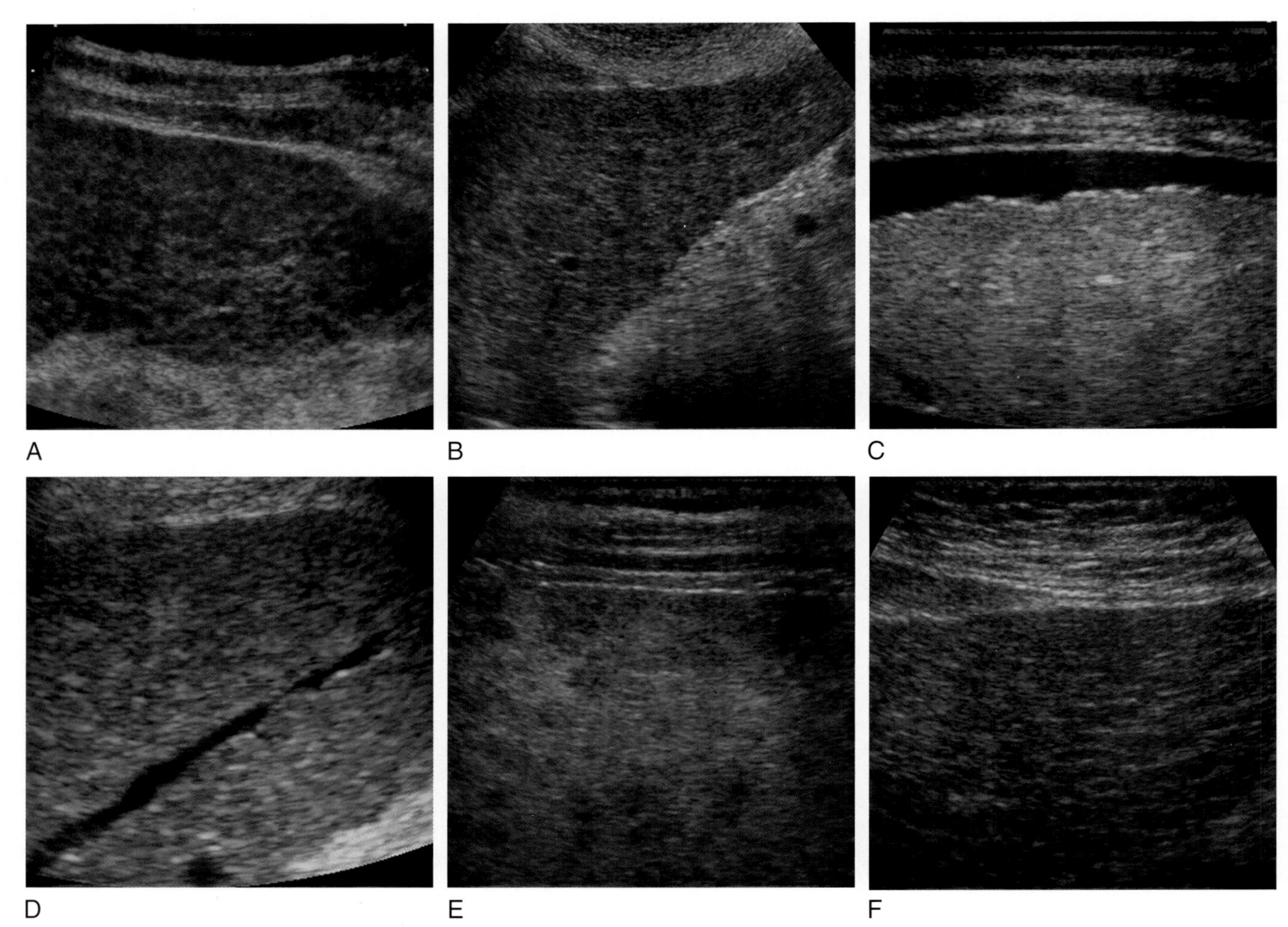

Figure 3-27 Cirrhosis in different patients. **A** and **B**, Conventional views show diffuse heterogeneity and nodularity to the liver parenchyma. **C**, High-resolution view of the liver surface shows surface nodularity. **D**, View of a hepatic vein shows multiple nodular impressions on the hepatic vein lumen. **E**, High-resolution view of the superficial liver parenchyma demonstrates scattered multifocal hypoechoic nodules. **F**, High-resolution view of the liver surface demonstrates diffuse heterogeneity and hyperechoic strands of parenchymal fibrosis.

surface and the liver parenchyma. Unless there is associated fatty infiltration, cirrhosis does not typically result in significant attenuation of sound.

VASCULAR DISEASE

Normal Hemodynamics

The portal vein normally supplies 75% of the blood flow to the liver. Because it is isolated from the systemic veins and the right atrium, it is relatively unaffected by the pressure changes that occur during cardiac contraction and relaxation. Therefore, portal flow is usually characterized by little or no pulsatility (Fig. 3-28). However, portal vein pulsatility can be normal, especially in thin individuals. Normal flow velocities average 20 to 30 cm/sec. Antegrade portal flow into the liver is referred to as hepatopetal.

The hepatic veins drain into the IVC near the right atrium, and the flow is very dependent on right atrial activity. Figure 3-29 illustrates the normal hepatic venous waveform and describes its relationship to atrial contraction and relaxation. Because the waveform is pulsatile with two antegrade pulses and one retrograde pulse, it is referred to as triphasic. A deep inspiration can cause blunting and occasionally complete loss of hepatic vein pulsatility, so hepatic vein waveforms should be obtained at normal end expiration. Antegrade hepatic venous flow is away from the liver and is referred to as hepatofugal.

Hepatic arterial flow is similar to arterial flow to other solid organs such as the kidney and brain. It has a low-resistance arterial waveform with well-maintained antegrade flow throughout diastole.

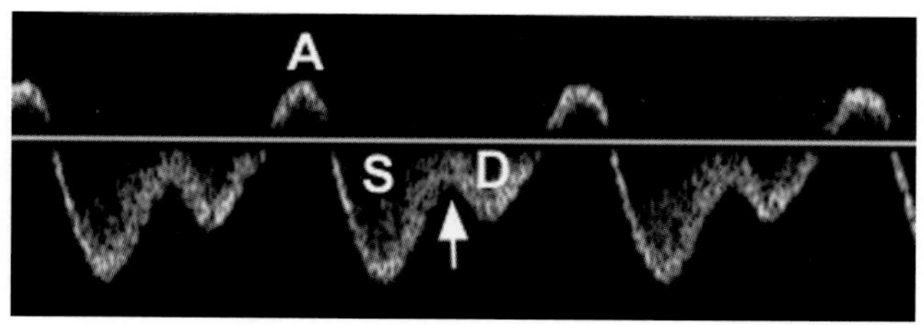

Figure 3-29 Normal hepatic vein waveform. During right atrial contraction (A), flow is in a retrograde direction back into the liver. After right atrial contraction, there is a phase of rapid right atrial filling and rapid outflow of blood from the hepatic veins into the right atrium, which is visualized as a large pulse below the baseline, referred to as the S wave (because it occurs during ventricular systole). As the right atrium gets progressively fuller, flow out of the hepatic vein starts to slow and the waveform starts to return to the baseline. When the tricuspid valve opens *(arrow)*, blood from the right atrium starts to flow into the right ventricle, promoting a second pulse of flow out of the hepatic veins and into the right atrium called the D wave (because it occurs during ventricular diastole). This second antegrade pulse is usually smaller than the first. After the D wave, the right atrium contracts again and the cycle repeats itself.

Portal Hypertension

Portal hypertension can be divided into intrahepatic, extrahepatic, and hyperdynamic categories (Box 3-5).

Intrahepatic portal hypertension is the most common type in North America, owing to the prevalence of alcoholic cirrhosis. In this disease, hepatocellular death results in scarring, which causes increased resistance to flow in the hepatic sinusoids and the small centrilobular veins that drain the sinusoids. Initially, the portal venous pressure increases so that total portal flow to the liver is maintained. However, the resistance to flow into the liver eventually becomes equal to resistance in potential portosystemic collaterals and some of the portal flow becomes diverted into those collaterals. As portal flow decreases, hepatic arterial flow increases to partially compensate for the diminished portal inflow. Eventually, resistance to flow in the sinusoids and central veins becomes so great that even the high-pressure hepatic

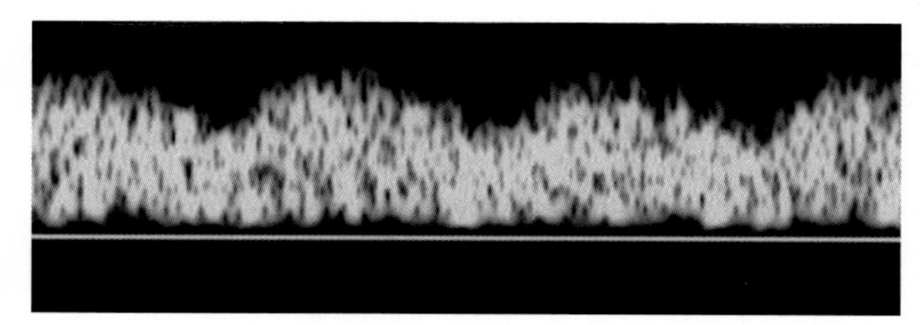

Figure 3-28 Normal portal vein waveform. Minimal pulsatility is identified and is related to the cardiac cycle.

Box 3-5 Classification of Portal Hypertension

INTRAHEPATIC	EXTRAHEPATIC	HYPERDYNAMIC
Postsinusoidal	**Prehepatic**	**Arterioportal Fistula**
Cirrhosis	Portal vein thrombosis	Post-traumatic
Veno-occlusive disease	Portal vein compression	Congenital
		Atherosclerotic
Presinusoidal	**Posthepatic**	
Hepatic fibrosis	Hepatic vein thrombosis	
Schistosomiasis	IVC obstruction	
Lymphoma	Constrictive pericarditis	
Sarcoidosis		

IVC, inferior vena cava.

arterial flow has difficulty getting through the normal channels into the hepatic veins. At this point, some hepatic artery flow gets diverted into the portal system through microscopic collaterals in the peribiliary plexus and vasa vasorum of the portal vein. When this occurs, flow in the portal vein reverses.

There are a number of sonographic findings seen with portal hypertension. On gray-scale imaging, they include enlargement of the portal vein, splenomegaly, and ascites. Portal vein diameter is an attractive measurement because it is easy to obtain. Unfortunately, there is a wide range of accepted normal values (10 to 17 mm) and variations occur with patient positioning, respiration, and fasting status. One commonly quoted figure is 13 mm measured in the anteroposterior direction where the portal vein crosses the IVC in a supine patient during quiet respiration. Detection of portosystemic collaterals is relatively sensitive and is the most specific sign of portal hypertension. The easiest collateral to detect with ultrasound is the umbilical vein (Fig. 3-30). This communicates with the umbilical segment of the left portal vein located between the medial and lateral segment of the left lobe of the liver. It travels in the ligamentum teres and communicates with periumbilical collaterals in the ligamentum teres and the abdominal wall. It ultimately drains into the inferior epigastric veins or less commonly the superior epigastric veins. In some patients the fibrous band of the obliterated umbilical vein can be seen as a hypoechoic tubular structure in the ligamentum teres (see Fig. 3-1F). Therefore, detection of hepatofugal venous flow on Doppler analysis is required to establish patency of this potential collateral. On gray-scale imaging, this structure should not exceed 3 mm in diameter.

The next most easily detected collateral on sonography is the coronary vein. It can be seen behind the left lobe of the liver arising from the splenic vein (near the portosplenic confluence) and extending superiorly and usually toward the left (Fig. 3-31). It typically travels over the branches of the celiac bifurcation, although it may be identified posterior to the bifurcation. In normal patients it should not exceed 6 mm. Reversed coronary

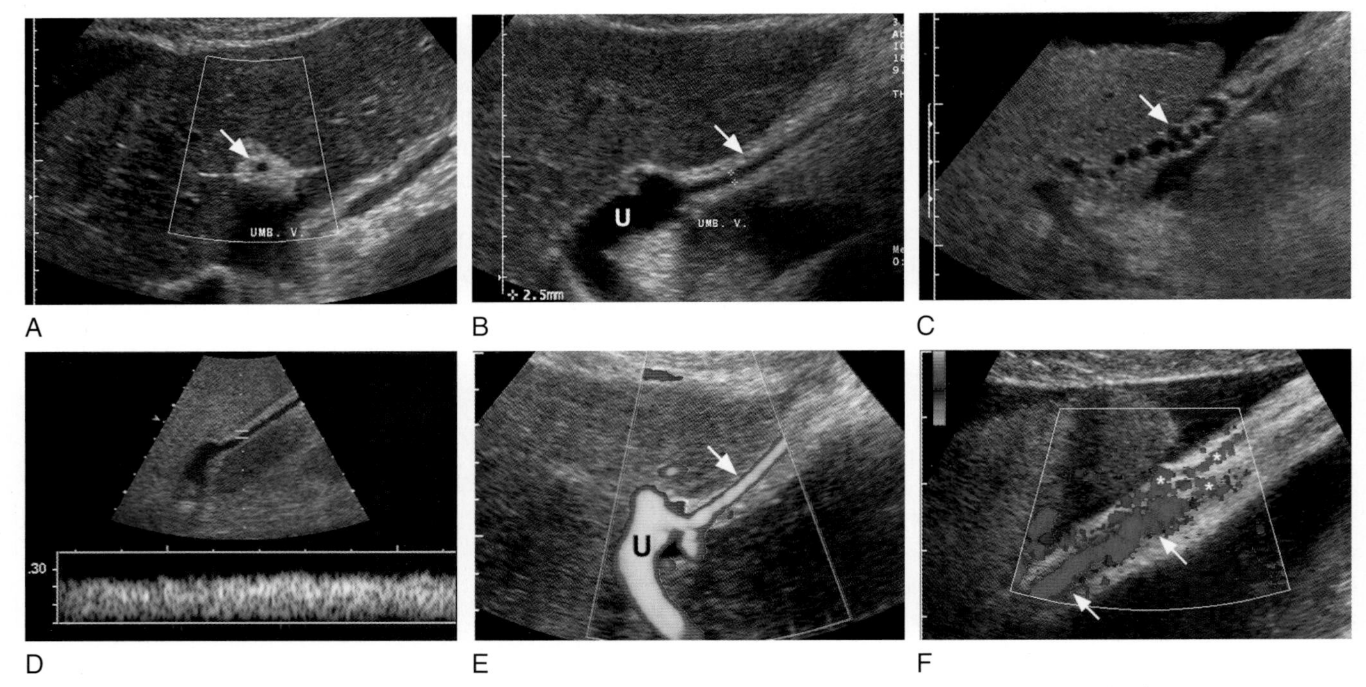

Figure 3-30 Umbilical vein collateral in different patients. **A,** Transverse view of the left lobe of the liver demonstrates the echogenic ligamentum teres *(arrow)*. It contains an umbilical collateral that appears as a small central hypoechoic, round structure. **B,** Longitudinal view of the left lobe of the liver shows the ligamentum teres *(arrow)* and an umbilical collateral seen as a small, 2.5 mm, central vessel *(cursors)*. Note that the umbilical vein collateral communicates with the umbilical segment of the left portal vein (U). **C,** Longitudinal view of the ligamentum teres *(arrow)* shows a very tortuous vascular structure within the ligament consistent with a paraumbilical collateral. **D,** Pulsed Doppler waveform from an umbilical vein collateral shows hepatofugal venous flow directed out of the liver. **E,** Power Doppler view shows blood flow within the umbilical segment of the left portal vein (U) communicating with an umbilical vein collateral *(arrow)*. **F,** Color Doppler view shows an umbilical collateral *(arrows)* as it starts to supply multiple periumbilical collaterals (*).

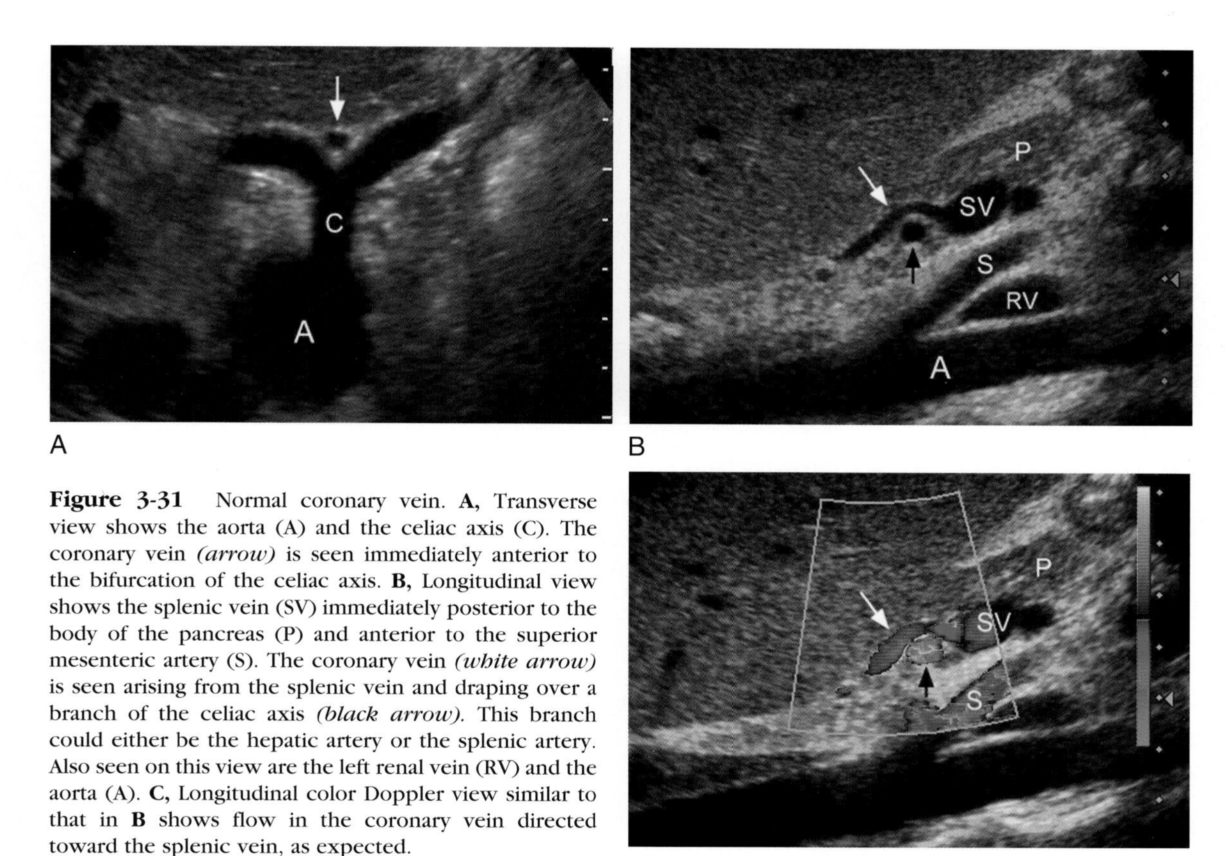

Figure 3-31 Normal coronary vein. **A,** Transverse view shows the aorta (A) and the celiac axis (C). The coronary vein *(arrow)* is seen immediately anterior to the bifurcation of the celiac axis. **B,** Longitudinal view shows the splenic vein (SV) immediately posterior to the body of the pancreas (P) and anterior to the superior mesenteric artery (S). The coronary vein *(white arrow)* is seen arising from the splenic vein and draping over a branch of the celiac axis *(black arrow).* This branch could either be the hepatic artery or the splenic artery. Also seen on this view are the left renal vein (RV) and the aorta (A). **C,** Longitudinal color Doppler view similar to that in **B** shows flow in the coronary vein directed toward the splenic vein, as expected.

vein flow (i.e., away from the splenic vein and toward the gastroesophageal junction) and enlargement indicate portal hypertension (Fig. 3-32). In fact, reversed flow in any tributary of the portal or splenic vein is a sign of portal hypertension. Many other potential portosystemic collaterals exist but are more difficult to detect sonographically. These include splenorenal, splenoretroperitoneal, superior mesenteric, and inferior mesenteric venous collaterals.

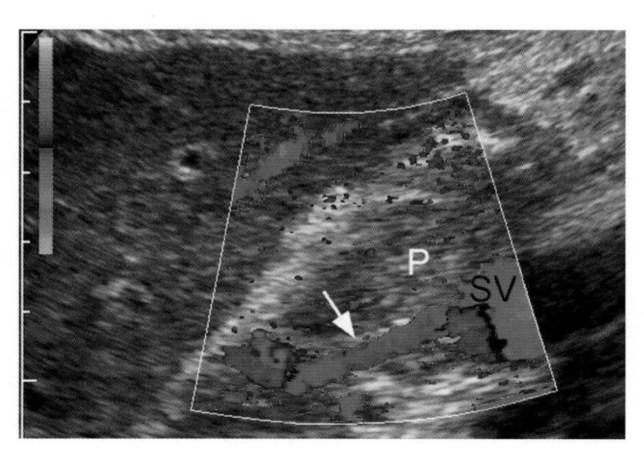

Figure 3-32 Abnormal coronary vein. Longitudinal view shows the splenic vein (SV) immediately posterior to the body of the pancreas (P). The coronary vein *(arrow)* has flow directed away from the splenic vein.

Detection of hepatofugal (retrograde) flow in the portal vein is another relatively specific sign of portal hypertension that occurs in more advanced cases. Initially, it occurs in isolated peripheral branches of the portal vein (Fig. 3-33A). With more advanced disease, it involves the central right and left portal branches and eventually the main portal vein itself (see Fig. 3-33B). It can be recognized on Doppler waveforms when portal flow is on the opposite side of the baseline from the hepatic arteries (see Fig. 3-33C). In patients with large umbilical collaterals, it is common to have reversed flow in the right portal vein that crosses the bifurcation and supplies antegrade flow to the left portal vein and ultimately to the umbilical vein. Box 3-6 reviews the sonographic findings in portal hypertension.

Extrahepatic causes of portal hypertension are divided into prehepatic and posthepatic. Prehepatic causes include portal vein thrombosis and portal vein compression. Portal vein compression usually occurs owing to tumors in adjacent organs or lymphadenopathy (Fig. 3-34). Portal vein thrombosis frequently occurs in patients with slow portal flow caused by portal hypertension. It also occurs in patients with hypercoagulable

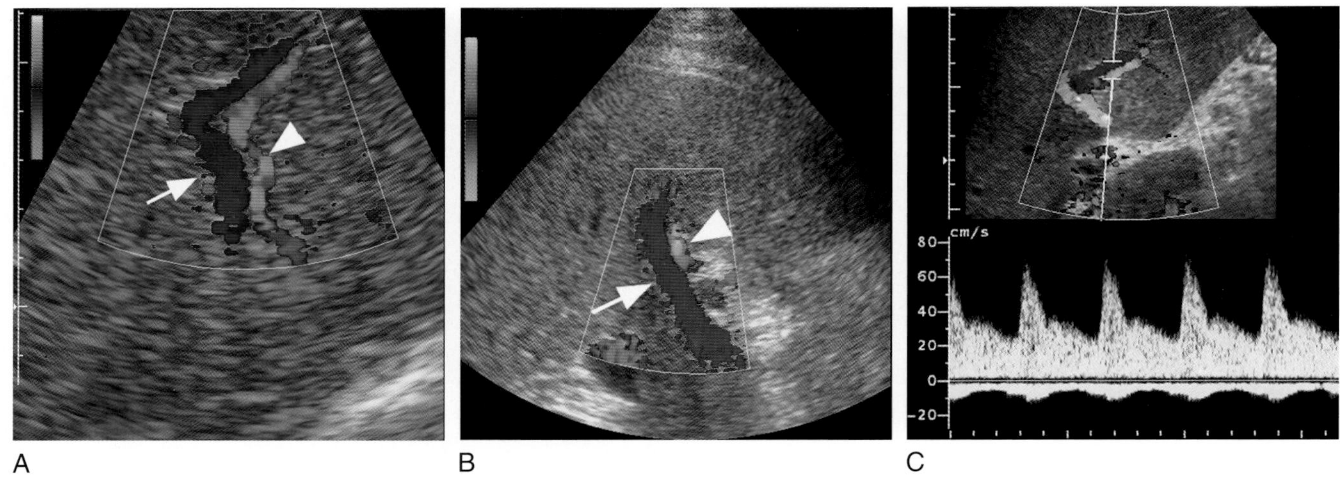

Figure 3-33 Portal vein flow reversal in different patients. **A,** Magnified color Doppler view of the peripheral aspect of the right lobe of the liver shows a portal vein *(arrow)* adjacent to a hepatic artery *(arrowhead).* Flow direction in these two vessels is different. Hepatic arterial flow is directed toward the periphery of the liver, and portal vein flow is directed away from the periphery of the liver. **B,** Longitudinal view of the porta hepatis shows the main portal vein *(arrow)* and adjacent hepatic artery *(arrowhead).* As in **A,** hepatic arterial flow is directed into the liver and portal vein flow is directed out of the liver. **C,** Pulsed Doppler waveform from an adjacent intrahepatic portal vein and hepatic artery shows arterial flow above the baseline and portal venous flow below the baseline indicating reversal of portal vein flow.

states and intestinal infection or inflammation (i.e., appendicitis, diverticulitis, inflammatory bowel disease). On gray-scale imaging, detection of thrombosis depends on identification of an intraluminal filling defect or abnormal intraluminal echoes. The latter finding may be difficult to distinguish from the artifactual low-level echoes that often appear in the portal vein. Thrombus can appear hyperechoic, isoechoic, hypoechoic (Fig. 3-35), or rarely anechoic. In the latter case it will be undetectable with gray-scale sonography; therefore, color and duplex Doppler imaging studies are important adjunctive tools. On color Doppler analysis, portal vein thrombosis appears as a localized flow void or as complete lack of detectable intraluminal flow. When no flow is detected but no thrombus is seen on gray-scale imaging, then the possibility of a patent vein with very slow flow should be considered (Fig. 3-36). Because portal flow increases after a meal, rescanning after eating may convert slow undetectable flow to faster flow that is detectable. If this fails, another imaging study using an intravenous contrast agent (CT, MRI or US) should be performed to document thrombosis or establish portal vein patency. The overall accuracy of color Doppler imaging in diagnosing portal vein thrombosis is high, with a sensitivity and specificity of approximately 90%. False-negative results are very uncommon, and the negative predictive value is 98%. One potential cause of a false-negative examination is when a single, isolated, large, periportal collateral is confused with a patent portal vein (Fig. 3-37). The clue to this diagnosis is that the

Box 3-6 Sonographic Signs of Portal Hypertension

Ascites
Splenomegaly
Portal vein enlargement
Portosystemic collaterals
Enlarged hepatic arteries
Hepatofugal (reversed) portal flow

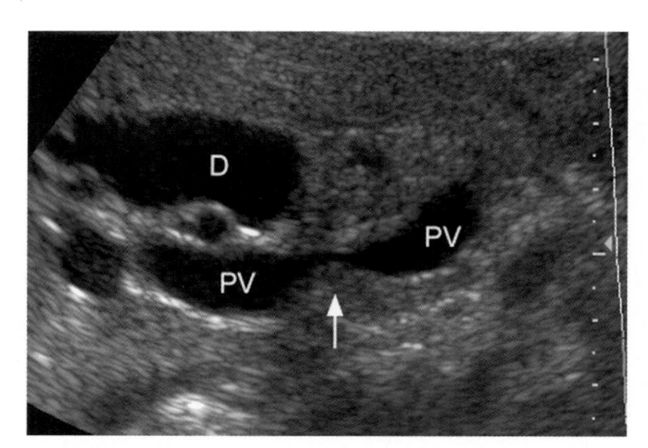

Figure 3-34 Extrahepatic portal hypertension secondary to portal vein compression. Longitudinal view of the porta hepatis shows the portal vein (PV) with an area of marked narrowing *(arrow).* This was due to a cholangiocarcinoma that encased the portal vein. Also noted is a markedly dilated bile duct (D).

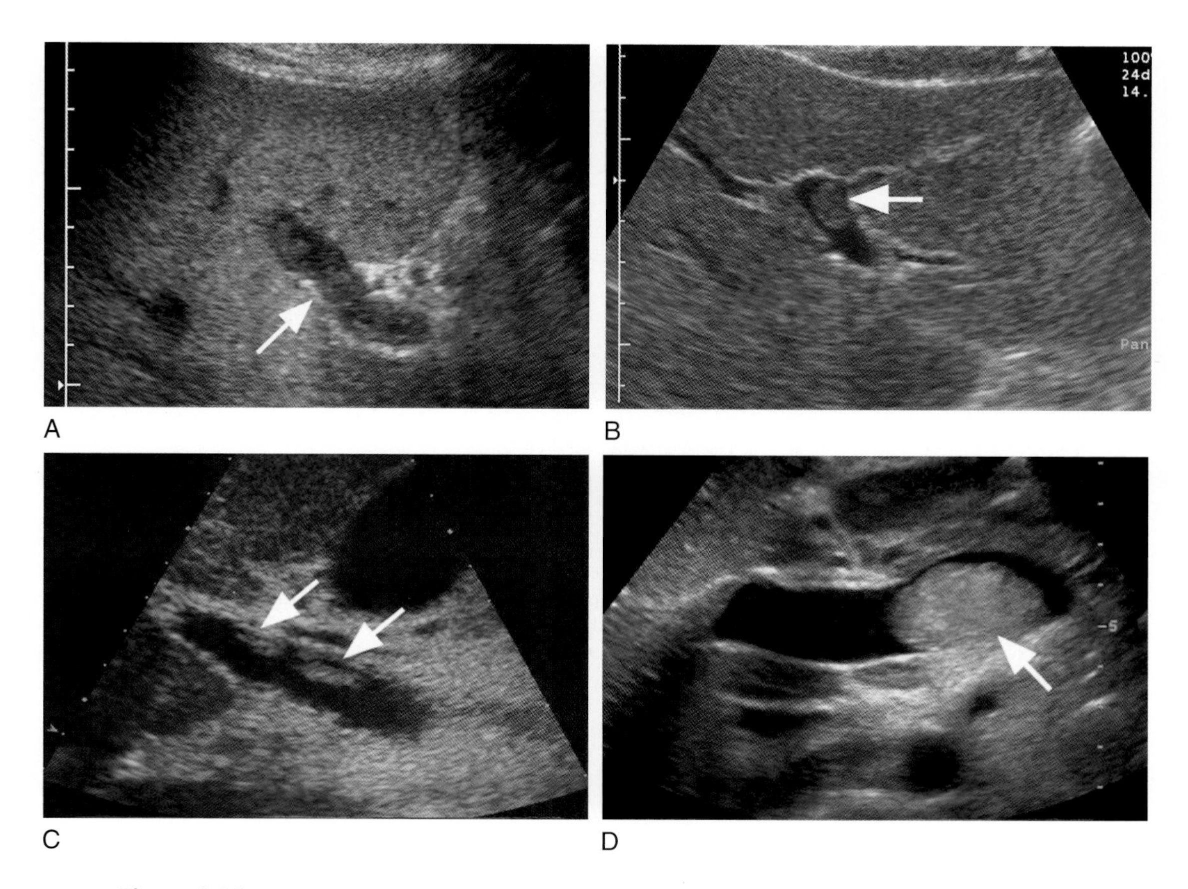

Figure 3-35 Portal vein thrombosis in different patients. **A,** Longitudinal view of the main portal vein *(arrow)* shows hypoechoic thrombus throughout the venous lumen. **B,** Transverse view of the left portal vein shows focal isoechoic thrombus *(arrow)* within the lumen. **C,** Longitudinal view of the main portal vein shows focal hyperechoic thrombus *(arrows)* within the lumen. **D,** Transverse view of the main portal vein shows a large hyperechoic thrombus *(arrow)* near the splenic vein confluence.

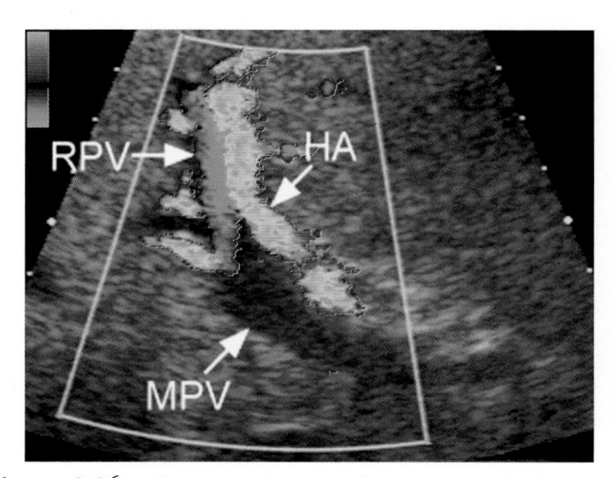

Figure 3-36 Slow portal venous flow. Longitudinal view of the portal vein shows flow in the hepatic artery (HA) and detectable but reversed flow in the right portal vein (RPV). No flow is detected in the main portal vein (MPV). Subsequent MRI examination showed slow flow in a patent main portal vein.

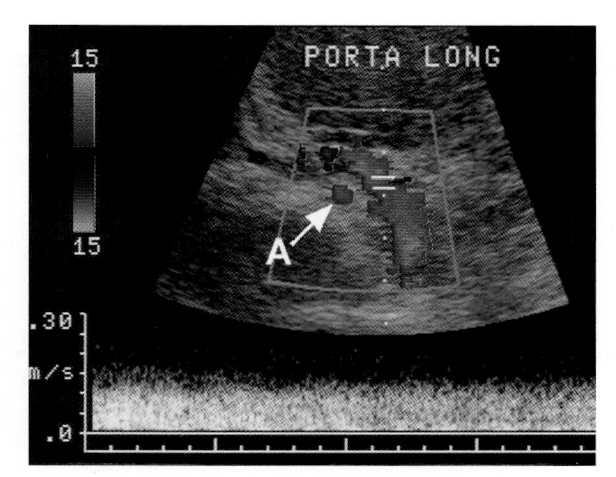

Figure 3-37 Periportal collateral simulating a patent portal vein. Longitudinal color and pulsed Doppler view demonstrates a large vessel in the porta hepatis with hepatopetal venous flow. This could easily be mistaken for a patent portal vein. However, it is located anterior to the hepatic artery (A). This patient had chronic portal vein thrombosis, and the portal vein was small and fibrotic and could not be visualized.

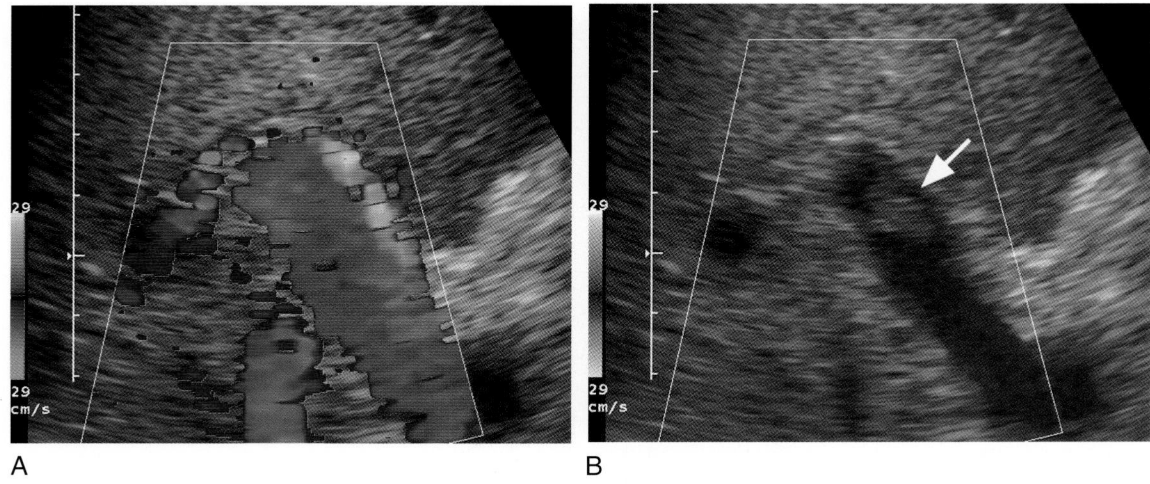

Figure 3-38 Color Doppler blooming artifact obscuring focal portal vein thrombosis. Longitudinal color Doppler views of the portal vein with the color Doppler information displayed (**A**) and not displayed (**B**). **A,** With the color Doppler signals being displayed on the image, there is no evidence of a filling defect within the portal vein. **B,** When the color Doppler signal is not displayed, so that the background gray-scale image can be seen, a focal nonocclusive thrombus *(arrow)* is seen in the portal vein lumen.

collateral is almost always located anterior to the hepatic artery. Another potential pitfall is when focal non-occlusive thrombus is obscured by blooming artifact on color Doppler analysis (Fig. 3-38). Therefore, it is important to perform a careful gray-scale evaluation as well as a Doppler evaluation. As mentioned earlier, false-positive results can occur because of slow portal vein flow. Fortunately, modern Doppler techniques have made this uncommon. Intravenous contrast agents will undoubtedly make the sonographic diagnosis of portal vein thrombosis easier.

Because of the dual arterial and portal blood supply, liver infarcts are uncommon even in the setting of total portal vein thrombosis. They usually occur only in the setting of advanced underlying vascular disease of the liver. The sonographic appearance of liver infarcts depends on their age: acute infarcts are hypoechoic, and chronic infarcts are hyperechoic. Although a wedge shape is characteristic, it is not always seen sonographically (Fig. 3-39).

In addition to bland thrombus, tumors can invade the portal vein and produce intraluminal tumor thrombus. Expansion of the portal vein suggests tumor thrombus.

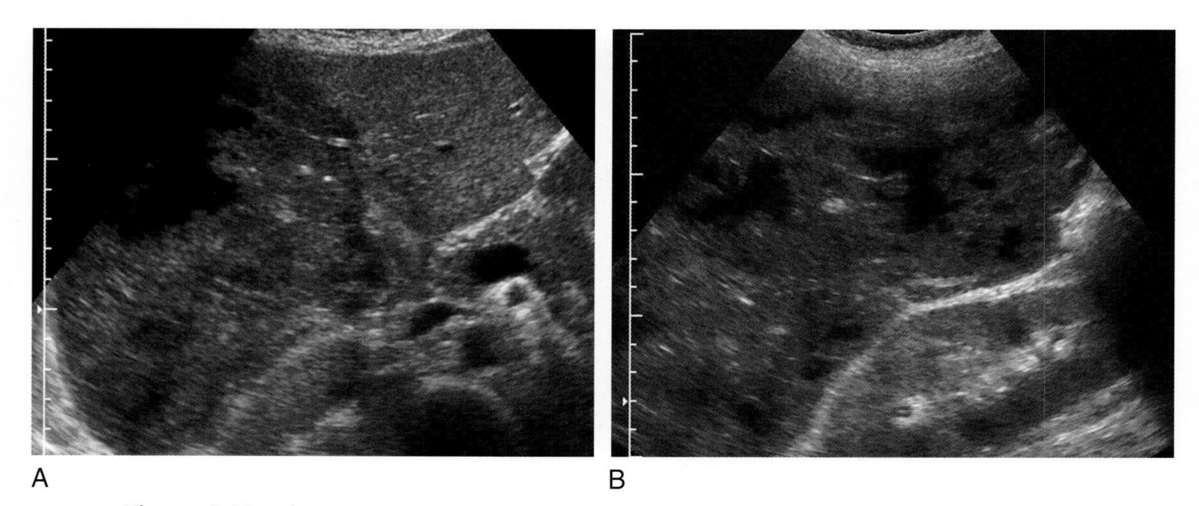

Figure 3-39 Hepatic infarction in a patient with HELLP (hemolysis, elevated liver enzymes, and low platelets) syndrome. **A,** Transverse view of the liver demonstrates diffuse decreased echogenicity and areas of liquefaction throughout the right lobe of the liver. The left lobe of the liver is normal. **B,** Longitudinal view through the right lobe of the liver shows multiple areas of liquefaction secondary to hepatic necrosis.

Tumor thrombus can confidently be diagnosed if blood flow is seen within the thrombus on color Doppler imaging (Fig. 3-40). As mentioned earlier, HCC is the tumor most likely to invade the portal vein.

In some cases of portal vein thrombosis, prominent periportal collaterals with hepatopetal flow will develop anterior to the portal vein. The collaterals typically form in the hepatoduodenal ligament (Fig. 3-41), but they have also been identified in the wall of the common bile duct. This is referred to as cavernous transformation of the portal vein, which is actually a misnomer and should not be confused with recanalized portal vein thrombosis.

Posthepatic causes of portal hypertension include hepatic vein thrombosis, IVC thrombosis, IVC membranes, and constrictive pericarditis. Hepatic vein thrombosis can potentially produce all the signs of portal hypertension described earlier. On gray-scale imaging, thrombus can occasionally be seen in the hepatic veins (Fig. 3-42A). In addition, it can cause several characteristic changes in the hepatic vein flow. The most obvious is lack of flow in the hepatic veins despite clear identification of the veins on gray-scale imaging (see Fig. 3-42D). In some cases the hepatic veins cannot be identified on gray-scale imaging and no flow is detected on color Doppler imaging. In many cases, collateral drainage will develop to compensate for the occluded hepatic veins. This drainage may flow into a main hepatic vein or accessory hepatic vein that has been spared into normal veins that drain the caudate lobe (see Fig. 3-42E), or into subcapsular veins. When collaterals develop, the hepatic vein that supplies the collateral will have reversed flow (see Fig. 3-42B). In addition, because the hepatic veins are isolated from the right atrium, pulsatility will be blunted, and in most cases the waveform will be monophasic and flat (Fig. 3-42C). Other causes of blunted hepatic vein pulsatility include cirrhosis, diffuse metastatic disease, extrinsic compression of the vein, liver transplant rejection, other diffuse parenchymal diseases, and a deep inspiration. The sensitivity of Doppler ultrasound in making the diagnosis of hepatic vein thrombosis is quite high when relying on two criteria: (1) hepatic vein(s) seen on gray-scale imaging with no detectable flow or reversed flow on color Doppler, and (2) hepatic vein(s) not seen on either gray-scale imaging or color Doppler ultrasound analysis.

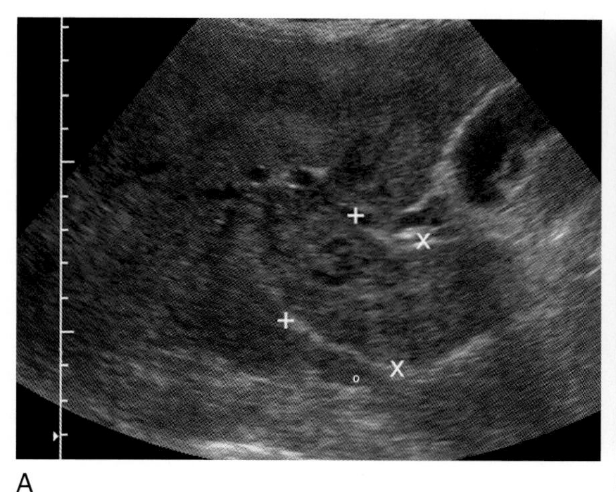

A

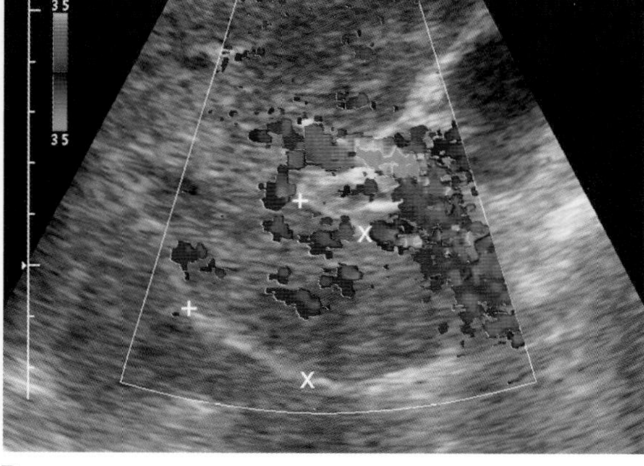

B

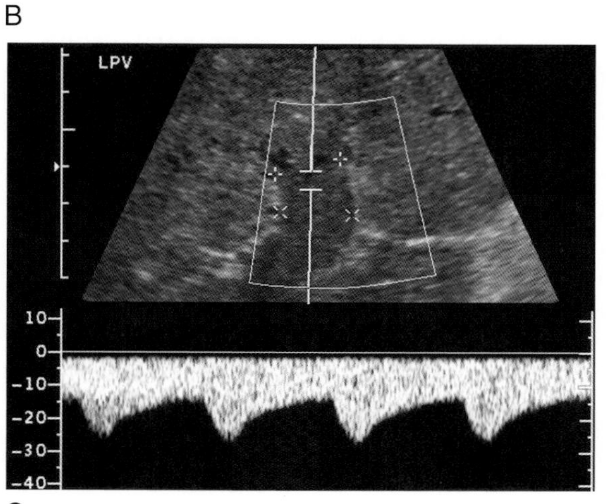

C

Figure 3-40 Portal vein tumor thrombus. Longitudinal gray-scale (**A**) and color Doppler (**B**) views of the porta hepatis show a markedly expanded portal vein *(cursors)* filled with solid tumor. In **B**, there is internal blood flow within the thrombus confirming that this represents vascularized tissue and thus tumor thrombus. **C**, In a different patient, pulsed Doppler analysis of thrombus in the left portal vein *(cursors)* shows hepatofugal arterial flow.

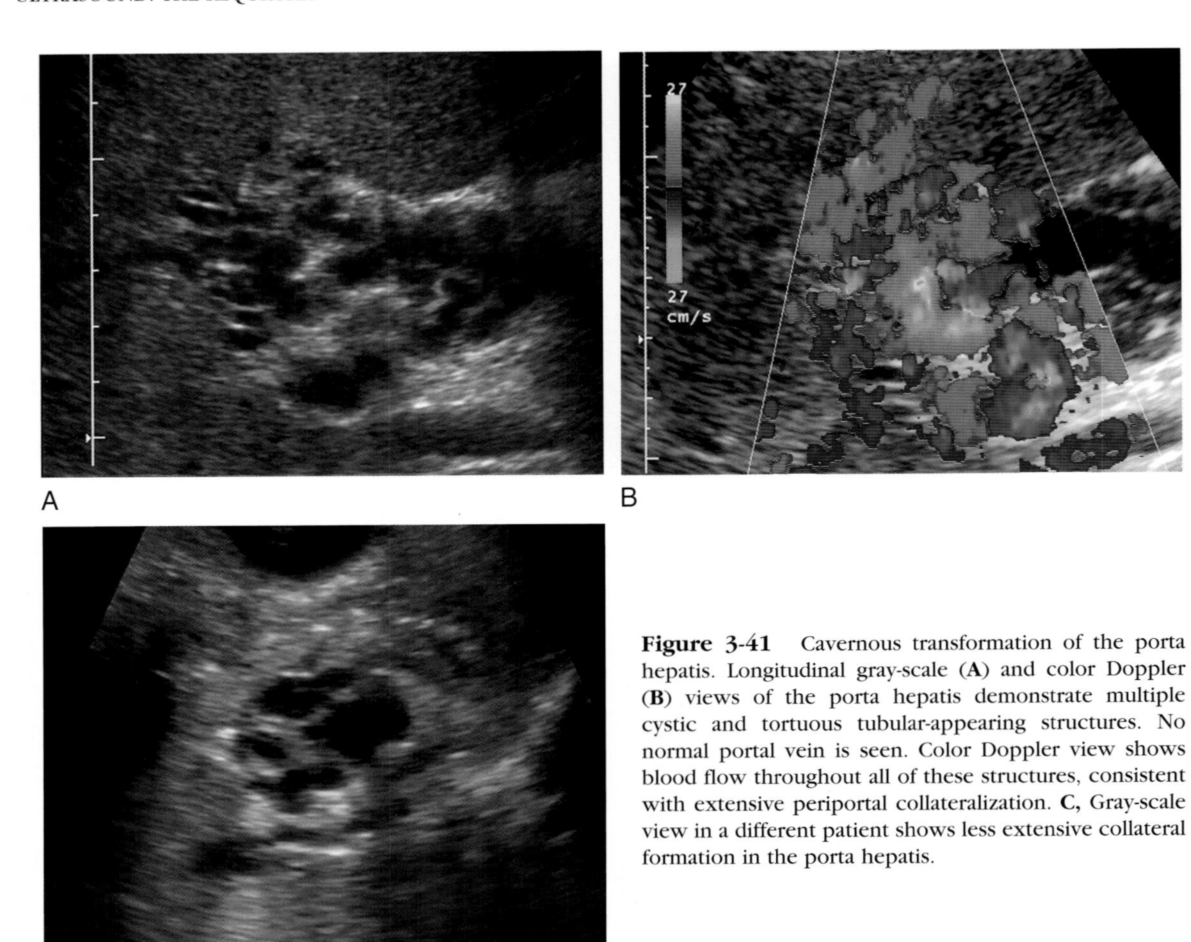

Figure 3-41 Cavernous transformation of the porta hepatis. Longitudinal gray-scale (**A**) and color Doppler (**B**) views of the porta hepatis demonstrate multiple cystic and tortuous tubular-appearing structures. No normal portal vein is seen. Color Doppler view shows blood flow throughout all of these structures, consistent with extensive periportal collateralization. **C,** Gray-scale view in a different patient shows less extensive collateral formation in the porta hepatis.

Unfortunately, approximately 15% of patients with advanced cirrhosis but no hepatic vein thrombosis will have one or more hepatic veins that cannot be identified on either gray-scale or color Doppler imaging. Therefore, the specificity of ultrasound is not as good as its sensitivity.

The last category of portal hypertension is called hyperdynamic, and it refers to arterioportal fistulas. These fistulas may be congenital or post-traumatic (e.g., following liver biopsy) and can also result from a hepatic artery aneurysm that erodes into the adjacent portal vein. They generally appear as a multilobulated, multicystic mass in the liver. Doppler analysis will reveal arterial flow within the lesion and reversal of flow and arterialization of the draining portal vein. In patients with hereditary hemorrhagic telangiectasia (Osler-Weber-Rendu syndrome), tiny arterioportal fistulas may occur. These are usually not detectable with either gray-scale or color Doppler imaging. However, the hemodynamic consequences of localized peripheral portal vein flow reversal and enlargement of the hepatic arteries are visible (Fig. 3-43).

Passive Hepatic Congestion

Heart failure can result in passive congestion of the liver, causing right upper quadrant pain and liver function abnormalities. It can be suggested on gray-scale imaging by noting hepatomegaly, enlarged hepatic veins, and an enlarged IVC. Pulsed Doppler waveforms from the portal vein will show prominent pulsatility related to the cardiac cycle. The minimum degree of portal vein pulsatility required to diagnose right-sided heart dysfunction is not uniformly agreed upon. However, most would agree that when pulsatile portal flow either reaches or goes below the Doppler baseline, right-sided heart dysfunction is very likely to be present (Fig. 3-44A).

Right-sided heart failure will also produce increased pulsatility in the hepatic veins so that the antegrade and retrograde components are more equalized and the waveform has a "W"-shaped appearance (see Fig. 3-44B). Tricuspid regurgitation causes the normally antegrade systolic hepatic vein flow to invert and produces a waveform with only one antegrade pulse that occurs during diastole (see Fig. 3-44C).

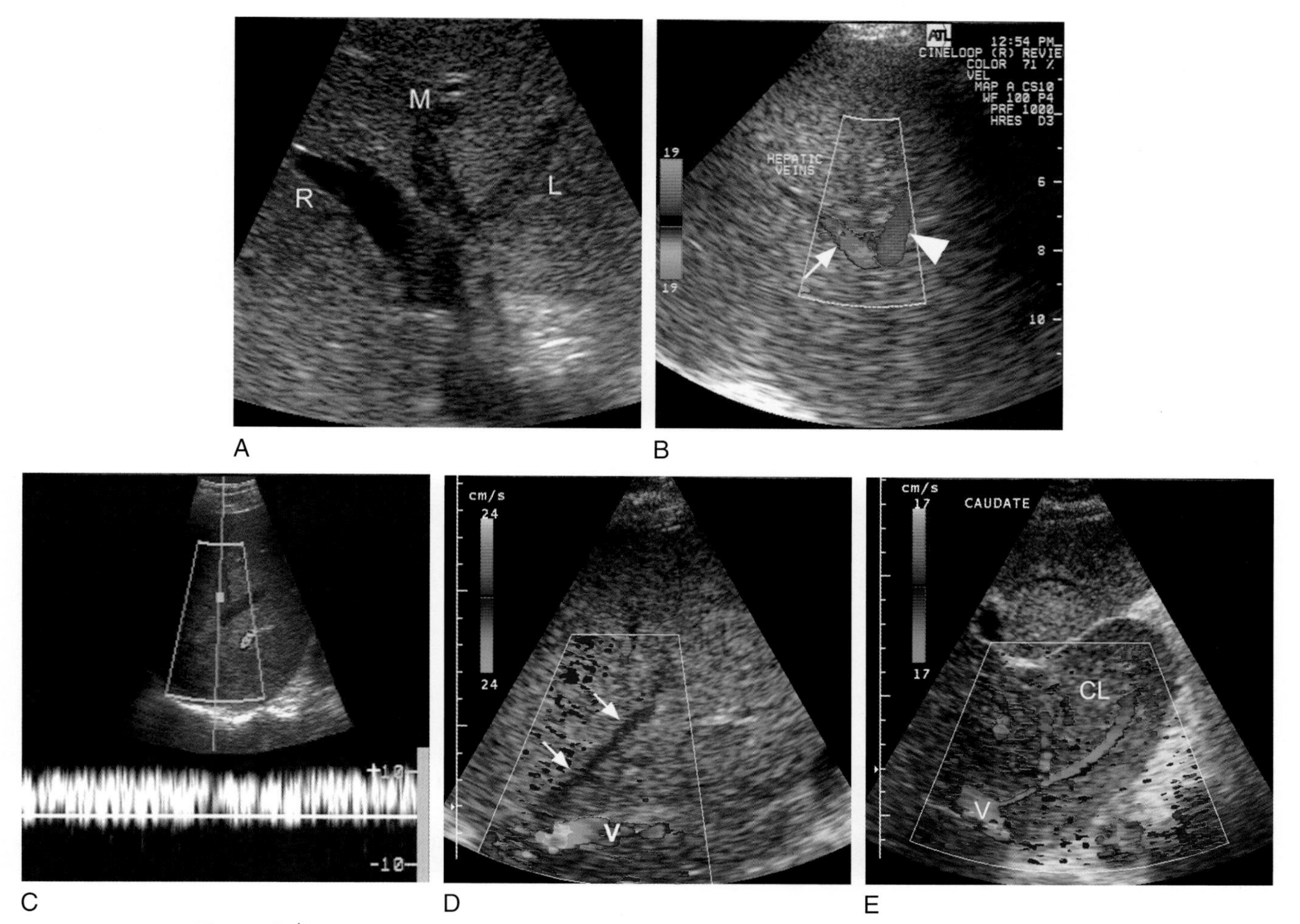

Figure 3-42 Hepatic vein thrombosis in different patients. **A,** Transverse gray-scale view of the hepatic vein confluence demonstrates hypoechoic thrombus within the left (L) and middle (M) hepatic veins. The right hepatic vein (R) remains patent. **B,** Color Doppler view of a hepatic vein bifurcation demonstrates normal direction flow in one branch *(arrow)* and reverse flow in the other branch *(arrowhead)*. The vessel with reversed flow must be supplying a collateral somewhere in the liver. **C,** Pulsed Doppler waveform from a hepatic vein shows reversed flow that has lost all of its normal pulsatility. **D,** Color Doppler view showing flow in the inferior vena cava (V) but no detectable flow within the middle hepatic vein *(arrows)*. **E,** Transverse color Doppler view shows an enlarged caudate lobe (CL). Multiple venous collaterals are seen draining from the caudate lobe into the vena cava (V).

Hepatic Transplant Complications

Improvements in surgical techniques have decreased, but not eliminated, the incidence of complications after liver transplantation. The major complications that sonography is capable of detecting are vascular and biliary. Identification of biliary obstruction and bile leaks depends on the same principles that apply to the native bile ducts (see Chapter 4).

Vascular thrombosis and stenosis can affect the hepatic artery, portal vein, hepatic veins, and the IVC after transplantation. Arterial lesions are especially critical because the bile ducts are supplied exclusively by the hepatic arteries, and significant interruption of arterial flow results in biliary necrosis. Hepatic artery thrombosis is suspected when no arterial signal is detected on either duplex or color Doppler imaging. Because thrombosis can affect the main hepatic artery or the right or left branch, all three vessels should be studied. Collateral arterial flow can develop and result in an arterial signal despite complete thrombosis of the main hepatic artery. Arterial stenosis can also be detected. Peak systolic velocities greater than 200 cm/sec or focal increases in velocity of greater than threefold suggest a

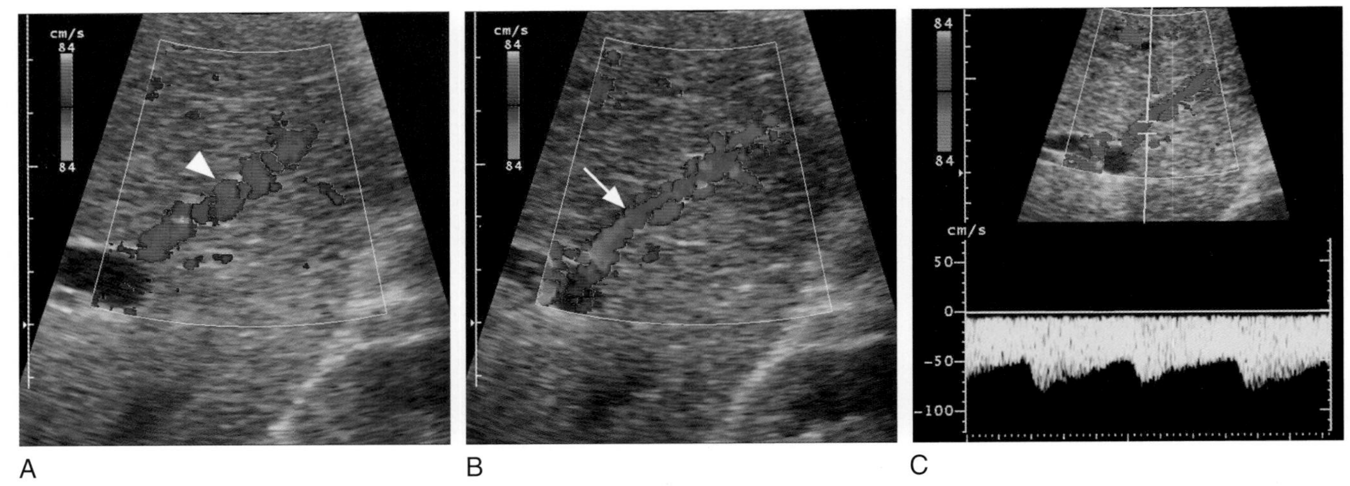

Figure 3-43 Arterial portal fistula secondary to Osler-Weber-Rendu syndrome. **A,** Magnified view of the peripheral aspect of the liver shows an enlarged tortuous intrahepatic artery *(arrowhead).* **B,** Similar view immediately adjacent to the hepatic artery shown in **A** shows an adjacent portal vein *(arrow)* with reversed flow, opposite in direction to the hepatic artery. **C,** Pulsed Doppler waveform from the portal vein shows arterialization of the portal vein flow as well as reversal of flow. This indicates a more distal arteriovenous fistula.

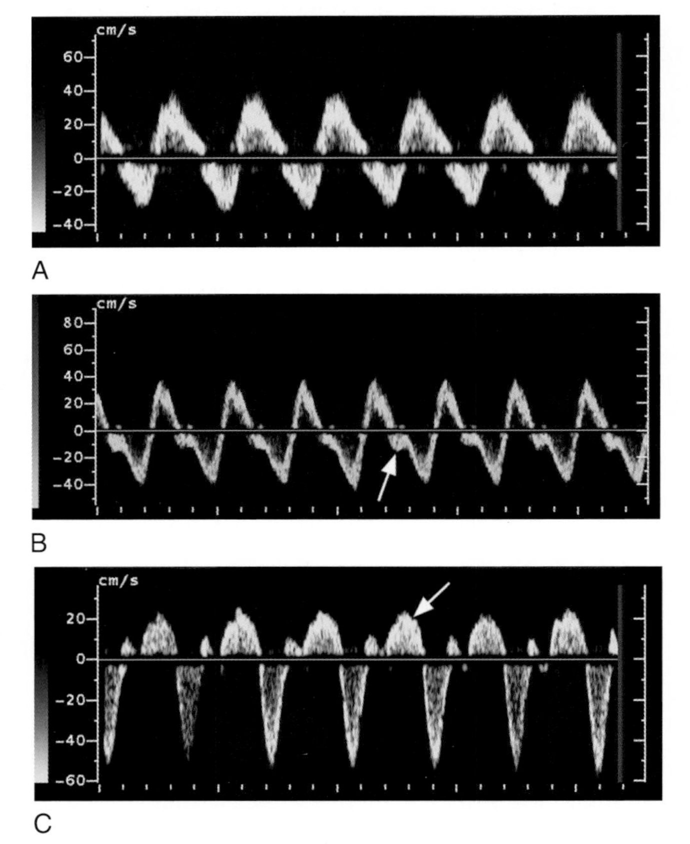

Figure 3-44 Passive congestion in different patients. **A,** Portal vein waveform showing markedly abnormal venous pulsatility. **B,** Hepatic vein waveform demonstrating increased pulsatility and a diminished systolic pulse *(arrow).* **C,** Hepatic vein waveform showing inversion of the systolic pulse *(arrow).*

stenosis of greater than 50%. Waveforms obtained distal to the stenosis demonstrate blunting of the systolic peak that can be quantified with resistive index measurements. Values less than 0.4 are almost always due to arterial obstruction, and values between 0.4 and 0.5 are suspicious. Blunting of the intrahepatic arterial waveforms occurs with both a proximal stenosis and complete thrombosis with collateral flow (Fig. 3-45). Reversal of arterial flow is a sign of collateral flow and indicates thrombosis or severe stenosis. As with other stenotic arteries, turbulent flow can cause perivascular soft tissue vibration that may be visible both on color Doppler and on pulsed Doppler.

Portal vein, hepatic vein, and IVC thrombosis appear as they would in native livers. Portal vein stenosis can occur at the anastomosis and should be suspected when there is a threefold to fourfold focal increase in the flow velocity in the portal vein. Stenosis of the IVC at the superior anastomosis causes focal velocity elevation, loss of pulsations in the hepatic veins and in the proximal IVC, and hepatic vein flow reversal. Loss of hepatic vein pulsatility has also been reported in rejection.

Portosystemic Shunts

A variety of portosystemic shunts can be created surgically to decompress the portal system in patients with portal hypertension. These generally involve a shunt between the portal vein or superior mesenteric vein and the IVC or between the splenic vein and the left renal

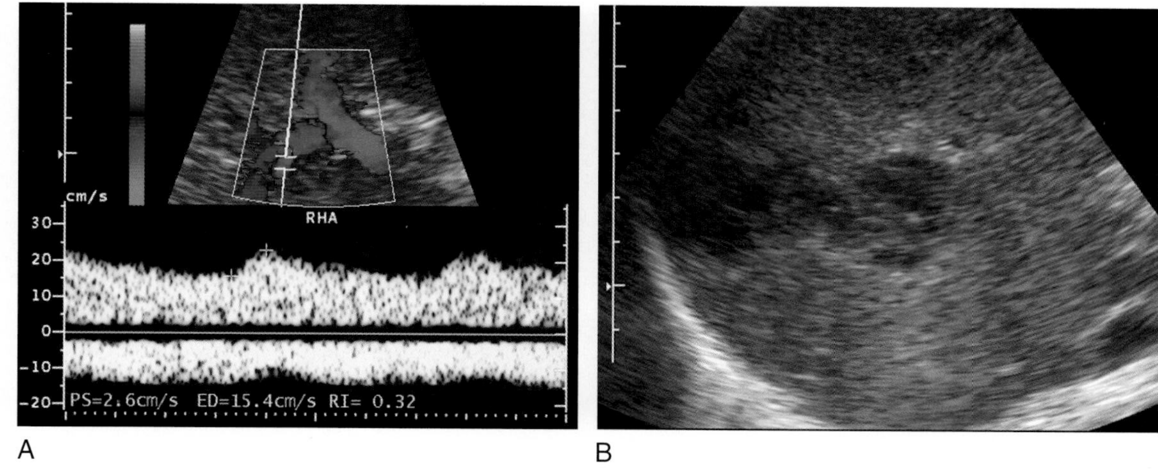

Figure 3-45 Post liver transplant hepatic artery thrombosis. **A,** Color Doppler image and pulsed Doppler waveform of the right posterior segment hepatic artery shows an extremely blunted hepatic arterial waveform with a resistive index value of 0.32. Also note that hepatic arterial flow is on the opposite side of the baseline from the portal venous flow. This implies that the right hepatic artery is functioning as a collateral vessel and has reversal of flow. **B,** Gray-scale view of the liver parenchyma demonstrates a complex fluid collection due to a biloma. This occurred because of bile duct necrosis related to the hepatic artery thrombosis.

vein. Of the surgical shunts, the portocaval shunts are in general the easiest to evaluate sonographically for shunt patency. Splenorenal shunts are more difficult to visualize, owing to left upper quadrant bowel gas.

A transjugular intrahepatic portosystemic shunt (TIPS) is now used commonly in patients with complications of portal hypertension. These shunts are very easy to evaluate for patency because the liver provides an acoustic window and overlying bowel gas is rarely a problem. The normal stent should have detectable flow throughout its lumen. Because the stent decompresses the portal system directly into the low pressure hepatic venous system, portal flow in the right and left portal vein usually reverses after stent placement and is directed into the stent instead of into the liver (Fig. 3-46A). Flow velocities in the stent are higher than typical for venous structures and range between 90 and 190 cm/sec (see Fig. 3-46B). Common problems with

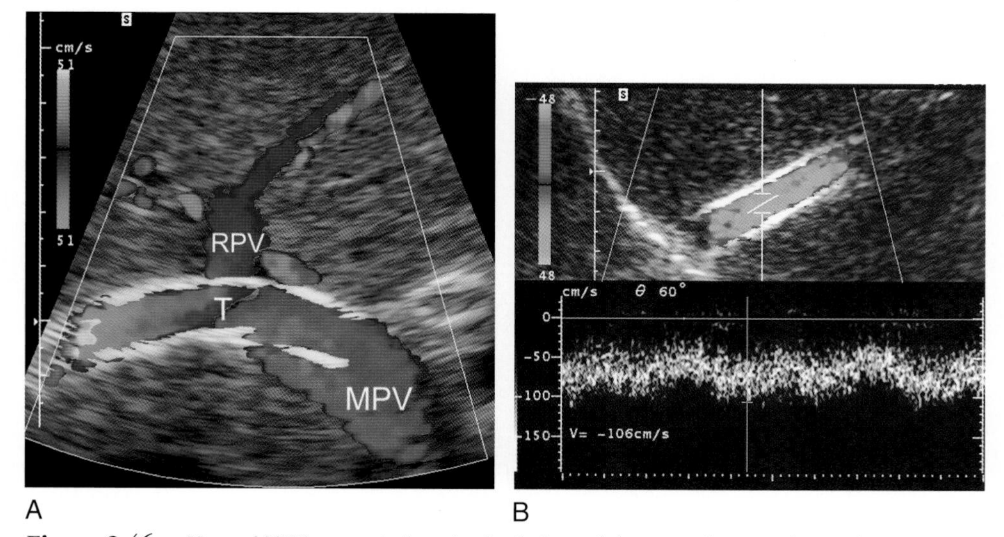

Figure 3-46 Normal TIPS stent. **A,** Longitudinal view of the porta hepatis shows the TIPS stent (T) entering the portal vein near the junction of the main portal vein (MPV) and right portal vein (RPV). Note that flow is seen throughout the lumen of the stent and note the reversal of flow in the right portal vein. **B,** Pulsed Doppler waveform from the middle aspect of a TIPS stent shows mild pulsatility and normally high velocity of 106 cm/sec.

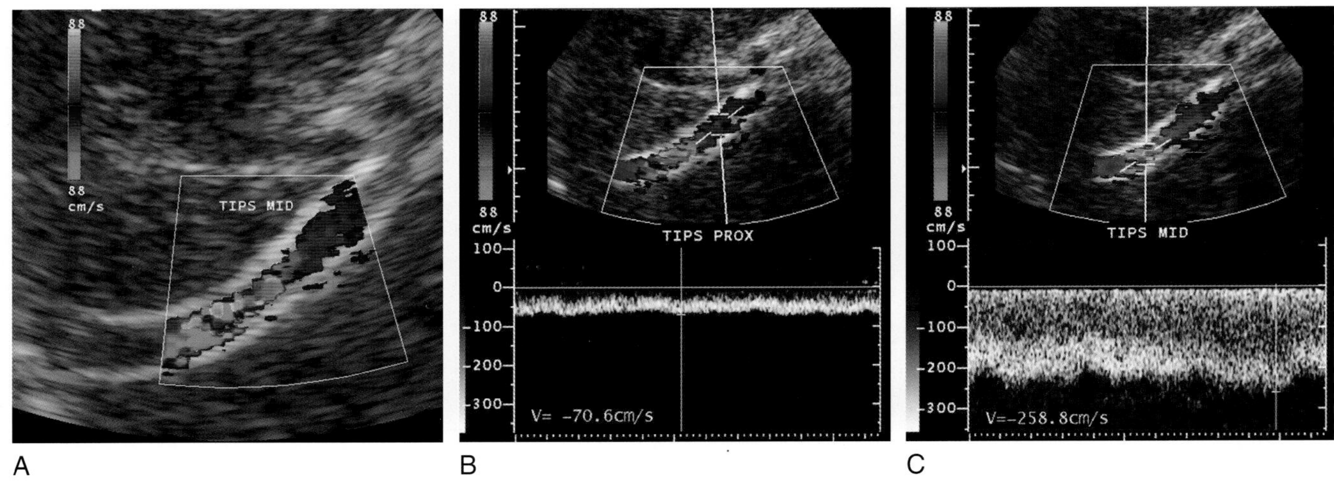

Figure 3-47 TIPS stenosis. **A,** Longitudinal color Doppler view of the stent shows a focal area of color aliasing manifest as a red color assignment in the middle aspect of the stent. This indicates elevated frequency shifts in this region and, because the Doppler angle is relatively constant, must be due to elevated velocities. **B,** Pulsed Doppler waveform from the proximal aspect of the stent shows an abnormally low velocity of 70.6 cm/sec. **C,** Pulsed Doppler waveform from the area of aliasing in the mid aspect of the stent shows abnormally elevated velocity of 258.8 cm/sec.

TIPS are stenoses of the stent or the hepatic vein. In most cases it is possible to detect these stenoses in asymptomatic patients by performing regular Doppler evaluations of the shunt and the portal veins. This allows for intervention before symptomatic decompensation. Signs of stenosis include elevated velocities across the narrowed segment, typically seen on color Doppler imaging as focal areas of color aliasing (Fig. 3-47A). When an abnormality is seen on color Doppler analysis, pulsed Doppler waveforms can be obtained through the stenotic and non-stenotic segments and velocities can be calculated. Elevated maximum and depressed minimum stent velocities are signs of stent stenosis (see Fig. 3-47B and C). One system uses 90 cm/sec and 190 cm/sec as the lower and upper limits, of normal stent velocities. Additional signs of dysfunction are low portal vein velocity, a temporal increase or decrease in maximum and minimum stent velocities on sequential examinations, and reversal of flow in the draining hepatic vein. Conversion of left and/or right portal flow from the normal pattern of flow toward the stent to a pattern of flow away from the stent on follow-up scans indicates decreased flow going through the shunt. This type of flow conversion in the right and left portal veins is usually a late manifestation of shunt dysfunction. In some patients neointimal hyperplasia and hepatic vein stenosis can also be imaged directly. It is seen as a narrowing in the flow lumen on color or power Doppler imaging (Fig. 3-48). Minimal deviations from normal in single Doppler parameters usually do not indicate a

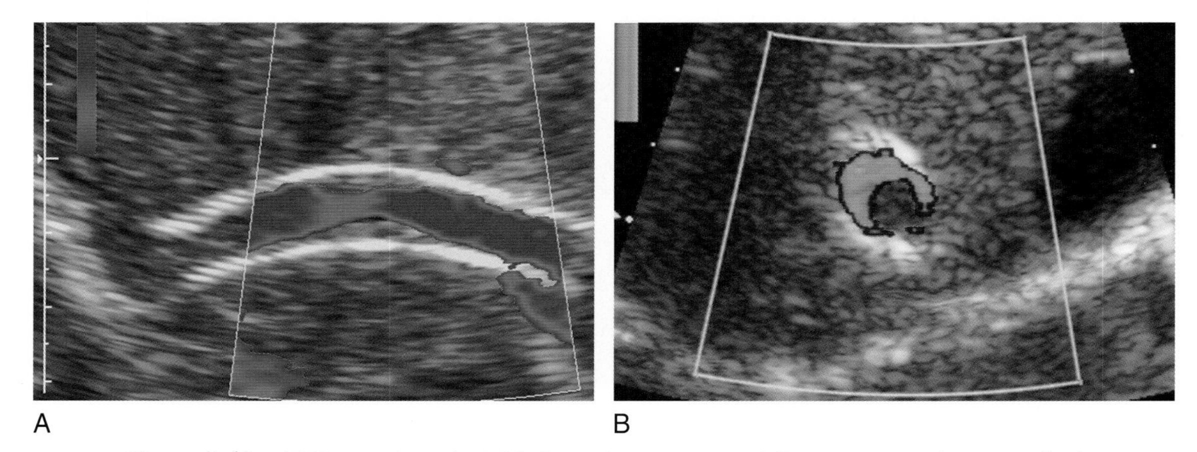

Figure 3-48 TIPS stenosis with visible luminal narrowing in different patients. **A,** Longitudinal power Doppler view of the stent shows an area of narrowing in the middle aspect of the stent. **B,** Transverse power Doppler view shows partial occlusion and only eccentric blood flow in the lumen of the stent.

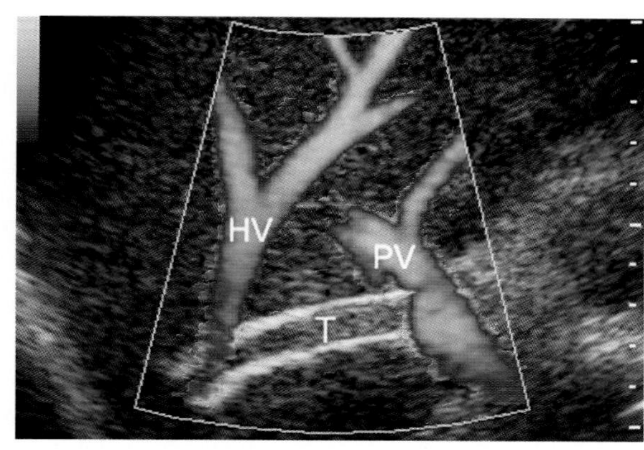

Figure 3-49 TIPS thrombosis. Longitudinal power Doppler view of the TIPS (T) shows no detectable flow within the stent. Readily detectable flow is seen in the right portal vein (PV) and in the hepatic vein (HV).

significant stenosis. However, when multiple parameters are abnormal, a stenosis is likely and intervention should be considered. When stent stenosis is not detected, it can progress to complete thrombosis. This is usually easy to diagnose with Doppler analysis because normal stent flow is relatively easy to detect (Fig. 3-49).

SUGGESTED READINGS

Abu-Judeh HH: The "starry sky" liver with right-sided heart failure. AJR Am J Roentgenol 178:78, 2002.

Abu-Yousef MM: Duplex Doppler sonography of the hepatic vein in tricuspid regurgitation. AJR Am J Roentgenol 156:79-83, 1991.

Abu-Yousef MM: Normal and respiratory variations of the hepatic and portal venous duplex Doppler waveforms with simultaneous electrocardiographic correlation. J Ultrasound Med 11:263-268, 1992.

Abu-Yousef MM, Milam SG, Farner RM: Pulsatile portal vein flow: A sign of tricuspid regurgitation on duplex Doppler sonography. AJR Am J Roentgenol 155:785-788, 1990.

Atri M, et al: Incidence of portal vein thrombosis complicating liver metastasis as detected by duplex ultrasound. J Ultrasound Med 9:285-289, 1990.

Avva R, Shah HR, Angtuaco TL: US case of the day: Giant hemangiomas of the liver. Radiographics 19:1689-1692, 1999.

Bennett GL, Krinsky GA, Abitbol RJ, et al: Sonographic detection of hepatocellular carcinoma and dysplastic nodules in cirrhosis: Correlation of pretransplantation sonography and liver explant pathology in 200 patients. AJR Am J Roentgenol 179:75-80, 2002.

Key Features

Echogenicity of the liver should be equal or slightly greater than that of the right kidney, equal or less than that of the pancreas, and less than that of the spleen.

The segments of the liver are divided by the hepatic veins, the gallbladder, the interlobar fissure, the fissure for the ligamentum venosum, and the ligamentum teres.

Hepatic cysts are easily seen and characterized with sonography. They frequently have partial septations and peripheral wall puckering.

Hemangiomas are typically homogeneous and hyperechoic. In a patient at low risk for malignancy, this type of lesion requires no further evaluation.

Focal nodular hyperplasia is usually nearly isoechoic to the liver. The classic vascularity seen on color and power Doppler analysis is a spoke-wheel pattern.

Hepatic adenomas are rare and exhibit a variety of sonographic appearances.

Target lesions are masses with a hypoechoic peripheral halo. These are very likely to be malignant.

Most liver metastases are target lesions, but there is a wide range of appearances.

Hepatocellular cancer should be suspected whenever a solid mass is seen in a patient with chronic liver disease (especially cirrhosis and chronic hepatitis). There is a propensity to invade the portal vein and, to a lesser extent, the hepatic veins.

Lymphoma typically appears as a hypoechoic mass or masses. Rarely it can appear anechoic and simulate a cyst.

Acute hepatitis may cause a "starry sky" appearance. This is often a subtle finding and is not specific for hepatitis.

Fatty infiltration is usually diffuse and causes increased hepatic echogenicity. When more severe, it attenuates the sound pulse and makes it difficult to see the diaphragm and the hepatic vessels. Fatty infiltration often localizes adjacent to the ligamentum teres or portal bifurcation. Focal sparing frequently localizes around the gallbladder and portal bifurcation.

Cirrhosis causes the hepatic parenchyma to be coarsened and inhomogeneous and the liver surface to be nodular. High-resolution views often show distinct small nodules.

The sonographic signs of portal hypertension are splenomegaly, ascites, portosystemic collaterals, and reversal of portal venous flow.

The umbilical vein and the coronary vein are the easiest portosystemic collaterals to visualize.

The diagnosis of portal vein thrombosis requires the combined use of gray-scale analysis and color-Doppler imaging and relies on the absence of detectable blood flow or the visualization of intraluminal filling defects.

Hepatic vein thrombosis may appear as an intraluminal hepatic vein thrombus, reversal of hepatic vein flow, no detectable hepatic vein flow, and hepatic vein collaterals.

Brancatelli G, Federle MP, Grazioli L, et al: Benign regenerative nodules in Budd-Chiari syndrome and other vascular disorders of the liver: Radiologic-pathologic and clinical correlation. Radiographics 22:847-862, 2002.

Buetow PC, Pantograg-Brown L, Buck JL, et al: From the Archives of the AFIP: Focal nodular hyperplasia of the liver: Radiologic-pathologic correlation. Radiographics 16:369-388, 1996.

Buetow PC, Buck JL, Ros PR, Goodman ZD: From the Archives of the AFIP: Malignant vascular tumors of the liver: Radiologic-pathologic correlation. Radiographics 14:153-166, 1994.

Birnbaum BA, et al: Definitive diagnosis of hepatic hemangiomas: MR imaging versus Tc-99m-labeled red blood cell SPECT. Radiology 176:95-101, 1990.

Bolondi L, et al: Liver cirrhosis: Changes of Doppler waveform of hepatic veins. Radiology 178:513-516, 1991.

Bree RL, et al: The varied appearances of hepatic cavernous hemangiomas with sonography, computed tomography, magnetic resonance imaging, and scintigraphy. Radiographics 7:1153-1175, 1987.

Casillas VJ, Amendola MA, Gascue A, et al: Imaging of nontraumatic hemorrhagic hepatic lesions. Radiographics 20:363-378, 2000.

Caturelli E, Pompili M, Bartolucci F, et al: Hemangioma-like lesions in chronic liver disease: Diagnostic evaluation in patients. Radiology 220:337-342, 2001.

Cerri GG, de Oliveira IRS, Machado MM: Hepatosplenic schistosomiasis: Ultrasound evaluation update. Ultrasound Q 15(4):210-215, 1999.

Chehida FB, Gharbi HA, Hammou A, et al: Ultrasound findings in hydatid cyst. Ultrasound Q 15(4):216-222, 1999.

Cho KJ, Lunderquist A: The peribiliary vascular plexus: The microvascular architecture of the bile duct in the rabbit and in clinical cases. Radiology 147:357-364, 1983.

Cronan JJ, et al: Cavernous hemangioma of the liver: Role of percutaneous biopsy. Radiology 166:135-138, 1988.

Dodd GD III, et al: Detection of malignant tumors in end-stage cirrhotic livers: Efficacy of sonography as a screening technique. AJR Am J Roentgenol 159:727-733, 1992.

Dodd GD III, et al: Hepatic artery stenosis and thrombosis in transplant recipients: Doppler diagnosis with resistive index and systolic acceleration time. Radiology 192:657-661, 1994.

Dodd GD III, Baron RL, Oliver JH III, Federle MP: Pictorial review: Spectrum of imaging findings of the liver in end-stage cirrhosis: I. Gross morphology and diffuse abnormalities. AJR Am J Roentgenol 173:1031-1036, 1999.

Dodd GD III, Baron RL, Oliver JH III, Federle MP: Pictorial review: Spectrum of imaging findings of the liver in end-stage cirrhosis: II. Focal abnormalities. AJR Am J Roentgenol 173:1185-1192, 1999.

Dodd GD III, Baron RL, Oliver JH, Federle MP: End-stage primary sclerosing cholangitis: CT findings of hepatic morphology in 36 patients. Radiology 211:357-362, 1999.

Dodd GD III, Memel DS, Baron RL, et al: Portal vein thrombosis in patients with cirrhosis: Does sonographic detection of intrathrombus flow allow differentiation of benign and malignant thrombus? AJR Am J Roentgenol 165:573, 1995.

Duerinckx AJ, et al: The pulsatile portal vein in cases of congestive heart failure: Correlation of duplex Doppler findings with right atrial pressures. Radiology 176:655-658, 1990.

Feldstein VA, Patel MD, LaBerge JM: TIPS shunts: Accuracy of Doppler US in determination of patency and detection of stenoses. Radiology 201:141-147, 1996.

Freedman AM, Sanyal AJ, Tisnado J, et al: Complications of transjugular intrahepatic portosystemic shunt: A comprehensive review. Radiographics 13:1185-1210, 1993.

Filly RA, Reddy SG, Nalbandian AB, et al: Sonographic evaluation of liver nodularity: Inspection of deep versus superficial surfaces of the liver. J Clin Ultrasound 30: 399-407, 2002.

Gallix BP, Taourel P, Dauzat M, et al: Flow pulsatility in the portal venous system: A study of Doppler sonography in healthy adults. AJR Am J Roentgenol 169:141-144, 1997.

Gazelle GS, Lee MJ, Mueller PR: Cholangiographic segmental anatomy of the liver. Radiographics 14:1005-1013, 1994.

Gibney RG, Hendin AP, Cooperberg PL: Sonographically detected hepatic hemangiomas: Absence of change over time. AJR Am J Roentgenol 149:953-957, 1987.

Gibson PR, et al: A comparison of duplex Doppler sonography of the ligamentum teres and portal vein with endoscopic demonstration of gastroesophageal varices in patients with chronic liver disease or portal hypertension, or both. J Ultrasound Med 11:327-331, 1992.

Gibson RN, et al: Identification of a patent paraumbilical vein by using Doppler sonography: Importance in the diagnosis of portal hypertension. AJR Am J Roentgenol 153:513-516, 1989.

Glockner JF, Forauer AR: Pictorial essay: Vascular or ischemic complications after liver transplantation. AJR Am J Roentgenol 173:1055-1059, 1999.

Goyal AK, Pokharna DS, Sharma SK: Ultrasonic measurements of portal vasculature in diagnosis of portal hypertension: A controversial subject reviewed. J Ultrasound Med 9:45-48, 1990.

Grazioli L, Federle MP, Brancatelli G, et al: Hepatic adenomas: Imaging and pathologic findings. Radiographics 21:877-894, 2001.

Herold C. Reck T, Ott R, et al: Changes in hepatic hemodynamics after orthotopic liver transplantation: Color Doppler sonography. Abdom Imaging 26:32-35, 2001.

Hung C-H, Changchien C-S, Lu S-N, et al: Sonographic features of hepatic adenomas with pathologic correlation. Abdom Imaging 26:500-506, 2001.

Ichikawa T, Federle MP, Grazioli L, et al: Fibrolamellar hepatocellular carcinoma: Imaging and pathologic findings in 31 recent cases. Radiology 21:352-361, 1999.

Ito K, Honjo K, Fujita T, et al: Liver neoplasms: Diagnostic pitfalls in cross-sectional imaging. Radiographics 16:273-293, 1996.

Kane R, Eustace S: Diagnosis of Budd-Chiari syndrome: Comparison between sonography and MR angiography. Radiology 195:117-121, 1995.

Kanterman RY, Darcy MD, Middleton WD, et al: Doppler sonographic findings associated with transjugular intrahepatic portosystemic shunt (TIPS) malfunction. AJR Am J Roentgenol 168:467-472, 1997.

Keogan MT, McDermott VG, Price SK, et al: Pictorial essay: The role of imaging in the diagnosis and management of biliary complications after liver transplantation. AJR Am J Roentgenol 173:215-219, 1999.

Kliewer MA, Sheafor DH, Paulson EK, et al: Percutaneous liver biopsy: A cost-benefit analysis comparing sonographic and CT guidance. AJR Am J Roentgenol 173:1199-1202, 1999.

Konno K, Ishida H, Sato M, et al: Liver tumors in fatty liver: Difficulty in ultrasonographic interpretation. Abdom Imaging 26:487-491, 2001.

Kruskal JB, Thomas P, Nasser I, et al: Hepatic colon cancer metastases in mice: Dynamic in vivo correlation with hypoechoic rims visible at US. Radiology 215:852-857, 2000.

Kudo M, Tomita S, Tochio H, et al: Hepatic focal nodular hyperplasia: Specific findings at dynamic contrast-enhanced US with carbon dioxide microbubbles. Radiology 179:377-382, 1991.

Kurtz AB, Rubin CS, Cooper HS, et al: Ultrasound findings in hepatitis. Radiology 136:717-723, 1980.

Lafortune M, Patriquin HB: The hepatic artery: Studies using Doppler sonography. Ultrasound Q 15(1):9-26, 1999.

Liefer DM, Middleton WD, Teefey SA, et al: Follow-up of patients at low risk for hepatic malignancy with a characteristic hemangioma at US. Radiology 214:167-172, 2000.

Marn CS, Bree RL, Silver TM: Ultrasonography of the liver: Technique and focal and diffuse disease. Radiol Clin North Am 29:1151-1170, 1991.

Marsh JI, Gibney RG, Li DK: Hepatic hemangioma in the presence of fatty infiltration: An atypical sonographic appearance. Gastrointest Radiol 14:262-264, 1989.

McKenney KL: Role of US in the diagnosis of intraabdominal catastrophes. Radiographics 19:1332-1339, 1999.

McLarney JK, Rucker PT, Bender GN, et al: From the archives of the AFIP: Fibrolamellar carcinoma of the liver: Radiologic-pathologic correlation. Radiographics 19:453-471, 1999.

Mergo PJ, Ros PR, Buetow PC, Buck JL: Diffuse disease of the liver: Radiologic-pathologic correlation. Radiographics 14:1291-1307, 1994.

Middleton WD, Hiskes H, Teefey SA, Boucher LD: Small (1.5 cm or less) liver metastases: US-guided biopsy. Radiology 205:729-732, 1997.

Millener P, et al: Color Doppler imaging findings in patients with Budd-Chiari syndromes: Correlation with venographic findings. AJR Am J Roentgenol 161:307-312, 1993.

Moody AR, Wilson SR: Atypical hepatic hemangiomas: A suggestive sonographic morphology. Radiology 188:413-417, 1993.

Mostbeck GH, et al: Hemodynamic significance of the paraumbilical vein in portal hypertension: Assessment with duplex US. Radiology 170:339-342, 1989.

Nascimento AB, Mitchell DG, Rubin R, Weaver E: Diffuse desmoplastic breast carcinoma metastases to the liver simulating cirrhosis at MR imaging: Report of two cases. Radiology 221:117-121, 2001.

Nelson RC, Chezmar JL: Diagnostic approach to hepatic hemangiomas. Radiology 176:11-13, 1990.

Nghiem HV, Bogost GA, Ryan JA, et al: Cavernous hemangiomas of the liver: Enlargement over time. AJR Am J Roentgenol 169:137-140, 1997.

Nghiem HV, Tran Khai, Winter TC III, et al: Imaging of complications in liver transplantation. Radiographics 16:825-840, 1996.

Pedrosa I, Saiz A, Arrazola J, et al: Hydatid disease; radiologic and pathologic features and complications. Radiographics 20:795-817, 2000.

Pena CS, Chew FS, Keel SB: Posttransplantation lymphoproliferative disorder of the liver. AJR Am J Roentgenol 171:192, 2000.

Platt JF, Yutzy GG, Bude RO, et al: Use of Doppler sonography for revealing hepatic artery stenosis in liver transplant recipients. AJR Am J Roentgenol 168:473-476, 1997.

Quinn SF, Gosink BB: Characteristic sonographic signs of hepatic fatty infiltration. AJR Am J Roentgenol 145:753-755, 1985.

Ralls PW: Color Doppler sonography of the hepatic artery and portal venous system. AJR Am J Roentgenol 155:517-525, 1990.

Richards JR, McGahan JP: Ultrasound for blunt abdominal trauma in the emergency department. Ultrasound Q 15(2): 60-72, 1999.

Rosenthal SJ, Harrison LA, Baxter KG, et al: Doppler US of helical flow in the portal vein. Radiographics 15:1103-1111, 1995.

Schneck CD: Embryology, histology, gross anatomy and normal imaging anatomy of the liver. In Friedman AC, Dachman AH (eds): Radiology of the Liver, Biliary Tract, and Pancreas. St. Louis, Mosby, 1994, pp 1-25.

Singh, Y, Winic AB, Tabbara SO: Residents' teaching files: Multiloculated cystic liver lesions: Radiologic-pathologic differential diagnosis. Radiographics 17:219-224, 1997.

Smith D, Downey D, Spouge A, Soney S: Sonographic demonstration of Couinaud's liver segments. J Ultrasound Med 17:375-381, 1998.

Stoopen ME, Kimura-Fujikami K, Quiroz y Ferrari FA, Barois-Boullard V: Ultrasound imaging of hepatic amebic abscess. Ultrasound Q 15(4):189-200, 1999.

Stoupis C, Taylor HM, Paley MR, et al: The rocky liver: Radiologic-pathologic correlation of calcified hepatic masses. Radiographics 18:675-685, 1998.

Tchelepi H, Ralls PW, Radin R, Grant E: Sonography of diffuse liver disease. J Ultrasound Med 21:1023-1032, 2002.

Teefey SA, Hildebolt CC, Dehdashti F, et al: Detection of primary hepatic malignancy in liver transplant candidates: Prospective comparison of CT, MR imaging, US and PET. Radiology 226:533-542, 2003.

Teefey SA, Middleton WD, Crowe TM, Peters MG: Doppler evaluation of the portal vein: Effects of intravenous DDFP. J Ultrasound Med 16:641-645, 1997.

Tessler FN, et al: Diagnosis of portal vein thrombosis: Value of color Doppler imaging. AJR Am J Roentgenol 157:293-296, 1991.

Tessler FN, Tublin ME, Purdy S, Rifkin MD: US case of the day: Diffuse large B-cell lymphoma (posttransplant lymphoproliferative disorder [PTLD]). Radiographics 18:1307-1309, 1998.

Uggowitzer MM, Kugler C, Mischinger HJ, et al: Echo-enhanced Doppler sonography of focal nodular hyperplasia of the liver. J Ultrasound Med 18:445-451, 1999.

Vilgrain V, Boulos L, Vullierme MP, et al: Imaging of atypical hemangiomas of the liver and pathologic correlation. Radiographics 20:379-397, 2000.

VanSonnenberg E. Simeone JF, Mueller PR, et al: Sonographic appearance of hematoma in liver, spleen and kidney: A clinical, pathologic and animal study. Radiology 147:507-510, 1983.

Wachsberg RH: Sonography of liver transplants. Ultrasound Q 14(2):76-94, 1998.

Wachsberg RH, Simmons MZ: Coronary vein diameter and flow direction in patients with portal hypertension: Evaluation with duplex sonography and correlation with variceal bleeding. AJR Am J Roentgenol 162:637-641, 1994.

Wagner RC, Koenigsberg M, Wexler JP: US case of the day: Focal nodular hyperplasia (FNH). Radiographics 16:974-978, 1996.

Want SS, et al: Focal hepatic fatty infiltration as a cause of pseudotumors: Ultrasonographic patterns and clinical differentiation. J Clin Ultrasound 18:401-409, 1990.

Warshauer DM, Molina PL, Hamman SM, et al: Nodular sarcoidosis of the liver and spleen: Analysis of 32 cases. Radiology 195:757-762, 1995.

Weltin G, et al: Duplex Doppler: Identification of cavernous transformation of the portal vein, AJR Am J Roentgenol 144:999-1001, 1985.

Wernecke K, et al: Pathologic explanation for hypoechoic halo seen on sonograms of malignant liver tumors: An in vitro correlative study. AJR Am J Roentgenol 159:1011-1016, 1992.

Wernecke K, et al: The distinction between benign and malignant liver tumors on sonography: Value of a hypoechoic halo. AJR Am J Roentgenol 159:1005-1009, 1992.

White EM, et al: Focal periportal sparing in hepatic fatty infiltration: A cause of hepatic pseudomass on US. Radiology 162:57-59, 1987.

Yates CK, Streight RA: Focal fatty infiltration of the liver simulating metastatic disease. Radiology 159:83-84, 1986.

Yoshikawa J, et al: Focal fatty change of the liver adjacent to the falciform ligament: CT and sonographic findings in five surgically confirmed cases. AJR Am J Roentgenol 149:491-494, 1987.

Zweibel WJ: Sonographic diagnosis of diffuse liver disease. Semin US CT MRI 16:8-16, 1995.

CHAPTER 4

Bile Ducts

ANATOMY

The bile ducts are generally divided into the intrahepatic and extrahepatic portions. The intrahepatic ducts run in the portal triads with the portal veins and hepatic arteries. The right and left hepatic ducts are anterior to the adjacent portal veins. The peripheral intrahepatic ducts run parallel and adjacent to the hepatic arteries and portal veins, but the relative anterior and posterior relationship of the three structures is more variable than that of the extrahepatic ducts.

The extrahepatic portion of the bile ducts includes the common hepatic duct, common bile duct, and a portion of the central right and left ducts. The common hepatic duct is the segment located above the cystic duct insertion, and the common bile duct is the segment below. In most cases the cystic duct insertion is not seen, so it is not possible to distinguish the common hepatic from the common bile duct. Because of this, many people simply refer to the duct as the common duct and divide it subjectively into the proximal, mid, and distal segments. At the porta hepatis the proximal common duct runs anterior to the right and main portal vein and the right hepatic artery (Fig. 4-1A). The mid duct runs posterior to the duodenum. In those situations where the cystic duct insertion is visible, it is seen posterior to the common duct (see Fig. 4-1B). Inferiorly, the distal common duct enters the head of the pancreas and travels along the most posterior aspect of the pancreatic head (see Fig. 4-1C).

The hepatic artery arises from the celiac axis and travels in the hepatoduodenal ligament anterior to the portal vein and medial to the common duct (see Fig. 4-1D). On transverse views of the porta hepatis, this configuration produces the "Mickey Mouse" appearance with the head being the portal vein, the ear to the patient's left being the artery, and the ear to the right being the bile duct (see Fig. 4-1E). The relationship of the bile duct and hepatic artery can be remembered by noting that the bile duct comes from the liver (a right-sided structure) and the hepatic artery arises from the aorta (a left-sided structure). The right hepatic artery passes between the common duct and the portal vein in 85% to 90% of patients (see Fig. 4-1A). Ten to 15 percent of individuals have a normal variant in which the artery passes anterior to the common duct (Fig. 4-2A). In a very small percentage of patients, two arteries are seen anterior and/or posterior to the duct (see Fig. 4-2 B and C). This can be due to either two branches of the right hepatic artery or the right hepatic artery and the cystic artery.

Compared with the common duct, the hepatic artery is relatively tortuous, so it is difficult to display more than 2 to 3 cm of its long axis in any plane. In addition, the hepatic artery maintains a relatively similar diameter throughout its course. Finally, the hepatic artery may cause an extrinsic impression on the bile duct and/or the portal vein. On the other hand, the common duct is relatively straight, has a diameter that varies along its course, and does not produce an impression on adjacent vessels (see Figs. 4-1 and 4-2 and Table 4-1).

A replaced right hepatic artery arising from the superior mesenteric artery is a common normal variant that alters the anatomy of the porta hepatis. As described earlier in Chapter 3, a replaced or accessory right hepatic

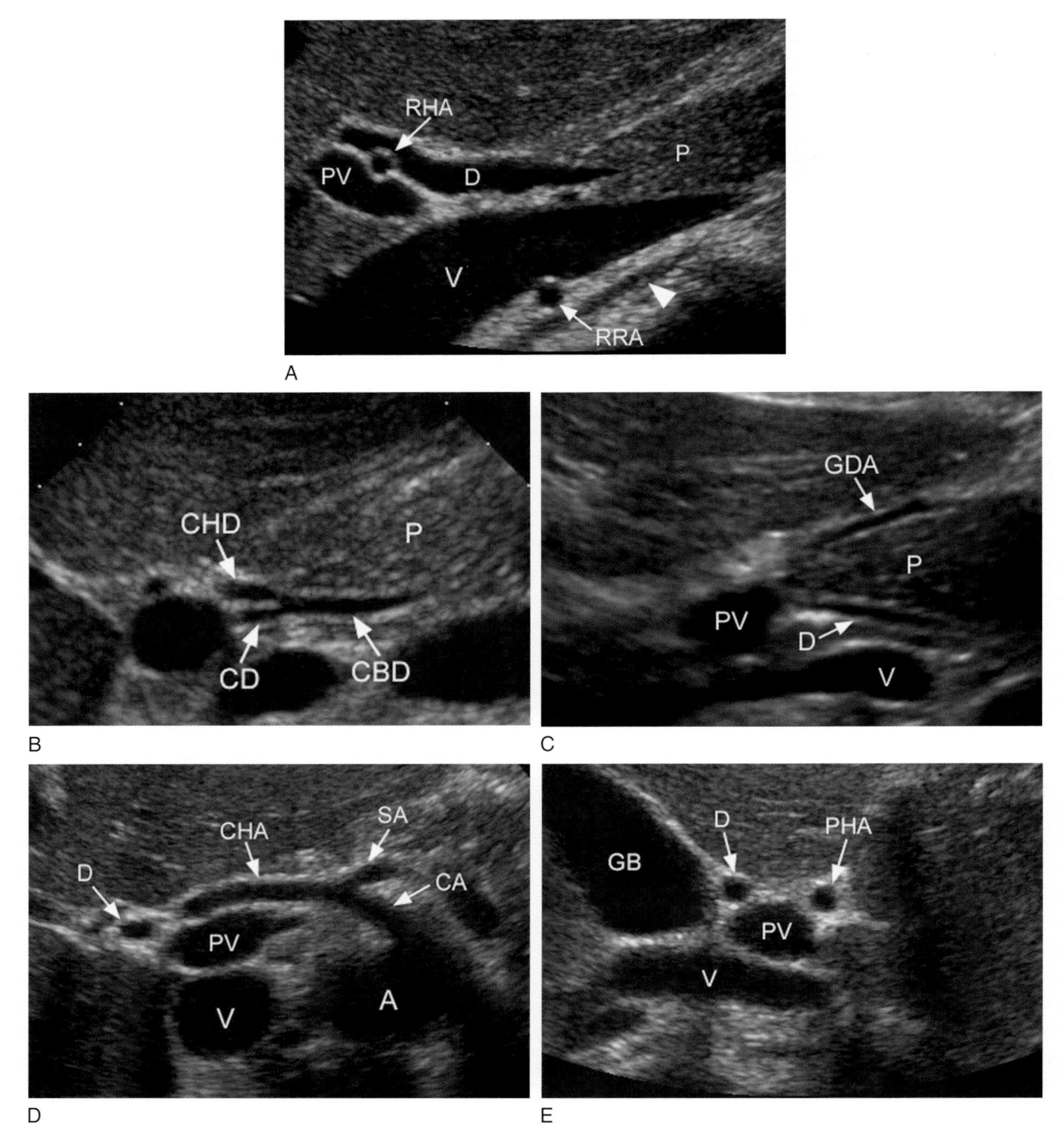

Figure 4-1 Normal anatomy. **A,** Longitudinal view shows the classic anatomy with the bile duct (D) located anterior to the portal vein (PV) and the right hepatic artery (RHA) located between these two structures. The distal duct enters the head of the pancreas (P). The inferior vena cava (V), the right renal artery (RRA), and the crus of the right hemidiaphragm *(arrowhead)* are often seen on this view. **B,** Longitudinal view shows the cystic duct insertion (CD) at the junction of the common hepatic duct (CHD) and the common bile duct (CBD). The pancreatic head (P) is also seen. **C,** Longitudinal view of the head of the pancreas (P) shows the distal common bile duct (D) running through the posterior pancreas. This is opposed to the gastroduodenal artery (GDA), which runs along the anterior pancreatic head. Also seen are the portal vein (PV) and the vena cava (V). **D,** Transverse view of the inferior porta hepatis shows the celiac axis (CA) arising from the aorta (A) and dividing into the splenic artery (SA) and common hepatic artery (CHA). The hepatic artery travels anterior to the portal vein (PV) and medial to the common duct (D). Note the close relationship between the portal vein and the vena cava (V). **E,** Transverse view of the superior porta hepatis shows the classic "Mickey Mouse" view with the common duct (D) located anterior to the portal vein (PV) and to the right of the proper hepatic artery (PHA). The gallbladder (GB) and the vena cava (V) are often seen on this view.

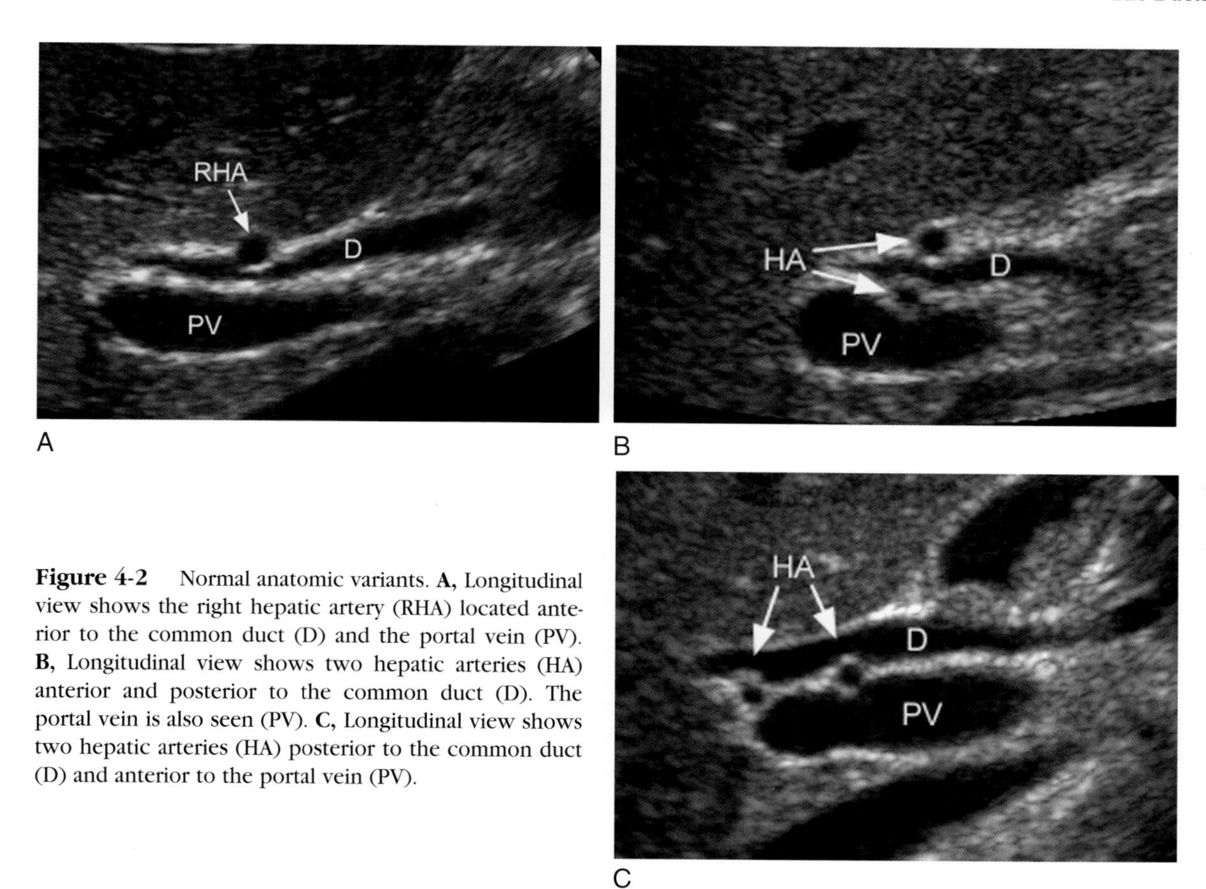

Figure 4-2 Normal anatomic variants. **A,** Longitudinal view shows the right hepatic artery (RHA) located anterior to the common duct (D) and the portal vein (PV). **B,** Longitudinal view shows two hepatic arteries (HA) anterior and posterior to the common duct (D). The portal vein is also seen (PV). **C,** Longitudinal view shows two hepatic arteries (HA) posterior to the common duct (D) and anterior to the portal vein (PV).

artery runs between the inferior vena cava and the portal vein and is situated on the right lateral aspect of the portal vein. It can be distinguished from the bile duct by following it to its origin or by Doppler analysis. Another potentially confusing anatomic variant in this area is a cystic duct that inserts unusually low. In such cases the cystic and common hepatic duct travel in a common sheath and appear as parallel tubular structures before they join to form the common bile duct (Fig. 4-3). Occasionally, a tortuous gallbladder neck simulates the appearance of the proximal common duct (Fig. 4-4). Careful scanning in multiple obliquities usually reveals the continuity of a tortuous neck with the rest of the gallbladder. In addition, it is not possible for a tortuous gallbladder neck to elongate to the same extent as the common duct.

Table 4-1 Differentiation between Common Duct and Hepatic Artery

Characteristics	Duct	Artery
Location	Anterior to right hepatic artery (85%)	Posterior to duct (85%)
	Posterior to right hepatic artery (15%)	Anterior to duct (15%)
	Lateral to proper hepatic artery	Medial to duct
Visible length	Long	Short
Diameter	Variable	Constant
Compression of nearby structures	No	Yes
Doppler signal	Absent	Present

TECHNIQUE

The proximal common duct is usually best seen by placing the patient in a left lateral decubitus or left posterior oblique position and by scanning from a right subcostal approach during a deep inspiration. Because of its size and ease of visualization, the portal vein is a valuable landmark for the common duct. As the portal vein and bile duct exit from the liver, they separate from each other, with the portal vein heading toward the left and the bile duct heading more inferiorly. Therefore, if the main portal vein can first be imaged in its long axis, the mid bile duct can then be visualized by rotating the transducer slightly in a clockwise direction.

Most pathologic processes affecting the bile duct occur distally. The distal common duct is located in the

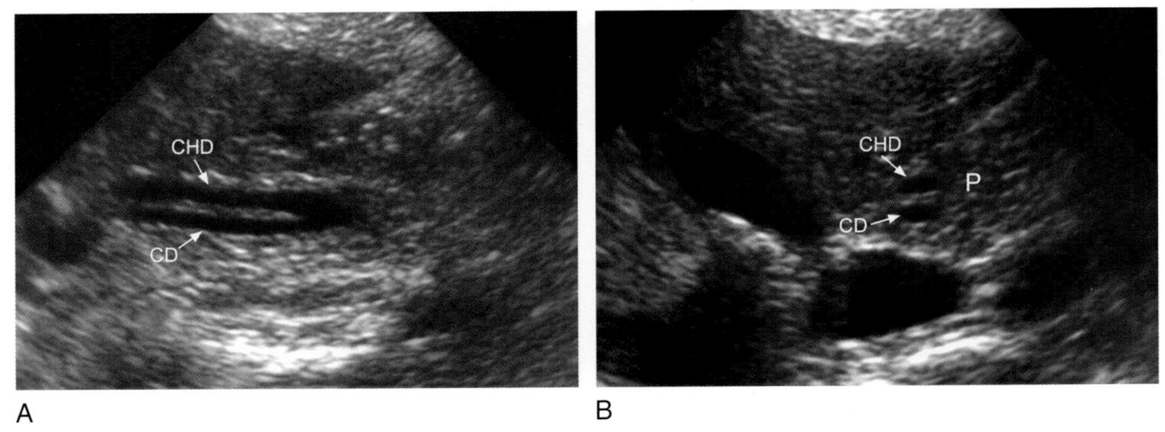

Figure 4-3 Low inserting cystic duct. **A,** Longitudinal view shows the common hepatic duct (CHD) and cystic duct (CD). Note the long parallel course that they assume when the cystic duct inserts low. **B,** Transverse view of the head of the pancreas (P) shows the anterior common hepatic duct (CHD) and the posterior cystic duct (CD).

posterior and right lateral aspect of the head of the pancreas. From an anterior epigastric approach, the superior mesenteric vein can usually be seen in a longitudinal plane, running posterior to the body of the pancreas. Angling the transducer to the patient's right will then visualize the pancreatic head and eventually the bile duct. If overlying bowel gas is a problem, pressure can be applied with the transducer to push the gas out of the way. In some cases it is necessary to have the patient drink water to displace gas out of the stomach and duodenum. Changing the patient from a supine to an upright position is also occasionally useful. When the anterior epigastric approach fails to allow visualization of the distal common duct, a right lateral or anterolateral approach with the patient in a left posterior oblique position frequently allows the distal common duct to be visualized in a semicoronal plane. Another useful technique is to position the patient (usually in a left posterior oblique or left lateral decubitus position) so that the gallbladder is directly over the head of the pancreas. This allows the gallbladder to be used as an acoustic window. Another technique used to deal with overlying gastric or duodenal gas is to position the patient in a right lateral decubitus position until the gas moves out of these structures. Then the patient can be moved into a supine or left lateral decubitus position to re-image the bile duct.

BILIARY OBSTRUCTION

Obstructed bile ducts are diagnosed sonographically by finding ductal dilatation. The normal intrahepatic bile ducts can be seen in many patients as parallel channels adjacent to portal veins. Normal intrahepatic ducts should not be more than 40% of the diameter of the adjacent portal vein, and peripheral ducts should not be

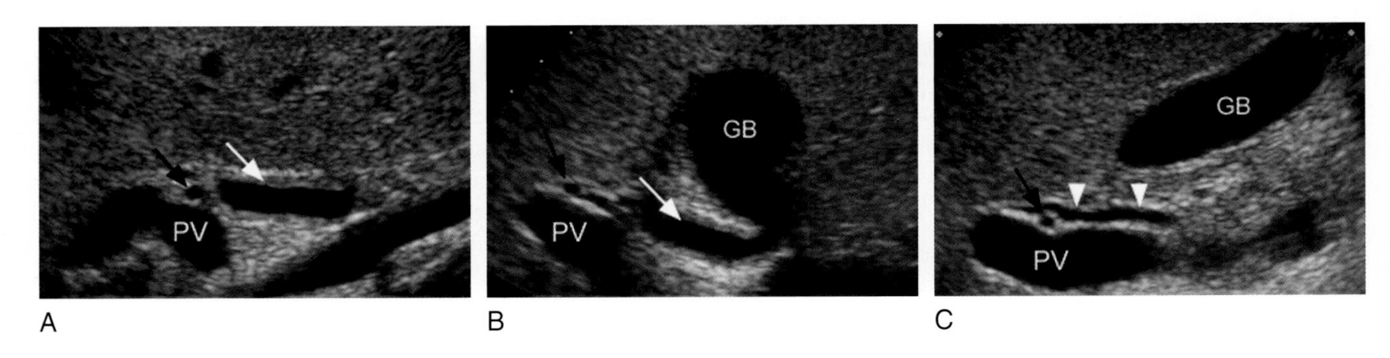

Figure 4-4 Gallbladder neck simulating the common duct. **A,** Longitudinal view of the porta hepatis shows a tubular structure *(white arrow)* simulating the common duct. **B,** At a slightly different plane, it is evident that this structure communicates with the gallbladder (GB) and is the gallbladder neck. **C,** At another plane, the real common duct is identified *(arrowheads)*. Also seen on these views are the portal vein (PV) and the right hepatic artery *(black arrow)*.

more than 2 mm in diameter (Fig. 4-5A and B). Dilated intrahepatic ducts can be distinguished from portal veins by their tortuosity or wall irregularity, by the presence of increased through transmission, and by a stellate configuration centrally (Fig. 4-5C and D). Doppler analysis is useful for confirmation and as an aid in equivocal cases. Doppler analysis is also helpful for distinguishing between an enlarged hepatic artery and a dilated duct (see Fig. 4-5E and F). Confusion occurs most often in the setting of portal hypertension when hepatic arterial flow increases to compensate for decreased portal venous flow (Box 4-1).

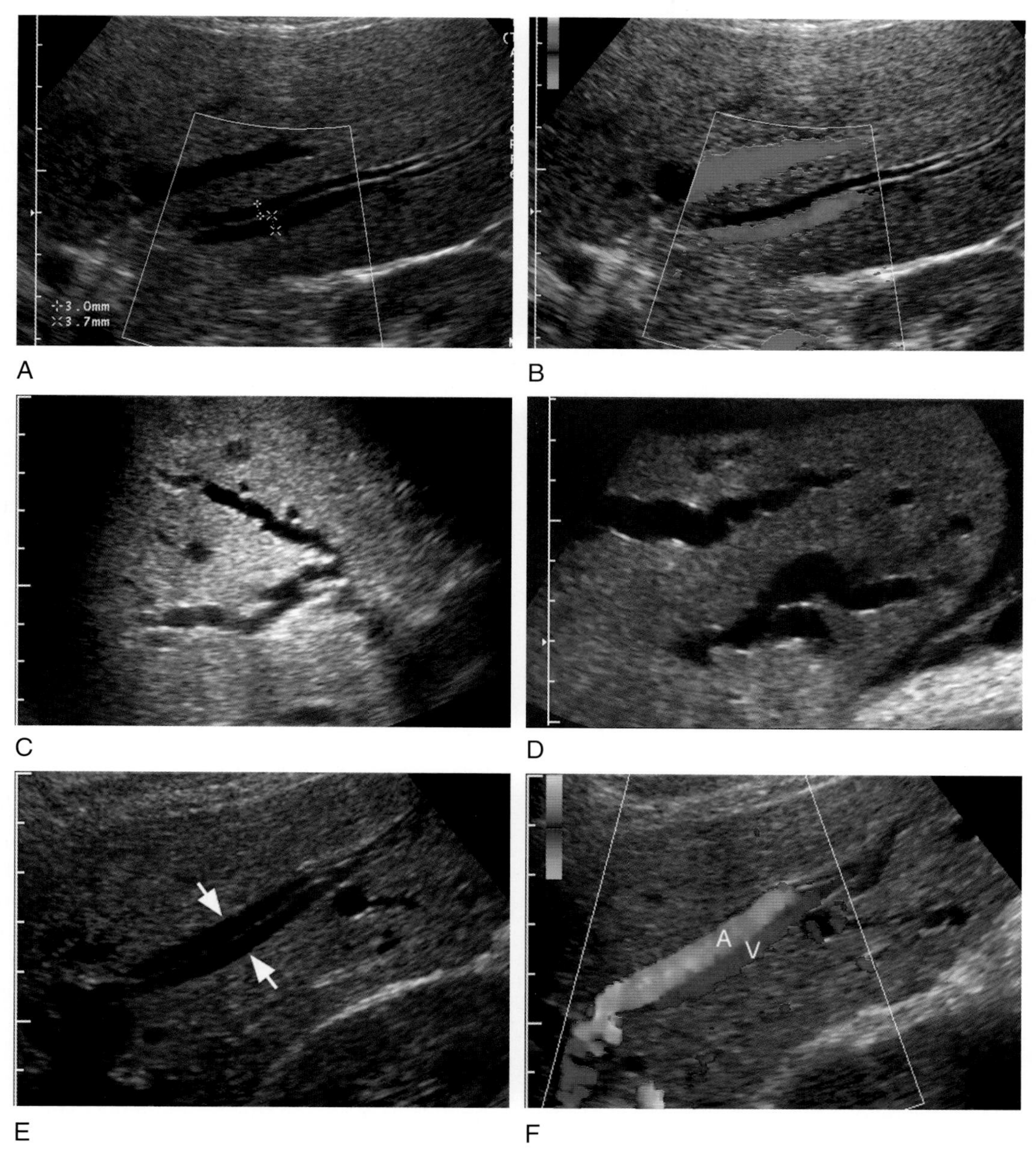

Figure 4-5 Dilated intrahepatic ducts in different patients. Gray-scale (**A**) and color Doppler (**B**) views of the liver show the parallel channel sign with adjacent tubular structures measuring 3.0 and 3.7 mm. Color Doppler view shows that the larger posterior structure is vascular, and further analysis indicated it was an intrahepatic portal vein. The anterior structure is not vascular and consistent with a bile duct. Because it exceeds 2 mm and 40% of the diameter of the adjacent portal vein, it is dilated. **C,** Single dilated duct with an irregular appearance and with some posterior enhancement. **D,** Multiple dilated ducts assuming a tortuous configuration. Gray-scale (**E**) and color Doppler (**F**) views show a parallel channel sign *(arrows)* owing to a portal vein (V) and a dilated hepatic artery (A). This potential pitfall should be considered in patients with conditions that can lead to dilated hepatic arteries. This patient had hereditary hemorrhagic telangiectasia (Osler-Weber-Rendu disease) and multiple intrahepatic arterioportal fistulas.

Box 4-1 Criteria for Dilated Intrahepatic Ducts

Larger than 2 mm diameter
More than 40% of diameter of adjacent portal vein
Increased through transmission
Irregular, tortuous walls
Stellate configuration centrally
Lack of Doppler signal

There is not a universally accepted approach to the detection of extrahepatic ductal dilatation. The least restricted segment of the bile duct is the mid segment (between the right hepatic artery and pancreas), so this is the segment that dilates first in the setting of obstruction. This segment is generally considered dilated when it is 7 mm or greater in inner diameter. However, this measurement is not universally applicable in all situations. In particular, the common duct enlarges with age and, although it remains somewhat controversial, most sonologists believe that the duct enlarges after a cholecystectomy. Therefore, mid-duct diameters that exceed 7 mm may be normal in elderly patients and in postcholecystectomy patients.

Another approach is to measure the proximal duct where it crosses the right hepatic artery. At this level, the duct is usually considered dilated when it exceeds 4 mm in diameter. The advantage of this approach is that the proximal duct is more reliably visualized than the mid duct. The disadvantage is that this segment may not dilate as early as the mid duct. Another complicating factor is that acute, intermittent, and partial obstruction may be present in the absence of ductal dilatation at any level.

Because a dilated common duct may not be obstructed and an obstructed duct may not be dilated, unequivocal reliance on a specified upper limit of normal is a mistake. A better approach is to detect an obstructing lesion that is responsible for the dilated ducts or for the patient's clinical symptoms. It is also helpful to analyze the morphology of the duct. For instance, a duct that is mildly dilated at all levels is more likely to be obstructed than a duct that is mildly dilated at the mid level but tapers in the proximal and distal segment.

Evaluation of the ductal response to a fatty meal has also been reported to be helpful in patients with equivocal duct diameters. In normal patients a fatty meal will produce either no change or a decrease in the common duct diameter. This occurs because fatty meals cause the sphincter of Oddi to relax and allows bile to drain from unobstructed bile ducts. In patients with obstructed ducts, relaxation of the sphincter has no effect on biliary drainage and the other effects of fatty meals—increased bile production and gallbladder contraction—cause the common duct diameter to increase by 1 mm or more. Although response to fatty meals has theoretical advantages, this technique has not gained widespread acceptance, primarily owing to difficulties in reproducing the exact level of measurement and the acoustic window used before and after a fatty meal.

In addition to distinguishing obstructive from nonobstructive jaundice, another major role of sonography is to determine the level and cause of obstruction. In jaundiced patients, sonography can determine the level of obstruction in more than 90% of the patients and can identify the cause of obstruction in approximately 80%. In patients with nonobstructive jaundice, liver biopsy and clinical data are generally used to determine the exact cause.

CHOLEDOCHOLITHIASIS

Choledocholithiasis is one of the most common causes of biliary obstruction. As with gallbladder stones, ductal stones classically appear as hyperechoic, shadowing, intraductal structures (Fig. 4-6A and B). Unlike gallbladder stones, in approximately 20% of the cases it is not possible to demonstrate an acoustic shadow behind a ductal stone (see Fig. 4-6C and D). This likely is related to the lack of a significant amount of bile surrounding ductal stones. In addition, it is usually not possible to show mobility of ductal stones.

Most stones are located in the most distal portion of the intrapancreatic duct near the ampulla of Vater. Methods for visualizing this segment include scanning after the oral administration of water, scanning with the patient in an upright or right posterior oblique position, and using the gallbladder as a window when the patient is in a left posterior oblique position (see Fig. 4-6E). In some cases it is difficult to determine if an echogenic focus is in the duct or adjacent to the duct on longitudinal images. Sequential transverse images can be very helpful in resolving this problem (see Fig. 4-6F).

The reported sensitivity of sonography for detecting ductal stones varies greatly. The best sensitivity that has been reported is approximately 75%. Most false-negative results are due to failure to visualize the distal common bile duct. Although 25% or more of ductal stones may not be visualized sonographically, most of these patients will have dilated ducts and will eventually undergo some form of cholangiography to establish the cause of obstruction. False-positive results also occur but are less

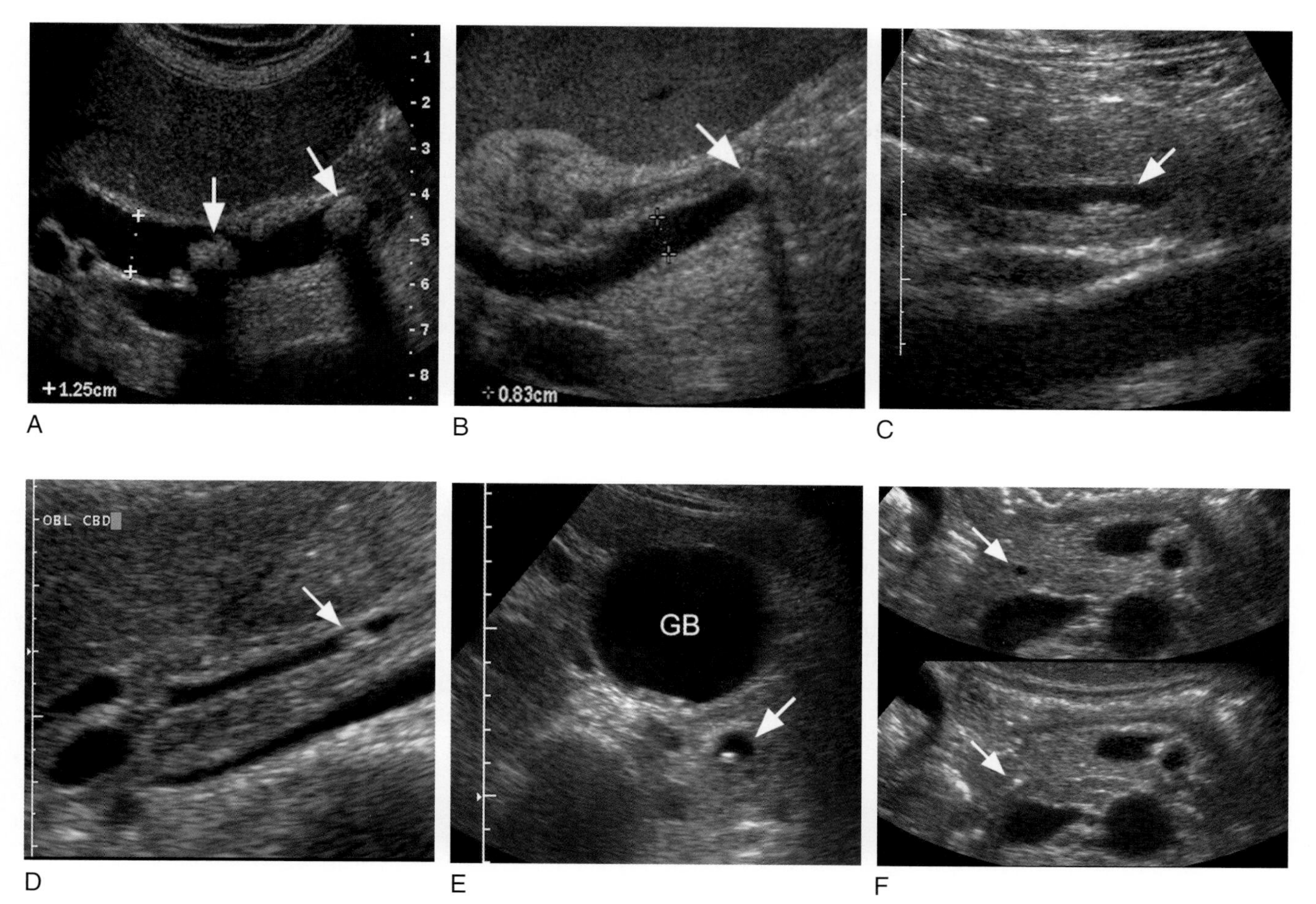

Figure 4-6 Common bile duct stones in different patients. **A,** Dilated (1.25 cm) bile duct *(cursors)* containing two large shadowing stones *(arrows)*. **B,** Dilated (0.83 cm) bile duct *(cursors)* with a shadowing stone *(arrow)* impacted in the distal aspect. This is the most common location for bile duct stones. **C,** Dilated distal duct with several small non-shadowing stones *(arrow)*. **D,** Non-dilated distal duct with a single small non-shadowing stone *(arrow)*. **E,** Transverse view using the gallbladder (GB) as a window shows a small bile duct stone *(arrow)*. **F,** Dual adjacent transverse views of the pancreatic head show the non-dilated bile duct *(arrow)* on the upper image and the small stone *(arrow)* on the lower image.

common than false-negative results. Calcifications in the hepatic artery and pancreatic head (Fig. 4-7A), and gas in duodenal diverticula can sometimes be confused with ductal stones (see Fig. 4-7B). In all these instances transverse views of the duct are valuable for distinguishing between an intraductal and periductal abnormality. In rare instances the cystic duct insertion can simulate a stone. Recognition of the possibility of this pitfall is usually enough to avert misinterpretation.

Intrahepatic duct stones are much less common than common bile duct stones. Unlike extrahepatic duct stones that form in the gallbladder and pass into the duct, intrahepatic duct stones tend to form primarily in the bile ducts and typically are a complication of some other biliary tract abnormality. Most primary biliary stones are pigment stones that form from bacterial deconjugation of bilirubin diglucuronide. Predisposing factors are bile stasis and bacterial infection (usually enteric organisms). Recurrent pyogenic cholangitis (also known as oriental cholangiohepatitis) is a common cause of primary duct stones in Asian populations. Biliary flukes such as *Clonorchis sinensis* or *Ascaris lumbricoides* result in superimposed bacterial infection, and this leads to stone formation. Intrahepatic duct stones may be single, but they are often multiple and literally pack the lumen of the duct. They are softer than common bile duct stones and are even less likely to produce a shadow (Fig. 4-8).

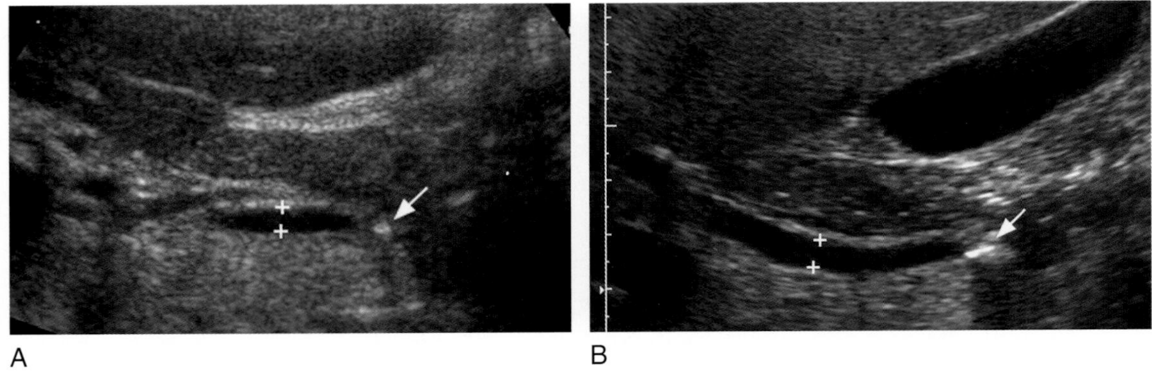

Figure 4-7 Pitfalls for common duct stones in different patients. **A,** Longitudinal view of the distal bile duct *(cursors)* shows a small pancreatic calcification *(arrow)* immediately adjacent to the duct. **B,** Longitudinal view of the distal duct *(cursors)* shows gas in a duodenal diverticulum *(arrow)* immediately adjacent to the duct.

Intrabiliary gas is occasionally indistinguishable from stones (Fig. 4-9). In most cases gas produces a brighter reflection and dirtier shadow than do stones. A ring-down artifact is only seen behind gas and, when found, can be used to confirm the diagnosis of pneumobilia (see Fig. 4-9B). Gas is also more likely to move. Extensively calcified intrahepatic arteries can also simulate ductal stones. In many cases the double line from the anterior and posterior wall can be seen with calcified arteries (Fig. 4-10). When this is not evident, a survey of the kidneys and spleen will usually show extensive arterial calcification as well and assist in the diagnosis.

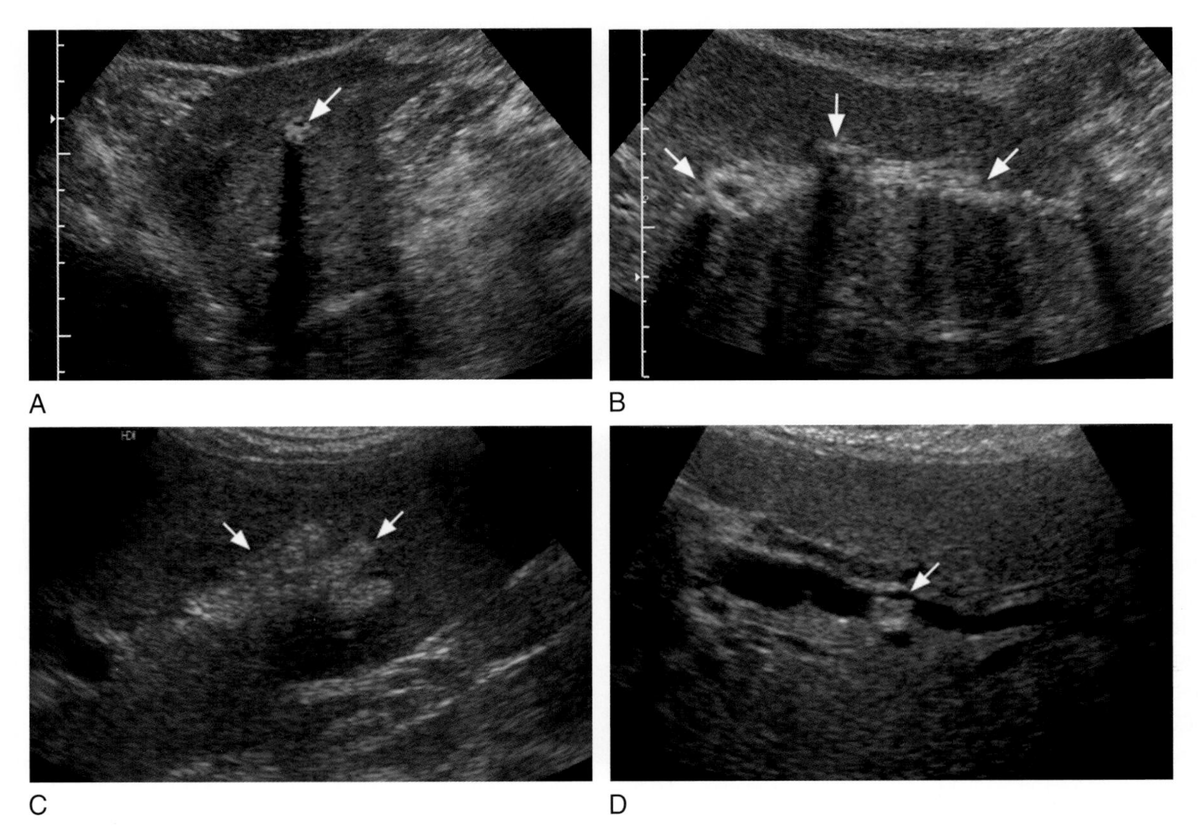

Figure 4-8 Intrahepatic duct stones in different patients. Longitudinal (**A**) and transverse (**B**) views of the left lobe of the liver show shadowing echogenic structures *(arrows)* in a linear pattern typical of stones. **C,** View of the liver shows markedly dilated, branching ducts completely filled with slightly shadowing stones *(arrows)*. **D,** View of a dilated intrahepatic duct shows a single non-shadowing stone *(arrow)*.

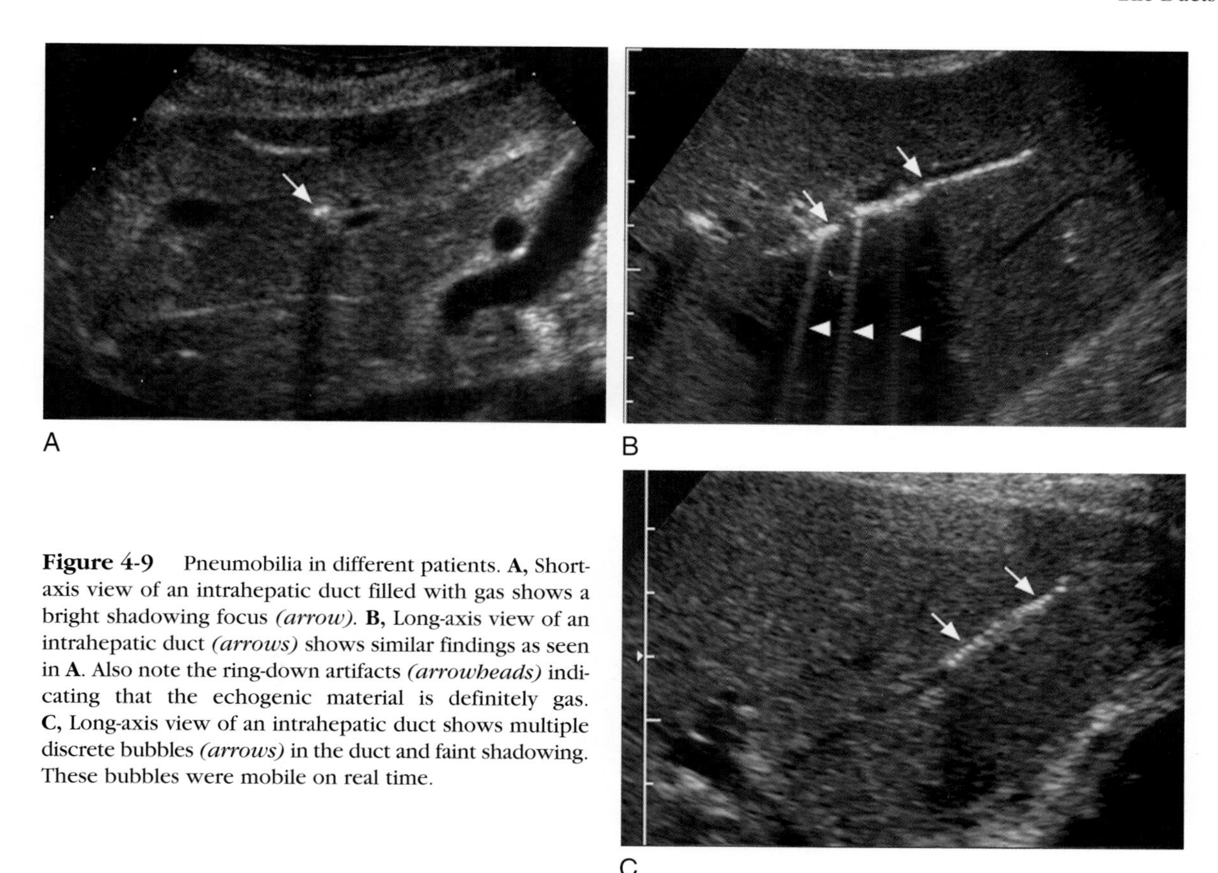

Figure 4-9 Pneumobilia in different patients. **A,** Short-axis view of an intrahepatic duct filled with gas shows a bright shadowing focus *(arrow)*. **B,** Long-axis view of an intrahepatic duct *(arrows)* shows similar findings as seen in **A**. Also note the ring-down artifacts *(arrowheads)* indicating that the echogenic material is definitely gas. **C,** Long-axis view of an intrahepatic duct shows multiple discrete bubbles *(arrows)* in the duct and faint shadowing. These bubbles were mobile on real time.

Abdominal radiographs can also assist in distinguishing bile duct stones, pneumobilia, and hepatic artery calcification.

CHOLANGIOCARCINOMA

Cancer of the bile ducts occurs most commonly at the bifurcation of the common hepatic duct, with involvement of both the central left and right duct. Tumors at this location are referred to as Klatskin tumors. Bile duct cancer occurs less frequently in the distal and mid duct. Approximately 5% of cholangiocarcinomas are multicentric. In the most common pattern of growth, the tumor infiltrates the duct wall and produces a focal stricture. Much less commonly, cholangiocarcinomas grow either as an intraluminal polypoid mass or in a diffuse sclerosing pattern. In many patients the tumors are unresectable because of invasion of the liver, involvement of more peripheral ductal branches, or vascular invasion.

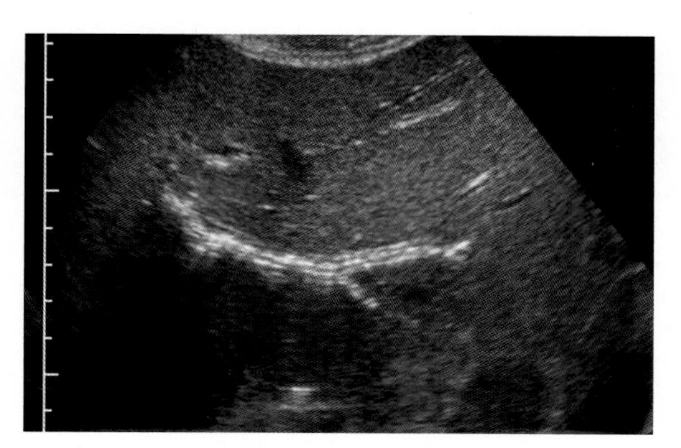

Figure 4-10 Intrahepatic arterial calcification. View of the liver shows a linear echogenic structure with some shadowing. Note the anterior and posterior wall of the artery producing two bright parallel lines. In some cases this will distinguish arterial calcification from pneumobilia and ductal stones.

The sonographic appearance of cholangiocarcinoma is illustrated in Figure 4-11. In most cases cholangiocarcinomas appear as a dilated duct that abruptly terminates at the level of the tumor. A mass may or may not be seen to explain the obstruction. When detected, the tumor itself is usually poorly marginated and is close to the same echogenicity as the liver. Klatskin tumors classically appear as dilated intrahepatic ducts with no communication between the left and right duct system. Focal thickening of the bile duct wall without a mass is an uncommon but well-described sonographic appearance of cholangiocarcinoma. Polypoid intraluminal masses are only rarely encountered. The differential diagnosis of cholangiocarcinoma depends on its location. Lesions

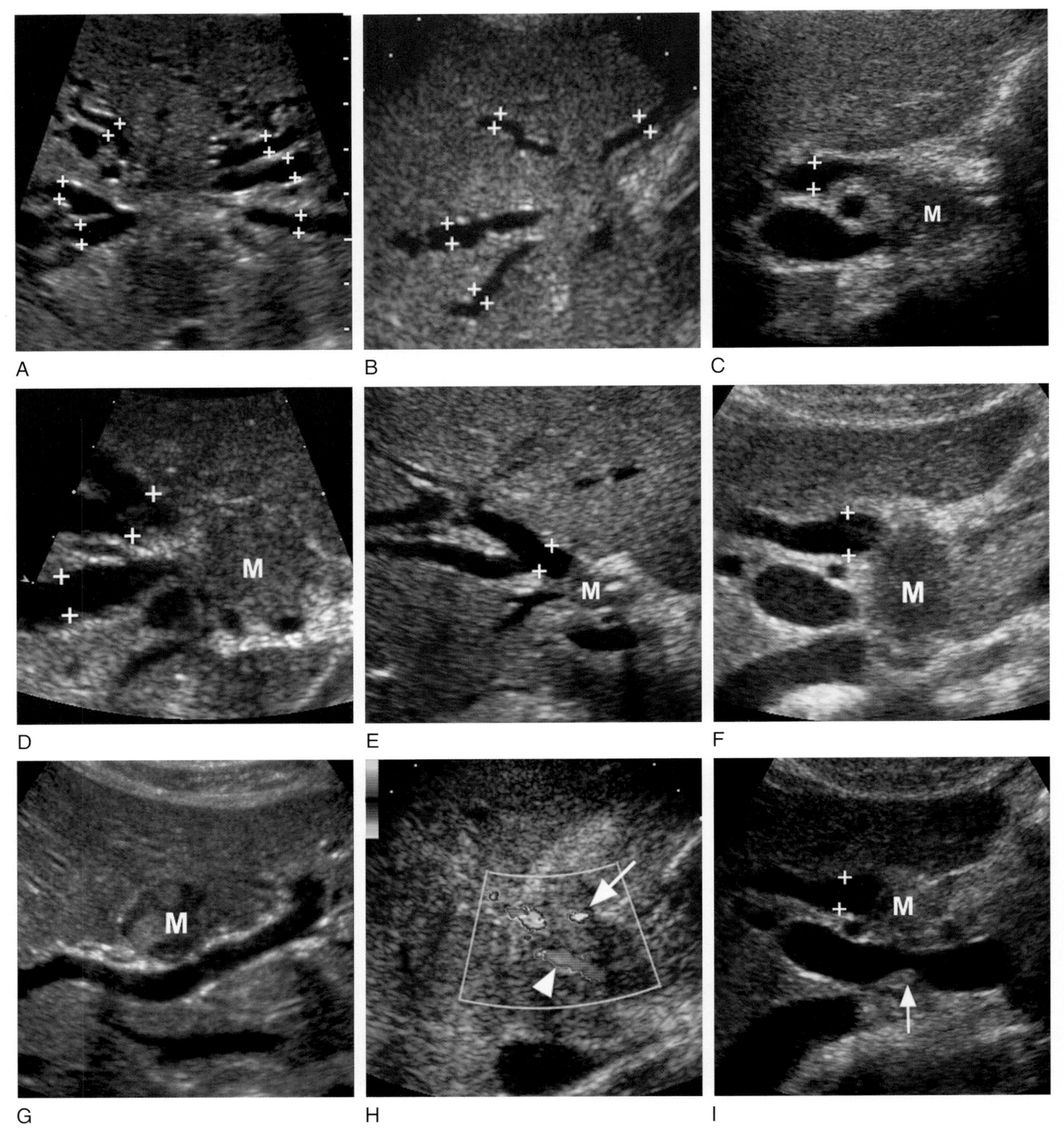

Figure 4-11 Cholangiocarcinoma in different patients. **A** and **B,** Multiple ducts *(cursors)* from the right and left lobe terminate abruptly near their confluence without communicating with each other. The site of termination defines a central isoechoic mass. **C** to **F,** Views showing obstructed, dilated ducts *(cursors)*, all of which terminate at the level of a soft tissue mass (M). **G,** View of the liver shows an intrahepatic cholangiocarcinoma as a heterogeneous solid mass (M) anterior to the portal bifurcation. There are no associated obstructed ducts. **H,** Doppler view of the porta hepatis shows a soft tissue mass encasing the hepatic artery *(arrow)* and narrowing the portal vein *(arrowhead)*. This indicates vascular invasion. **I,** View of the porta hepatis shows a poorly defined hyperechoic mass (M) causing dilatation of the duct *(cursors)* and encasing and narrowing the portal vein *(arrow)*.

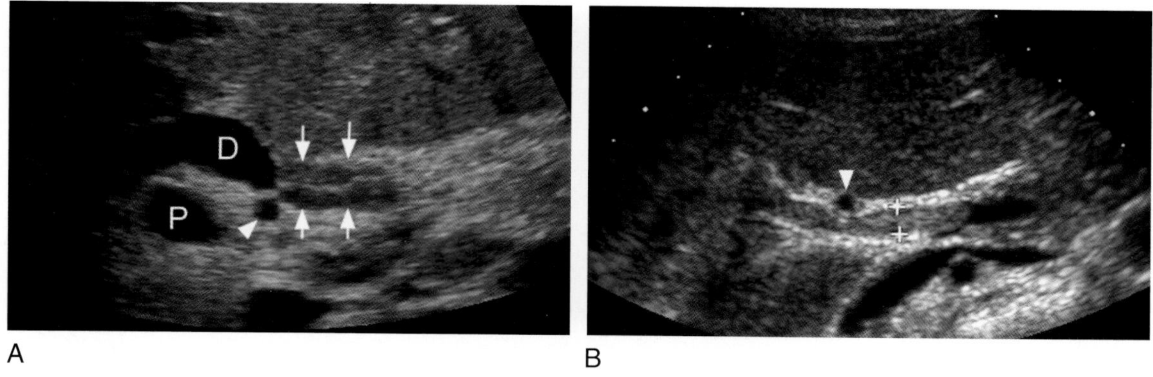

Figure 4-12 Metastatic disease to the bile duct in different patients. **A,** Longitudinal view of the common duct (D) shows ductal dilatation with abrupt wall thickening *(arrows)* that obliterates the lumen and produces a thin central white line. This was due to metastatic bronchogenic cancer. This appearance can also be seen with primary bile duct cancer. The portal vein (P) and hepatic artery *(arrowhead)* are also seen. **B,** Longitudinal view of the common duct shows a polypoid hyperechoic filling defect *(cursors)* in the lumen that arose from a more peripheral colon cancer hepatic metastasis. The duct is posterior to the hepatic artery *(arrowhead).*

at the ductal confluence can be due to gallbladder carcinoma and hepatocellular cancer. Pancreatic or ampullary cancer can cause lesions in the distal duct. Metastatic disease to the duct (Fig. 4-12) or adjacent nodes can simulate cholangiocarcinoma at any level.

Obtaining histologic proof of the diagnosis of cholangiocarcinoma can be difficult. Biopsies obtained endoluminally at the time of endoscopic retrograde cholangiography are usually attempted but are often negative. When the lesion is visible on sonography, ultrasound-guided biopsies can be a valuable way of obtaining a tissue diagnosis.

Once the diagnosis is suspected or confirmed, sonography and Doppler imaging can serve as complementary tools to CT and MRI in determining the resectability of the lesion. Hepatic metastases, invasion of the portal vein, and encasement of the hepatic artery located in strategic locations are all generally regarded as signs of nonresectability (see Fig. 4-11H and I). Intraoperative sonography and laparoscopic sonography are also both helpful in detecting signs of nonresectability.

BILE DUCT WALL THICKENING

Thickening of the bile duct wall is a nonspecific finding that is becoming more evident with continuing improvements in image resolution. The bile duct walls are normally displayed as single bright lines, which actually represent the reflection between the wall and the bile in the lumen. When the wall becomes thick, it may be resolved as a layer of tissue separate from the luminal reflection. This layer is almost always hypoechoic (Fig. 4-13).

An important cause of bile duct thickening is sclerosing cholangitis, which is characterized by fibrotic thickening of the bile ducts and adjacent fibrofatty tissues. Patients initially exhibit a cholestatic picture, and cirrhosis and its complications may then ensue. It most frequently affects young men and is strongly associated with inflammatory bowel disease, especially ulcerative colitis. It affects the intrahepatic and extrahepatic ducts in the majority of patients and occasionally involves the gallbladder and cystic duct. The wall thickening may appear smooth or irregular. In addition, multifocal strictures and beading develop in the intrahepatic ducts. These are optimally displayed by cholangiography and are difficult to see on sonography. Sonography more reliably detects intrahepatic disease when the strictures are associated with ductal dilatation.

Patients with sclerosing cholangitis are predisposed to the development of cholangiocarcinoma. It is generally not possible to detect coexistent sclerosing cholangitis and cholangiocarcinoma sonographically. However, cancer should be suspected whenever biliary centered or hepatic parenchymal mass lesions are detected in a patient with sclerosing cholangitis. Duct wall thickening greater than 5 mm and disproportionately dilated intrahepatic ducts should also raise the suspicion of cholangiocarcinoma. It is not uncommon to see prominent nodes in the porta hepatis in patients with uncomplicated sclerosing cholangitis. This is therefore not a reliable sign of metastatic disease stemming from superimposed cholangiocarcinoma.

Other causes of bile duct wall thickening include choledocholithiasis, indwelling stents, AIDS cholangiopathy, pancreatitis, and recurrent pyogenic cholangitis (Box 4-2). AIDS cholangiopathy is most often due to

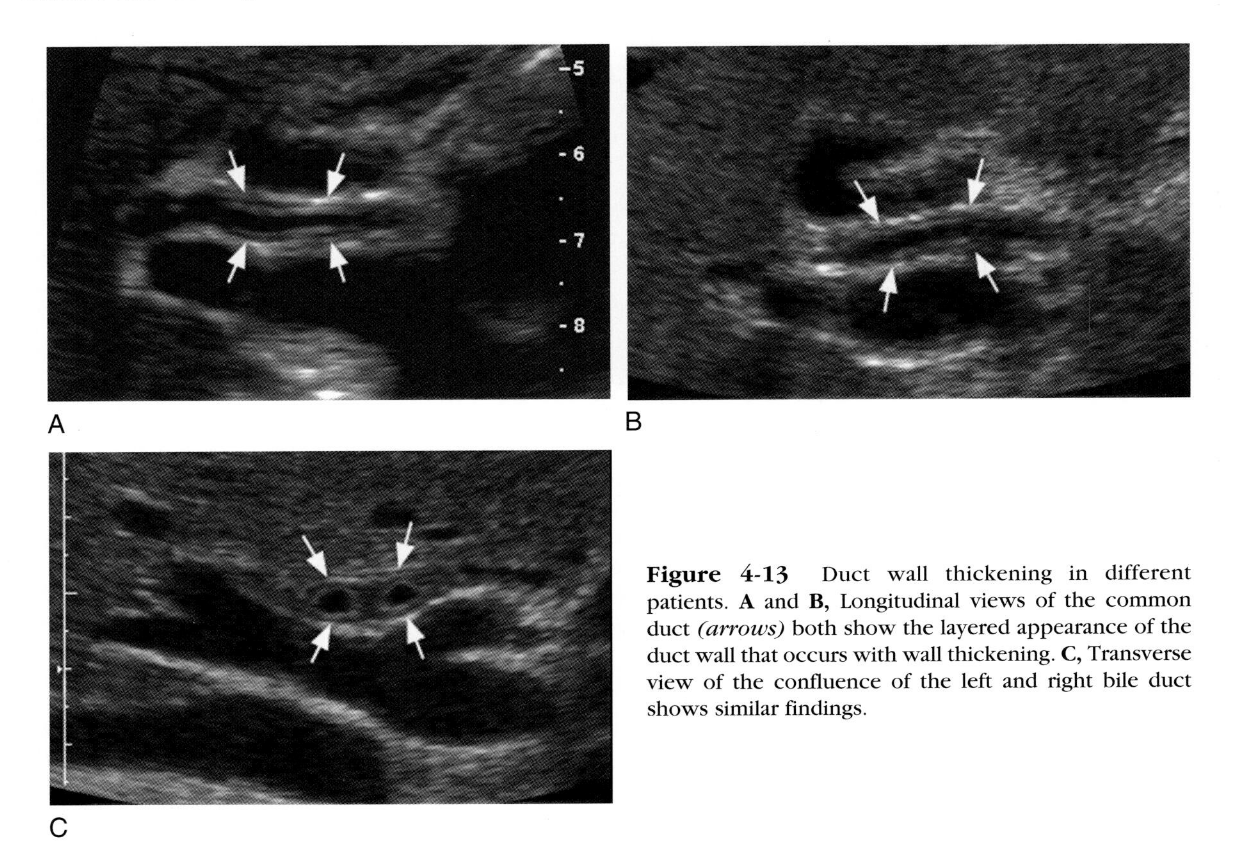

Figure 4-13 Duct wall thickening in different patients. **A** and **B,** Longitudinal views of the common duct *(arrows)* both show the layered appearance of the duct wall that occurs with wall thickening. **C,** Transverse view of the confluence of the left and right bile duct shows similar findings.

infection with cytomegalovirus or *Cryptosporidium* organisms. There are two forms: one that exactly mimics sclerosing cholangitis and one that produces isolated papillary stenosis (Fig. 4-14). An unusual cause of duct wall thickening is portal vein thrombosis with intramural collaterals (Fig. 4-15). This is important to recognize because interventional procedures carry a much higher risk of hemorrhage.

Box 4-2 Causes of Bile Duct Wall Thickening

- Sclerosing cholangitis
- Common bile duct stones
- Pancreatitis
- Ascending cholangitis
- AIDS cholangiopathy
- Cholangiocarcinoma
- Recurrent pyogenic cholangitis
- Biliary stents
- Intramural venous collaterals

CYSTIC DISEASE

Cystic lesions of the bile ducts are very unusual and occur more commonly in girls and women. They are believed to develop as the result of an anomalous connection of the common bile duct and pancreatic duct, such that pancreatic secretions can reflux into the biliary tract. Classification schemes vary, but all agree on the

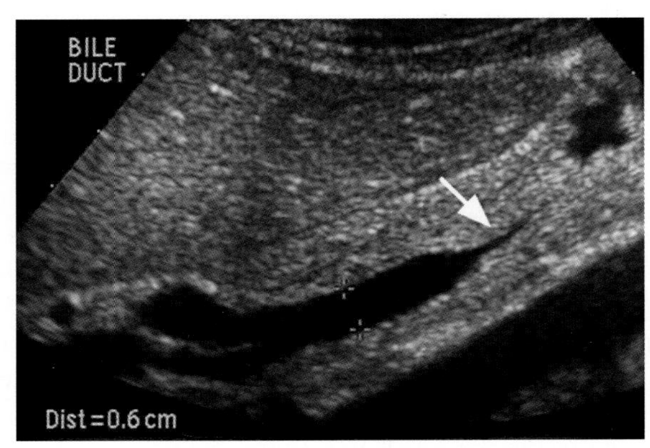

Figure 4-14 AIDS cholangitis. Longitudinal view of the common bile duct *(cursors)* in a young HIV-positive man shows mild duct dilatation and abrupt narrowing at the level of the ampulla *(arrow).*

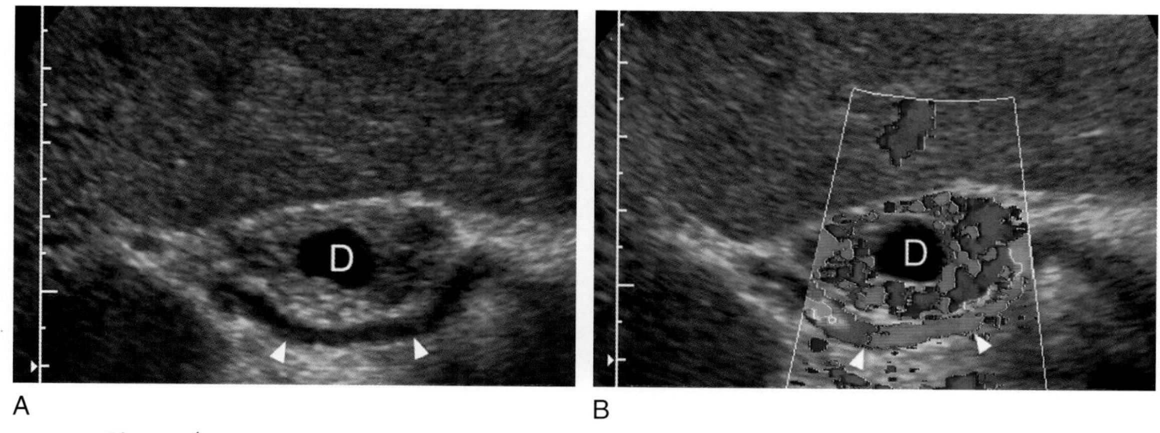

Figure 4-15 Choledochal collaterals due to portal vein thrombosis. **A,** Transverse view of a dilated common duct (D) shows marked thickening of the duct wall. The hepatic artery *(arrowheads)* is seen posterior to the duct. **B,** Color Doppler view shows multiple collateral veins in the duct wall.

definitions of types 1 through 3. The most common is type 1, which is a fusiform dilatation of the extrahepatic duct (Fig. 4-16). Type 2 is a diverticular outpouching of the extrahepatic duct. Type 3 is a choledochocele, which is a dilatation of the distal intramural portion of the common bile duct that protrudes into the duodenum. Some authorities define type 4 as multifocal dilatations of the intrahepatic and extrahepatic bile ducts and type 5 as Caroli's disease.

The classic clinical triad of choledochal cysts is jaundice (occurring in approximately 80%), a palpable mass (occurring in approximately 50%), and abdominal pain (occurring in approximately 50%). Although choledochal cysts are typically thought of as pediatric lesions, they are occasionally first detected during adulthood. The differential diagnosis includes cysts of the liver, right kidney, duodenum, mesentery, and omentum, as well as pancreatic pseudocysts and hepatic artery aneurysms (Box 4-3).

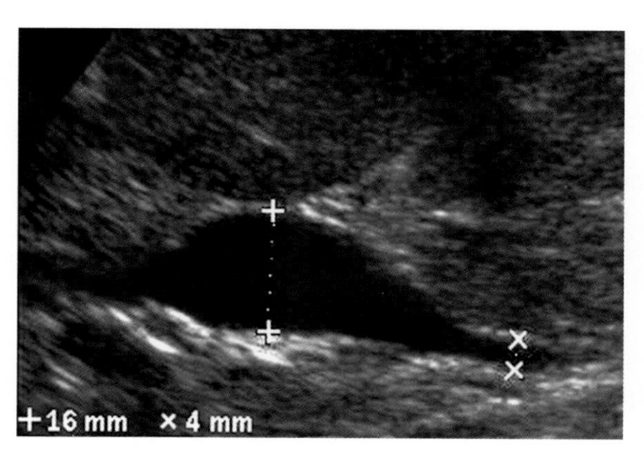

Figure 4-16 Choledochal cyst. Longitudinal view of the common bile duct shows fusiform dilatation of the mid duct (+ *cursors,* diameter 16 mm) and normal tapering in the distal duct (× *cursors,* diameter 4 mm).

Caroli's disease is characterized by multifocal saccular dilatation of the intrahepatic bile ducts with sparing of the extrahepatic ducts. In its classic form, patients exhibit multiple complications of biliary stasis, including ductal stones and obstruction, cholangitis, and liver abscesses. More commonly it is associated with hepatic fibrosis, which leads to portal hypertension and variceal bleeding. Cystic disease of the kidney, including medullary sponge disease (tubular ectasia), is also strongly associated with Caroli's disease. In fact, the dominant clinical feature may be renal failure rather than biliary disease.

The sonographic features of Caroli's disease are illustrated in Figure 4-17. Cystic intrahepatic lesions are the hallmark. In most cases it is possible to document communication with the bile ducts and the diagnosis is straightforward. A very specific sonographic sign of Caroli's disease is the "central dot" sign, which occurs when the dilated segment of the bile duct surrounds the adjacent hepatic artery and portal vein so that these vascular structures produce a small focus in the middle of the dilated duct. Sonographically detectable complications such as intrahepatic duct stones and secondary signs of portal hypertension should be searched for in

Box 4-3 Differential Diagnosis of Choledochal Cysts

Duplication cyst of duodenum
Dilated cystic duct remnant
Omental or mesenteric cyst
Pancreatic pseudocyst
Right renal cyst
Hepatic cyst
Aneurysm/pseudoaneurysm

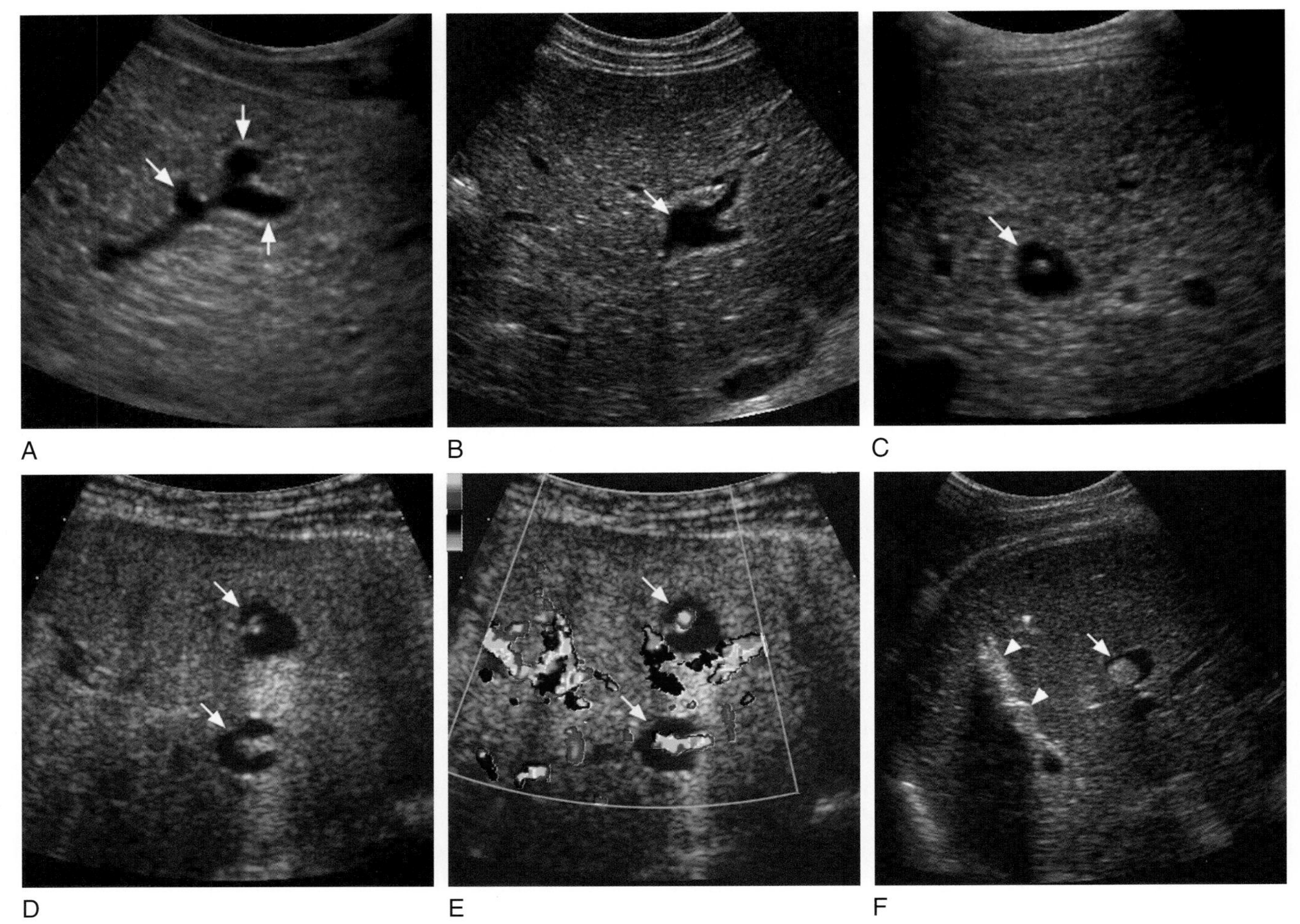

Figure 4-17 Caroli's disease in different patients. **A** and **B**, Views of the liver show areas of saccular dilatation *(arrows)* of the bile ducts. **C**, Central dot sign *(arrow)*. **D** and **E**, Gray-scale and color Doppler views show two central dot signs *(arrows)* with blood flow identified within the central vessels. **F**, Shadowing stones complicating a case of Caroli's disease are seen filling one duct *(arrowheads)*, and a single large non-shadowing stone is seen in another duct *(arrow)*.

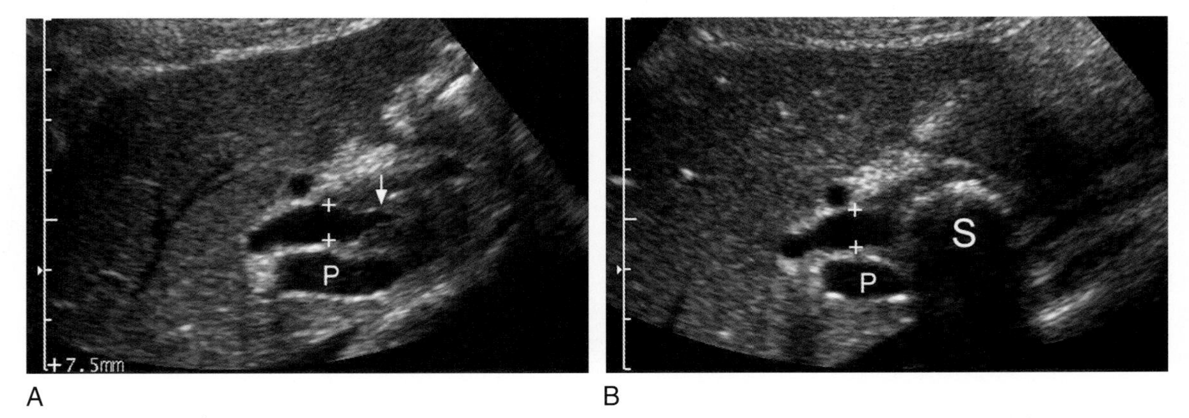

Figure 4-18 Mirrizi's syndrome. **A**, Longitudinal view of a dilated common duct *(cursors)* shows gradual tapering *(arrow)* at the porta hepatis. The portal vein (P) is seen posteriorly. **B**, Longitudinal view adjacent to the view in **A** shows a shadowing stone (S) at the level of tapering. Other views showed that the stone was in the neck of the gallbladder.

patients with Caroli's disease. Occasionally, Caroli's disease can be confused with biliary obstruction or multiple hepatic cysts. When the diagnosis is in doubt, cholangiography or hepatobiliary scintigraphy can then be used to document the communication between the cystic lesions and the bile ducts.

MIRIZZI'S SYNDROME

Mirizzi's syndrome is a rare abnormality that consists of a common duct obstruction caused by a gallstone in the cystic duct or the gallbladder neck. This is more likely to occur with a low inserting cystic duct that travels in a common sheath with the common duct. The obstruction may be caused by the actual mass effect of the stone or by an associated inflammatory reaction in the hepatoduodenal ligament. It is a particular problem for the surgeon because it may be difficult to distinguish the cystic duct from the common duct, resulting in inappropriate ligation of the common duct. Therefore, preoperative knowledge of this condition is extremely valuable.

Sonographic findings can occasionally suggest the diagnosis in the setting of dilated ducts if an extrinsic mass effect from a shadowing stone is seen at the level of obstruction (Fig. 4-18). Often this is not possible, however, and the patient will need to undergo cholangiography for the diagnosis to be established. Cholangiography is also valuable for detecting the fistulas that often complicate the condition.

Key Features

The proximal common duct normally runs anterior to the portal vein and right hepatic artery. A common variant occurs when the hepatic artery runs anterior to the common duct.

The proximal common duct normally runs to the right of the proper hepatic artery. These structures form the ears and the portal vein forms the head in the "Mickey Mouse" view.

Biliary obstruction is suspected when the bile ducts are dilated. There is no magic diameter that distinguishes an obstructed common duct from an unobstructed duct. The patient's age, history of cholecystectomy, and the location of the diameter measurements are important factors in interpreting the significance of common duct size.

Dilated intrahepatic ducts produce the "parallel channel" sign. With more severe dilatation, the intrahepatic ducts become tortuous and irregular and produce posterior enhancement.

Enlarged intrahepatic arteries can simulate dilated ducts.

The detection of choledocholithiasis is improved by concentrating on the most distal intrapancreatic portion of the common bile duct. At best, the sensitivity is 75%.

Bile duct stones are less likely to shadow than gallstones.

Cholangiocarcinoma should be suspected when there is abrupt termination of a dilated duct with no visible mass or a mass that is nearly isoechoic to liver. It is most frequently located at the confluence of the right and left hepatic ducts.

Duct wall thickening is seen as a hyperechoic inner layer and a hypoechoic outer layer.

Choledochal cysts should be considered when cystic lesions are detected in the hepatoduodenal ligament. The most common appearance is focal fusiform dilatation of the common bile duct.

Caroli's disease produces segmental saccular dilatation of the intrahepatic ducts and is usually associated with hepatic fibrosis and renal cystic disease.

The "central dot" sign is classic for Caroli's disease and is caused by the dilated bile duct surrounding the adjacent hepatic artery and portal vein.

Mirizzi's syndrome consists of a common bile duct obstruction resulting from a stone in the cystic duct or gallbladder neck.

SUGGESTED READINGS

Babbit DP, Starshak RJ, Clemett AR: Choledochal cyst: A concept of etiology. AJR Am J Roentgenol 119:57, 1973.

Becker CD, Hassler H, Terrier F: Preoperative diagnosis of Mirizzi syndrome: Limitations of sonography and computed tomography. AJR Am J Roentgenol 143:591, 1984.

Bloom CM, Langer B, Wilson SR: Role of US in the detection, characterization, and staging of cholangiocarcinoma. Radiographics 19:1199-1218, 1999.

Brandt DJ, et al: Gallbladder disease in patients with primary sclerosing cholangitis. AJR Am J Roentgenol 150:571, 1988.

Bressler EL, Rubin JM, McCracken S: Sonographic parallel channel sign: A reappraisal. Radiology 164:343, 1987.

Bret PM, deStempel JV, Atri M, et al: Intrahepatic bile duct and portal vein anatomy revisited. Radiology 169:405, 1988.

Buck JL, Elsayed AM: Ampullary tumors: Radiologic-pathologic correlation. Radiographics 13:193-212, 1993.

Bude RO, Bowerman RA: Biliary ascariasis. Radiology 214:844-847, 2000.

Carroll BA, Oppenheimer DA: Sclerosing cholangitis: Sonographic demonstration of bile duct wall thickening. AJR Am J Roentgenol 139:1016, 1982.

Choi BI, et al: Hilar cholangiocarcinoma: Comparative study with sonography and CT. Radiology 172:689, 1989.

Choi BI, Yeon KM, Kim SH, Han MC: Caroli disease: Central dot sign in CT. Radiology 174:161, 1990.

Coffey RJ, Wiesnet RH, Beaver SJ: Bile duct carcinoma: A late complication of end-stage primary sclerosing cholangitis. Hepatology 4:1056, 1984.

Darweesh R, et al: Fatty-meal sonography for evaluating patients with suspected partial common duct obstruction. AJR Am J Roentgenol 151:63, 1988.

Dolmatch BL, et al: AIDS-related cholangitis: Radiographic features in nine patients. Radiology 163:313, 1987.

Fulcher AS, Turner MA, Sanyal AJ: Case 38: Caroli disease and renal tubular ectasia. Radiology 220:720-723, 2001.

Gibson RN, et al: Bile duct obstruction: Radiologic evaluation of level, cause, and tumor resectability. Radiology 160:43, 1986.

Harvey RT, Miller WT Jr: Acute biliary disease: Initial CT and follow-up US versus initial US and follow-up CT. Radiology 213:831-836, 1999.

Hilger DJ, VerSteeg KR, Beaty PJ: Mirizzi syndrome with common septum: Ultrasound and computed tomography findings. J Ultrasound Med 7:409, 1988.

Kim OH, Chung HJ, Choi BG: Imaging of the choledochal cyst. Radiographics 15:69-88, 1995.

Kirby, CL, Horrow MM, Rosenberg HK, Oleaga JA: US case of the day: Oriental cholangiohepatitis. Radiographics 15:1503-1506, 1995.

Klatskin G: Adenocarcinoma of the hepatic duct at its bifurcation within the portal hepatis: An unusual tumor with distinctive clinical and pathological features. Am J Med 38:241, 1965.

Laing FC, et al: Biliary dilatation: defining the level and cause by real-time US. Radiology 160:39, 1986.

Laing FC, Jeffrey RB, Wing VW: Improved visualization of choledocholithiasis by sonography. AJR Am J Roentgenol 143:949, 1984.

Laing FC, London LA, Filly RA: Ultrasonographic identification of dilated intrahepatic bile ducts and their differentiation from portal venous structures. J Clin Ultrasound 6:73, 1978.

Levy AD, Murakata LA, Abbott RM, Rohrmann CA Jr: Benign tumors and tumorlike lesions of the gallbladder and extrahepatic bile ducts: Radiologic-pathologic correlation. Radiographics 22:387-413, 2002.

Lim JH: Oriental cholangiohepatitis: Pathologic, clinical, and radiologic features. AJR Am J Roentgenol 157:1-8, 1991.

Lim JH, et al: Oriental cholangiohepatitis: Sonographic findings in 48 cases. AJR Am J Roentgenol 155:511, 1990.

Li-Yeng C, Goldberg HI: Sclerosing cholangitis: Broad spectrum of radiographic features. Gastrointest Radiol 9:39, 1984.

MacCarty RL, et al: Cholangiocarcinoma complicating primary sclerosing cholangitis: Cholangiographic appearances. Radiology 156:43, 1985.

Marchal GJ, et al: Caroli disease: High-frequency US and pathologic findings. Radiology 158:507, 1986.

Meyer DG, Weinstein BJ: Klatskin tumors of the bile ducts: Sonographic appearance. Radiology 148:803, 1983.

Middleton WD: The bile ducts. In Goldberg BB (ed): Diagnostic Ultrasound. Baltimore, Williams & Wilkins, 1993, pp 146-172.

Miller DR, Egbert RM, Braunstein P: Comparison of ultrasound and hepatobiliary imaging in the early detection of acute total common bile duct obstruction. Arch Surg 119:1233, 1984.

Miller WJ, Sechtin AG, Campbell WL, Pieters PC: Imaging findings in Caroli's disease. AJR Am J Roentgenol 165:333-337, 1995.

Nagorney DM, McIlrath DC, Adson MA: Choledochal cysts in adults: Clinical management. Surgery 96:656, 1984.

Nesbit GM, et al: Cholangiocarcinoma: Diagnosis and evaluation of resectability by CT and sonography as procedures complementary to cholangiography. AJR Am J Roentgenol 151:933, 1988.

Parulekar SG: Transabdominal sonography of bile ducts. Ultrasound Q 18:187-202, 2002.

Ralls PW, et al: The use of color Doppler sonography to distinguish dilated intrahepatic ducts from vascular structures. AJR Am J Roentgenol 152:291, 1989.

Rizzo RJ, Szucs RA, Turner MA: Congenital abnormalities of the pancreas and biliary tree in adults. Radiographics 15:49-68, 1995.

Romano AJ, et al: Gallbladder and bile duct abnormalities in AIDS: Sonographic findings in eight patients. AJR Am J Roentgenol 150:123, 1988.

Rosenthal SJ, Cox GG, Wetzel LH, Batnitzky S: Pitfalls and differential diagnosis in biliary sonography. Radiographics 10:285-311, 1990.

Sato M, Ishida H, Donno K, et al: Choledochal cyst due to anomalous pancreatobiliary junction in the adult; sonographic findings. Abdom Imaging 26:395-400, 2001.

Schulte SJ, et al: CT of the extrahepatic bile ducts: Wall thickness and contrast enhancement in normal and abnormal ducts, AJR Am J Roentgenol 154:79, 1990.

Simeone JF, et al: The bile ducts after a fatty meal: Further sonographic observations. Radiology 154:763, 1985.

Subramanyam BR, et al: Ultrasonic features of cholangiocarcinoma. J Ultrasound Med 3:405, 1984.

Takasan H, et al: Clinicopathologic study of seventy patients with carcinoma of the biliary tract. Surg Gynecol Obstet 150:721, 1980.

Teixidor HS, Godwin TA, Ramirez EA: Cryptosporidiosis of the biliary tract in AIDS. Radiology 180:51, 1991.

Todani T, et al: Congenital bile duct cysts: Classification, operative procedures, and review of thirty-seven cases including cancer arising from choledochal cyst. Am J Surg 134:263, 1977.

Tublin ME, Tessler FN, Rifkin MD: US case of the day: Acquired immunodeficiency syndrome (AIDS)-related *(Cryptosporidium)* cholangitis and *Cryptosporidium* colitis. Radiographics 18:1043-1045, 1998.

Turner MA, Fulcher AS: The cystic duct: Normal anatomy and disease processes. Radiographics 21:3-22, 2001.

Wiesner RH, LaRusso NF: Clinicopathologic features of the syndrome of primary sclerosing cholangitis. Gastroenterology 79:200, 1980.

Wu CC, Ho Y-H, Chen C-Y: Effect of aging on common bile duct diameter: A real-time ultrasonographic study. J Clin Ultrasound 12:473, 1984.

Yeung EYC, et al: The ultrasonographic appearance of hilar cholangiocarcinoma (Klatskin tumours). Br J Radiol 61:991, 1988.

CHAPTER 5

Kidney

For Key Features summary see p. 148

ANATOMY

Unlike the other solid abdominal organs, the kidneys have a very complex internal architecture that is responsible for producing a variety of internal echogenicities. The central renal sinus is composed of fibrofatty tissue that appears echogenic on sonograms. The renal vessels and collecting system are occasionally seen as thin anechoic, fluid-containing structures located within the echogenic tissues of the renal sinus. The lymphatics also pass through the renal sinus but cannot be resolved sonographically. Each kidney consists of multiple functional units called lobes. The archetypical lobe contains a calyx, a medullary pyramid, cortical tissue, and vessels. In adults there is an average of eleven pyramids and nine calices, with some compound calices draining more than one pyramid. Sonographically, the pyramids are cone- or heart-shaped hypoechoic structures (Fig. 5-1). The cortex is slightly more echogenic than the pyramids, although this distinction is not always apparent. The cortical echogenicity of the kidney should be equal or slightly less than that of the liver and substantially less than that of the spleen. The kidneys are slightly ovoid in cross section, with the longest dimension directed from anteromedial to posterolateral. Therefore, longitudinal views of the kidney will demonstrate a different shape depending on how the view was obtained.

The external contour of the kidney is generally smooth. A common normal variant, called the junctional parenchymal defect (or the interrenuncular junction), produces a wedge-shaped hyperechoic defect in the anterior aspect of the kidney near the junction of the upper and middle thirds. It occurs because of incomplete embryologic fusion of the upper and lower poles. It can be distinguished from a scar or mass by its typical triangular shape and location. In addition, the junctional parenchymal defect communicates with the renal sinus medially at the level where the renal vessels exit the hilum (Fig. 5-2). Slight lobulation of the external contour of the kidney can also be seen as a result of persistent fetal lobation (Fig. 5-3). A prominent column of cortical tissue occasionally protrudes into the renal sinus and can simulate a mass. These are called columns of Bertin and are located in the mid third of the kidney. Columns of

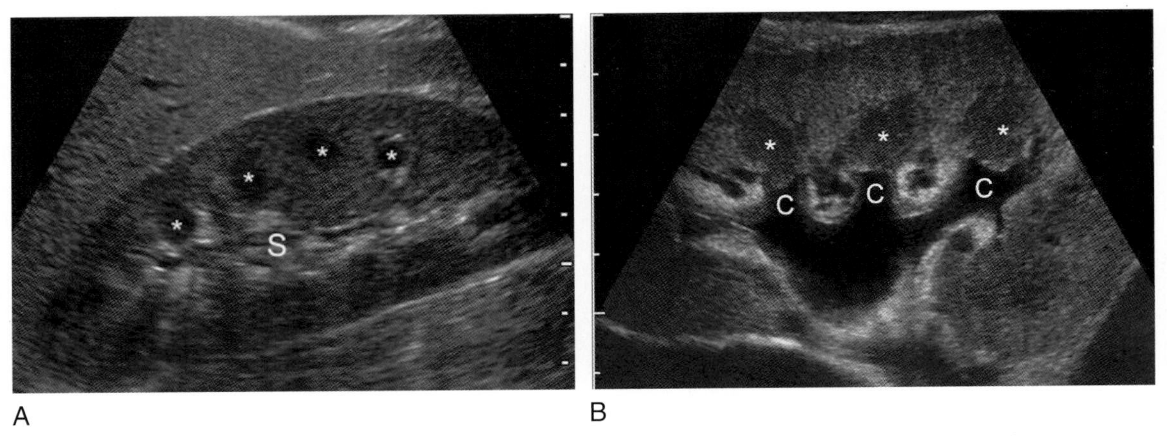

Figure 5-1 Normal kidney in different patients. **A**, Longitudinal view of the right kidney shows a central echogenic renal sinus (S) and a peripheral hypoechoic renal cortex. Between the sinus and the cortex are several hypoechoic pyramids (*). **B,** High-resolution view of a renal transplant shows a slightly distended collecting system with multiple calices (C) and their corresponding pyramids (*).

Bertin have similar echogenicity to the rest of the cortex and occasionally contain a small hypoechoic region due to an associated pyramid (Fig. 5-4). Duplication of the intrarenal collecting system is a relatively common variant that produces a separate central echogenic complex in the upper and lower pole (Fig. 5-5).

The size of the kidney varies with the age, sex, height, and weight of the person. In adults the average length of the kidney is 10.5 to 11 cm. The lower and upper limits of normal are 9 and 13 cm, respectively. The renal anteroposterior thickness and renal width can also be measured to calculate the renal volume based on the formula for an ellipsoid: volume = (length × thickness × width)/2. (See Table 5-1 for a summary of the characteristics of the normal kidney.)

A number of congenital anomalies of the kidneys can be detected sonographically. Agenesis is associated with an empty renal fossa and an elongated ipsilateral adrenal. The latter is much easier to detect in the neonatal period than later in life. Hypertrophy of the contralateral kidney is also usually present in cases of renal agenesis. Detection of renal agenesis should prompt a search for other anomalies in the genitourinary tract, such as duplication anomalies of the uterus and anomalies of the seminal vesicles and vas deferens. Ectopic kidneys can also appear as an empty renal fossa. Most ectopic kidneys are found inferior to the renal fossa, often in the pelvis. They have also been reported to occur in the thorax. Crossed, fused renal ectopy also occurs and may appear as an unusually large kidney with a duplicated renal sinus or as a mass arising from the lower pole. Fusion anomalies in general are relatively common (1 in 250). The most common fusion anomaly is the horseshoe kidney. It appears as a variably thick band of renal tissue (or rarely

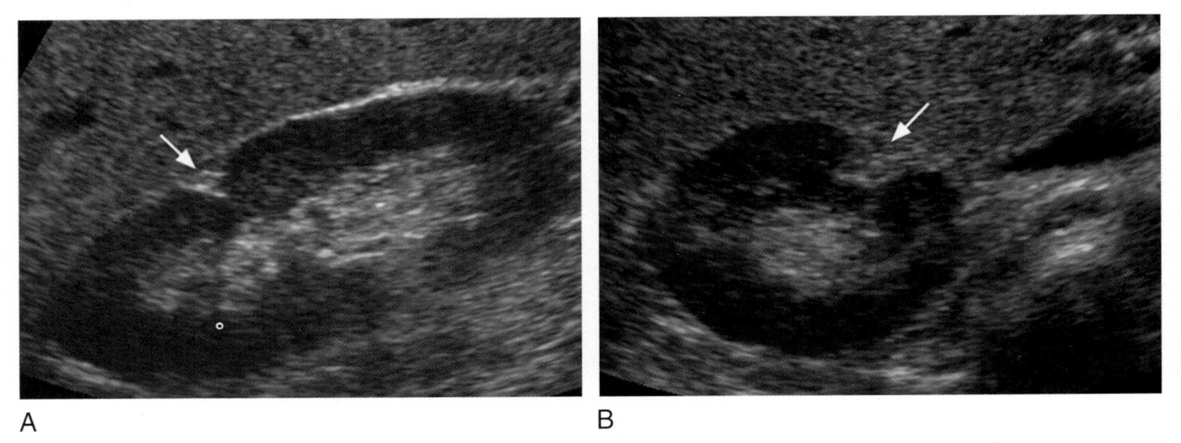

Figure 5-2 Junctional parenchymal defect. **A,** Longitudinal view shows a triangular echogenic defect *(arrow)* in the anterior aspect of the kidney near the junction of the upper and middle thirds typical of a junctional parenchymal defect. **B,** Transverse view shows similar defect.

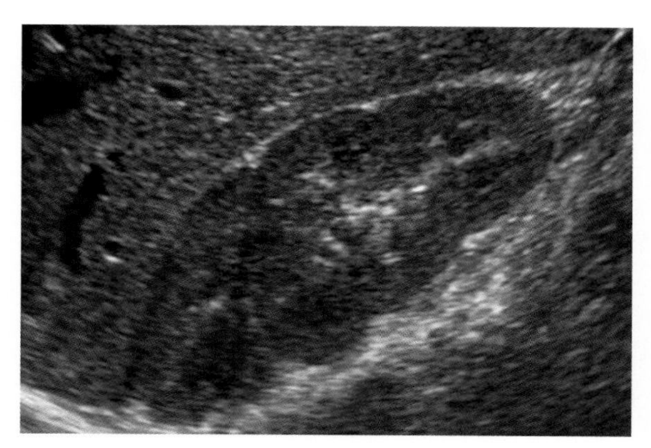

Figure 5-3 Fetal lobation. Longitudinal view shows slight indentations on the external surface of the kidney.

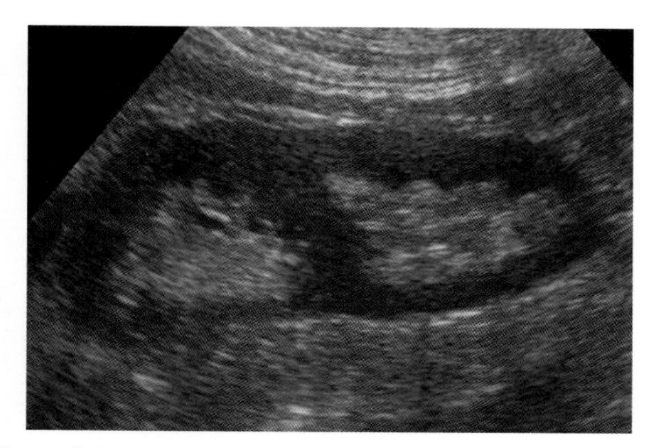

Figure 5-5 Renal duplication. Longitudinal view shows a band of cortical tissue separating the renal sinus into a superior and an inferior component.

as a thin fibrous band) extending from both lower poles to connect anterior to the aorta below the level of the inferior mesenteric artery (Fig. 5-6). It should be suspected when the axis of the kidney is distorted and the lower poles of the kidneys are hard to image sonographically. It should also be suspected on longitudinal scans of the aorta when an oval hypoechoic mass is seen anterior to the aorta. A rare variation of horseshoe kidney is the pancake kidney, where fusion occurs in both the lower and upper poles (Fig. 5-7).

TECHNIQUE

The native kidneys are best imaged with a 2- to 5-MHz transducer, depending on the patient's body habitus and the depth of the kidney. Higher frequencies can usually be used in renal transplants. Sector-type probes or curved arrays are generally best for imaging native kidneys, and linear arrays or curved arrays are best for imaging renal transplants.

The native kidneys can be viewed from a variety of approaches. The upper poles of each kidney are often seen best with the patient supine and using a high, posterior, intercostal approach and the liver or spleen as a window. Failure to go high enough and posterior enough is the most common reason for inadequate visualization of the upper pole, especially on the left. The lower poles can be seen best using a subcostal approach, usually during a deep inspiration. The transducer location should be varied from anterior to lateral to posterior, and the patient position should be varied from supine to decubitus until the best view is obtained. In some people the lower pole of the left kidney can be seen best from an anterolateral approach with the patient in a right lateral decubitus position. This view seems to be especially advantageous in obese patients. It is important to compare renal echogenicity to the liver and spleen. This allows for detection of abnormally echogenic kidneys, as well as abnormalities in hepatic and splenic echogenicity. Therefore, views including a portion of the liver and spleen are important to obtain. It is equally important to visualize the kidneys from a posterior or posterolateral approach without using the liver or spleen as a window. A posterior approach

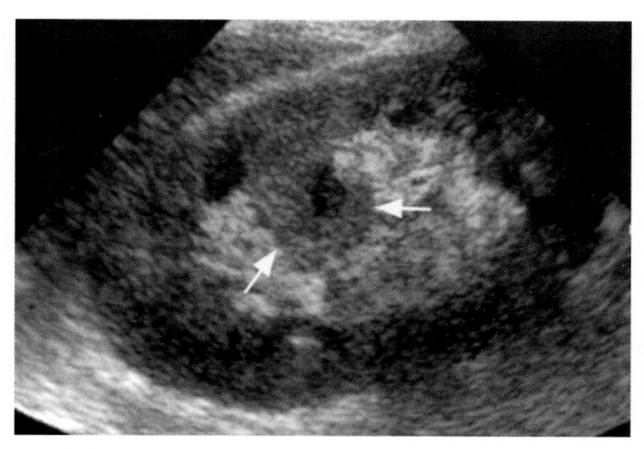

Figure 5-4 Hypertrophied column of Bertin. Longitudinal view of the kidney obtained from a lateral approach demonstrates a rounded mass-like structure *(arrows)* protruding into the renal sinus. This is isoechoic to the renal cortex, which is typical of a hypertrophied column of Bertin. In addition, a central hypoechoic region is also seen, consistent with a renal pyramid. Renal pyramids are not always identified within columns of Bertin but are a very characteristic finding when they are seen.

Table 5-1 Characteristics of Normal Kidney

Characteristic	Appearance
Size	Average, 11 cm (range, 9-13 cm)
Echogenicity	Right, ≤liver; left, <spleen
Parenchyma	Homogeneous (except for hypoechoic pyramids)
Renal sinus	Hyperechoic
Surface	Smooth

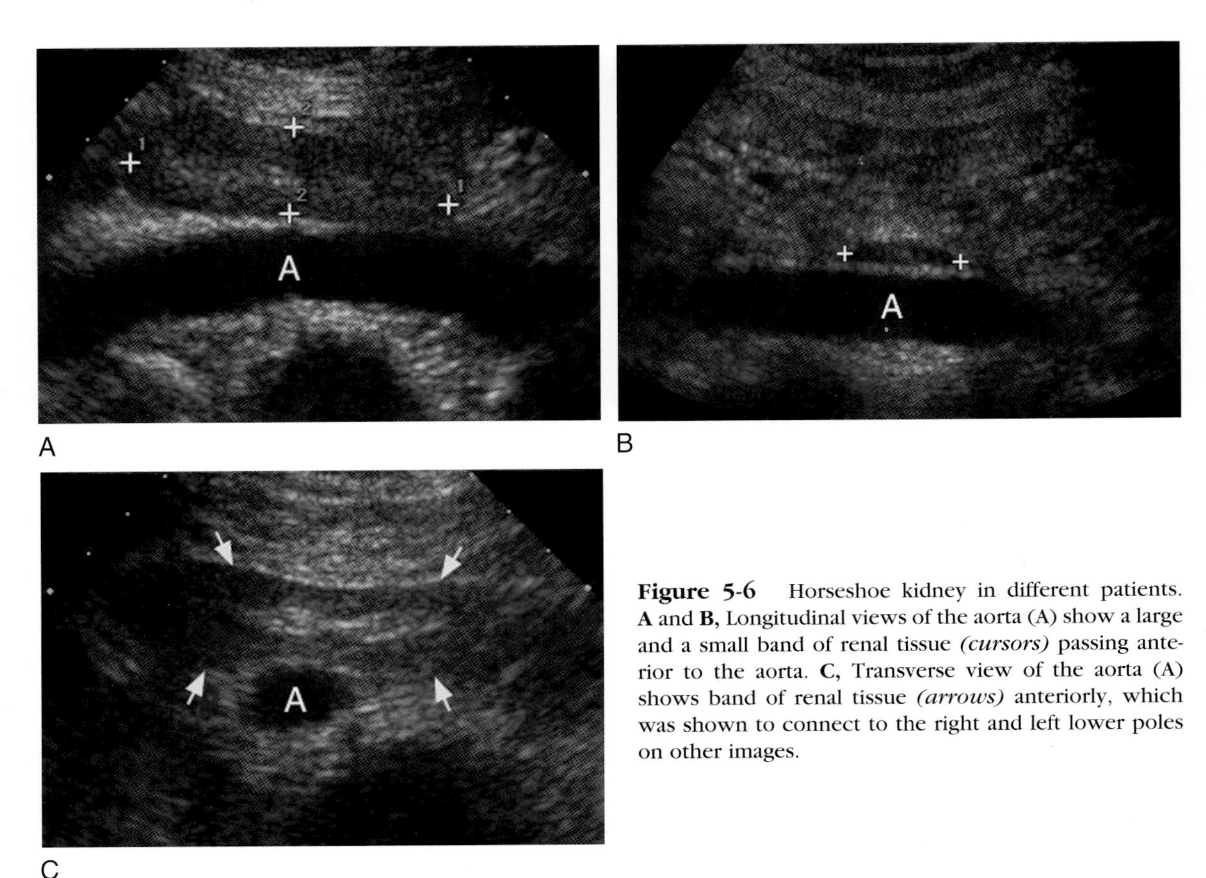

Figure 5-6 Horseshoe kidney in different patients. **A** and **B,** Longitudinal views of the aorta (A) show a large and a small band of renal tissue *(cursors)* passing anterior to the aorta. **C,** Transverse view of the aorta (A) shows band of renal tissue *(arrows)* anteriorly, which was shown to connect to the right and left lower poles on other images.

usually gets the transducer closer to the kidney and often will allow for better visualization of common abnormalities such as cysts and stones.

OBSTRUCTION

Approximately 5% of patients with renal failure suffer from urinary obstruction. In most cases bilateral obstruction is required for renal insufficiency to develop. Early detection is important, because untreated obstruction can lead to irreversible renal damage. The degree of long-term functional loss depends on both the degree and duration of obstruction. In dogs, complete ureteral obstruction lasting 7 days results in an average long-term recovery of only 70% of function. If an obstructed kidney is also infected, permanent renal damage can occur much more rapidly. Patients with signs of infection who are suspected to have renal obstruction should be treated as emergencies, with immediate renal sonography and urgent drainage performed if hydronephrosis is detected. In general, uninfected patients with suspected renal obstruction are not considered emergencies and are scanned as soon as is reasonable.

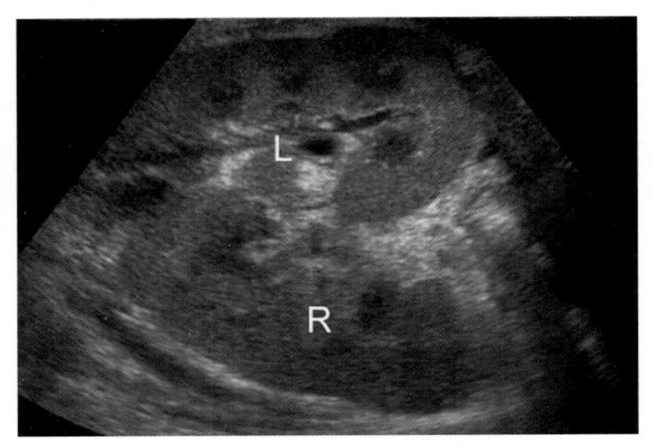

Figure 5-7 Pancake kidney. Coronal view from the left side shows broad connection between the left (L) and right (R) kidney.

The likelihood of sonographic detection of hydronephrosis in patients with renal failure depends on the patient's history. In patients with no risk factors for urinary obstruction, only 1% will have hydronephrosis detected sonographically. In many of these low-risk patients, an ultrasound finding of hydronephrosis will ultimately prove to be incorrect, or the patient will receive no therapy despite the ultrasound results. Although the yield of sonography is very low in these patients, it is an easy procedure to perform and is almost always included in the work-up. On the other hand, approximately 30% of the patients with known risk factors such as a known pelvic tumor, a palpable abdominal or pelvic mass, a history of renal stone disease, renal colic, sepsis, recent surgery, or history of bladder outlet obstruction will have hydronephrosis.

The sonographic diagnosis of obstruction has traditionally relied on the detection of a dilated collecting system (Fig. 5-8). This appears as anechoic spaces that conform to the expected location and shape of the renal calices and infundibula and generally communicate with a dilated renal pelvis. Communication with the renal pelvis is best shown on coronal or semicoronal views. Marked hydronephrosis (sometimes called grade 3) refers to severe dilatation that is associated with cortical thinning. Moderate hydronephrosis (grade 2) refers to dilatation of the collecting system that is readily evident but not associated with cortical thinning. Neither moderate nor marked hydronephrosis is difficult to identify or interpret correctly on sonograms. Mild hydronephrosis (grade 1) refers to minimal amounts of urine producing slight distention of the collecting system. Detecting the various grades of hydronephrosis is much less difficult than determining their significance. In general, the more distended the renal collecting system, the more likely it is caused by a clinically significant obstruction. However, repeated or long-standing obstruction may cause a dilated, ectatic collecting system that persists even when obstruction is relieved, and acute obstruction may produce minimal hydronephrosis or may be imaged before any hydronephrosis develops. For this reason, comparison with old studies is extremely valuable. Mild hydronephrosis is much more likely to be due to obstruction if it is a new finding. On the other hand, even moderate hydronephrosis is less likely to be due to obstruction when it is a chronic unchanged finding.

In addition to obstruction, there are a number of other processes that can cause a dilated renal collecting system (Box 5-1). They include very active physiologic diuresis, diuresis related to diabetes insipidus, overdistention of the urinary bladder, pregnancy, vesicoureteral reflux, an extrarenal pelvis, and previous episodes of obstruction. The best way to show that sonographically detected hydronephrosis is actually due to obstruction is to identify an obstructing lesion. Most obstructing lesions, such as prostatic hypertrophy, gynecologic masses, and bladder tumors, occur in the pelvis and are relatively easy to detect with sonography. When the pelvis is normal, one should scan along the course of the ureters, searching for masses, fluid collections, or stones. In many cases the ureters themselves are not seen, even though the obstructing process can be identified. Small retroperitoneal masses and mid-ureteral stones will not be seen on most sonograms; and in such patients, CT or urography is required.

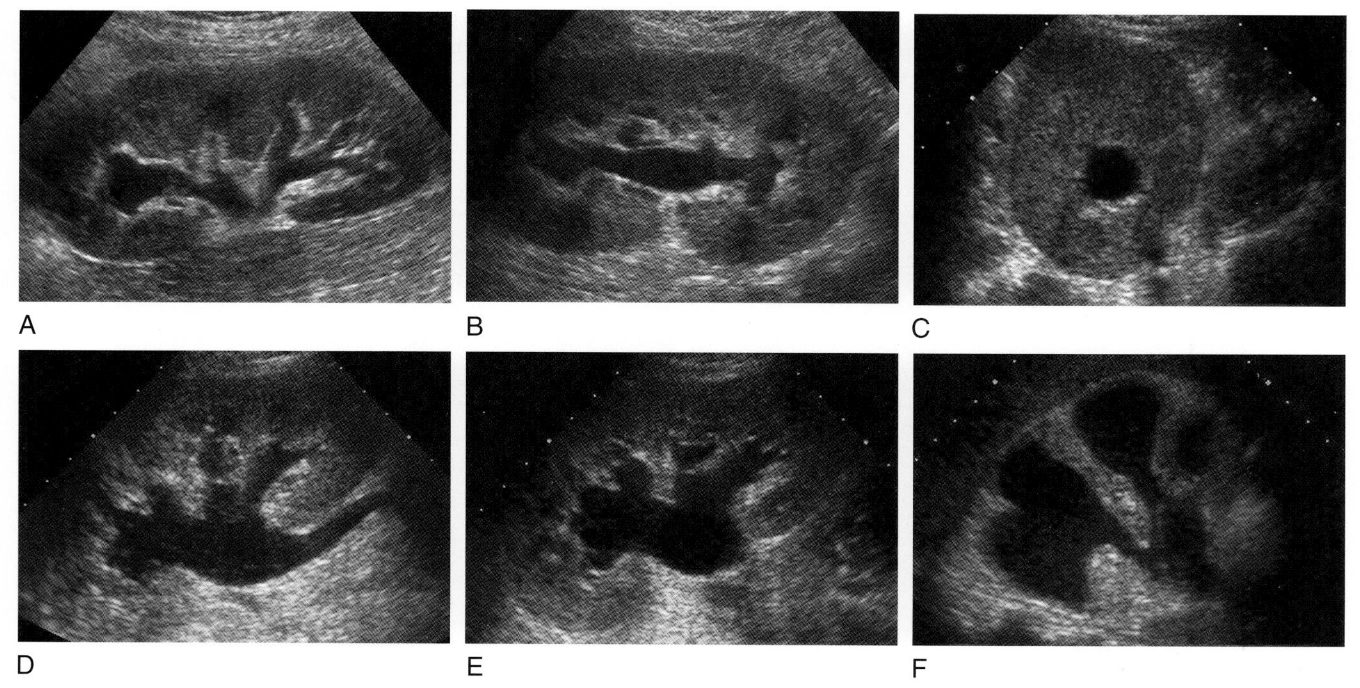

Figure 5-8 Hydronephrosis in different patients. Multiple longitudinal (**A** and **B**, **D** to **F**) and transverse (**C**) views of the kidney with different grades of hydronephrosis. Cortical thinning in **F** indicates severe hydronephrosis.

Box 5-1 Causes of Hydronephrosis

COMMON	UNCOMMON
Obstruction	Active diuresis
Previous obstruction	Diabetes insipidus
Extrarenal pelvis	Reflux nephropathy
Distended bladder	
Pregnancy	

When evaluating suspected renal obstruction, Doppler analysis can assist in several ways. Prominent renal vessels (usually veins) occasionally mimic a dilated renal collecting system and can be mistaken for mild hydronephrosis. Doppler analysis can distinguish these patients from those with true renal pelvis dilation (Fig. 5-9). In addition, resistance to renal arterial flow is increased in the setting of obstruction owing to the release of vasoactive substances and vasoconstriction. This produces an elevated resistive index (>0.7) or asymmetry between the ipsilateral and contralateral resistive index (a difference of 0.08 to 0.10 or more) (Fig. 5-10). Therefore, in patients with clinically suspected obstruction, a unilateral elevated resistive index suggests obstruction even when the hydronephrosis is mild or when there is no hydronephrosis. On the other hand, normal or bilaterally symmetric resistive indices in the setting of obvious hydronephrosis do not imply that the hydronephrosis is nonobstructive. Although the results of initial studies indicated that analysis of renal resistive indices was both sensitive and specific in its ability to detect renal obstruction, the results have not been difficult to reproduce, and this method remains controversial and not widely utilized. One of the difficulties with renal resistive indices is that they may not detect either acute or partial obstruction and they may remain abnormal for a variable length of time after obstruction is relieved. In addition, many processes other than obstruction cause abnormal resistive indices.

Analysis of ureteral jets is a third way Doppler studies can assist in the evaluation of the potentially obstructed kidney. Although ureteral jets are visible on gray-scale sonography, they are only seen intermittently and are often subtle. Jets are much more apparent on color Doppler imaging (Fig. 5-11), and it is possible to obtain useful information by scanning the bladder in the region of the trigone and looking for intermittent bursts of urine flowing from the ureteral orifices. Ureteral jets are absent in the presence of urinary obstruction but are maintained in the presence of nonobstructive hydronephrosis. Occasionally, a low-level but continuous jet is seen in the setting of obstruction. The advantage of this technique over resistive index analysis is that ureteral jets are affected immediately when obstruction develops and when obstruction resolves. However, as with renal resistive index measurements, a low-grade partial obstruction may not eliminate ureteral jets and may result in a false-negative examination. The detection of ureteral jets depends on differences in density between urine in the bladder and urine exiting the ureters. Because the density of urine in the bladder is the average density of urine collected over long periods, it usually differs from the density of urine exiting the ureter at any point in time. This may not be the case in a well-hydrated patient who has recently voided because the fresh urine collecting in the bladder may have the

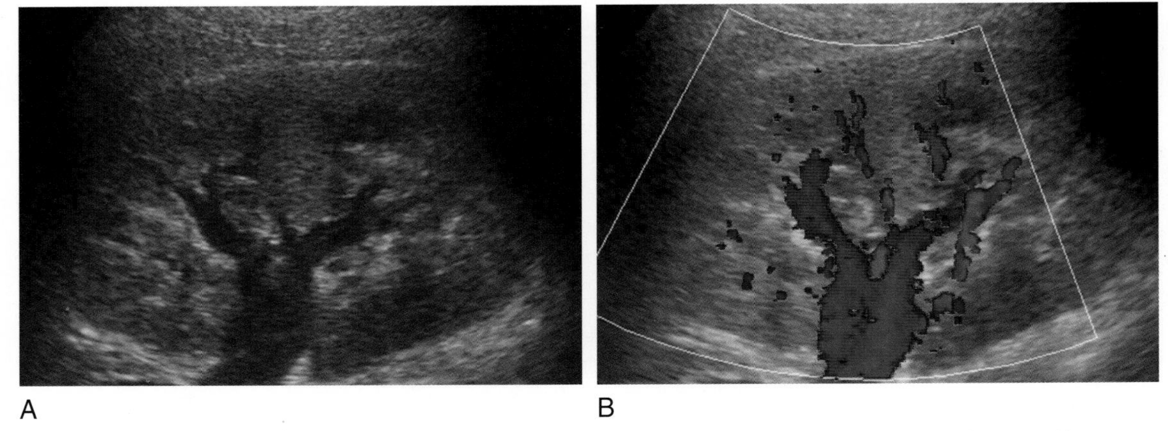

Figure 5-9 Prominent renal veins simulating hydronephrosis. **A,** Longitudinal view shows mild separation of the central sinus by hypoechoic branching structures. Although the branching pattern is slightly different than the collecting system, this appearance is easy to confuse with hydronephrosis. **B,** Color Doppler view confirms that this is prominent vessels rather that the collecting system.

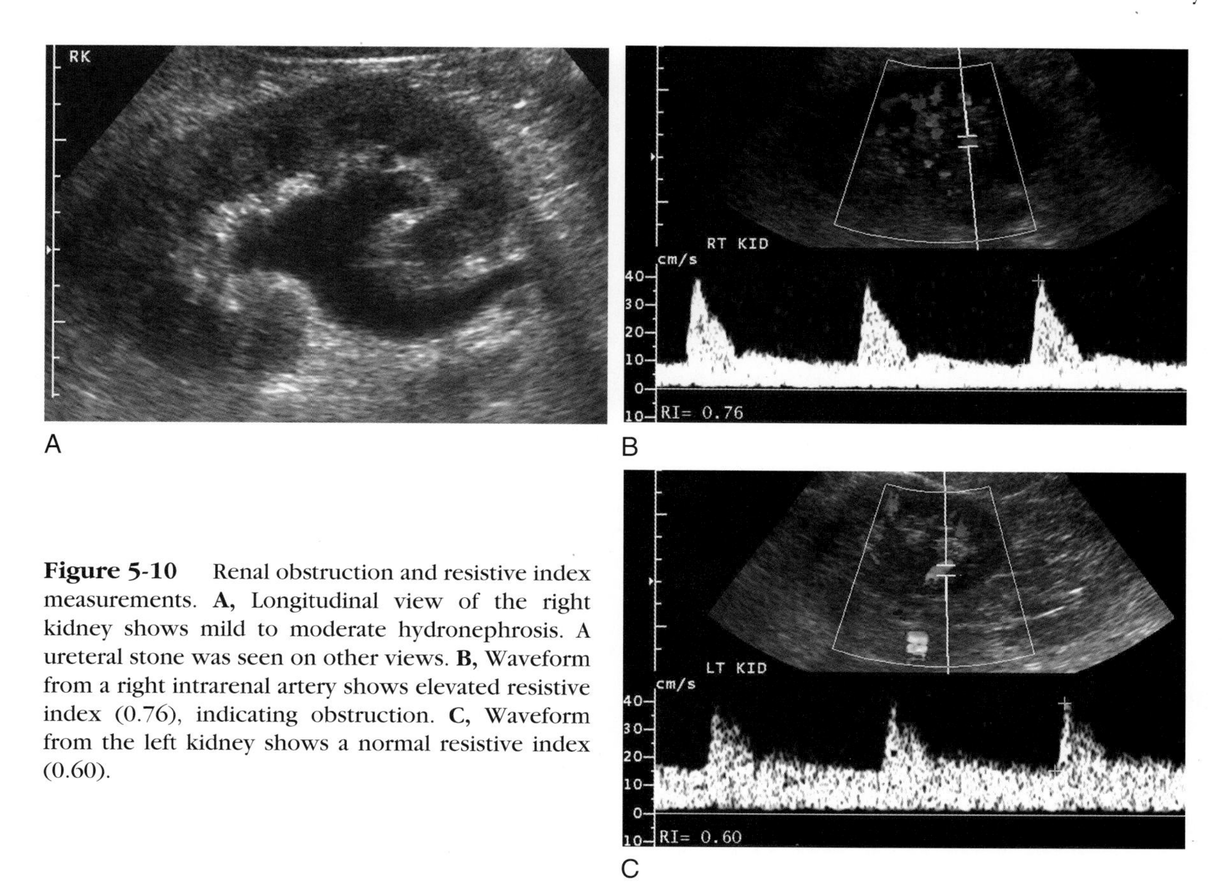

Figure 5-10 Renal obstruction and resistive index measurements. **A,** Longitudinal view of the right kidney shows mild to moderate hydronephrosis. A ureteral stone was seen on other views. **B,** Waveform from a right intrarenal artery shows elevated resistive index (0.76), indicating obstruction. **C,** Waveform from the left kidney shows a normal resistive index (0.60).

same density as the urine exiting the ureters. Therefore, patients should not be allowed to void completely before the examination.

The sensitivity of ultrasound studies in detecting obstruction is approximately 95%. Sources of false-negative findings include acute or partial obstruction, obstruction in a dehydrated patient, and lack of recognition of mild hydronephrosis. A number of abnormalities can be mistaken for hydronephrosis and lead to a false-positive diagnosis of obstruction. These include dilated renal vessels, peripelvic cysts, chronic reflux nephropathy, and severe papillary necrosis. In most cases, gray-scale sonography is capable of distinguishing these other abnormalities from hydronephrosis. Chronic

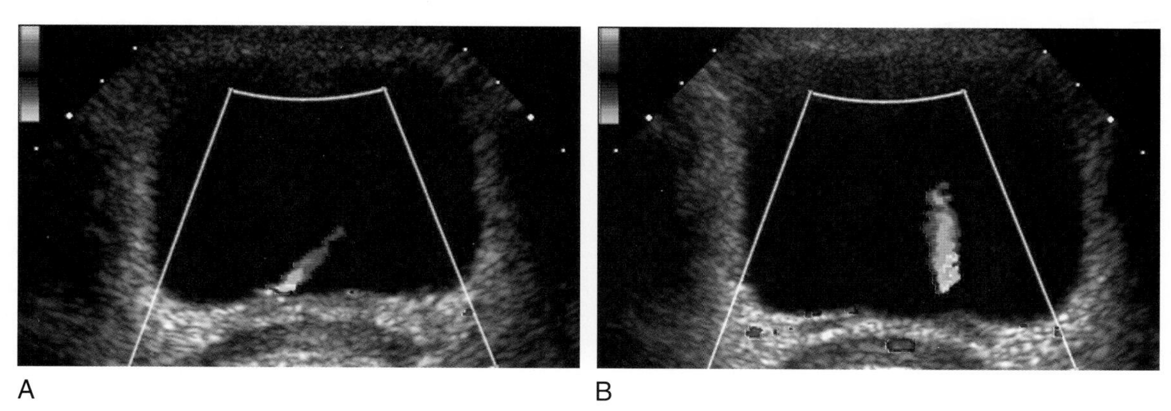

Figure 5-11 Ureteral jets. **A,** Transverse color Doppler view of the bladder shows a ureteral jet exiting the right ureteral orifice and entering the bladder. The angle of flow is typical. **B,** Similar view in the same patient shows the left jet. The angle of flow is straighter than is typically seen.

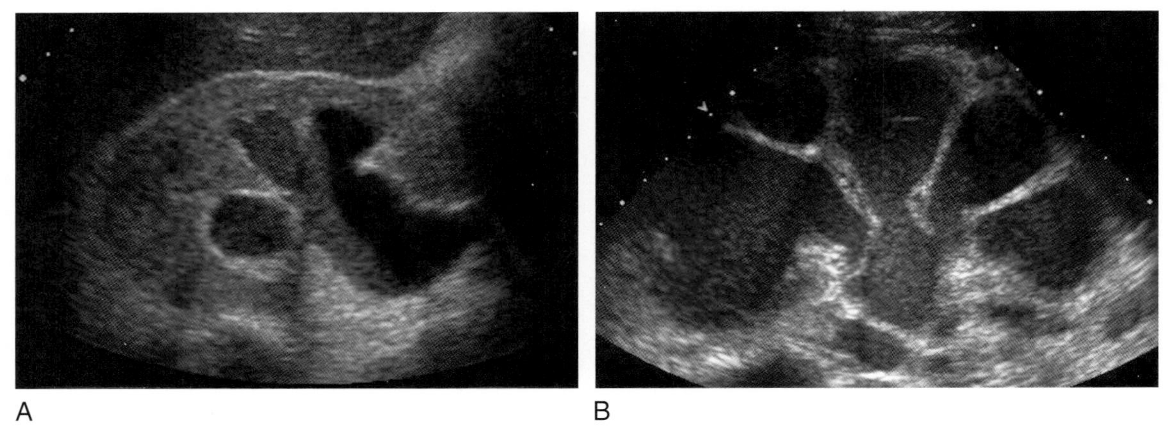

Figure 5-12 Pyonephrosis in different patients. **A,** Oblique view shows moderate hydronephrosis and echogenic material layering in the dependent portion of the collecting system. **B,** Longitudinal view shows marked hydronephrosis and echogenic material throughout the collecting system. Note that echogenic urine is not always seen in pyonephrosis.

reflux nephropathy affects the calices and produces cortical thinning but spares the renal pelvis. Severe papillary necrosis causes the papillae to be replaced with urine-filled sacs that simulate dilated calices, but again the renal pelvis and infundibula are spared.

Pyonephrosis refers to an obstructed and infected collecting system. In some cases echogenic pus can be seen filling the collecting system or layering in the dependent portion of the collecting system (Fig. 5-12). However, pus may not be evident in patients with pyonephrosis, so the diagnosis should be suspected in any patient with hydronephrosis and clinical evidence of urinary tract infection. As mentioned earlier, pyonephrosis can cause rapid and permanent deterioration of renal function and should be decompressed as soon as it is detected.

CYSTIC DISEASES (TABLE 5-2)

Benign Cysts

Renal cysts are the most common renal mass. Their frequency increases with age, and they are present in half the population above the age of 50. The etiology of renal cysts is not known, but it is possible that they form from the epithelial overgrowth of tubules or collecting ducts, with resulting distention of the nephron. This would explain why cysts enlarge over time, and the involvement of adjacent nephrons might explain why thin septations develop.

Sonography is the most accurate way to evaluate cystic lesions in the kidney. When indeterminate but probable cystic lesions are seen on urography, CT, or MRI, sonography is the appropriate way to confirm that the lesion is a cyst. To qualify as a simple cyst, the lesion should have the following characteristics.

1. Anechoic lumen
2. Well-defined back wall
3. Acoustic enhancement deep to the lesion
4. No measurable wall thickness

Figure 5-13 shows several simple cysts. Note that not all features need to be evident on every view. Small cysts may have low-level artifactual internal echoes owing to slice thickness limitations or to degradation of the ultrasound beam by overlying soft tissues such as fat. Imaging from multiple different approaches will vary the composition of overlying tissues and often helps to clear out the internal artifacts. Harmonic imaging and real-time compounding also assist in minimizing these artifacts. Small cysts may also not have demonstrable posterior acoustic enhancement. Almost all cysts, regardless of size, should have a well-defined back wall because of the high acoustic impedance mismatch between cyst fluid and the cyst wall.

A cyst can still be considered benign if it contains a limited number of thin internal septations, provided it satisfies the other criteria. Septations are seen in approximately 5% of benign renal cysts. Thick septations should be considered suspicious for a cystic neoplasm such as cystic renal cell carcinoma, but they can also be seen in benign cystic neoplasms and complicated nonneoplastic cysts. Cysts are complicated by intraluminal hemorrhage approximately 5% of the time. Hemorrhage may cause diffuse low-level internal echoes, fibrinous membranes, internal echogenic clots, or a fluid-debris level (Fig. 5-14). These appearances can overlap with those of cystic renal cell cancer, and patients may require CT or MRI for further evaluation. Follow-up sonograms are also useful if they show resolution or improvement of abnormalities

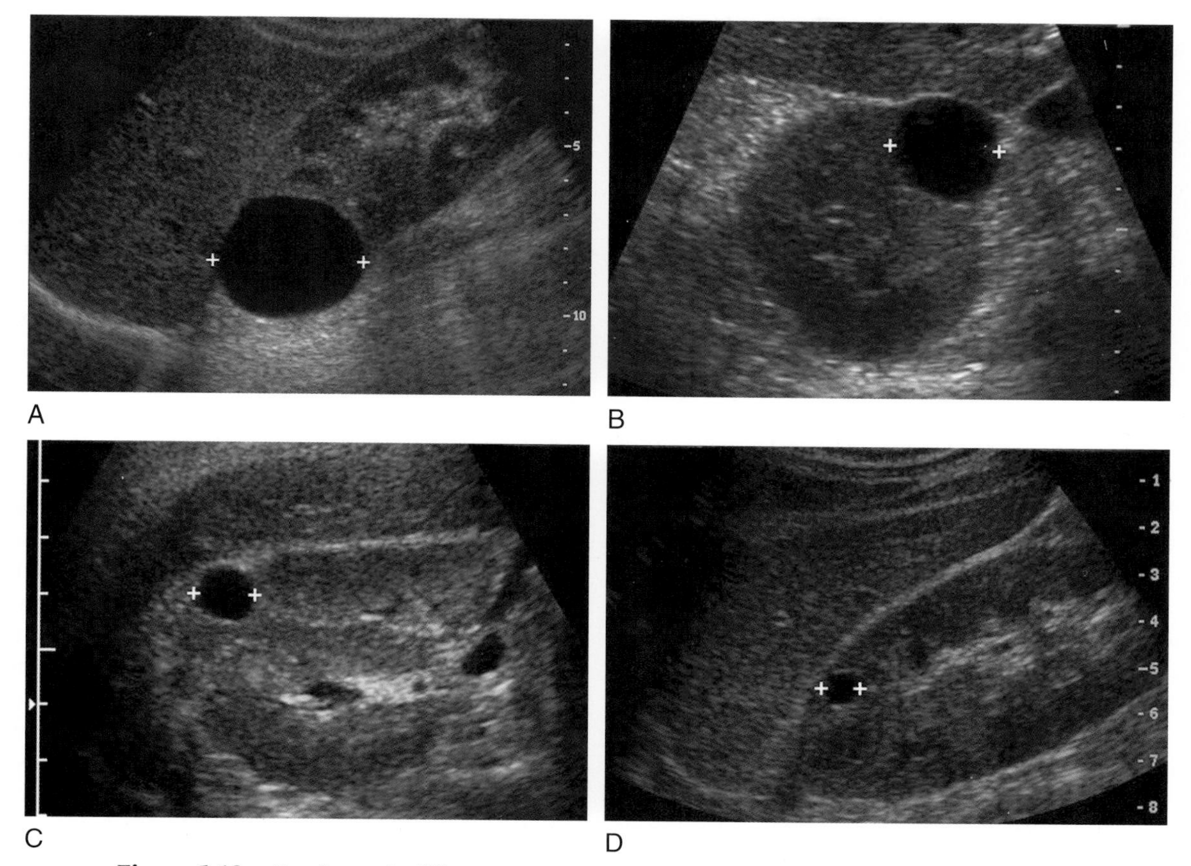

Figure 5-13 Renal cysts in different patients. **A** to **D,** Various-sized simple renal cysts *(cursors).* The detection of posterior enhancement and the presence of intraluminal echoes depend on the size of the cyst and the nature and thickness of the overlying tissues.

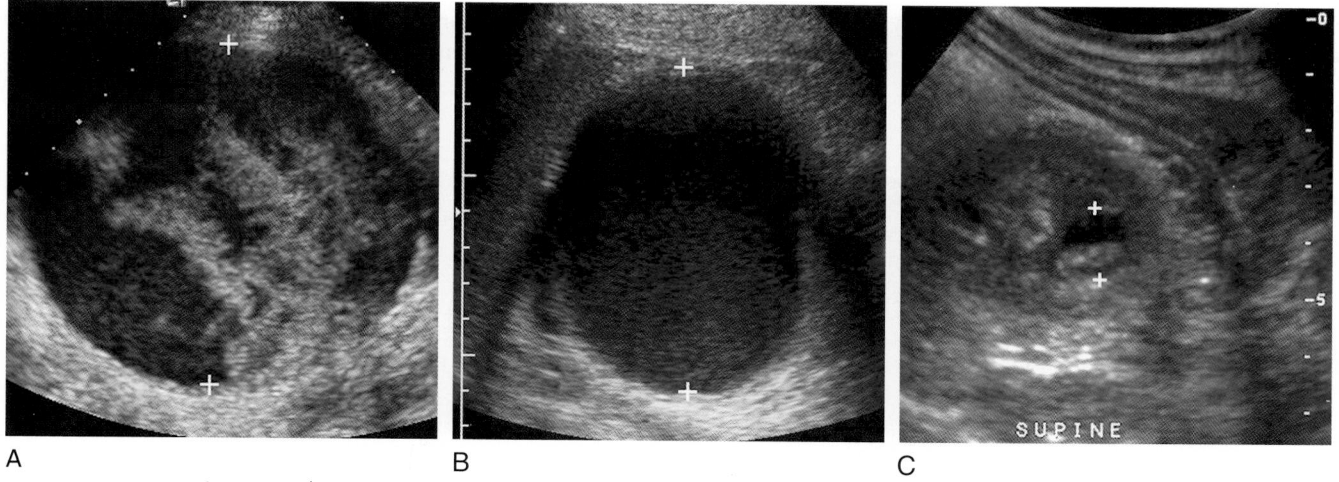

Figure 5-14 Hemorrhagic cysts in different patients. **A,** Large cyst *(cursors)* with blood and solid clot within the lumen. This appearance simulates a cystic renal cell cancer. **B,** Large cyst *(cursors)* with low-level internal reflections caused by cellular material floating in the lumen. **C,** Small cyst *(cursors)* with a fluid-cellular level similar to a hematocrit effect.

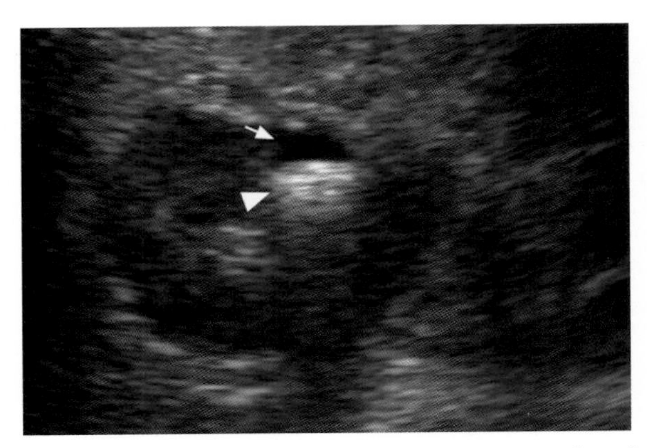

Figure 5-15 Milk of calcium cyst. Cyst contains clear fluid *(arrow)* in the non-dependent aspect and highly echogenic, partially shadowing crystalline material *(arrowhead)* in the dependent aspect.

in a few months. The characteristics of hemorrhagic cysts also overlap with those of infected renal cysts, and this distinction can only be made on the basis of clinical findings and the findings yielded by cyst aspiration. A common clinical problem is a hyperdense mass seen on CT, usually due to hemorrhage or high protein content in the fluid of a cyst. Sonography is extremely useful in excluding the less likely possibility of a solid mass because most hyperdense cysts appear simple and anechoic on sonography.

Calcifications occur in 1% to 3% of cysts and usually result from prior hemorrhage, infection, or ischemia. Thin, curvilinear, peripheral calcifications should not raise the suspicion of carcinoma, but thick, globular calcification may indicate an underlying malignancy. Crystalline material can accumulate in cysts and produce shadowing, echogenic material that may or may not layer in the dependent aspect of the lumen (Fig. 5-15). If this crystalline material is visible on radiographs, it is called milk of calcium. In some cases, crystals may form in cysts that are too small to resolve sonographically. In these cases the echogenic crystals are all that is detected. Small ring-down artifacts detectable on gray-scale and color Doppler imaging can form posterior to this crystalline material.

The differential diagnosis of cysts includes caliceal diverticula, papillary necrosis, obstructed upper pole duplications, and lymphoma. Vascular abnormalities such as aneurysms, pseudoaneurysms, and arteriovenous malformations (Fig. 5-16) should also be considered in the differential diagnosis of cystic renal lesions.

Cysts that form in the renal sinus are called peripelvic cysts. These cysts are probably lymphatic in origin. They are frequently bilateral and often are multiple (Fig. 5-17). They are important primarily because they can be confused with hydronephrosis (see Fig. 5-17C and D). On coronal views, true hydronephrosis is usually very typical with a dilated renal pelvis that extends into dilated infundibula that extend into the upper, mid, and lower zones of the kidney. Because peripelvic cysts do not communicate with each other, they lack the typical appearance of hydronephrosis. Nevertheless, the walls that separate peripelvic cysts may be subtle and the cysts may elongate and herniate out of the renal sinus. Whenever there is doubt, intravenous urography is a good method to distinguish the two possibilities. If the patient has renal dysfunction, gadolinium-enhanced MRI or scintigraphy can be used. In general, it is more difficult to demonstrate the classic criteria of a cyst for peripelvic cysts than for cortically based cysts, possibly because of the renal sinus fat that surrounds the peripelvic cyst.

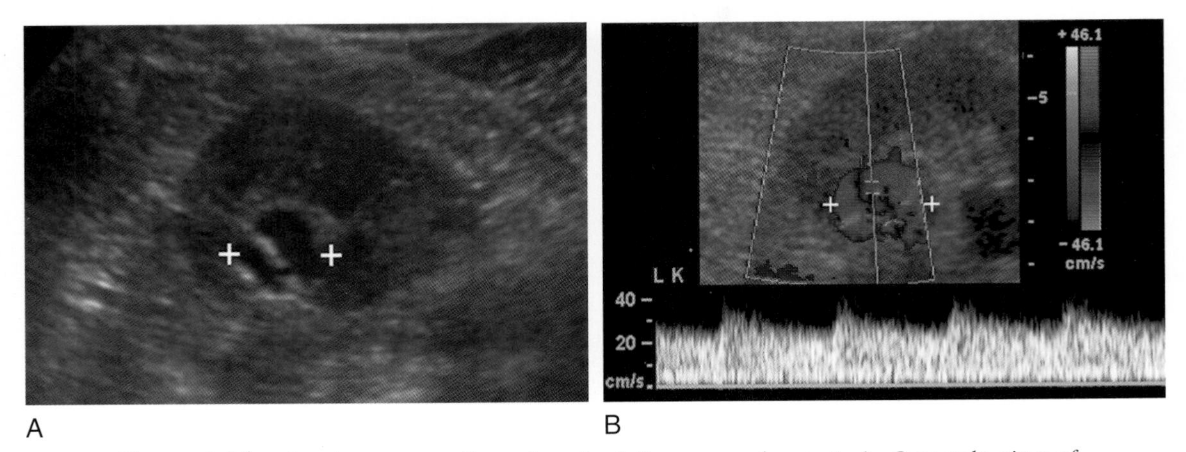

Figure 5-16 Arteriovenous malformation simulating a complex cyst. **A,** Gray-scale view of the kidney shows what appears to be a septated cyst *(cursors)*. **B,** Color and pulsed Doppler show internal flow throughout the lumen of the lesion with a low vascular resistance typical of an arteriovenous malformation.

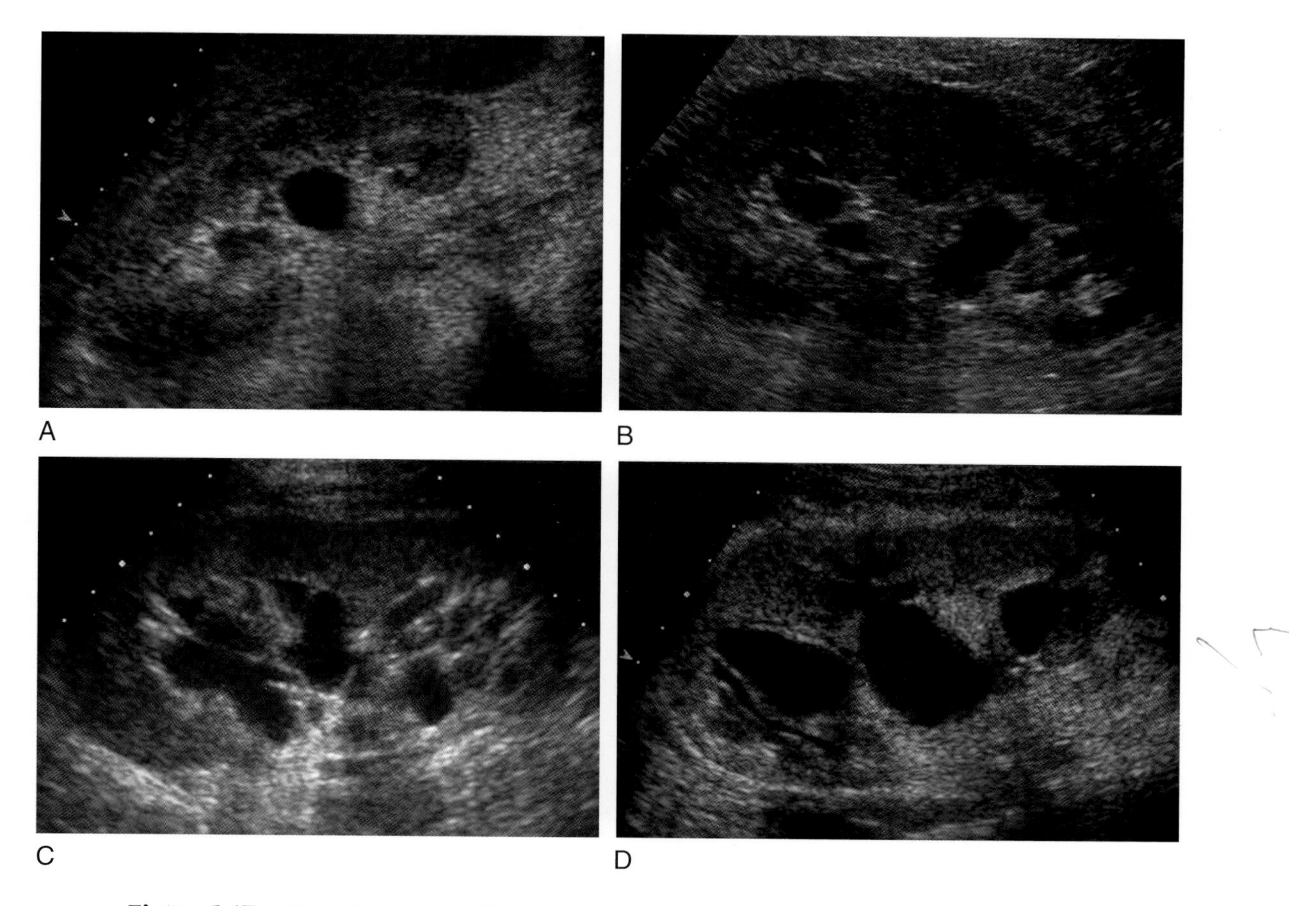

Figure 5-17 Peripelvic cysts in different patients. **A,** Single cyst located within the renal sinus. **B,** Multiple renal cysts in the renal sinus. **C** and **D,** Multiple peripelvic cysts, some of which have assumed an oval configuration and have started to extend into the renal hilum. When this happens, the appearance can be confused with hydronephrosis.

Autosomal Dominant Polycystic Disease

Autosomal dominant polycystic disease affects the kidneys to a greater degree than any other organ. For this reason it is commonly referred to as adult polycystic kidney disease (PCKD). However, the liver is involved in approximately 50% of patients, the pancreas in up to 5% of patients, and other organs in an even smaller percentage. Cerebral aneurysms occur in approximately 20% or more of the patients and are the cause of death in up to 10%. Up to 10% of cases of end-stage renal disease in North America and Europe are due to PCKD. If untreated, patients survive approximately 10 years from the onset of symptoms.

Despite the autosomal dominant pattern of inheritance, up to 50% of the patients have no family history of the disease. This is due to the variable expression of the disorder and the occurrence of spontaneous mutations. PCKD arises from two different genetic defects. Type 1 is most common (90% of cases) and presents earlier than type 2. The disease generally becomes clinically apparent in the fourth or fifth decade, but it can cause renal failure in utero or may not become clinically evident until the eighth or ninth decade. It is unusual for affected patients to reach age 60 without renal failure. The classic signs and symptoms of the disease are hypertension and renal failure. Others include a palpable mass, abdominal pain, hematuria, renal infection, and polycythemia.

The most conspicuous sonographic feature of autosomal dominant polycystic disease are multiple, variably sized cortical- and medullary-based cysts in the kidneys (Fig. 5-18). The process affects the kidneys bilaterally in almost all instances, but it may be asymmetric. Early in the disease it is possible to detect normal renal parenchyma, but with time the kidney becomes completely replaced by cysts and no normal parenchyma is identified. As the cysts become more numerous and enlarge, the kidney itself enlarges. The mass effect of the cysts can cause compression and partial obstruction of the collecting system. The resulting urinary stasis likely explains the increase in stone formation in these patients.

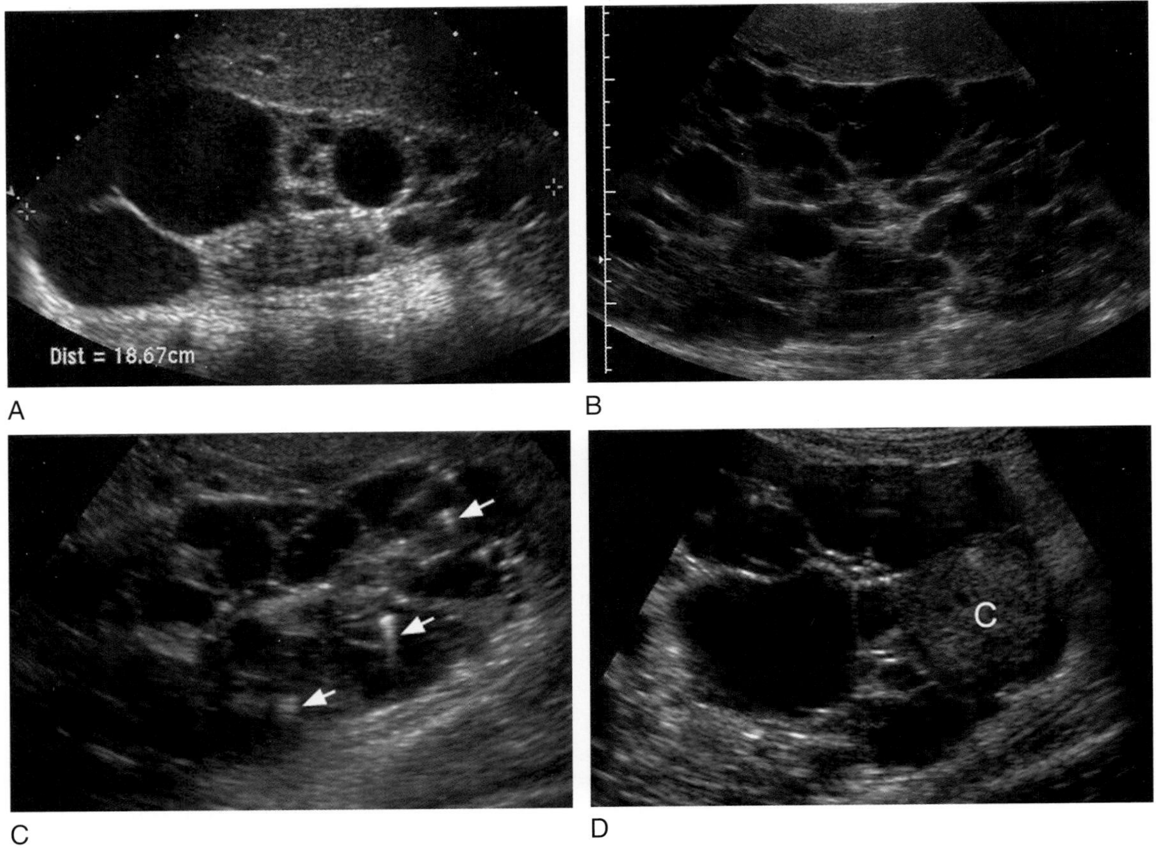

Figure 5-18 Polycystic kidney disease in different patients. **A,** Multiple cysts within an enlarged (18.67 cm) kidney. Some solid renal parenchyma can still be seen. **B,** Multiple cysts completely replacing the kidney. No normal parenchyma is detected. **C,** Short ring-down artifacts *(arrows)* indicate crystals have precipitated in some of the cysts. **D,** Solid clot (C) is present in one of the cysts. This is common and should not be confused with a neoplasm unless there are worrisome features on other modalities or unless there is detectable vascularity on Doppler.

Detectable calcification may also be located in the walls of the cysts. In addition, crystals frequently form in the cysts and produce comet tail artifacts. Hemorrhage into the cysts is common and assumes the appearance of a solid-appearing mass, a complex cyst, or a cyst with a fluid-debris level. Hemorrhagic cysts are much more common than neoplasms in patients with autosomal dominant polycystic disease, so a complex-appearing mass should be monitored rather than removed. Unlike many other cystic diseases of the kidney, PCKD does not have a significant increased risk of renal cell cancer.

Sonography is often used to screen the family members of affected patients. Criteria that have been established include the presence of at least two cysts in one kidney or one cyst in each kidney in an at-risk person younger than 30 years of age, the presence of at least two cysts in each kidney in an at-risk person between 30 and 59 years of age, and at least four cysts in each kidney for those persons at risk aged 60 years and above. It is important to realize that these criterion do not apply to the population in general. In most patients with PCKD, there are many cysts present bilaterally and the diagnosis is not in doubt. If cysts are not detected by age 30, it is very unlikely that the patient has the disease. When ultrasound results are indeterminate or are confusing, DNA linkage analysis can be performed if it is available.

Acquired Cystic Disease

Multiple renal cysts develop in patients on long-term dialysis if they live long enough. This process is called acquired cystic disease and occurs in up to 90% of the patients who have been on dialysis for 3 years or more. Rarely, it can occur in patients with chronic renal failure who are not receiving dialysis treatment. The etiology is unknown, although it seems likely that dialysis fails to clear renotropic substances that accumulate and promote cyst formation. The cysts range in size and are usually seen in the setting of a small echogenic kidney (Fig. 5-19A). Occasionally, the cysts become so numerous

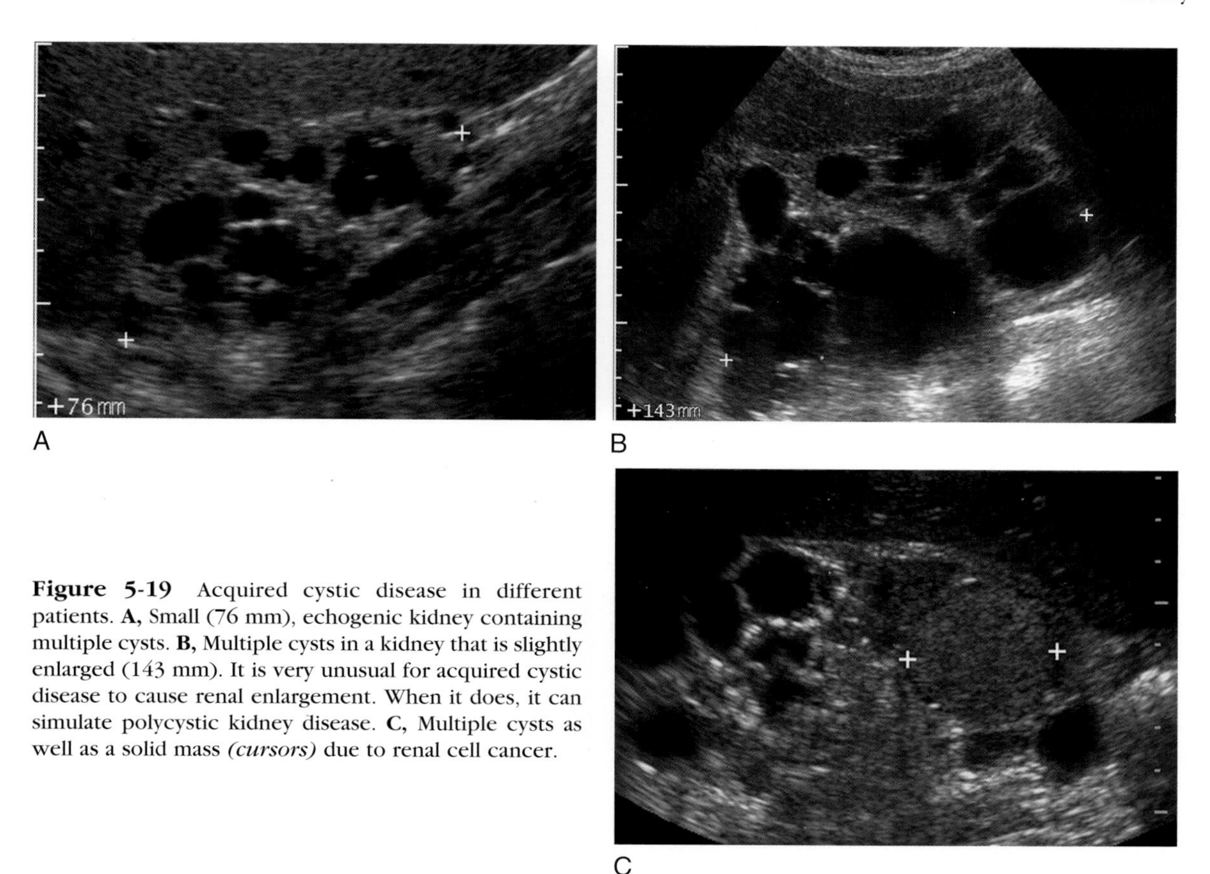

Figure 5-19 Acquired cystic disease in different patients. **A,** Small (76 mm), echogenic kidney containing multiple cysts. **B,** Multiple cysts in a kidney that is slightly enlarged (143 mm). It is very unusual for acquired cystic disease to cause renal enlargement. When it does, it can simulate polycystic kidney disease. **C,** Multiple cysts as well as a solid mass *(cursors)* due to renal cell cancer.

that the kidney is actually enlarged. As with polycystic disease, cyst hemorrhage is common. Major hemorrhage into the retroperitoneum is the most serious complication of acquired cystic disease.

Solid renal neoplasms occur in approximately 7% of patients with acquired cystic disease, but most are small (<3 cm) and exhibit benign behavior (see Fig. 5-19C). The risk of invasive or metastatic renal cell carcinoma is three to six times that for the general population, but it is not clear that screening for neoplasms is truly cost-effective.

von Hippel-Lindau Disease

von Hippel-Lindau disease is inherited as an autosomal dominant trait. It usually becomes clinically evident by the third to the fifth decade of life. In affected patients, neoplasms or cysts, or usually both, form in a variety of organs. The significant lesions that are most common are renal cell carcinoma (25% to 50%), retinal angioma (60%), central nervous system hemangioblastoma (>50%), and pheochromocytoma (20%). Most commonly the presenting symptoms are those produced by cerebellar or spinal cord hemangioblastomas or retinal angiomas. Occasionally, abdominal manifestations arise before central nervous system problems.

Thirty to 70 percent of the patients with von Hippel-Lindau disease have renal involvement in the form of multiple renal cysts. Despite their multiplicity, the cysts do not cause renal failure or hypertension and do not generally cause renal enlargement. There is, however, an increased incidence of tumors developing in the cyst walls. Therefore, even benign-appearing cysts should be monitored.

Renal cell carcinoma occurs in up to 75% of the patients with von Hippel-Lindau disease whose kidneys are involved. These tumors are most often multiple (90%) and bilateral (75%), and they occur at a much earlier age than does the sporadic form of renal cell carcinoma. They may either develop in the walls of cysts or as separate solid tumors (Fig. 5-20).

The overall incidence of pheochromocytomas is increased in patients with von Hippel-Lindau disease and occurs in up to 20%, although most cases are isolated to certain kindreds in which the incidence is even higher. Pheochromocytomas produce symptoms less frequently in this population than do sporadic varieties, despite the fact that they are more frequently multiple and located in extra-adrenal sites.

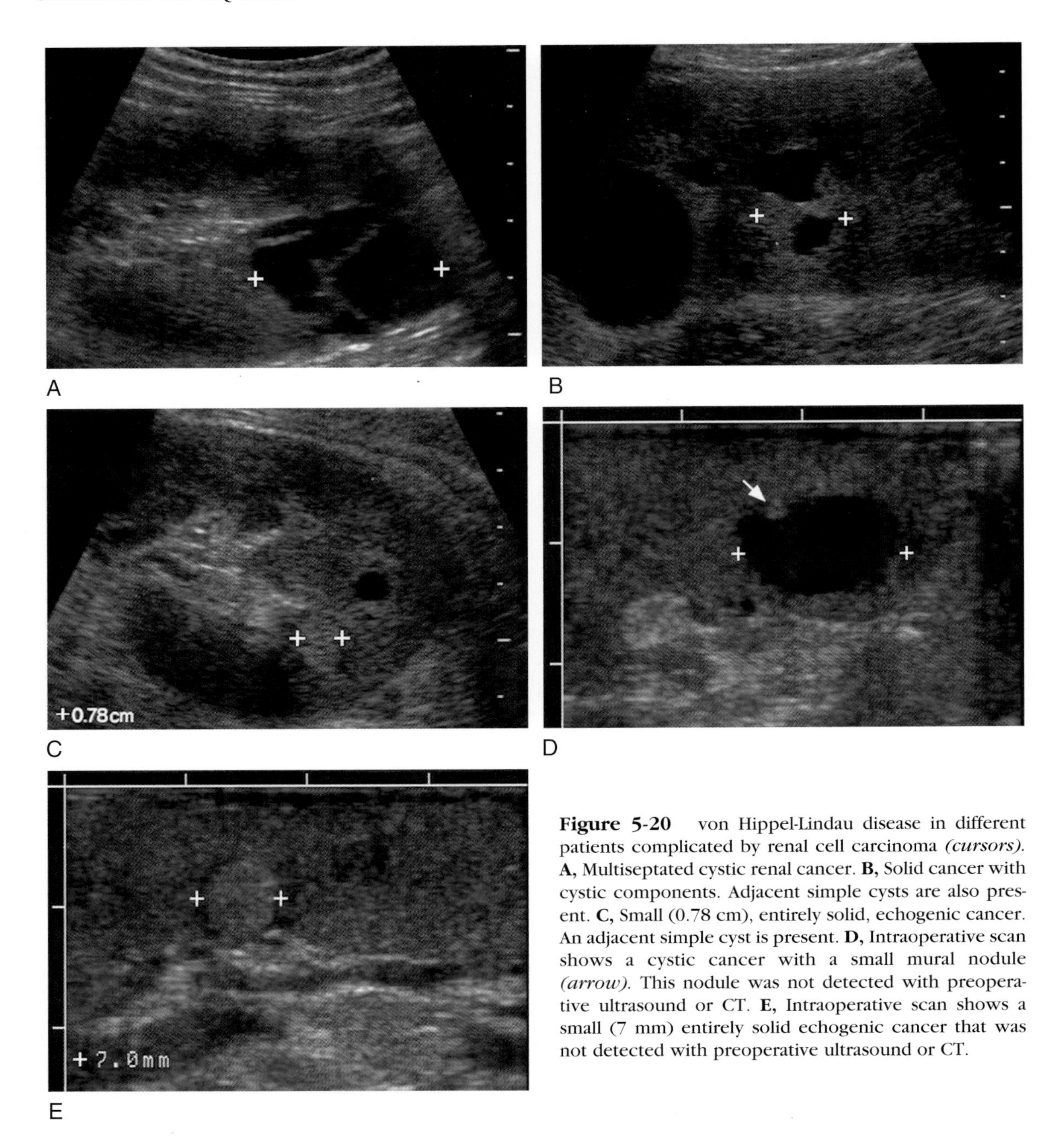

Figure 5-20 von Hippel-Lindau disease in different patients complicated by renal cell carcinoma *(cursors).* **A,** Multiseptated cystic renal cancer. **B,** Solid cancer with cystic components. Adjacent simple cysts are also present. **C,** Small (0.78 cm), entirely solid, echogenic cancer. An adjacent simple cyst is present. **D,** Intraoperative scan shows a cystic cancer with a small mural nodule *(arrow).* This nodule was not detected with preoperative ultrasound or CT. **E,** Intraoperative scan shows a small (7 mm) entirely solid echogenic cancer that was not detected with preoperative ultrasound or CT.

The pancreas is also affected, with an increased incidence of simple cysts that are generally asymptomatic. There is also an increased risk of islet cell tumors and cystic pancreatic neoplasms.

The diagnosis is made by finding a hemangioblastoma and at least one other lesion of the VHL complex, or at least one lesion in a patient in whom a family member has a hemangioblastoma. Family members at risk of inheriting the disease should be evaluated in late adolescence for both genetic counseling and therapeutic reasons. The brain, spinal cord, orbit, and abdomen should all be imaged in some fashion to search for the major manifestations of the disease. CT is the best means of initially evaluating the abdomen and is preferred for following the progress of the disease in affected patients. Sonography is valuable as a means of evaluating indeterminate masses in the kidney and pancreas. Intraoperative ultrasound examination is quite useful in patients undergoing partial nephrectomy for renal cell carcinoma. It is very sensitive for both detecting additional solid lesions and characterizing the nature of indeterminate lesions (see Fig. 5-20D and E).

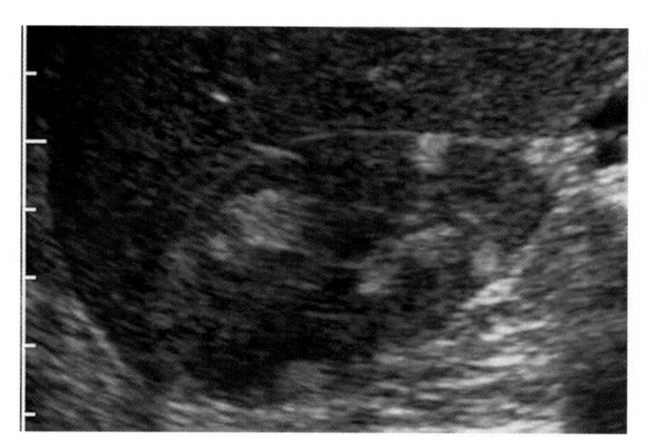

Figure 5-21 Tuberous sclerosis. Oblique view of the right kidney shows multiple hyperechoic masses due to multifocal angiomyolipomas.

Tuberous Sclerosis

Tuberous sclerosis is another multisystem disorder that is associated with the formation of renal cysts and neoplasms. Its classic clinical triad consists of mental retardation, seizures, and cutaneous lesions. In addition to the renal abnormalities, central nervous system lesions (cortical hamartomas, periventricular subependymal glial nodules, subependymal giant cell astrocytomas, and retinal hamartomas), cardiovascular lesions (cardiac rhabdomyomas), pulmonary lesions (lymphangiomyomatosis), and skeletal lesions (sclerotic patches and cystic lesions) may develop.

The kidneys are affected in up to 95% of adult patients, with 50% to 80% having multiple bilateral angiomyolipomas. These are usually small (Fig. 5-21), but they can become quite large and eventually replace most of the renal parenchyma. Their sonographic characteristics are identical to those of sporadic isolated angiomyolipomas. Renal cysts occur in 20% to 40% of patients. Cysts are a more common renal manifestation in infancy and childhood.

Table 5-2 compares and contrasts the different features of polycystic kidney disease, acquired cystic disease, von Hippel Lindau disease, and tuberous sclerosis.

MALIGNANT RENAL NEOPLASMS

Renal Cell Carcinoma

Renal cell carcinoma constitutes approximately 90% of the primary renal malignancies and is the most common solid renal mass in adults. Each year 15,000 new cases are detected in the U.S. population. Risk factors include advanced age, smoking, von Hippel-Lindau disease, and long-term dialysis. The male-to-female ratio is approximately 2:1. Hematuria occurs in approximately 60% of patients. Other signs and symptoms include weight loss, anemia, and fatigue. Paraneoplastic or hormonally related symptoms such as fever, erythrocytosis, and anorexia are also well described. One percent of the renal cell carcinomas are bilateral at presentation, and 1% of the patients will be found to have a contralateral renal cell carcinoma on follow-up. Ten percent of renal cell cancers are multifocal within the same kidney at the time of presentation. Histologically, they can be described in terms of the cell

Table 5-2 Renal Cystic Disease

	Kidney Size	Kidney Tumors	Extrarenal Cysts	Extrarenal Lesions
APKD	Large	None	Liver	Cerebral aneurysms
VHL	Normal/large	RCC	Pancreas	Pancreas cystic neoplasms Pancreas islet cell tumors Pheochromocytomas CNS hemangioblastomas Retinal angiomas
ACD	Small	RCC	None	None
TS	Normal/large	AML	None	Cerebral hamartomas Periventricular nodules Subungual fibromas Cardiac rhabdomyomas Lung lymphangiomyomatosis

APKD, adult polycystic kidney disease; VHL, von Hippel-Lindau disease; RCC, renal cell carcinoma; CNS, central nervous system; ACD, acquired cystic disease; TS, tuberous sclerosis; AML, angiomyolipoma.

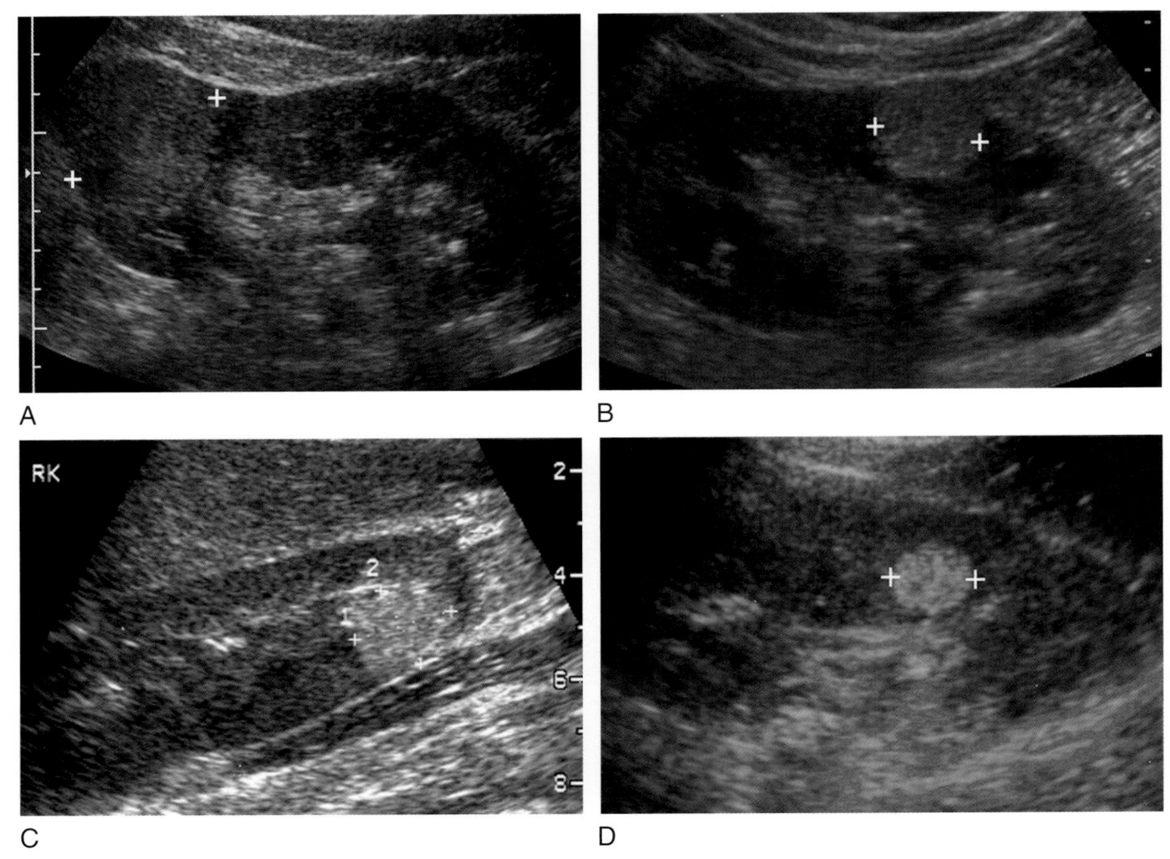

Figure 5-22 Hyperechoic renal cell cancer. Different patients with solid cancers *(cursors)* that are all more echogenic than renal cortex. **A,** Mildly echogenic mass. **B,** Moderately echogenic mass. **C** and **D,** Very echogenic masses that could simulate angiomyolipomas.

type (clear cell or granular cytoplasm), cellular organization (papillary, tubular, or medullary), and cellular morphology (well differentiated, poorly differentiated, or undifferentiated).

Renal cell cancer is a surgical lesion. Traditionally, it has been treated with radical nephrectomy. However, improvements in surgical techniques and follow-up data indicating similar survival have led to an increased percentage of patients being treated with partial nephrectomies. Cryoablation and other ablative techniques are also gaining acceptance for small renal cancers. Percutaneous needle biopsy of suspected renal cell cancer is rarely indicated because a negative biopsy does not exclude the diagnosis and the results of the biopsy rarely influence the need for surgical management. Exceptions to this rule include masses seen in patients with a history of extrarenal malignancies, lymphoma, or suspected infectious lesions, because surgery is not indicated in any of these conditions.

Fifty percent of renal cell carcinomas are hyperechoic compared with the normal adjacent renal parenchyma (Fig. 5-22). Forty percent are only slightly more echogenic than the renal parenchyma, but 10% are markedly hyperechoic, to the point that they are similar to the echogenicity of the renal sinus. Lesions that are this echogenic are even more common among small cancers, and these lesions can potentially be confused with angiomyolipomas. Thirty percent of renal cell cancers are isoechoic to the renal parenchyma (Fig. 5-23), and

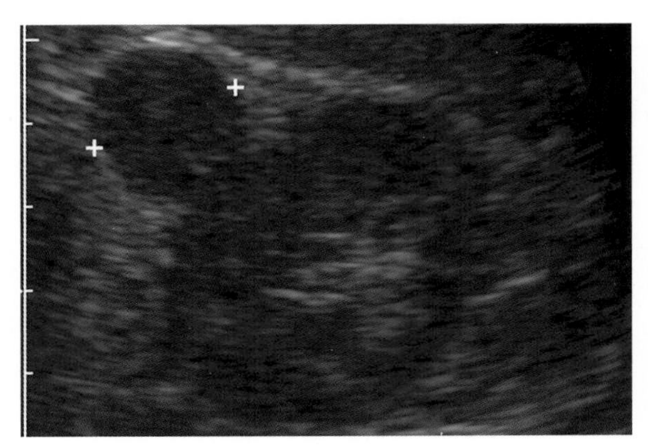

Figure 5-23 Isoechoic renal cell cancer. Transverse scan shows an exophytic mass *(cursors)* that is similar in echogenicity to the rest of the renal cortex.

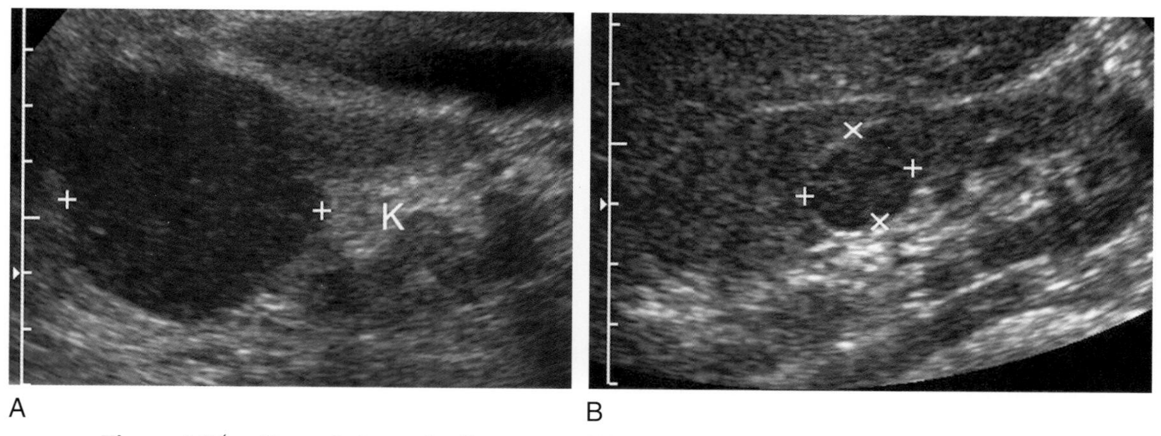

Figure 5-24 Hypoechoic renal cell cancer in different patients. **A**, Large mass *(cursors)* arising from the periphery of the kidney (K). **B**, Smaller mass *(cursors)* arising in the central renal cortex.

10% are hypoechoic (Fig. 5-24). Isoechoic tumors are detected when they are exophytic or when they distort the renal contour. Many renal cancers will be complex, either solid with scattered cystic components or solid with hemorrhagic or necrotic regions (Fig. 5-25). Twenty percent of renal cell cancers contain identifiable calcification that may appear punctate, amorphous, or mottled (Fig. 5-26A). It is very unusual for renal cell tumors to have peripheral rim-like calcification. Lesions that are so densely calcified that portions are obscured by shadowing should be evaluated with follow-up CT (see Fig 5-26B).

All solid renal masses in adults should be assumed to be renal cell carcinoma unless there is unequivocal evidence to the contrary. For practical purposes the only way to prove that a solid mass is not a renal cancer is to document the presence of fat in the mass. This is best done with nonenhanced CT or MRI, using thin sections when necessary.

Although it is not uncommon for renal cell carcinoma to contain cystic components and areas of necrosis or hemorrhage, predominantly cystic renal cell carcinomas are unusual and account for less than 5% of the total cases (Fig. 5-27). They may assume the form of a cyst with multiple thick septations, a thick or irregular wall, or a cyst with a solid mural nodule. In general the likelihood of malignancy increases with an increasing number and thickness of septations and with increased wall thickness or irregularity. Detection of blood flow within solid-appearing areas of a complex cystic lesion should be taken as strong evidence of malignancy. Predominantly cystic lesions that are well seen sonographically and have features worrisome for malignancy should be considered potentially malignant regardless of the

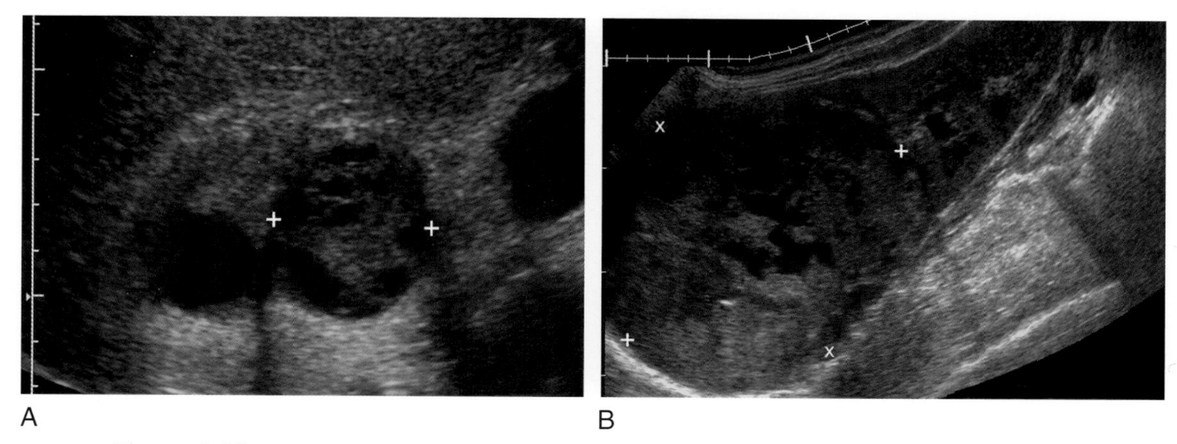

Figure 5-25 Complex renal cell cancer in different patients. **A**, Predominantly solid mass *cursors)* with scattered cystic components. **B**, Large mass *(cursors)* with central areas of liquefaction likely due to hemorrhage or necrosis.

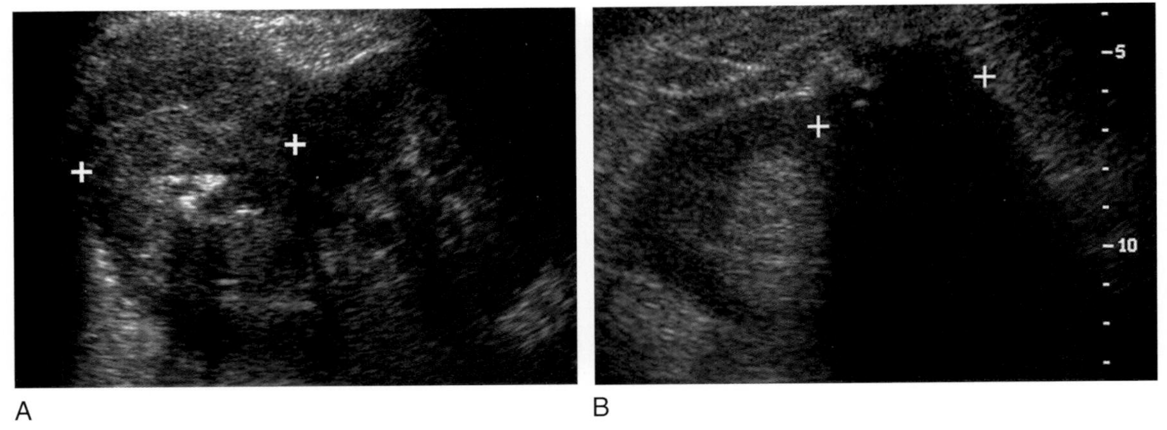

Figure 5-26 Renal cell cancer with calcification in different patients. **A,** Solid mass *(cursors)* with punctate areas of central, shadowing calcification. **B,** Lesion *(cursors)* with irregular peripheral, densely shadowing calcification. Because the shadow precluded evaluation of the deeper aspects of the mass, this lesion was evaluated with CT, which showed extensive irregular calcification that was both central and peripheral.

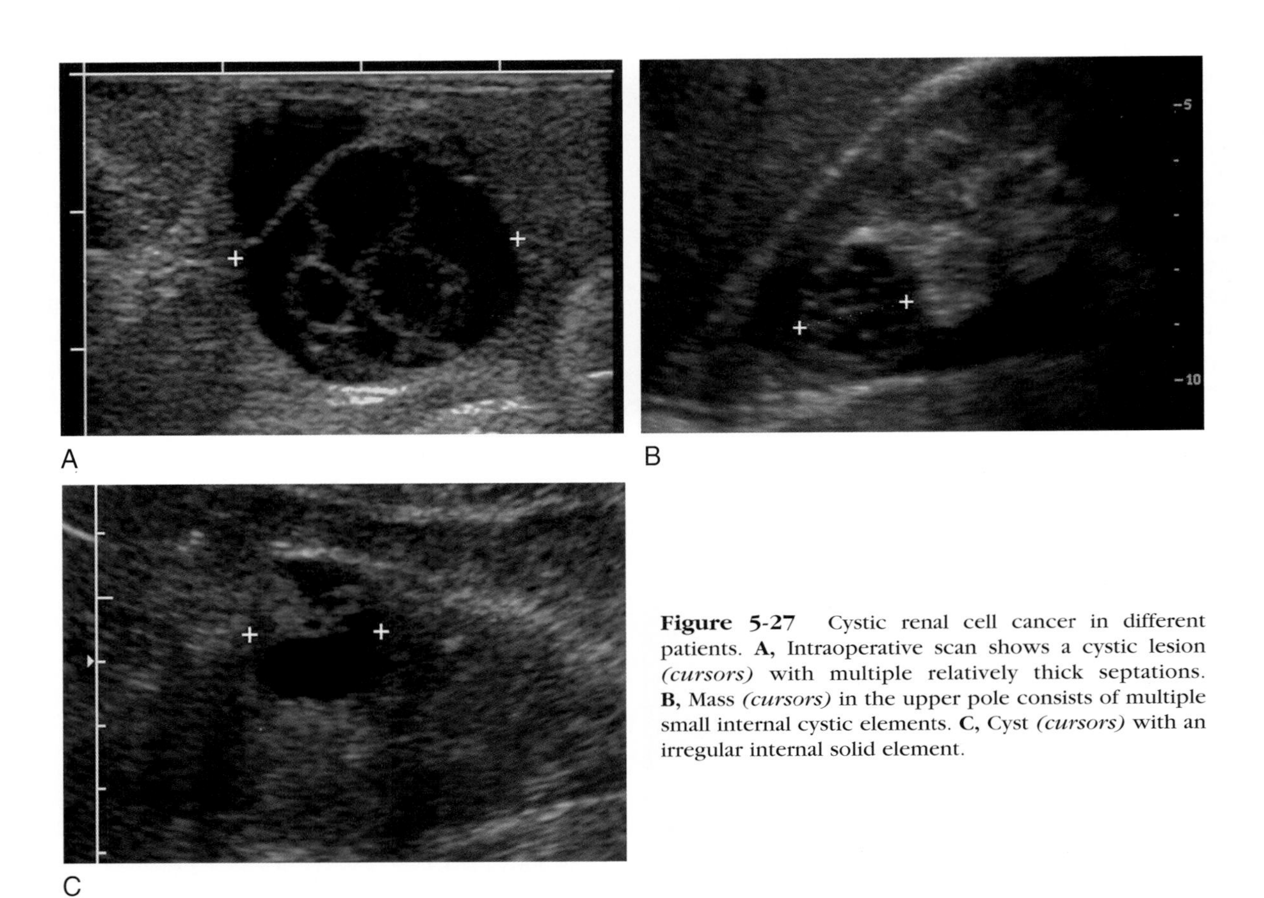

Figure 5-27 Cystic renal cell cancer in different patients. **A,** Intraoperative scan shows a cystic lesion *(cursors)* with multiple relatively thick septations. **B,** Mass *(cursors)* in the upper pole consists of multiple small internal cystic elements. **C,** Cyst *(cursors)* with an irregular internal solid element.

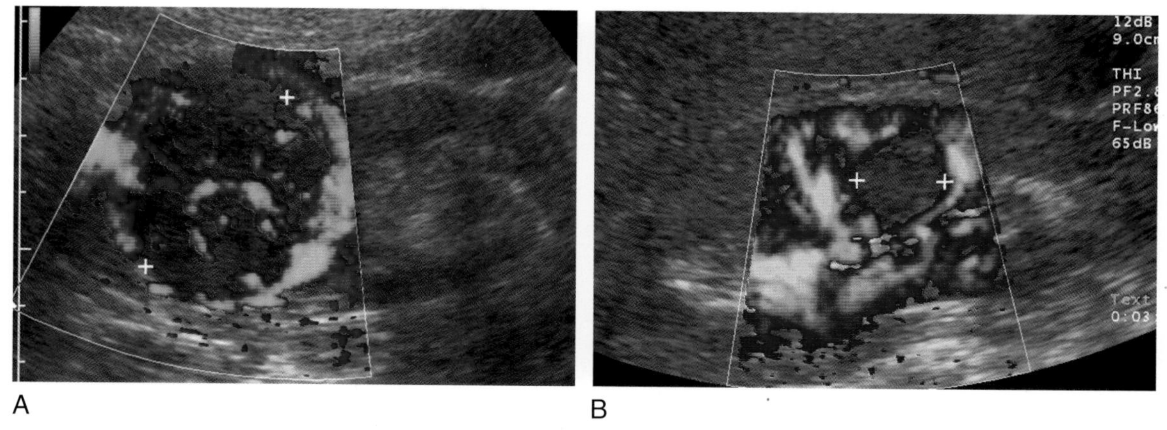

Figure 5-28 Vascularity of renal cell cancer in different patients. **A,** Power Doppler scan shows a solid mass *(cursors)* with readily detectable internal vascularity. **B,** Power Doppler scan shows a solid mass *(cursors)* with no detectable internal vascularity.

findings from other imaging studies such as CT or MRI. On the other hand, the findings of these other studies are very useful in excluding malignancy in lesions that are truly indeterminate or are poorly visualized sonographically.

Renal cell carcinoma is a vascular tumor, and in many instances it is possible to detect tumor vascularity on color or power Doppler analysis (Fig. 5-28A). For indeterminate lesions, detection of vascularity is helpful because it indicates that the lesion contains soft tissue and is almost certainly a tumor. Even when tumor vascularity is seen, it is rarely as vascular as the normal renal parenchyma. Failure to detect vascularity is not helpful because some tumors are hypovascular and detection of flow is difficult in deep lesions (see Fig. 5-28B). Intravenous contrast agent administration will undoubtedly assist in the detection of vascularity by documenting enhancement, similar to post-contrast CT scans (Fig. 5-29).

The most widely used staging system for renal cell carcinoma is the Robson system. Stage I is confined to the kidney. Stage II is invasion of the perinephric fat. Stage IIIA is invasion of the renal vein, IIIB is regional nodal metastases, and IIIC is combined venous and nodal involvement. Stage IV is invasion of adjacent organs (IVA) or distant metastases (IVB).

In the past, approximately 10% of patients with renal cell carcinoma have had caval involvement and 20% have had renal vein involvement at the time of presentation. Nowadays, the majority of renal cell cancers are discovered as small incidental masses on CT and ultrasound examinations, and venous invasion is much less common in these instances. Usually, tumor invades the lumen of the vein but does not invade the vessel wall.

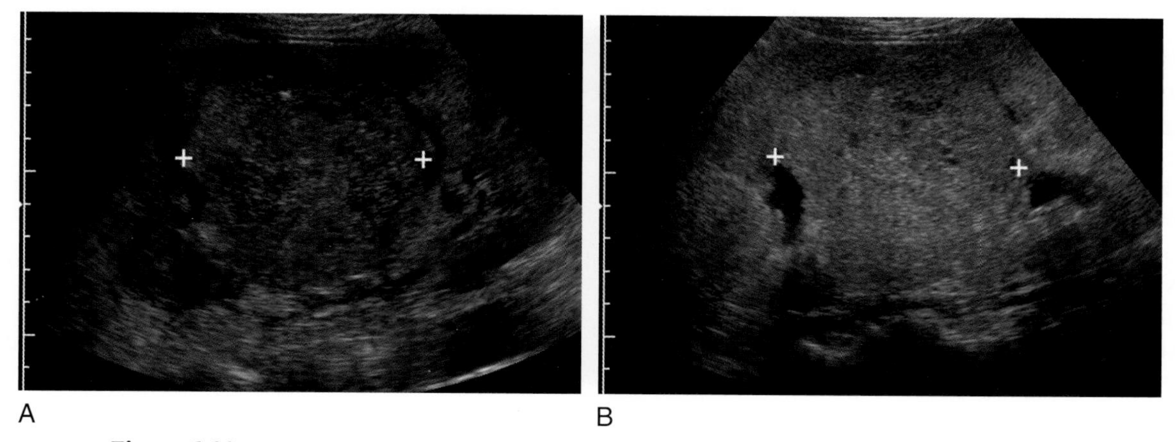

Figure 5-29 Contrast enhancement of renal cell cancer. **A,** Noncontrast scan shows a large solid mass *(cursors)* that is slightly hyperechoic. **B,** Postcontrast scan shows enhancement of the mass to a degree similar to renal cortex.

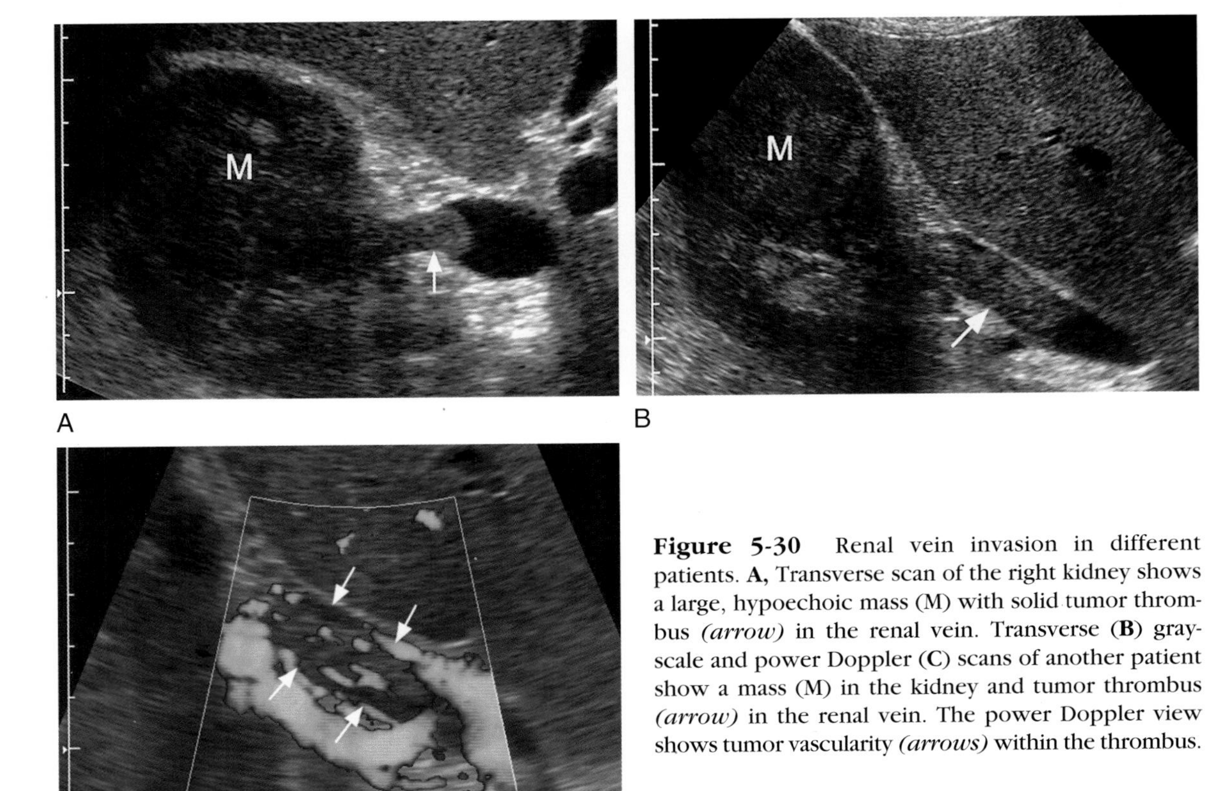

Figure 5-30 Renal vein invasion in different patients. **A,** Transverse scan of the right kidney shows a large, hypoechoic mass (M) with solid tumor thrombus *(arrow)* in the renal vein. Transverse **(B)** grayscale and power Doppler **(C)** scans of another patient show a mass (M) in the kidney and tumor thrombus *(arrow)* in the renal vein. The power Doppler view shows tumor vascularity *(arrows)* within the thrombus.

Sonography is an excellent means of identifying venous invasion (Fig. 5-30), especially invasion of the inferior vena cava (Fig. 5-31). In many cases, the internal vascularity of tumor thrombus can be detected with color or power Doppler imaging. Venous invasion has little effect on prognosis but does effect the surgical approach. When tumor thrombus extends above the diaphragm, especially when the heart is involved, a combined thoracoabdominal approach is needed. In most cases, CT or MRI is used to stage renal cell carcinoma and sensitivity for venous invasion is similar to sonography.

A variant of renal cell carcinoma that is becoming more widely recognized is medullary cancer. This is an aggressive cancer that affects patients with sickle cell trait. It is seen at an earlier age, is more commonly associated with metastases at the time of presentation, and has a much worse prognosis than typical renal cell cancer (Fig. 5-32).

Occasionally, normal renal parenchyma can assume a mass-like appearance and be confused with a renal cell carcinoma (Box 5-2). Hypertrophied columns of Bertin are common variants that have been described previously (see Fig. 5-4). Residual functioning renal parenhyma can also be confused with a solid mass when it is surrounded by atrophic renal parenchyma (Fig. 5-33). In most cases knowledge of these potential pitfalls is enough to allow for a confident diagnosis to be made. When there is doubt, scintigraphy, CT, and MRI are useful tools for further evaluation.

Box 5-2 Differential Diagnosis of Solid Renal Masses

Renal cell carcinoma
Angiomyolipoma
Transitional cell carcinoma
Oncocytoma
Lymphoma
Metastasis
Juxtaglomerular cell tumor
Column of Bertin
Focal parenchymal hypertrophy
Focal pyelonephritis

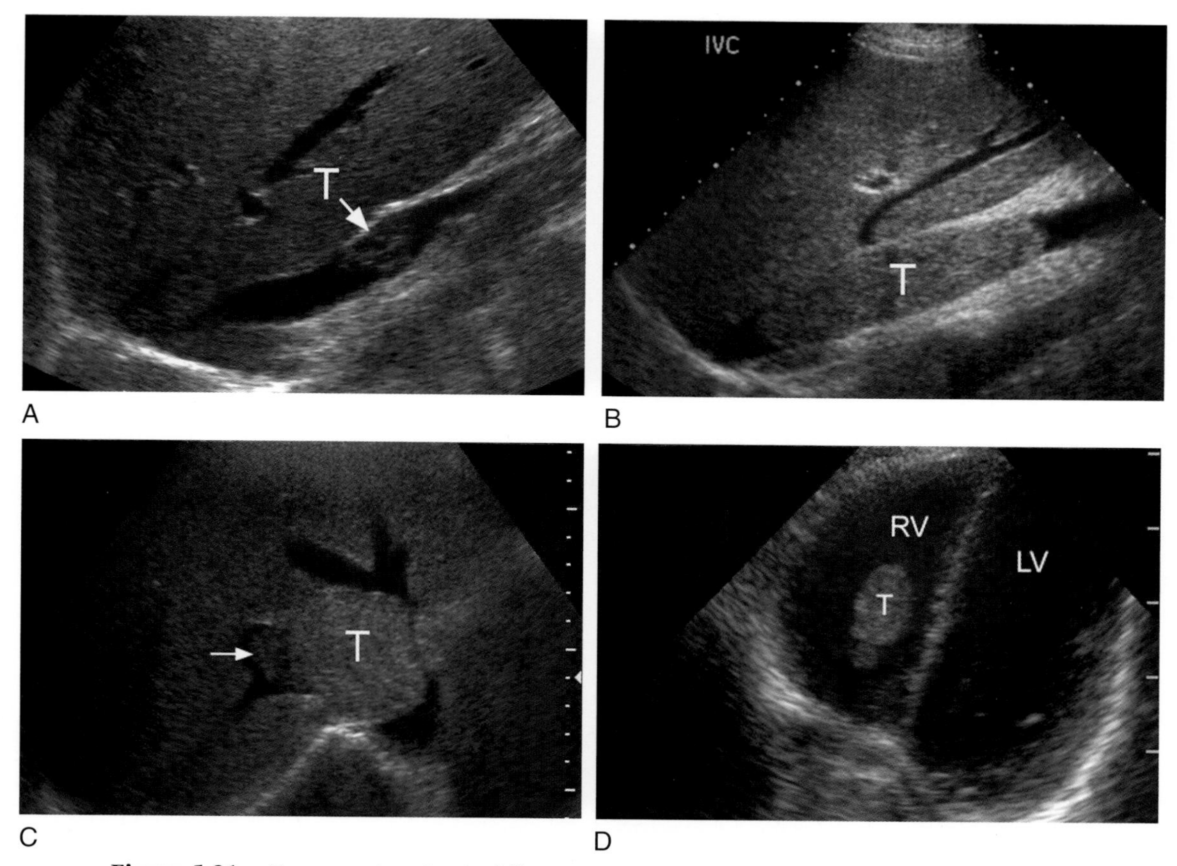

Figure 5-31 Vena cava invasion in different patients. **A,** Longitudinal view of the inferior vena cava shows localized, solid tumor thrombus (T) entering the cava at the level of the renal vein. **B,** Longitudinal view of the cava shows more extensive tumor thrombus (T) entering the cava and growing superiorly but remaining below the diaphragm. **C,** Transverse view of the cava at the level of the hepatic vein confluence shows a large tumor thrombus (T) at this level. Thrombus is also seen entering the right hepatic vein *(arrow)*. **D,** View of the heart shows the right ventricle (RV) and the left ventricle (LV). A solid tumor thrombus (T) extended from the vena cava into the right atrium and the right ventricle.

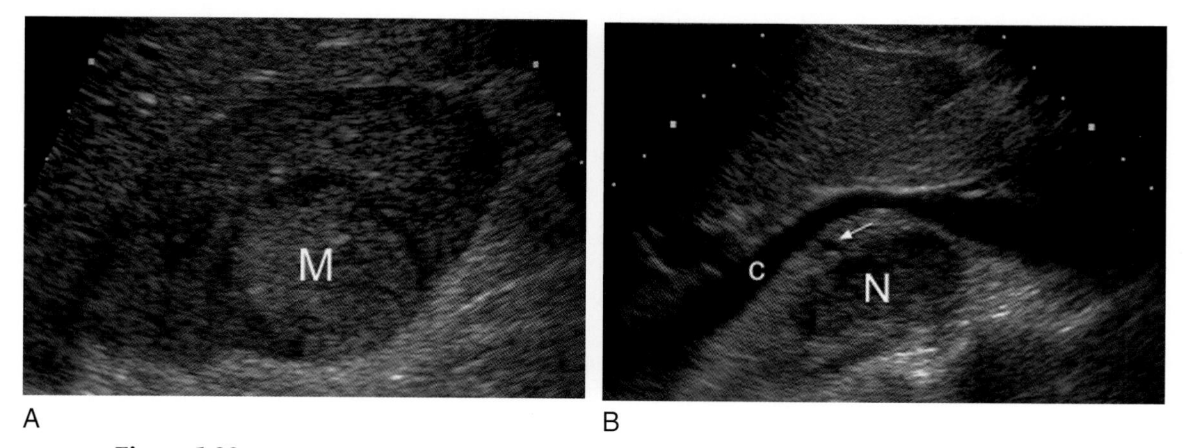

Figure 5-32 Medullary renal cancer. **A,** Longitudinal view of the lateral aspect of the right kidney shows a solid, slightly hyperechoic mass (M). **B,** Longitudinal view of the inferior vena cava (C) shows a large retroperitoneal nodal metastasis (N) deviating the vena cava and the right renal artery *(arrow)* anteriorly. A liver metastasis was also seen on other images.

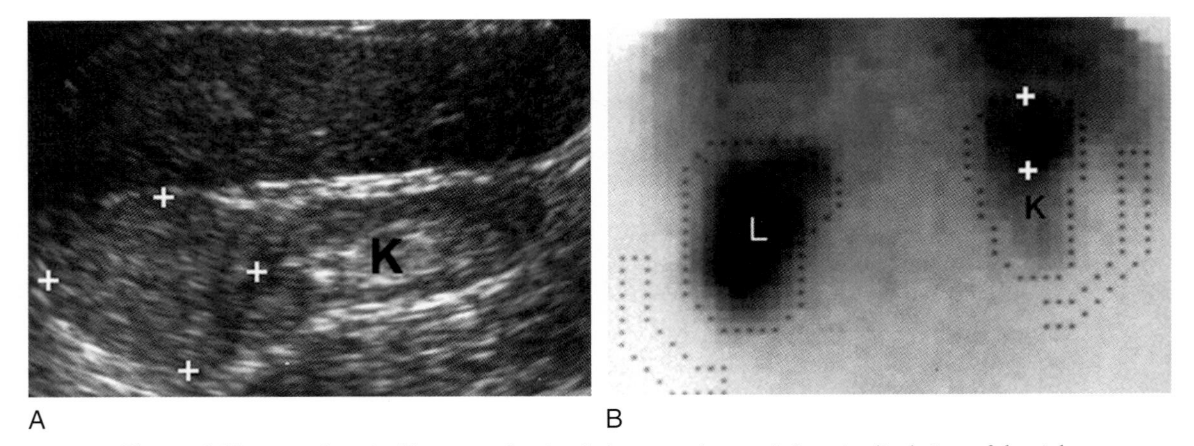

Figure 5-33 Focal cortical hypertrophy simulating a renal mass. **A,** Longitudinal view of the right kidney demonstrates an isoechoic mass-like lesion *(cursors)* arising from the upper pole of the kidney (K). The kidney itself is atrophic and echogenic. **B,** Renal scintigraphy from a posterior view shows functioning parenchyma *(cursors)* in the upper pole of the right kidney (K). The normal left kidney (L) is also seen.

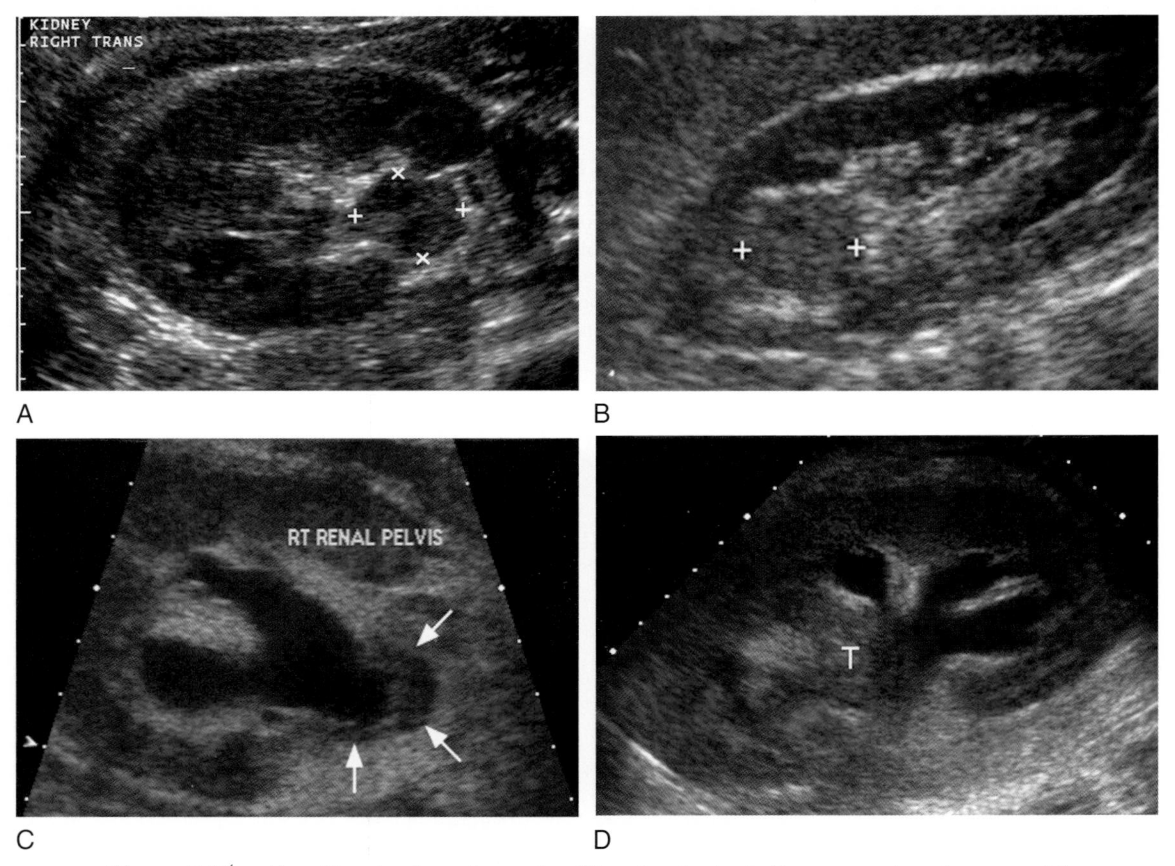

Figure 5-34 Transitional cell carcinoma in different patients. **A,** Transverse view shows a solid mass *(cursors)* located in the renal hilum. **B,** Longitudinal view shows a solid mass centered in the upper pole renal sinus *(cursors)*. **C,** Transverse view shows hydronephrosis and focal thickening of the renal pelvis *(arrows)*. **D,** Longitudinal view shows solid tissue (T) filling the superior renal collecting system and hydronephrosis of the rest of the collecting system.

Transitional Cell Carcinoma

Transitional cell carcinoma accounts for more than 90% of the urothelium-based tumors. Most of the remainder are squamous cell carcinomas. Transitional cell carcinoma of the intrarenal collecting system is five to ten times less frequent than renal cell carcinoma. Multiplicity and bilaterality are relatively common, and up to 10% of the patients have bilateral metachronous or synchronous primary tumors. The presence of a transitional cell carcinoma indicates that the entire urothelium is at risk, with the bladder at greatest risk followed by the renal pelvis and the ureter.

Most transitional cell carcinomas in the kidney are too small to be detected by sonography. Intravenous urography and retrograde pyelography are the main methods used to detect this carcinoma in the kidney and ureter. The sonographic appearance of more bulky transitional cell carcinoma includes an intraluminal polypoid mass, thickening of the urothelium, and an otherwise nonspecific solid mass centered in the renal sinus (Fig. 5-34). Infiltration of the adjacent renal parenchyma can occur, and in such cases it is not possible to distinguish transitional cell carcinoma from renal cell carcinoma. However, transitional cell cancer that invades the kidney typically has a more infiltrative appearance than renal cell cancer. Besides transitional cell carcinoma, other lesions that appear as intraluminal masses in the collecting system include blood clots (Fig. 5-35), fungus balls, fibroepithelial polyps, malakoplakia, and calculi. Sonography is good at distinguishing stones in the collecting system from the other lesions. Detection of internal vascularity excludes clot and fungus balls, but lack of detectable vessels is not helpful.

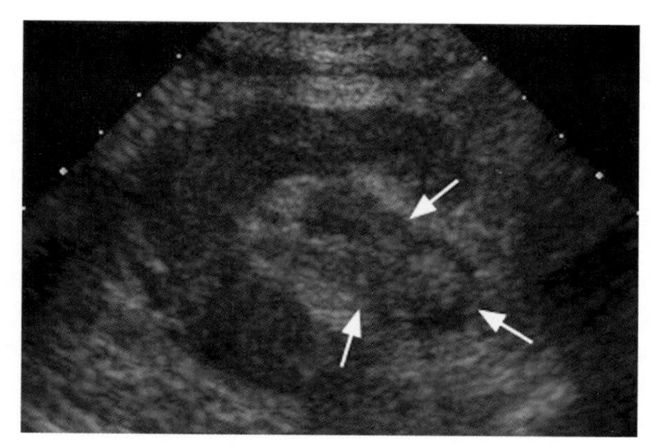

Figure 5-35 Blood clot. Transverse view shows solid clot filling the renal pelvis *(arrows)*. This occurred immediately after a renal biopsy and was accompanied by gross hematuria.

One potential pitfall in the diagnosis of transitional cell carcinoma is mistaking prominent renal papillae as filling defects in the calices. This can occur in the setting of hydronephrosis (Fig. 5-36). The primary distinguishing feature of papillae is that they appear in all the calices, but other lesions such as transitional cell carcinoma appear only in one or a very limited number of calices.

Lymphoma

The vast majority of renal lymphomas occur in the setting of more widespread disease and are caused by hematogenous spread or by direct invasion from adjacent involved lymph nodes. Renal involvement is most often bilateral and occurs much more commonly in patients with non-Hodgkin's lymphomas than in those

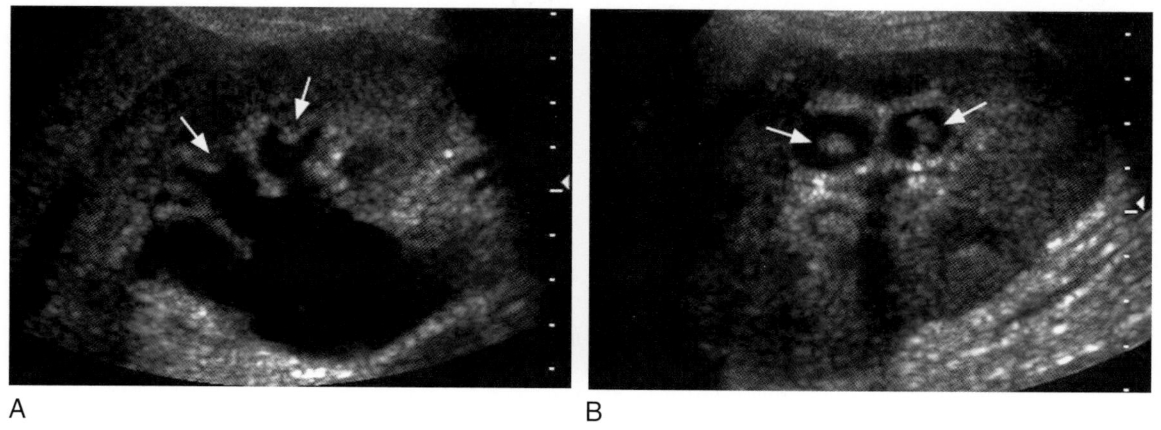

Figure 5-36 Prominent papillary tips. **A,** Longitudinal view shows moderate hydronephrosis and distention of the calyces. The tips of the papillae *(arrows)* are seen protruding into the calyces. **B,** Oblique view shows the papillary tips *(arrows)* appearing to be isolated solid lesions within the lumen of the calyx. These should not be confused with tumors, blood clots, or other filling defects.

with Hodgkin's disease. It is found at autopsy in up to one third of the patients with lymphoma but is not noted this frequently on imaging studies, owing to the small size of the nodules or occasionally to the diffusely infiltrating nature of the process. It is unusual for renal lymphoma to produce symptoms.

The most common sonographic finding is multiple bilateral hypoechoic masses (Fig. 5-37A). Unifocal, unilateral disease occurs but is unusual. Diffuse infiltration and smooth renal enlargement may also be seen. Because lymphoma is a very homogeneous tumor with a monotonous histologic composition and little stromal tissue, there are very few internal reflectors. This can result in an anechoic or near-anechoic appearance that simulates cysts in the kidney (see Fig. 5-37B) and elsewhere in the body. In most cases the lack of acoustic enhancement deep to the mass provides a clue that it is solid and not cystic. In rare instances a certain amount of acoustic enhancement can be seen despite the solid nature of the tumor. One fairly characteristic pattern of growth is for the tumor to grow into the perinephric space so that it partially or completely surrounds the kidney (see Fig. 5-37C and D). As with parenchymal involvement, perinephric involvement can simulate fluid.

Metastatic Disease

Metastatic disease to the kidney generally occurs in the setting of known metastases elsewhere in the body. The most common primary tumors that spread to the kidneys are those of the lung, colon, breast, stomach, prostate, pancreas, and melanoma. The incidence of renal metastases in cancer patients is as high as 20% in

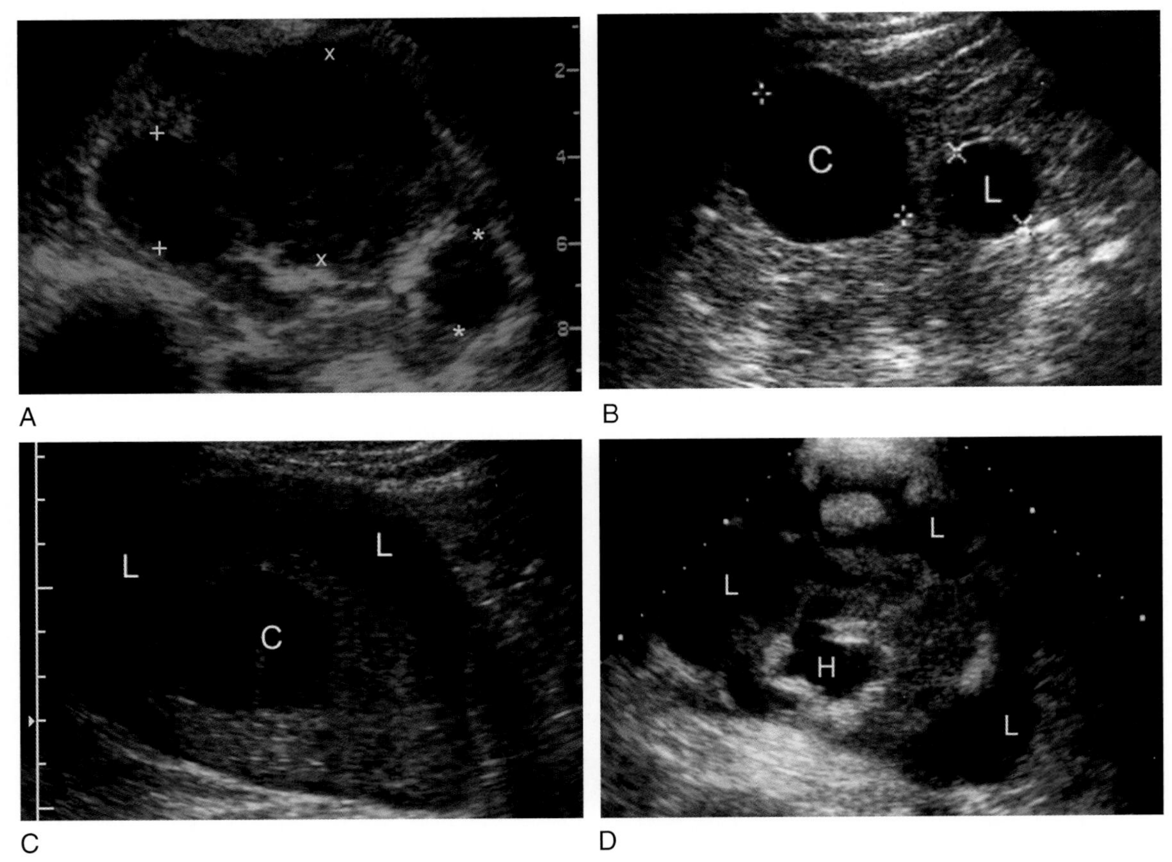

Figure 5-37 Lymphoma in different patients. **A,** Longitudinal view shows several hypoechoic masses *(cursors).* **B,** Longitudinal view shows a large renal cyst (C) and a smaller lymphomatous lesion (L) that closely simulates a cyst. Contrast medium–enhanced CT showed that the smaller lesion was enhancing and follow-up scans showed interval growth. **C,** Transverse view shows hypoechoic and anechoic lymphomatous tissue (L) infiltrating in the perinephric space. A septated renal cyst (C) is also present. **D,** Transverse view shows anechoic and hypoechoic lymphomatous tissue (L) infiltrating the echogenic fat within the perinephric space. Hydronephrosis (H) is also present. In **C** and **D**, the lymphomatous infiltration of the perinephric space could be confused with perinephric fluid.

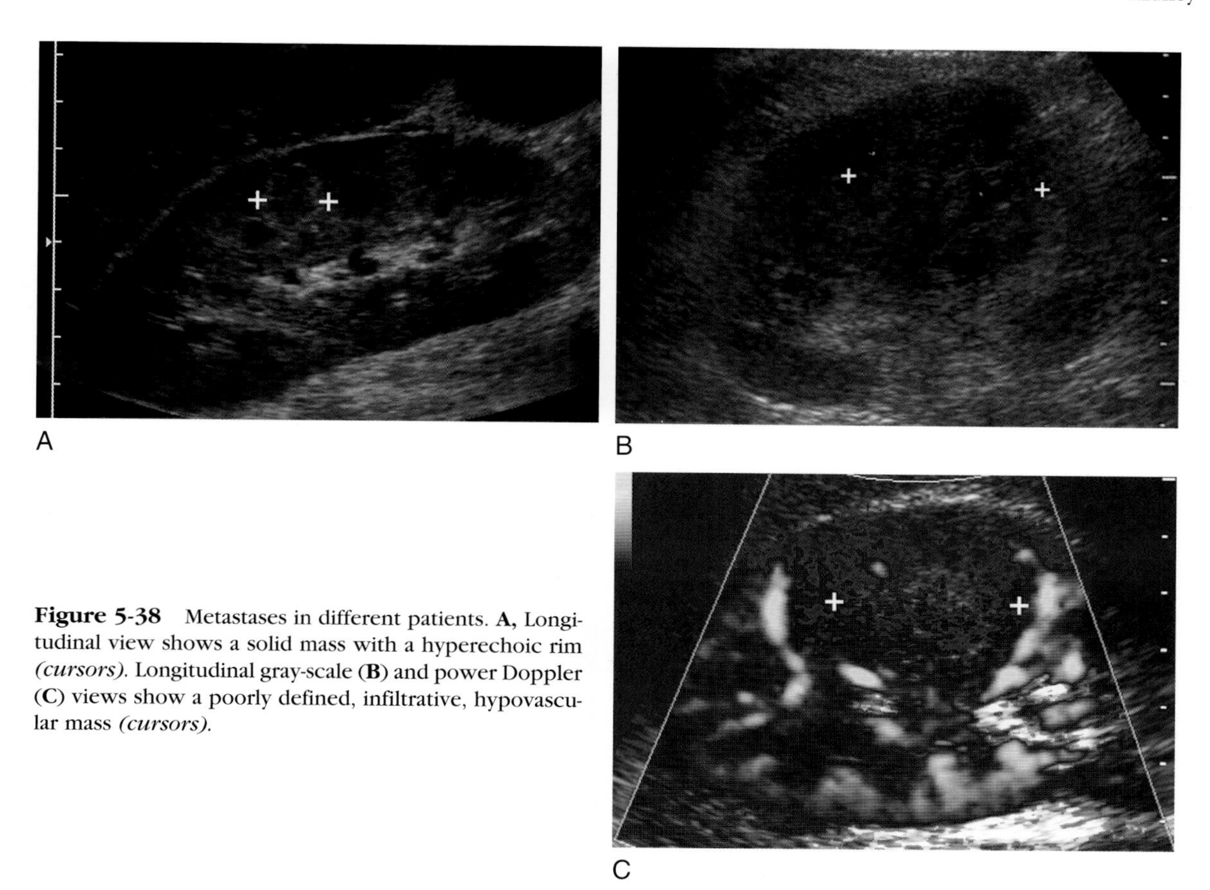

Figure 5-38 Metastases in different patients. **A,** Longitudinal view shows a solid mass with a hyperechoic rim *(cursors).* Longitudinal gray-scale (**B**) and power Doppler (**C**) views show a poorly defined, infiltrative, hypovascular mass *(cursors).*

autopsy series. The improved detection of smaller renal lesions with current state-of-the-art ultrasound and CT equipment has allowed us to detect a larger number of renal metastases. Renal metastases are typically solid and are often infiltrative. Unlike renal cell carcinoma, it is unusual for metastases to be complex and cystic. Because the sonographic characteristics of renal cell carcinoma and renal metastases overlap, the diagnosis depends on biopsy findings (Fig. 5-38).

BENIGN RENAL NEOPLASMS

Angiomyolipoma

As the name implies, angiomyolipomas are tumors composed of vessels, muscles, and fat. They are the most common benign renal neoplasm and are second only to renal cell carcinoma in overall frequency of renal tumors. These tumors occur most frequently in middle-aged women. They have no malignant potential and rarely cause symptoms. Bleeding is the only serious complication, but it is rare and tends to occur only when lesions exceed 4 cm. For this reason, some urologists advocate removal of asymptomatic angiomyolipomas larger than 4 cm.

The classic sonographic appearance, seen approximately 80% of the time, is a homogeneous, well-defined cortical mass that is as echogenic as renal fat (Fig. 5-39). Although this is very suggestive of angiomyolipoma, approximately 10% of renal cell carcinomas can mimic this appearance (see Fig. 5-22). One distinguishing feature, seen in 20% to 30% of angiomyolipomas, is some degree of acoustic shadowing. In the absence of calcification, this is almost never a feature of renal cell carcinoma. The shadowing associated with angiomyolipomas is probably due to attenuation of the sound beam by the mixture of fatty and soft tissue elements of the tumor. Another useful feature to look for are cystic components, because these are rare in angiomyolipomas but are not uncommon in renal cell carcinoma. Hyperechoic renal masses that show no partial shadowing require further evaluation. If an angiomyolipoma is 1 cm or larger, thin-section CT or MRI should be able to detect fat. Volume-averaging effects may make it difficult to detect fat in very small angiomyolipomas, and it is reasonable to monitor such masses with periodic ultrasound studies. If fat is not detected on CT or MRI in a lesion larger than 1 cm, renal cell carcinoma should be a strong consideration and it should be handled accordingly.

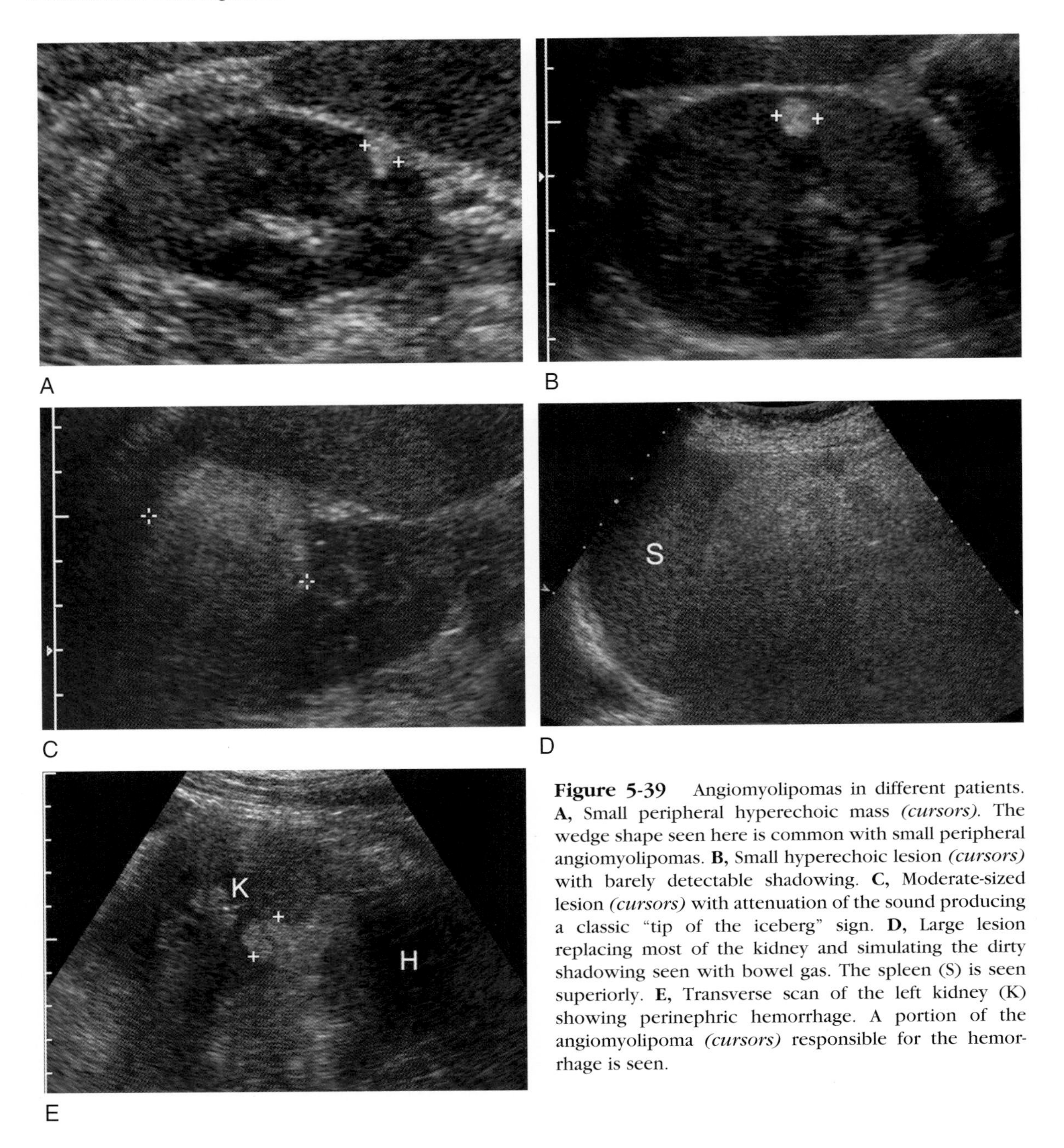

Figure 5-39 Angiomyolipomas in different patients. **A,** Small peripheral hyperechoic mass *(cursors).* The wedge shape seen here is common with small peripheral angiomyolipomas. **B,** Small hyperechoic lesion *(cursors)* with barely detectable shadowing. **C,** Moderate-sized lesion *(cursors)* with attenuation of the sound producing a classic "tip of the iceberg" sign. **D,** Large lesion replacing most of the kidney and simulating the dirty shadowing seen with bowel gas. The spleen (S) is seen superiorly. **E,** Transverse scan of the left kidney (K) showing perinephric hemorrhage. A portion of the angiomyolipoma *(cursors)* responsible for the hemorrhage is seen.

Other lesions that can simulate an angiomyolipoma are deep cortical scars or cysts that are nearly completely filled with crystals. In most cases scars are filled with perinephric fat, and this is evident sonographically (Fig. 5-40). Crystal-filled cysts will produce a color Doppler ring-down artifact that is not seen with angiomyolipomas.

Oncocytoma

Oncocytomas are a type of renal adenoma with large epithelial cells rich in granular eosinophilic cytoplasm. They account for approximately 5% of renal neoplasms. Their sonographic appearance is generally nonspecific and overlaps with renal cell cancer (Fig. 5-41). A stellate central scar is characteristic of oncocytomas on CT, but it is rarely seen without contrast medium enhancement and only occasionally even seen then. Unfortunately, renal cell carcinomas can also have central necrosis or hemorrhage that simulates a central scar, so these lesions almost always must be surgically removed to determine if they are malignant. A partial nephrectomy or cryoablation can be substituted for radical nephrectomy if the diagnosis of oncocytoma is suspected preoperatively.

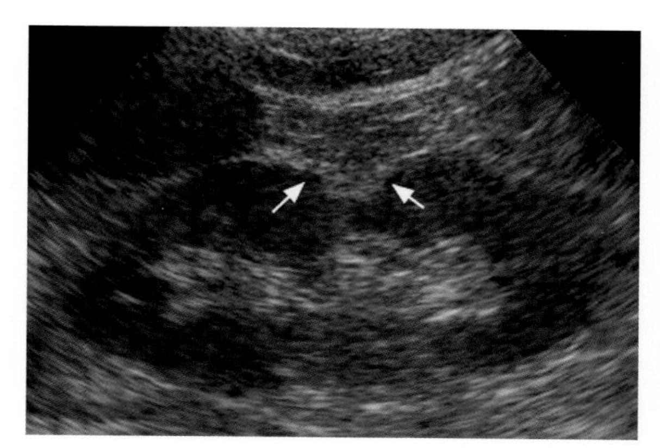

Figure 5-40 Cortical scar. Longitudinal view of the kidney shows an echogenic region *(arrows)* replacing the normal cortex. The continuity with the echogenic perinephric fat and the smooth transition of the renal capsule help to distinguish this from an echogenic mass such as an angiomyolipoma.

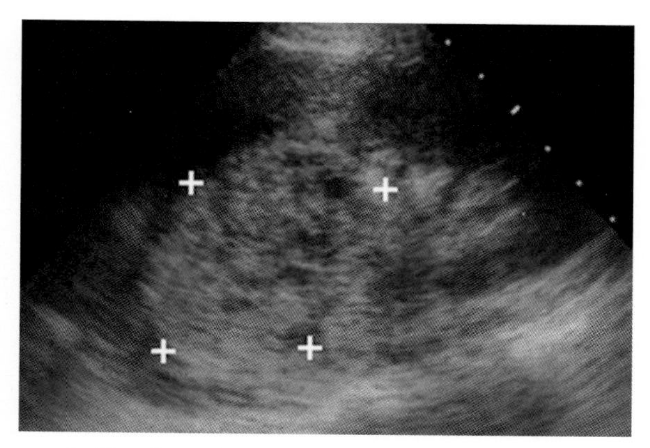

Figure 5-42 Juxtaglomerular cell tumor. Longitudinal view of a young woman with hypertension shows a complex echogenic mass *(cursors)* in the left kidney.

Juxtaglomerular Cell Tumor

A juxtaglomerular cell tumor is a rare benign tumor that is also called a reninoma because it secretes renin. It occurs most often in young women, and patients typically initially exhibit signs and symptoms relating to severe hypertension. The sonographic characteristics of this lesion are variable, but they are most often hyperechoic (Fig. 5-42).

Multilocular Cystic Nephroma

Multilocular cystic nephroma goes by a variety of names, and this has resulted in a certain amount of

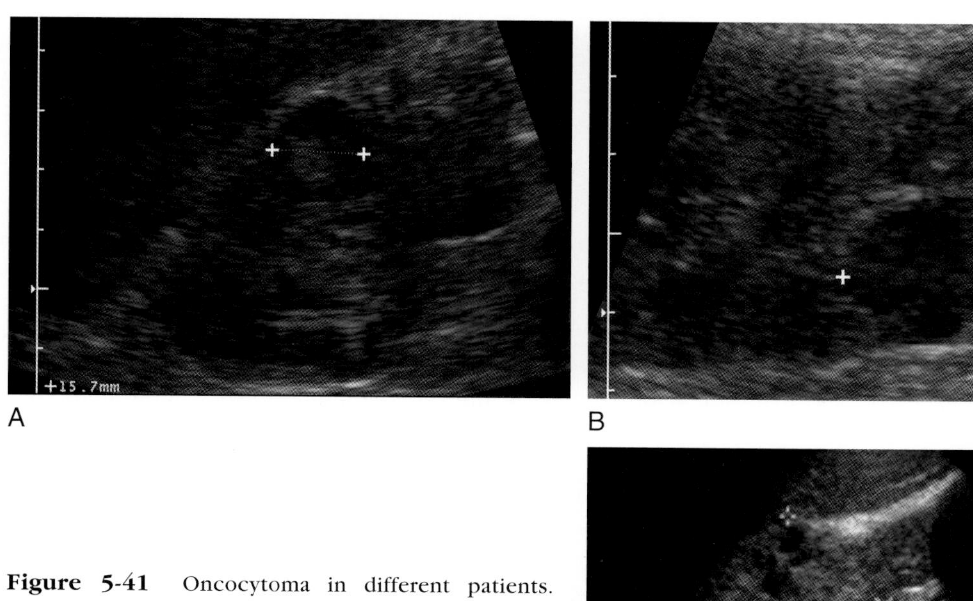

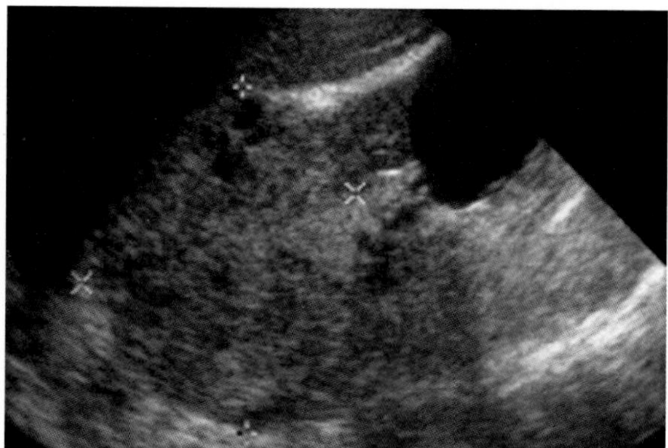

Figure 5-41 Oncocytoma in different patients. **A,** Longitudinal view shows a solid, heterogeneous mass *(cursors)*. **B,** Longitudinal view shows a solid, uniformly hypoechoic mass *(cursors)*. **C,** Longitudinal view shows a solid, hyperechoic mass *(cursors)*. In all cases, the appearance is indistinguishable from a renal cell cancer.

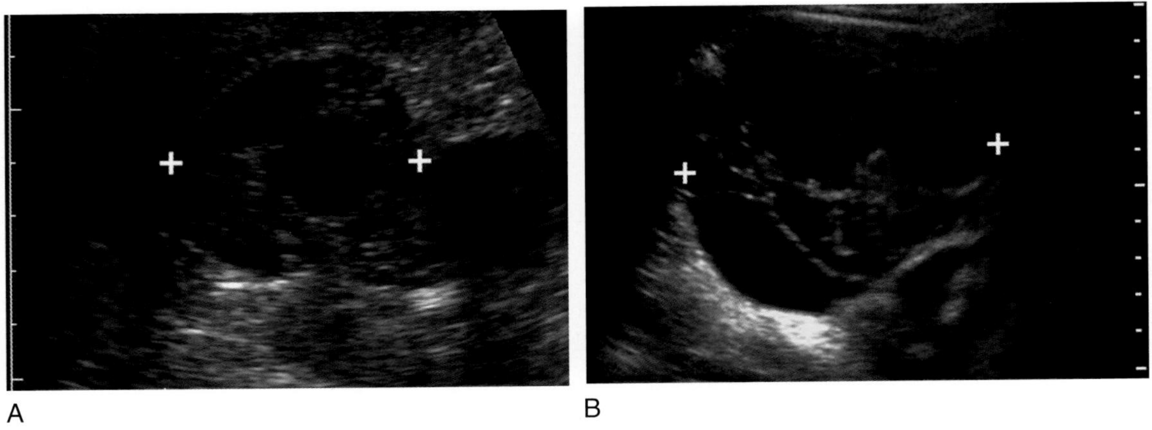

Figure 5-43 Multilocular cystic nephroma in different patients. **A** and **B,** Views show complex, predominantly cystic masses *(cursors)* that contain both large and small cystic regions.

Box 5-3 Differential Diagnosis of Complex Cystic Masses

- Hemorrhagic cyst
- Infected cyst
- Multiseptated cyst
- Abscess
- Hematoma
- Cystic renal cell carcinoma
- Multilocular cystic nephroma

confusion about its characteristics. Most experts consider it to be a benign renal neoplasm composed of multiple large, noncommunicating cystic spaces. It is an encapsulated lesion that contains no differentiated renal tissue and tends to afflict young boys and older women. Although a mass composed of multiple, various-sized cysts is characteristic of multilocular cystic nephroma (Fig. 5-43), this finding can also be exhibited by cystic renal cell carcinoma (see Fig. 5-27) and by cystic Wilms' tumors occurring in childhood (Box 5-3). For practical purposes, masses composed of multiple cysts or multiple loculations must be removed surgically because of the possibility of malignancy. If the preoperative diagnosis of multilocular cystic nephroma is suggested, a partial nephrectomy may be performed rather than a radical nephrectomy.

INFECTION

Pyelonephritis, as the name implies, refers to infection of the renal collecting system and renal parenchyma. It usually stems from the retrograde migration of bacteria up the ureter and into the kidney. This classically is associated with the reflux of urine from the bladder to the ureter, but in most adults and some children there is no evidence of vesicoureteral reflux and presumably bacteria ascend the ureter against the persistent antegrade flow of urine. Hematogenous transmission of infection to the kidneys also occurs generally in the setting of intravenous drug abuse or endocarditis and occasionally originates from some other extraurinary site of infection.

As bacteria travel from the collecting system into the tubules, leukocytes migrate from the interstitium into the affected tubules. The subsequent release of enzymes destroys tubular integrity and allows the bacteria to enter the interstitium. Casts of inflammatory cells in the tubules produce a focal microscopic obstruction that, when coupled with focal vasoconstriction, causes regions of decreased function and ischemia. Generally, the process extends from the tip of the papilla to the periphery of the cortex and involves the kidney in a patchy manner. The demarcation between infected and normal parenchyma is usually sharp.

Clinically, patients present with flank pain, fever, leukocytosis, pyuria, bacteremia, and positive urine culture results. Uncomplicated cases of pyelonephritis treated with appropriate antibiotic therapy usually resolve within 72 hours. Chronic scarring may occur, particularly when there is associated vesicoureteral reflux. Severe forms of pyelonephritis may persist beyond 72 hours, and these are the patients who benefit from imaging studies such as ultrasound, mostly to look for complications such as abscess formation, obstruction, or other confounding abnormalities such as stones.

The ultrasound findings in most cases of uncomplicated pyelonephritis are normal. Occasionally, the involvement of the collecting system produces urothelial thickening that is detectable on sonograms (Fig. 5-44A and B).

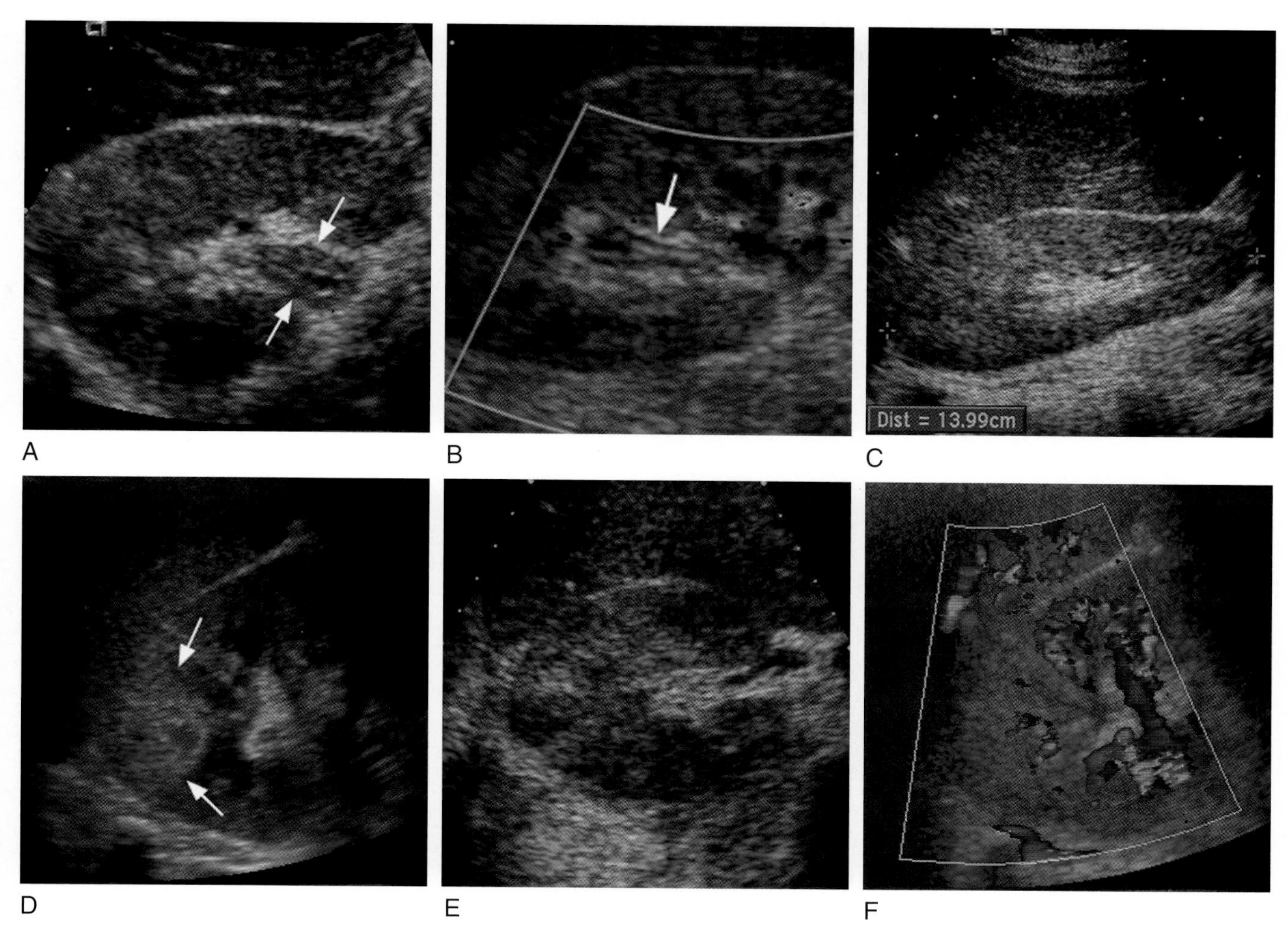

Figure 5-44 Pyelonephritis in different patients. **A,** Transverse view shows thickening of the renal pelvis *(arrows)*. **B,** Longitudinal view shows thickening of the infundibulum *(arrow)* to the upper pole producing the white line sign. **C,** Longitudinal view shows enlargement of the kidney (13.99 cm) and diffuse increased echogenicity. **D,** Longitudinal view of the upper pole shows a wedge-shaped region of increased echogenicity *(arrows)*. **E,** Transverse view shows patchy areas of increased and decreased cortical echogenicity. **F,** Longitudinal color Doppler view shows a focal area of decreased perfusion in the upper pole.

In the proper clinical setting this is a reliable sign of infection. However, it is nonspecific and can also be seen in association with calculi and stents, after bouts of obstruction, with transitional cell carcinoma, and in renal transplants with rejection and ischemia (Box 5-4). Renal enlargement is another finding of infection (see Fig. 5-44C). Pyelonephritis can alter the echogenicity of the renal parenchyma, producing areas of both increased and decreased echogenicity (see Fig. 5-44D), which may be isolated or multifocal and produce a patchy appearance to the cortex (see Fig. 5-44E). The associated vasoconstriction may produce focal areas of decreased perfusion. These will occasionally be seen as decreased vascularity on color or power Doppler analysis (see Fig. 5-44F). There may also be focal areas of enlargement that can simulate a mass.

The primary role of sonography in evaluating patients with pyelonephritis is to identify possible complications, including obstruction, renal abscess, or perinephric abscess. Identification of stones is also important, because they may form the nidus for persistent infection. Renal abscesses appear as complex fluid collections or complex cystic masses (Fig. 5-45). The treatment of large and moderately sized renal abscesses generally consists of percutaneous drainage or occasionally surgery. However, small abscesses can be effectively treated with antibiotics. Perinephric abscesses appear as complex perinephric fluid collections. Many patients with uncomplicated pyelonephritis have small anechoic perinephric fluid collections, and these should not be misinterpreted as abscesses. In addition, the perinephric fat can occasionally appear very hypoechoic and should

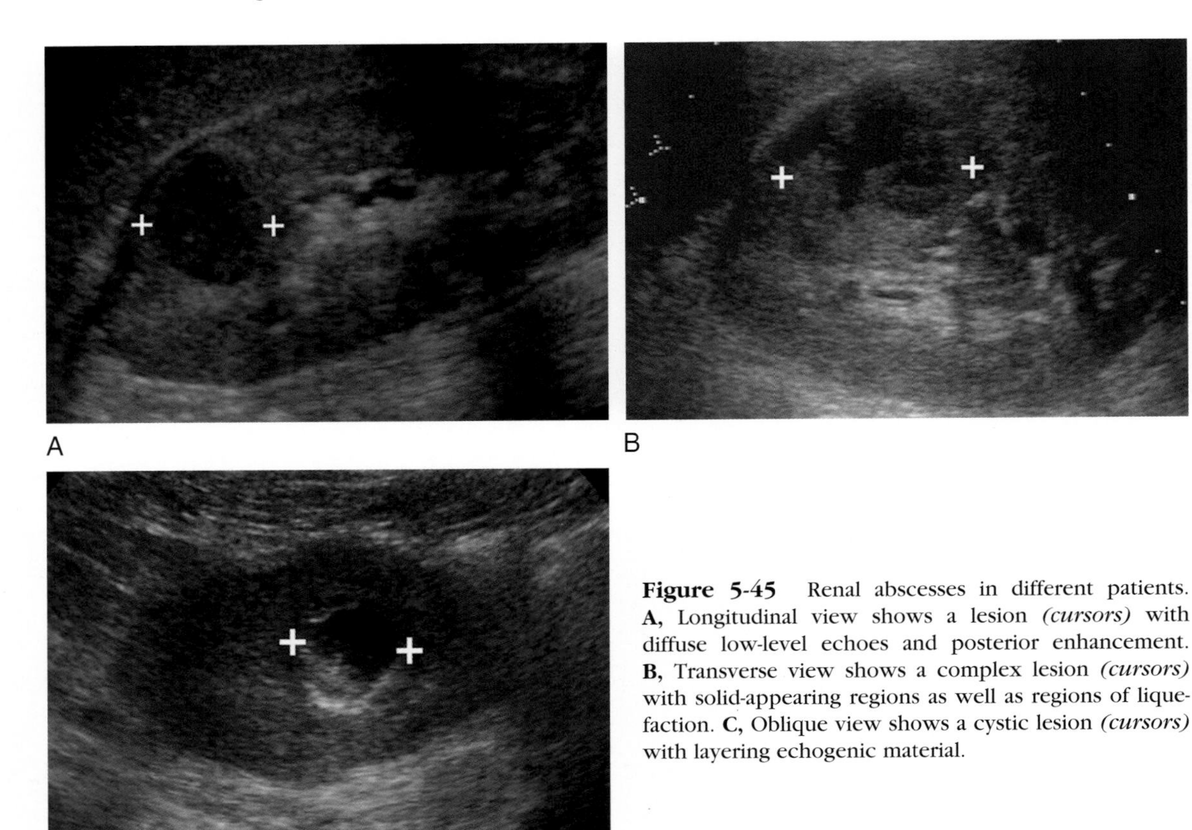

Figure 5-45 Renal abscesses in different patients. **A,** Longitudinal view shows a lesion *(cursors)* with diffuse low-level echoes and posterior enhancement. **B,** Transverse view shows a complex lesion *(cursors)* with solid-appearing regions as well as regions of liquefaction. **C,** Oblique view shows a cystic lesion *(cursors)* with layering echogenic material.

also not be confused with perinephric fluid or abscesses. Hypoechoic perinephric fat tends to occur in patients with renal atrophy and is bilateral in the vast majority of cases (Fig. 5-46).

One unusual type of renal infection is xanthogranulomatous pyelonephritis. This is a chronic inflammatory process usually associated with long-standing urinary obstruction. The pathologic response to the infection is the formation of yellow inflammatory masses composed of lipid-laden macrophages. The most common organisms are *Proteus mirabilis* and *Escherichia coli.* More than 75% of patients will have a stone, and most will be of the staghorn variety. The classic radiologic triad is a stone, renal enlargement, and lack of function. Sonographic findings include a shadowing stone in the renal pelvis together with dilated renal calices, perinephric fluid collection, and perinephric inflammatory tissue (Fig. 5-47).

Emphysematous pyelonephritis is a serious renal infection that typically occurs in diabetic women. It results

Box 5-4 Causes of Urothelial Thickening

- Pyelonephritis
- Ureteral calculi
- Ureteral stents
- Relieved obstruction
- Transplant rejection
- Transplant ischemia
- Transitional cell carcinoma

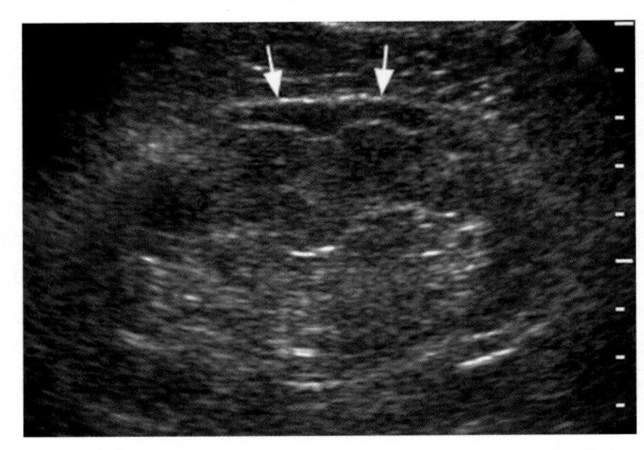

Figure 5-46 Hypoechoic perinephric fat. Longitudinal view of the kidney shows very hypoechoic fat *(arrows)* in the perinephric space. This should not be confused with fluid.

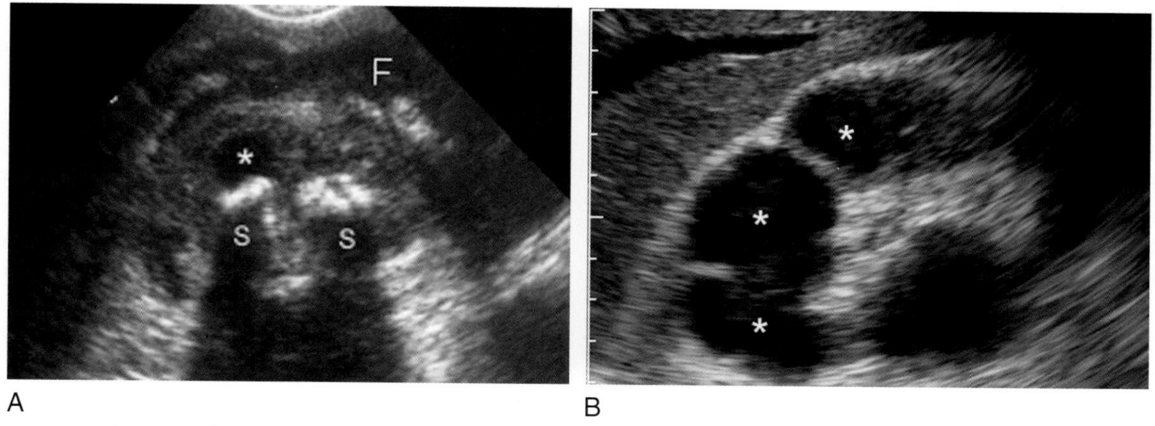

Figure 5-47 Xanthogranulomatous pyelonephritis in different patients. **A,** Transverse view of the kidney shows shadowing stones (S), a distended calyx (*), and perinephric fluid (F). **B,** Longitudinal view of the kidney shows distended upper pole calices (*) containing some echogenic material. This case is unusual because there was not a stone and the lower pole of the kidney was not involved.

from the formation of gas in the renal parenchyma stemming from high tissue glucose concentrations, vascular disease, and a necrotizing infection with a gas-forming organism such as *E. coli.* Nephrectomy is usually required for treatment. Emphysematous pyelitis is a less serious condition in which gas forms in the collecting system but not the renal parenchyma. The sonographic diagnosis of gas-forming infections depends on the detection of bright reflectors with dirty shadows or ring-down artifacts (Fig. 5-48). It may be difficult to determine whether the gas is confined to the collecting system or involves the parenchyma. CT is helpful for making this distinction.

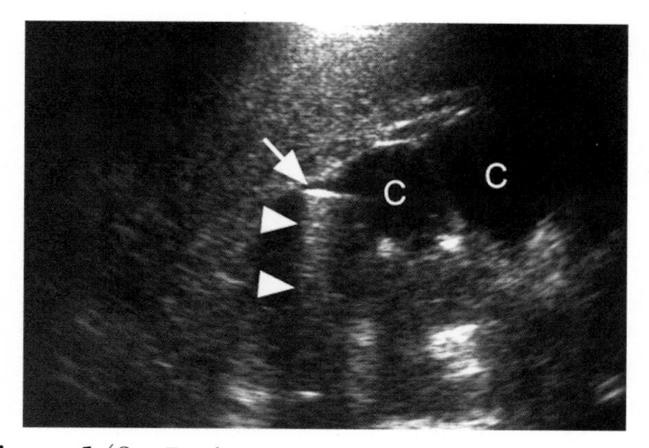

Figure 5-48 Emphysematous pyelonephritis. Longitudinal view of the kidney shows markedly dilated calices (C) and a very bright reflector *(arrow)* with associated ring-down artifact *(arrowheads)* due to gas.

RENAL CALCULI

Urolithiasis is an extremely common problem, affecting 12% of the population by age 70. It affects men up to three times more often than women and is more common in whites than other racial groups. Risk factors include low fluid intake and diets high in animal protein. The latter factor may explain why stones are more common in affluent patients. Conditions that promote urinary stasis also predispose to the formation of stones; these include ureteropelvic junction obstruction, autosomal dominant polycystic disease, caliceal diverticula, tubular ectasia, and horseshoe kidneys. Stones can have a variety of compositions. Calcium-containing stones are most common (80% to 85%), and the calcium usually occurs in the form of calcium oxalate or calcium phosphate. Most calcium stones arise idiopathically in the absence of associated metabolic abnormalities. Uric acid stones account for 5% to 10% of all calculi. They are commonly thought to be associated with gout, but only 25% of patients with gout have uric acid stones and only 25% of patients with uric acid stones have gout. Other conditions that predispose to the formation of uric acid stones include Crohn's disease and other small bowel abnormalities, as well as myeloproliferative diseases that are being treated with chemotherapy. Pure uric acid stones are radiolucent. Cistine stones account for less than 5% of all renal calculi and are related to cistinuria, a rare metabolic disorder. They are relatively radiolucent. Approximately 10% of stones are associated with infection by urea-splitting bacteria such as *Proteus, Pseudomonas, Staphylococcus aureus,* and *Klebsiella.*

These stones are composed of struvite (magnesium-ammonium-phosphate) or apatite (calcium phosphate), or both. They often develop into staghorn calculi.

As with gallstones, the sonographic appearance of renal stones depends on their size and not their composition. Stones of sufficient size produce an echogenic focus in the renal sinus with an associated acoustic shadow (Fig. 5-49). Smaller stones may just appear as an echogenic focus without a shadow. Small stones present a diagnostic problem because they are hard to separate from the echogenic renal sinus itself. Efforts should therefore be made to identify a shadow by using a high-frequency transducer that is focused at the appropriate depth and by viewing the stone from a variety of locations. Color Doppler imaging can help because some stones will produce a short color ring-down artifact, called a "twinkle" artifact (see Fig. 5-49E).

A pitfall in the sonographic diagnosis of stones is refractive shadowing arising from the renal sinus (see Chapter 1 for a discussion of sound refraction). This occurs as the result of differences in the speed of sound between soft tissue, fluid, and fat. Because all three of these substances are present in the renal sinus, refractive shadowing is common. Therefore, a shadow should not

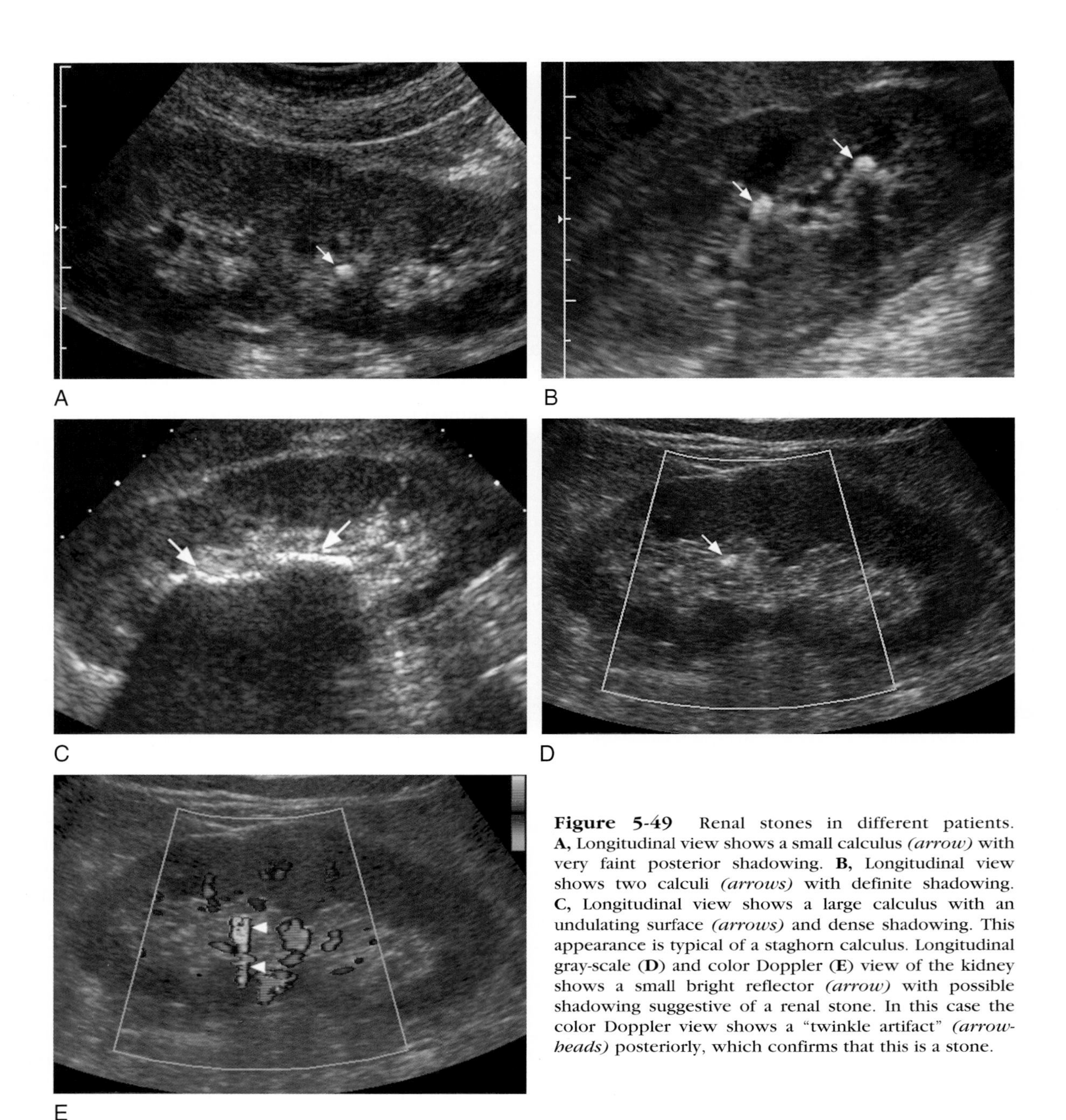

Figure 5-49 Renal stones in different patients. **A,** Longitudinal view shows a small calculus *(arrow)* with very faint posterior shadowing. **B,** Longitudinal view shows two calculi *(arrows)* with definite shadowing. **C,** Longitudinal view shows a large calculus with an undulating surface *(arrows)* and dense shadowing. This appearance is typical of a staghorn calculus. Longitudinal gray-scale (**D**) and color Doppler (**E**) view of the kidney shows a small bright reflector *(arrow)* with possible shadowing suggestive of a renal stone. In this case the color Doppler view shows a "twinkle artifact" *(arrowheads)* posteriorly, which confirms that this is a stone.

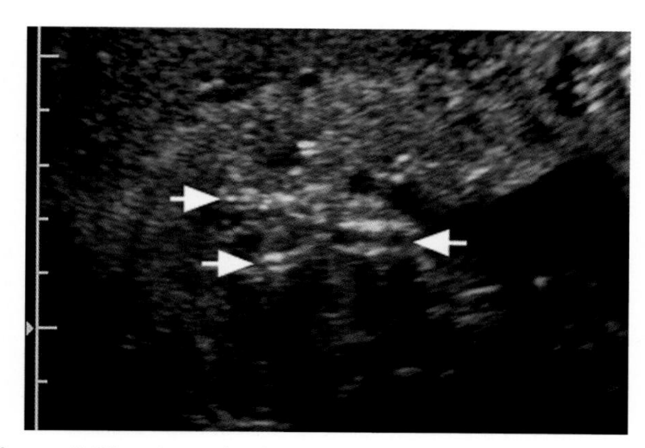

Figure 5-50 Arterial calcification. Transverse view of the right kidney shows several bright linear reflectors arranged as parallel lines *(arrows)* with associated posterior shadowing. This is typical of arterial calcification.

be taken as evidence of a stone unless it is arising from a definite echogenic focus. False-positive results can also occur in patients with renal arterial calcification and should be suspected if the echogenic focus is linear or composed of parallel, closely spaced reflectors (Fig. 5-50).

The sensitivity of ultrasound in detecting renal calculi is superior to that of abdominal radiography but inferior to CT. Sensitivity depends primarily on the size of the stones, with stones that are larger than 5 mm detected with a high sensitivity whereas smaller stones are detected less reliably. Stone composition has little affect on sensitivity. Sonography is not accurate in determining stone size.

Sonographic sensitivity for detecting ureteral calculi depends on their location. Although stones can be seen in the mid ureter, they are considerably easier to detect at the proximal ureter and ureteropelvic junction and especially in the distal ureter and ureterovesical junction (Fig. 5-51A and B). Most ureteral stones impact in the distal ureter near the ureterovesical junction so scans looking at the distal ureter through a moderately distended urinary bladder should always be obtained in someone suspected of passing a stone. In women, transvaginal sonography can visualize distal ureteral stones extremely well (see Fig. 5-51C). The exact role of sonography in evaluating patients with renal colic and suspected ureteral calculi is somewhat controversial. The combined use of gray-scale sonography to detect the morphologic changes of hydronephrosis, perinephric fluid collections, and ureteral calculi, along with Doppler analysis of intrarenal resistive indexes and ureteral jets to estimate the degree of obstruction, is relatively effective and can provide adequate information

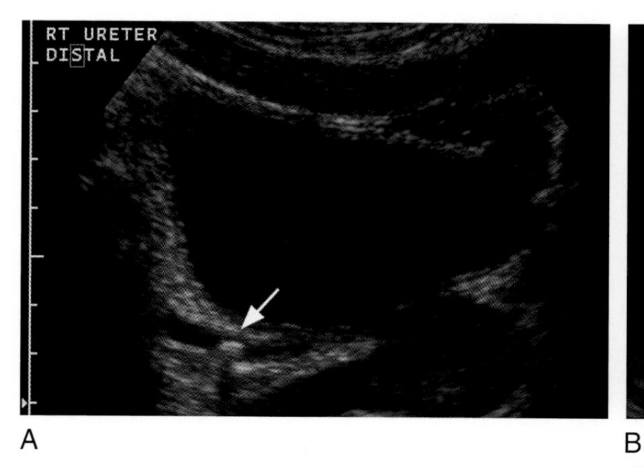

A

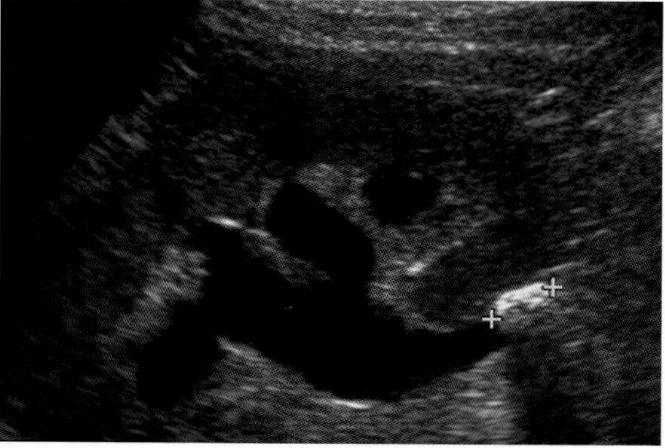

B

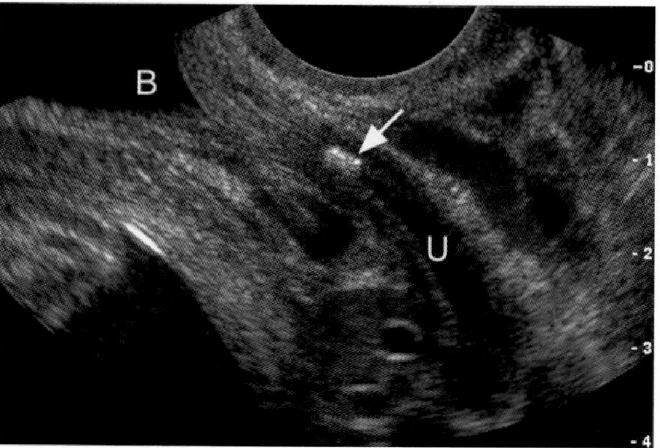

C

Figure 5-51 Ureteral stones in different patients. **A,** Longitudinal view through the bladder shows a stone *(arrow)* in the distal ureter. **B,** Longitudinal view of the kidney shows a stone *(cursors)* at the ureteropelvic junction. **C,** Transvaginal scan in a pregnant patient shows the distal ureter (U), the bladder (B), and a ureteral stone *(arrow)*.

to guide management in most cases. Despite this, nonenhanced CT is now the recommended first test because it is faster, easier, and in most practices more reliable than sonography. Sonography and intravenous urography are used mostly in a problem-solving mode. Sonography should be the initial test in pregnant patients in whom radiation needs to be avoided.

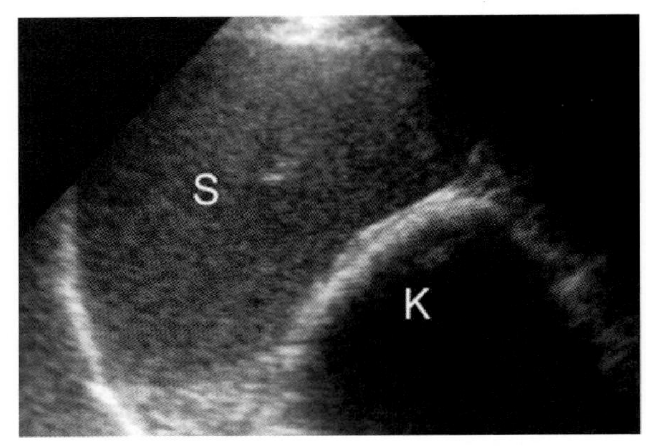

Figure 5-53 Cortical nephrocalcinosis. Longitudinal view of the left kidney (K) shows complete dense shadowing and no visible renal tissue. The spleen is also seen (S).

NEPHROCALCINOSIS

Medullary nephrocalcinosis refers to calcification in the medullary pyramids rather than the renal collecting system. It is caused by a number of processes, but the three most common are medullary sponge kidney (tubular ectasia), renal tubular acidosis, and hyperparathyroidism. In its early stages it causes increased medullary echogenicity at the periphery of the pyramids and eventually involves the entire pyramids (Fig. 5-52A to C). With progressive calcification, shadowing begins to develop (see Fig. 5-52D). Sonography is unusually sensitive in detecting this condition, and the sonographic changes predate any visible calcification on plain films and are generally more dramatic than the abnormalities seen on CT. Diffuse cortical nephrocalcinosis is rare and

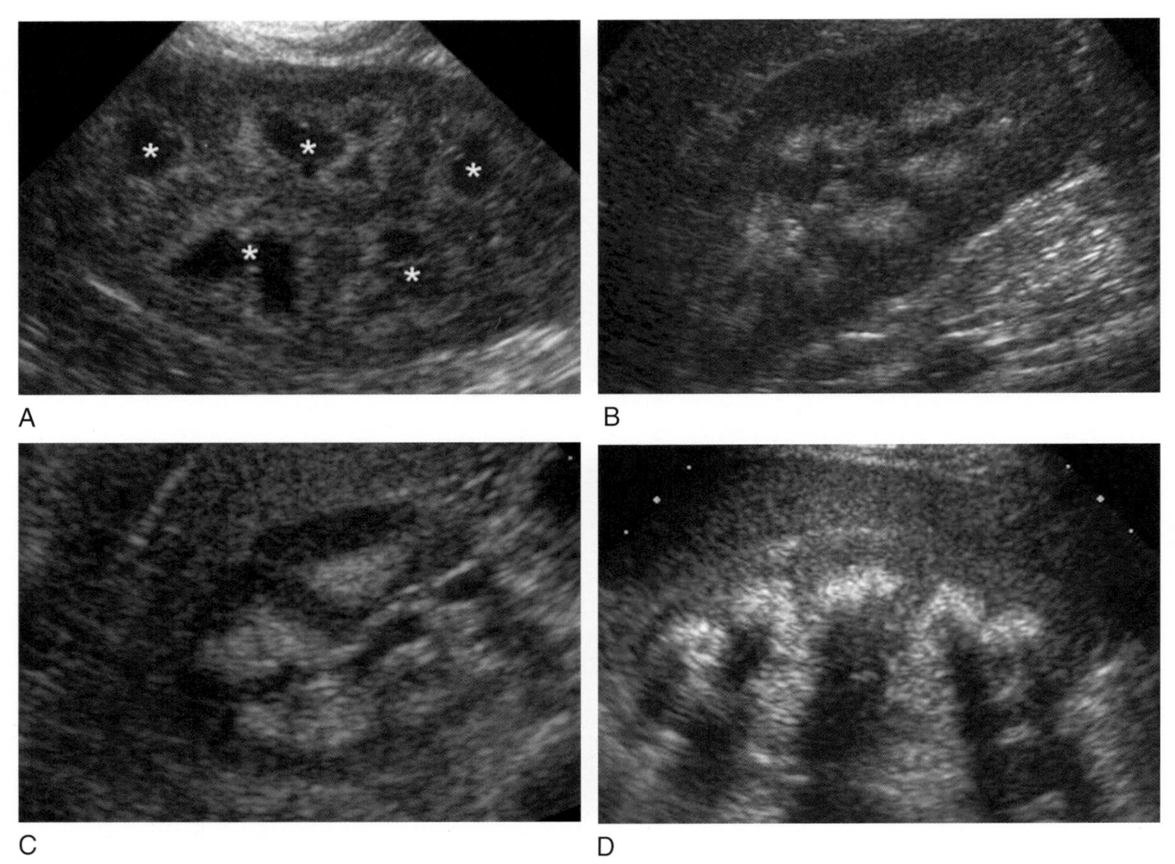

Figure 5-52 Medullary nephrocalcinosis in different patients. **A,** Longitudinal view of the kidney just lateral to the renal sinus shows multiple renal pyramids (*) with increased echogenicity peripherally. Longitudinal (**B**) and transverse (**C**) views in another patient shows diffusely echogenic pyramids without posterior shadowing. **D,** Longitudinal view in a third patient shows echogenic pyramids with multiple areas of shadowing consistent with more dense calcification.

usually secondary to cortical necrosis and hyperoxaluria (Fig. 5-53).

RENAL PARENCHYMAL DISEASE

A large number of diseases affect the renal parenchyma and produce renal failure. The term "medical renal disease" is often used but is not truly appropriate because some of these patients will benefit from a surgical procedure (i.e., renal transplantation). Increased parenchymal echogenicity is often seen in the setting of renal parenchymal disease (Fig. 5-54). The degree of echogenicity correlates loosely with the severity of, but not the type of, histopathologic change. Therefore, although an underlying parenchymal abnormality is suggested by increased echogenicity, the cause cannot be determined. Echogenicity is considered increased when the right kidney is more echogenic than the liver or when the echogenicity of the left kidney is equal or greater than that of the spleen. If images are not available to show the relative echogenicity of the kidneys and the liver or spleen, echogenicity is considered increased if the pyramids are unusually hypoechoic with respect to the renal cortex. In most cases, patients with parenchymal disease are scanned because of acute renal failure. In this setting, it is not uncommon to see a trace amount of perinephric fluid, and this should not be misinterpreted as a sign of infection or trauma (see Fig. 5-54D). The main role of sonography in these patients is to exclude urinary obstruction and determine renal size. Renal biopsy of normal sized or enlarged kidneys may then be done to determine the underlying histologic diagnosis. Small kidneys usually indicate a chronic process with end-stage changes, and biopsy is often not indicated because the histopathologic findings cannot distinguish the possible causes.

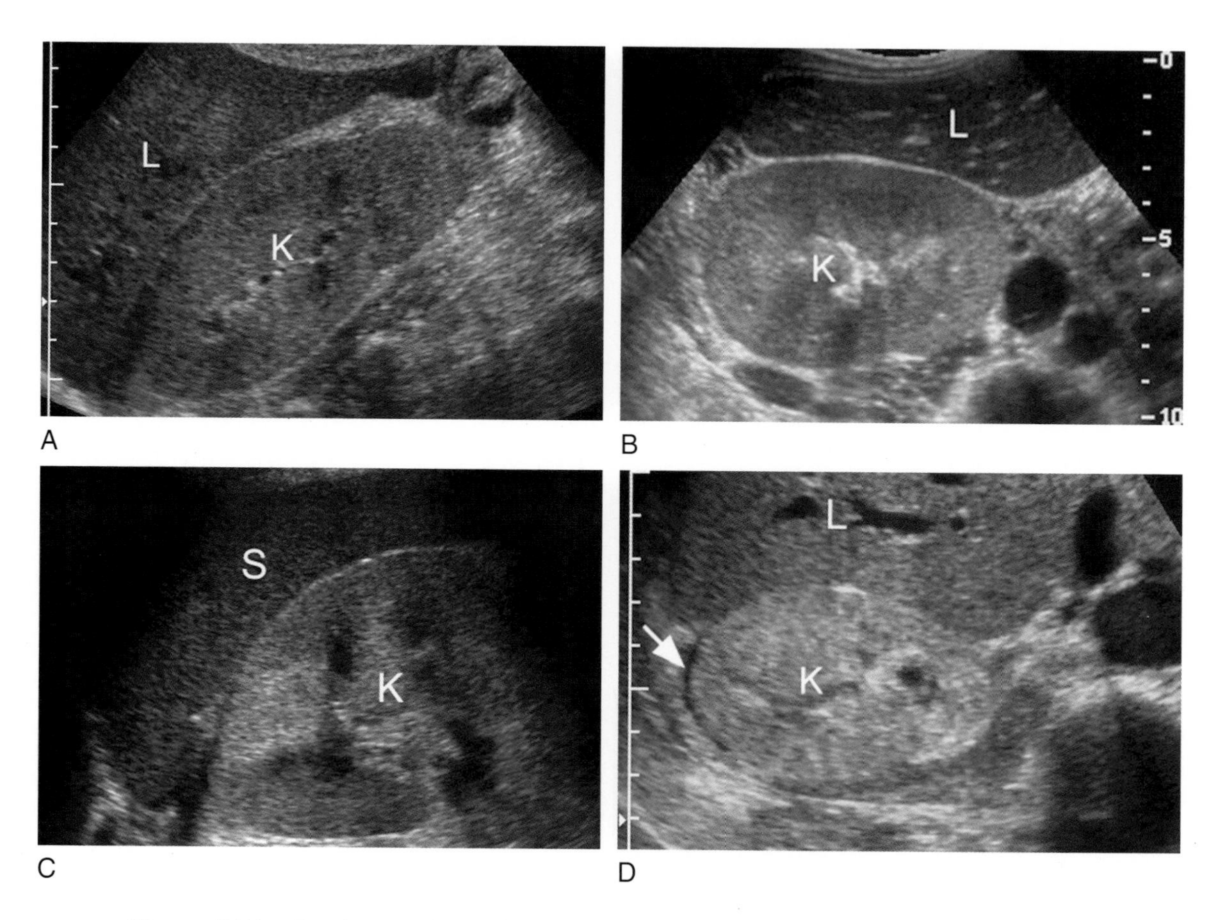

Figure 5-54 Renal parenchymal disease in different patients. **A,** Longitudinal view of the right kidney (K) shows that it is slightly more echogenic than the liver (L). **B,** Transverse view of the right kidney (K) shows that it is much more echogenic than the liver (L). **C,** Longitudinal view of the left kidney (K) shows that it is more echogenic than the adjacent spleen (S). It also shows prominent renal pyramids. **D,** Transverse view of the liver (L) and right kidney (K) shows hyperechoic renal parenchyma and a small amount of perinephric fluid *(arrow)*. Small amounts of perinephric fluid may be seen with acute renal failure.

RENAL TRAUMA

Sonography is generally not recommended as a means of evaluating renal trauma, because contrast medium-enhanced CT is superior for detecting and determining the extent of post-traumatic abnormalities. Nevertheless, certain post-traumatic lesions are encountered frequently during the sonographic evaluations of other problems, so their sonographic appearance should be recognized. Renal hematomas go through the same stages as do hematomas elsewhere, evolving from echogenic, to heterogeneous and mixed, to predominantly liquefied, to purely cystic. Subcapsular hematomas are particularly difficult to detect in the acute stages because they may be almost isoechoic to the kidney and they tend to distort the kidney so that the renal margins are difficult to discern (Fig. 5-55). Because subcapsular hematomas are in a contained space, they exert significant mass effect on the kidney and reduce blood flow, sometimes dramatically. Primary vascular lesions are usually well evaluated with CT, but sonography is helpful at problem solving when the CT is equivocal or suboptimal. It is also useful in the follow-up of post-traumatic pseudoaneurysms and arteriovenous fistulas.

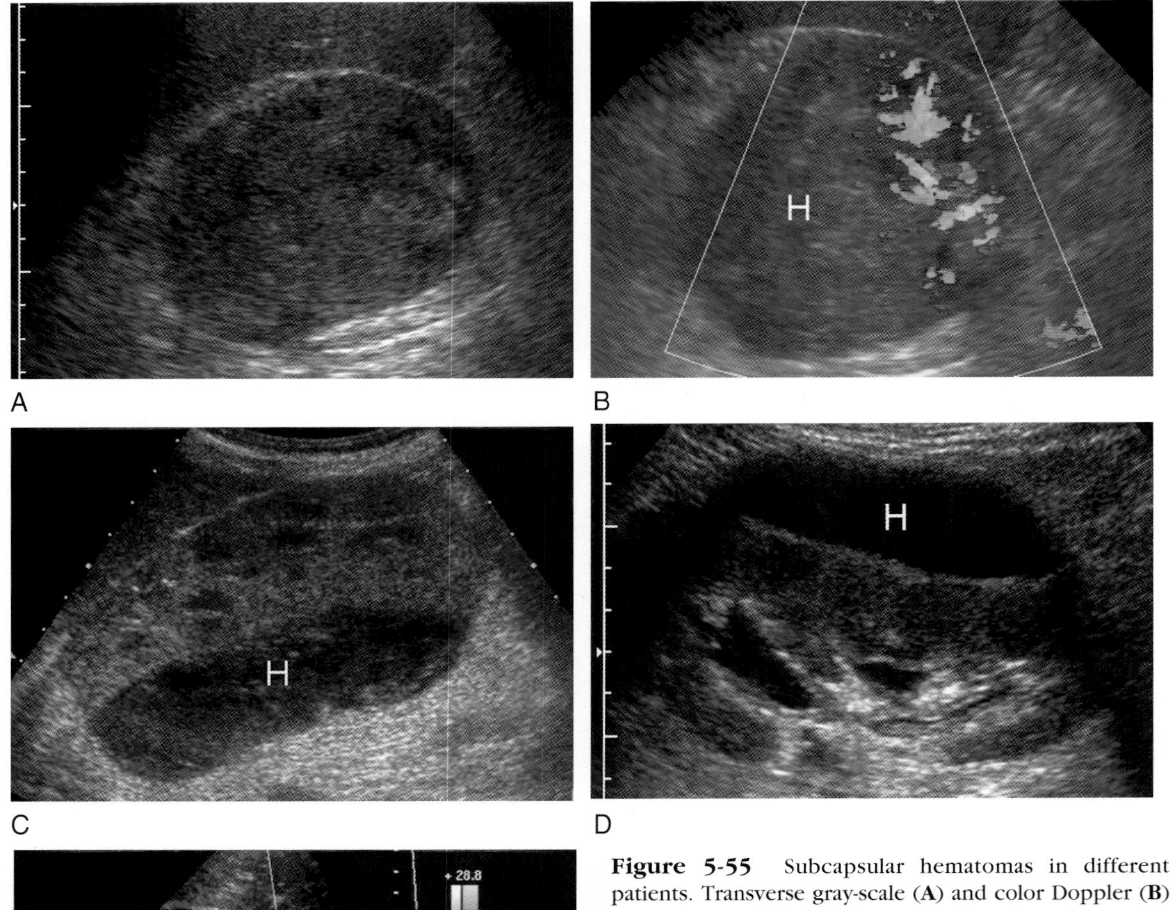

Figure 5-55 Subcapsular hematomas in different patients. Transverse gray-scale (**A**) and color Doppler (**B**) views show a globular kidney with distortion of the architecture and loss of the echogenic sinus. The color Doppler image indicates where the renal parenchyma is and contrasts the compressed kidney to the isoechoic hematoma (H). **C,** Longitudinal view shows a partially liquefied, subacute hematoma (H). **D,** Longitudinal view shows a completely liquefied and simple-appearing hematoma (H). In **C** and **D**, the compression of the kidney produced by the hematoma is evident. **E,** Pulsed Doppler waveform from a kidney with a subcapsular hematoma shows a "to and fro" waveform with pandiastolic flow reversal. This reflects markedly increased renal vascular resistance due to the compression of the renal parenchyma.

VASCULAR DISEASE

Normal Anatomic Characteristics and Hemodynamic Function

The kidneys are usually supplied by a single main renal artery that arises from the aorta just inferior to the origin of the superior mesenteric artery (Fig. 5-56). The main renal arteries travel posterior to the corresponding vein and the right renal artery passes posterior to the inferior vena cava as well. Accessory renal arteries occur in approximately 20% of the kidneys (Fig. 5-57). They usually originate near the origin of the main renal artery (either above or below), but this is variable. They are usually smaller than the main renal artery, but this is also variable. The renal arteries branch into multiple segmental arteries that travel from the renal hilum into the renal sinus. The segmental arteries subsequently branch into the interlobar arteries and arcuate arteries (Fig. 5-58). The normal intrarenal arteries are rarely visible on gray-scale sonography but are routinely visible with color Doppler analysis. The amount of detectable flow depends on the depth of the kidney and the type of Doppler technique and transducer used. With modern equipment using both color and power Doppler techniques, blood flow should be seen throughout the cortex to the capsular margin of the kidney in most superficial native kidneys and most renal transplants. The difference in perfusion between the cortical tissues and the medullary pyramids is generally well displayed on color and power Doppler studies (see Fig. 5-58B and C). The pulsed Doppler waveforms from the renal arteries show findings typical of a parenchymal organ with a low-resistance pattern (Fig. 5-59).

The right renal vein is short and relatively constant in location and appearance. It is generally easily seen on both gray-scale and color Doppler scans (Fig. 5-60A). The left renal vein is approximately three times longer than the right and is considerably more difficult to see along its entire length. It travels between the superior

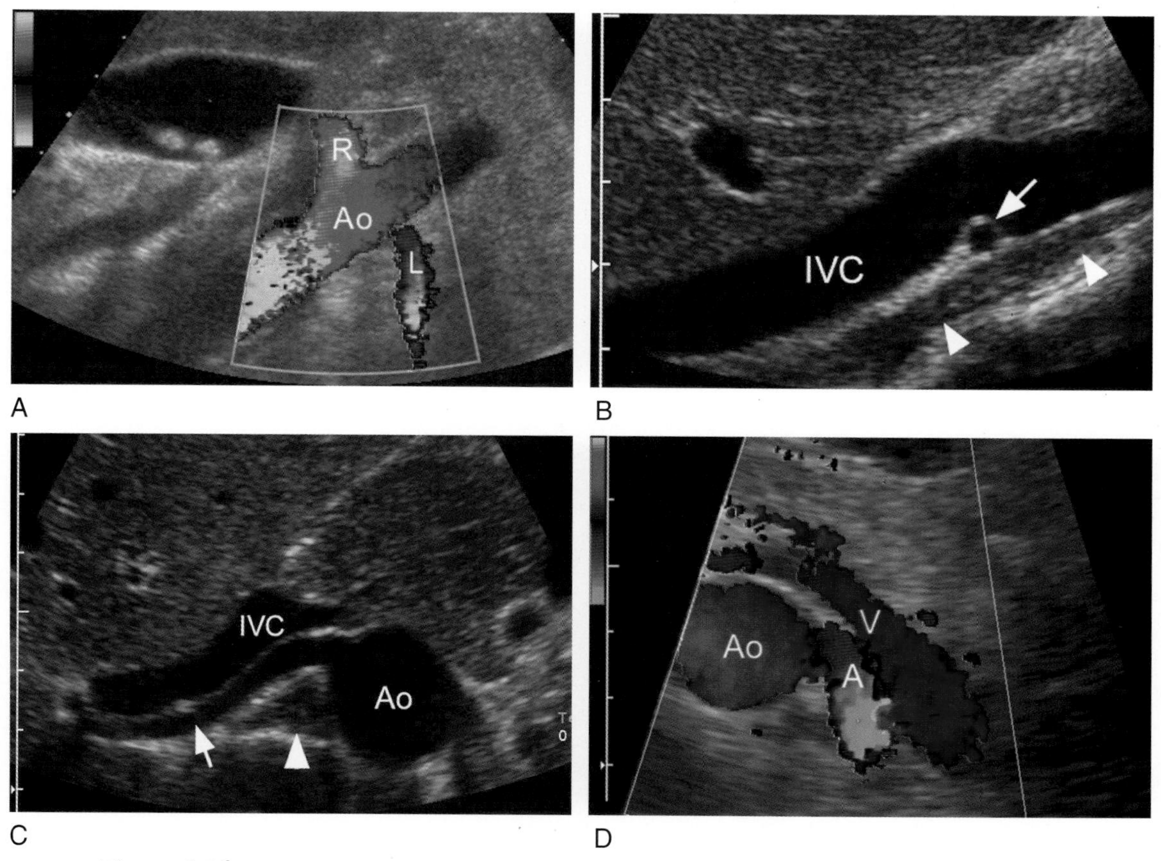

Figure 5-56 Normal renal arteries in different patients. **A,** Coronal color Doppler view of the aorta (Ao) from a right lateral approach ("banana peel view") shows a single right renal artery (R) and a single left renal artery (L). Stones are also seen in the gallbladder. Longitudinal (**B**) and transverse (**C**) views show the right renal artery *(arrow)* posterior to the inferior vena cava (IVC) and anterior to the crus of the right hemidiaphragm *(arrowheads)*. **D,** Transverse color Doppler view of the aorta (Ao) shows the origin of the left renal artery (A) passing posterior to the left renal vein (V).

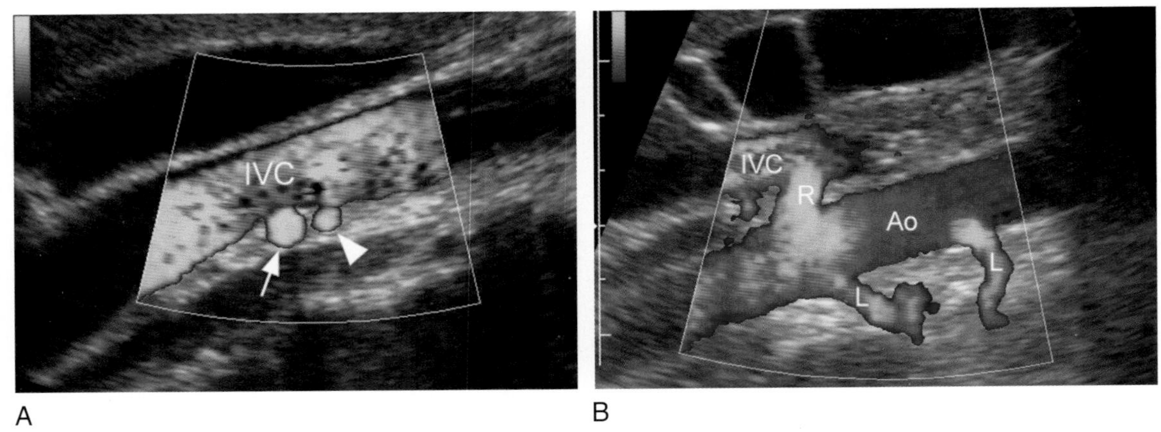

Figure 5-57 Accessory renal arteries in different patients. **A,** Longitudinal power Doppler view shows two arteries posterior to the inferior vena cava (IVC). The larger artery is the main renal artery *(arrow),* and the smaller artery is an accessory renal artery *(arrowhead)* supplying the lower pole. **B,** Coronal power Doppler view obtained from the right side shows the aorta (Ao) and two similarly sized left renal arteries (L). The origin of the right renal artery (R) and the inferior vena cava (IVC) are also seen.

mesenteric artery and aorta in most subjects (see Fig. 5-60B). A retroaortic or circumaortic left renal vein is present in 3% and 17% of individuals, respectively (Fig. 5-61). The segment of left renal vein immediately to the left of the superior mesenteric artery and aorta is often relatively dilated and can simulate a periaortic mass. In addition, it may communicate with prominent lumbar veins that can also simulate a mass. Doppler techniques are effective in determining the nature of questionable lesions in this area.

Renal Artery Stenosis

Hypertension affects up to 60 million people in the United States and is one of the most common diseases in the world. Three fourths of the cases are mild and controlled by diet and diuretics. Almost all of these patients have primary hypertension. Severe hypertension that is poorly controlled or controlled only with multiple medications is more likely to be caused by a secondary factor such as renal artery stenosis. Although

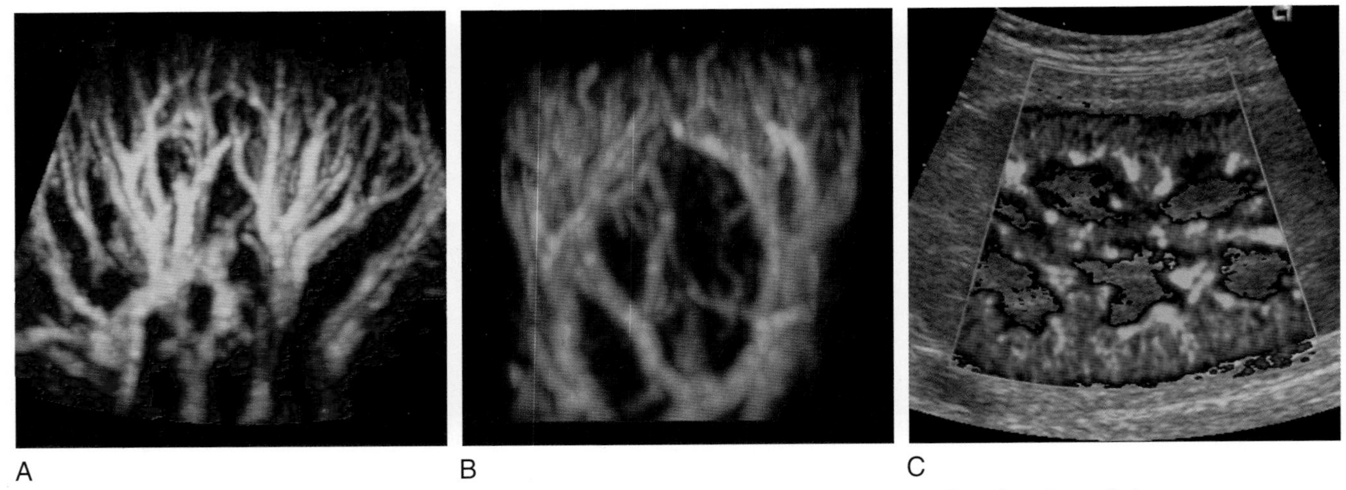

Figure 5-58 Intrarenal arteries in different patients. **A,** A 3D power Doppler view of the intrarenal arteries shows multiple segmental arteries in the renal hilum branching into lobar and interlobular arteries. **B,** Magnified 3D power Doppler view of the renal cortex shows multiple interlobular and arcuate arteries surrounding a relatively avascular renal pyramid. **C,** Longitudinal 2D power Doppler view shows intense cortical vascularity and no detectable flow in the renal pyramids.

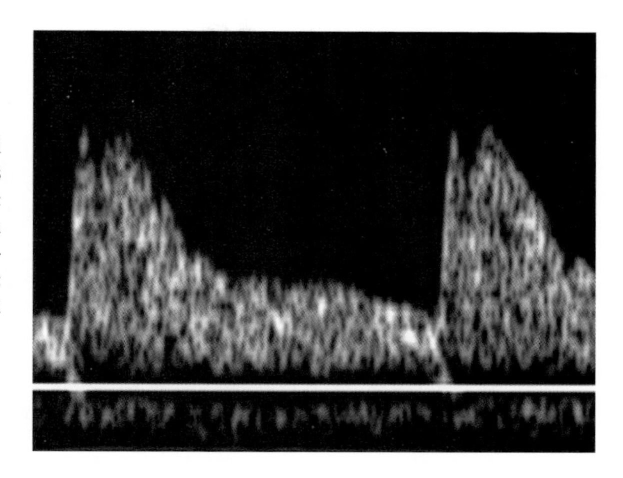

Figure 5-59 Normal renal artery waveform. Arterial flow to the kidney shows typical low-resistance features with well-maintained diastolic flow throughout the cardiac cycle, a broad systolic peak, and a gradual transition between systole and diastole. Also note the sharp, well-defined early systolic peak and the steep early systolic slope. Faint venous flow from an adjacent vein is seen below the baseline.

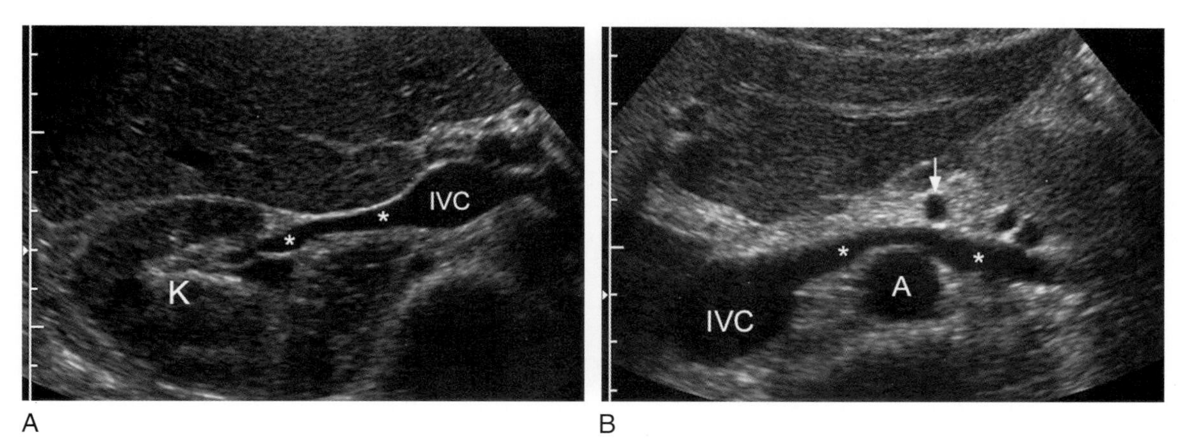

Figure 5-60 Normal renal veins. **A,** Transverse view of the right upper quadrant shows the right kidney (K) and the right renal vein (*) draining into the inferior vena cava (IVC). **B,** Transverse view of the mid abdomen shows the aorta (A) and the inferior vena cava (IVC) with the left renal vein (*) passing anterior to the aorta and posterior to the superior mesenteric artery *(arrow)*.

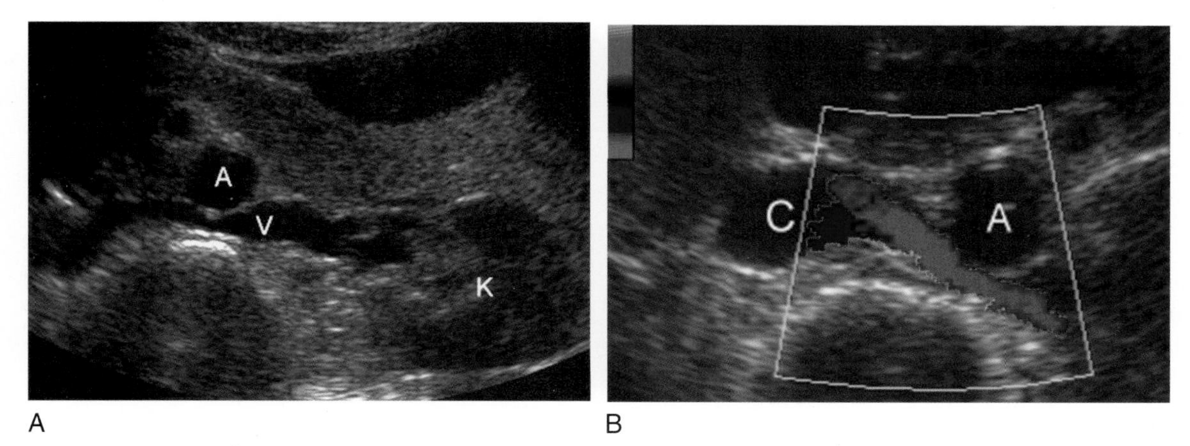

Figure 5-61 Retroaortic left renal vein. **A,** Transverse view shows the left kidney (K) and the left renal vein (V) traveling from the renal hilum behind the aorta (A). **B,** Transverse color Doppler view shows the left renal vein (V) traveling behind the aorta (A) before reaching the inferior vena cava (C).

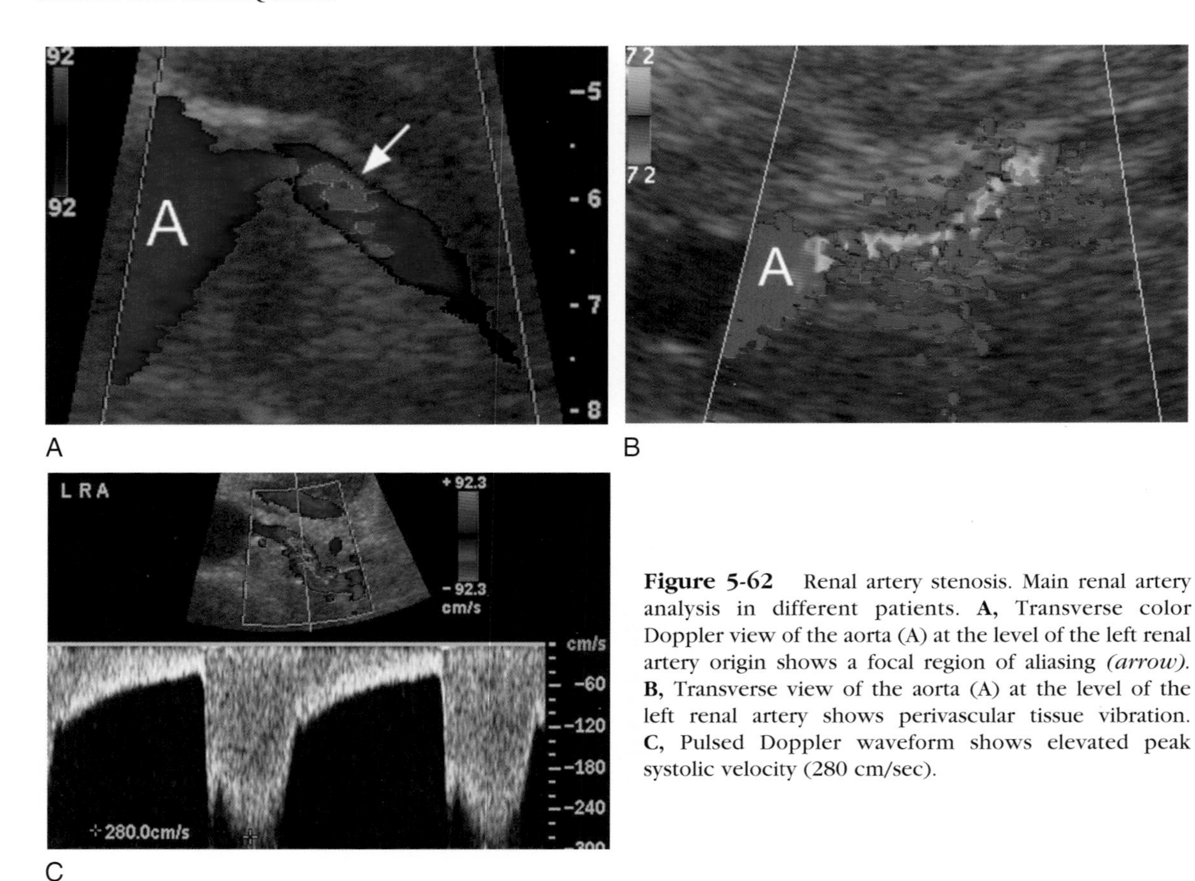

Figure 5-62 Renal artery stenosis. Main renal artery analysis in different patients. **A,** Transverse color Doppler view of the aorta (A) at the level of the left renal artery origin shows a focal region of aliasing *(arrow)*. **B,** Transverse view of the aorta (A) at the level of the left renal artery shows perivascular tissue vibration. **C,** Pulsed Doppler waveform shows elevated peak systolic velocity (280 cm/sec).

renal artery stenosis accounts for only 5% of the total number of patients with hypertension, it is potentially curable. Therefore, noninvasive screening tests that can identify patients with renal artery stenosis are important.

Doppler ultrasound examination is among the methods used to detect renal artery stenosis. Abnormalities seen on color Doppler include focal areas of aliasing and localized perivascular tissue vibration (Fig. 5-62). Pulsed Doppler analysis of abnormal areas identified on color Doppler imaging will reveal a peak systolic velocity exceeding 200 cm/sec (see Fig. 5-62) and a peak renal artery velocity-to-peak aortic velocity ratio of greater than 3.5. With experience, the main renal arteries can be effectively visualized with color Doppler imaging and sampled with pulsed Doppler imaging in 80% to 90% of patients. Obesity, dyspnea, and overlying bowel gas can all make it impossible to complete the study successfully. Because of bowel gas, patients should be fasting before the examination. Other difficulties include Doppler angles that are greater than 60 degrees, extensive arterial calcification that shadows the Doppler signal, distal lesions (e.g., fibromuscular dysplasia), cardiac arrhythmias, and accessory renal arteries.

A proximal stenosis will also cause blunting of the waveform from distal arteries. This dampening of the distal arterial waveforms has been referred to as the parvus-tardus effect (slowed systolic upstroke and a delayed time to peak systole). In severe cases this effect is detectable subjectively (Fig. 5-63). In less severe cases, the effect can be detected quantitatively by measuring the early systolic acceleration. Values less than 300 cm/sec^2 are considered abnormal. The potential advantage of this method is that the intrarenal arteries

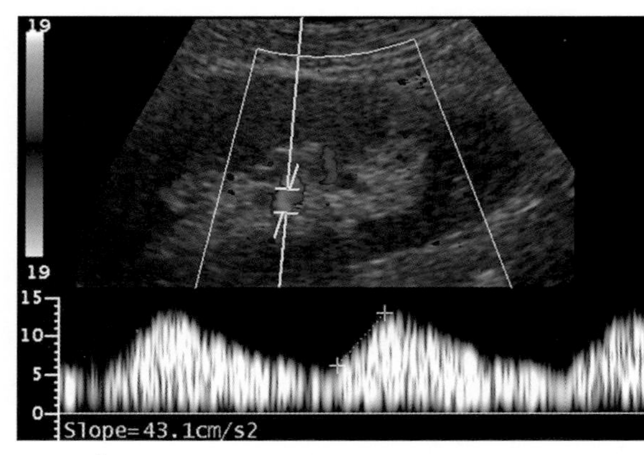

Figure 5-63 Renal artery stenosis. Intrarenal artery analysis. Pulsed Doppler waveform from a segmental renal artery shows a parvus-tardus appearance with slowed early systolic acceleration (43.1 cm/sec^2).

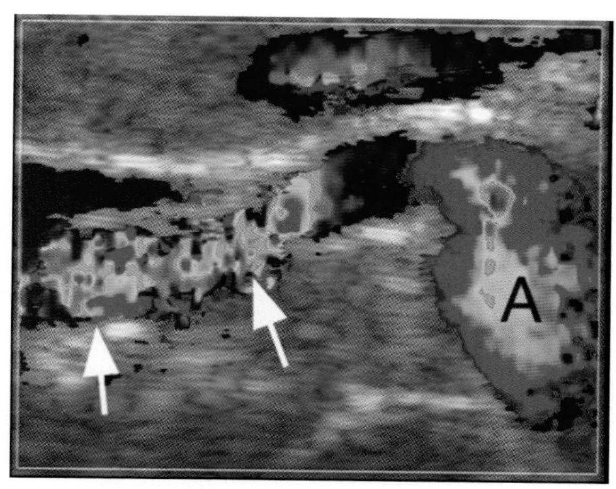

Figure 5-64 Fibromuscular dysplasia. Transverse color Doppler view of the aorta (A) and the right renal artery shows a normal appearance of flow in the origin of the renal artery but a marked break up and disorganization of flow in the mid renal artery *(arrows).*

are more easily and reproducibly imaged than the main renal arteries. However, difficulties include decreased sensitivity to borderline stenosis, inability to distinguish high-grade stenosis from complete occlusion, inability to localize the site of stenosis, variation in cursor location for measurement of systolic acceleration, and dependence on compliant vessels. Studies focusing on renal arterial Doppler analysis show widely discrepant results, so it is not possible to recommend Doppler imaging as the screening test of choice other than at facilities with well-trained personnel who have abundant experience.

In most patients, renal artery stenosis is caused by atherosclerotic disease and is located at or near the origin. Fibromuscular dysplasia (FMD) predominantly affects middle-aged women and is the next most common cause of renal artery hypertension. FMD affects the mid and distal renal artery and is more difficult to visualize than atherosclerotic disease (Fig. 5-64).

Renal Vein Thrombosis

Bland renal vein thrombosis is a relatively rare event in adults. It occurs in the settings of dehydration, coagulopathy, trauma, and certain renal parenchymal processes that cause the nephrotic syndrome such as membranous glomerulonephritis. It may also occur secondary to inferior vena cava thrombosis or ovarian vein thrombosis.

The imaging characteristics of renal vein thrombosis depend on the rapidity of onset and the completeness of occlusion. Totally occlusive acute renal vein thrombosis produces an enlarged kidney on gray-scale images. A defect in the renal vein may or may not be detected on gray-scale images, but no venous flow will be identified on pulsed or color Doppler studies. The venous outflow obstruction will result in diminished arterial inflow and cause a high-resistance arterial waveform. In some instances, pandiastolic flow reversal occurs, and this should always raise a suspicion of underlying renal vein thrombosis.

In most cases of native renal vein thrombosis, the clot develops slowly, which allows venous collaterals to form. In these cases the kidney remains normal in size and intrarenal arterial and venous flow is maintained. Because of this, the detection of venous flow in the kidney or renal hilum does not exclude renal vein thrombosis (Fig. 5-65). In fact, detection of venous flow in the vein itself does not exclude thrombosis because the thrombus is frequently nonocclusive. The only way to establish the diagnosis in such cases is to identify the thrombus as a filling defect in the renal vein on either gray-scale or color Doppler studies. In most cases it is possible to detect or exclude renal vein thrombosis on the right side because the vein is short and the liver provides an adequate acoustic window. As mentioned earlier, evaluation of the left renal vein is considerably more difficult because the vein is long and overlying bowel gas often obscures segments. Unless the entire left renal vein is seen and appears normal on both gray-scale and color-Doppler images, renal vein thrombosis cannot be excluded.

Pseudoaneurysms

Pseudoaneurysms are almost always caused by trauma, especially penetrating trauma such as percutaneous biopsies. Blunt trauma with renal lacerations is a less common cause. Pseudoaneurysms appear as cystic spaces on gray-scale images and can easily be mistaken for renal cysts. Doppler analysis can be performed to prove the presence or absence of internal blood flow. Realistically this is not necessary in routine examinations of native kidneys because cysts are so common and pseudoaneurysms so rare. However, it is definitely necessary in renal transplants because cysts are much less common and pseudoaneurysms are more frequent.

The color Doppler characteristics of renal pseudoaneurysms are similar to those of pseudoaneurysms elsewhere in the body: a swirling pattern of internal blood flow (Fig. 5-66). With an isolated pseudoaneurysm, a "to and fro" pattern of flow is present in the neck because flow entering the aneurysm during systole must exit the aneurysm during diastole. Because of the deeper location, this pattern of flow is more difficult to detect on Doppler waveforms in the kidney than in peripheral arteries. In addition, renal pseudoaneurysms are often associated with an arteriovenous fistula, so the flow progresses from the feeding artery, to the pseudoaneurysm, and then to the draining vein. Therefore, the "to-and-fro" flow pattern is replaced by a low-resistance, high-velocity pattern.

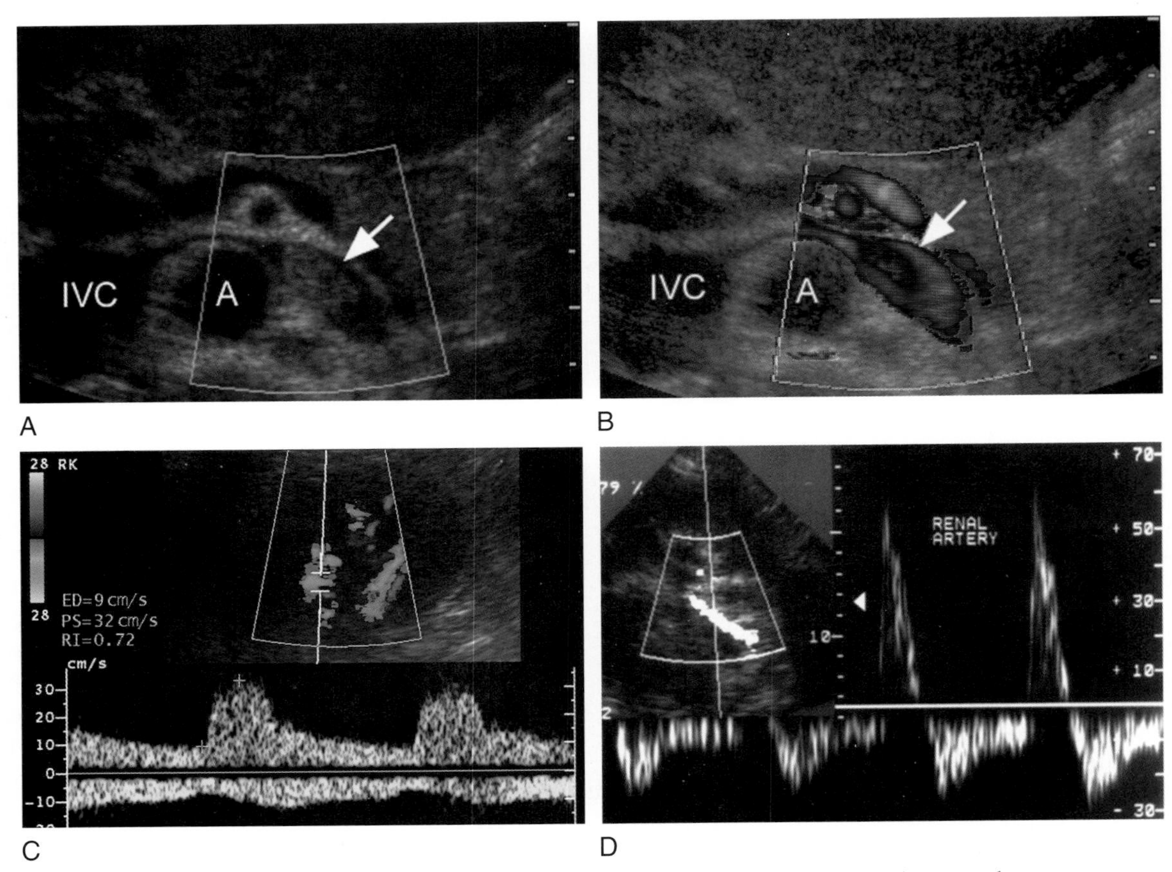

Figure 5-65 Renal vein thrombosis in different patients. Transverse gray-scale (**A**) and power Doppler view (**B**) of the left renal vein show an intraluminal thrombus *(arrow)* that only partially occludes the vessel. The aorta (A) and the inferior vena cava (IVC) are also seen. **C,** Intrarenal pulsed Doppler waveform from a patient with native kidney renal vein thrombosis shows intact venous flow below the baseline. The arterial flow above the baseline has a slightly elevated resistive index (0.72). **D,** Pulsed Doppler waveform from a renal transplant shows a "to-and-fro" pattern of arterial inflow with pandiastolic flow reversal. This classic pattern is usually seen in renal transplants because there are no available collateral veins. It is rarely seen in native kidney venous thrombosis.

Arteriovenous Fistulas

Like pseudoaneurysms, arteriovenous fistulas generally result from penetrating trauma, with percutaneous renal biopsy being the most common cause. Small fistulas are probably fairly common after biopsies, but they rarely cause symptoms. Occasionally, persistent bleeding occurs with or without associated urinary obstruction. Large fistulas are a rare cause of high-output cardiac failure, renal ischemia, and renal hypertension. Most renal arteriovenous fistulas resolve spontaneously without treatment. Persistent symptomatic fistulas can be embolized from a transarterial approach.

In most cases there are no morphologic changes detectable with gray-scale sonography unless there is an associated pseudoaneurysm. Hemodynamic changes that can be detected with Doppler analysis include increased velocity and decreased resistance to flow in the supplying artery, increased velocity and arterialization of the draining vein, and perivascular soft tissue vibration in the region of the fistula (Fig. 5-67).

RENAL TRANSPLANTS

The main role of sonography in the evaluation of renal transplants is to identify hydronephrosis and peritransplant fluid collections. Hydronephrosis has the same appearance in transplants as it does in native kidneys. However, because transplants are more superficially located and can be imaged with higher-resolution transducers, it is often possible to identify urine in the normal renal pelvis and even in the calices and infundibula. This improved visualization of the normal renal collecting system should not be confused with hydronephrosis. In addition, mild distention of the renal pelvis and intrarenal collecting system is common in transplants and should not be construed as functionally

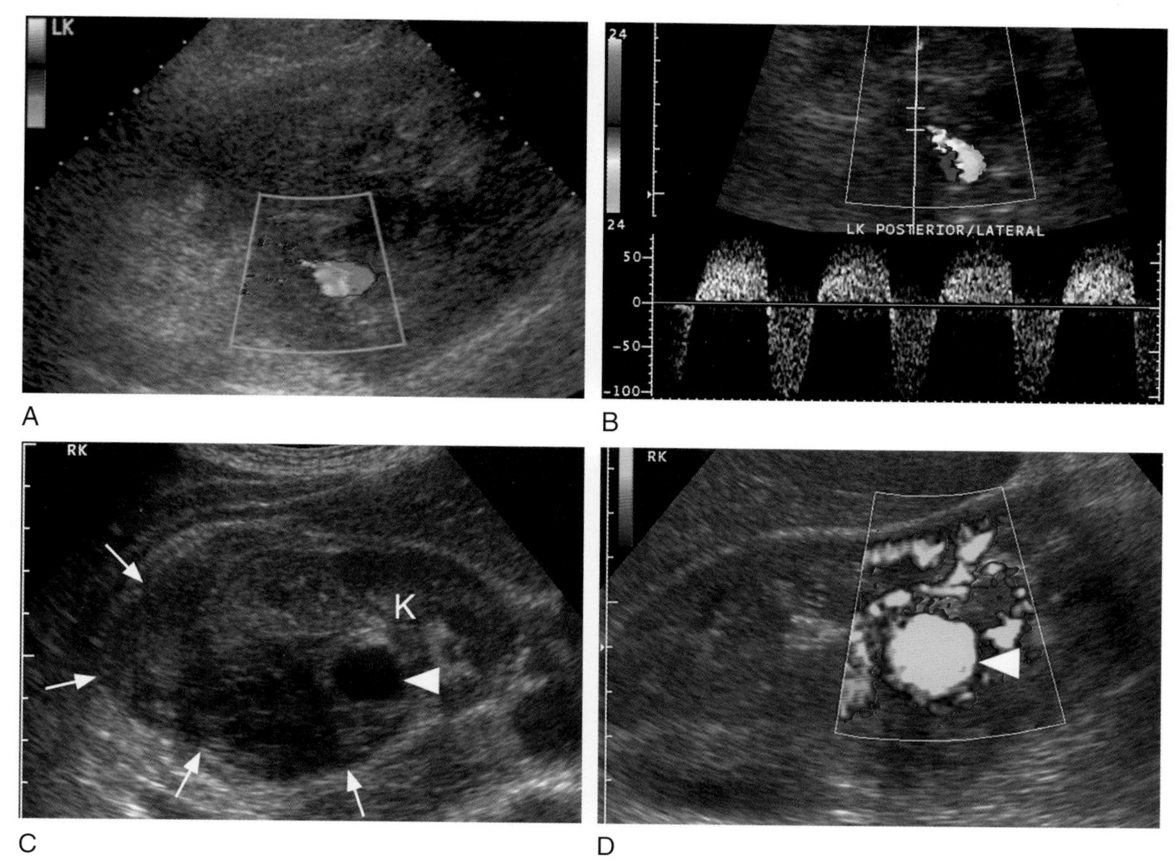

Figure 5-66 Post-traumatic pseudoaneurysms in different patients. Transverse color Doppler view (**A**) and pulsed Doppler waveform (**B**) of the left kidney shows a rounded area with a swirling pattern of intraluminal flow typical of a pseudoaneurysm. Pulsed Doppler waveform shows a "to and fro" pattern arising from the neck of the pseudoaneurysm reflecting flow into the aneurysm during systole and out of the aneurysm during diastole. It is often difficult to show this "to and fro" pattern in renal pseudoaneurysms. Transverse gray-scale (**C**) and power Doppler (**D**) views of the right kidney (K) in another patient who had blunt abdominal trauma shows a hematoma as a complex fluid collection *(arrows)* in the perinephric region. A pseudoaneurysm is seen as a cyst-like structure *(arrowhead)* at the periphery of the kidney. The power Doppler view shows flow throughout the lumen of the pseudoaneurysm.

significant obstruction. It may stem from mild edema at the ureteroneocystostomy site in the early postoperative period and from a redundancy in the collecting system in the later postoperative period. Comparison with old studies is very helpful for eliminating doubt about the significance of mild collecting system dilatation. When old studies are not available, scintigraphy can be used to determine the functional significance of the dilatation.

Peritransplant fluid collections are very common and readily visualized sonographically. Small hematomas are seen frequently in the early postoperative period and are of no importance. Larger hematomas may develop and become important if they compress the ureter and produce urinary obstruction. Compression of the renal parenchyma can also occur, especially with subcapsular hematomas, and this may cause a substantial reduction in renal blood flow. The sonographic appearance of peritransplant hematomas varies depending on their age, just as with hematomas in the native kidney and elsewhere in the body.

Lymphoceles are the most common fluid collection encountered in transplant recipients. These typically arise 1 to 3 weeks postoperatively and are of concern only if they compress the ureter or cause local symptoms of pain and tenderness. They may or may not be septated, and they can vary in size from a few centimeters to massive collections that surround much of the kidney (Fig. 5-68).

Urinomas typically occur as the result of a breakdown in the ureteral implantation into the bladder. Ureteric ischemia can be another cause. Urinomas tend to form in the first 2 postoperative weeks. They are due to urine extravasation and under most circumstances require surgical repair. Because they usually arise from the ureteral anastomosis, they generally occur in continuity with the bladder and often produce a mass effect on the bladder.

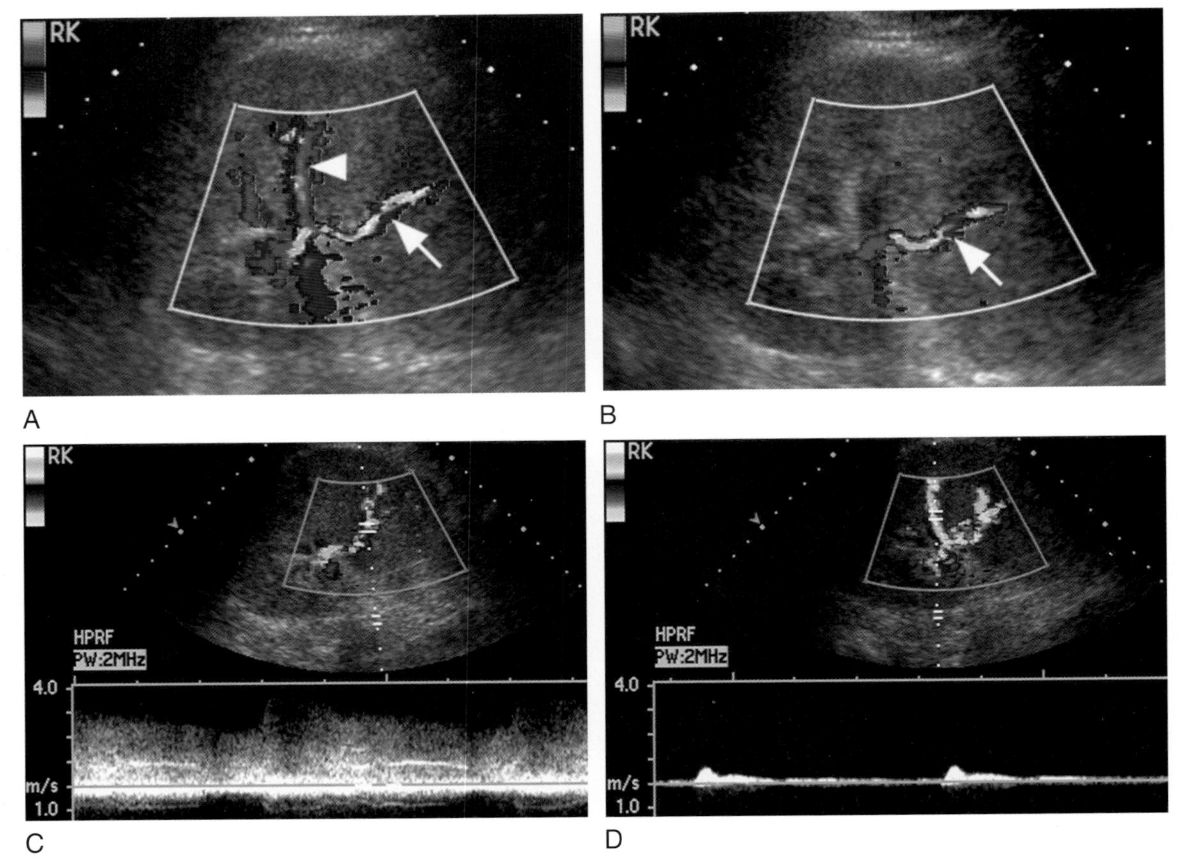

Figure 5-67 Post-biopsy arteriovenous fistula. **A** and **B,** Longitudinal color Doppler views of the right kidney in systole (**A**) and diastole (**B**). In systole, the artery supplying the fistula *(arrow)* is brighter than the artery supplying normal parenchyma *(arrowhead)*. This reflects higher velocity and higher volume flow in the artery to the fistula. In diastole, there is no flow in the uninvolved artery while flow persists in the artery supplying the fistula. **C** and **D,** Pulsed Doppler waveforms from the two arteries confirm the high velocity and low-resistance flow to the artery supplying the fistula compared with the normal artery.

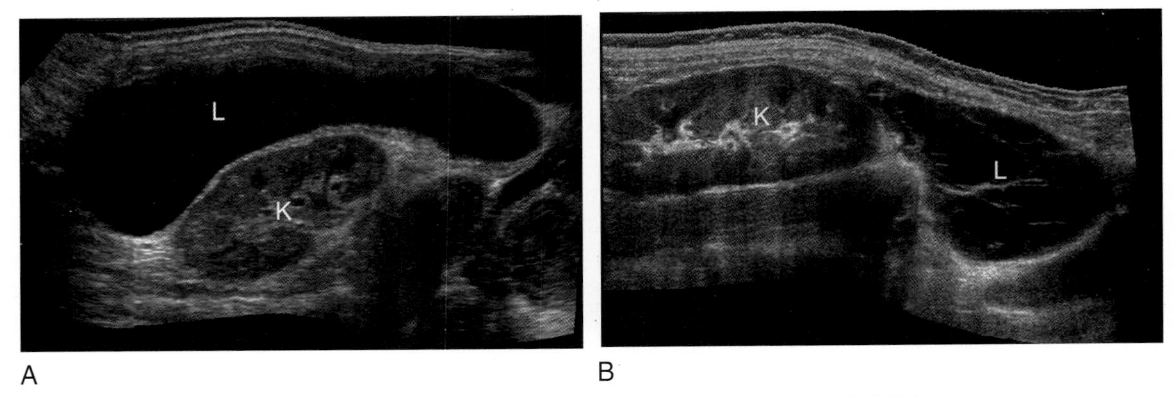

Figure 5-68 Lymphoceles in different patients. **A,** Longitudinal extended field of view scan shows an anechoic unilocular lymphocele (L) anterior to the kidney transplant (K). **B,** Similar view in another patient shows a multi-septated lymphocele (L) inferior to the kidney transplant (K).

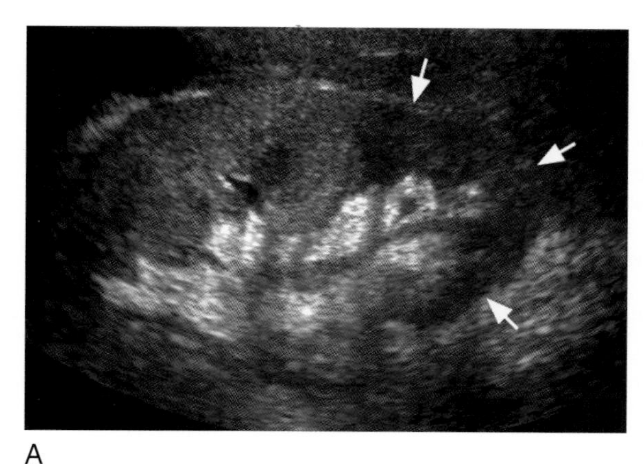

A

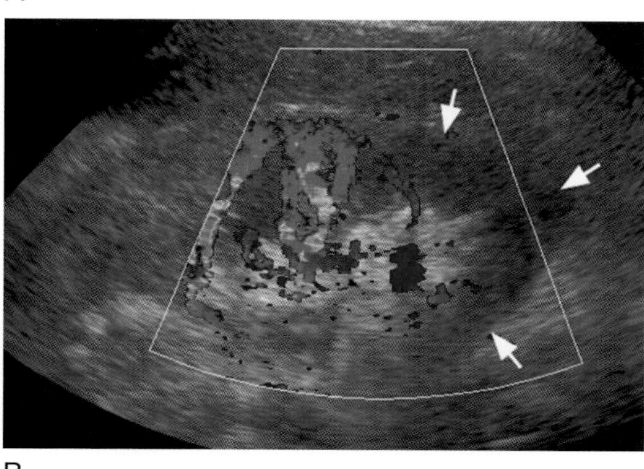

B

Figure 5-69 Transplant infarction. **A,** Longitudinal view of a renal transplant shows decreased echogenicity to the lower pole *(arrows)*. **B,** Color Doppler view shows lack of detectable flow in the lower pole *(arrows)* confirming the infarct.

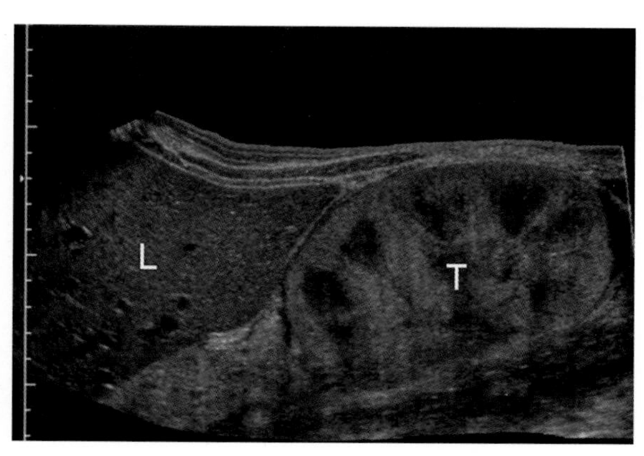

Figure 5-70 Transplant rejection. Longitudinal extended field of view scan shows the transplant kidney (T) and the liver (L). The kidney is swollen, the central sinus fat is poorly visualized, and the pyramids are prominent. These are all signs of rejection.

As they enlarge, they fill in the space between the lower pole of the transplant and the bladder. Their sonographic characteristics are nonspecific and overlap with those of resolving hematomas and lymphoceles. Therefore diagnosis depends on the findings yielded by aspiration and analysis of the fluid or the demonstration of urinary extravasation on scintigraphy or contrast studies.

Abscesses may result from infection involving a preexisting fluid collection or may develop de novo. They typically appear as complex fluid collections containing internal debris, just as they do elsewhere in the body. They are difficult to distinguish from other fluid collections, especially hematomas, so diagnosis depends on a high index of clinical suspicion coupled with the findings from analysis of the fluid aspirated.

Vascular complications of renal transplants include stenosis and thrombosis of the artery and vein, arteriovenous fistula, pseudoaneurysm, and segmental infarction. Most of these complications and their sonographic findings have been discussed already. Segmental infarcts have traditionally been difficult to detect with sonography, but with the development of color and power Doppler analysis, moderate and large segmental infarcts can now be reliably documented (Fig. 5-69). Enhancement with intravenous injection of a contrast agent will almost certainly further improve the detection of small segmental infarcts. As with native kidneys, capsular collaterals form in areas of infarction and produce rim perfusion to the kidney.

Parenchymal processes affecting renal transplants are best diagnosed by ultrasound-guided percutaneous biopsy. Sonography can often show gray-scale changes, but in most cases they are not specific enough on which to base management decisions. Transplant rejection causes renal swelling that affects both the parenchyma and the urothelium. It may also produce enlarged hypoechoic pyramids, cortical regions of decreased echogenicity, and decreased visibility of the renal sinus (Fig. 5-70). The more of these abnormalities that are present, the more likely is the diagnosis of rejection. However, acute tubular necrosis, cyclosporin toxicity, and infection can also produce one or more of these abnormalities. Parenchymal disease also causes an increase in the resistance to blood flow that can be detected by measurement of resistive indices. Normally, the resistive index is less than 0.7. Rejection tends to have the most severe effect and causes the highest resistive indices, but as with the gray-scale changes there is significant overlap; and in an individual patient, it is hard to rely on Doppler waveforms for management decisions.

Post-transplant lymphoproliferative disorder (PTLD) is the result of immunosuppression that accompanies organ transplants. It frequently spares the lymph nodes and affect the larger organs. It is less common with renal transplants than with most of the other organ transplants. In addition to masses in the liver, lung, and spleen, solid hypoechoic infiltration of the soft tissue around the renal transplant hilum should suggest PTLD (Fig. 5-71).

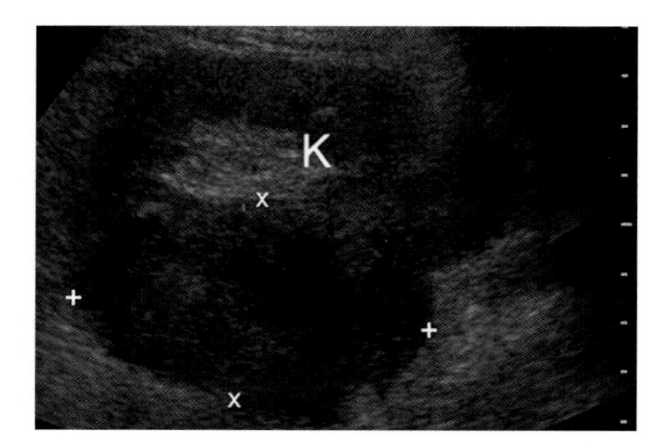

Figure 5-71 Post-transplant lymphoproliferative disease. Oblique view of the transplant kidney (K) shows a slightly heterogeneous, solid, predominantly hypoechoic mass *(cursors)* located in the region of the renal hilum. The major differential diagnoses are an acute hematoma and lymphoproliferative disease. Percutaneous biopsies were nondiagnostic, but surgical exploration and biopsy confirmed lymphoproliferative disease.

Key Features

The detection of urinary obstruction is one of the most common indications for abdominal sonography. Diagnosis relies on the detection of hydronephrosis and/or increased resistance to renal arterial flow and/or loss of ureteral jets.

Pyonephrosis should be suspected in patients with infected urine and hydronephrosis.

Renal cysts are seen frequently. Patients with simple cysts require no further evaluation. Patients with complex cystic lesions require surgical treatment, evaluation with CT or MRI, or periodic follow-up examinations.

Multiple renal cysts can occur in the settings of autosomal dominant polycystic disease, acquired cystic disease of dialysis, von Hippel-Lindau syndrome, and tuberous sclerosis.

Renal cell cancer is most often a solid mass that is slightly more echogenic than adjacent renal cortex. However, it ranges in echogenicity from very hyperechoic to hypoechoic.

Renal cell cancer may have significant cystic elements and may contain calcifications.

Solid and complex renal masses in adults should be considered renal cell carcinoma until proved otherwise.

When a renal cell carcinoma is suspected, a prospective search should be made for renal vein and inferior vena cava invasion.

Small, homogeneous, very hyperechoic masses are most likely to be angiomyolipomas, which can be confirmed with CT or MRI or monitored sonographically, depending on size.

Transitional cell carcinoma is usually occult sonographically. When seen, it is typically located in the renal sinus, is solid, and is often associated with hydronephrosis.

Lymphoma usually involves the kidneys in a multifocal manner and can be very difficult to detect sonographically. It is usually very hypoechoic and on rare occasions may mimic a renal cyst. It may infiltrate the perinephric space.

Pyelonephritis may cause focal areas of increased and decreased cortical echogenicity, renal enlargement, urothelial thickening, and focal areas of decreased blood flow. However, sonographic findings are often normal in patients with pyelonephritis.

Renal calculi appear as echogenic reflectors with acoustic shadows and often with a twinkle artifact.

Sonography is a relatively effective means of detecting intrarenal calculi. It is also effective for ureteral stones located near the ureteropelvic junction and in the distal ureter. Nonenhanced CT is a more reliable means of detecting renal and ureteral calculi. Sonography should be used to search for calculi in pregnant patients or patients who have confusing or nondiagnostic CT scans.

Nephrocalcinosis produces hyperechoic pyramids with or without shadowing.

Increased renal cortical echogenicity is a nonspecific finding that in general is associated with renal parenchymal diseases.

Renal artery stenosis can be detected with Doppler analysis on the basis of an elevated main renal artery velocity, an elevated renal-to-aortic velocity ratio, or slowed segmental renal artery systolic acceleration. However, the use of sonography for this purpose requires much experience and is not possible in up to 20% of patients.

The detection and exclusion of renal vein thrombosis is relatively easy on the right side but relatively difficult on the left side. Arterial inflow is usually only minimally altered in the native kidneys.

In the evaluation of renal transplant dysfunction, sonography is most valuable in detecting the following surgical complications: urinary obstruction, postoperative fluid collections, and renal vascular thrombosis or stenosis. It is not effective at distinguishing rejection from other parenchymal processes that cause dysfunction.

SUGGESTED READINGS

al-Murrani B, et al: Echogenic rings—an ultrasound sign of early nephrocalcinosis. Clin Radiol 44:49, 1991.

Agrons GA, Wagner BJ, Davidson AJ, Suarez ES: From the Archives of the AFIP: Multilocular cystic renal tumor in children: Radiologic-pathologic correlation. Radiographics 15:653-669, 1995.

Banner MP, et al: Multilocular renal cysts: Radiologic-pathologic correlation. AJR Am J Roentgenol 136:239, 1981.

Baker S, Middleton WD: In vivo color Doppler sonographic analysis of ureteral jets in normal volunteers: Importance of the relative specific gravity of urine in the ureter and bladder. AJR Am J Roentgenol 59:773-775, 1992.

Baumgarten DA, Baumgarten BR: Imaging and radiologic management of upper urinary tract infections. Urol Clin North Am 24:545-569,1997.

Bechtold RE, Zagoria RJ: Imaging approach to staging of renal cell carcinoma. Urol Clin North Am 24:507-522, 1997.

Berland LL, et al: Renal artery stenosis: Prospective evaluation of diagnosis with color Doppler ultrasound compared with angiography. Radiology 174:421, 1990.

Bosniak MA, et al: CT diagnosis of renal angiomyolipoma: The importance of detecting small amounts of fat. AJR Am J Roentgenol 151:497, 1988.

Brown ED, Chen MYM, Wolfman NT, et al: Complications of renal transplantation: evaluation with US and radionuclide imaging. Radiographics 20:607-622, 2000.

Bude RO, Rubin JM, Platt JF, et al: Pulsus tardus: Its cause and potential limitations in detection of arterial stenosis. Radiology 190:779-784, 1994.

Burge JH, Middleton WD, McClennan BL, Hildeboldt CF: Ureteral jets in healthy subjects and in patients with unilateral ureteral calculi: Comparison with color Doppler ultrasound. Radiology 180:437-442, 1991.

Carter AR, et al: The junctional parenchymal defect: A sonographic variant of renal anatomy. Radiology 154:499, 1985.

Chamorro HA, Forbes TW, Padowsky GO, Wholey MH: Multi-imaging approach in the diagnosis of Page kidney. AJR Am J Roentgenol 136:620-621, 1981.

Charnsangavej C: Lymphoma of the genitourinary tract. Radiol Clin North Am 28:865, 1990.

Cho KJ, Thornbury JR, Prince MR: Renal arteries and veins: Normal variants. In Pollack HM, McClennan BL (eds): Clinical Urography, 2nd ed. Philadelphia, WB Saunders, 2000, pp 2476-2489.

Choyke PL, et al: The natural history of renal lesions in von Hippel-Lindau disease: A serial CT study in 28 patients. AJR Am J Roentgenol 159:1229, 1992.

Choyke PL, et al: Renal metastases: Clinicopathologic and radiologic correlation. Radiology 162:359, 1987.

Choyke PL, Glenn GM, Walther MM, et al: Von Hippel-Lindau disease: Genetic, clinical, and imaging features. Radiology 194:626-642, 1995.

Cronan JJ, et al: Peripelvic cysts: An imposter of sonographic hydronephrosis. J Ultrasound Med 1:229, 1982.

Curry NS, Bissada NK: Radiologic evaluation of small and indeterminant renal masses. Urol Clin North Am 24:493-505, 1997.

Dalla Palma L, Stacul F, Bazzocchi M, et al: Ultrasonography and plain film versus intravenous urography in ureteric colic. Clin Radiol 47:333, 1993.

Dillard JP, Talner LB, Pinckney L: Normal renal papillae simulating caliceal filling defects on sonography. AJR 148:895, 1987.

Dodd GD III, Tublin ME, Shah A, Zajko AB: Imaging of vascular complications associated with renal transplants. AJR Am J Roentgenol 157:449, 1991.

Dunnick NR, et al: The radiology of juxtaglomerular tumors. Radiology 147:321, 1983.

Ellenbogen PH, Scheible FW, Talner LB, Leopold GR: Sensitivity of gray scale ultrasound in detecting urinary tract obstruction. AJR Am J Roentgenol 130:731-733, 1978.

Forman HP, Middleton WD, Melson GL, McClennan BL: Increasing frequency of detection of hyperechoic renal cell carcinomas. Radiology 188:431, 1993.

Genkins SM, Sanfilippo FP, Carroll BA: Duplex Doppler sonography of renal transplants: Lack of sensitivity and specificity in establishing pathologic diagnosis. AJR Am J Roentgenol 152:535, 1989.

Glazer GM, Callen PW, Filly RA: Medullary nephrocalcinosis: Sonographic evaluation. AJR Am J Roentgenol 138:55, 1992.

Goiney RC, et al: Renal oncocytoma: Sonographic analysis of 14 cases. AJR Am J Roentgenol 143:1001, 1984.

Goldman SM, Fishman EK: Upper urinary tract infection: The current role of CT, ultrasound, and MRI. Semin Ultrasound CT MR 12:355, 1991.

Grant DC, et al: Sonography in transitional cell carcinoma of the renal pelvis. Urol Radiol 8:1, 1986.

Hartman DS, et al: Renal lymphoma: Radiologic-pathologic correlation of 21 cases. Radiology 144:759, 1982.

Hartman DS, et al: Angiomyolipoma: Ultrasonic-pathologic correlation. Radiology 139:451, 1981.

Hartman DS, et al: Xanthogranulomatous pyelonephritis: Sonographic-pathologic correlation of 16 cases. J Ultrasound Med 3:481, 1984.

Hayes WS, Hartman DS, Sesterhenn IA: From the Archives of the AFIP: Xanthogranulomatous pyelonephritis. Radiographics 11:485, 1991.

Heiken JP, McClennan BL, Gold RP: Renal lymphoma. Semin Ultrasound CT MR 7:58, 1986.

Hoddick W, Filly RA, Backman U, et al: Renal allograft rejection: US evaluation. Radiology 161:469, 1986.

House MK, Dowling RJ, King P, Gibson RN: Using Doppler sonography to reveal renal artery stenosis: An evaluation of optimal imaging parameters. AJR Am J Roentgenol 173:761-765, 1999.

Hricak H, et al: Renal parenchymal disease: Sonographic-histologic correlation. Radiology 144:141, 1982.

Jeffrey RB, et al: Sensitivity of sonography in pyonephrosis: A re-evaluation. AJR Am J Roentgenol 144:71, 1985.

Kawashima A, Goldman SM, Sandler CM: The indeterminate renal mass. Radiol Clin North Am 34:997-1015, 1996.

Kliewer MA, et al: Renal artery stenosis: Analysis of Doppler waveform parameters and tardus-parvus pattern. Radiology 189:779, 1993.

Koelliker SL, Cronan JJ: Acute urinary tract obstruction: Imaging update. Urol Clin North Am 24:571-582, 1997.

Lafortune M, et al: Sonography of the hypertrophied column of Bertin. AJR Am J Roentgenol 146:53, 1986.

Letourneau JG, Day DL, Ascher NL, Castaneda-Zuniga WR: Imaging of renal transplants. AJR Am J Roentgenol 150:833, 1988.

Levine E, Hartman DS, Smirniotopoulos JG: Renal cystic disease associated with renal neoplasms. In Pollack HM (ed): Clinical Urography. Philadelphia, WB Saunders, 1990.

Levine E, et al: Natural history of acquired renal cystic disease in dialysis patients: A prospective longitudinal CT study. AJR Am J Roentgenol 156:501, 1991.

Levine E, Hartman DS, Meilstrup JW, et al: Current concepts and controversies in imaging of renal cystic diseases. Urol Clin North Am 24:523-544, 1997.

Luscher TF, Lie JT, Stanson AW, et al: Arterial fibromuscular dysplasia. Mayo Clin Proc 62:931-952, 1987.

Madewell JE, et al: Multilocular cystic nephroma: A radiographic-pathologic correlation of 58 patients. Radiology 146:309, 1983.

Middleton WD, et al: Renal calculi: Sensitivity for detection with US. Radiology 167:239, 1988.

Middleton WD, et al: Postbiopsy renal transplant arteriovenous fistulas: Color Doppler ultrasound characteristics. Radiology 171:253, 1989.

Middleton WD, Melson GL: Renal duplication artifact in ultrasound imaging. Radiology 173:427, 1989.

Nicolet V, et al: Thickening of the renal collecting system: A nonspecific finding at ultrasound. Radiology 168:411, 1988.

Pagani JJ: Solid renal mass in the cancer patient: Second primary renal cell carcinoma versus renal metastasis. J Comput Assist Tomogr 7:444, 1983.

Patriquin H, Robitaille P: Renal calcium deposition in children: Sonographic demonstration of the Anderson-Carr progression. AJR Am J Roentgenol 146:1253, 1986.

Piccirillo M, Rigsby CM, Rosenfield AT: Sonography of renal inflammatory disease. Urol Radiol 9:66, 1987.

Platt JF, Rubin JM, Bowerman RA, Marn CS: The inability to detect kidney disease on the basis of echogenicity. AJR Am J Roentgenol 151:317-319, 1988.

Platt JF, Ellis JH, Rubin JM: Intrarenal arterial Doppler sonography in the detection of renal vein thrombosis of the native kidney. AJR Am J Roentgenol 162:1367, 1994.

Platt JF, et al: Duplex Doppler ultrasound of the kidney: Differentiation of obstructive from nonobstructive dilatation. Radiology 171:515, 1989.

Platt JF, Ellis JH, Rubin JM: Intrarenal arterial Doppler sonography in the detection of renal vein thrombosis of the native kidney. AJR Am J Roentgenol 162:1367-1370, 1994.

Pollack HM, et al: The accuracy of gray-scale renal ultrasonography in differentiating cystic neoplasms from benign cysts. Radiology 143:741, 1982.

Ohnishi K, Watanabe H, Ohe H, Saitoh M: Ultrasound findings in urolithiasis in the lower ureter. Ultrasound Med Biol 12:577-579, 1986.

Pozniak MA, et al: Extraneous factors affecting resistive index. Invest Radiol 23:899, 1988.

Quinn MJ, et al: Renal oncocytoma: New observations. Radiology 153:49, 1984.

Radin DR, et al: Visceral and nodal calcification in patients with AIDS-related *Pneumocystis carinii* infection. AJR Am J Roentgenol 154:27, 1990.

Ravine D, Gibson RN, Walker RG, et al: Evaluation of ultrasonographic criteria for autosomal dominant polycystic kidney disease 1. Lancet 343:824, 1994.

Rifkin MD, et al: Evaluation of renal transplant rejection by duplex Doppler examination: Value of the resistive index. AJR Am J Roentgenol 148:759, 1987.

Ritchie WW, et al: Evaluation of azotemic patients: Diagnostic yield of ultrasound examination. Radiology 167:245, 1988.

Rosenberg ER, et al: The significance of septations in a renal cyst. AJR 144:593, 1985.

Rosenfield AT, Siegel NJ: Renal parenchymal disease: Histopathologic-sonographic correlation. AJR Am J Roentgenol 137:793, 1981.

Schwerk WB, Schwerk WN, Rodeck G: Venous renal tumor extension: A prospective ultrasound evaluation. Radiology 156:491, 1985.

Siegel CL, Middleton WD, Teefey SA, McClennan BL: Angiomyolipoma and renal cell carcinoma: Ultrasound differentiation. Radiology 198:789-793, 1996.

Strauss S, Duchnitsky T, Peer A, et al: Sonographic features of horseshoe kidney: Review of 34 patients. J Ultrasound Med 19:27-31, 2000.

Stavros AT, et al: Segmental stenosis of the renal artery: Pattern recognition of tardus and parvus abnormalities with duplex sonography. Radiology 184:487, 1992.

Stavros T, Harshfield D: Renal Doppler, renal artery stenosis, and renovascular hypertension: Direct and indirect duplex sonographic abnormalities in patients with renal artery stenosis. Ultrasound Q 12(4):217-263. 1994.

Taylor AJ, et al: Renal imaging in long-term dialysis patients: A comparison of CT and sonography. AJR Am J Roentgenol 153:765, 1989.

Taylor DC, et al: Duplex ultrasound scanning in the diagnosis of renal artery stenosis: A prospective evaluation. J Vasc Surg 7:363, 1988.

Taylor KJW, et al: Vascular complications in renal allografts: Detection with duplex Doppler ultrasound. Radiology 162:31, 1987.

Vrtiska TJ, et al: Role of ultrasound in medical management of patients with renal stone disease. Urol Radiol 14:131, 1992.

Warshauer DM, et al: Unusual causes of increased vascular impedance in renal transplants: Duplex Doppler evaluation. Radiology 169:367, 1988.

Wilson DA, Wenzl JE, Altshuler GP: Ultrasound demonstration of diffuse cortical nephrocalcinosis in a case of primary hyperoxaluria. AJR Am J Roentgenol 132:659, 1979.

Wong-You-Cheong JJ, Wagner BJ, Davis CJ Jr: From the Archives of the AFIP: Transitional cell carcinoma of the urinary tract: Radiologic-pathologic correlation. Radiographics 18:123-142, 1998.

Wood BP, et al: Tuberous sclerosis. AJR Am J Roentgenol 158:750, 1992.

Yamashita Y, et al: Small renal cell carcinoma: Pathologic and radiologic correlation. Radiology 184:493, 1992.

Yousem DM, et al: Synchronous and metachronous transitional cell carcinoma of the urinary tract: Prevalence, incidence, and radiographic detection. Radiology 167:613, 1988.

CHAPTER 6 Lower Genitourinary

For Key Features summary see p. 188

SCROTUM

Sonography is the primary method used to image the scrotum. Patients are usually examined in the supine position. A towel can be draped between the thighs to help support the scrotum. Warm gel should always be used because cold gel can elicit a cremasteric response and the resulting scrotal thickening makes it very difficult to perform a thorough examination.

The normal testes appear as homogeneous ovoid organs that are symmetric bilaterally. The normal testis measures 4 to 5 cm in length, 2 to 3 cm in width, and 2 to 2.5 cm in depth. The normal volume of the testis using the formula for an ellipsoid (length ×width × depth × 0.53) is 15 to 20 mL. Testicular size decreases with age. The seminiferous tubules converge to form the rete testes, which is located at the testicular mediastinum. The mediastinum itself appears as a peripherally located, elongated hyperechoic structure (Fig. 6-1A and B). The rete testes connects to the epididymal head via the efferent ductules. The head of the epididymis is semilunar with rounded edges, and its echogenicity is similar to that of the testis (see Fig. 6-1C). It rests directly on the upper pole of the testis and should be seen in almost all men. It continues inferiorly into the body and tail of the epididymis, which are hypoechoic to the testis (see Fig. 6-1D and E). The body and tail of the epididymis are more difficult to identify than the head, but, with practice, they can usually be seen along the anterolateral or posterior aspect of the testis.

The vascular supply of the testis is shown in Figure 6-2. Unlike other organs, the major arteries of the testis are located peripherally and are called capsular arteries. They supply blood to the testicular parenchyma by means of branches called centripetal arteries. The centripetal arteries enter the testis and travel toward the mediastinum. As they approach the mediastinum, they branch into recurrent rami that curve away from the mediastinum. In approximately 50% of testes, one or more major branches of the testicular artery enter the testis through the mediastinum. These transmediastinal arteries are often large enough to be seen by gray-scale sonography, and a transmediastinal vein often accompanies them. Like other solid parenchymal organs, the testicular arterial waveforms have a low resistance pattern. The veins of the testis drain through the mediastinum as well as through the capsule of the testis. They are more difficult to visualize than the arteries, but with continued improvement in Doppler sensitivity they are being seen with more regularity. Blood flow may or may not be seen in the normal epididymis, but it should not be as vascular as the testis. (See Table 6-1 for a summary of the characteristics of normal testes.)

One of the major roles of sonography is the evaluation of scrotal masses, and the most important determination is whether the mass is inside or outside the testis. The vast majority of extratesticular masses are benign, but intratesticular masses are much more likely to be malignant. In addition to location, it is also important to determine whether the mass is cystic or solid, whether it has detectable internal vascularity on color Doppler imaging, and whether it is palpable (Box 6-1).

The most common scrotal mass is the spermatocele. These are cystic lesions that form in the head of the epididymis and are filled with spermatozoa-containing fluid (Fig. 6-3). Low-level echoes can be seen in the lumen of some spermatoceles, especially when the gain is increased. Septations are occasionally seen with large

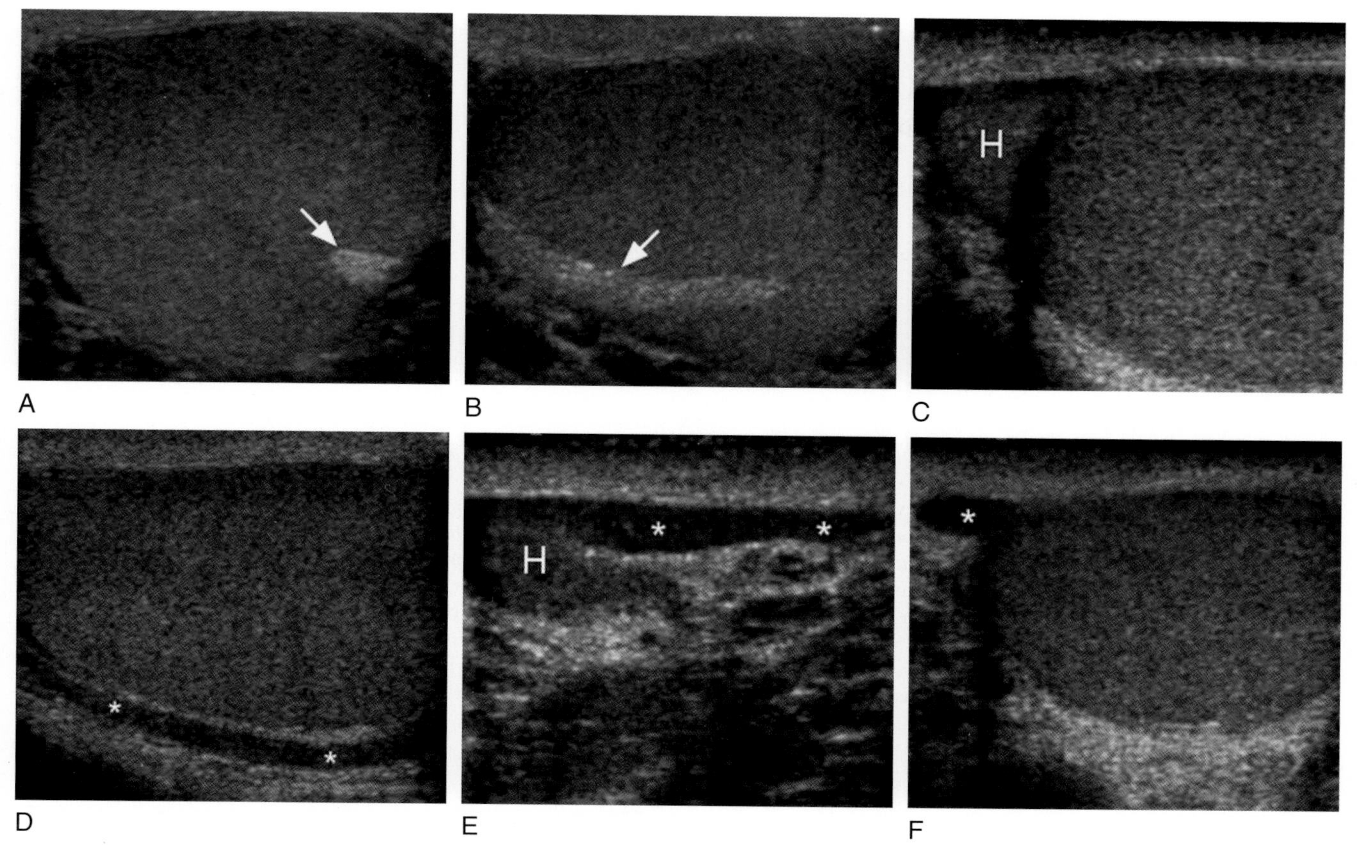

Figure 6-1 Normal scrotal anatomy. **A,** Transverse view of the testis shows normal homogeneous echogenicity throughout with the exception of the peripherally located hyperechoic mediastinum *(arrow)*. **B,** Longitudinal view of the testis shows the mediastinum *(arrow)* as an elongated hyperechoic structure. **C,** Longitudinal view shows the upper pole of the testis and the head of the epididymis (H). The head of the epididymis and testis have similar echogenicities. **D,** Longitudinal view shows the body of the epididymis (*) located posterior to the testis. **E,** Longitudinal view shows the head (H) and body (*) of the epididymis. Note that the body is less echogenic than the head. In this case the body of the epididymis is located anteriorly. **F,** Transverse view of the right testis shows the hypoechoic epididymal body (*) located along the anterior lateral aspect of the testis.

spermatoceles. Epididymal cysts may also form in the epididymal head as well as the body and tail. They contain serous fluid and are anechoic and indistinguishable from spermatoceles. Both are benign lesions that rarely produce symptoms other than those related to the mass effect. Cystic lesions are extremely common, and at least a small spermatocele can be seen in more than 70% of scans.

Hydroceles are collections of fluid that form in the potential space of the tunica vaginalis. Most large hydroceles are idiopathic. A variety of conditions, including scrotal inflammatory processes, testicular torsion, and testicular tumors, can cause small to moderate hydroceles. Although variable, hydroceles usually occur in the anterior aspect of the scrotum and displace the testis posteriorly (Fig. 6-4A and B). Crystals can precipitate in hydrocele fluid and produce mobile low-level reflectors (see Fig. 6-4C). When hydroceles are large and the testis is compressed posteriorly, it can be difficult to obtain high-resolution views of the testes. This can be overcome by positioning the transducer posteriorly to get closer to the testes. Rarely, hydrocele fluid will accumulate in the spermatic cord in an unobliterated portion of the tunica vaginalis. This type of hydrocele will appear superior to the testis and is referred to as a funiculocele or a hydrocele of the cord. It can be distinguished from a spermatocele because it does not arise from the epididymis (see Fig. 6-4D). Pyoceles and hematoceles are hydroceles that are complicated by infection or hemorrhage. They appear as complex collections with internal echoes and septations and often in conjunction with scrotal wall hyperemia (Fig. 6-5). They should be suspected on the basis of combined clinical and sonographic features.

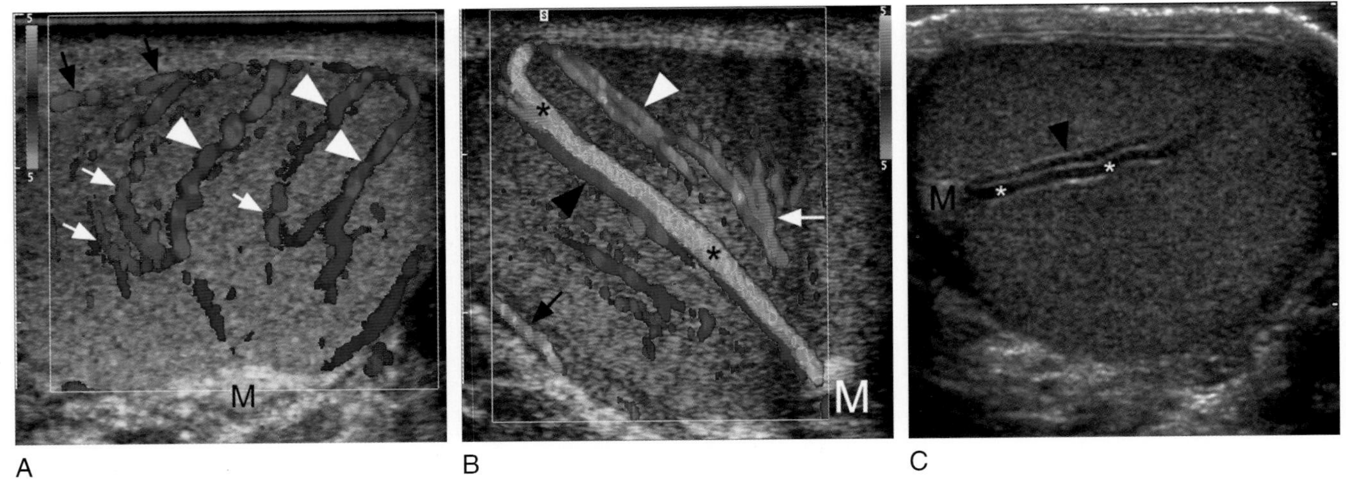

Figure 6-2 Testicular vascular anatomy. **A,** Transverse color Doppler view shows a peripherally located capsular artery *(black arrows)* supplying several centripetal arteries *(white arrowheads).* Several recurrent rami *(white arrows)* are seen arising from the centripetal arteries. M, mediastinum. **B,** Transverse color Doppler view of a different patient shows a large transmediastinal artery (*) passing through the mediastinum (M) and traveling to the opposite side of the testis. An adjacent transmediastinal vein *(black arrowhead)* is also seen. A centripetal artery *(white arrowhead),* recurrent ramus *(white arrow),* and a capsular artery *(black arrow)* are also seen. **C,** Grayscale view of a different patient shows a transmediastinal artery (*) as well as vein *(arrowhead)* and their relationship to the mediastinum (M).

Table 6-1 Characteristics of a Normal Testis

Characteristic	Appearance
Echogenicity	Medium level (except echogenic mediastinum)
Texture	Homogeneous
Surface	Smooth
Vascularity	Largest vessels on surface
Size	15-20 mL (average 4-5 × 2-3 × 2-3 cm)

Box 6-1 Appearance of Scrotal Lesion versus Chance of Neoplasm

FACTORS THAT DECREASE CHANCE OF NEOPLASM	FACTORS THAT INCREASE CHANCE OF NEOPLASM
Extratesticular	Intratesticular
Nonpalpable	Palpable
Simple cystic appearance	Solid or complex cystic
No detectable vascularity	Detectable internal vascularity

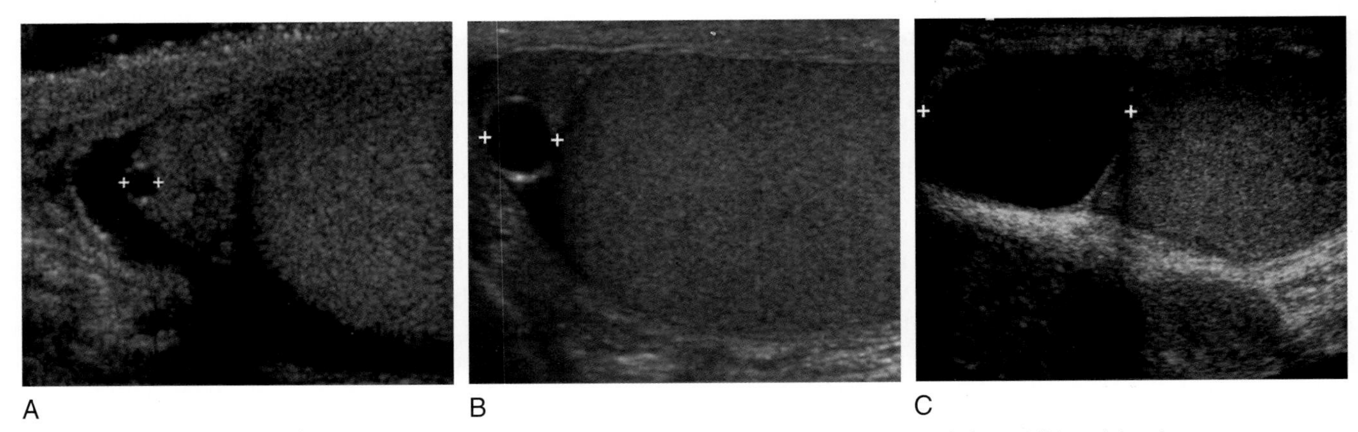

Figure 6-3 Spermatoceles in different patients. **A,** Longitudinal view of the epididymal head shows a small spermatocele *(cursors).* **B,** Longitudinal view shows a moderate-sized spermatocele *(cursors).* **C,** Longitudinal view shows a large spermatocele *(cursors)* that makes it difficult to visualize the adjacent epididymal head.

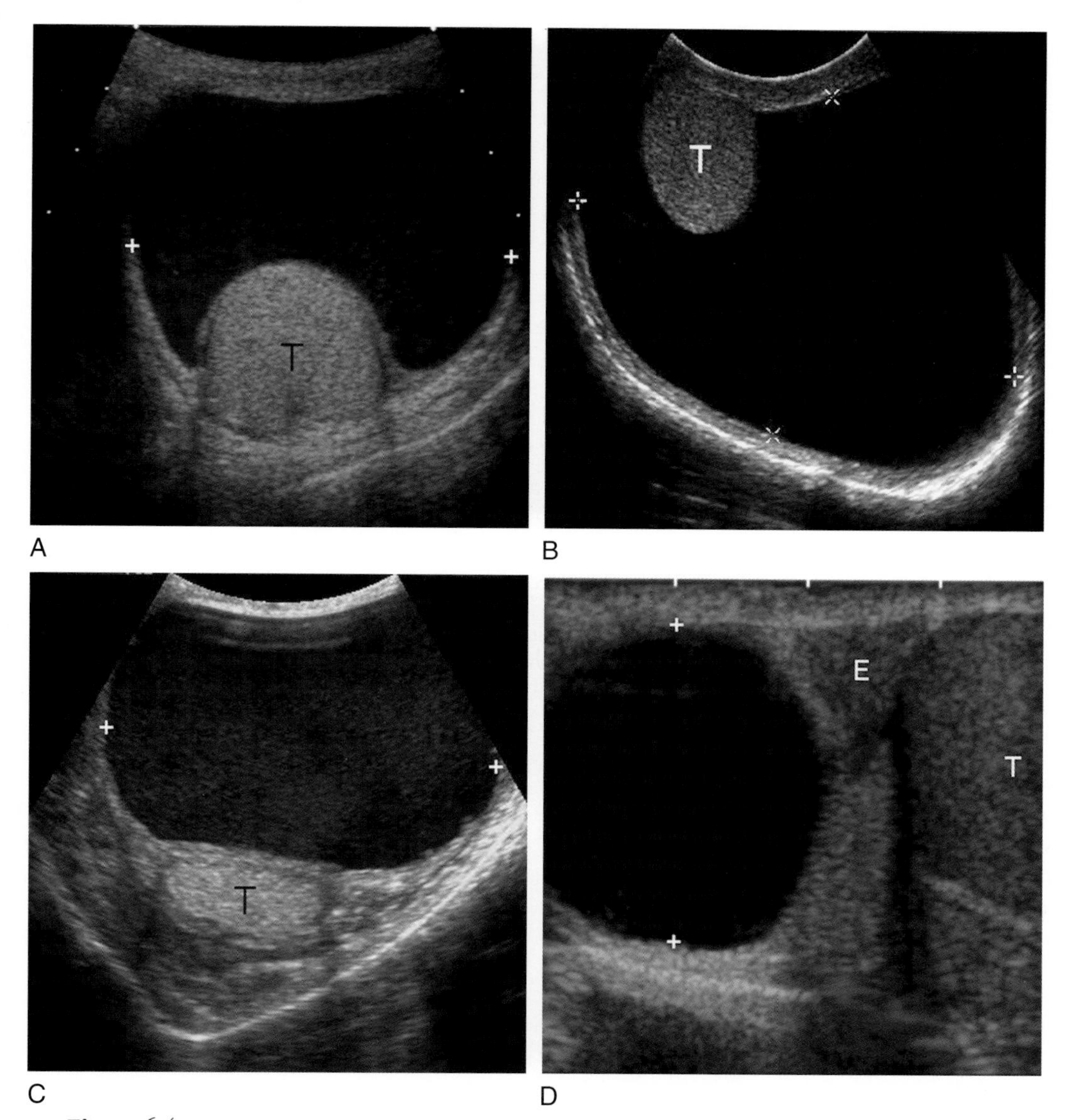

Figure 6-4 Hydroceles in different patients. **A,** Transverse view shows a large anechoic hydrocele *(cursors)* surrounding the testis (T). **B,** Transverse view shows a large hydrocele *(cursors)* surrounding the testis (T). This case is unusual because the testis is located anteriorly. **C,** Transverse view shows a hydrocele *(cursors)* with diffuse low-level echoes. The testis (T) is seen posteriorly. **D,** Longitudinal view shows a cystic lesion *(cursors)* in the scrotum located superior to the epididymal head (E). This is the expected location and appearance of a hydrocele of the spermatic cord.

Varicoceles are dilated peritesticular veins that form as the result of incompetent valves in the spermatic veins. The left spermatic vein drains into the left renal vein and the right spermatic vein drains into the inferior vena cava. Because the superior mesenteric artery compresses the left renal vein, the pressure on the left side is higher than that on the right, and this presumably explains why 85% of the varioceles are on the left. Most of the remaining 15% are bilateral. It is so unusual to have an isolated right-sided varicocele that compression of the right spermatic vein by retroperitoneal masses, or situs inversus should be considered whenever one is detected. Although the yield is very low, a sonographic survey of the upper abdomen should be performed whenever an isolated right-sided varicocele or an unusually large and asymmetric right-sided varicocele is detected.

Varicoceles generally do not cause pain or discomfort until they become large. However, even small nonpalpable varicoceles can potentially cause infertility. Therefore, a search for varicoceles is important in the evaluation of an infertile couple. Gray-scale sonography depicts varicoceles as numerous, dilated, tortuous, tubular channels in the peritesticular tissues (Fig. 6-6). They are usually located lateral, posterior and/or superior to the testis.

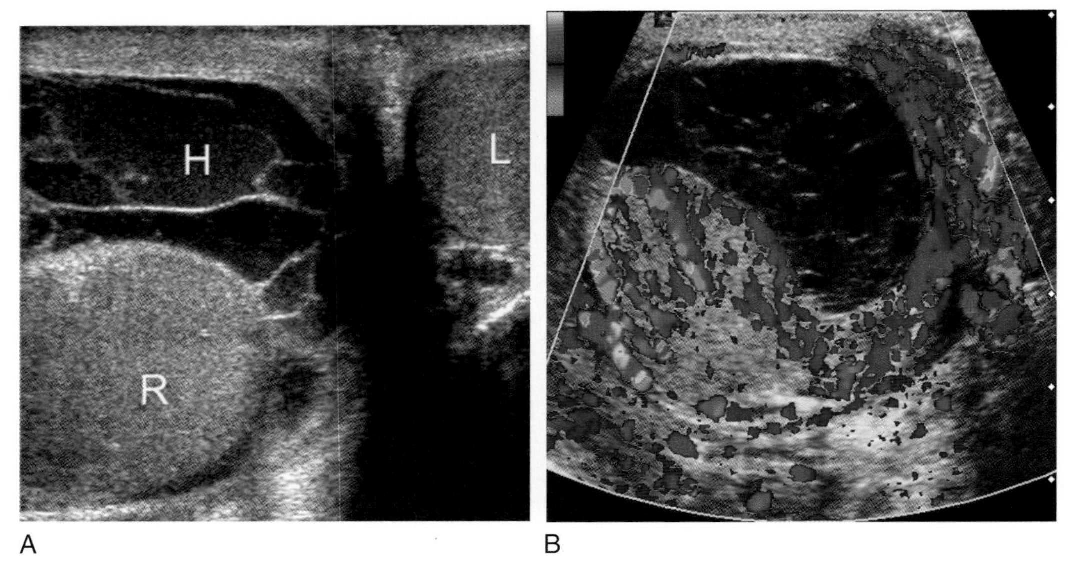

Figure 6-5 Complicated hydroceles in different patients. **A,** Transverse view of the scrotum shows a complex multi-septated hydrocele (H) containing low-level echoes. The right (R) and left (L) testes are also seen. This was a post-traumatic hematocele. **B,** Color Doppler view of the scrotum in a different patient with epididymitis shows a multi-septated collection in the scrotal sac with peripheral hyperemia. This is consistent with a pyocele.

Rarely, varicoceles will involve intratesticular veins. The upper limit of normal for the caliber of scrotal veins is 2 mm. At rest, blood flow in varicoceles is occasionally visible on gray-scale sonography, but it is usually too slow to be detected with color Doppler imaging. However, when the patient performs a Valsalva maneuver, the incompetent valves in the spermatic vein allow rapid retrograde blood flow into the pampiniform plexus, and this is detectable on color Doppler imaging (Fig. 6-7). In most patients this Valsalva-induced flow augmentation is readily detectable when the patient is supine. If the examination is normal with the patient supine, then the

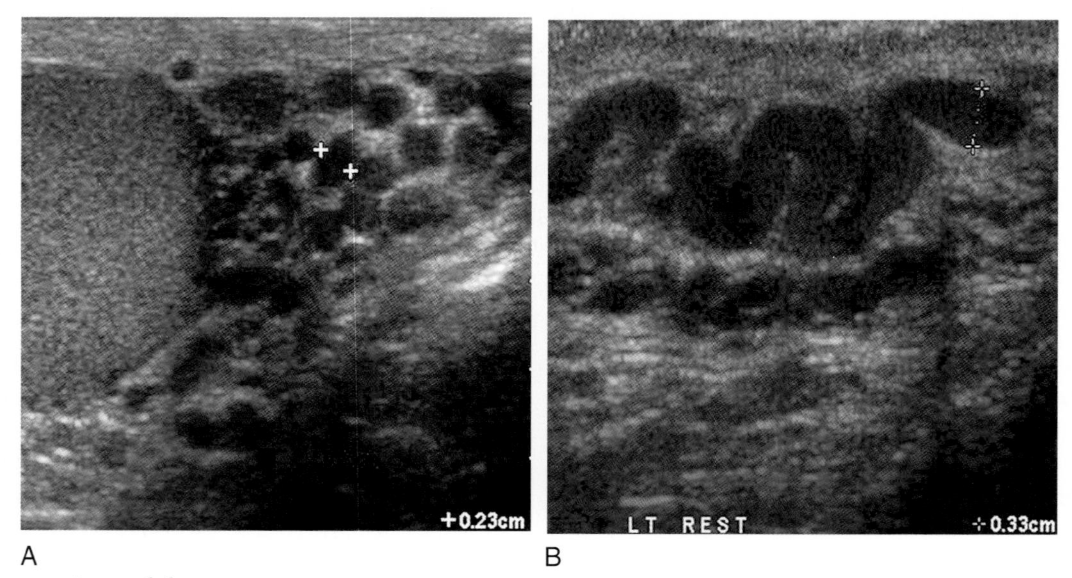

Figure 6-6 Varicoceles in different patients. **A,** Transverse view of the left testis shows multiple cystic-appearing spaces *(cursors)* lateral to the testis. During real-time scanning these could be shown to communicate with each other and are consistent with peritesticular veins. They all measure slightly greater than 2 mm in diameter *(cursors)*. **B,** Longitudinal view of the left scrotum shows a tortuous vein lateral to the left testis *(cursors)*. At rest, this vein measured 3.3 mm in diameter.

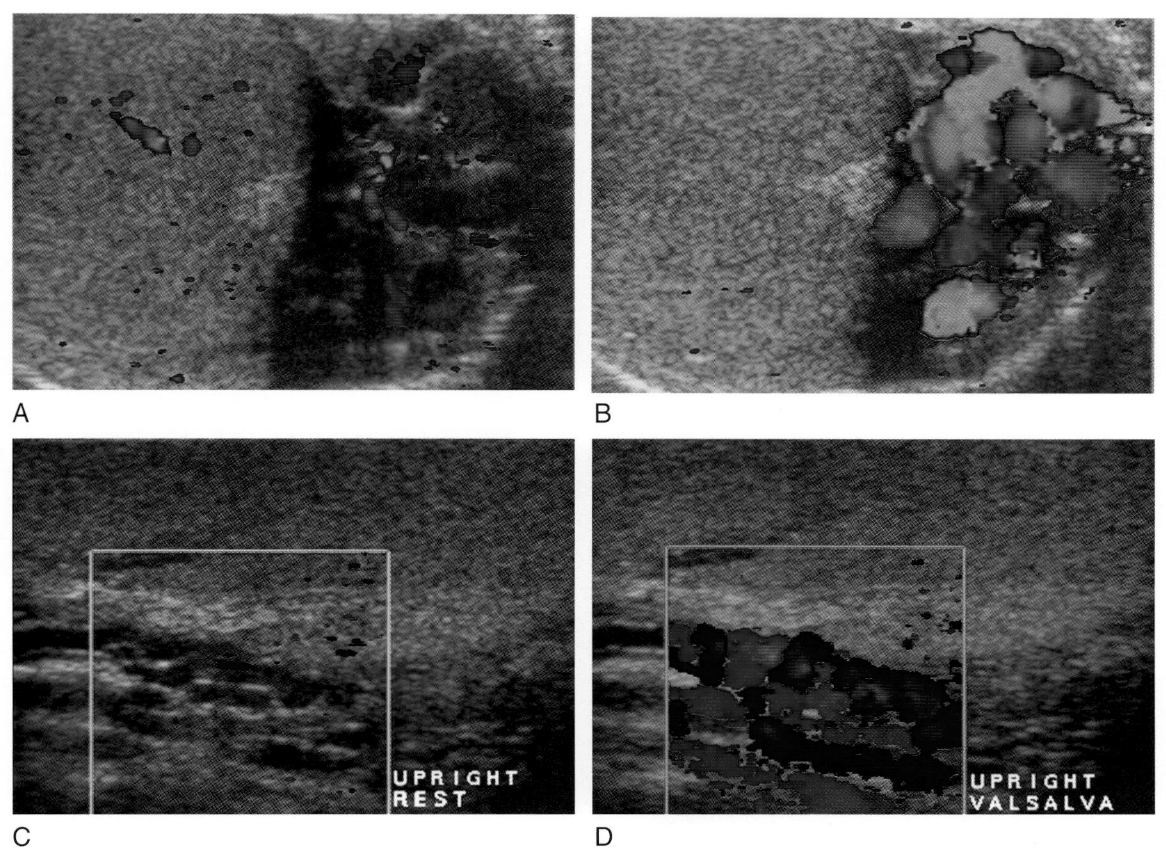

Figure 6-7 Varicoceles in different patients. **A** and **B,** Transverse color Doppler views of the left scrotum at rest (**A**) and during Valsalva maneuver (**B**) show dilated peritesticular veins with little detectable flow at rest but readily detectable augmented venous flow during Valsalva maneuver. **C** and **D,** Longitudinal views in the upright position at rest (**C**) and during Valsalva maneuver (**D**) show minimally dilated veins posterior to the testis that have augmented venous flow during Valsalva maneuver.

study should be repeated with the patient upright because the increased hydrostatic pressure may accentuate the varicocele's appearance. Short-duration Valsalva augmented peritesticular venous flow can occasionally be seen in normal men. The diagnosis of a varicocele should be made when the Valsalva-augmented flow is persistent (greater than 1 second) or the veins are dilated on gray-scale sonography.

Spermatoceles, hydroceles, and varicoceles account for the majority of extratesticular scrotal masses, and this explains why most extratesticular masses are benign. Other non-neoplastic peritesticular masses include exuberant scars, sperm cell granulomas, chronic hematomas (Fig. 6-8), hernias (Fig. 6-9), scrotal wall edema (Fig. 6-10), and scrotoliths (Fig. 6-11). Extratesticular tumors occur but are rare. The most common is the adenomatoid tumor. It is a benign lesion that arises

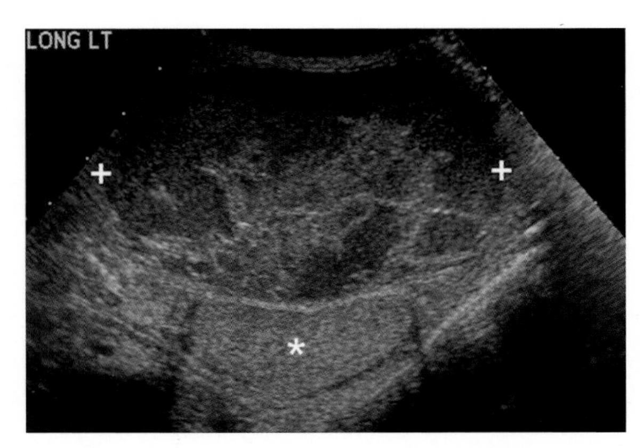

Figure 6-8 Scrotal hematoma. Longitudinal view of the left scrotum shows the testis posteriorly (*). A large complex fluid collection *(cursors)* with internal membranes and solid-appearing components is identified. This patient had undergone a hernia repair, and this is a typical appearance of an evolving hematoma.

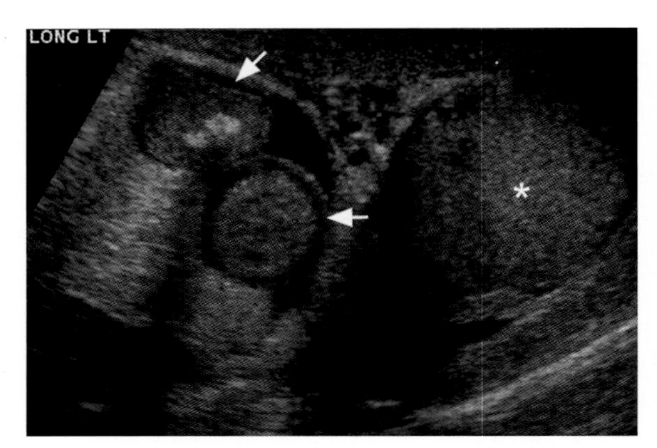

Figure 6-9 Hernia. Longitudinal view of the left scrotum shows the testis inferiorly (*) and a hernia sac containing loops of small bowel *(arrows)* superiorly. The typical target appearance of the small bowel is apparent, and peristalsis could be seen on real-time examination.

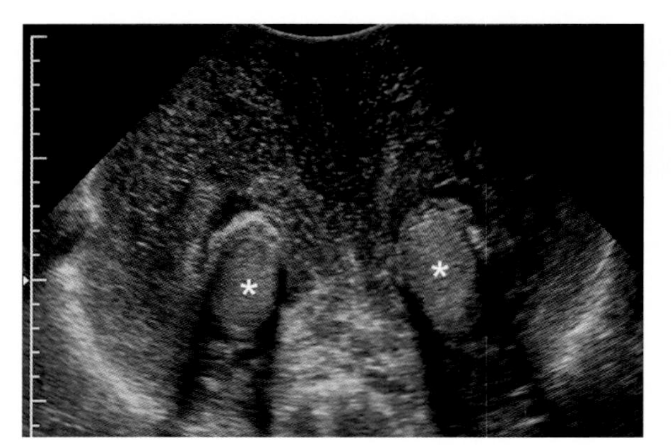

Figure 6-10 Severe scrotal edema. Transverse view of the scrotum shows the right and left testis (*) surrounded by markedly thickened scrotal wall bilaterally.

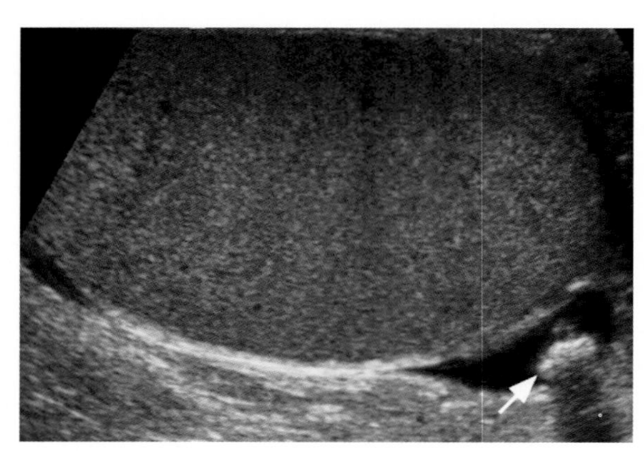

Figure 6-11 Scrotolith. Longitudinal view shows a small shadowing scrotolith *(arrow)* in the inferior aspect of the scrotum posterior to the testis.

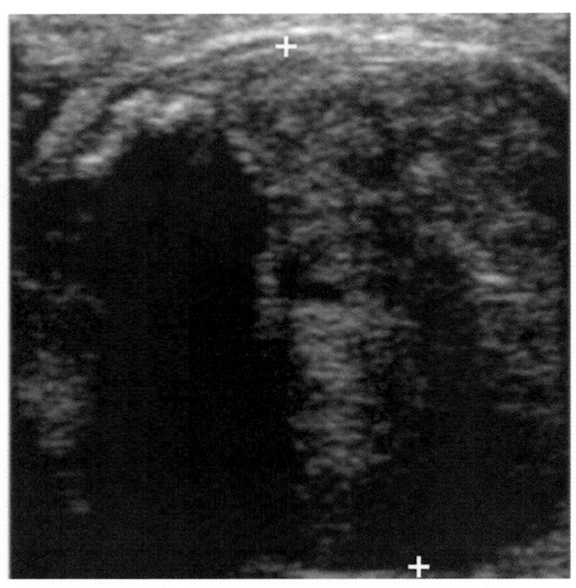

Figure 6-12 Leiomyosarcoma. Longitudinal view in the region of the spermatic cord shows a heterogeneous solid mass *(cursors)* with an area of shadowing calcification superiorly. Because of its size and appearance this was resected and shown to be a leiomyosarcoma.

from the epididymis or the tunica vaginalis and varies in its ultrasound appearance. Benign and malignant soft tissue tumors (lipomas/liposarcomas, leiomyomas/leiomyosarcomas) can arise in the scrotum (Fig. 6-12) and metastases can also develop in the scrotum (Fig. 6-13). Neoplasms should be suspected when large solid or complex masses are seen in the peritesticular region.

Intratesticular cysts are much less common than spermatoceles. Nonetheless, reports indicate that they can

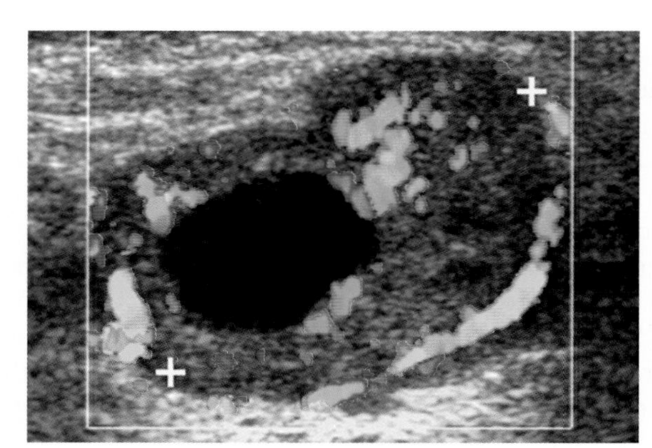

Figure 6-13 Scrotal metastasis. Longitudinal color Doppler view in the left supratesticular region shows a solid mass *(cursors)* with an internal cystic region and readily detectable internal and peripheral blood flow. Further evaluation in this patient showed peritoneal nodules and a supraclavicular node. The patient was subsequently shown to have metastatic bronchogenic carcinoma.

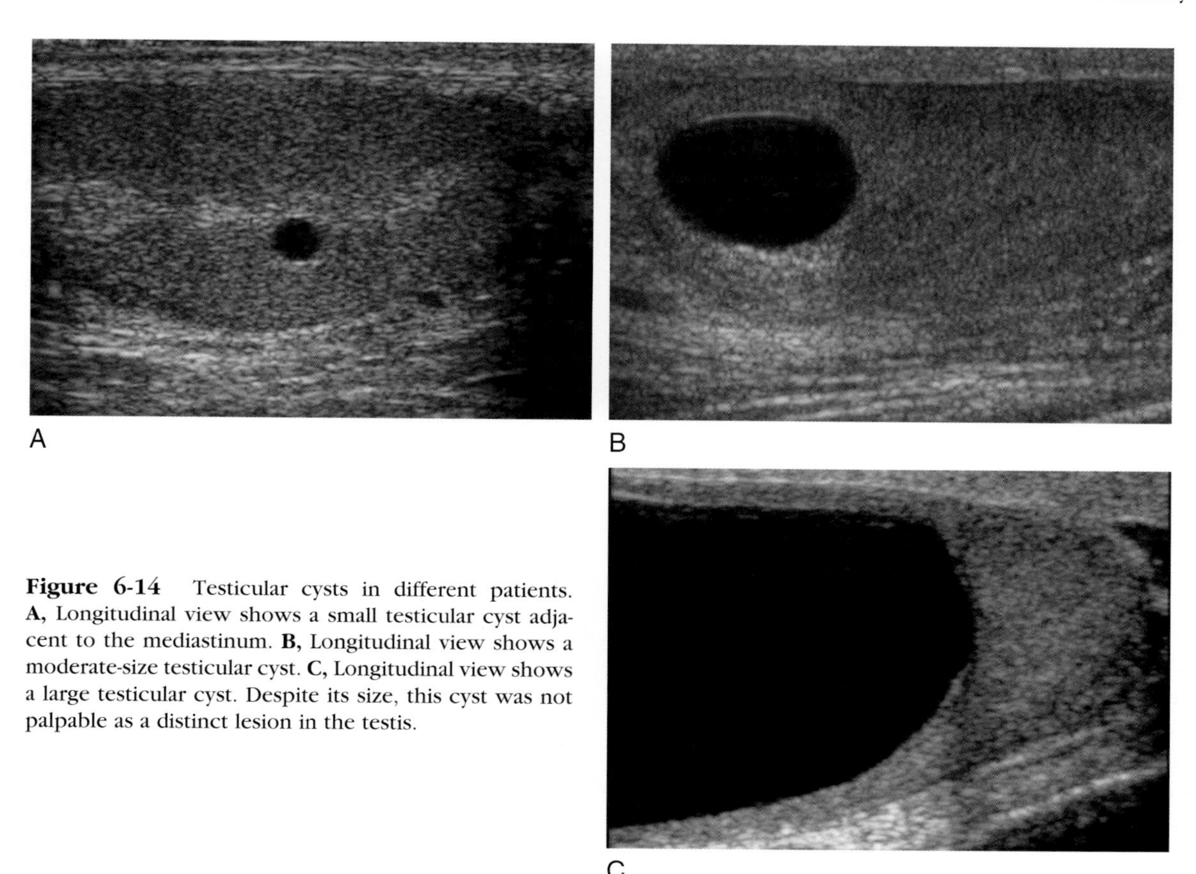

Figure 6-14 Testicular cysts in different patients. **A,** Longitudinal view shows a small testicular cyst adjacent to the mediastinum. **B,** Longitudinal view shows a moderate-size testicular cyst. **C,** Longitudinal view shows a large testicular cyst. Despite its size, this cyst was not palpable as a distinct lesion in the testis.

be found in as many as 10% of testicular sonograms (Fig. 6-14). They are most common in elderly patients and are often located near the mediastinum of the testis. Even when they are large they are usually not palpable. If they appear as simple cysts on sonography, they can be ignored. However, a cystic tumor such as a teratoma should be considered if they are multiseptated, contain intraluminal internal echogenicity, exhibit solid components, have a thick wall, or have detectable internal vascularity. Unlike simple cysts, complex cystic tumors are usually palpable.

A variant of simple testicular cysts that are very firm and easily palpable are cysts of the tunica albuginea. Despite their firmness, if they satisfy the sonographic criteria for a simple cyst, they can also be ignored (Fig. 6-15). Typically they are solitary and very small, but

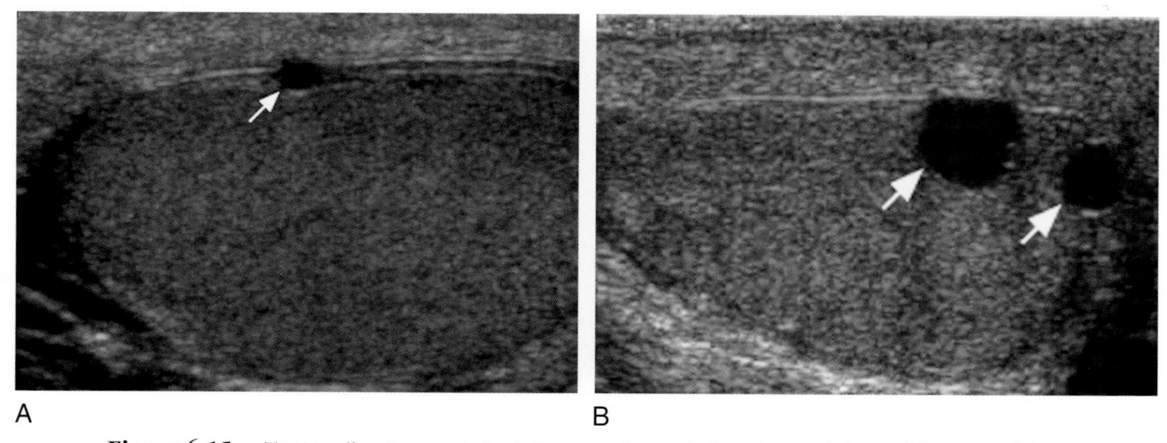

Figure 6-15 Tunica albuginea cysts in different patients. **A,** Longitudinal view of the testis shows a typically small, peripherally located cyst *(arrow)*. **B,** Oblique view shows two peripherally located cysts *(arrows)* that are slightly larger than typical for tunica albuginea cysts.

Box 6-2 Testicular Neoplasms

Germ cell tumors
- Seminoma
- Embryonal cell
- Teratoma
- Choriocarcinoma
- Yolk sac
- Mixed germ cell

Stromal tumors
- Leydig cell tumor
- Sertoli cell tumor

Lymphoma/leukemia

Metastases

Epidermoid cyst

they may be larger and multiple. Because they arise within the tunica albuginea, they are always located at the periphery of the testis.

Tubular ectasia of the rete testis can also produce tiny cystic-appearing changes in the mediastinum. This is usually bilateral, although it can be quite asymmetric and in a minority of cases can be unilateral. It is often associated with spermatoceles and with intratesticular cysts. Like testicular cysts, it is not palpable. Sonographically it has the appearance of multiple small cystic or tubular spaces that replace and enlarge the mediastinum (Fig. 6-16). This is a very characteristic appearance and should not be mistaken for a testicular tumor and does not require any further evaluation or follow-up.

The primary reason for scanning a patient with a scrotal mass is to determine if the mass is a testicular tumor. Germ cell tumors of the testis are the most common neoplasm in young adult men. They usually present as a nontender palpable mass. Approximately 10% will present with pain, and an even smaller percentage will present with symptoms related to metastatic disease. The most common germ cell tumors are pure seminomas and mixed germ cell tumors. Seminomas typically are homogeneous and hypoechoic (Fig. 6-17) until they become large, at which point they may become heterogeneous. Calcifications and cystic changes are rare in seminomas. They are highly sensitive to irradiation and carry a good prognosis. Mixed germ cell tumors include various combinations of seminoma, teratoma, embryonal cell carcinoma, and choriocarcinoma. They are usually heterogeneous and often have calcification and cystic elements (Fig. 6-18). The

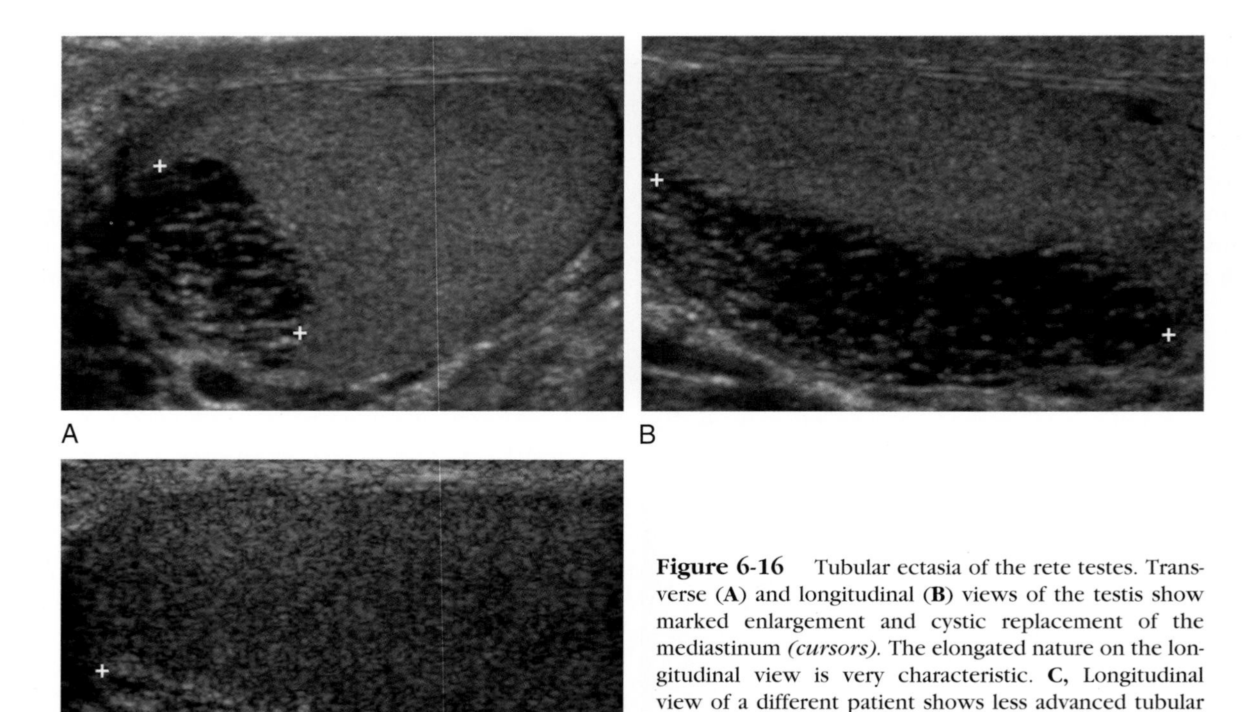

Figure 6-16 Tubular ectasia of the rete testes. Transverse (**A**) and longitudinal (**B**) views of the testis show marked enlargement and cystic replacement of the mediastinum *(cursors)*. The elongated nature on the longitudinal view is very characteristic. **C,** Longitudinal view of a different patient shows less advanced tubular ectasia *(cursors)*.

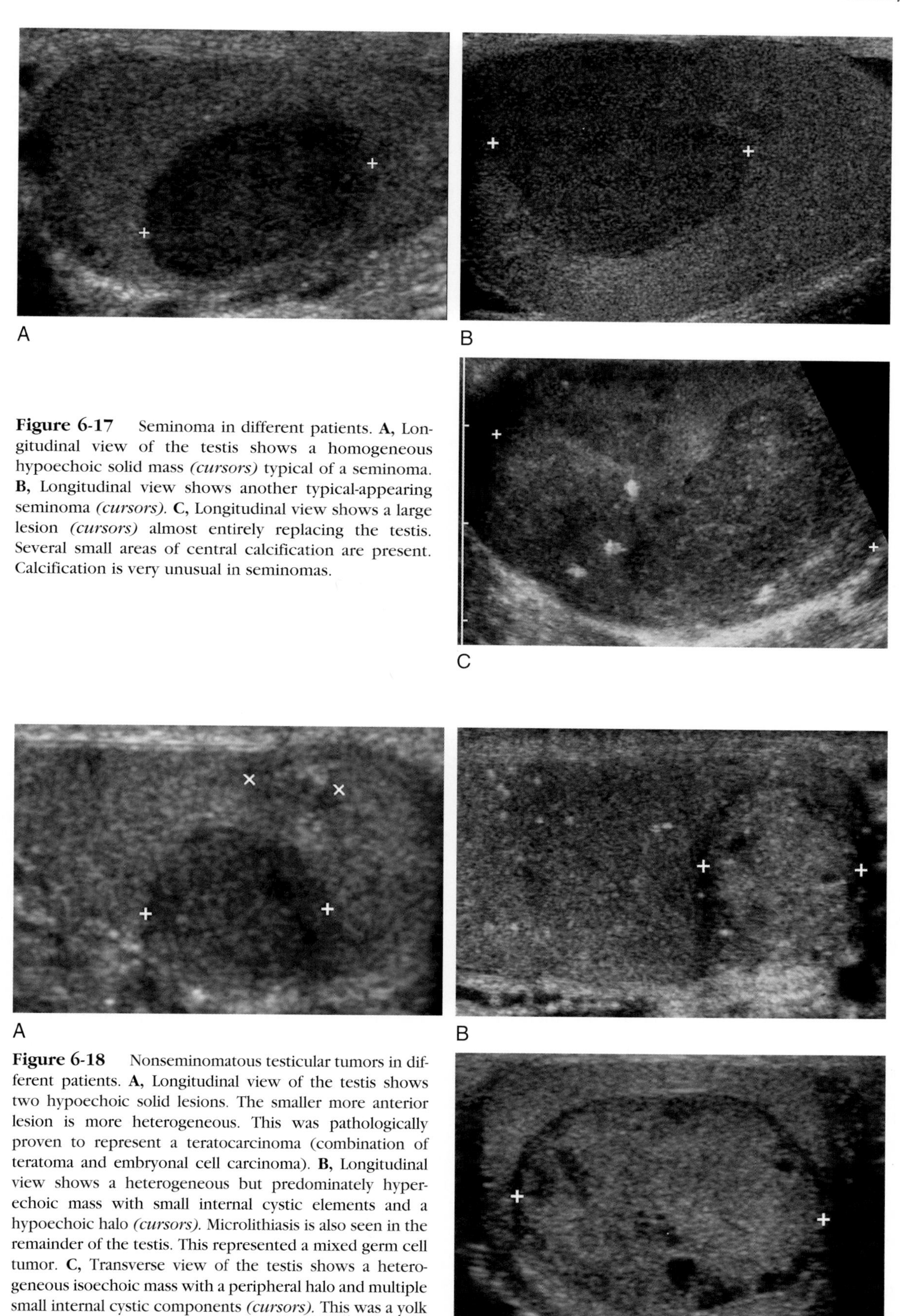

Figure 6-17 Seminoma in different patients. **A,** Longitudinal view of the testis shows a homogeneous hypoechoic solid mass *(cursors)* typical of a seminoma. **B,** Longitudinal view shows another typical-appearing seminoma *(cursors).* **C,** Longitudinal view shows a large lesion *(cursors)* almost entirely replacing the testis. Several small areas of central calcification are present. Calcification is very unusual in seminomas.

Figure 6-18 Nonseminomatous testicular tumors in different patients. **A,** Longitudinal view of the testis shows two hypoechoic solid lesions. The smaller more anterior lesion is more heterogeneous. This was pathologically proven to represent a teratocarcinoma (combination of teratoma and embryonal cell carcinoma). **B,** Longitudinal view shows a heterogeneous but predominately hyperechoic mass with small internal cystic elements and a hypoechoic halo *(cursors).* Microlithiasis is also seen in the remainder of the testis. This represented a mixed germ cell tumor. **C,** Transverse view of the testis shows a heterogeneous isoechoic mass with a peripheral halo and multiple small internal cystic components *(cursors).* This was a yolk sack tumor.

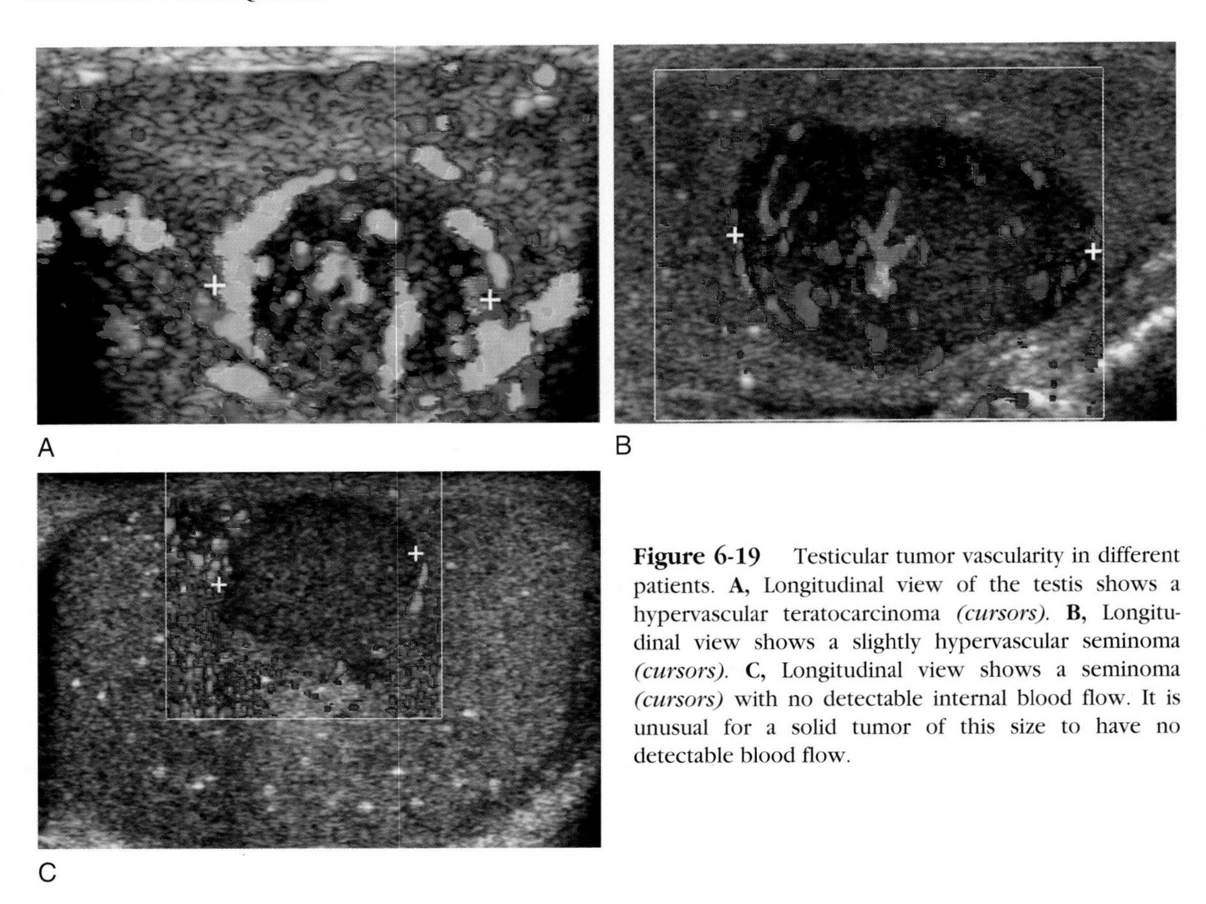

Figure 6-19 Testicular tumor vascularity in different patients. **A,** Longitudinal view of the testis shows a hypervascular teratocarcinoma *(cursors).* **B,** Longitudinal view shows a slightly hypervascular seminoma *(cursors).* **C,** Longitudinal view shows a seminoma *(cursors)* with no detectable internal blood flow. It is unusual for a solid tumor of this size to have no detectable blood flow.

majority of germ cell tumors will have detectable internal vascularity on color Doppler imaging and some will be hypervascular (Fig. 6-19). When a lesion suspected to represent a germ cell tumor is detected in the testis, it is useful to scan the retroperitoneum near the level of the kidneys to look for nodal metastasis (Fig. 6-20A and B). When present, nodal metastases help to confirm that the testicular mass is a tumor and also upstage the tumor. Once the diagnosis is made, CT will be performed to more fully evaluate for metastatic disease. It is important to realize that this process also works in reverse. Whenever retroperitoneal adenopathy is detected in a young adult male, occult testicular tumors should be considered and a scan of the testes should be performed to look for an occult tumor (see Fig. 6-20C and D). If biopsies show that metastatic disease anywhere in the body is secondary to a germ cell tumor, sonography of the testes should also be performed. If a tumor is not identified with sonography, scrotal MRI should be considered.

Non-germ cell tumors account for 5% to 10% of testicular tumors. The most common are Leydig and Sertoli cell tumors (Fig. 6-21). Although the majority are benign, these stromal tumors can produce hormonal changes, and they are always removed because they cannot be distinguished from malignant germ cell tumors. They appear as solid masses, and their echogenicity ranges from hypoechoic to hyperechoic. Like germ cell tumors, internal vascularity is usually detectable on color Doppler analysis.

Epidermoid cysts are benign tumors similar to teratomas, but they contain only ectodermal derivatives. They appear as hypoechoic masses with a hyperechoic, calcified rim or multiple concentric internal laminations that simulate an onion slice (Fig. 6-22). Although these are virtually pathognomonic appearances, epidermoid cysts are typically enucleated while preserving the rest of the testis.

In addition to primary testicular tumors, the testes may be the site of metastatic disease. This usually appears as a focal testicular mass or masses with a variable echogenicity (Fig. 6-23). In elderly patients, metastatic disease is more common than primary germ cell tumors. The testes can also be involved with lymphoma and leukemia. Because chemotherapy does not cross a blood-testis barrier, the testes can serve as a sanctuary for lymphoma and leukemia when the patient's disease is in remission elsewhere in the body. Lymphoma and

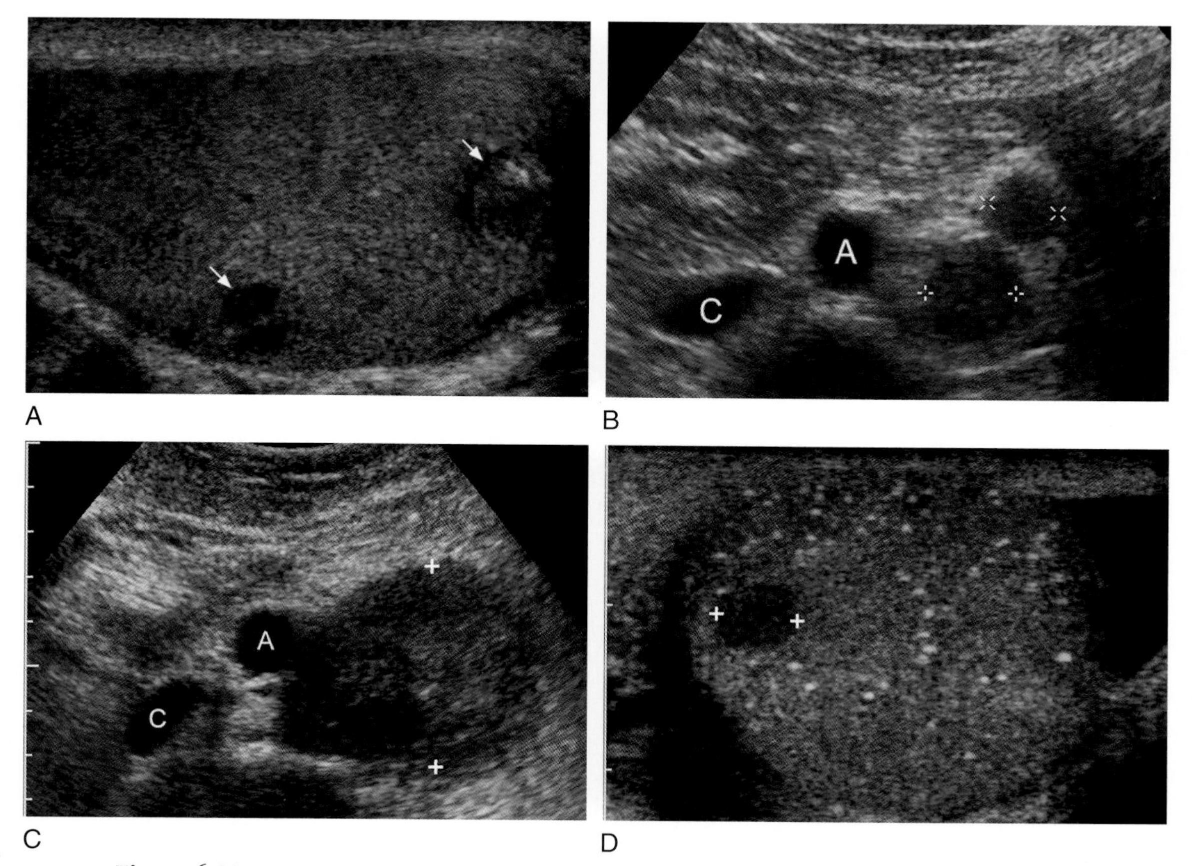

Figure 6-20 Mixed germ cell tumor with lymph node metastasis. Longitudinal view of the testis (**A**) and transverse view of the upper abdomen (**B**) show two small heterogeneous solid masses in the testis *(arrows)*. These are very suggestive of germ cell tumors, and a survey of the retroperitoneum should be performed for evaluation for possible lymph node metastasis. In this case, two enlarged periaortic nodes *(cursors)* were identified to the left of the aorta (A). The inferior vena cava (C) is also identified. Transverse view of the upper abdomen (**C**) and transverse view of the left testis (**D**) in a different patient who presented with back pain show a large retroperitoneal mass *(cursors)* deviating the aorta (A) anteriorly. The inferior vena cava (C) is also identified. Detection of retroperitoneal adenopathy in a young adult male should raise suspicion for a testicular tumor. In this case, subsequent scans of the testis confirmed the presence of a small solid germ cell tumor *(cursors)* in a testis with diffuse microlithiasis.

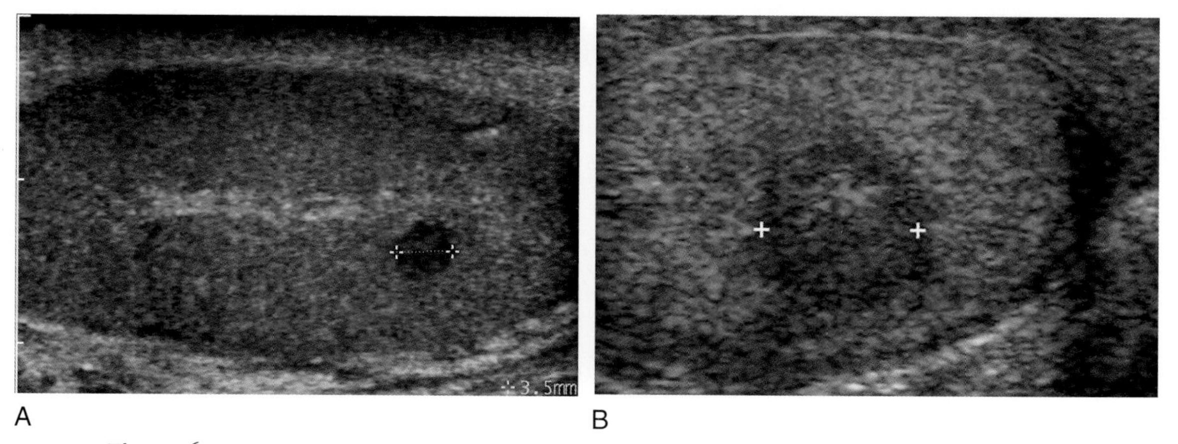

Figure 6-21 Leydig cell tumors in different patients. **A,** Longitudinal view of the testis shows a small 3.5-mm hypoechoic solid mass *(cursors)* adjacent to the mediastinum. This was detected incidentally. **B,** Longitudinal view shows a larger solid hypoechoic mass *(cursors)*.

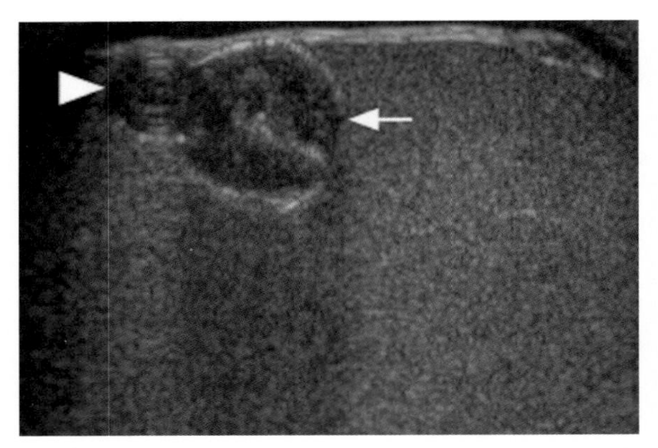

Figure 6-22 Epidermoid. Longitudinal view of the testis shows a bilobed solid lesion. The larger inferior component *(arrow)* has a thin rim of peripheral calcification and faint posterior acoustic shadowing. The superior component *(arrowhead)* shows an internal "onion peel" appearance.

leukemia can both appear either as focal unilateral or bilateral hypoechoic masses or as diffuse testicular infiltration (Fig. 6-24). When the testes are diffusely infiltrated in a symmetric and bilateral manner, the decreased echogenicity may be difficult to appreciate. In such cases color Doppler imaging can be helpful in detecting an abnormality because the testis will be hypervascular. MRI can also be useful for further evaluation because the signal characteristics will be abnormal.

Sonography is highly sensitive (95% to 100%) in detecting testicular tumors. In fact, as mentioned earlier, an important role of sonography is to detect nonpalpable lesions in young adult men with metastatic disease from an unknown primary (see Fig. 6-20). The specificity of ultrasound varies depending on the referral patterns. There are numerous lesions that can simulate testis tumors (Box 6-3). These include infarcts, focal orchitis, focal fibrosis, hematomas, abscesses, sarcoid, tuberculosis, and adrenal rest tissue. In many cases the patient's history is useful in suggesting the correct diagnosis. The physical examination is also very important because most palpable intratesticular lesions are tumors, and most of the nonpalpable lesions larger than 1 cm in diameter are not tumors. Lesions smaller than 1 cm may be nonpalpable tumors or benign lesions. Color Doppler also plays a role because many of the non-neoplastic lesions will not have any internal vascularity whereas most tumors will have detectable vascularity (Fig. 6-25).

One relatively common abnormality that is easy to mistake for a tumor is testicular atrophy and fibrosis. In most patients these conditions can produce hypoechoic regions in the testis that are arranged in a linear pattern, producing a striated appearance to the testis that does not simulate a tumor (Fig. 6-26A). However, if these areas become more confluent, they can be misdiagnosed as tumors. This mistake can usually be avoided by scanning in multiple planes and noting the wedge shape of

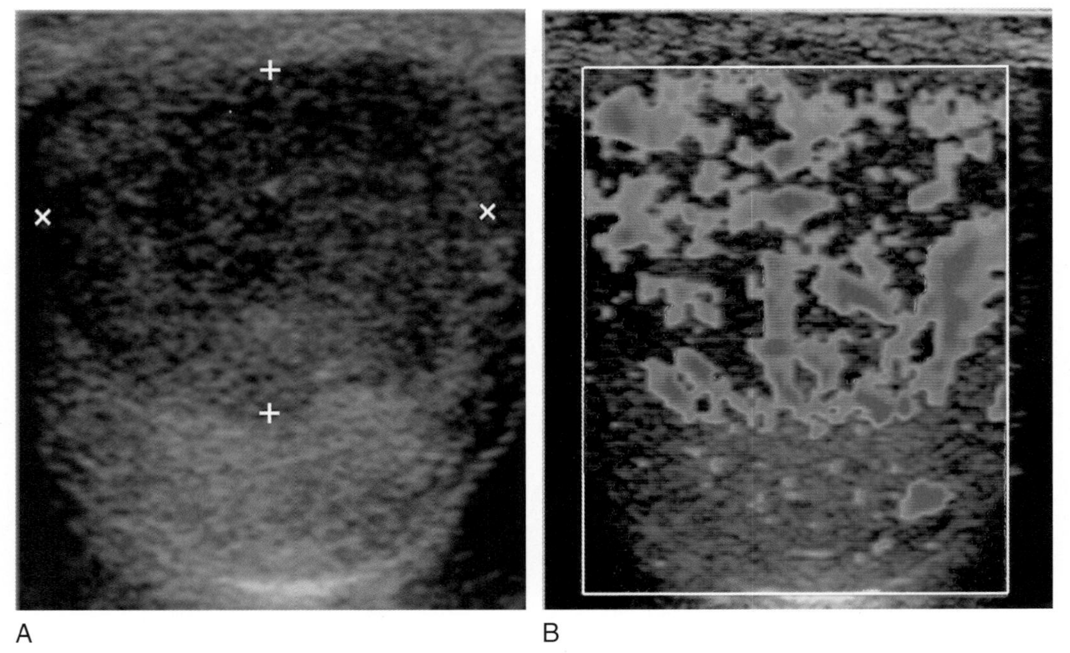

Figure 6-23 Metastasis to the testis from a rhabdomyosarcoma. **A,** Gray-scale view of the testis shows a large solid hypoechoic mass *(cursors)* in the anterior aspect of the testis. **B,** Color Doppler view shows intense hypervascularity throughout this metastatic lesion.

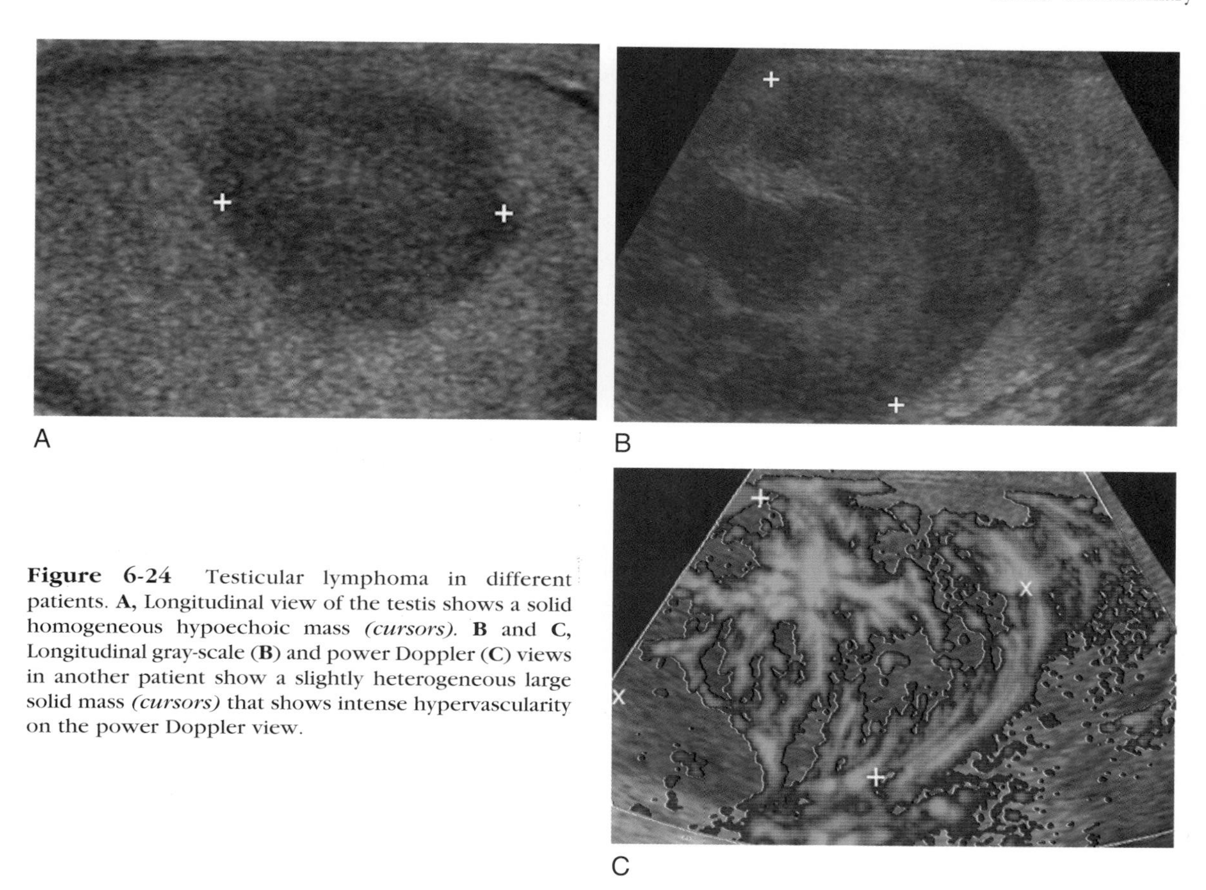

Figure 6-24 Testicular lymphoma in different patients. **A,** Longitudinal view of the testis shows a solid homogeneous hypoechoic mass *(cursors)*. **B** and **C,** Longitudinal gray-scale (**B**) and power Doppler (**C**) views in another patient show a slightly heterogeneous large solid mass *(cursors)* that shows intense hypervascularity on the power Doppler view.

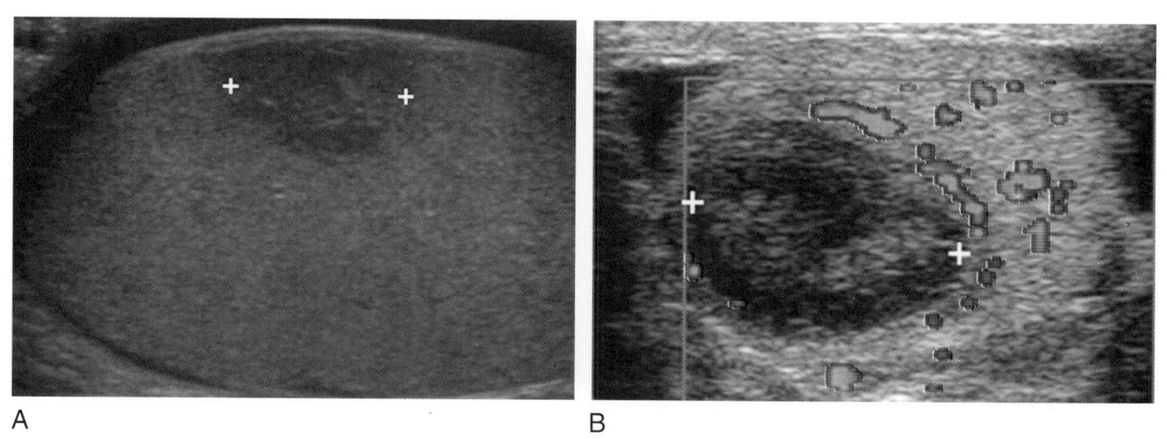

Figure 6-25 Testicular hematoma in different patients. **A,** Longitudinal view of the testis shows a slightly heterogeneous solid-appearing mass *(cursors)*. This is nonspecific appearing and could be mistaken for a testicular tumor. **B,** Color Doppler view shows a heterogeneous predominately hypoechoic solid-appearing mass *(cursors)* with no detectable internal blood flow. In a post-traumatic patient, lack of detectable blood flow in a lesion such as this should suggest a testicular hematoma rather than a testicular tumor. Follow-up scans confirmed slow resolution of this lesion.

Box 6-3 Testicular Lesions Mimicking Tumors

Focal orchitis
Focal atrophy/fibrosis
Infarcts
Abscess
Hematoma
Contusion
Sarcoid
Tuberculosis
Adrenal rest tissue

the abnormality and the way it radiates from the mediastinum (see Fig. 6-26B and C).

Testicular microlithiasis is a condition in which laminated concretions form in the lumen of the seminiferous tubules. On sonography they appear as tiny, nonshadowing, bright reflectors in the testicular parenchyma (Fig. 6-27). Classic testicular microlithiasis is defined as five or more microliths seen on at least one image of the testis. Microlithiasis with fewer than five microliths on all images is referred to as limited testicular microlithiasis. Microlithiasis has been reported to occur in association with numerous conditions, the most important of which is testicular tumors. Approximately 10% of patients with microlithiasis will have a testicular germ cell tumor detected sonographically at the time of their initial ultrasound examination (Fig. 6-28). Several case reports suggest that patients who initially present with isolated testicular microlithiasis (i.e., testicular microlithiasis with no tumor) may be predisposed to develop tumors in the future. However, longitudinal data in larger groups of patients suggest that the risk, if real, is probably quite low. Original recommendations for patients with classic testicular microlithiasis were to have yearly ultrasound examinations. However, the yield of annual sonographic screening is so low that it is probably more realistic to perform regular self-examinations and annual physical examinations.

When a patient initially presents with a testicular tumor in one testis and has microlithiasis in the contralateral testis, the risk of intratubular germ cell neoplasia (the equivalent of carcinoma in situ of the testis) developing in the contralateral testis is definitely increased. Therefore, a biopsy of the contralateral testis is necessary to obtain tissue for histologic study. This is

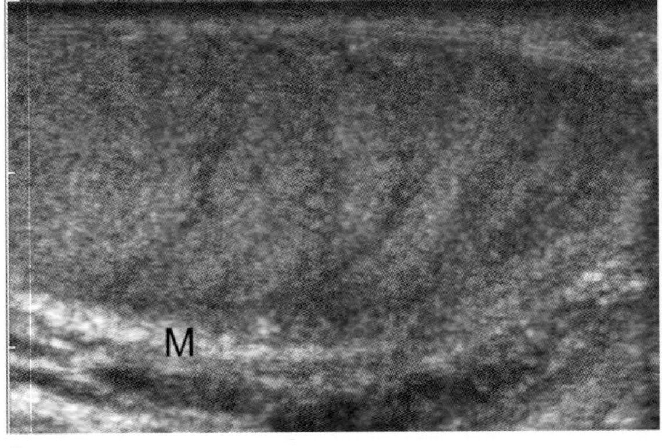

A

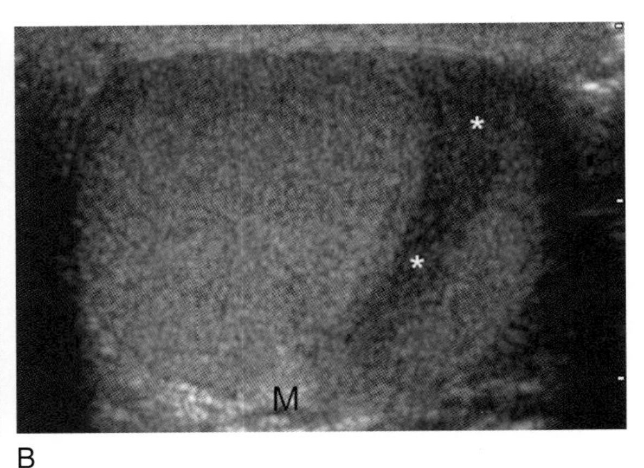

B

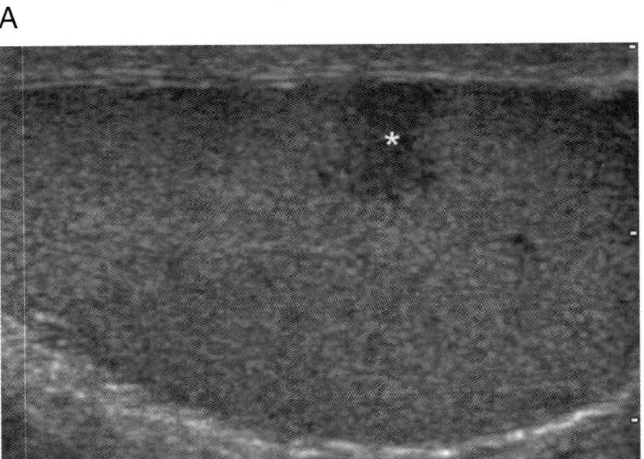

C

Figure 6-26 Focal testicular atrophy/fibrosis. **A,** Longitudinal view of the testis shows hypoechoic striations in the testicular parenchyma radiating toward the mediastinum (M). **B** and **C,** Transverse (**B**) and longitudinal (**C**) views in another patient show a confluent area of atrophy (*) again radiating toward the mediastinum (M). On the transverse view the typical geometry of the lesion is seen. However, on the longitudinal view this lesion could be mistaken for a testicular neoplasm.

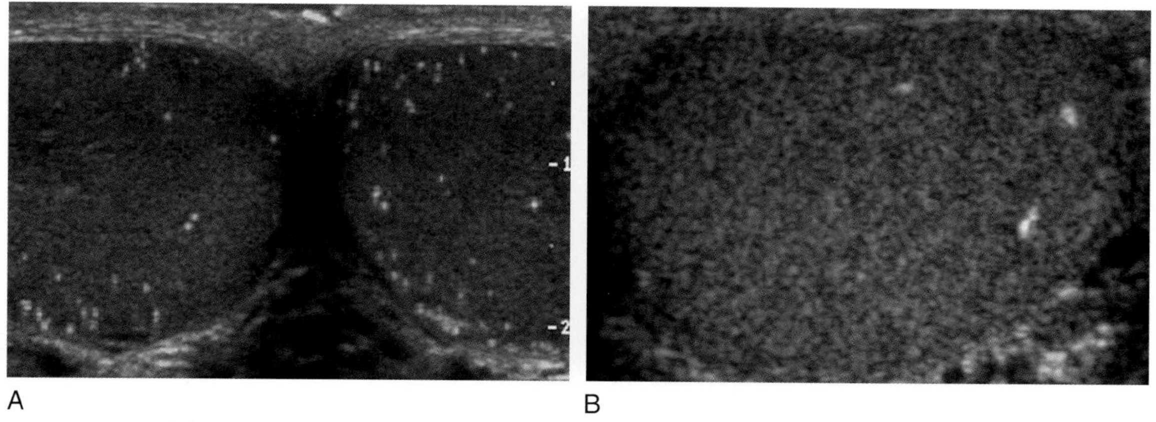

Figure 6-27 Testicular microlithiasis in different patients. **A,** Transverse view of both testes shows scattered bilateral small bright reflectors without acoustic shadowing. Because there are more than five detectable microliths in both testes, this meets the definition for bilateral classic microlithiasis. **B,** Transverse view shows three microliths in the testis. This is classified as limited microlithiasis.

usually done at the time orchiectomy is performed for removal of the ipsilateral tumor (see Fig. 6-28).

Calcification can also develop on the tunica albuginea of the testis and can present as a palpable mass. It is referred to as a plaque of the tunica and it usually occurs due to previous episodes of trauma or infection. When it is calcified it can be identified readily with sonography (Fig. 6-29A and B). Noncalcified plaques appear as thickening of the tunica but are much harder to see with sonography (see Fig. 6-29C).

Another condition that is associated with testicular tumors is undescended testes. Approximately 80% of undescended testes are located within the inguinal canal and are easily visualized with sonography (Fig. 6-30A). Intra-abdominal testes occur in the retroperitoneum from the level of the kidneys to the internal inguinal ring (see Fig. 6-30B). The risk of germ cell tumors is as much as 40 times greater than the general population, and the risk is even higher for intra-abdominal testes (Fig. 6-31). The risk of cancer is eliminated if the testis is surgically relocated to the scrotum prior to age 5. Between ages 5 and 10, orchiopexy has a diminishing effect on the rate of cancer. After age 10, orchiectomy is usually performed.

In addition to evaluating scrotal masses, ultrasound is helpful in the work-up of patients with acute scrotal pain and swelling. In the adult patient population, this primarily involves differentiating testicular torsion from

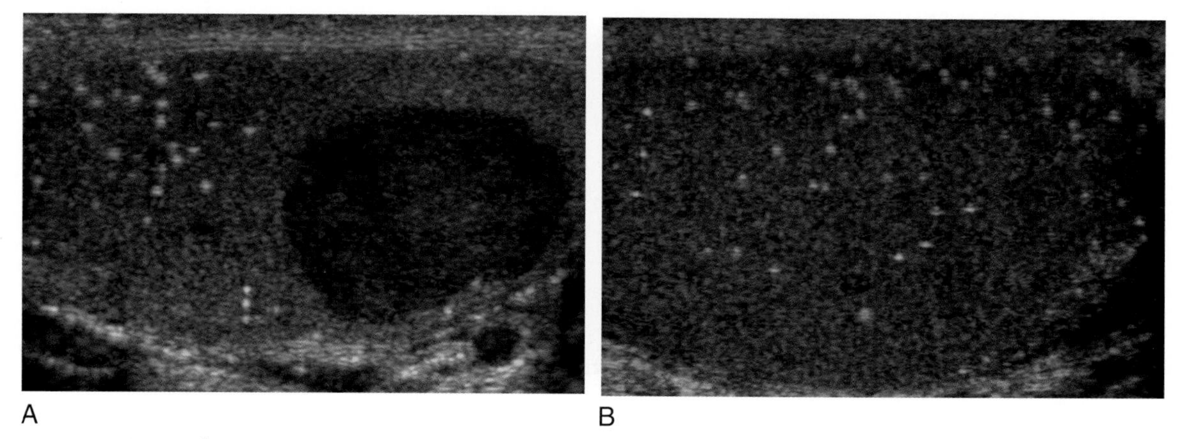

Figure 6-28 Microlithiasis associated with a testicular tumor. **A,** Longitudinal view of the symptomatic testis shows a hypoechoic mass in the lower pole due to a germ cell tumor. Classic microlithiasis is seen in the upper pole of the testis. **B,** Longitudinal view of the contralateral testis shows classic microlithiasis here as well. At the time of orchiectomy, this contralateral testis was sampled and intratubular germ cell neoplasia was detected.

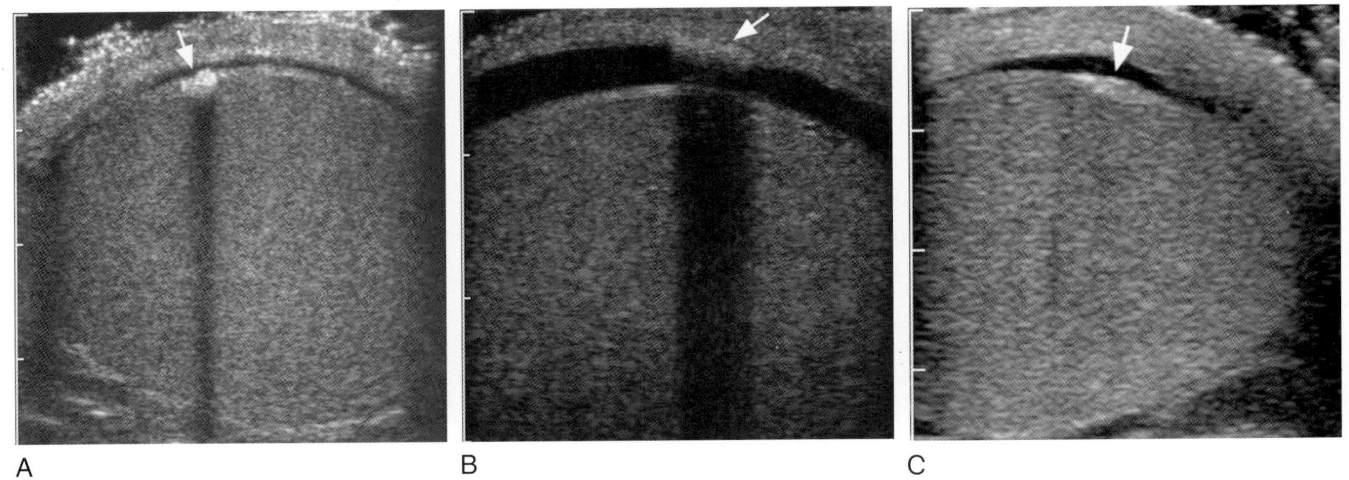

Figure 6-29 Fibrous plaques in different patients. **A,** Transverse view of the testis shows a small calcified plaque *(arrow)* of the tunica albuginea. **B,** Transverse view shows a small calcified plaque *(arrow)* of the tunica vaginalis of the scrotal wall. **C,** Transverse view shows a noncalcified plaque *(arrow)* of the tunica albuginea that manifests as a focal area of hyperechoic thickening of the tunica.

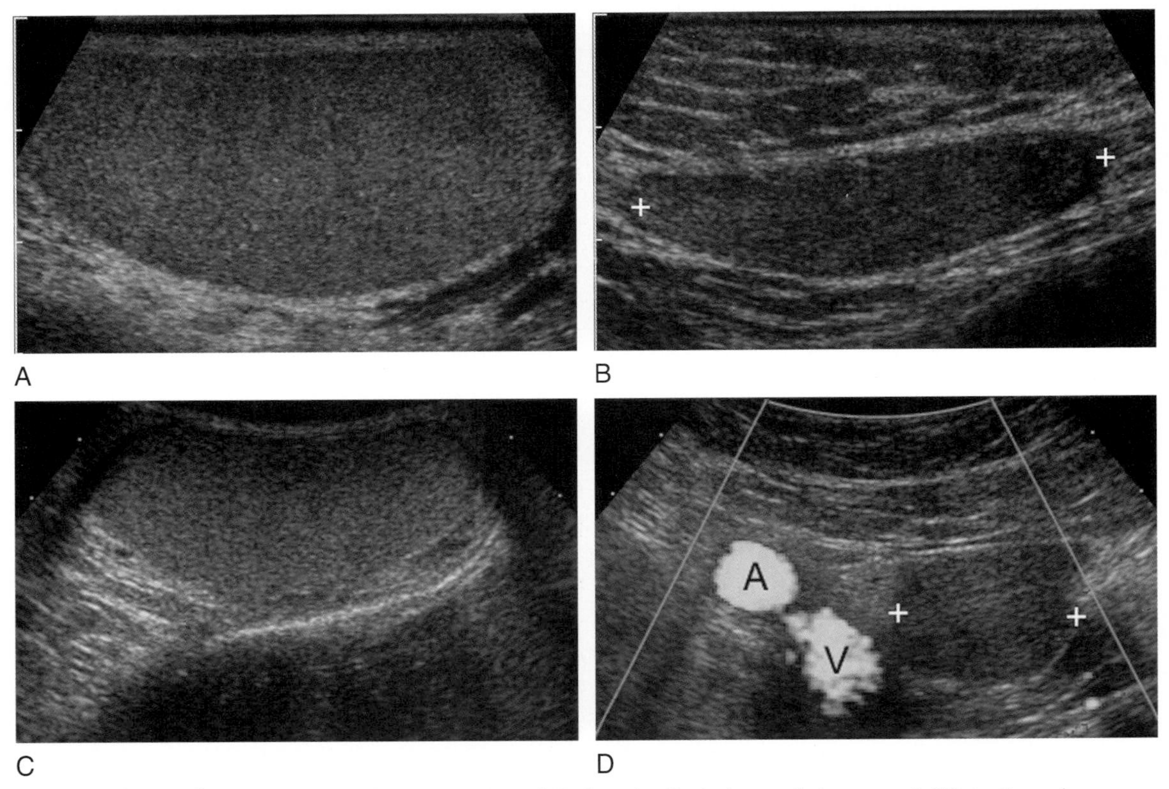

Figure 6-30 Undescended testes. **A** and **B,** Longitudinal views of the normal (**A**) testis and undescended (**B**) show that the undescended testis *(cursors)* that is located in the inguinal canal is smaller and has a more elongated appearance. It also has significantly thicker overlying tissues than the normal intrascrotal testis. **C** and **D,** Longitudinal view of the normal testis (**C**) and transverse view of the undescended testis (**D**) in another patient show the right external iliac artery (A) and vein (V) and the adjacent intrapelvic undescended right testis *(cursors).*

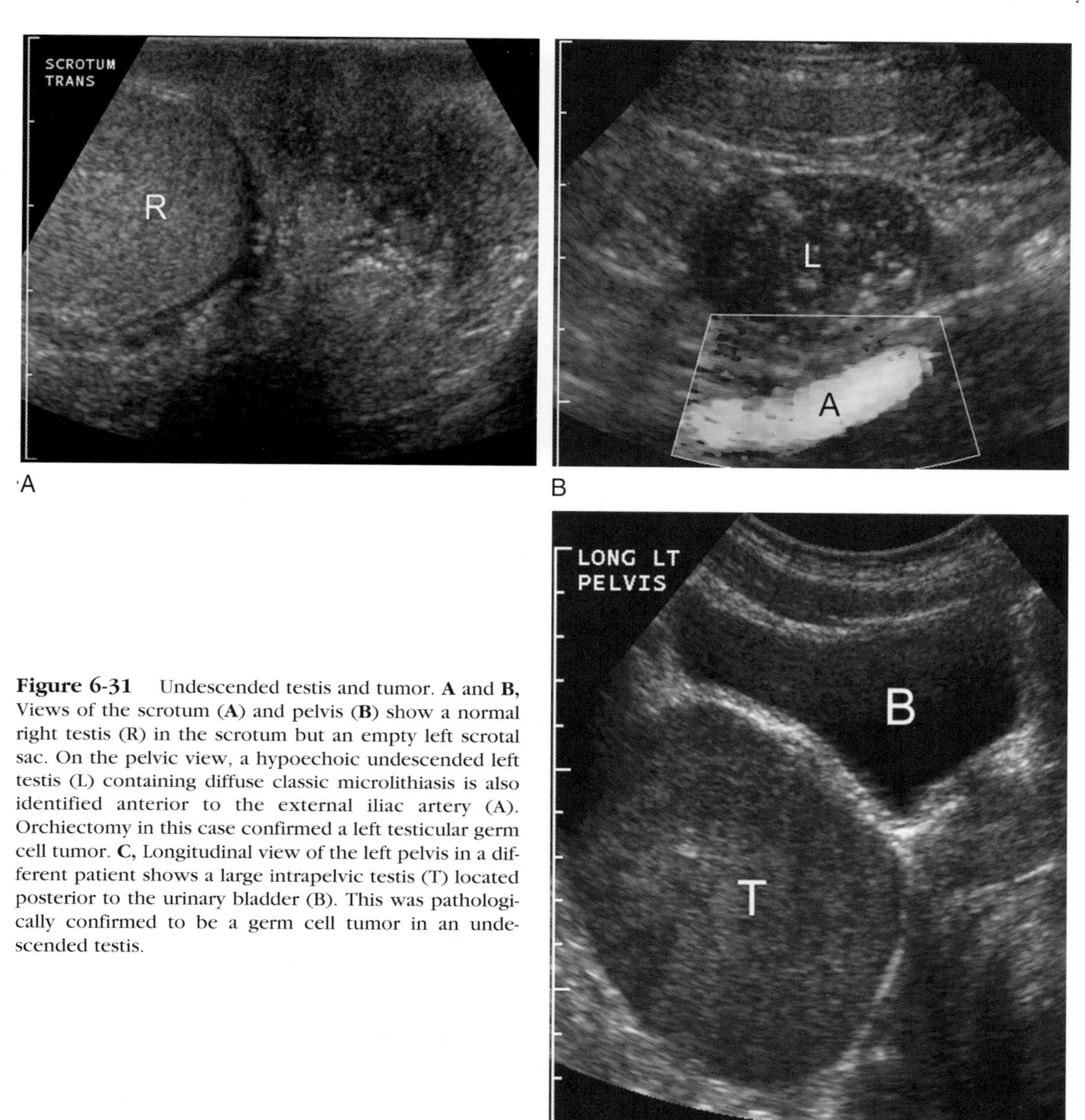

Figure 6-31 Undescended testis and tumor. **A** and **B,** Views of the scrotum (**A**) and pelvis (**B**) show a normal right testis (R) in the scrotum but an empty left scrotal sac. On the pelvic view, a hypoechoic undescended left testis (L) containing diffuse classic microlithiasis is also identified anterior to the external iliac artery (A). Orchiectomy in this case confirmed a left testicular germ cell tumor. **C,** Longitudinal view of the left pelvis in a different patient shows a large intrapelvic testis (T) located posterior to the urinary bladder (B). This was pathologically confirmed to be a germ cell tumor in an undescended testis.

inflammatory conditions such as epididymitis. Testicular torsion occurs as the result of the faulty attachment of the testis to the scrotal wall. The most common anatomic anomaly producing this faulty attachment is the bell-clapper deformity. It consists of a tunica vaginalis that completely surrounds the testis, causing the testis to be attached only to the spermatic cord and otherwise freely suspended in the scrotal sac like the clapper in a bell. The first hemodynamic consequence of testicular torsion is venous obstruction, followed rapidly by obstruction of arterial inflow and testicular ischemia. The viability of the testis depends on the duration of the torsion as well as the number of twists of the spermatic cord. Infarction can occur as soon as 4 hours after the appearance of symptoms. However, if the degree of torsion is low (180 to 360 degrees), the testes can remain viable for more than 24 hours. In general, urologists try to operate before the symptoms have lasted for 6 hours.

Gray scale sonography is not very valuable in diagnosing torsion because there may be no abnormalities (Fig. 6-32A). Nonspecific abnormalities that sometimes occur include decreased testicular echogenicity, testicular swelling, and reactive hydroceles (see Fig. 6-32B). A torsion knot due to the twisted spermatic cord is occasionally seen superior to the testis (see Fig. 6-32C). In rare instances, there is enough of a hydrocele so that it is possible to identify a bell clapper deformity (see Fig. 6-32D).

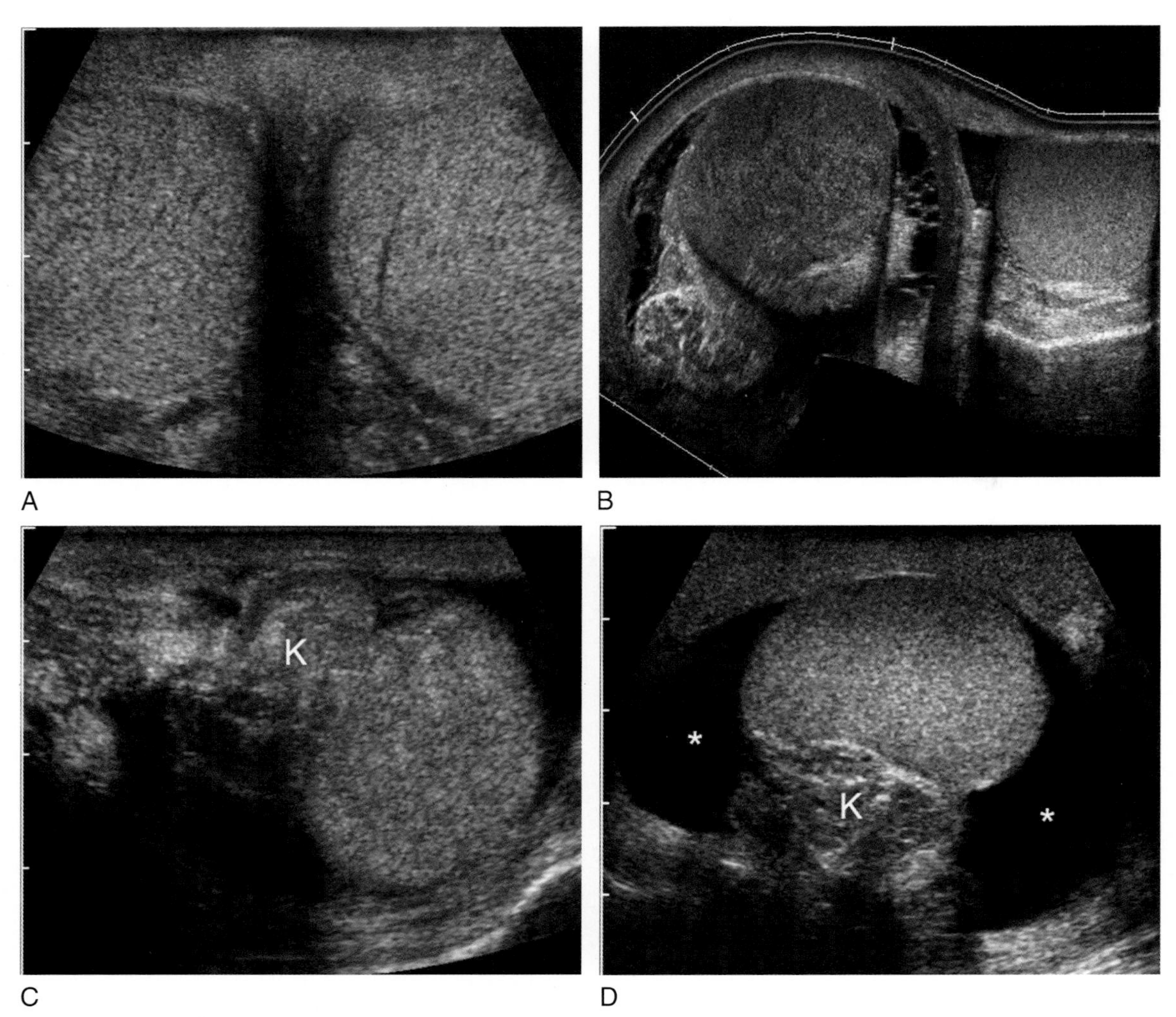

Figure 6-32 Gray-scale appearance of testicular torsion in different patients. **A,** Transverse view shows normal symmetric-appearing right and left testes. In this case the left testis was torsed. **B,** Extended field of view scan in a patient with right testicular torsion shows an enlarged hypoechoic right testis with a reactive hydrocele. The left testis is normal. **C,** Longitudinal view shows a torsion knot (K) in the spermatic cord located superior to the testis. **D,** Longitudinal view shows the torsion knot (K), posterior to the testis. A reactive hydrocele (*) is also identified. The acute angle between the hydrocele and the testis in all scanning planes indicated lack of attachment of the testis to the scrotal wall consistent with a bell clapper deformity.

Although gray-scale sonography is not good at identifying torsion in most patients, it can provide useful information about testicular viability. If the testis is normal on gray-scale analysis, then it is very likely viable regardless of the duration of symptoms. If the testis is hypoechoic or inhomogeneous, it is very likely to be infarcted and nonviable.

Fortunately color Doppler imaging is an effective way to detect testicular ischemia because it can show absent (Fig. 6-33A and B) or asymmetrically decreased testicular vascularity (see Fig. 6-33C). In prolonged torsion, there is an inflammatory reaction that develops in the soft tissue around the infarcted testis. This produces a hyperemic scrotal wall (see Fig. 6-33D). It is also an effective way of documenting the success or failure of manual detorsion (see Fig. 6-33E and F). In adults, color Doppler analysis is better than scintigraphy in the diagnosis of testicular torsion. Given its speed, lower cost, lack of radiation, and better depiction of scrotal morphology, color Doppler imaging is the preferred way to evaluate these patients.

Although color Doppler imaging is quite good at evaluating patients with suspected testicular torsion, false-positive and false-negative results can occur. A false-positive finding means that the patient will undergo surgery, which he would have anyway if the ultrasound evaluation had not been performed. False-negative findings are more of a problem because most of these patients will then go on to suffer infarction of the testis.

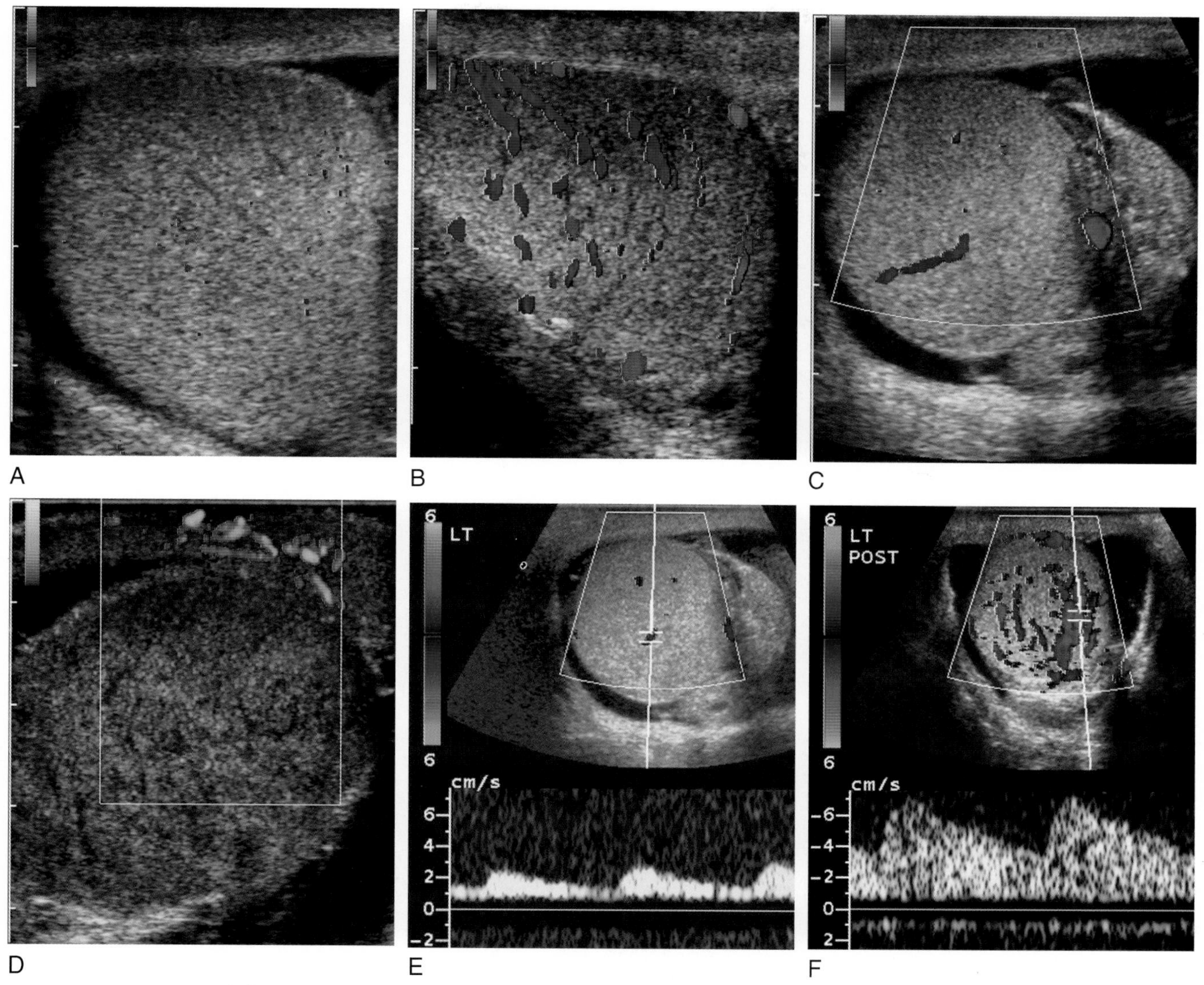

Figure 6-33 Color Doppler appearance of testicular torsion in different patients. **A** and **B**, Transverse views of a torsed testis (**A**) and the normal contralateral testis (**B**) shows no detectable blood flow in the torsed testis and readily detectable blood flow in the contralateral normal testis. **C**, Transverse view shows detectable but diminished blood flow in the testis. **D**, Transverse view shows a hypoechoic, heterogeneous testis with no detectable blood flow and increased flow in the wall of the scrotum. **E** and **F**, Color and pulse Doppler views of a torsed testis before (**E**) and after (**F**) manual detorsion. Note the detectable but diminished flow before manual detorsion and the reactive hyperemia immediately after manual detorsion.

False-negative findings can occur when the torsion is intermittent, is low grade, or spontaneously resolves. No technique that relies on blood flow determinations can establish the diagnosis if the blood flow is not decreased when the examination is performed.

Scrotal inflammatory disease usually involves the epididymis initially and spreads from there to the testis, scrotal sac, or scrotal wall. The hallmark of epididymitis on gray-scale studies is enlargement and decreased echogenicity of the epididymis (Fig. 6-34). Involvement of the epididymis may be diffuse but also is frequently focal. Therefore, it is important to scan the entire epididymis in patients with suspected epididymitis. With advanced epididymitis, small abscesses are occasionally seen as complex hypoechoic collections in the epididymis (see Fig. 6-34E and F). Color Doppler imaging is valuable when the gray-scale findings are equivocal or normal because it can detect inflammatory hyperemia as increased epididymal vascularity.

Orchitis usually occurs in conjunction with epididymitis. Isolated orchitis is less common and generally is

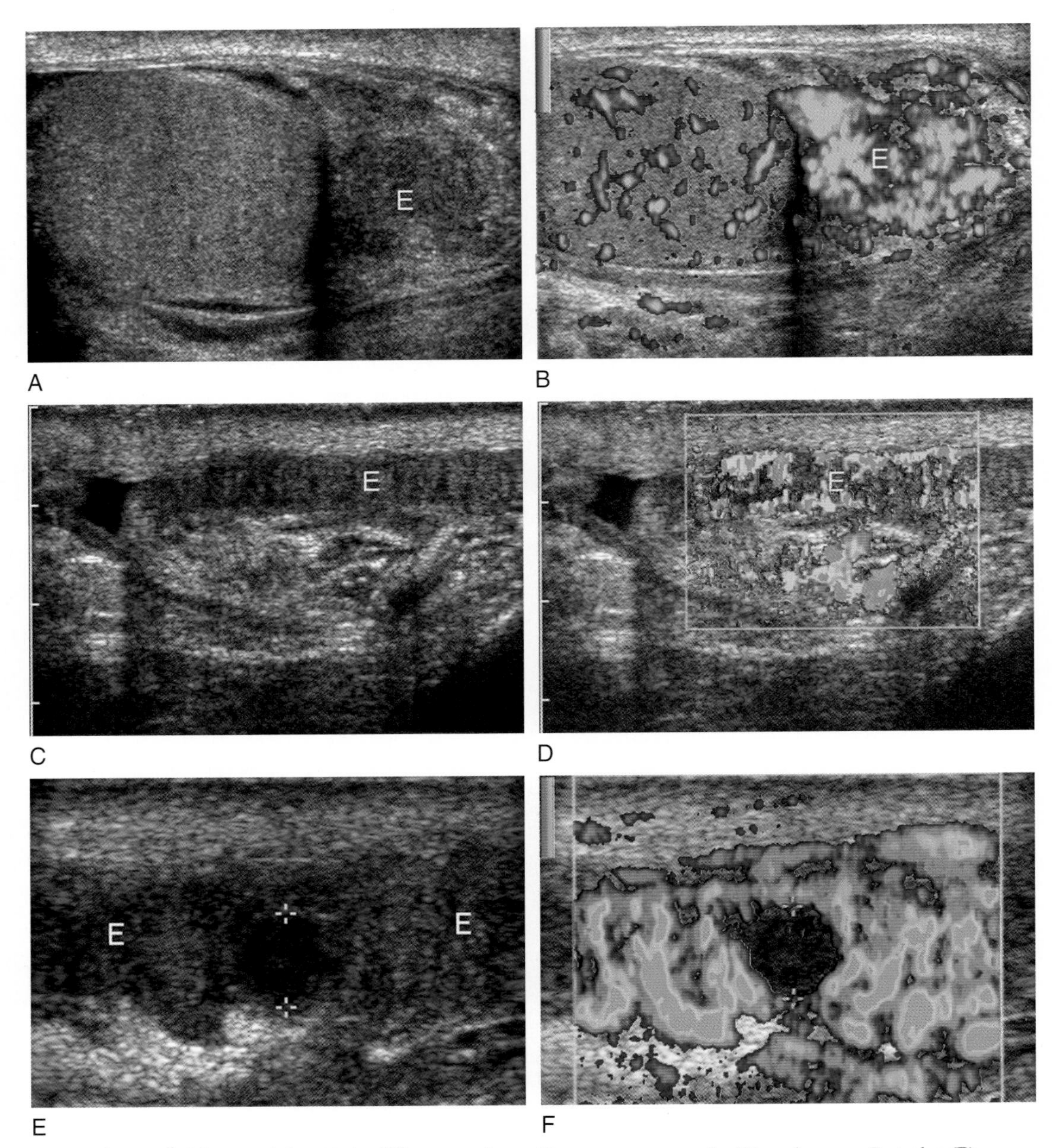

Figure 6-34 Epididymitis in different patients. Transverse gray-scale (**A**) and power Doppler (**B**) views show an enlarged hypoechoic body of the epididymis (E) adjacent to the left testis. Marked hyperemia of the epididymis is evident on power Doppler. Longitudinal gray-scale (**C**) and color Doppler (**D**) views of the epididymis show a slightly enlarged epididymis (E) with intense hypervascularity on the color Doppler view. Longitudinal gray-scale (**E**) and power Doppler (**F**) views of the epididymis (E) show epididymal enlargement and a small hypoechoic lesion *(cursors)* due to an epididymal abscess. Power Doppler shows intense hypervascularity of the epididymis but no detectable flow in the abscess.

viral (i.e., mumps). Testicular enlargement, decreased echogenicity, and hypervascularity are all typical findings (Fig. 6-35A and B). As with epididymitis, hypervascularity may be the only abnormal finding, so color Doppler analysis is more sensitive in the diagnosis of orchitis than is gray-scale sonography alone (see Fig. 6-35C and D). In addition to orchitis, the differential diagnosis for an enlarged, hypoechoic testis includes torsion, diffuse lymphoma or leukemia, and diffuse seminoma (Table 6-2). Orchitis is much less frequently focal than is epididymitis. In such cases it can be difficult to distinguish a hypoechoic hypervascular tumor from focal orchitis (see Fig. 6-35E and F). Clues to look for that make orchitis more likely include the finding of

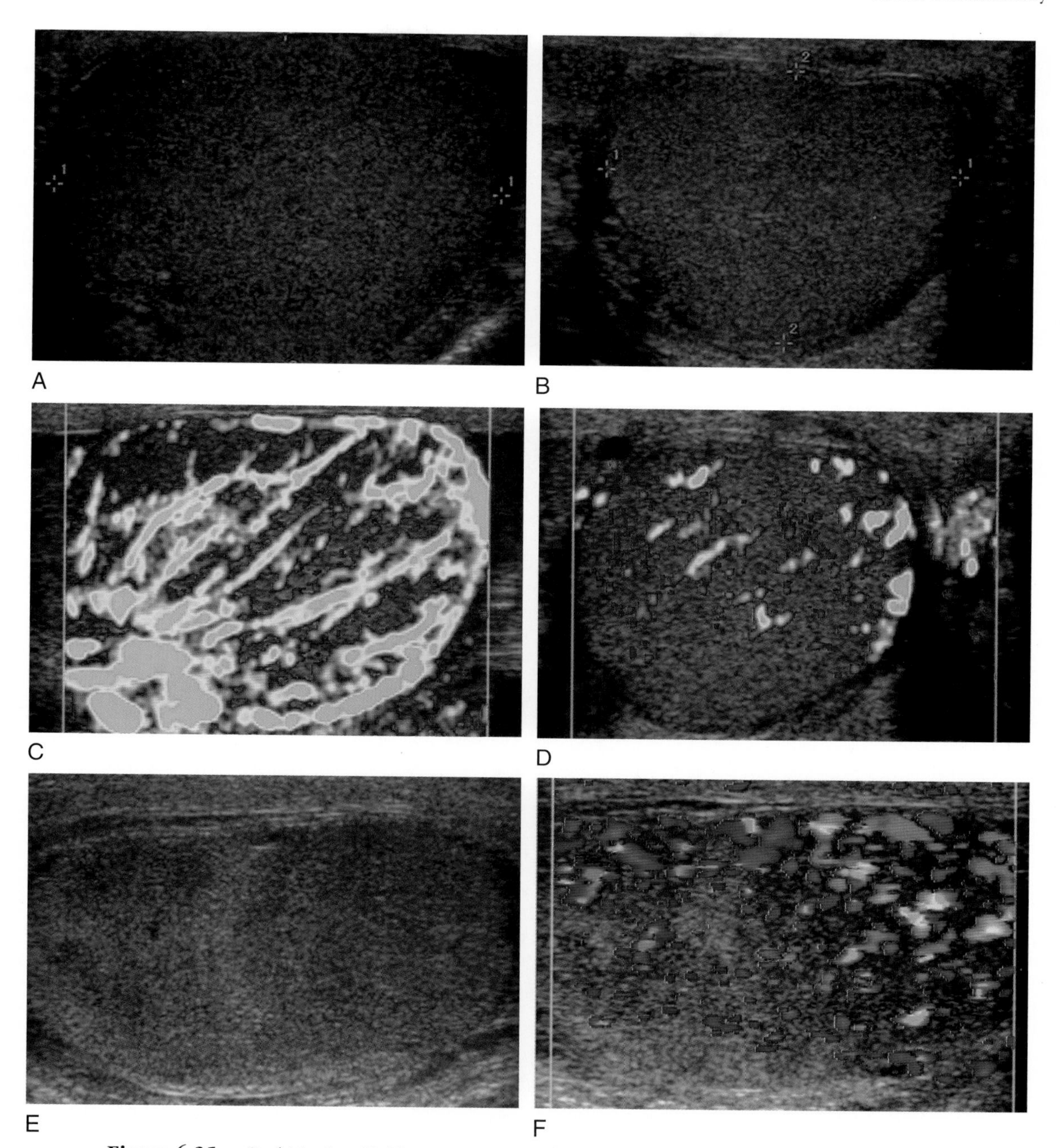

Figure 6-35 Orchitis. **A** to **D**, Transverse gray-scale and color Doppler views of the symptomatic (**A** and **C**) and asymptomatic (**B** and **D**) testes in a patient with orchitis. The symptomatic testis is enlarged and slightly hypoechoic compared with the asymptomatic testis. It is also markedly hyperemic compared with the asymptomatic testis. **E** and **F**, Longitudinal gray-scale (**E**) and color Doppler (**F**) views in another patient show a focal area of orchitis most prominent in the lower pole that appears as a poorly defined region of decreased echogenicity on gray scale and a region of increased vascularity on color Doppler. This type of lesion should be followed to resolution to ensure that it is not an occult neoplasm.

Table 6-2 Causes of an Enlarged Hypoechoic Testis

Abnormality	Blood Flow	Physical Examination
Orchitis	Increased	Tender
Torsion	Decreased	Tender
Lymphoma	Increased	Nontender
Seminoma	Increased	Nontender

pain and tenderness without a palpable mass on physical examination and the sonographic finding of associated involvement of the epididymis. Orchitis may progress to a testicular abscess if appropriate therapy is not instituted. Testicular abscesses will appear as complex fluid collections that are avascular but have intense peripheral hyperemia (Fig. 6-36). Scrotal wall abscesses may develop from testicular abscesses, or they may arise primarily within the soft tissues of the scrotum (Fig. 6-37).

One other role of sonography is in the evaluation of testicular trauma. An important clinical question is the status of the tunica albuginea. If it is intact, surgery is usually not indicated. If it is ruptured, surgery is required within 72 hours to maintain testicular viability. Fractures of the testis rarely appear as linear testicular defects on sonography. More commonly, nonspecific-appearing areas of increased or decreased echogenicity are seen within the testis or the testis becomes misshapen and distorted (Fig. 6-38). This is usually due to a combination of hemorrhage and extrusion of seminiferous tubules.

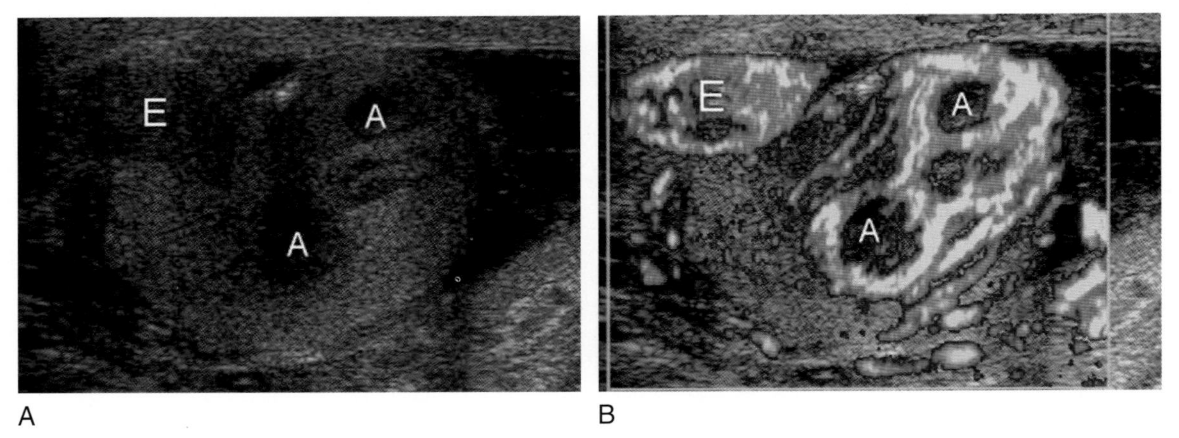

Figure 6-36 Testicular abscess. **A,** Transverse gray-scale view of the right testis shows two small intratesticular abscesses (A) and an enlarged epididymis (E). A reactive hydrocele is also identified. **B,** Power Doppler view shows marked hyperemia of the epididymis (E) and peripheral hyperemia surrounding the testicular abscesses (A).

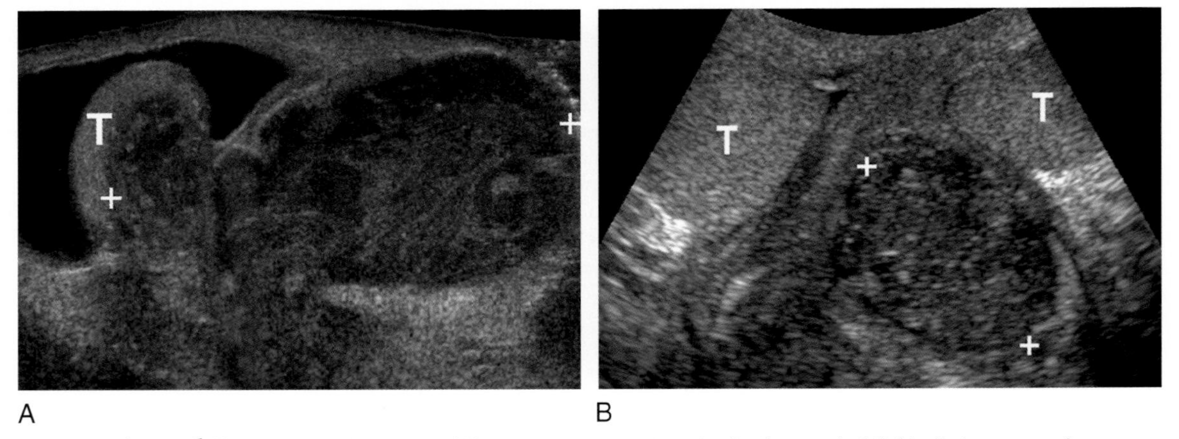

Figure 6-37 Scrotal abscess in different patients. **A,** Longitudinal extended field of view scan of the testis shows a hypoechoic lesion that arises in the testis (T) and extends into the scrotal soft tissues *(cursors)*. This complex fluid collection represented a rapidly enlarging abscess. **B,** Transverse view of the scrotum shows a normal right and left testis (T). A complex hypoechoic fluid collection *(cursors)* is seen in the scrotum posterior to the left testis.

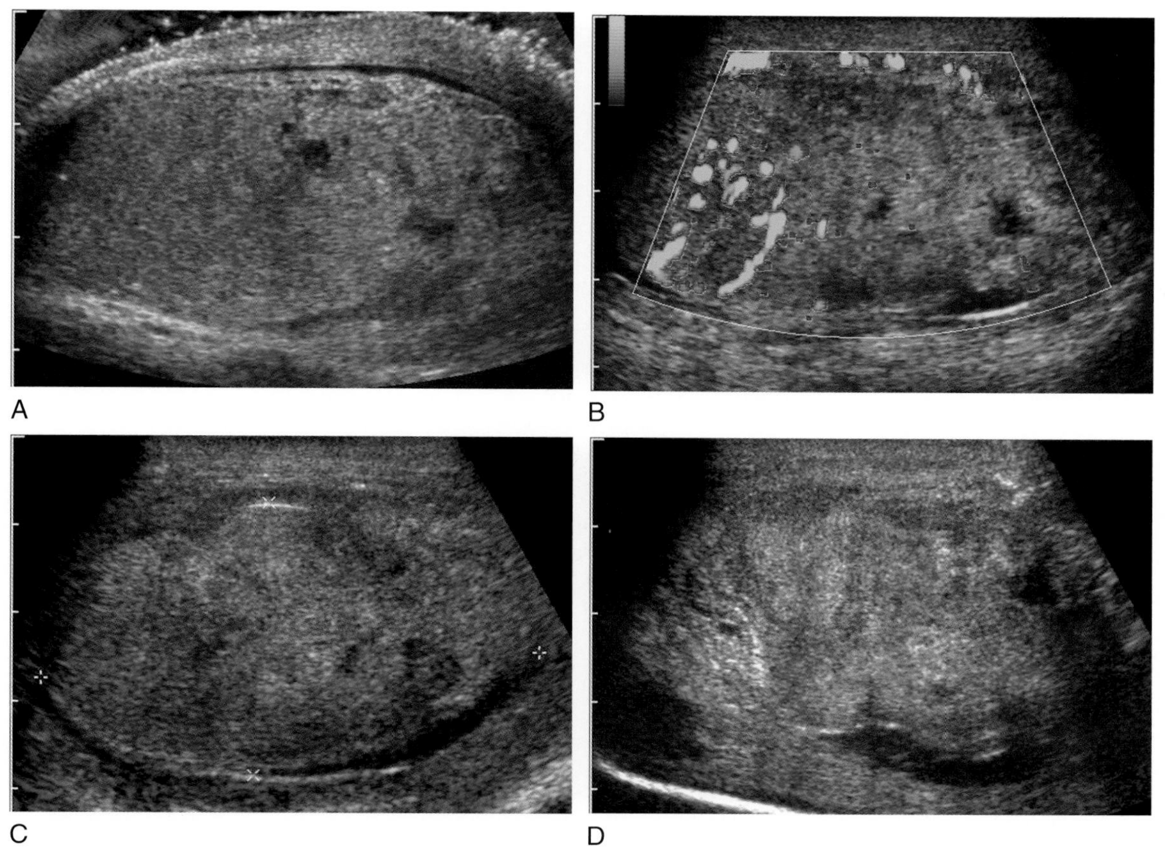

Figure 6-38 Testicular rupture. **A** and **B,** Longitudinal gray-scale (**A**) and power Doppler (**B**) views show slight increased echogenicity and heterogeneity of the lower pole of the testis with decreased blood flow to this region. At surgery, a lower pole hematoma and extruded seminiferous tubules were identified. **C,** Longitudinal view of another patient shows a diffusely heterogeneous testis with some irregularity of the anterior surface. At surgery, there was a large rupture of the tunica albuginea with extruded seminiferous tubules. **D,** Longitudinal view in another patient shows an extremely distorted testis that is misshapen and diffusely heterogeneous. At surgery, there was extensive disruption of the tunica albuginea and little detectable normal testicular parenchyma.

It is important to keep in mind that trauma can serve as an event that leads to a careful self-examination and uncovers a preexisting testicular tumor. Therefore, post-traumatic intratesticular abnormalities whose sonographic characteristics overlap with tumors should be viewed with suspicion and either evaluated surgically or with careful ultrasound follow-up. Trauma can also induce testicular torsion. Therefore, a careful Doppler examination should be a routine part of the evaluation of the traumatized patient.

BLADDER

The urinary bladder is usually well seen with sonography and determination of post-void residuals, using the formula for an ellipsoid (length × width × height × 0.53), is a common request. However, a number of other abnormalities can be visualized.

The most common abnormality seen on sonography is bladder wall thickening. This is most commonly due to bladder outlet obstruction. Other causes include neurogenic bladder, cystitis, edema from adjacent inflammatory processes, radiation, and primary or secondary neoplasms. Detection with cross-sectional imaging is somewhat subjective because thickening will vary with the degree of bladder distention (Fig. 6-39). Reasonable guidelines for upper limits of normal are 3 mm for a well-distended bladder and 5 mm for a poorly distended bladder.

Bladder tumors are frequently detected on sonography, usually in patients who are having renal sonograms for hematuria. Ninety percent are transitional cell carcinoma. Smoking, analgesic abuse, and industrial carcinogen exposure all predispose to transitional cell

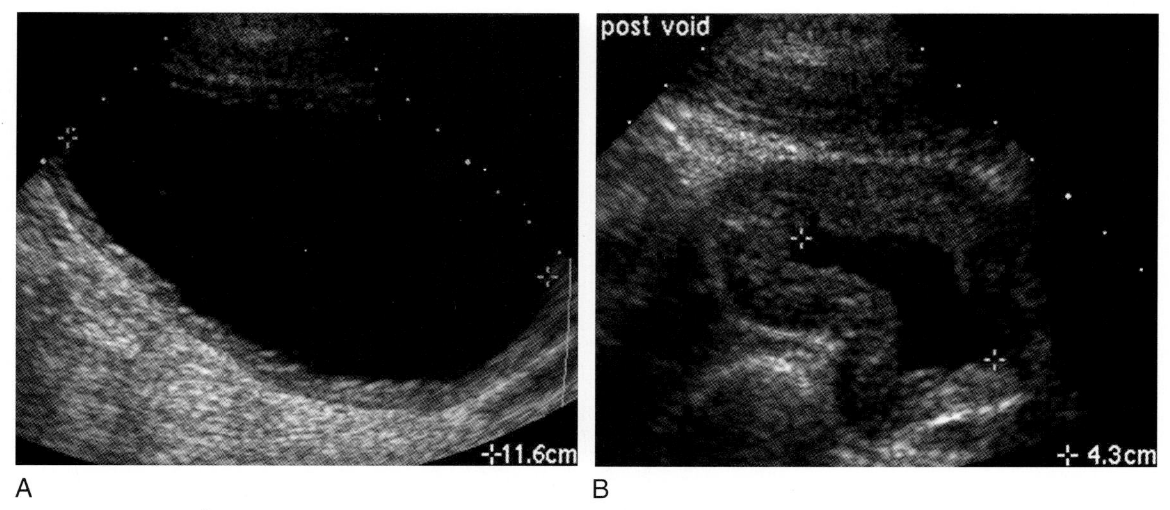

Figure 6-39 Bladder wall thickening. **A,** Longitudinal view of the bladder in a relatively distended state (length of 11.6 cm) shows apparent mild thickening of the bladder wall *(cursors).* **B,** In the same patient following voiding, the decompressed bladder (measuring 4.3 cm in length) shows what appears to be more dramatic bladder wall thickening *(cursors).*

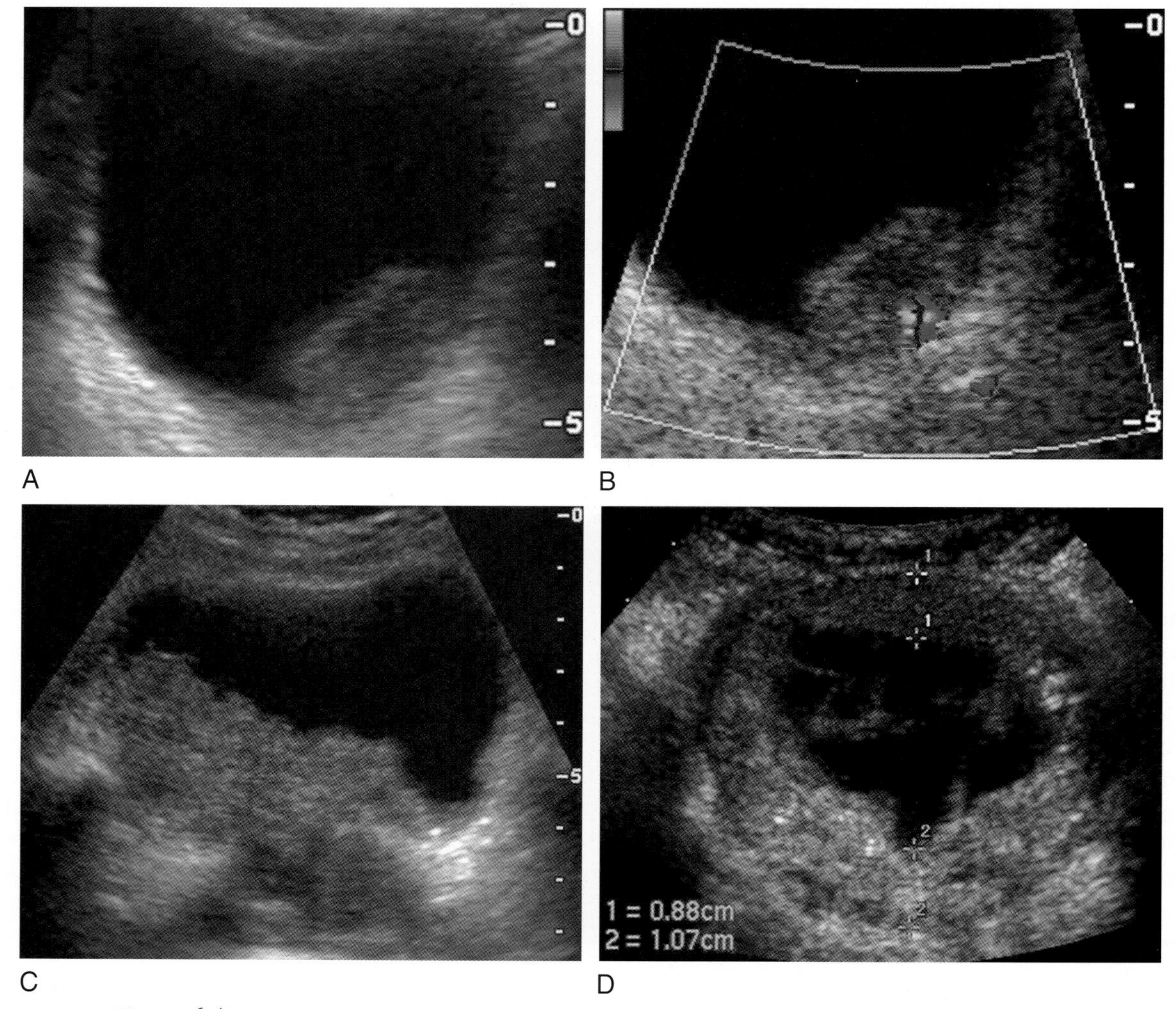

Figure 6-40 Transitional cell cancer in different patients. **A** and **B,** Transverse gray-scale (**A**) and color Doppler (**B**) views of the bladder show a polypoid mass rising from the left posterior bladder wall. Detectable blood flow is seen at the base of the mass on the color Doppler view. **C,** Transverse view shows a more diffuse region of localized bladder wall thickening predominantly along the right lateral bladder wall. **D,** Transverse view of the bladder shows diffuse wall thickening *(cursors).*

cancer. Five percent are squamous cell cancer. These occur in patients with bladder schistosomiasis, neurogenic bladders, or chronic inflammatory conditions of the bladder. Two percent of bladder tumors are adenocarcinoma, which tend to occur in urachal remnants and in bladder exstrophy. Bladder carcinoma is three times more common in men and tends to occur in middle-aged and older populations. The prognosis is dependent on the depth of invasion and, in particular, the degree of involvement of the muscularis.

The majority of transitional cell cancers of the bladder arise along the posterior wall, in the region of the trigone. Sonographically, the majority are polypoid with a mass arising from the bladder wall extending into the bladder lumen (Fig. 6-40A and B). Less often they are infiltrative with diffuse or localized thickening of the bladder wall (see Fig. 6-40C). The presence of a transitional cell cancer in the bladder or in the upper tracts places the entire urothelium at risk and periodic imaging is required.

The primary differential diagnosis for bladder cancer is blood clots (Fig. 6-41). The useful findings that distinguish bladder cancer from blood clot are immobility and presence of blood flow. The differential diagnosis also includes other intraluminal lesions such as stones and fungus balls; other causes of focal wall thickening such as invasion by adjacent tumors (prostate, rectum, cervix), involvement by adjacent inflammatory processes, fistulas with adjacent organs, wall trabeculation, benign prostatic hypertrophy, endometriosis, malakoplakia, leukoplakia, tuberculosis, and schistosomiasis; and rare tumors such as adenocarcinoma, squamous cell carcinoma, and pheochromocytoma. Bladder stones are easily distinguished from other abnormalities by the combination of shadowing and mobility (Fig. 6-42). Benign prostatic hypertrophy may produce a prominent mass in the base of the bladder that simulates a transitional cell cancer (Fig. 6-43). In most cases, lesions of benign prostatic hypertrophy will be located in the midline and continuity with the prostate will be apparent.

Bladder diverticula are other common abnormalities that are visible on sonography. They usually occur due to outlet obstruction and often coexist with a thick bladder wall. They appear as a fluid-filled structure adjacent to the bladder. In the majority of cases, careful scanning will demonstrate the connection between the bladder and the diverticulum (Fig. 6-44A and B). When the connection is not visible on gray-scale sonography, compression of the bladder with the transducer may demonstrate urine flow between the bladder and diverticulum on color Doppler imaging (see Fig. 6-44C and D).

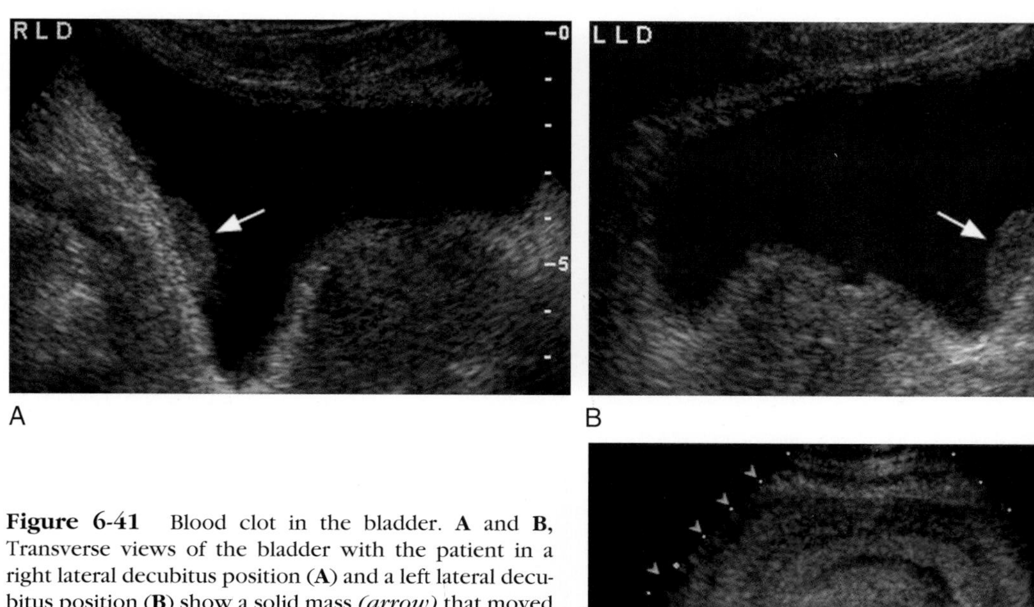

Figure 6-41 Blood clot in the bladder. **A** and **B,** Transverse views of the bladder with the patient in a right lateral decubitus position (**A**) and a left lateral decubitus position (**B**) show a solid mass *(arrow)* that moved from the right to the left wall of the bladder with patient repositioning. **C,** Transverse view of another patient shows a mass completely filling the bladder lumen. This developed immediately after a percutaneous kidney biopsy.

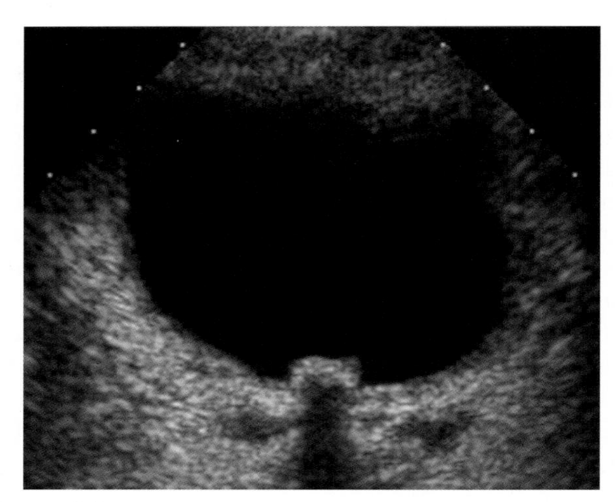

Figure 6-42 Bladder calculus. Transverse view of the bladder shows a hyperechoic intraluminal lesion with a posterior acoustic shadow located along the dependent aspect of the bladder.

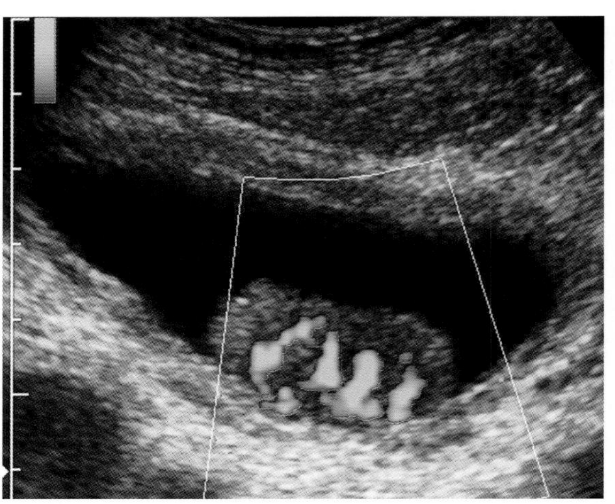

Figure 6-43 Prostatic hypertrophy simulating a bladder cancer. Longitudinal power Doppler view of the bladder shows a polypoid intraluminal mass similar in appearance to the transitional cell carcinoma seen in Fig. 6-40A. Readily detectable internal blood flow indicates that this is vascularized soft tissue and not a blood clot. Continuity with an enlarged prostate was identified on other views.

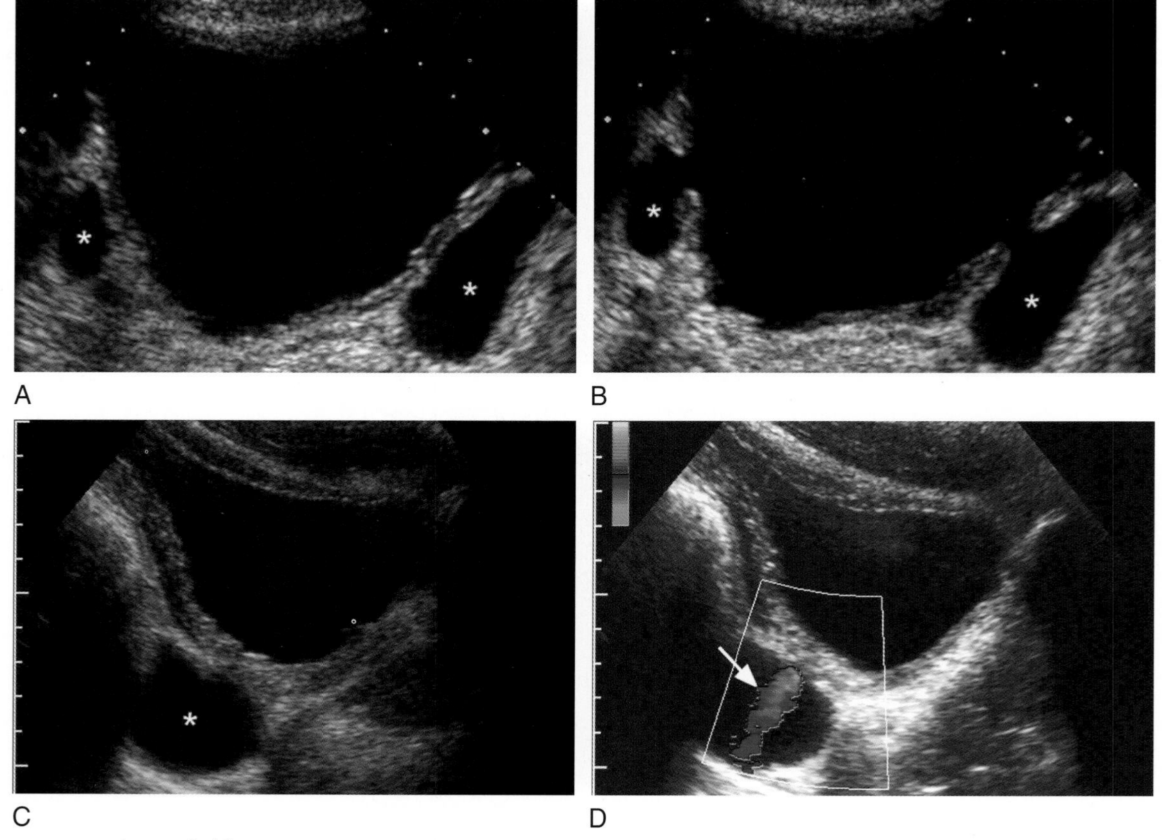

Figure 6-44 Bladder diverticulum. **A** and **B,** Adjacent transverse views of the bladder show two retrovesicular fluid collections (*). With careful scanning it was possible to show the communication between the fluid collections and the bladder. **C** and **D,** Longitudinal gray-scale (**A**) and color Doppler (**B**) views of the bladder in another patient show a retrovesicular fluid collection (*). Despite careful scanning, a definite communication between the collection and the bladder could not be documented on gray-scale imaging. However, with compression of the bladder, urine flow *(arrow)* could be documented between the bladder and the diverticulum on color Doppler scanning.

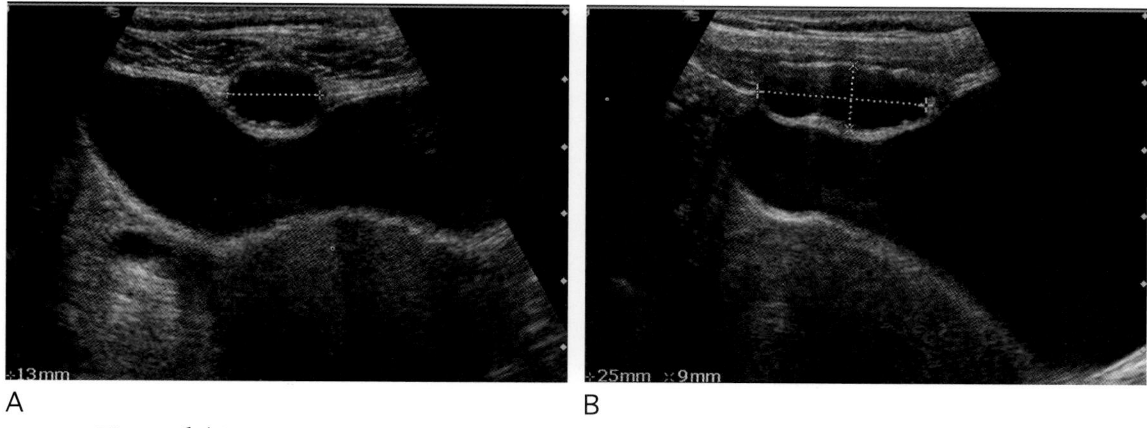

Figure 6-45 Urachal cyst. **A,** Transverse view of the bladder shows a cyst *(cursors)* along the anterior wall of the bladder. **B,** Longitudinal view confirms the presence of the cyst and localizes it to the superior aspect of the bladder.

Urinary stasis in the diverticulum predisposes to infection, stone formation, and cancer. Because it may be difficult for the urologist to pass a cystoscope through the neck of a diverticulum, it is important to scan them carefully to exclude these potential complications.

Another unusual perivesicular fluid collection is the urachal diverticulum or cyst. These form if there is incomplete closure of the urachus. If the umbilical segment closes but the vesicular segment does not, a diverticulum is formed. If the segment between the bladder and umbilicus fails to close then a urachal cyst forms (Fig. 6-45). Both abnormalities are characterized by their location adjacent to the anterior dome of the bladder.

Simple ureteroceles are easy to detect with sonography. They are caused by dilatation of the intramural portion of the distal ureter protruding into the bladder lumen. In adults, they are usually incidental findings and are located in the expected location of the ureteral orifice. They are formed by mild stenosis of the ureteral orifice presumably due to limited resorption of Chwalla's membrane during embryologic ureteral recanalization. On sonography they appear as round or oval, thin-walled cystic structures on the posterior wall of the bladder. On real-time scanning they can be observed to change size as they fill and empty and ureteral jets can be observed intermittently emanating from their orifice (Fig. 6-46). Pseudoureteroceles caused by some pathologic process that obstructs the ureteral orifice, such as stones, tumors, and recent manipulation, can mimic simple ureteroceles, but the wall is usually thicker and the obstructing lesion should be visible. Box 6-4 reviews the causes of bladder wall lesions.

Box 6-4 Causes of Bladder Wall Lesions

- Primary neoplasms
  - Transitional cell
  - Adenocarcinoma
  - Squamous cell
  - Pheochromocytoma
- Invasion from adjacent neoplasms
  - Rectum
  - Prostate
  - Cervix
  - Uterus
- Inflammation from adjacent organs
  - Diverticulitis
  - Crohn's disease
  - Pelvic inflammatory disease
  - Appendicitis
- Ureteroceles
- Urachal cysts
- Cystitis cystica
- Endometriomas
- Fistulas
- Malakoplakia
- Leukoplakia
- Tuberculosis
- Schistosomiasis

URETHRA

Sonography is not a primary modality used to evaluate most urethral abnormalities. However, it can be quite valuable in some instances. The normal female urethra

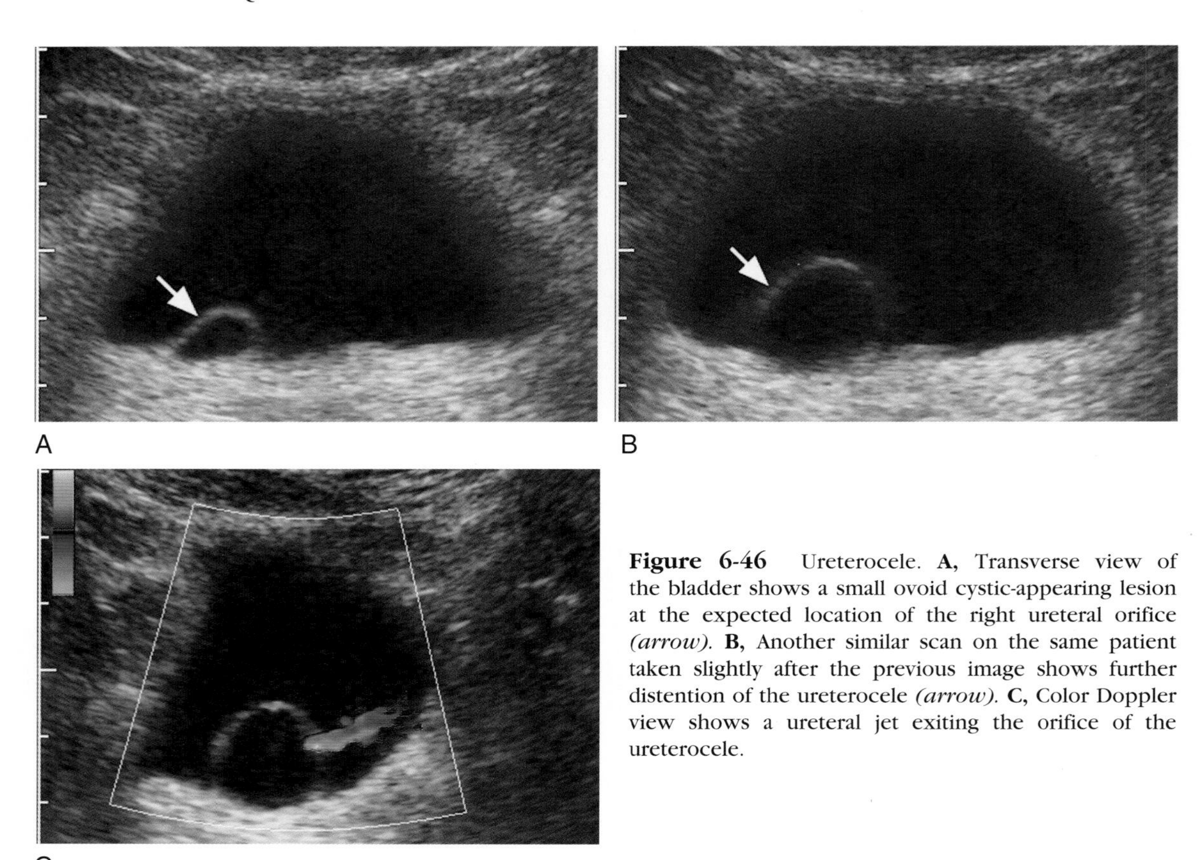

Figure 6-46 Ureterocele. **A,** Transverse view of the bladder shows a small ovoid cystic-appearing lesion at the expected location of the right ureteral orifice *(arrow).* **B,** Another similar scan on the same patient taken slightly after the previous image shows further distention of the ureterocele *(arrow).* **C,** Color Doppler view shows a ureteral jet exiting the orifice of the ureterocele.

can routinely be identified on transvaginal and transperineal scans as a hypoechoic linear structure arising from the base of the bladder and passing inferior to the symphysis pubis (Fig. 6-47). Because of the anisotropic properties of the urethral wall muscles, the urethral wall may appear very hypoechoic or even anechoic when it is oriented parallel to the direction of the sound. This should not be confused with urine in the lumen of the urethra.

A combination of transvaginal and transperineal scanning is very effective in identifying urethral diverticula in women. These appear as simple or complex collections of fluid that are intimately related to the urethra. They usually arise from the mid urethra and initially extend posteriorly. However, they frequently wrap around one or both lateral aspects of the urethra (Fig. 6-48). They can be complicated by both stones and cancer. Periurethral abscesses simulate diverticula but are more remote from the urethra and are usually associated with a hyperemic inflammatory reaction (Fig. 6-49).

In men, sonography is occasionally used to evaluate urethral strictures. The main purpose is to accurately

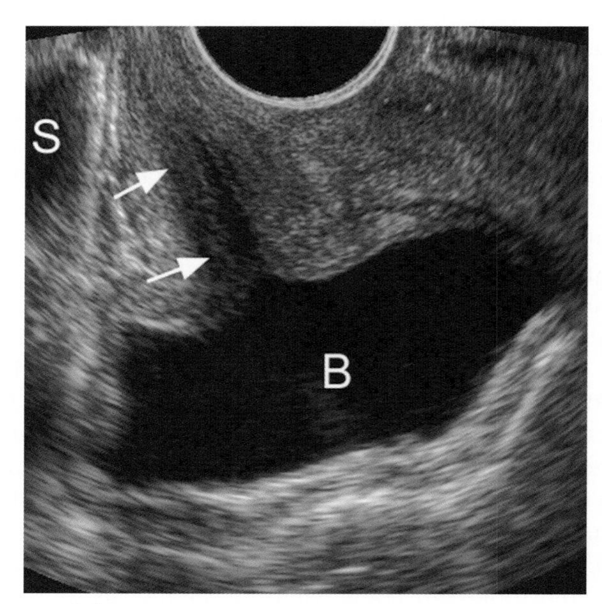

Figure 6-47 Normal female urethra. Sagittal transvaginal scan in the pelvic midline shows the urinary bladder (B) in the deep aspect of the field of view. The urethra *(arrows)* is seen as a hypoechoic linear structure exiting from the base of the bladder and traveling inferior to the synthesis pubis (S).

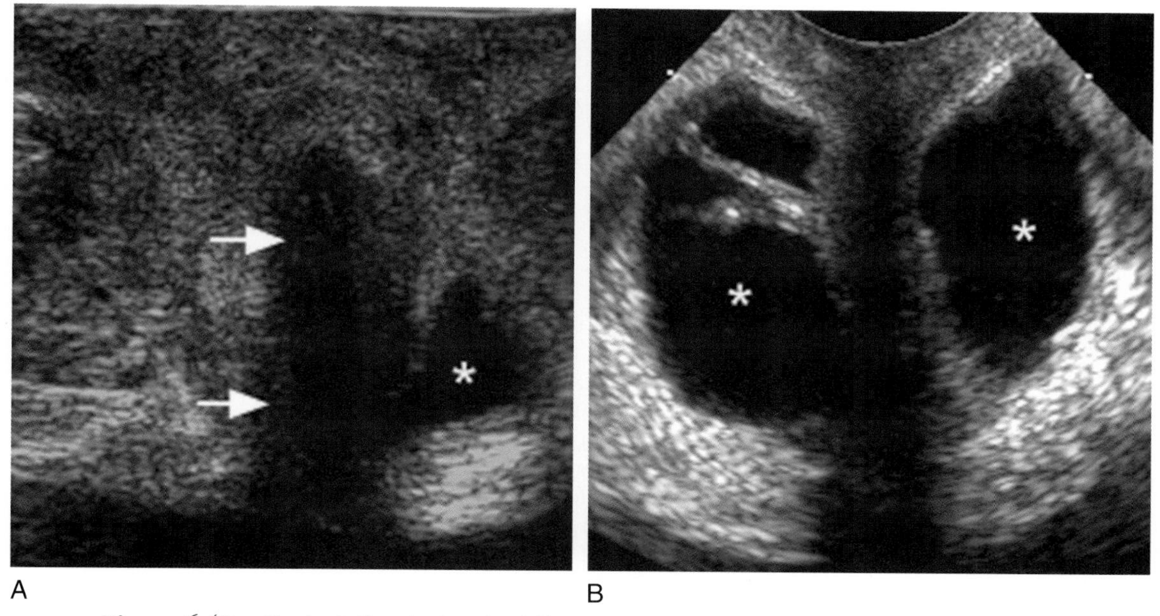

Figure 6-48 Urethral diverticulum in different patients. **A,** Sagittal transperineal view of the urethra *(arrows)* shows a small fluid collection (*) posterior to the urethra and in intimate contact to the urethra consistent with a small urethral diverticulum. **B,** Coronal transvaginal view of the urethra shows a large diverticulum (*) that extends to the right and left aspect of the urethra.

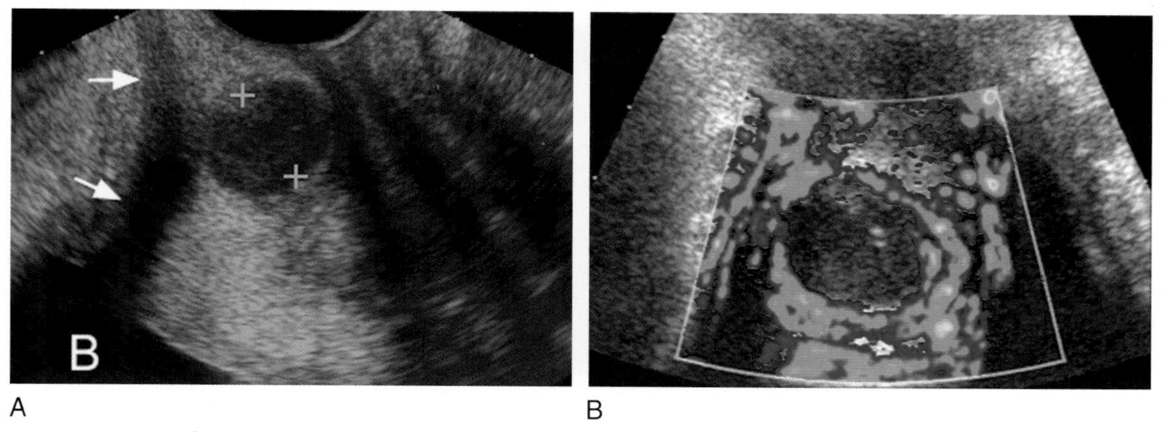

Figure 6-49 Periurethral abscess. **A,** Sagittal transvaginal view shows a hypoechoic complex fluid collection *(cursors)* posterior to the urethra *(arrows).* The base of the urinary bladder (B) is seen in the deep field of view. **B,** Power Doppler view of the same patient shows intense hypervascularity surrounding the abscess but no internal blood flow.

determine the location and measure the length and thickness of the stricture to determine the type of treatment that is required. To visualize the stricture, the urethra must be injected with saline or with viscous lidocaine at the time of the examination (Fig. 6-50).

PENIS

Several penile abnormalities can be evaluated with sonography. One primary role of sonography is diagnosing vascular causes of erectile dysfunction. This can be done with pulsed Doppler analysis after the injection of vasoactive drugs such as papaverine and prostaglandin E into the corpora cavernosa. In normal men, there is an increase in arterial flow to the bilateral cavernosal arteries that can be quantified by measuring systolic velocities. The recommended criteria for a normal response vary somewhat. Most would agree that systolic velocities exceeding 35 cm/sec can be considered normal (Fig. 6-51) and that maximum velocities below 25 cm/sec indicate arterial insufficiency. Velocities

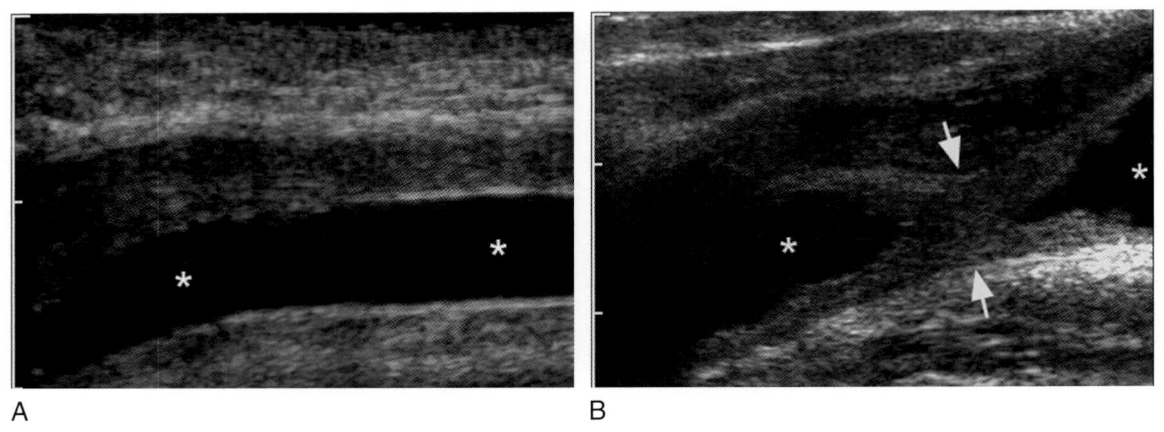

Figure 6-50 Urethral stricture in a man. **A,** Longitudinal view of the anterior urethra during injection of saline shows a normal uniform urethral lumen (*). **B,** Longitudinal view of the posterior urethra shows a localized stricture *(arrows)* with a normal urethral lumen both proximal and distal (*).

between 25 and 35 cm/sec are indeterminate. In addition, as the venous outflow mechanism starts to prevent outflow of blood from the corpora cavernosa, diastolic arterial inflow starts to drop and may even reverse. This can be quantified by measuring the arterial resistive index. If arterial inflow is adequate and the resistive index stays below 0.8 for 15 to 20 minutes after the injection, venous leak should be suspected.

Priapism is another condition that can be evaluated with Doppler. This is done primarily to search for an occult arteriovenous fistula (high-flow priapism), which occurs most often in patients with a history of penile or perineal trauma, or thrombosis of the dorsal penile vein (low-flow priapism).

Peyronie's disease is fibrosis of the tunica albuginea of the corpora cavernosa. It is an idiopathic condition that typically affects men older than 45 years old. Lack of expansion of the tunica albuginea in the area of fibrosis causes the penis to bend toward the plaque during erection. The associated pain and penile curvature can make intercourse impossible. On physical examination, an area of thickening corresponding to the plaque is typically palpable. On sonography, the plaques appear as a localized area of thickening of the tunica albuginea, often with calcification (Fig. 6-52). The typical location is along the dorsum of the penis near the base, but it can also involve other areas.

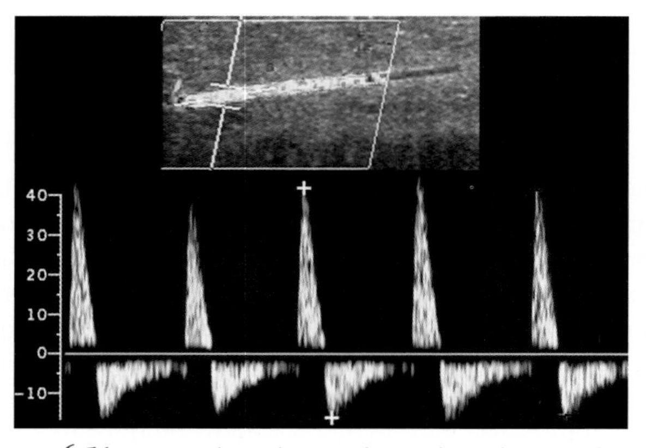

Figure 6-51 Normal penile Doppler study. Color Doppler and pulse Doppler waveform from the cavernosal artery after injection of prostaglandin E shows a high resistance waveform with a systolic velocity slightly greater than 40 cm/sec. Diastolic flow reversal indicates intact venous outflow mechanism.

Penile masses can occasionally be evaluated with sonography. As in the testes, soft tissue masses with internal blood flow should raise the suspicion of a tumor (Fig. 6-53). Lesions with no flow or lesions that are cystic are less likely to be neoplastic.

PROSTATE

Prostate cancer is the most common malignant tumor and is the second most common cause of cancer-related mortality in men. It is most common in blacks, less common in whites, and uncommon in Asians. As many as 50% of men in their 50s and 80% of men in their 80s will have at least microscopic foci of prostate cancer. Despite the relatively ubiquitous nature of prostate cancer in elderly men, there is only a 5% to 10% chance of their exhibiting symptoms from the disease. Therefore, most of these cancers are clinically occult.

The prostate is composed of four zones. In the normal gland, the peripheral zone is the largest. It is located posteriorly and extends to both lateral margins (Fig. 6-54). It becomes thicker in the apex (inferior aspect of the gland) and thinner in the base (superior aspect of the gland). Approximately 70% of the cases of prostate cancer occur in the peripheral zone. The central zone is the next largest

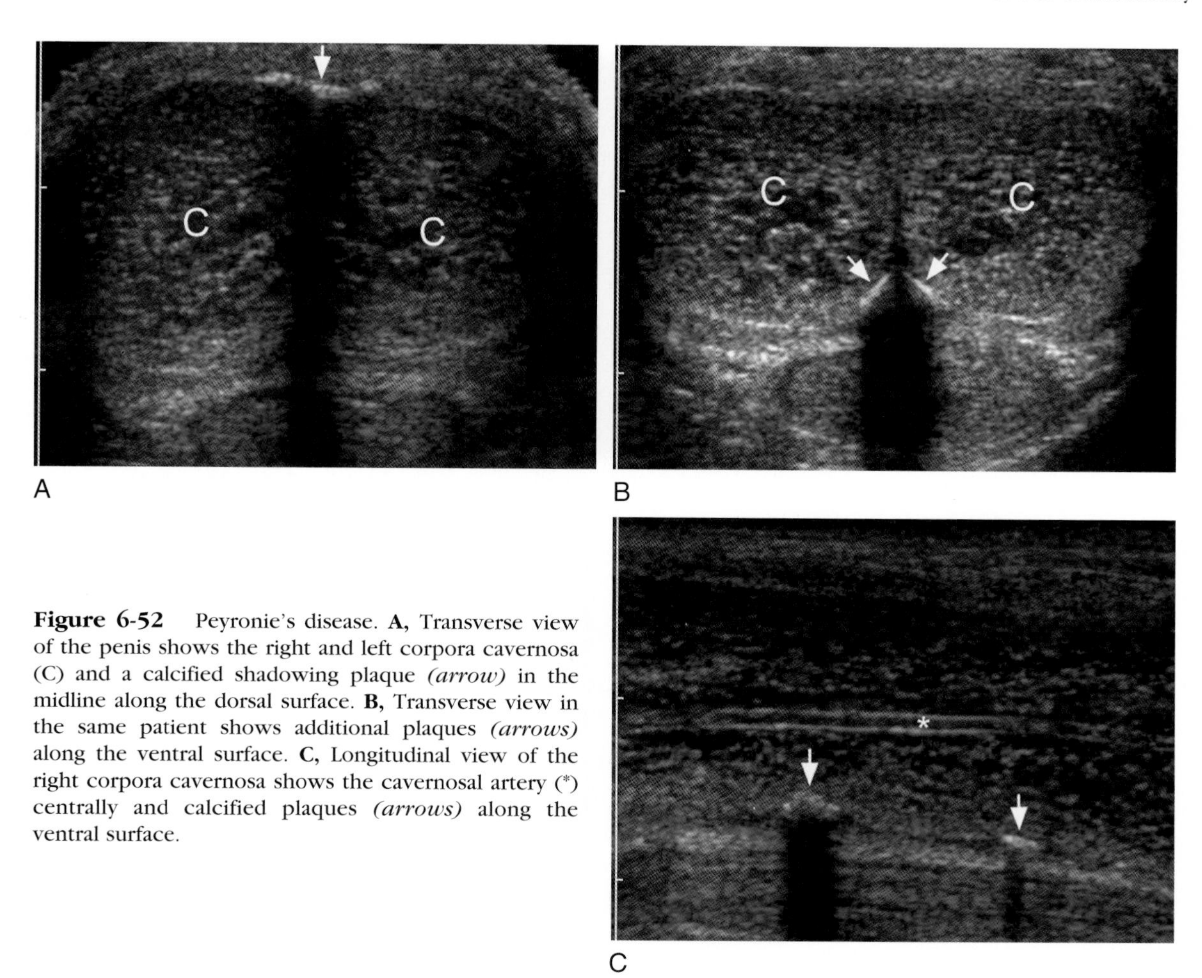

Figure 6-52 Peyronie's disease. **A,** Transverse view of the penis shows the right and left corpora cavernosa (C) and a calcified shadowing plaque *(arrow)* in the midline along the dorsal surface. **B,** Transverse view in the same patient shows additional plaques *(arrows)* along the ventral surface. **C,** Longitudinal view of the right corpora cavernosa shows the cavernosal artery (*) centrally and calcified plaques *(arrows)* along the ventral surface.

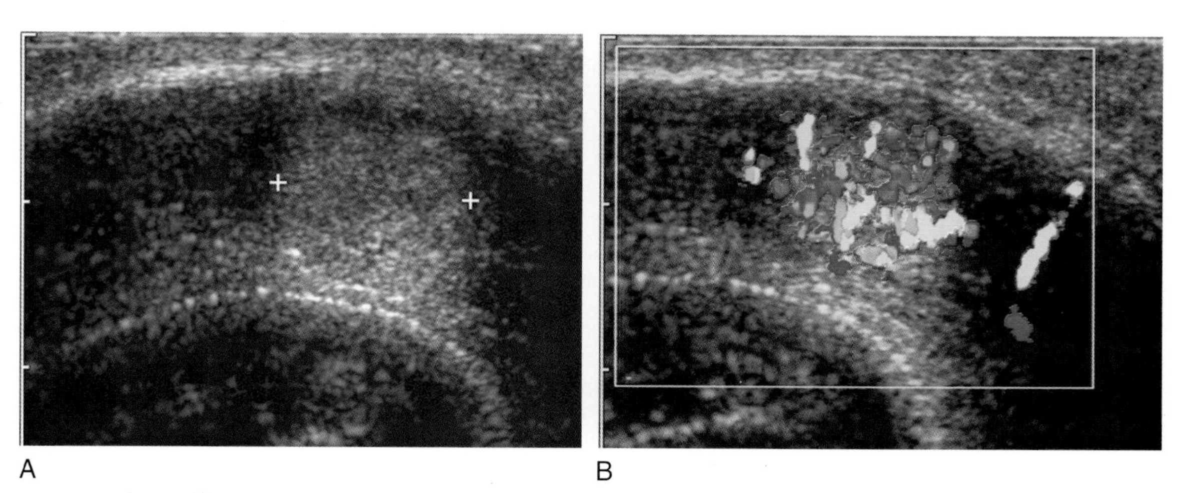

Figure 6-53 Penile metastasis from renal cell carcinoma. **A,** Longitudinal gray-scale view of the base of the penis shows a hyperechoic solid mass *(cursors)* within the corpora cavernosa. **B,** Color Doppler view shows marked hypervascularity within the mass. This was the only identified site of metastasis in this patient with a history of renal cell carcinoma.

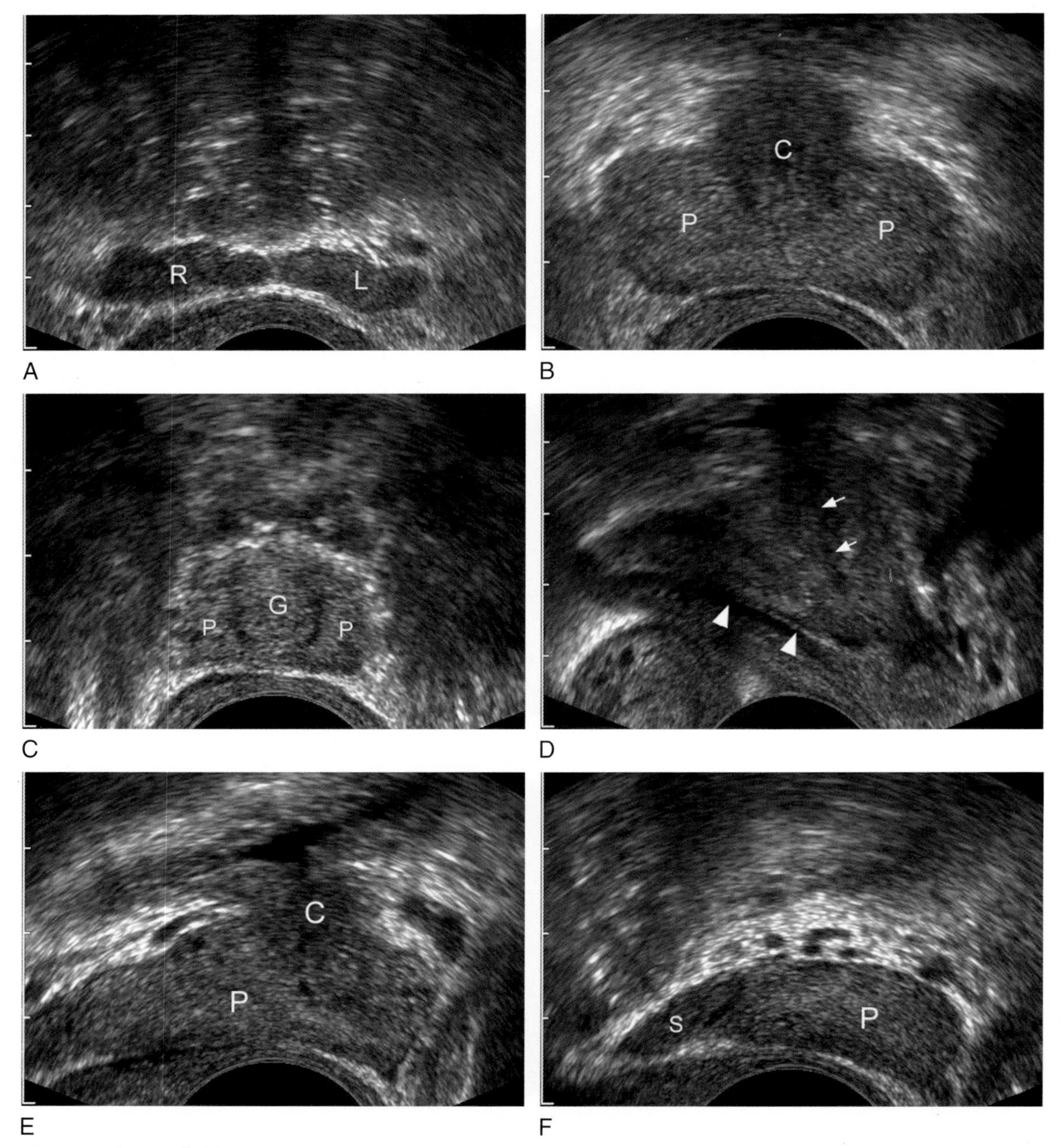

Figure 6-54 Normal prostate. **A,** Transverse view through the level of the seminal vesicles shows the hypoechoic oblong symmetric-appearing solid right (R) and left (L) seminal vesicles. **B,** Transverse scan through the base (superior aspect) of the prostate shows the slightly hyperechoic peripheral zone (P) and the slightly less echogenic central gland (C). **C,** Transverse view at the apex (inferior aspect) of the prostate shows the inferior aspect of the peripheral zone (P) and the periurethral glandular area (G). **D,** Midline sagittal view shows the ejaculatory duct *(arrowheads)* and the proximal urethra *(arrows)*. **E,** Sagittal view just lateral to the midline shows mostly peripheral zone (P) and a smaller central gland (C). **F,** Sagittal view through the lateral aspect of the prostate shows peripheral zone (P) and the seminal vesicle (S).

zone and is positioned immediately deep to the peripheral zone. It is located predominantly in the base (see Fig. 6-54). Five percent of the cases of cancer are located in the central zone. The transitional zone is located in the periurethral region between the base and apex. It is the smallest zone in the normal gland, but because benign prostatic hypertrophy arises in the transitional zone, it is rarely seen in its normal state. Twenty percent of the cases of cancer occur in the transitional zone. The anterior aspect of the prostate is composed of nonglandular tissue and is called the fibromuscular stroma. The seminal vesicles are bilaterally symmetric structures situated immediately above the prostate. They are bulbous laterally and taper medially (see Fig. 6-54). (See Table 6-3 for a summary of the characteristics of prostate cancer.)

The primary role of sonography in evaluation of the prostate is to guide biopsies. With modern transrectal transducers it is very easy to direct core biopsy needles into a specified area of the prostate. When focal lesions are visualized sonographically or palpated on rectal examinations, they should be sampled and random biopsy specimens from at least all four quadrants should be obtained. These random biopsy specimens are very important because cancer is found in up to 20% of such cases. If the prostate-specific antigen (PSA) level is elevated, then random biopsy specimens should be obtained even when there are no focal lesions.

It was originally hoped that transrectal sonography would be sensitive enough at detecting prostate carcinoma to serve as a screening test. Unfortunately, its sensitivity is only 60% to 70% at best. In addition, the specificity of sonography is not such that a focal lesion of any type can be assumed to be a cancer. Therefore, there is very little reason to perform prostate sonography without performing prostate biopsies at the same time.

The sonographic appearance of prostate cancer varies, but 70% are hypoechoic with respect to the peripheral zone (Fig. 6-55A to C). The remainder that can be seen with ultrasound are hyperechoic (see Fig. 6-55D) or mixed. Cancer may appear either as a discrete nodule or as an infiltrative hypoechoic region (see Fig. 6-55C). Cystic cancer is very rare. Although the classic appearance of prostate cancer is that of a hypoechoic nodule in the peripheral zone, only 20% to 30% of such nodules are actually cancers. The rest are benign conditions such as prostatitis, atrophy, fibrosis, infarct, and benign prostatic hyperplasia (Fig. 6-56). Most prostate cancers appear hypervascular on color Doppler analysis, and in a limited number of cases the hypervascularity is detectable even when a focal nodule is not seen on gray-scale studies (see Fig. 6-55E and F).

Table 6-3 Characteristics of Prostate Cancer

Characteristic	Frequency
Location	
Peripheral zone	75%
Transitional zone	20%
Central zone	5%
Echogenicity	
Hypoechoic	70%
Hyperechoic/mixed	30%

The American Cancer Society currently recommends that screening for prostate cancer consist of both the digital rectal examination and determination of the PSA level. This should be started at age 50, unless the patient is at high risk (African American or strong family history). The PSA level is considered normal if it is 0 to 4 ng/mL, borderline if it is 4 to 10 ng/ml, and abnormal if it exceeds 10 ng/ml. Besides prostate cancer, benign prostatic hypertrophy, prostatitis, and prostate infarcts can also cause the PSA level to be elevated. On the other hand, not all patients with prostate cancer have abnormal PSA levels. Additional factors that are helpful in determining the significance of the PSA value are the age of the patient, the degree of benign prostatic hypertrophy, and the rate of change from one determination to the next. Elevated or borderline levels are more worrisome in young men, men without significant benign prostatic hypertrophy, and men who have had previously normal levels.

Benign prostatic hypertrophy involves the transitional zone and produces enlargement, inhomogeneity, calcification, and occasionally cystic changes. These changes make it very difficult to detect cancer in the transitional zone.

Prostatic cysts are occasionally encountered and can occur from a variety of causes. Cysts that arise in or near the midline of the prostatic base include utricle cysts, müllerian duct cysts, and ejaculatory duct cysts (Fig. 6-57). They are difficult to differentiate with sonography alone, although ultrasound-guided aspiration of the cyst will reveal spermatozoa only in ejaculatory duct cysts. Cysts may also arise as the result of obstruction of the seminal vesicle. Retention cysts can occur anywhere in the prostate. Cystic changes can also occur in the settings of prostatitis and benign prostatic hypertrophy.

Seminal vesicle cysts and agenesis are rare anomalies that are occasionally encountered during sonography of the bladder or prostate (Fig. 6-58). Both are associated with other genitourinary anomalies, especially renal agenesis and agenesis of the vas deferens.

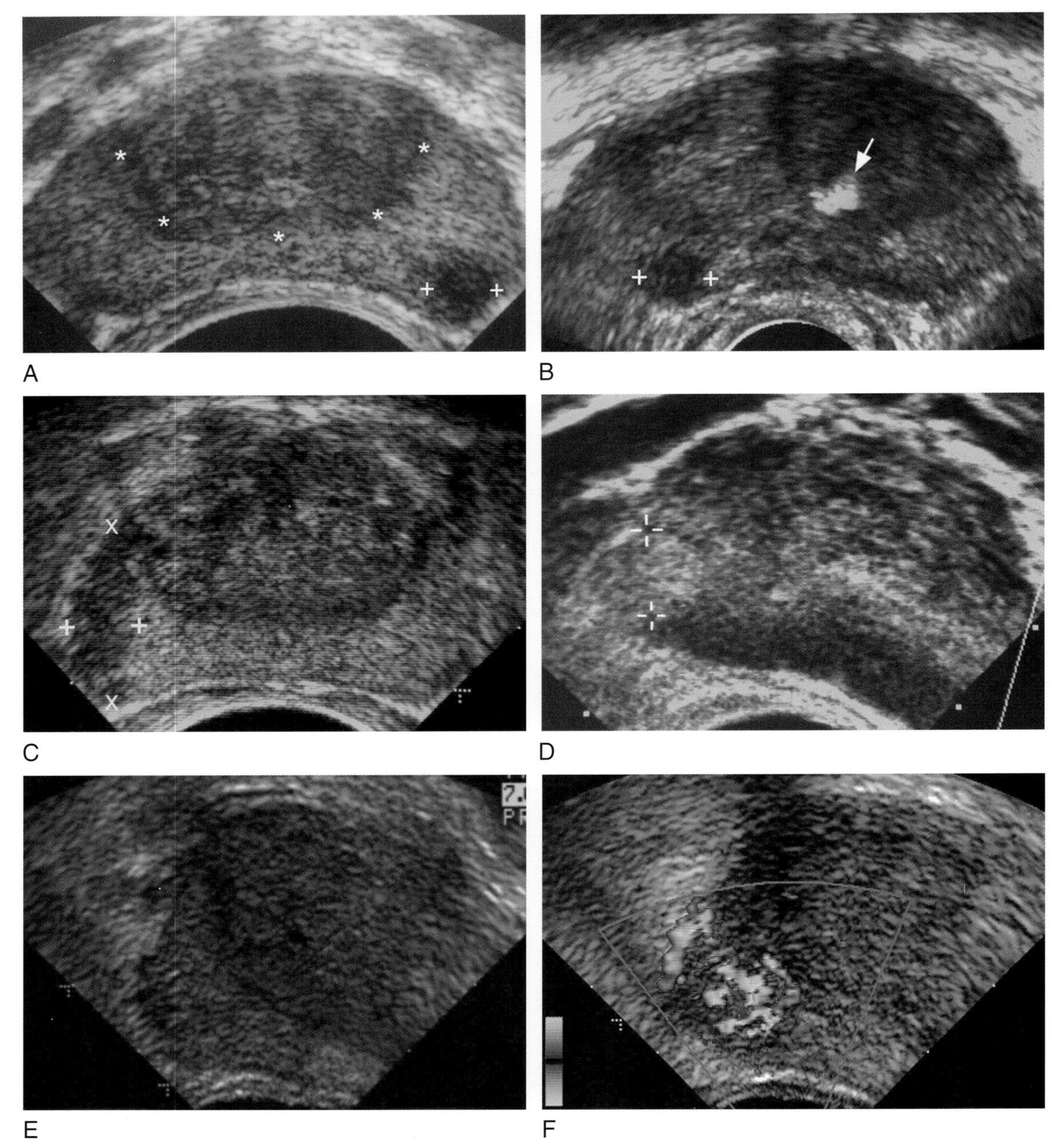

Figure 6-55 Prostate cancer in different patients. **A,** Transverse view through the mid gland shows a focal hypoechoic solid nodule in the left peripheral zone *(cursors).* The demarcation between the central gland and the peripheral zone (*) is well illustrated in this prostate. **B,** Transverse view through the mid gland shows a peripheral hypoechoic solid nodule in the right side of the prostate *(cursors).* A focus of calcification *(arrow)* is seen in the central gland. (Case courtesy of Steve Winn, Maine Medical Center.) **C,** Transverse view through the mid gland shows an infiltrative region of decreased echogenicity in the right peripheral zone *(cursors).* **D,** A transverse view through the right side of the prostate shows a solid hyperechoic nodule in the peripheral zone *(cursors).* This is an unusual appearance for prostate cancer. **E** and **F,** Transverse gray-scale (**E**) and color Doppler (**F**) views of the right side of the prostate show a focal area of hypervascularity *(cursors)* in the peripheral zone that was biopsy proven to represent prostate cancer. Because this cancer was isoechoic, no abnormality was identified in this region on gray-scale imaging.

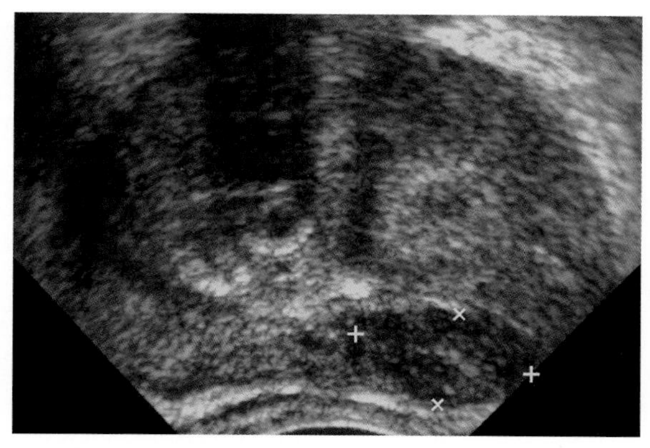

Figure 6-56 Benign nodule. Transverse view of the prostate shows a hypoechoic nodule *(cursors)* in the left peripheral zone. Some calcification is noted in the central zone. Biopsy showed no evidence of malignancy in the region of the focal peripheral zone nodule.

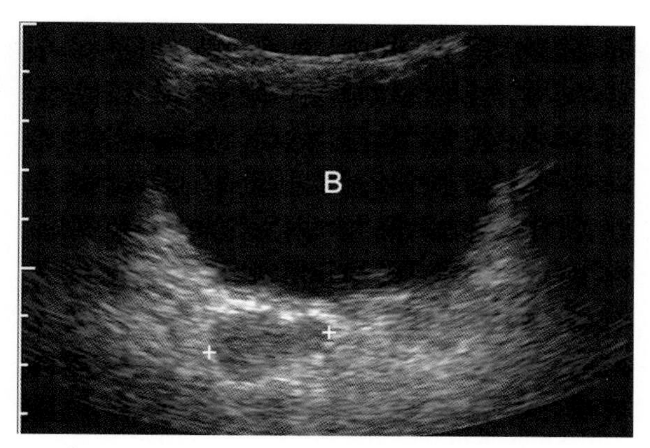

Figure 6-58 Agenesis of the seminal vesicle. Transverse transabdominal view of the pelvis through the filled urinary bladder (B) shows a normal-appearing right seminal vesicle *(cursors)*. No left seminal vesicle is identified. This patient also had congenital bilateral absence of the vas deferens.

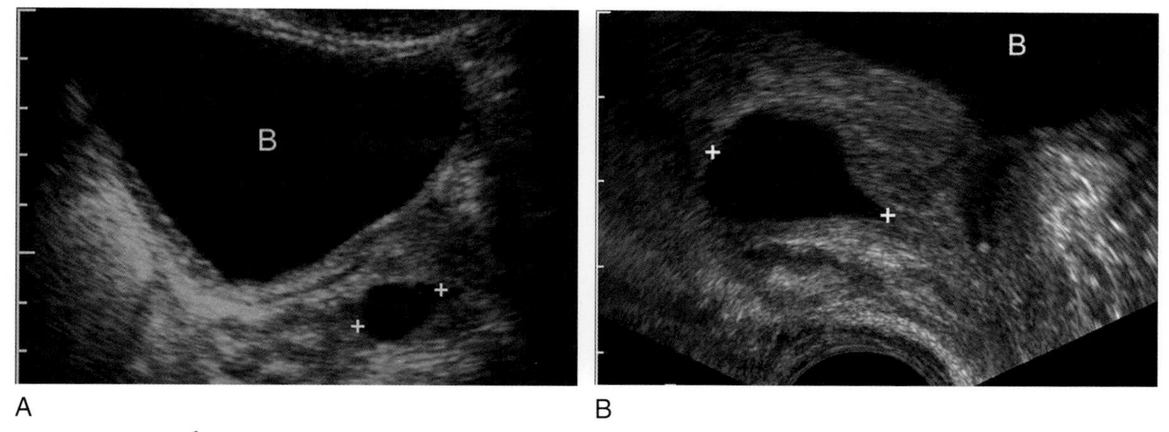

Figure 6-57 Prostatic utricle cyst. **A,** Transabdominal view through the filled urinary bladder (B) shows an ovoid cyst in the midline of the prostate *(cursors)*. **B,** Midline transrectal view in another patient shows a teardrop-shaped cyst in the superior aspect of the prostate *(cursors)*. The bladder (B) is seen superiorly.

Key Features

- The most important characteristics of a scrotal mass from the standpoint of determining its neoplastic vs. non-neoplastic nature is its location (intratesticular vs. extratesticular), tissue characteristics (cystic vs. solid/mixed), vascularity (detectable vs. nondetectable), and physical examination findings (palpable vs. nonpalpable).
- Seminomas are usually hypoechoic and homogeneous.
- Nonseminomatous germ cell tumors are usually heterogeneous and frequently have cystic components and calcifications.
- The most common scrotal mass is the spermatocele.
- Most hydroceles, especially large ones, are idiopathic. Hydroceles also occur with tumors, torsion, inflammatory disorders, and trauma.
- Varicoceles are very common and appear as enlarged, multiple, tortuous veins in the peritesticular region. Eighty-five percent are on the left, and 15% are bilateral. Isolated right varicoceles are rare.
- Epidermoid cysts typically have peripheral calcification or an "onion peel" appearance.
- The testis can act as a sanctuary site for lymphoma and leukemia.
- Testicular microlithiasis is seen in many patients with germ cell tumors. Isolated microlithiasis likely increases the risk of germ cell tumors but only minimally. Patients with isolated microlithiasis should have annual physical examinations and perform periodic self-examinations. Repeated follow-up sonograms have a very low yield and are probably not warranted.
- Testicular torsion may appear normal on gray-scale imaging. Detectable gray-scale abnormalities seen in some patients include an enlarged hypoechoic testis, a torsion knot, a reactive hydrocele, and scrotal wall thickening. The diagnosis is made by detecting decreased or absent blood flow to the testis.
- Epididymitis and orchitis can produce an enlarged, hypoechoic, and hypervascular epididymis and testis. Epididymitis is frequently focal. Orchitis is usually diffuse.
- Bladder cancer and blood clots can be distinguished by looking for mobility and detectable vascularity.
- Transvaginal and transperineal sonography are effective ways to evaluate women with suspected urethral diverticula and periurethral abnormalities.
- Normal penile Doppler should have a deep cavernosal velocity that exceeds 35 cm/sec after injection of a vasoactive substance.
- Peyronie's disease causes plaque formation in the tunica albuginea of the corpora cavernosa.
- The main role of prostate sonography is to help guide transrectal prostate biopsies. Screening for prostate cancer currently consists of measuring the PSA levels and digital rectal examinations.
- Seventy percent of prostate cancers are hypoechoic and located in the peripheral zone.

SUGGESTED READINGS

Atkinson GO Jr, et al: The normal and abnormal scrotum in children: Evaluation with color Doppler sonography. AJR Am J Roentgenol 158:613, 1992.

Backus ML, Mack LA, Middleton WD, et al: Testicular microlithiasis: Imaging appearances and pathologic correlation. Radiology 192:781-785, 1994.

Balconi G, Angeli E, Nessi R, et al: Ultrasonographic evaluation of Peyronie's disease. Urol Radiol 10:85-88, 1988.

Bennett HF, Middleton WD, Bullock AF, Teefey SA: Sonographic follow-up of patients with testicular microlithiasis. Radiology 218:359-363, 2001.

Berman LH, Bearcroft PW, Spector S: Ultrasound of the male anterior urethra. Ultrasound Q 18:123-133, 2002.

Brown DL, et al: Cystic testicular mass caused by dilated rete testis: Sonographic findings in 31 cases. AJR Am J Roentgenol 158:1257, 1992.

Burks DD, et al: Suspected testicular torsion and ischemia: Evaluation with color Doppler sonography. Radiology 175:815, 1990.

Cannon ML, Finger MJ, Bulas DI: Case report: Manual testicular detorsion aided by color Doppler ultrasonography. J Ultrasound Med 14:407-409, 1995.

Cass AS, Cass BP, Veeraraghavan K: Immediate exploration of the unilateral acute scrotum in young male subjects. J Urol 124:829, 1980.

Catalona WJ, et al: Measurement of prostate-specific antigen in serum as a screening test for prostate cancer. N Engl J Med 324:1156, 1991.

Cheng S, Rifkin MD: Color Doppler imaging of the prostate: Important adjunct to endorectal ultrasound of the prostate in the diagnosis of prostate cancer. Ultrasound Q 17:185-189, 2001.

Choyke PL: Imaging of prostate cancer. Abdom Imaging 20:505-515, 1995.

Dubin L, Amelar RD: Varicocele. Urol Clin North Am 5:563, 1978.

Dyke CH, Toi A, Sweet JM: Value of random US-guided transrectal prostate biopsy. Radiology 176:345, 1990.

Eskey CJ, et al: Malignant lymphoma of the testis. AJR Am J Roentgenol 169:822.

Fournier GR Jr, et al: High resolution scrotal ultrasonography: A highly sensitive but nonspecific diagnostic technique. J Urol 134:490, 1985.

Frauscher F, Klauser A, Halpern EJ: Advances in ultrasound for the detection of prostate cancer. Ultrasound Q 18: 135-142, 2002.

Gooding GAW, Leonhardt W, Stein R: Testicular cysts: US findings. Radiology 163:537, 1987.

Gooding GAW, et al. Cholesterol crystals in hydroceles: Sonographic detection and possible significance. AJR Am J Roentgenol 169:527-529, 1997.

Gordon LM, et al. Traumatic epididymitis: Evaluation with color Doppler sonography. AJR Am J Roentgenol 166: 1323-1325, 1996.

Halpern EJ, Frauscher F, Strup SE, et al: Prostate: high-frequency Doppler US imaging for cancer detection. Radiology 225:71-77, 2002.

Hamm B, Fobbe F, Loy V: Testicular cysts: Differentiation with US and clinical findings. Radiology 168:19, 1988.

Hamper UM, et al: Cystic lesions of the prostate gland: A sonographic-pathologic correlation. J Ultrasound Med 9: 395, 1990.

Horstman WG, et al: Color Doppler US of the scrotum. Radiographics 11:941, 1991.

Horstman WG, et al: Testicular tumors: Findings with color Doppler US. Radiology 185:733, 1992.

Horstman WG, Haluszka MM, Burkhard TB: Management of testicular masses incidentally discovered by ultrasound. J Urol 151:1263-1265, 1994.

Horstman WG, Middleton WD, Melson GL: Scrotal inflammatory disease: Color Doppler US findings. Radiology 179:55, 1991.

Horstman WG: Scrotal imaging. Urol Clin North Am 24: 653-671, 1997.

Karcnik TJ, Simmons MZ, Abujudea HA: Ultrasound imaging of the adult urinary bladder. Ultrasound Q 15:135-147, 1999.

Kaye KW, Richter L: Ultrasonographic anatomy of the normal prostate gland: reconstruction by computer graphics. Urology 35:12-17, 1990.

Kuligowska E, Barish MA, Fenlon HM, Blake M: Predictors of prostate carcinoma: Accuracy of gray-scale and color Doppler US and serum markers. Radiology 220:757-764, 2001.

Lerner RM, et al: Color Doppler US in the evaluation of acute scrotal disease. Radiology 176:355, 1990.

Leung ML, Gooding GA, Williams RD: High-resolution sonography of scrotal contents in asymptomatic subjects. AJR Am J Roentgenol 143:161, 1984.

Marsman JW: Clinical versus subclinical varicocele: Venographic findings and improvement of fertility after embolization. Radiology 155:635, 1985.

Martinez-Berganza MT, Sarria L, Cozcolluela R, et al: Cysts of the tunica albuginea: Sonographic appearance. AJR Am J Roentgenol 170:183-185, 1998.

Middleton WD, et al: Acute scrotal disorders: Prospective comparison of color Doppler US and testicular scintigraphy. Radiology 177:177, 1990.

Middleton WD, Bell MW: Analysis of intratesticular arterial anatomy with emphasis on transmediastinal arteries. Radiology 189:157, 1993.

Middleton WD, Melson GL: Testicular ischemia: Color Doppler sonographic findings in five patients. AJR Am J Roentgenol 152:1237, 1989.

Middleton WD, Middleton MA, Dierks M, et al: Sonographic prediction of viability in testicular torsion. J Ultrasound Med 16:23-27, 1997.

Middleton WD, Thorne DA, Melson GL: Color Doppler ultrasound of the normal testis. AJR Am J Roentgenol 152:293, 1989.

Middleton WD, Teefey SA, Santillan C: Testicular microlithiasis: Prospective analysis of prevalence and associated tumor. Radiology 224:425-428, 2002.

Moghe PK, Brady AP: Ultrasound of testicular epidermoid cysts. Br J Radiol 72:942-945, 1999.

Morey AF, McAninch JW: Ultrasound evaluation of the male urethra for assessment of urethral stricture. J Clin Ultrasound 24:473-479, 1996.

Morey AF, McAninch JW: Sonographic staging of anterior urethral strictures. J Urol 163:1070-1075, 2000.

Ngheim HT, Kellman GM, Sandberg SA, Craig BM: Cystic lesions of the prostate. Radiographics 10:635-650, 1990.

Nghiem HT, et al: Cystic lesions of the prostate. Radiographics 10:635, 1990.

Pavlica P, Barozzi L: Ultrasound of penile tumors and trauma. Ultrasound Q 14:95-109, 1998.

Phillips G, Kumari-Subaiya S, Sawitsky A: Ultrasonic evaluation of the scrotum in lymphoproliferative disease. J Ultrasound Med 6:169, 1987.

Rifkin MD, et al: Comparison of magnetic resonance imaging and ultrasonography in staging early prostate cancer: Results of a multi-institutional cooperative trial. N Engl J Med 323:621, 1990.

Rifkin MD, McGlynn ET, Choi H: Echogenicity of prostate cancer correlated with histologic grade and stromal fibrosis: Endorectal US studies. Radiology 170:549, 1989.

Rifkin MD: Biopsy techniques of the prostate. Ultrasound Q 15:162-183, 1999.

Schwerk WB, Schwerk WN, Rodeck G: Testicular tumors: Prospective analysis of real-time US patterns and abdominal staging. Radiology 164:369, 1987.

Shawker TH, et al: Intratesticular masses associated with abnormally functioning adrenal glands. J Clin Ultrasound 2:51-58, 1992.

Siegel C, Middleton WD, Teefey SA, et al: Sonography of the female urethra. AJR Am J Roentgenol 170:1269-1272, 1998.

Silverberg E: Cancer in young adults (ages 15 to 34). CA Cancer J Clin 32:32, 1982.

Steinfeld AD: Testicular germ cell tumors: Review of contemporary evaluation and management. Radiology 175:603, 1990.

Tackett RE, et al: High resolution sonography in diagnosing testicular neoplasms: Clinical significance of false positive scans. J Urol 135:494, 1986.

Thornbury JR, Ornstein DK, Choyke PL, et al: Review: Prostate cancer: What is the future role for imaging? AJR Am J Roentgenol 176:17-22, 2001.

Weingarten BJ, Kellman GM, Middleton WD, Gross ML: Tubular ectasia within the mediastinum testis. J Ultrasound Med 11:349-353, 1992.

Williamson RC: Torsion of the testis and allied conditions. Br J Surg 63:465, 1976.

Woodward PJ, Sohaey R, O'Donoghue MJ, Green DE: Tumors and tumorlike lesions of the testis: Radiologic-pathologic correlation. Radiographics 22:189-216, 2002.

Wong-You-Cheong JJ, Wagner BJ, Davis CJ Jr: From the Archives of the AFIP: Transitional cell carcinoma of the urinary tract: Radiologic-pathologic correlation. Radiographics 18: 123-142, 1998.

CHAPTER 7

Pancreas

ANATOMY

The pancreas is a retroperitoneal organ that develops from a large dorsal embryologic anlage and a smaller ventral anlage. The dorsal pancreatic anlage communicates by means of its central duct with the duodenum, and the ventral anlage communicates with the biliary tract. During embryologic development these pancreatic anlagen rotate with the intestinal structures and ultimately fuse together so that the dorsal pancreas is located anterior and superior to the ventral pancreas. The associated pancreatic ductal structures rotate with the parenchymal structures so that the dorsal pancreatic duct empties into the duodenum several centimeters above the ventral duct. The ventral duct connects to the distal common bile duct at the ampulla. In 15% to 20% of persons these embryologic ductal anatomic characteristics persist, with a short ventral duct that drains the head of the pancreas by way of the major papilla and a long dorsal duct that drains the remainder of the pancreas through the minor papilla. This is referred to as pancreas divisum. In most individuals the two ducts join and the minor papilla regresses so that the entire gland is drained through one duct that empties into the major papilla. Several other ductal patterns exist, but none are visible sonographically.

The pancreas is divided into a head, neck, body, tail, and uncinate process. The uncinate process extends inferiorly and medially from the head and is the only part of the pancreas that is located posterior to the superior mesenteric vein. The head is located to the right of the mesenteric vessels, and the neck and body are located anterior to these vessels. The tail of the pancreas is located to the left of the mesenteric vessels and extends superiorly and posteriorly to the region of the splenic hilum. In some references the tail of the pancreas is said to be that part that extends to the left of the vertebral column.

Because of its size, location, and echogenicity, the pancreas is one of the more difficult abdominal organs to image sonographically. For this reason adjacent vascular landmarks are used to help in the localization of the pancreas (Fig. 7-1). The head of the pancreas is located immediately anterior to the inferior vena cava. However, when patients are in the left lateral decubitus or left posterior oblique position, the head of the pancreas may slide somewhat to the left so that it is located over the aorta. The body and tail of the pancreas are located anterior to the splenic vein and the portal splenic confluence. The trifurcation of the celiac axis is located just superior to the pancreas, and the splenic artery generally runs near the superior aspect of the pancreas. The gastroduodenal artery arises from the common hepatic artery and travels inferiorly directly over the anterior and lateral aspects of the pancreatic head. The superior mesenteric vein is immediately adjacent to the posterior aspect of the pancreatic neck and body and to the medial aspect of the pancreatic head. There is no retroperitoneal fat between the superior mesenteric vein or the portosplenic confluence and the pancreas. There is, however, a prominent ring of retroperitoneal fat that separates the superior mesenteric artery from the pancreas.

The pancreatic duct is seen segmentally in 85% of patients. It is most commonly seen in the body, where its walls are perpendicular to the sound beam (see

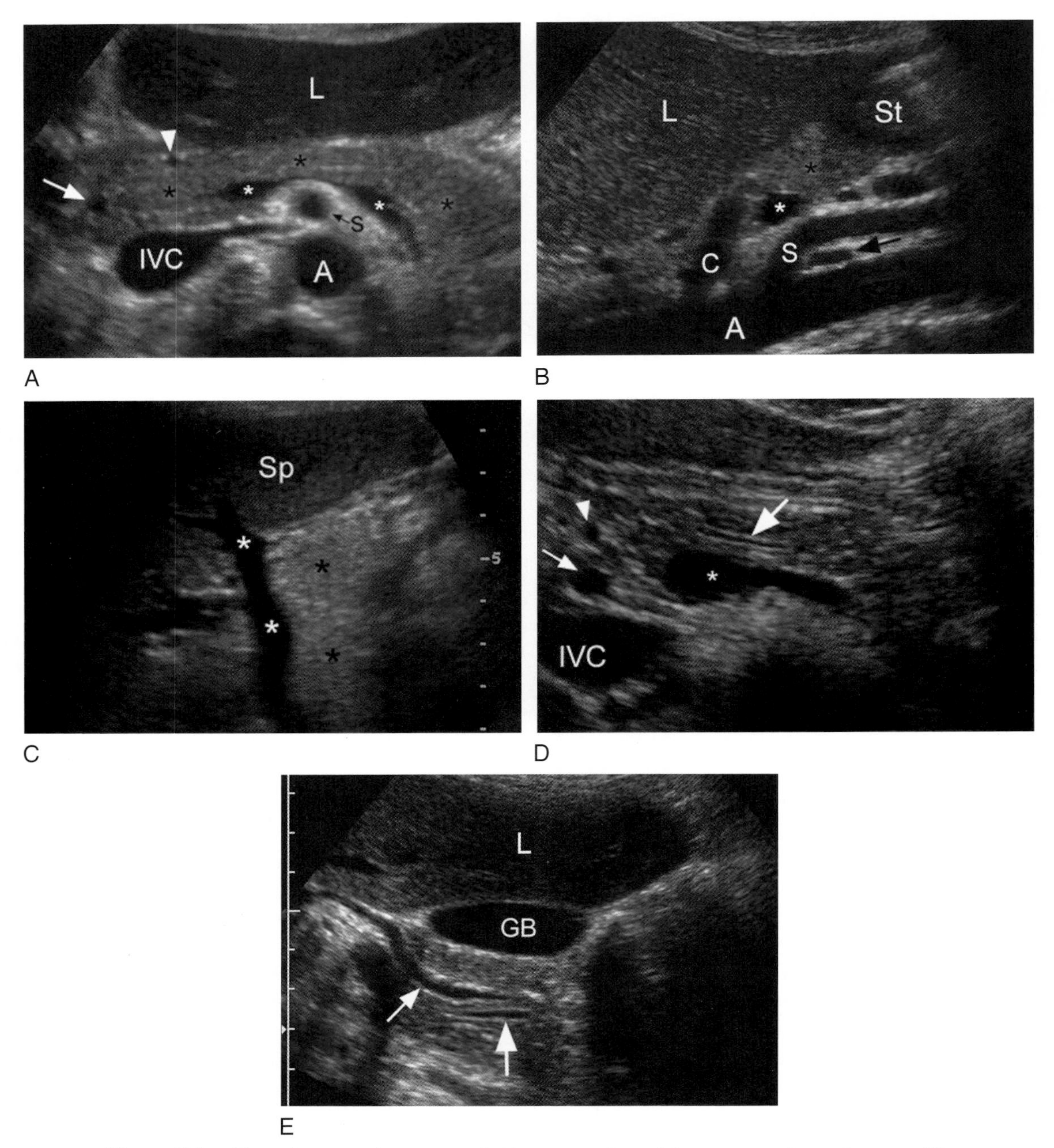

Figure 7-1 Normal pancreatic anatomy. **A,** Transverse view of the pancreas shows the aorta (A), inferior vena cava (IVC), superior mesenteric artery (S), portal splenic confluence *(white asterisks),* head, body, and tail of the pancreas *(black asterisks),* left lobe of the liver (L), common bile duct *(arrow),* and gastroduodenal artery *(arrowhead).* **B,** Longitudinal view of the body of the pancreas shows aorta (A), superior mesenteric artery (S), celiac axis (C), splenic vein *(white asterisk),* body of pancreas *(black asterisk),* left lobe of liver (L), stomach (St), and left renal vein *(black arrow).* **C,** Coronal view of the left upper quadrant shows the spleen (Sp), splenic vein *(white asterisks),* and pancreatic tail *(black asterisks).* **D,** Transverse view of the pancreas shows the pancreatic duct *(large arrow).* Also seen is the portal splenic confluence *(white asterisk),* inferior vena cava (IVC), common bile duct *(small white arrow),* and gastroduodenal artery *(arrowhead).* **E,** Right semicoronal view of the pancreatic head shows the distal common bile duct *(small arrow)* and the pancreatic duct *(large arrow).* Also seen are the liver (L) and the gallbladder (GB).

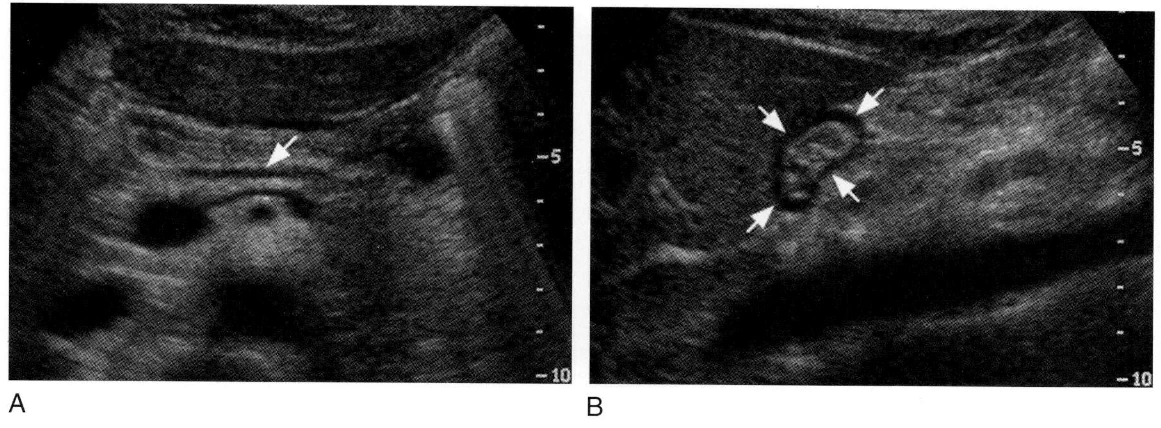

Figure 7-2 Pseudoduct caused by posterior gastric wall. **A,** Transverse view of the epigastrium shows what appears to be a hypoechoic tubular structure *(arrow)* running in the expected location of the main pancreatic duct. **B,** Longitudinal view through the same region shows that the structure actually represents the hypoechoic muscular layer of the wall of the stomach *(arrows).* It communicates with the superior, inferior, and anterior aspects of the gastric wall and forms the typical bull's eye appearance of an intestinal structure.

Fig. 7-1D). The portion of the pancreatic duct that travels through the head is more difficult to visualize sonographically. However, it is occasionally seen medial to the distal common bile duct and should not be confused with the bile duct or with a low-inserting cystic duct (see Fig. 7-1E). When the luminal diameter is very small, the pancreatic duct may appear as a single bright line. In most cases the diameter is sufficient to allow for resolution of both the anterior and posterior duct walls. The walls of the pancreatic duct should be smooth and parallel. Three millimeters is commonly used as the upper limit of normal for duct diameter in the body of the pancreas. However, the duct enlarges with age, and this should be considered when scanning young and elderly patients. In some patients the hypoechoic wall of the posterior surface of the stomach rests on the anterior surface of the pancreas and can be confused with the pancreatic duct on transverse views (Fig. 7-2). This potential pitfall is easy to avoid by scanning in the sagittal plane where the posterior wall of the stomach can be seen in continuity with the rest of the stomach wall.

Pancreatic echogenicity is variable, depending on the amount of fatty replacement. The normal pancreas is equal to, or more echogenic than, the normal liver. The pancreas may be hypoechoic, isoechoic, or hyperechoic with respect to the spleen. With age, pancreatic echogenicity increases as the result of fatty replacement. In general, the pancreas is homogeneous in echotexture. When the head is seen well, it is often possible to identify a focal area of decreased echogenicity in the posterior half of the pancreatic head. This is related to the lower fat content of the ventral embryologic anlage. This normal variant can be distinguished from pathologic processes that cause decreased pancreatic echogenicity (e.g., cancer and pancreatitis) by its straight border, lack of mass effect, and lack of biliary or pancreatic ductal dilation (Fig. 7-3).

The anteroposterior dimension of the pancreas varies throughout the gland, and the upper limit of normal for pancreatic measurements varies greatly from study to study. For practical purposes one can generally assume that the pancreas is abnormally enlarged when the thickness of the head, body, and tail is equal to or greater

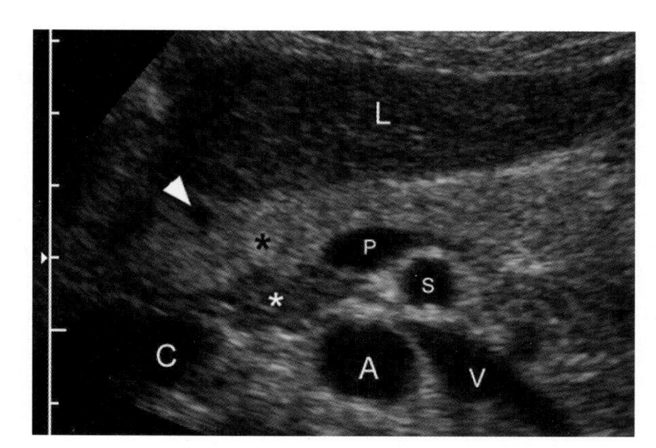

Figure 7-3 Normal pancreatic head variant due to differential fat infiltration. Transverse view of the pancreas shows the normal hyperechoic appearance to the anterior head *(black asterisk)* and a hypoechoic appearance to the posterior pancreatic head and uncinate process *(white asterisk).* Also seen is the aorta (A), inferior vena cava (C), left renal vein (V), superior mesenteric artery (S), portal splenic confluence (P), left lobe of the liver (L), and gastroduodenal artery *(arrowhead).*

Table 7-1 Normal Characteristics

Characteristic	Normal Finding
Size	Head, <3 cm; body, <2.5 cm; tail, <2.5 cm
Pancreatic duct	Smooth, diameter <3 mm
Echogenicity	>Liver, > or < or = spleen
Echotexture	Homogeneous
Surface	Smooth to slightly lobular

than 3.0, 2.5, and 2.0 cm, respectively. (See Table 7-1 for the normal characteristics of the pancreas.)

TECHNIQUE

The pancreas should be scanned with the patient in a fasting state to minimize the interference caused by overlying bowel gas. In most patients the body of the pancreas is well seen from an anterior subxiphoid approach using the left lobe of the liver as an acoustic window (see Fig. 7-1A and B). This is generally aided by a deep inspiration. In some cases visualization of the body of the pancreas is improved by having the patient try to push the abdomen out and make a "beer belly." Portions of the head of the pancreas are usually seen when the same anterior approach is employed as that used to see the body. However, it is often necessary to scan from a right subcostal approach with the transducer angled slightly medially to see the lateral portions of the pancreatic head that are not well seen from an anterior approach. This view can be aided by positioning the patient in a left posterior oblique position. When this approach is used, the relationship of the pancreatic head to the adjacent structures will differ from that visualized by the more familiar anterior approach.

The tail of the pancreas is difficult to see in its entirety using an anterior approach. To see the pancreatic tail well, it may be necessary to have the patient drink water and to use the resulting fluid-filled stomach as a window. Scanning from a left lateral intercostal approach and using the spleen as a window also helps to image the region of the pancreatic tail. The tail of the pancreas is located in the splenic hilum, immediately anterior to the left kidney and inferior to the splenic vein. Therefore, by scanning in a coronal plane and starting with a transplenic view of the upper pole of the kidney, an anterior angulation of the probe will bring the tail of the pancreas into view (see Fig. 7-1C).

The uncinate process of the pancreas should be viewed in a manner similar to that used for the pancreatic head. It is important to remember that the uncinate process extends quite inferiorly with respect to the pancreatic head and body; therefore, uncinate abnormalities can be easily overlooked if the scans are not extended inferiorly enough.

PANCREATITIS

Acute pancreatitis can be caused by a wide variety of abnormalities. The most common are alcohol abuse and gallstones. Less common causes include biliary crystals/sludge, peptic ulcers, trauma, pregnancy, drugs, mumps, endoscopic retrograde cholangiopancreatography (ERCP), tumors, hypercalcemia, hyperlipoproteinemia, and familial pancreatitis. The typical presenting features are upper abdominal and back pain and elevated levels of pancreatic enzymes in the blood or urine. The disease may be mild and respond well to supportive therapy, or it may progress to severe multisystem failure. Unfortunately, there are no pathognomonic clinical or laboratory findings that permit a definitive diagnosis of pancreatitis to be made.

One of the major roles of sonography in patients with pancreatitis is to evaluate the biliary tract for stone disease. This not only can identify the cause of the pancreatitis, but the findings can also be used to determine what the appropriate management should be, such as cholecystectomy and, if necessary, preoperative ERCP. The detection of biliary obstruction is also quite important, because many of these patients have coexistent liver disease and the source of abnormal liver function tests may be difficult to sort out clinically. Obstruction of the bile ducts in patients with pancreatitis may be caused by either a stone or a stricture in the distal common bile duct or by compression of the common bile duct by either a pseudocyst or the inflammatory swelling of the pancreatic head.

The pancreas itself may appear normal in mild cases of acute pancreatitis, and sonography should not be used to exclude the diagnosis. Nevertheless, when the pancreas does appear normal, other upper abdominal structures should be evaluated carefully to try and establish an alternative diagnosis such as cholecystitis.

Pancreatic enlargement, decreased pancreatic echogenicity, and heterogeneous echogenicity are the sonographic hallmarks of acute pancreatitis (Fig. 7-4A, B). The determination of pancreatic echogenicity relies on comparison with the echogenicity of the liver. When the liver is fatty infiltrated and abnormally echogenic, the pancreas may appear hypoechoic even though it is normal.

Alteration in the size and echogenicity of the pancreas is often subtle, and the diagnosis of pancreatitis is frequently based on the visualization of peripancreatic fluid collections in a patient with an appropriate clinical

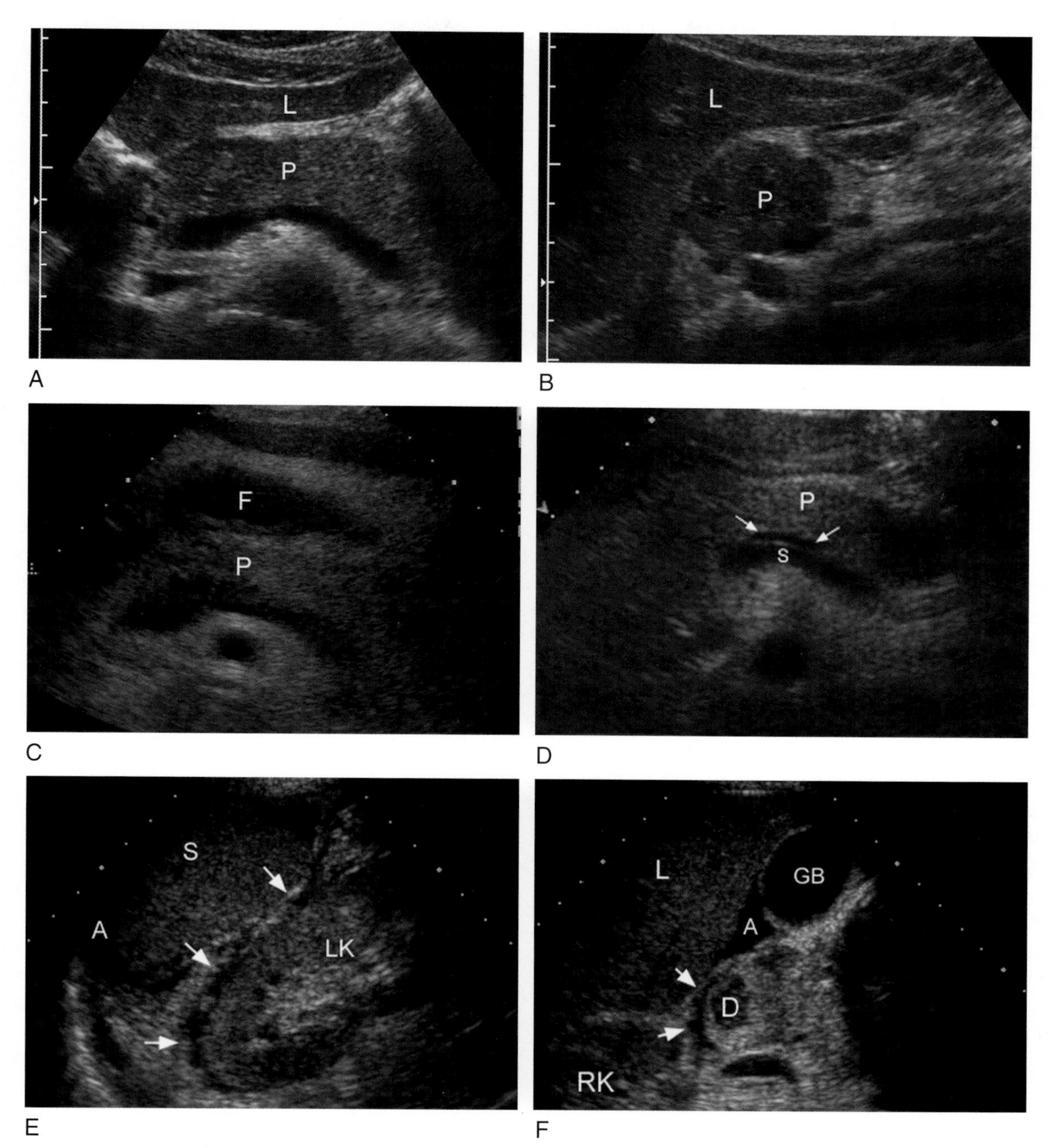

Figure 7-4 Acute pancreatitis in different patients. **A,** Transverse view shows an enlarged swollen pancreas (P) that is isoechoic to the adjacent liver (L). **B,** Longitudinal view shows an enlarged pancreas (P) that is isoechoic to the adjacent liver (L). On longitudinal views the body of the pancreas should be oval with an anteroposterior diameter that is less than its craniocaudal diameter. In this case the pancreas appears round. **C,** Transverse view of the pancreas (P) shows a localized peripancreatic fluid collection (F). **D,** Transverse view of the pancreas (P) shows a small collection of fluid *(arrows)* in the perivascular space anterior to the splenic vein (S). **E,** Coronal view of the left upper quadrant shows retroperitoneal fluid *(arrows)* in the perirenal region around the left kidney (LK). A small amount of ascites (A) is also seen around the spleen (S). **F,** Transverse view of the right upper quadrant shows a small amount of retroperitoneal fluid *(arrows)* between the duodenum (D) and the right kidney (RK). Also seen is ascites (A) between the gallbladder (GB) and liver (L).

history. Using an anterior subxiphoid approach, sonography can visualize fluid collections around the body of the pancreas in many patients (see Fig. 7-4C). Fluid may accumulate in a mantle anterior, superior, and inferior to the pancreas. It may also dissect along the portal splenic confluence and the superior mesenteric vein, producing so-called perivascular cloaking (see Fig. 7-4D). By using a left lateral approach and the spleen as a window, sonography can identify fluid in the left anterior pararenal space, the left perirenal space, and the interfascial plane (see Fig. 7-4E). Similar collections can be seen from a right lateral approach using the liver as a window (see Fig. 7-4F). Identifying fluid collections around the left and right kidneys and the duodenum is extremely useful when visualization of the pancreas is limited or when the pancreas appears normal. Therefore, these areas should be scanned carefully whenever pancreatitis is a consideration. (See Box 7-1 for a summary of the sonographic signs of acute pancreatitis.)

The changes seen with pancreatitis are usually diffuse but can, on occasion, be focal. Focal pancreatitis usually involves the pancreatic head (Fig. 7-5). It can be extremely difficult to distinguish focal pancreatitis from pancreatic cancer. Vascular invasion or other evidence of metastatic disease helps to establish the diagnosis of cancer, and history and clinical features help to establish the diagnosis of focal pancreatitis. Follow-up studies, ERCP, and biopsies are all necessary in some patients.

There are a number of complications that can occur in conjunction with acute pancreatitis (Box 7-2). One of the most common is pseudocyst formation. Pseudocysts are walled-off fluid collections that have a capsule composed of fibrous tissue rather than true epithelial cells. They can form virtually anywhere, but most are located within or near the pancreas. Their sonographic appearance differs from that of other fluid collections in patients with pancreatitis in that they have well-defined smooth margins and are loculated (Fig. 7-6). Their internal contents are usually anechoic, but the presence of debris can result in low-level internal echoes. Hemorrhage and infection can also produce complex internal echoes within a pseudocyst.

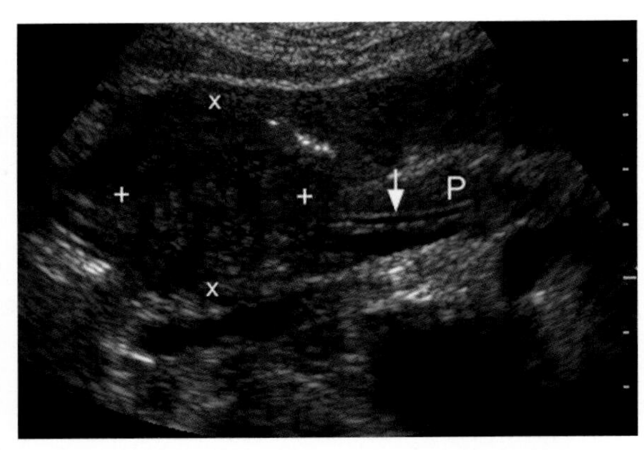

Figure 7-5 Focal pancreatitis. Transverse view of the pancreas shows a mass *(cursors)* in the region of the pancreatic head and a normal-appearing pancreatic body (P). Note that the pancreatic duct *(arrow)* is not dilated (pancreatic cancer in this location would typically result in pancreatic ductal obstruction). This patient had a history of recurrent pancreatitis.

The differential diagnosis of cystic pancreatic lesions is relatively broad. Besides pancreatitis, other causes of pancreatic cysts include cystic neoplasms, cysts related to autosomal dominant polycystic disease, von Hippel-Lindau disease (Fig. 7-7), and cystic fibrosis. In addition, pancreatic cysts can be mimicked by vascular lesions such as tortuous splenic arteries, splenic artery or splenic vein aneurysms (Fig. 7-8), and splenic artery pseudoaneurysms. Because of this, Doppler evaluation of suspected pancreatic cysts should always be performed, particularly if percutaneous drainage is being considered for treatment.

A number of vascular complications can occur in conjunction with pancreatitis. Thrombosis of the peripancreatic veins can arise as the result of compression and flow stasis. The splenic vein is involved most frequently, but the superior mesenteric vein may also be affected. Extension into the portal vein is also well described. Splenic vein thrombosis should be suspected whenever gastric varices are seen in the absence of associated esophageal varices. This stems from the formation of collaterals that extend from the short gastric veins to

Box 7-1 Sonographic Signs of Acute Pancreatitis

Decreased or heterogeneous pancreatic echogenicity
Pancreatic enlargement
Peripancreatic fluid collections
Perivascular fluid collections
Periduodenal fluid collections
Pararenal fluid collections

Box 7-2 Complications of Pancreatitis

Pseudocyst formation
Bile duct obstruction
Pancreatic abscess
Pancreatic necrosis
Venous thrombosis
Pseudoaneurysm

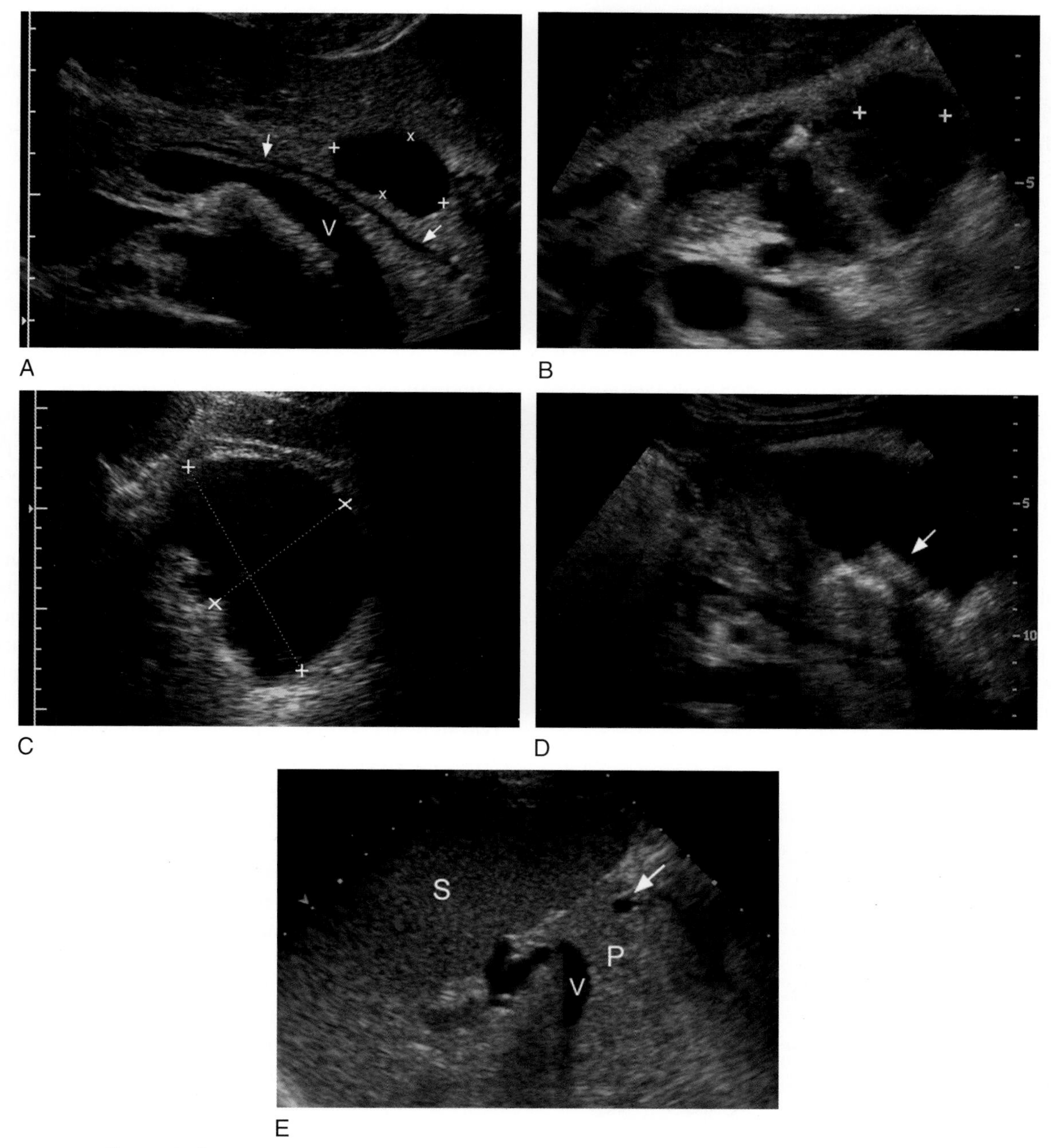

Figure 7-6 Pancreatic pseudocysts in different patients. **A,** Transverse view of the pancreas shows a well-defined fluid collection *(cursors)* anterior to the pancreatic tail typical of a pseudocyst. Also seen are a normal pancreatic duct *(arrows)* and the splenic vein (V). **B,** Transverse view in the region of the pancreatic body and tail shows complex peripancreatic fluid collection with one area that is beginning to liquefy and wall off *(cursors)* consistent with a developing pseudocyst. **C,** View of the left upper quadrant shows a minimally complex, slightly irregularly marginated fluid collection *(cursors)* with no identifiable adjacent anatomic structures. Pseudocysts should be considered when abdominal fluid collections are seen in patients with known pancreatitis. **D,** Transverse view of the epigastrium and left upper quadrant shows a pseudocyst with internal echogenic debris *(arrow)*. **E,** Coronal view of the left upper quadrant using a transplenic (S) view. Within the pancreatic tail (P) is a small cyst *(arrow)* that is nonspecific but in a patient with a history of pancreatitis most likely represents a pseudocyst. Also seen is the splenic vein (V). The small cyst seen in this image could not be seen from standard anterior views and illustrates the value of the transplenic view of the pancreatic tail.

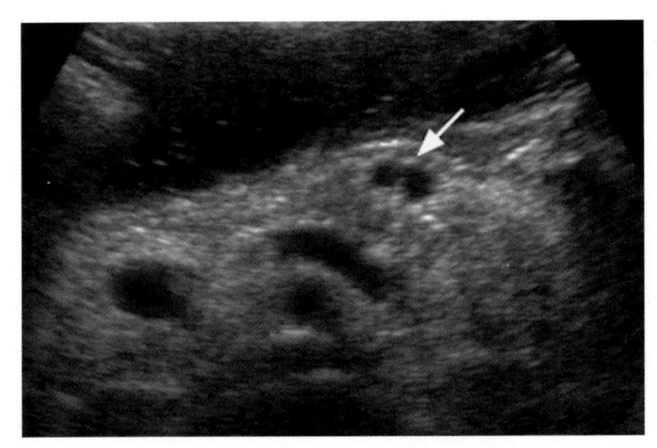

Figure 7-7 Pancreatic cyst in Von Hippel-Lindau disease. Transverse view of the pancreas using a fluid-filled stomach as a window shows a small bilobed cyst *(arrow)* in the pancreatic body.

the coronary vein and gastroepiploic veins. Pseudoaneurysms can also form as the result of erosion of the adjacent arteries produced by the proteolytic pancreatic enzymes. The splenic artery is involved most commonly, but any branch of the celiac axis can be affected. The gray-scale appearance of many pseudoaneurysms is similar to that of pseudocysts (Fig. 7-9). Detecting them sonographically requires a high level of suspicion combined with Doppler evaluation of any cystic mass in or around the pancreas. Predominantly thrombosed

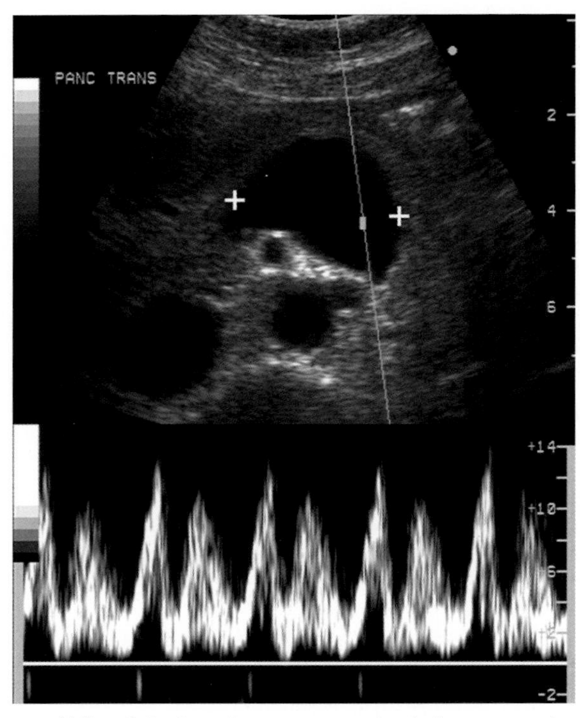

Figure 7-8 Splenic vein aneurysm simulating a pseudocyst. Transverse view shows an anechoic lesion *(cursors)* in the region of the pancreatic body. Although this mimics a cyst, pulsed Doppler waveform shows pulsatile venous flow, confirming the vascular nature of this lesion.

pseudoaneurysms can be very difficult to diagnose correctly, because they can closely simulate the characteristics of solid pancreatic masses. When the solid material appears laminated, this may indicate sequential development of thrombus and a pseudoaneurysm should be suspected. However, in most cases there are no distinguishing characteristics other than the presence of blood flow somewhere within the lumen.

Chronic pancreatitis is the permanent impairment of exocrine pancreatic function and permanent morphologic change in the gland as the result of persistent pancreatic inflammation. Pain may or may not be present, and acute exacerbations may or may not occur.

The classic sonographic sign of chronic pancreatitis is pancreatic calcifications (Fig. 7-10A to C). These typically appear as multifocal, punctate, hyperechoic foci in the pancreas. Shadowing may or may not be present, depending on the size and extent of calcification. Calcifications form as a consequence of increased pancreatic protein secretion and the subsequent calcification of intraductal protein plugs. Pancreatic calcifications occur commonly in the setting of alcoholic pancreatitis (20% to 40%) but rarely in the setting of gallstone pancreatitis (<2%). Although the pancreatic calcifications are intraductal, this is generally not apparent on imaging studies, which show them to be scattered in the pancreatic parenchyma. When calcifications erode from the small side branches into the main pancreatic duct, or form primarily in the main duct, they can cause pancreatic ductal obstruction and lead to persistent recurrent pancreatitis (see Fig. 7-10D).

Dilatation of the pancreatic duct is another sign of chronic pancreatitis (see Fig. 7-10E and F). In many cases associated short strictures produce alternating areas of narrowing and dilatation that are referred to as a chain of lakes. Tortuosity of the pancreatic duct is also typical of chronic pancreatitis. However, both of these patterns can be seen in patients with ductal obstruction due to pancreatic cancer. Therefore, a tortuous or beaded-appearing dilated duct should not be viewed as a pathognomonic sign of chronic pancreatitis.

As with acute pancreatitis, chronic pancreatitis can cause focal masses to develop that may be difficult to distinguish from cancers. The presence of calcifications is helpful in suggesting the diagnosis of focal pancreatitis, and an appropriate clinical history is also valuable. Nevertheless, other diagnostic studies such as CT, ultrasound-guided biopsies, or ERCP are often required.

PANCREATIC CARCINOMA

Pancreatic carcinoma is an adenocarcinoma arising from the ductal epithelium and constitutes more than 90% of all pancreatic tumors. Epithelial tumors arising

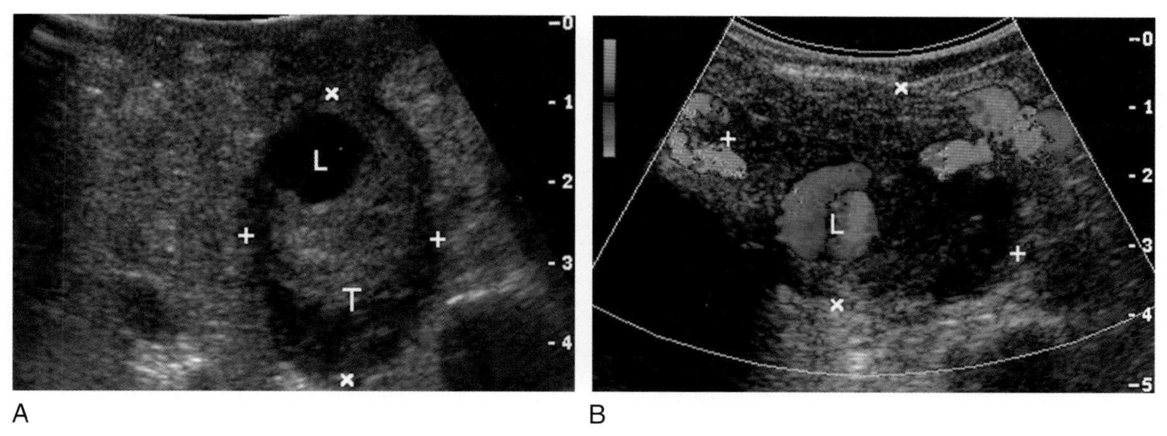

Figure 7-9 Pancreatic pseudoaneurysm seen on intraoperative scans. **A,** Transverse intraoperative scan of the pancreatic head region shows a complex lesion *(cursors).* There is hyperechoic and hypoechoic thrombus (T) as well as a well-defined residual pseudoaneurysm lumen (L). **B,** Semicoronal color Doppler view shows typical swirling pattern of intraluminal flow (L) in the aneurysm lumen. This case illustrates the need for performing Doppler analysis of cystic lesions in patients with pancreatitis.

from the acini are rare. Pancreatic carcinoma accounts for approximately 5% of all cancer deaths and is the fourth most common cause of cancer-related mortality, after lung, breast, and colon cancer. The 1-year survival is approximately 10%, with median survivals ranging from 3 to 8 months. Pancreatic carcinoma occurs primarily in elderly patients and is rare in those younger than the age of 40.

Most of the tumors arise in the pancreatic head, and the typical presenting symptom is painless jaundice. Thirty percent of the tumors occur in the body and tail, and in this setting nonspecific symptoms such as weight loss and pain tend to be the presenting features. Tumors in the head may be detected when small and potentially resectable because of the early biliary tract obstruction and jaundice that occur. On the other hand, tumors in the body and tail tend to present as larger masses and are only rarely resectable.

Sonographically, the vast majority of pancreatic cancers appear as hypoechoic masses when compared with the echogenicity of adjacent pancreatic parenchyma (Fig. 7-11A and B). They may or may not distort the contour of the pancreas, depending on their size and location. Obstruction of the common bile duct is common. Usually the dilated duct can be followed distally, and abrupt narrowing can be seen at the level of the pancreatic mass (see Fig. 7-11C and D). Obstruction of the pancreatic duct is a common finding in patients with pancreatic carcinoma (see Fig. 7-11E and F). In general, the duct appears less irregular and tortuous than does the ductal dilatation that is due to chronic pancreatitis. However, as mentioned earlier, there is overlap in the appearance of these diseases, and a careful search for a mass should be conducted in any patient with a dilated pancreatic duct. Pancreatic atrophy may be present in the segment of pancreas distal to the tumor. Although sonography is similar to CT in its ability to identify cancer in those portions of the pancreas that can be well visualized sonographically (typically the head and body), it cannot visualize the entire pancreas as consistently as does CT. Therefore, CT is the preferred imaging technique in patients with suspected pancreatic carcinoma. However, sonography is an extremely useful problem-solving tool in patients with equivocal CT results or in those with normal CT findings and a high suspicion of pancreatic carcinoma. ERCP is quite sensitive in detecting pancreatic cancer, but it is an invasive, costly procedure and can precipitate pancreatitis. In general, it can be reserved for those patients whose CT and ultrasound findings are nondiagnostic or for patients requiring the placement of biliary or pancreatic duct stents.

In addition to detecting the primary tumor, sonography should be directed at identifying tumor spread. Although the criteria for determining resectability vary among surgeons, typical contraindications to surgery include the presence of hepatic or peritoneal metastases, the involvement of extrapancreatic vessels, invasion of adjacent organs other than the duodenum, and the presence of malignant ascites. Invasion of adjacent vessels generally takes the form of vascular encasement by hypoechoic soft tissue. This can be detected by gray-scale sonography supplemented by color Doppler imaging (Fig. 7-12).

The differential diagnosis of hypoechoic pancreatic masses primarily includes pancreatic carcinoma and focal pancreatitis (Box 7-3). Focal pancreatitis can be

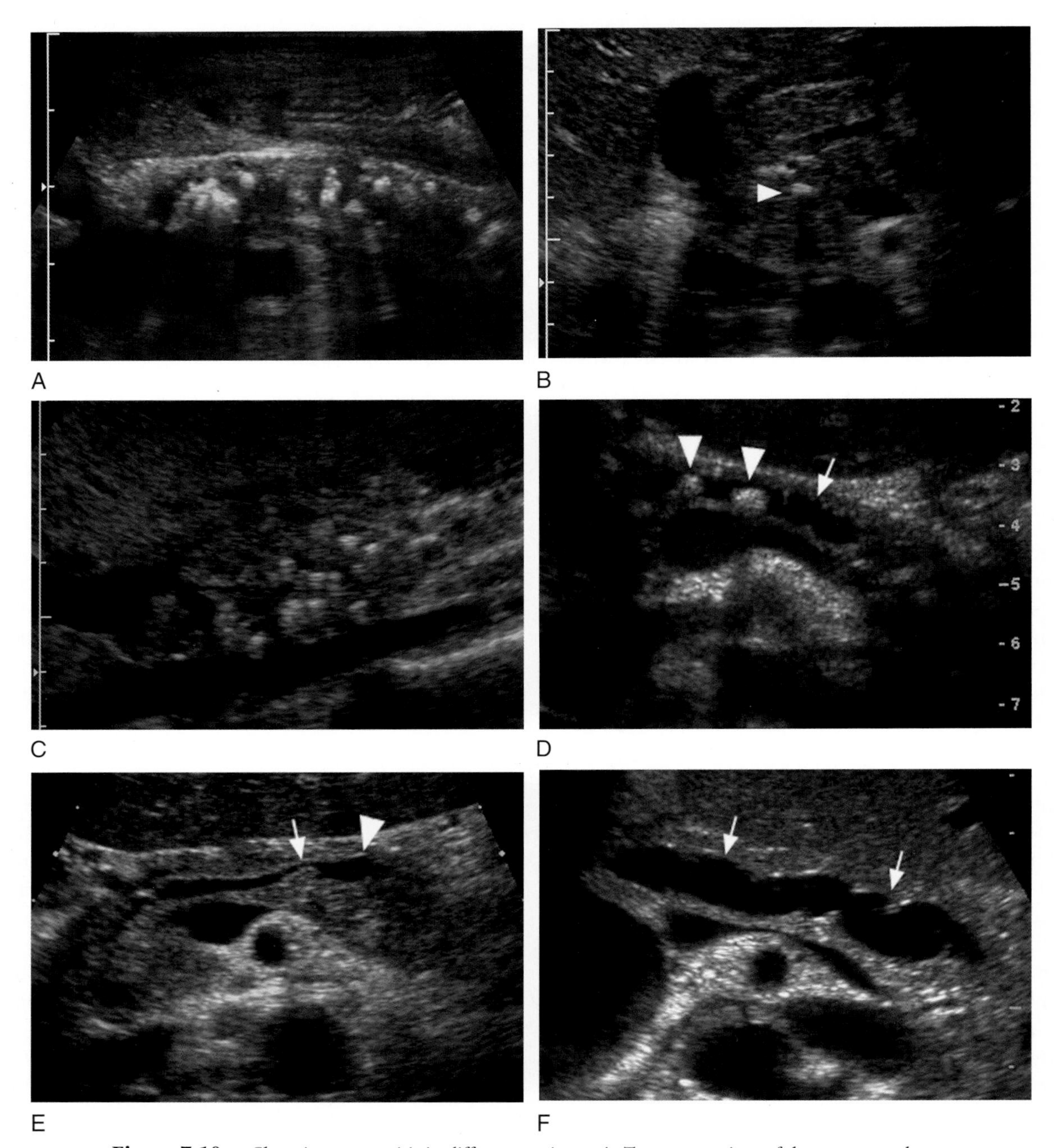

Figure 7-10 Chronic pancreatitis in different patients. **A,** Transverse view of the pancreas shows multiple shadowing calcifications spread throughout the pancreatic parenchyma secondary to calcific pancreatitis. **B,** Transverse view of the pancreatic head shows a single, shadowing parenchymal calcification *(arrowhead).* **C,** Longitudinal view of the pancreatic head shows multiple bright reflectors without associated acoustic shadows. **D,** Transverse view of the body of the pancreas shows a dilated pancreatic duct *(arrow)* containing two intraluminal stones *(arrowheads).* **E,** Transverse view of the pancreas shows a stricture *(arrow)* in the pancreatic duct with dilatation of the duct proximal to the stricture *(arrowhead).* **F,** Transverse view of the pancreas shows a dilated pancreatic duct *(arrows)* with tortuosity and irregularity of the duct wall.

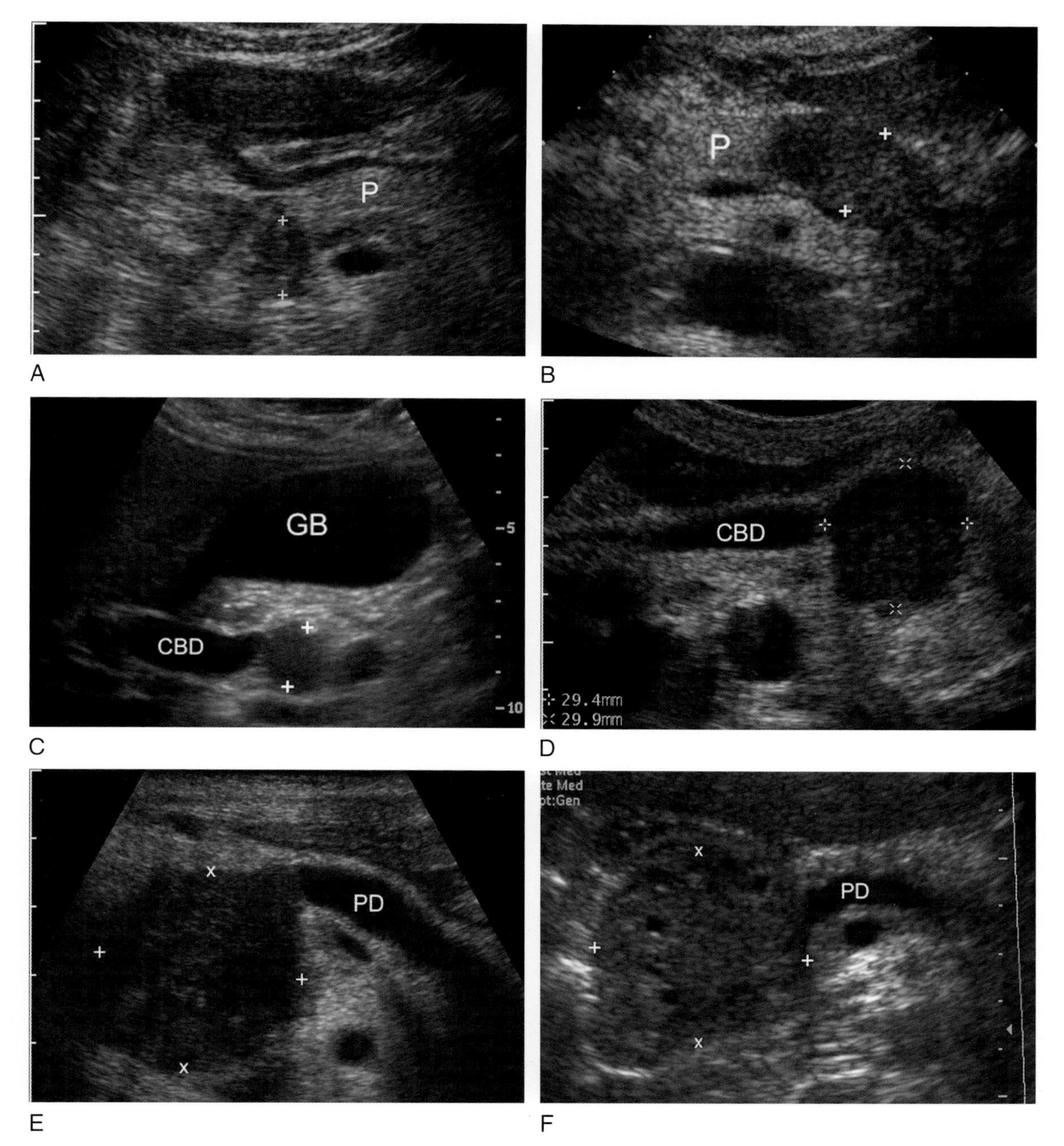

Figure 7-11 Pancreatic carcinoma in different patients. **A,** Transverse view of the pancreas (P) shows a small hypoechoic solid mass *(cursors)* in the head of the pancreas immediately to the right of the portal splenic confluence. **B,** Transverse view of the pancreas (P) shows a hypoechoic mass *(cursors)* replacing the pancreatic parenchyma at the junction of the body and the tail. **C,** Longitudinal view of the porta hepatis using the gallbladder (GB) as a window shows a dilated common bile duct (CBD) terminating abruptly at the level of a hypoechoic mass *(cursors)* in the pancreatic head. **D,** Longitudinal view of the common bile duct (CBD) shows abrupt termination of the duct at the level of a hypoechoic mass *(cursors)* in the pancreatic head. **E,** Transverse view of the pancreas shows a markedly dilated pancreatic duct (PD) being obstructed by a hypoechoic solid mass *(cursors)* in the pancreatic head. **F,** Transverse view of the pancreatic head shows a predominately solid mass *(cursors)* causing a dilated pancreatic duct (PD). This lesion is atypical because several small cystic spaces are seen within the mass.

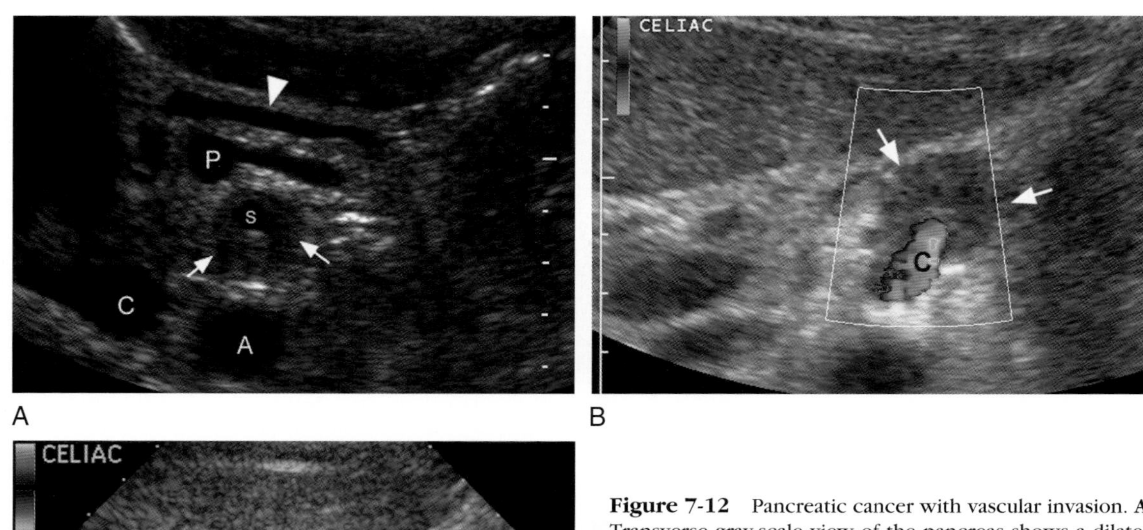

Figure 7-12 Pancreatic cancer with vascular invasion. **A,** Transverse gray-scale view of the pancreas shows a dilated pancreatic duct *(arrowhead)*. Soft tissue *(arrows)* is seen encasing the origin of the superior mesenteric artery (S). Also seen is the portal splenic confluence (P), aorta (A), and inferior vena cava (C). **B,** Transverse color Doppler view of the upper abdomen at the level of the celiac axis (C) shows hypoechoic soft tissue *(arrows)* encasing the anterior aspect of the artery. **C,** Longitudinal color Doppler view of the upper abdomen at the level of the celiac axis (C) shows similar findings as seen in the previous image. Also seen is the abdominal aorta (A).

excluded by the detection of metastases or vascular encasement. As mentioned earlier, the identification of scattered calcific foci in the hypoechoic mass makes focal chronic pancreatitis more likely. ERCP can provide useful information when the morphologic features revealed by ultrasound or CT studies overlap. Percutaneous biopsy findings are helpful when histologic analysis reveals malignancy, but normal biopsy findings do not exclude carcinoma. In addition to pancreatic carcinoma and focal pancreatitis, other uncommon lesions that produce hypoechoic masses are other pancreatic tumors, metastases to the pancreas (Fig. 7-13), pancreatic lymphoma, and peripancreatic lymph nodes.

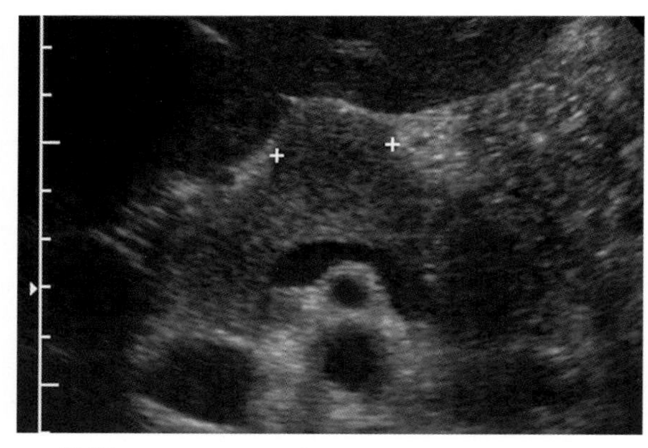

Figure 7-13 Metastasis to the pancreas. Transverse view of the pancreas shows an isoechoic solid mass *(cursors)* arising from the anterior aspect of the pancreatic body. This patient also had lung, liver, and brain metastases from an extratesticular germ cell tumor.

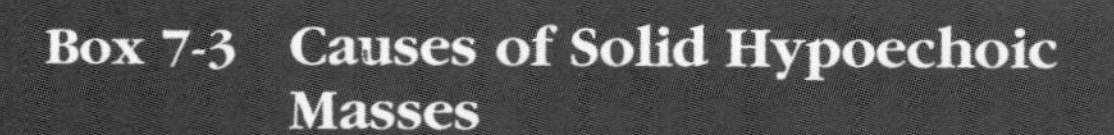

Box 7-3 Causes of Solid Hypoechoic Masses

Carcinoma
Focal pancreatitis
Lymphoma
Metastases
Islet cell tumors
Thrombosed aneurysms

ISLET CELL TUMORS

Endocrine tumors of the pancreas arise from the islets of Langerhans. They affect patients either because they are malignant and metastasize or because they produce excessive amounts of polypeptide hormones such as insulin, gastrin, glucagon, pancreatic polypeptide, and vasoactive intestinal peptide. Multiple islet cell tumors develop in patients with multiple endocrine neoplasm syndrome type I.

Insulinomas account for 70% to 75% of islet cell tumors. They are usually small (<2 cm) and solitary, and 90% to 95% of them are benign. Patients exhibit symptoms related to hypoglycemia and are found to have elevated fasting levels of insulin. Like other islet cell tumors, insulinomas appear as hypoechoic solid masses (Fig. 7-14A). They can be located anywhere in the pancreas. The reported sensitivity of ultrasound in published studies varies widely, but in experienced hands ultrasound can detect up to 60% of insulinomas preoperatively. Intraoperative ultrasound is the most sensitive means of identifying and localizing insulinomas and can detect some tumors that are not palpable at surgery (see Fig. 7-14B).

Gastrinomas account for approximately 20% of islet cell tumors. Unlike insulinomas, most gastrinomas are malignant, with up to 40% of affected patients having metastatic disease at the time of diagnosis. Symptoms are due to excessive gastrin secretion and include severe peptic ulcer disease and secretory diarrhea. Gastrinomas are small tumors, and preoperative localization with sonography is limited. Intraoperative ultrasound is useful for detecting lesions in the pancreas but is significantly less sensitive in detecting extrapancreatic lesions that typically occur in the wall of the duodenum (Fig. 7-15).

Islet cell tumors that are nonfunctioning present as larger masses, usually with evidence of metastases at the time of diagnosis (Fig. 7-16). Approximately 20% of nonfunctioning islet cell tumors contain areas of calcification.

CYSTIC PANCREATIC NEOPLASMS

Cystic neoplasms of the pancreas account for less than 5% of pancreatic tumors. There are two types. Microcystic adenoma (also called serous cystadenoma and glycogen-rich cystadenoma) is a benign tumor seen predominantly in middle-aged and elderly women. It is a well-circumscribed and usually large mass (mean diameter, 10 cm) that contains multiple small cysts. A central stellate scar that may calcify is characteristic. Macrocystic adenoma (also called mucinous cystadenoma/cystadenocarcinoma) is either malignant or has malignant potential. It occurs predominantly in middle-aged women, usually in the body or tail of the pancreas.

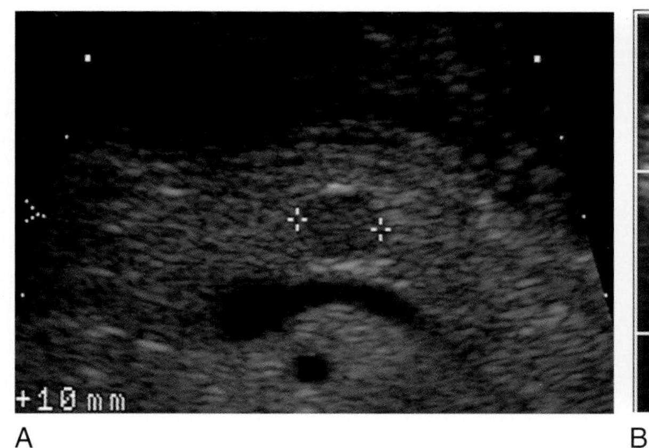

A

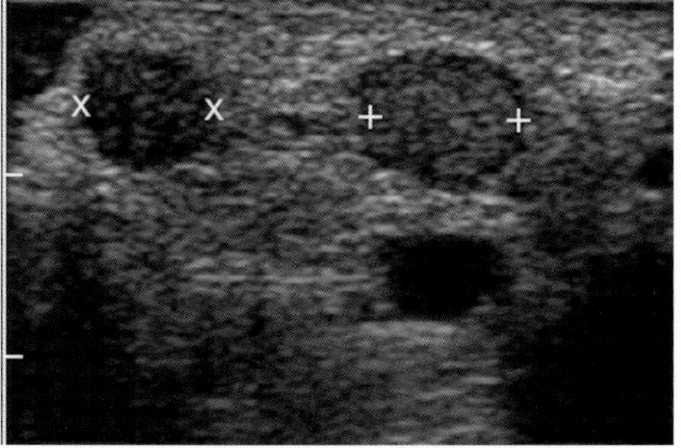

B

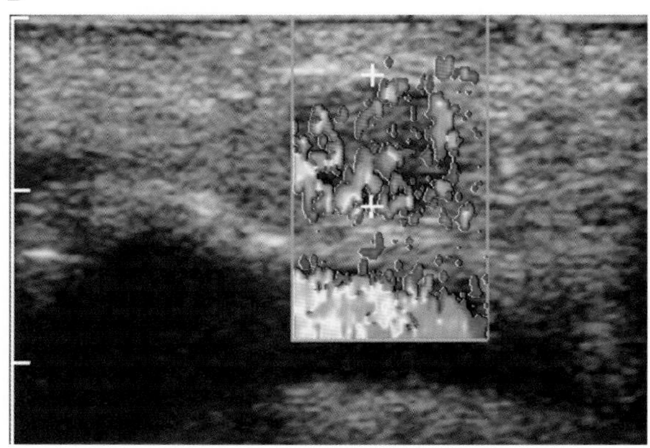

C

Figure 7-14 Insulinoma. **A,** Transverse view of the pancreas using a fluid-filled stomach as a window shows a small (10 mm) hypoechoic solid mass *(cursors)*. **B,** Intraoperative ultrasound of the pancreas shows two solid hypoechoic masses *(cursors)* in the pancreas. **C,** Intraoperative color Doppler view of the pancreas shows a hypervascular mass *(cursors)*.

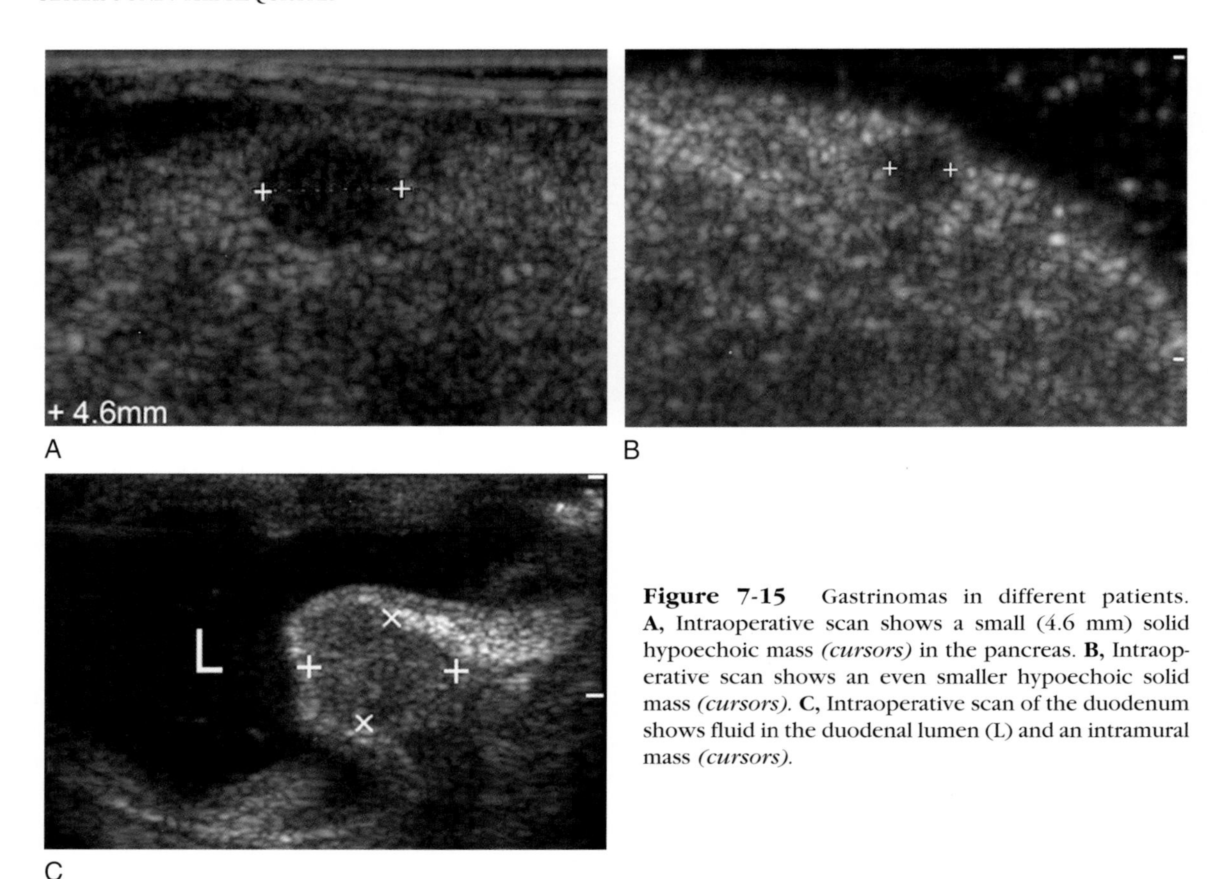

Figure 7-15 Gastrinomas in different patients. **A,** Intraoperative scan shows a small (4.6 mm) solid hypoechoic mass *(cursors)* in the pancreas. **B,** Intraoperative scan shows an even smaller hypoechoic solid mass *(cursors)*. **C,** Intraoperative scan of the duodenum shows fluid in the duodenal lumen (L) and an intramural mass *(cursors)*.

It is typically made up of well-defined cysts containing thick mucinous fluid, internal septations, or mural nodules.

Because macrocystic tumors are malignant or premalignant, it is important to distinguish them from microcystic tumors. On sonograms, macrocystic adenomas/cystadenocarcinomas generally appear as well-defined, predominantly cystic masses (Figs. 7-17). Internal septations are common but not uniformly present. Mural nodules and solid components may be seen, particularly in the frankly malignant lesions (see Fig. 7-17). Peripheral calcification in the cyst wall is detected occasionally.

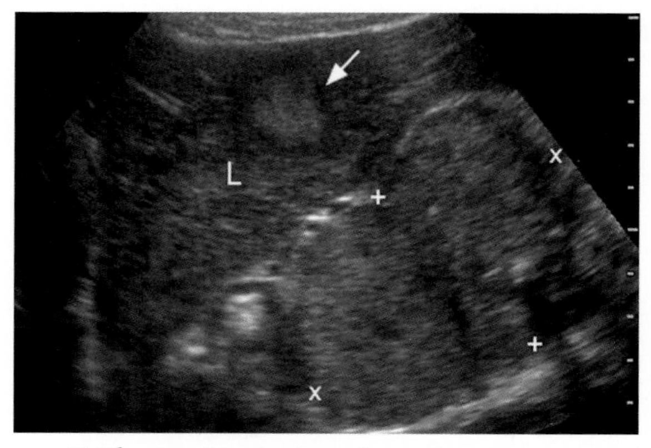

Figure 7-16 Nonfunctioning islet cell tumor. Longitudinal view of the epigastrium shows a large solid mass *(cursors)* arising from the body of the pancreas. A target lesion *(arrow)* due to a metastasis is seen in the left lobe of the liver (L).

The sonographic appearance of microcystic adenomas depends on the size of the cystic elements within the mass. When the internal cysts are very small, the mass itself will appear solid and may even be hyperechoic. When the internal cysts reach 5 to 10 mm in diameter, the mass itself appears multicystic (Fig. 7-18). Generally, the individual cysts are less than 2 cm in diameter and number more than six. The central stellate scar that may be seen on pathologic studies is generally difficult to identify sonographically.

Although sonography is relatively accurate in terms of the diagnosis and categorization of cystic pancreatic neoplasms, there is overlap and it is sometimes difficult to distinguish the neoplasms from one another or from pancreatic pseudocysts (Box 7-4). Necrotic pancreatic adenocarcinomas, adenocarcinomas with associated pseudocysts, solid and papillary epithelial neoplasms, and intraductal papillary mucinous tumors are also considerations. The clinical history is valuable in favoring a diagnosis of pseudocyst, because these patients frequently

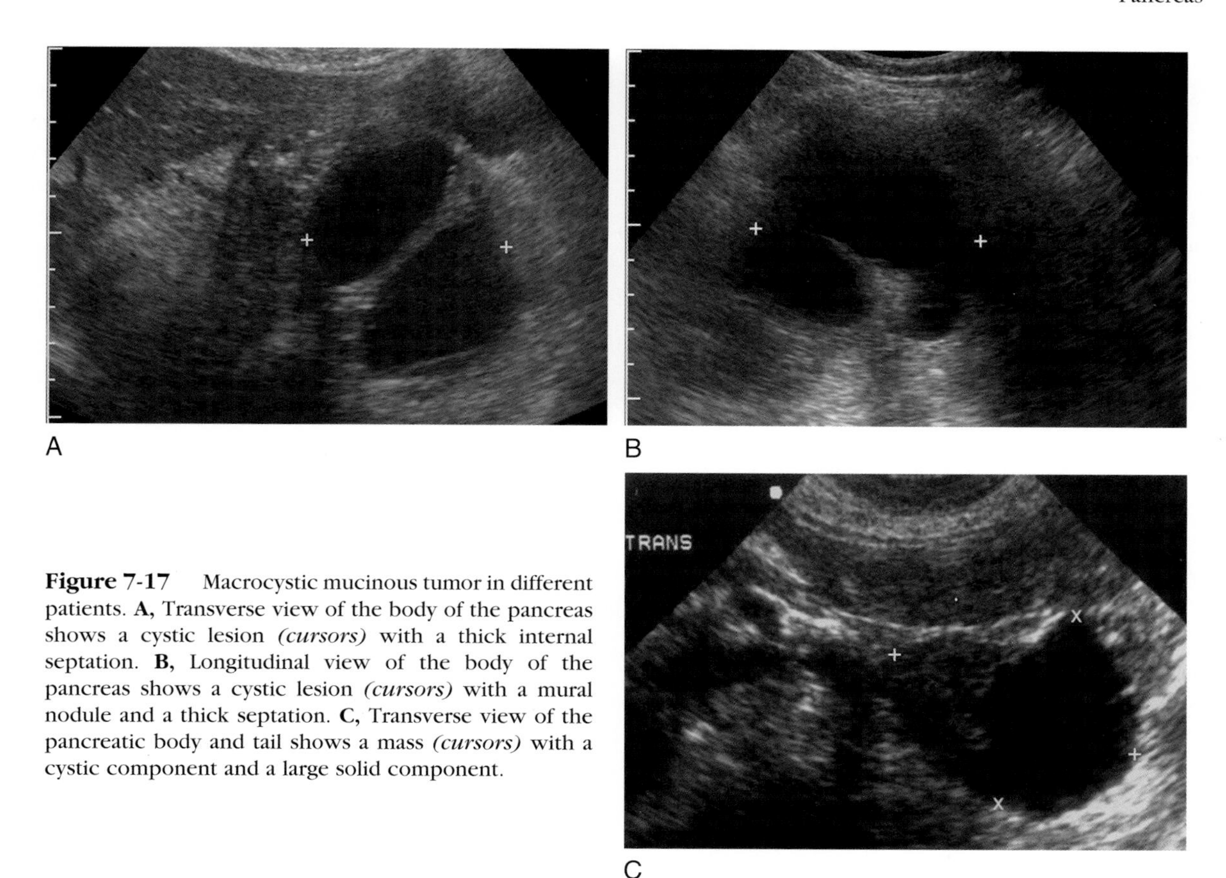

Figure 7-17 Macrocystic mucinous tumor in different patients. **A,** Transverse view of the body of the pancreas shows a cystic lesion *(cursors)* with a thick internal septation. **B,** Longitudinal view of the body of the pancreas shows a cystic lesion *(cursors)* with a mural nodule and a thick septation. **C,** Transverse view of the pancreatic body and tail shows a mass *(cursors)* with a cystic component and a large solid component.

have a history of pancreatitis. Extrapancreatic signs of malignancy that are seen on imaging studies or are identified clinically are also useful because they would make the diagnosis of a macrocystic tumor much more likely.

Percutaneous biopsy and aspiration of pancreatic cystic tumors can be useful. When mucin is detected either within the cells or in the fluid background of the tissue obtained, a macrocystic lesion can be diagnosed. Because pancreatic pseudocysts often communicate with the ducts, and cystic neoplasms rarely do so, ERCP can be useful in identifying these features.

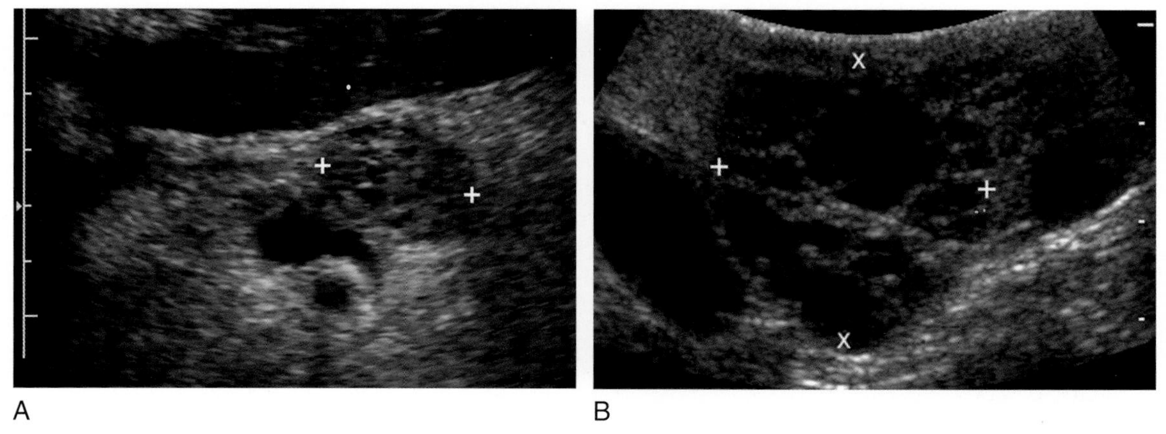

Figure 7-18 Microcystic adenoma in different patients. **A,** Transverse view of the pancreas shows a hypoechoic mass *(cursors)* containing multiple small internal cystic components. **B,** Intraoperative scan shows a complex approximately 3-cm lesion *(cursors)* containing multiple small internal cystic elements.

Box 7-4 Pancreatic Cystic Lesions

Pseudocyst
Macrocystic (mucinous) tumor
Microcystic (serous) tumor
Intraductal papillary mucinous tumor
Solid and papillary epithelial neoplasm
Autosomal dominant polycystic disease
von Hippel-Lindau disease
Cystic fibrosis
Aneurysm/pseudoaneurysm

RARE NEOPLASMS

Intraductal papillary mucinous tumor (IPMT) (also known as ductectatic neoplasm, cystadenocarcinoma, and ductectatic mucinous tumor) is characterized by the massive mucinous distention of side branches of the pancreatic duct. The involved ductal epithelium is either hyperplastic and atypical or overtly malignant. It is generally a low-grade malignancy, and the prognosis is much better than in adenocarcinoma. The tumor usually occurs in the head and uncinate process of the pancreas. Unlike macrocystic neoplasms, there is no female predominance. Patients often present with pain and elevated amylase levels and are initially thought to have pancreatitis. The tumor appears as nonspecific unilocular or multilocular cysts on sonography and CT. The ERCP findings can be diagnostic when mucinous material is seen draining from the pancreatic duct and dilated side branches are seen on a pancreatogram. When the tumor spreads into the main pancreatic duct or originally arises in the main duct, the main duct becomes dilated by the excess mucin that is produced (Fig. 7-19). This has been referred to as mucin-hypersecreting carcinoma of the pancreas.

Solid papillary epithelial neoplasms of the pancreas are tumors that predominantly afflict young women. They are usually large tumors with a low-grade malignancy. They are solid lesions but characteristically have sizable cystic components that are caused by hemorrhage and necrosis. They should be considered whenever a complex solid and cystic mass is seen in a young woman who has no history of pancreatitis (Fig. 7-20).

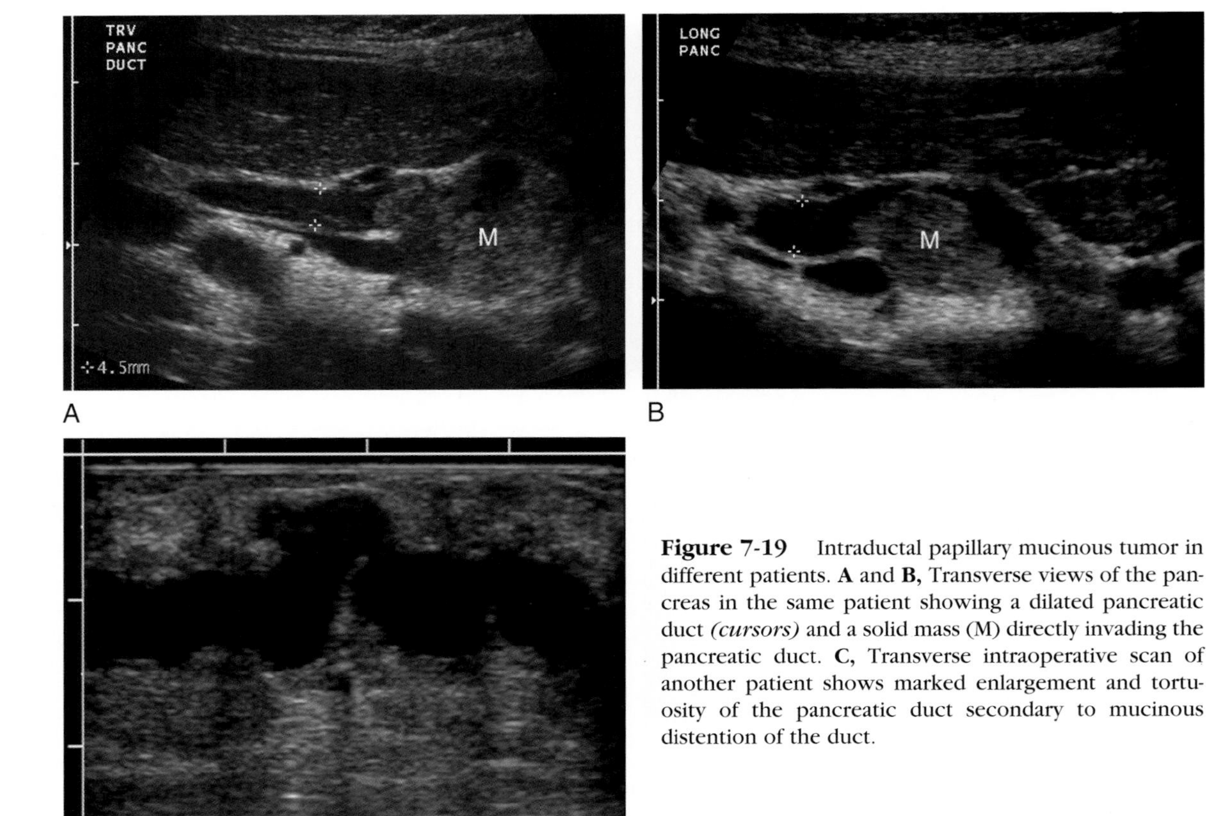

Figure 7-19 Intraductal papillary mucinous tumor in different patients. **A** and **B,** Transverse views of the pancreas in the same patient showing a dilated pancreatic duct *(cursors)* and a solid mass (M) directly invading the pancreatic duct. **C,** Transverse intraoperative scan of another patient shows marked enlargement and tortuosity of the pancreatic duct secondary to mucinous distention of the duct.

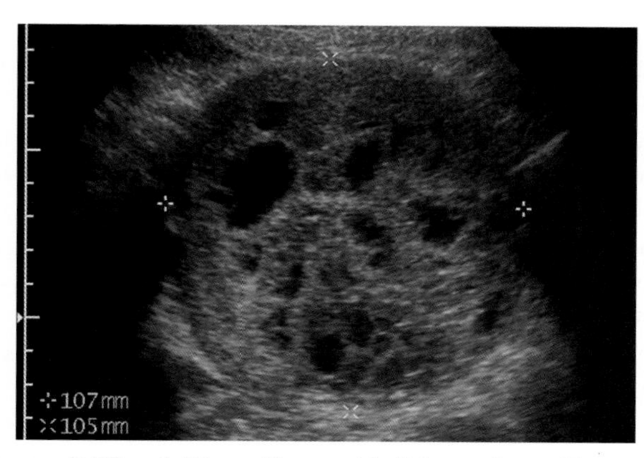

Figure 7-20 Solid papillary epithelial neoplasm. Transverse view of the left upper quadrant shows a large predominantly solid mass *(cursors)* containing multiple small internal cystic elements arising from the pancreatic tail.

Key Features

The echogenicity of the pancreas should be equal to or greater than that of the liver. It can be equal to, greater than, or less than the echogenicity of the spleen.

The pancreatic duct should be less than 3 mm in diameter, but it enlarges with age.

Acute pancreatitis is characterized by pancreatic enlargement, peripancreatic and retroperitoneal fluid collections, and decreased/heterogeneous pancreatic echogenicity.

Focal pancreatitis can simulate pancreatic cancer.

Complications of pancreatitis include biliary strictures, pseudocyst formation, splenic or portal vein thrombosis, splenic artery pseudoaneurysms, abscess, and pancreatic necrosis.

Chronic pancreatitis is characterized by pancreatic calcifications, ductal dilatation, ductal irregularity, and parenchymal atrophy.

Pancreatic cancer and islet cell tumors are both typically hypoechoic.

In addition to identifying pancreatic cancer, ultrasound and Doppler analysis should be used to stage the tumor, particularly the vascular involvement.

Intraoperative sonography is the most sensitive means of localizing islet cell tumors.

Microcystic adenomas contain serous fluid, consist of multiple small cystic elements, and are benign.

Macrocystic tumors contain mucinous fluid; consist of larger cystic elements, thick septations, and solid elements; and are either malignant or premalignant lesions.

SUGGESTED READINGS

Alpern MB, Sandler MA, Kellman GM, et al: Chronic pancreatitis: ultrasonic features. Radiology 155:215, 1985.

Angeli E, Venturini M, Vanzulli A: Color Doppler imaging in the assessment of vascular involvement by pancreatic carcinoma. AJR Am J Roentgenol 168:193-197, 1997.

Atri M, Nazarnia S, Mehio A, et al: Hypoechoic embryologic ventral aspect of the head and uncinate process of the pancreas: In vitro correlation of US with histopathologic findings. Radiology 190:441-444, 1994.

Balthazar EJ, Freeny PC, van Sonnenberg E: Imaging and intervention in acute pancreatitis. Radiology 193:297-306, 1994.

Bastid C, Sahel J, Sastre B, et al: Mucinous cystadenocarcinoma of the pancreas: Ultrasonographic findings in 5 cases. Acta Radiol 30:45, 1989.

Beutow PC, Miller DL, Parrino TV, Buck JL: Islet cell tumors of the pancreas: Clinical radiologic and pathologic correlation in diagnosis and localization. Radiographics 17:453-471, 1997.

Buetow PC, Rao P, Thompson LDR: From the Archives of the AFIP: Mucinous cystic neoplasms of the pancreas: Radiologic-pathologic correlation. Radiographics 18:433-449, 1998.

Bolondi L, LiBassi S, Saiani S, Barbara L: Sonography of chronic pancreatitis. Radiol Clin North Am 27:815, 1989.

Buck JL, Hayes WS: From the Archives of the AFIP. Microcystic adenoma of the pancreas. Radiographics 10:313, 1990.

Campagno J, Oertel JE, Krezmar M: Solid and papillary epithelial neoplasm of the pancreas, probably of small duct origin: A clinicopathologic study of 52 cases [abstract]. Lab Invest 40:248, 1979.

Campbell JP, Wilson SR: Pancreatic neoplasms: How useful is evaluation with US? Radiology 167:341, 1988.

DelMaschio A, Vanzulli A, Sironi S, et al: Pancreatic cancer versus chronic pancreatitis: Diagnosis with CA 19-9 assessment, US, CT and CT-guided fine-needle biopsy. Radiology 178:95, 1991.

Donald JJ, Shorvon PJ, Lees WR: Hypoechoic area within the head of the pancreas—a normal variant. Clin Radiol 41:337, 1990.

Falkoff GE, Taylor KJW, Morse SS: Hepatic artery pseudoaneurysm: Diagnosis with real-time and pulsed Doppler ultrasound. Radiology 58:55, 1986.

Freeny PC: Radiologic diagnosis and staging of pancreatic ductal adenocarcinoma. Radiol Clin North Am 27:121, 1989.

Friedman AC, Edmonds PR: Rare pancreatic malignancies. Radiol Clin North Am 27:15, 1989.

Friedman AC, Lichtenstein JE, Dachman AH: Cystic neoplasms of the pancreas: Radiological-pathological correlation. Radiology 149:45, 1983.

Friedman AC, Lichtenstein JE, Fishman EK, et al: Solid and papillary epithelial neoplasm of the pancreas. Radiology 154: 333, 1985.

Galiber AK, Reading CC, Charboneau JW, et al: Localization of pancreatic insulinoma: Comparison of pre- and intraoperative US with CT and angiography. Radiology 166:405, 1988.

Glazer HS, Lee JKT, Balfe DM, et al: Non-Hodgkin lymphoma: Computed tomographic demonstration of unusual extranodal involvement. Radiology 149:211, 1983.

Goekas MC: Etiology and pathogenesis of acute pancreatic inflammation: Acute pancreatitis. Ann Intern Med 103:86, 1985.

Itai Y, Kokubo T, Atomi Y, et al: Mucin-hypersecreting carcinoma of the pancreas. Radiology 165:51, 1987.

Itai Y, Ohhashi K, Nagai H, et al: "Ductectatic" mucinous cystadenoma and cystadenocarcinoma of the pancreas. Radiology 161:697, 1986.

Jeffrey RB Jr: Sonography in acute pancreatitis. Radiol Clin North Am 27:5, 1989.

Jeffrey RB Jr, Laing FC, Wing VW: Extrapancreatic spread of acute pancreatitis: New observations with real-time US. Radiology 159:707, 1986.

Johnson CD, Stephens DH, Charboneau JW, et al: Cystic pancreatic tumors: CT and sonographic assessment. AJR Am J Roentgenol 151:1133, 1988.

Jones SN, Lees WR, Frost RA: Diagnosis and grading of chronic pancreatitis by morphological criteria derived by ultrasound and pancreatography. Clin Radiol 39:43, 1988.

Karlson BM, Ekbom A, Lindgren PG, et al: Abdominal US for diagnosis of pancreatic tumor: Prospective cohort analysis. Radiology 213: 107-111, 1999.

Klein KA, Stephens DH, Welch TJ. CT characteristics of metastatic disease of the pancreas. Radiographics 18:369-378, 1998.

Lim JH, Lee G, Oh YL: Radiologic spectrum of intraductal papillary mucinous tumor of the pancreas. Radiographics 21:323-340, 2001.

McMahon PM, Halpern EF, Fernandez-del Castillo C, et al: Pancreatic cancer: Cost-effectiveness of imaging technologies for assessing resectability. Radiology 221:93-106, 2001.

Mathieu D, Guigui B, Valette PJ, et al: Pancreatic cystic neoplasms. Radiol Clin North Am 27:163, 1989.

Moser RP Jr: Microcystic adenoma of the pancreas. Radiographics 1990; 10:313-322.

Norton JA, Cromack DT, Shawker TH: Intraoperative ultrasonographic localization of islet cell tumors. Ann Surg 207:160, 1988.

Ormson MJ, Charboneau JW, Stephens DH: Sonography in patients with a possible pancreatic mass shown on CT. AJR Am J Roentgenol 148:551, 1987.

Paivansalo M, Suramo I: Ultrasonography of the pancreatic tail through the spleen and through the fluid-filled stomach. Eur J Radiol 6:113-115, 1986.

Procacci C, Megibow AJ, Carbognin G, et al: Intraductal papillary mucinous tumor of the pancreas: A pictorial essay. Radiographics 19:1447-1463, 1999.

Ros PR, Hamrick-Turner JE, Chiechi MV, et al: Cystic masses of the pancreas. Radiographics 12:673, 1992.

Rossi P, Allison DJ, Bezzi M, et al: Endocrine tumors of the pancreas. Radiol Clin North Am 27:129, 1989.

Schneck CD, Dabezies MA, Friedman AC: Embryology, histology, gross anatomy, and normal imaging anatomy of the pancreas. In Friedman AC, Dachman AH (eds): Radiology of the Liver, Biliary Tract, and Pancreas. St. Louis, Mosby, 1994, pp 715-742.

Taylor AJ, Bohorfoush AG (eds): Pancreatic duct in inflammation of the pancreas. In Interpretation of ERCP with Associated Digital Imaging Correlation. Philadelphia, Lippincott-Raven, 1997, pp 231-260.

Teefey SA, Stephens DH, Sheedy PF: CT appearance of primary pancreatic lymphoma. Gastrointest Radiol 11:41, 1987.

Warshaw AL, Compton CC, Lewandrowski K, et al: Cystic tumors of the pancreas: New clinical, radiologic, and pathologic observations in 67 patients. Ann Surg 212:432, 1990.

Warshaw AL, Swanson RS: Pancreatic cancer in 1988: Possibilities and probabilities. Ann Surg 208:541, 1988.

Wernecke K, Peters PE, Galanski M: Pancreatic metastases: Ultrasound evaluation. Radiology 160:339, 1986.

White AF, Barum S, Buranasiri S: Aneurysms secondary to pancreatitis. AJR Am J Roentgenol 127:393, 1976.

Wolfman NT, Ramquist NA, Karstaedt N, Hopkins MB: Cystic neoplasms of the pancreas: CT and sonography. AJR Am J Roentgenol 138:37, 1992.

Yeh HC, Stancato-Pasik A, Shapiro RS: Microcystic features at US: A nonspecific sign for microcystic adenomas of the pancreas. Radiographics 21:1455-1461, 2001.

CHAPTER 8

Spleen

For Key Features summary see p. 219

ANATOMY

The spleen is an intraperitoneal organ that occupies the superior, posterior, and lateral aspects of the left upper quadrant. It is normally in continuity with the diaphragm posteriorly, laterally, and superiorly. It contacts the kidney and splenic flexure inferiorly and the stomach and tail of the pancreas medially. The splenic artery arises from the celiac axis and travels along the posterosuperior aspect of the pancreas toward the splenic hilum. It often becomes quite tortuous with aging. The splenic vein exits the spleen at the hilum and initially travels superior to the tail of the pancreas. At the pancreatic body the vein travels along the posterior aspect of the pancreas to form a confluence with the superior mesenteric vein and portal vein. The splenic vein is located slightly inferior to the splenic artery.

The splenic parenchyma appears very homogeneous on sonograms, and it is more echogenic than the liver and is considerably more echogenic than the left kidney (Fig. 8-1). The measurement of splenic size in the detection of splenomegaly has been the subject of much research, and a variety of methods have been proposed for doing this. In actual practice a length that exceeds 13 cm in a coronal plane is a reasonable cut-off between normal and enlarged. A thickness of 6 cm, measured from the hilum to the opposite edge, is also a useful cut-off when the length is borderline. The shape of the spleen has a number of variations. The most common is a medial tubercle that extends as a tongue-shaped protrusion, usually positioned over the upper pole of the left kidney. On longitudinal scans this medial tubercle can occasionally be misconstrued to be a renal or adrenal mass. (See Table 8-1 for a summary of the normal characteristics of the spleen.)

Small nodules of splenic tissue are often located in the left upper quadrant adjacent to the spleen. These are referred to as splenules, accessory spleens, splenunculi, and supernumerary spleens. They are usually small (<3 cm) but can enlarge and become more evident when the spleen itself enlarges or when the spleen is removed. They are seen in approximately 30% of autopsy studies and are multiple in approximately 10% of cases. They are supplied by branches of the splenic artery and usually arise immediately adjacent to the spleen, often near the splenic hilum. They tend to be round or ovoid and are isoechoic to the spleen (Fig. 8-2). They can usually be distinguished from pancreatic tail masses and left renal masses by noting their echogenicity similar to the spleen. When there is doubt, a sulfur colloid scan or a heat-damaged tagged red blood cell scan can be useful. Splenic clefts are also relatively common. They appear as thin, bright, linear reflections that extend from the periphery of the spleen into the splenic parenchyma (Fig. 8-3).

TECHNIQUE

The spleen is generally best visualized from a high posterolateral intercostal approach with the patient supine. Failure to position the transducer superior and posterior enough is a common problem when sonographers and sonologists are inexperienced. In some

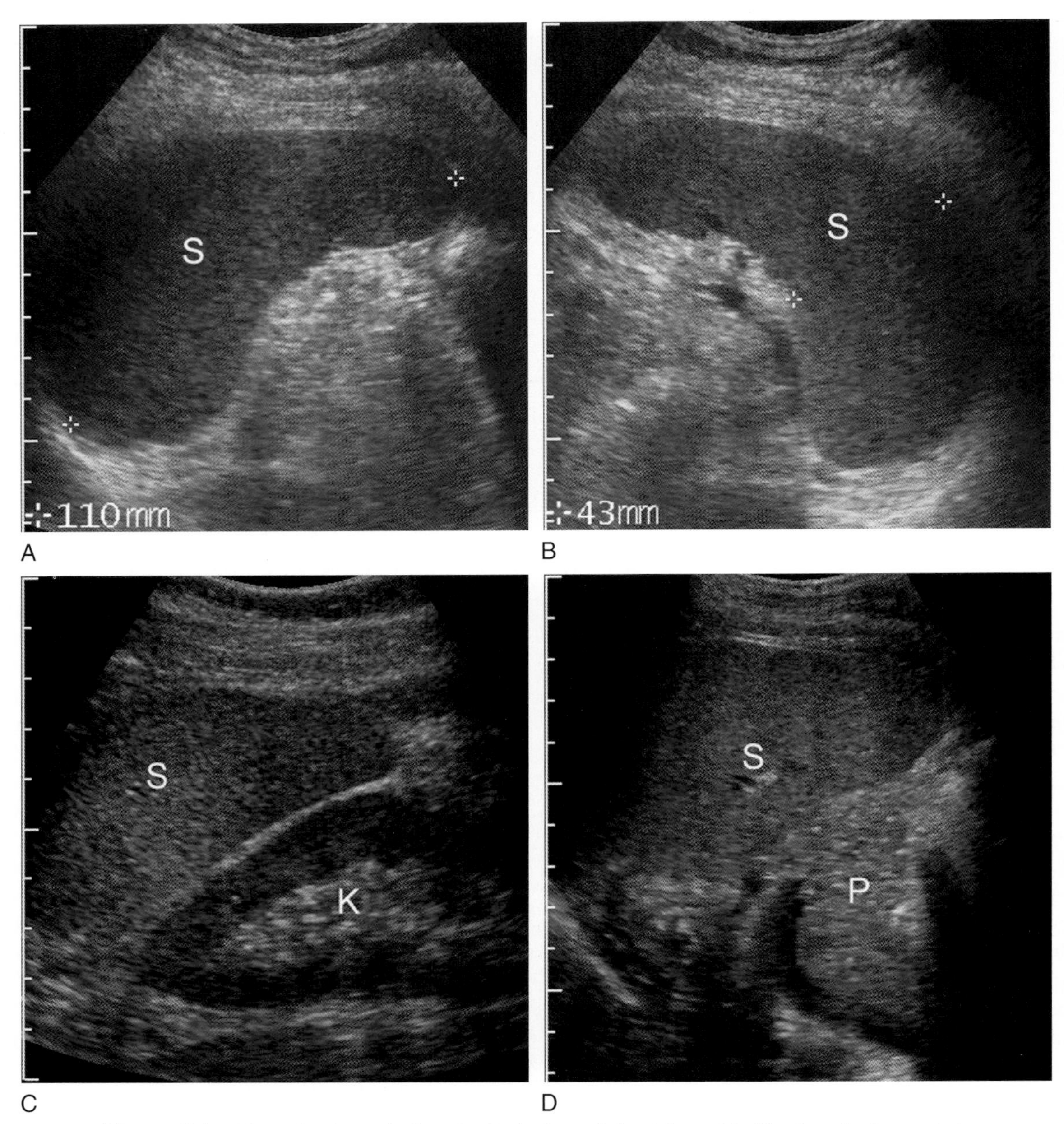

Figure 8-1 Normal spleen. **A,** Longitudinal view of the spleen (S). The length *(cursors)* is 11.0 cm. **B,** Transverse view of the spleen (S). The thickness *(cursors)* is 4.3 cm. **C,** Longitudinal view of the spleen (S) and left kidney (K) shows that the spleen is considerably more echogenic than the kidney. **D,** Longitudinal view of the spleen (S) and the tail of the pancreas (P) shows that in this patient the spleen is less echogenic than the pancreas.

patients the spleen is seen well from an anterolateral subcostal approach with the patient in a right lateral decubitus or right posterior oblique position. When scanning from a subcostal approach, a deep inspiration is often helpful in bringing the spleen farther into the field of view. The right lateral decubitus and right posterior oblique positions should generally not be used when scanning from an intercostal approach because this causes the spleen to fall away from the chest and abdominal wall and causes aerated lung to migrate inferiorly and obscure an otherwise acceptable acoustic window. As with the liver, diffuse or multifocal disease of the spleen can often be detected with high-resolution linear array probes when it is subtle or completely unapparent with conventional abdominal probes.

Table 8-1 Normal Characteristics

Characteristic	Normal Finding
Size	≤13 cm long, ≤6 cm thick
Echogenicity	>Left kidney, >liver, >/<pancreas
Echotexture	Homogeneous
Surface	Smooth
Shape	Crescentic

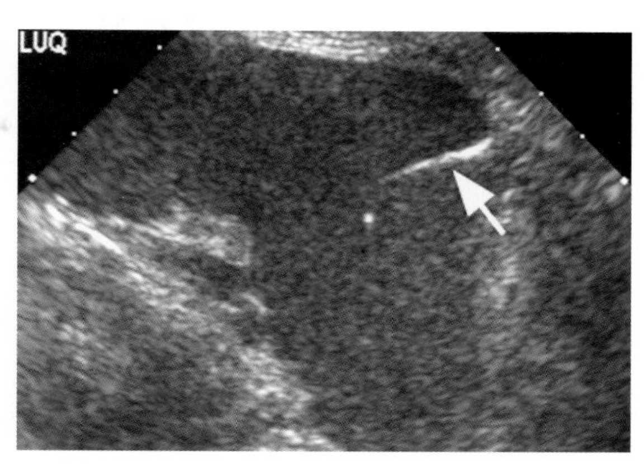

Figure 8-3 Splenic cleft. Transverse view of the spleen shows a thin, well-defined line *(arrow)* due to a peripheral splenic cleft.

CYSTS

Most splenic cysts result from trauma. They actually represent hematomas that have evolved into seromas and formed a pseudocapsule. They can also arise from prior infections and infarcts. Their appearance is similar to that of cysts in other organs (Fig. 8-4A). Cyst wall calcification is occasionally encountered and does not imply an increased risk of neoplasm (see Fig. 8-4B). True epithelial-lined cysts of the spleen are rare and are probably congenital. They are also referred to as epidermoid cysts because the wall generally contains squamous cells. Parasitic cysts can occur as the result of hydatid disease. These are an important consideration in persons living or traveling in endemic parts of the world. The sonographic appearance of splenic echinococcus is similar to that of liver disease (see Chapter 3), but is much less common.

Pseudocysts of the pancreas can erode into the spleen and simulate the appearance of splenic cysts. As in any parenchymal organ, aneurysms, pseudoaneurysms, venous collaterals, and vascular malformations can also mimic splenic cysts. All can be diagnosed with Doppler imaging, and aneurysms often have partially calcified walls (Fig. 8-5). Perisplenic cysts can arise from a variety of organs adjacent to the spleen. The most common are exophytic renal cysts and pancreatic pseudocysts. Peritoneal-based cystic lesions such as endometriomas (Fig. 8-6) and metastatic ovarian carcinoma can also arise next to the spleen.

TUMORS

Hemangiomas of the spleen are relatively common in autopsy series, but they are seen on imaging studies much less frequently than they are in the liver. They are typically hyperechoic and homogeneous (Fig. 8-7) but are more variable in appearance than they are in the liver. Hamartomas and lymphangiomas are even less

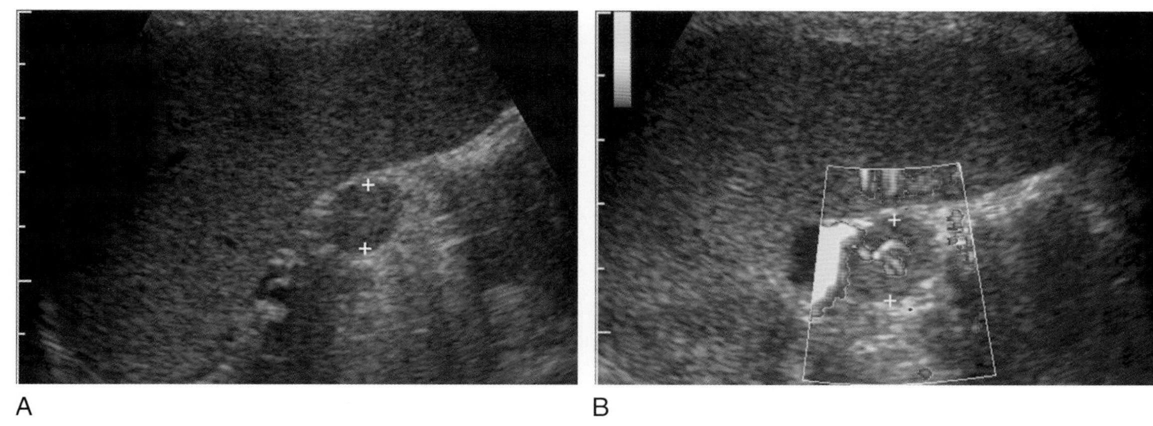

Figure 8-2 Splenule. **A,** Longitudinal view of the spleen shows an isoechoic mass *(cursors)* in the splenic hilum characteristic of a splenule. **B,** Power Doppler view shows internal blood flow arising from a branch of the splenic artery.

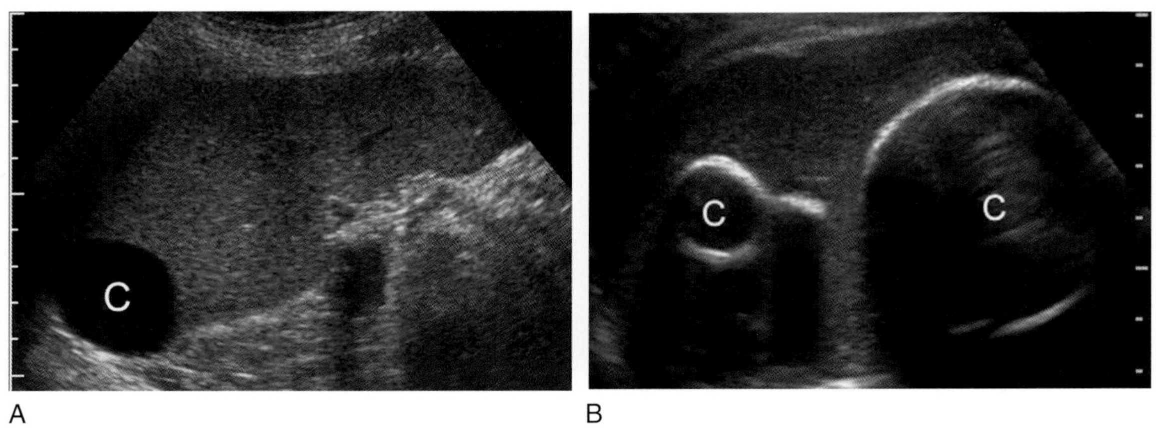

Figure 8-4 Splenic cysts in different patients. **A,** Longitudinal view of the spleen shows a well-defined anechoic mass (C) in the superior aspect of the spleen. There are no solid elements and good enhanced-through transmission. **B,** Longitudinal view shows two cysts (C) with peripheral wall calcification and some posterior shadowing.

common benign tumors. Lymphangiomas are composed of multiple cystic spaces that vary in size. When the cysts are large enough, they will be seen as anechoic spaces (Fig. 8-8), but collections of very small cysts will appear solid. Hamartomas have not been well described but are usually solid lesions. Hemangiosarcomas are primary splenic malignancies that are extremely rare. They tend to be inhomogeneous with hyperechoic and hypoechoic areas.

Splenic lymphoma commonly involves the spleen in a unifocal (Fig. 8-9A), multifocal (see Fig. 8-9B and C), or diffuse manner. The focal lesions are almost always hypoechoic. When large, they may become heterogeneous. Hyperechoic lesions are rare. Diffuse involvement may or may not produce splenomegaly and is difficult to detect with sonography or other modalities. Sonography is relatively insensitive in its ability to detect splenic lymphoma, but the detection of focal hypoechoic lesions is a relatively specific sign of splenic involvement in patients with known lymphoma.

Metastatic disease to the spleen is much less common than that to the liver. Overall, the spleen is the tenth most common organ involved by metastatic spread, and splenic metastases usually are a late manifestation of metastatic disease. Generally, splenic metastases are believed to arise from hematogenous routes. Melanoma is the primary tumor most likely to spread to the spleen, although the more common tumors such as lung, breast, and colon account for the majority of splenic metastases. In most cases splenic metastases occur in the setting of widespread metastases elsewhere in the body. The sonographic appearance of splenic metastases is quite variable,

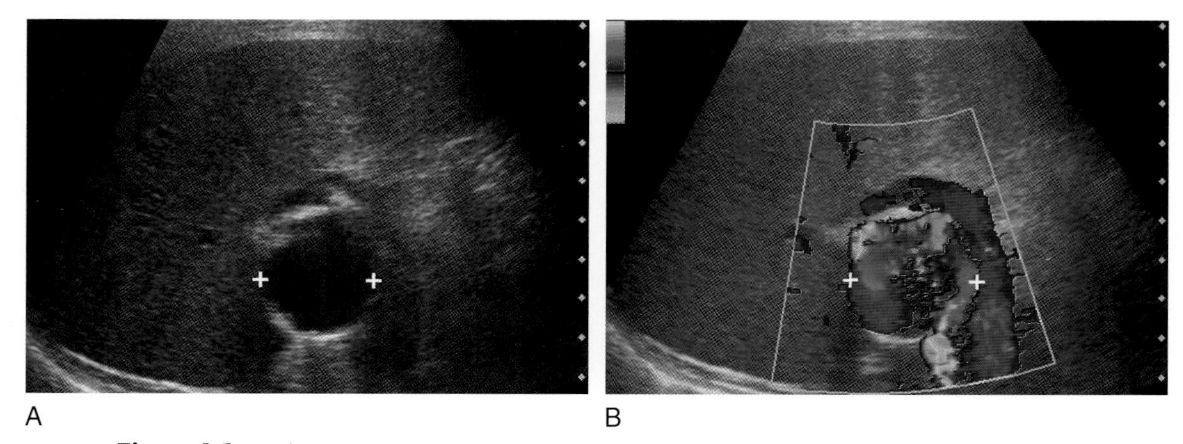

Figure 8-5 Splenic artery aneurysm. **A,** Longitudinal view of the spleen shows a well-defined cystic appearing lesion *(cursors)* in the splenic hilum. **B,** Color Doppler view shows internal blood flow in a swirling pattern typical of an aneurysm.

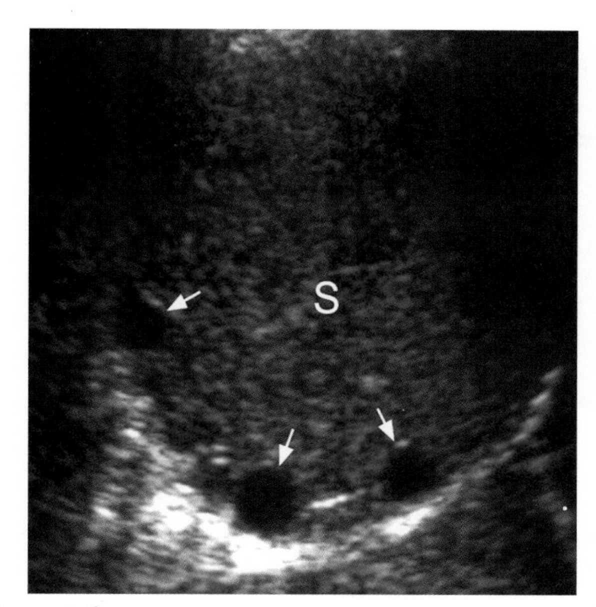

Figure 8-6 Perisplenic endometriosis. Transverse view of the left upper quadrant shows the superior aspect of the spleen (S) and multiple small cystic lesions *(arrows)* between the spleen and the diaphragm. Laparoscopic findings confirmed the diagnosis of endometriosis.

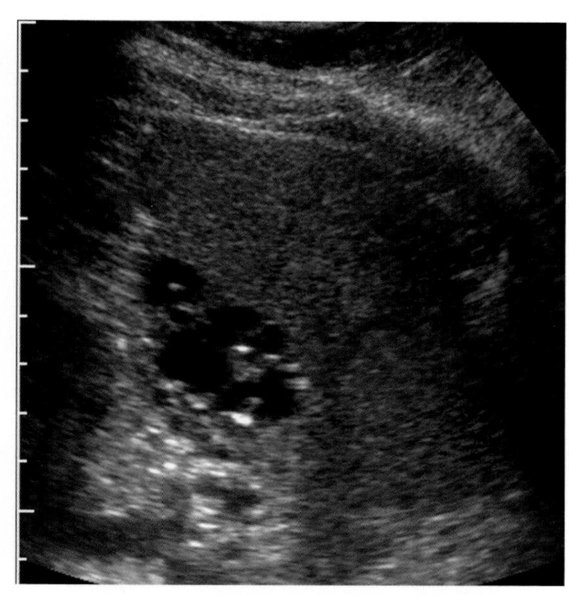

Figure 8-8 Lymphangioma. Transverse view of the spleen shows a multicystic mass in the medial aspect of the spleen. This lesion was stable over several years, and its appearance is most consistent with a lymphangioma.

and all of the patterns exhibited by hepatic metastases are also exhibited by splenic metastases (Fig. 8-10).

Besides tumors, other causes of multiple splenic masses include abscesses, granulomatous disease, extramedullary hematopoiesis, and Gaucher's disease. Because of the concave nature of the splenic hilum, partial volume effects can occasionally cause the higher-amplitude echoes from the perisplenic fat to appear intrasplenic and simulate a mass (Fig. 8-11). Correlating longitudinal and transverse images can avert this potential pitfall. (See Box 8-1 for a listing of solid spleen lesions.)

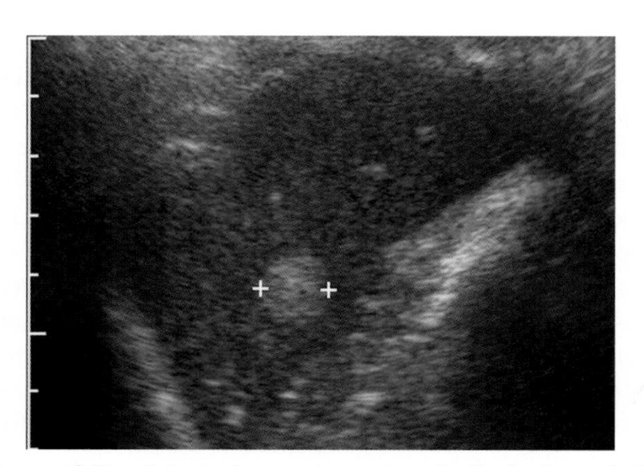

Figure 8-7 Splenic hemangioma. Longitudinal view of the spleen shows a homogeneous hyperechoic mass *(cursors)*. This mass was found to be stable over many years, and this behavior is most consistent with a hemangioma.

In most cases, focal splenic lesions can be diagnosed based on correlation with clinical history and the results of other imaging studies such as CT and MRI. Follow-up scans are useful to confirm that suspected benign lesions are stable over time. Ultrasound guided biopsies of splenic lesions are generally avoided because the spleen is a vascular organ and the possibility of bleeding is greater than with other organs. When a tissue diagnosis is required, it is usually possible to biopsy a site other than the spleen. Splenic biopsies can be performed when necessary; and if coagulation parameters are normal, the risk of bleeding is low (Fig. 8-12).

SPLENOMEGALY

A large number of processes can result in splenomegaly, and a partial list of them is given in Box 8-2. In most cases it is not possible to determine the cause of splenic enlargement based on sonographic analysis of the spleen itself. Analysis of associated findings may, however, provide clues to the cause of splenomegaly.

INFECTIONS/INFLAMMATION

Splenic abscesses are uncommon, probably due to the efficient phagocytic activity of its reticuloendothelial system leukocytes. However, these defenses may be insufficient in the settings of bacterial endocarditis,

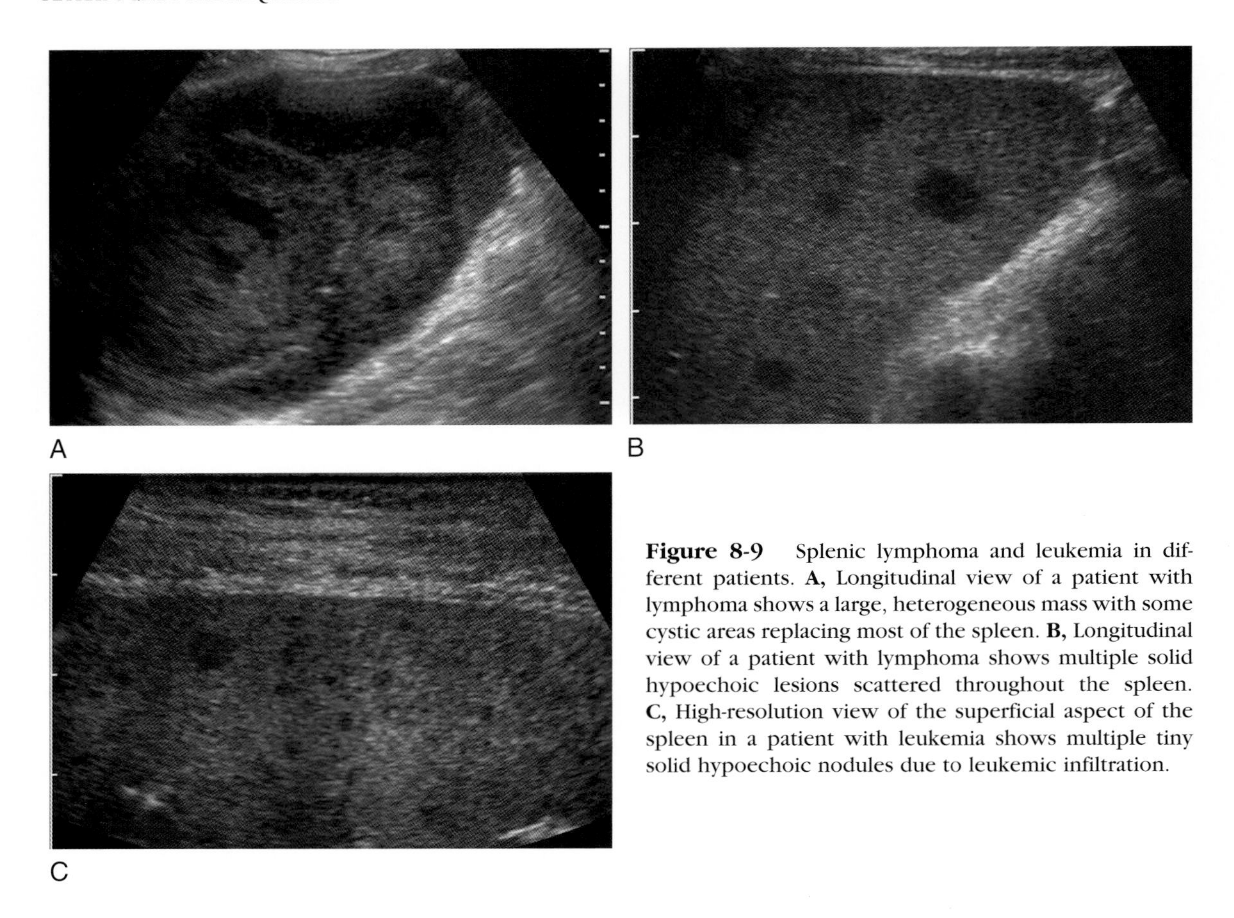

Figure 8-9 Splenic lymphoma and leukemia in different patients. **A,** Longitudinal view of a patient with lymphoma shows a large, heterogeneous mass with some cystic areas replacing most of the spleen. **B,** Longitudinal view of a patient with lymphoma shows multiple solid hypoechoic lesions scattered throughout the spleen. **C,** High-resolution view of the superficial aspect of the spleen in a patient with leukemia shows multiple tiny solid hypoechoic nodules due to leukemic infiltration.

septicemia, immunologic deficiencies, intravenous drug abuse, splenic trauma, and infarcts. Splenic abscesses are similar to abscesses elsewhere and typically appear as complex fluid-filled lesions. However, they can also appear as hypoechoic solid lesions (Fig. 8-13). The differential diagnosis primarily includes hematoma and necrotic tumor.

Fungal abscesses of the spleen have an appearance similar to that of fungal abscesses in the liver. They are usually small and may appear as a target lesion. Granulomatous infection of the spleen can occur in the settings of tuberculosis and histoplasmosis. In both situations multiple small punctate areas of increased echogenicity are seen, and these represent calcifications (Fig. 8-14). Sarcoidosis is another granulomatous disease that can affect the spleen. In fact, approximately 30% of patients with sarcoid will have splenic, liver, and/or abdominal lymph node involvement. Splenic involvement can be either diffuse or multifocal and appear as hypoechoic masses (Fig. 8-15).

TRAUMA

The spleen is the most commonly involved organ in victims of upper abdominal trauma. Splenic disruption can occur with or without capsular laceration. If the capsule remains intact, an intraparenchymal or subcapsular hematoma may develop. Laceration of the splenic capsule can result in hemoperitoneum as well as splenic hematomas. In a trauma patient, the finding of localized fluid around the spleen suggests splenic laceration regardless of the sonographic appearance of the spleen.

Splenic hematomas, subcapsular hematomas, and perisplenic hematomas all vary in their sonographic appearance, depending on their age. In the acute phase they appear complex and hypoechoic. However, it is very unusual for patients to present early enough to identify this appearance. With clot formation they appear more echogenic and may be isoechoic to the splenic parenchyma (Fig. 8-16). For this reason, splenic lacerations may not be apparent on sonography. With time the clot lyses and liquefies and becomes more hypoechoic to anechoic. Although sonography is capable of detecting splenic lacerations and ruptures, it is significantly less accurate than contrast medium–enhanced CT. Enhanced CT is also better at determining the size and extent of abnormalities related to splenic trauma. In addition, it is more difficult to assess the other upper abdominal organs with sonography than with enhanced CT. Therefore, sonography has not been used extensively in North America to evaluate parenchymal organs in the traumatized patient. As mentioned in

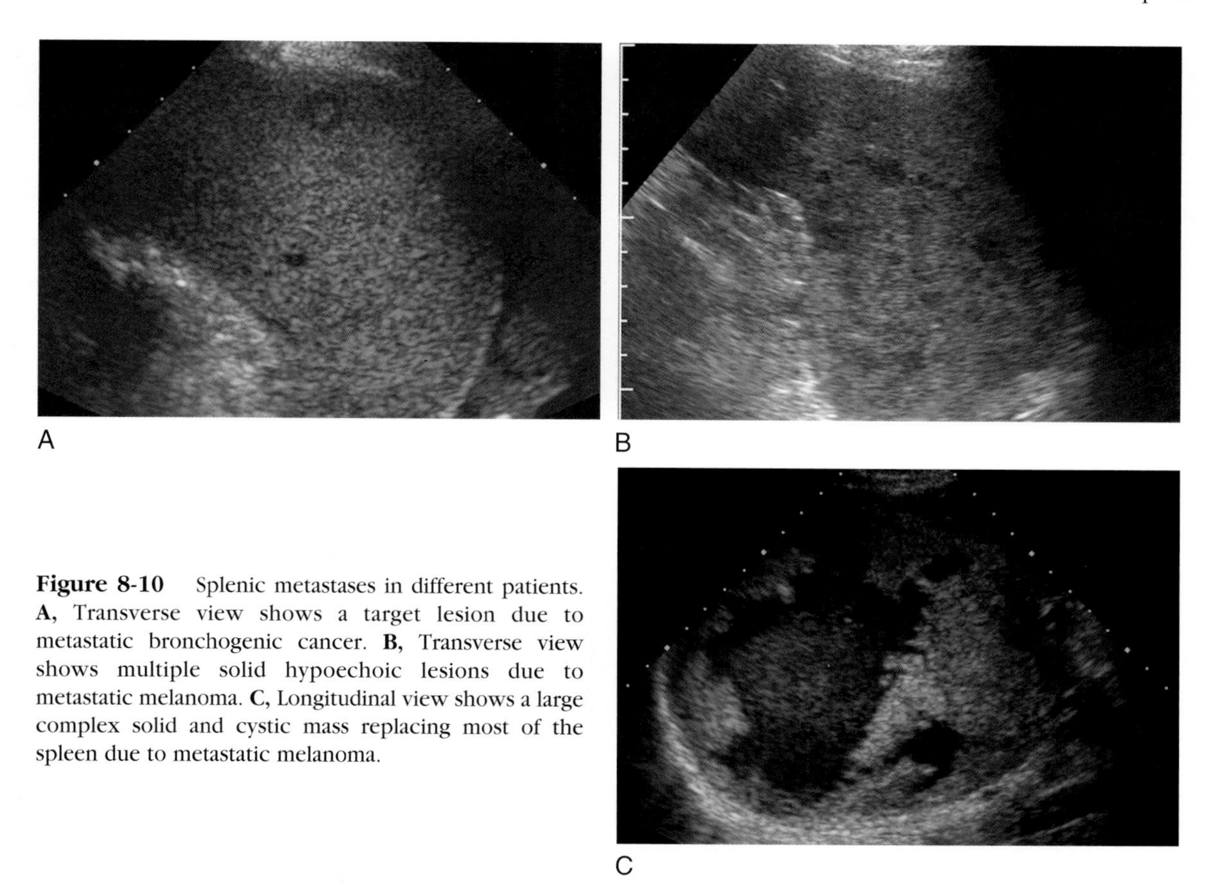

Figure 8-10 Splenic metastases in different patients. **A**, Transverse view shows a target lesion due to metastatic bronchogenic cancer. **B**, Transverse view shows multiple solid hypoechoic lesions due to metastatic melanoma. **C**, Longitudinal view shows a large complex solid and cystic mass replacing most of the spleen due to metastatic melanoma.

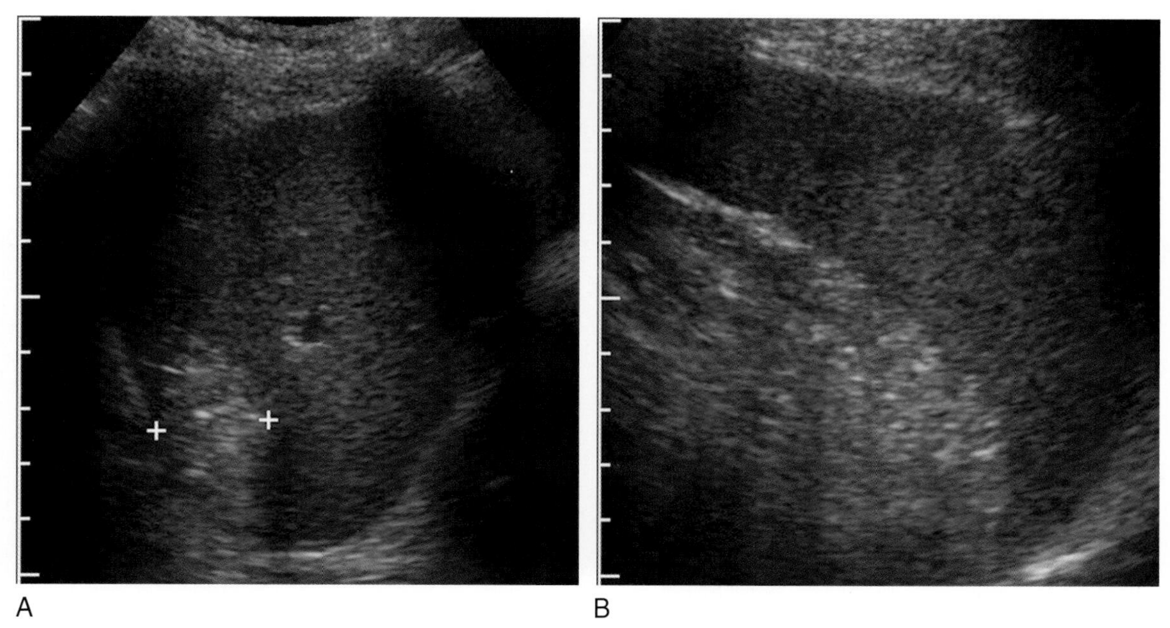

Figure 8-11 Splenic pseudolesion. **A**, Longitudinal view of the left upper quadrant shows an apparent hyperechoic mass *(cursors)* in the periphery of the spleen. **B**, Transverse view shows no corresponding lesion. Fibrofatty tissue in the splenic hilum appeared as an intrasplenic lesion on the longitudinal view because of the effects of volume averaging.

Box 8-1 Solid Spleen Lesions

Hemangiomas
Hamartomas
Lymphomas
Metastases
Infarcts
Abscesses
Sarcoidosis
Granulomas
Extramedullary hematopoiesis

Box 8-2 Causes of Splenomegaly

COMMON	UNCOMMON
Heart failure	Glycogen storage disease
Portal hypertension	Malaria
Leukemia	Myelofibrosis
Lymphoma	
Hepatitis	
Mononucleosis	
Generalized infections	
Hemolytic anemias	

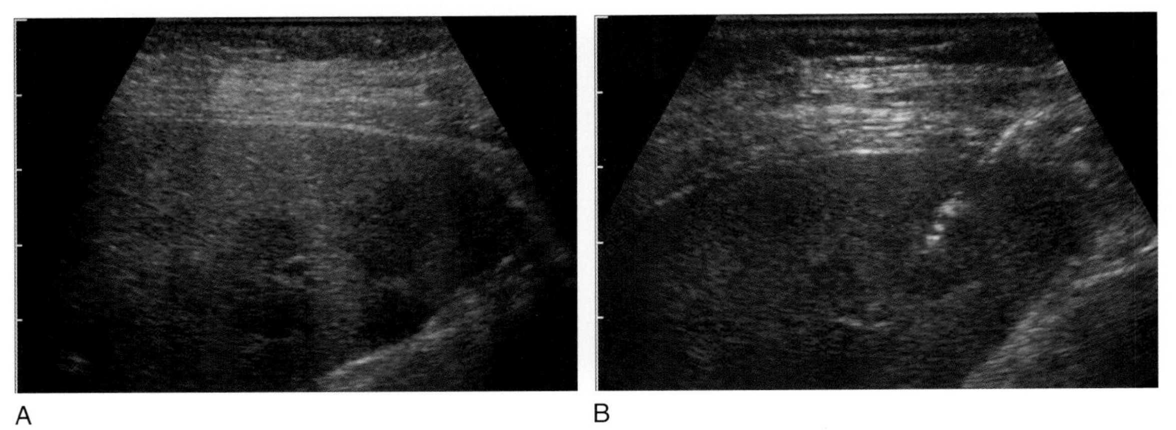

Figure 8-12 Ultrasound guided splenic biopsy. **A,** Longitudinal view of the spleen shows several solid hypoechoic lesions. This patient had no risk factors for malignancy, and a CT scan of the chest and abdomen showed no other lesions. **B,** Similar view shows a 25-gauge needle within the lesion. Fine-needle aspiration was performed primarily to rule out lymphoma. Cytology showed granulomas and no evidence of malignancy.

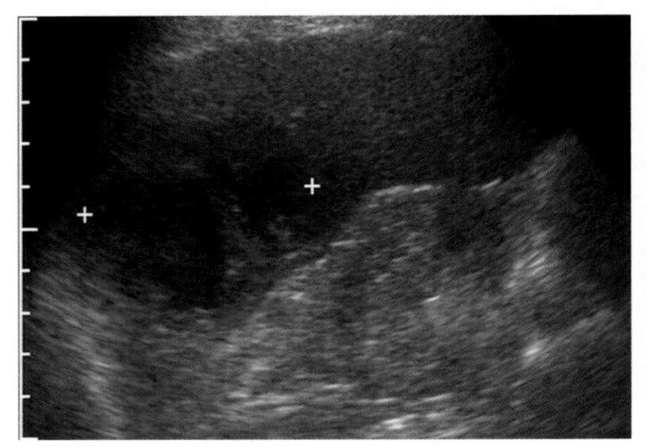

Figure 8-13 Splenic abscess. Longitudinal view shows a complex fluid collection *(cursors)* in the superior aspect of the spleen. This patient was a diabetic with peptic ulcer disease and concomitant liver abscesses documented by percutaneous aspiration.

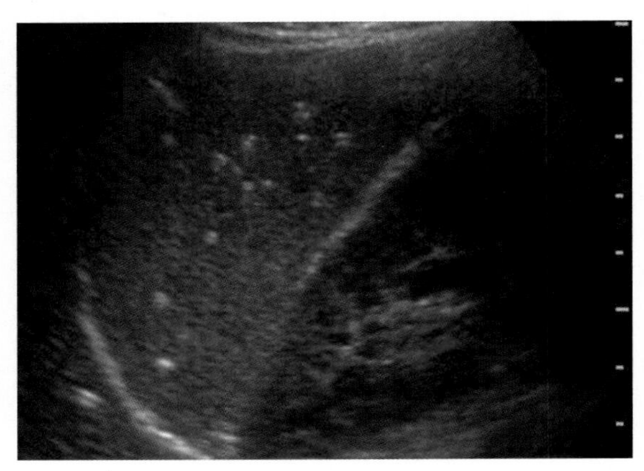

Figure 8-14 Granulomas. Longitudinal view shows multiple, small, non-shadowing, bright reflectors scattered throughout the spleen. CT done for other reasons confirmed that these were all tiny calcifications.

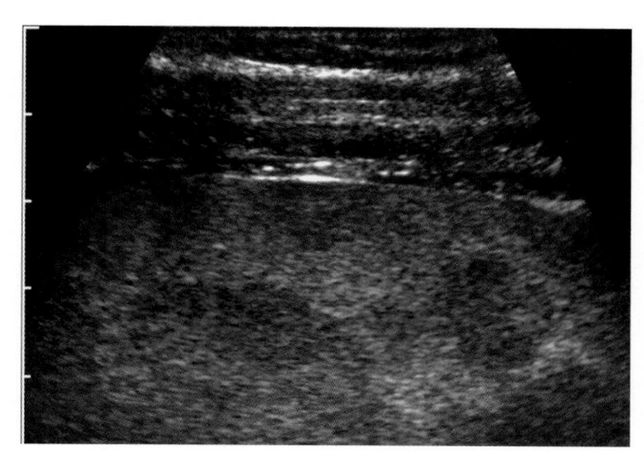

Figure 8-15 Sarcoidosis. High-resolution view of the superficial aspect of the spleen shows several solid, hypoechoic lesions in the spleen. This was not biopsy proven, but this patient had well-documented sarcoidosis in the chest.

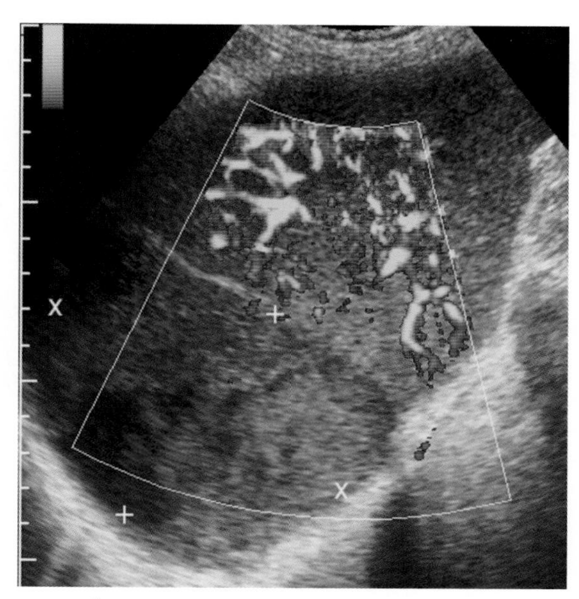

Figure 8-16 Hematoma. Longitudinal power Doppler view of the left upper quadrant shows a complex solid and liquefied mass *(cursors)* with no internal blood flow. Readily detectable flow is seen throughout the spleen.

Chapter 3, sonography is effective at detecting hemoperitoneum in the traumatized patient and can be used instead of the diagnostic peritoneal lavage. Therefore, sonography now is used in the triage of certain trauma patients in many emergency departments.

One important pitfall to be aware of is the elongated left hepatic lobe that crosses the midline and insinuates itself between the spleen and the diaphragm. Because the liver is less echogenic than the spleen, this anatomic variant can give the false impression of a perisplenic or splenic subcapsular fluid collection (Fig. 8-17). In general, knowledge of this pitfall is sufficient to avert a diagnostic error. In addition, the detection of vascular structures running through the hepatic parenchyma can help in distinguishing it from perisplenic fluid.

A condition that may develop after splenic trauma is splenosis. This consists of the implantation of splenic tissue onto intraperitoneal surfaces with subsequent vascularization and growth. The end result is the development of macroscopic nodules of splenic tissue. Like the spleen itself, these nodules are very homogeneous in their echogenicity and are usually round or ovoid

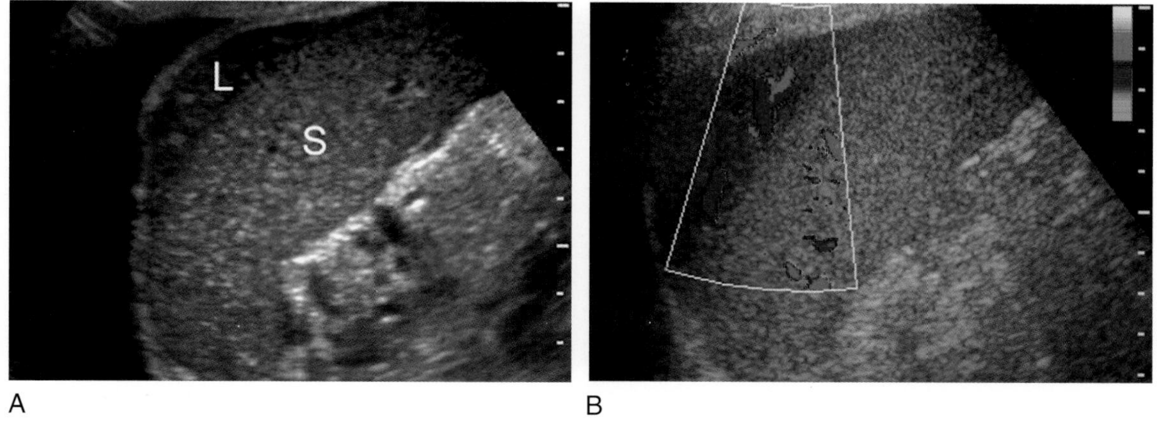

Figure 8-17 Pseudo-perisplenic fluid. A, Longitudinal view of the left upper quadrant shows the spleen (S) and an elongated left hepatic lobe (L) insinuating itself between the spleen and the diaphragm. The decreased echogenicity of the liver compared with the spleen often results in this anatomic variant being misinterpreted as perisplenic fluid. Note that there is a pleural effusion above the diaphragm. B, Color Doppler image shows multiple vessels within the hepatic parenchyma. This confirms that this is liver and not a perisplenic fluid collection.

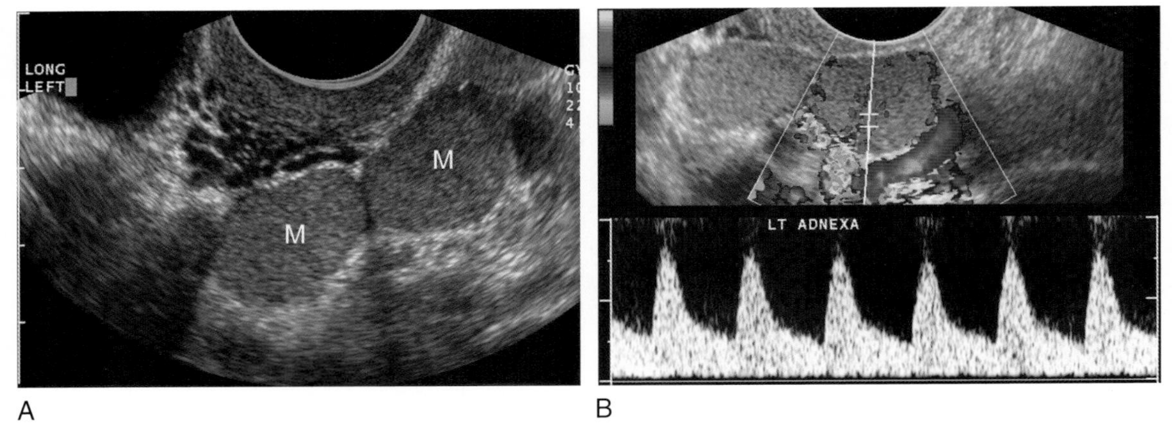

Figure 8-18 Splenosis. **A,** Transvaginal view of the left adnexa shows two adjacent solid masses (M) that were shown to be separate from a normal left ovary. **B,** Color and pulsed Doppler view shows detectable blood flow with an arterial signal similar to solid parenchymal organs. Multiple peritoneal based lesions were initially considered until additional views of the upper abdomen showed an absent spleen. The patient then revealed the history of prior splenectomy for a ruptured spleen. A heat-damaged red blood cell scan confirmed that this was ectopic splenic tissue.

(Fig. 8-18). The differential diagnosis includes other intraperitoneal masses such as metastasis and endometriosis. If there is a history of splenic trauma or splenic surgery, splenosis should be considered likely. Tagged damaged red blood cell scans or sulfur colloid scans can be used for confirmation in confusing cases.

INFARCTION

Splenic infarctions stem from an embolic phenomenon as well as from thrombosis of the splenic artery, splenic vein, and their branches. They are one of the most common causes of focal splenic lesions seen on

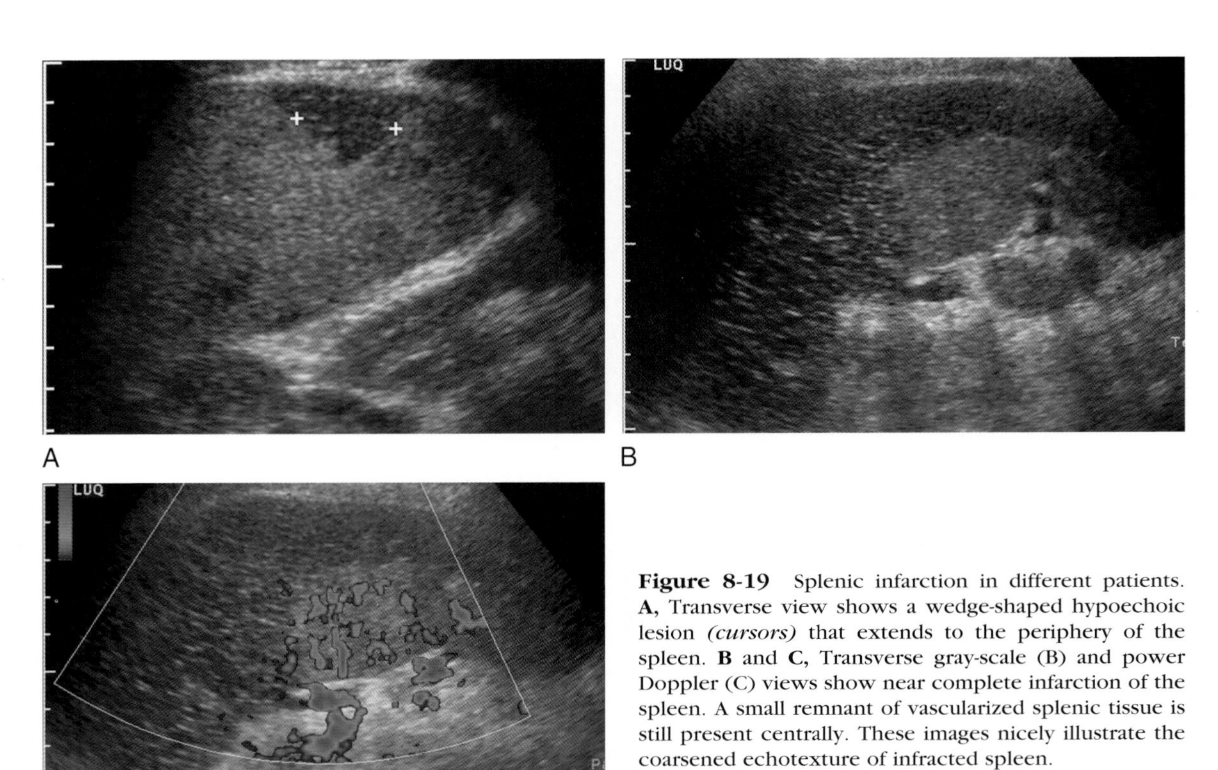

Figure 8-19 Splenic infarction in different patients. **A,** Transverse view shows a wedge-shaped hypoechoic lesion *(cursors)* that extends to the periphery of the spleen. **B** and **C,** Transverse gray-scale (B) and power Doppler (C) views show near complete infarction of the spleen. A small remnant of vascularized splenic tissue is still present centrally. These images nicely illustrate the coarsened echotexture of infracted spleen.

cross-sectional images. In approximately 50% of cases they are multiple. Infarcts usually appear hypoechoic and have a coarsened echotexture on sonography. With time, scar formation may cause infarcts to become hyperechoic. When a wedge-shaped, peripherally located splenic lesion is identified, an infarct should be considered (Fig. 8-19). Complete infarction of the spleen can be more difficult to detect sonographically. However, as with focal infarcts, an alteration in splenic echogenicity and echotexture can be a clue to an underlying infarct.

Key Features

The spleen is normally more echogenic than the liver and the kidney. It may be greater than, less than, or equal in echogenicity to the pancreas.

Splenules are very common, are isoechoic to the spleen, and should not be confused with other left upper quadrant masses.

Splenic cysts are most frequently the result of prior episodes of trauma and hematoma formation.

Splenic lymphoma and leukemia can appear as diffuse, focal, or multifocal involvement of the spleen. Lesions are almost always hypoechoic.

Metastases to the spleen are uncommon and usually represent a late manifestation of generalized metastatic disease.

Ultrasound is an effective means of detecting splenomegaly, but in the absence of associated findings it is not capable of distinguishing among the many potential causes.

Splenic abscesses share the sonographic characteristics of abscesses elsewhere in the body, ranging in appearance from solid-appearing masses to markedly or minimally complex fluid collections.

Splenic infarcts are common and typically have a hypoechoic and coarsened echotexture.

Granulomatous disease such as histoplasmosis and tuberculosis may produce multiple small calcifications in the spleen.

Detection of a hemoperitoneum can be used in the triage of patients with suspected splenic trauma.

SUGGESTED READINGS

Costello P, Kane RA, Oster J, et al: Focal splenic disease demonstrated by ultrasound and computed tomography. J Can Assoc Radiol 36:22, 1985.

Crivello MS, Peterson IM, Austin RM: Left lobe of the liver mimicking perisplenic collections. J Clin Ultrasound 14:697, 1986.

Dodds WJ, Taylor AJ, Erickson SJ, et al: Radiologic imaging of splenic anomalies. AJR Am J Roentgenol 155:805, 1990.

Goerg C, Schwerk WB: Splenic infarction: Sonographic patterns, diagnosis, follow-up, and complications. Radiology 174:803, 1990.

Goerg C, Schwerk WB, Goerg K: Splenic lesions: Sonographic patterns, follow-up, differential diagnosis. Eur J Radiol 13:59, 1991.

Goerg C, Schwerk WB, Goerg K: Sonography of focal lesions of the spleen. AJR Am J Roentgenol 156:949, 1991.

Li DK, Cooperberg PL, Graham MF, Callen P: Pseudo perisplenic "fluid collections": A clue to normal liver and spleen echogenic texture. J Ultrasound Med 5:397, 1986.

Maillard JC, Menu Y, Scherrer A, et al: Intraperitoneal splenosis: Diagnosis by ultrasound and computed tomography. Gastrointest Radiol 14:179, 1989.

Maresca G, Mirk P, DeGaetano AM, et al: Sonographic patterns in splenic infarction. J Clin Ultrasound 14:23, 1986.

Normand JP, Rioux M, Dumont M, Bouchard G: Ultrasonographic features of abdominal ectopic splenic tissue. Can Assoc Radiol J 44:179-184, 1993.

Pastakia B, Shawker TH, Thalar M, et al: Hepatosplenic candidiasis: wheels within wheels. Radiology 166:417, 1988.

Permutter GS: Ultrasound measurements of the spleen. In Goldberg BB, Kurtz AB (eds): Atlas of Ultrasound Measurements. Chicago, Year Book Medical, 1990, pp 126-138.

Richards JR, McGahan JP: Ultrasound for blunt abdominal trauma in the emergency department. Ultrasound Q 15(2): 60-72, 1999.

Ross PR, Moser RP, Dackman AH, et al: Hemangioma of the spleen: Radiologic-pathologic correlation in ten cases. AJR Am J Roentgenol 162:73, 1987.

Subramanyam BR, Balthazar EJ, Horii SC: Sonography of the accessory spleen. AJR Am J Roentgenol 143:47-49, 1984.

Warshaur , Molina PL, Hamman SM, et al: Nodular sarcoidosis of the liver and spleen: Analysis of 32 cases. Radiology 195: 757-762, 1995.

CHAPTER 9

General Abdomen

Bowel
Peritoneum
Abdominal Wall
Lymphadenopathy
Aorta
Inferior Vena Cava
Adrenal
For Key Features summary see p. 242

BOWEL

Sonography is not routinely used as a primary tool for evaluation of the bowel. Nevertheless, there are many patients with nonspecific bowel-related complaints who are initially scanned with ultrasound, and in these patients attention to the intestinal structures can often identify the abnormality and direct the work-up in the appropriate direction. Therefore, a quick survey of the bowel is a useful undertaking in patients undergoing abdominal sonography. When necessary, sonography can be performed after ingestion of water to improve evaluation of the stomach and proximal small bowel. Retrograde infusion of water can also be used to distend the colon (hydrocolonic sonography) and evaluate colonic lesions.

The normal bowel has a typical appearance on sonography. In general it has a bull's-eye or target-like appearance with a central hyperechoic component and an outer hypoechoic ring. In some cases, multiple layers are apparent (Fig. 9-1). Five layers have been described. The inner hyperechoic layer arises from the interface reflection between the lumen and the surface of the mucosa. The second layer is hypoechoic and arises from the combined deep mucosa and the muscularis mucosa. The third layer is hyperechoic and arises from the submucosa. The fourth layer is hypoechoic and arises from the muscularis propria. The final outer layer is hyperechoic and arises from the interface reflection between the muscularis propria and the serosa or adventitia (plus peri-intestinal fat). These five layers are routinely seen on endoscopic ultrasound and are intermittently seen on transcutaneous scans (Table 9-1).

One of the most common intestinal abnormalities seen on sonography is intestinal obstruction. Distended, fluid-filled, peristaltic loops are the hallmark of bowel obstruction (Fig. 9-2). In many cases, the gas-filled loops located in the nondependent anterior abdomen will obscure these findings. This pitfall can be avoided by scanning in the lateral flanks where dependent fluid-filled loops are located. When a bowel obstruction is detected, a search for the cause should be performed. Hernias, intrinsic bowel wall lesions, abdominal masses,

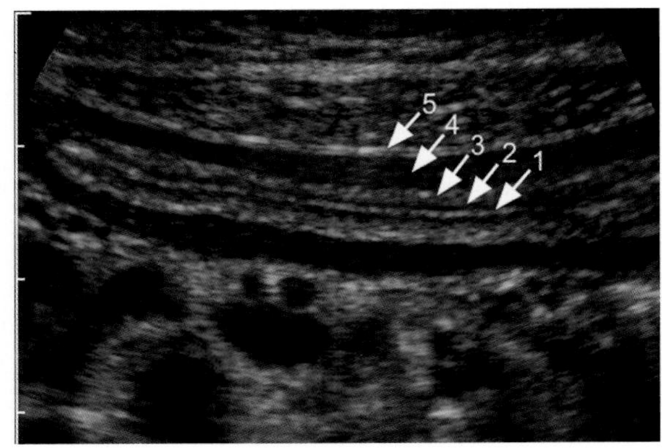

Figure 9-1 Normal bowel layers. Long-axis view of the gastric antrum shows the interface between the coapted anterior and posterior mucosal surfaces (1). The deep mucosa and muscularis mucosa is the next hypoechoic layer (2). The submucosa is the next hyperechoic layer (3). The muscularis propria is the next hypoechoic layer (4). The final layer is the interface between the muscularis propria and the serosa (5). Note that the same layers labeled on the anterior wall of the antrum are repeated on the posterior wall of the antrum.

Table 9-1 Layers of Bowel Seen on High-Resolution Sonography

Layer	Echogenicity
Mucosal interface	Echogenic
Deep mucosa and muscularis mucosa	Hypoechoic
Submucosa	Echogenic
Muscularis propria	Hypoechoic
Serosa interface	Echogenic

and abdominal fluid collections can all be detected with sonography.

The normal intestinal wall should be less than 5 mm in thickness. A wide variety of disorders can cause bowel wall thickening (Box 9-1). In almost all cases, thickened intestinal walls appear as a target-like lesion with the central echogenic mucosa surrounded by a hypoechoic layer. The major causes of bowel wall thickening are inflammation, infection, edema, ischemia, and neoplasms. Eccentric thickening (Fig. 9-3) or thickening

Box 9-1 Common Causes of Bowel Wall Thickening

Inflammation
Infection
Neoplasm
Ischemia
Edema
Hemorrhage

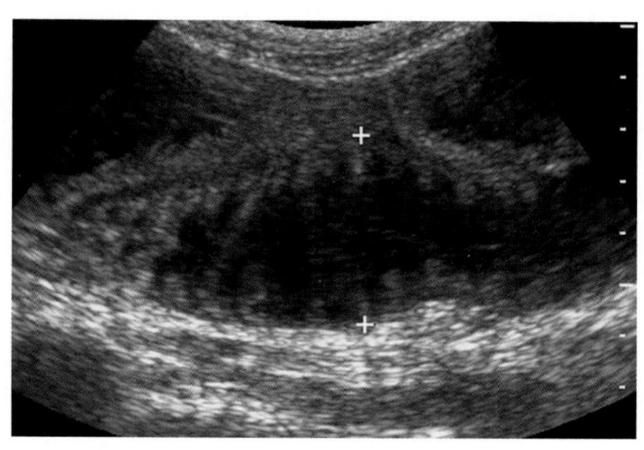

Figure 9-2 Small bowel obstruction. View of the left upper quadrant shows a dilated fluid-filled loop of small bowel *(cursors)* measuring more than 3 cm in diameter. Active peristalsis was seen during real-time examination, typical of small bowel obstruction.

associated with more focal masses (Fig. 9-4) is usually neoplastic. Carcinoma, lymphoma, and gastrointestinal stromal tumors are the most commonly encountered neoplasms. Lymphoma may also affect the bowel wall in a concentric and diffuse manner (Fig. 9-5). Gastrointestinal stromal tumors (also known as spindle cell tumors, leiomyomas, or leiomyosarcomas) range from small, homogeneous masses (Fig. 9-6A) to large lesions with central necrosis and calcification (see Fig. 9-6B). In most instances, it is possible to determine the type of tumor based on endoscopic biopsies. However, when endoscopic biopsies are nondiagnostic, percutaneous ultrasound-guided biopsies can be performed with a high level of success.

Inflammatory thickening of the intestines is generally diffuse and concentric (Fig. 9-7). Commonly encountered causes include diverticulitis, Crohn's disease, ischemia, pseudomembranous colitis, and ulcerative

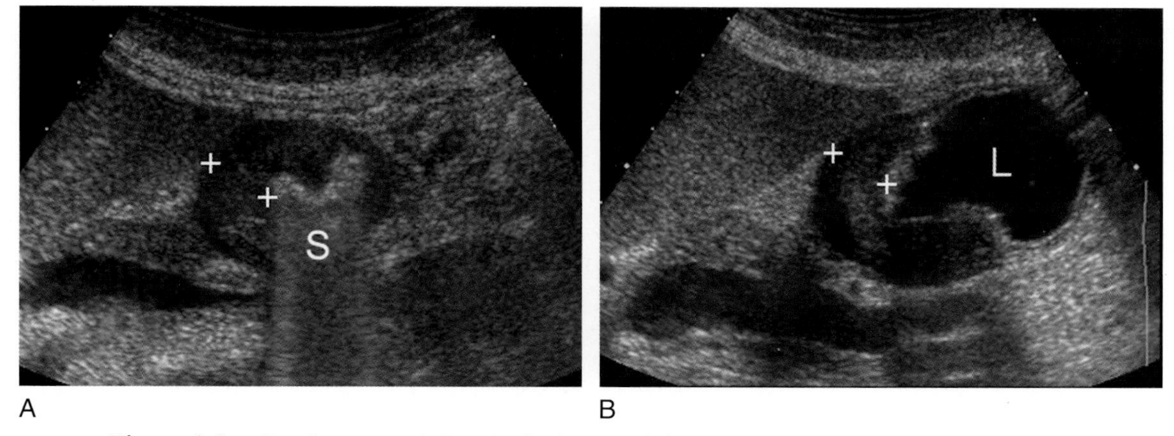

Figure 9-3 Gastric cancer. **A,** Longitudinal view of the gastric antrum shows eccentric thickening along the lesser curvature *(cursors)*. Dirty shadowing (S) is identified arising from air in the lumen of the stomach. **B,** Repeat scans of the same patient after water was ingested shows persistent thickening of the lesser curvature *(cursors)* while fluid in the lumen of the stomach (L) produces effacement of the greater curvature.

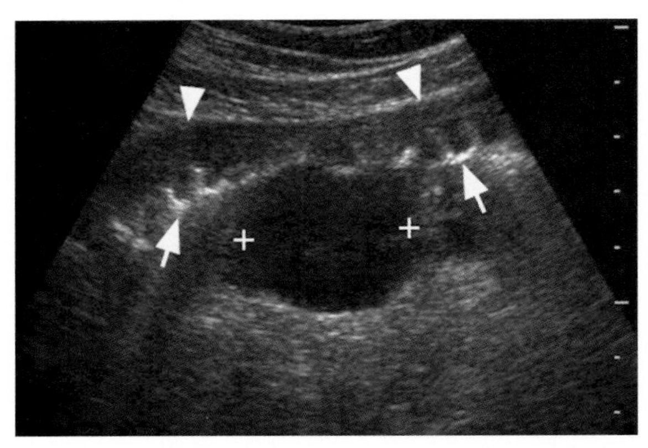

Figure 9-4 Small bowel lymphoma. A view of a loop of small bowel shows a focal hypoechoic solid mass *(cursors)* along the mesenteric wall of the bowel. Gas in the lumen *(arrows)* obscures most of the adjacent mesenteric wall of the bowel. The anti-mesenteric wall of the bowel *(arrowheads)* is thickened, as are the small bowel folds.

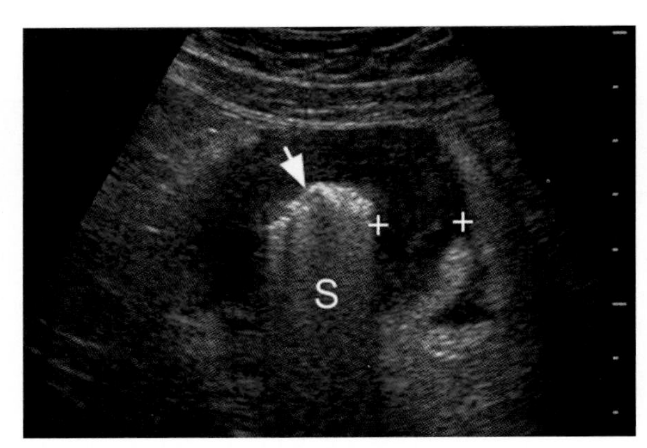

Figure 9-5 Small bowel lymphoma. Short-axis view of a loop of small bowel shows marked concentric thickening of the bowel wall *(cursors)*. Gas in the lumen *(arrow)* produces a dirty acoustic shadow (S).

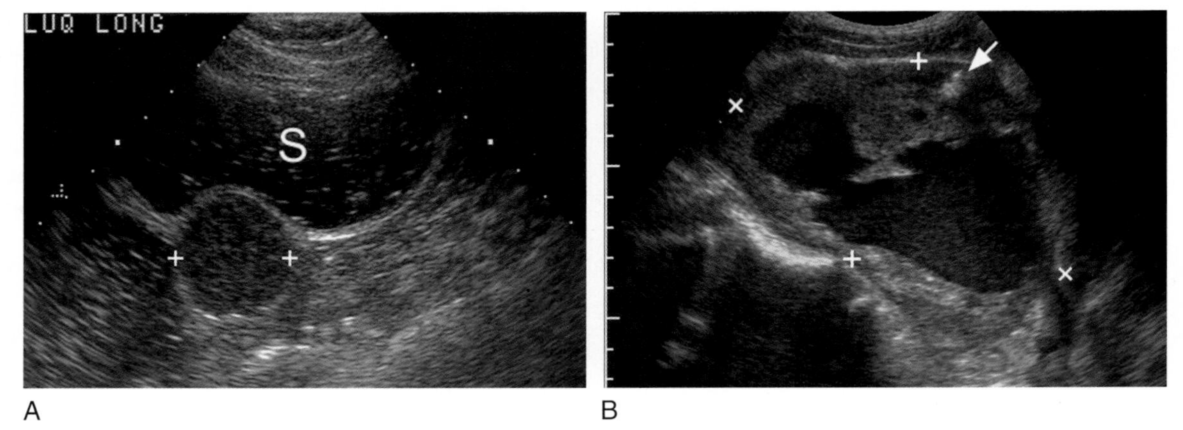

Figure 9-6 Gastrointestinal stromal tumor. **A,** View of the fluid-filled stomach (S) shows a hypoechoic solid submucosal mass arising from the posterior gastric wall *(cursors)*. This is a typical appearance for a small gastrointestinal stromal tumor. **B,** Longitudinal view of the lower abdomen in a different patient shows a complex mass *(cursors)* with a large area of central liquefaction. A small faintly shadowing calcification *(arrow)* is also identified. This is a common appearance for large gastrointestinal stromal tumors. At this size, it is difficult to determine the organ of origin with cross-sectional imaging.

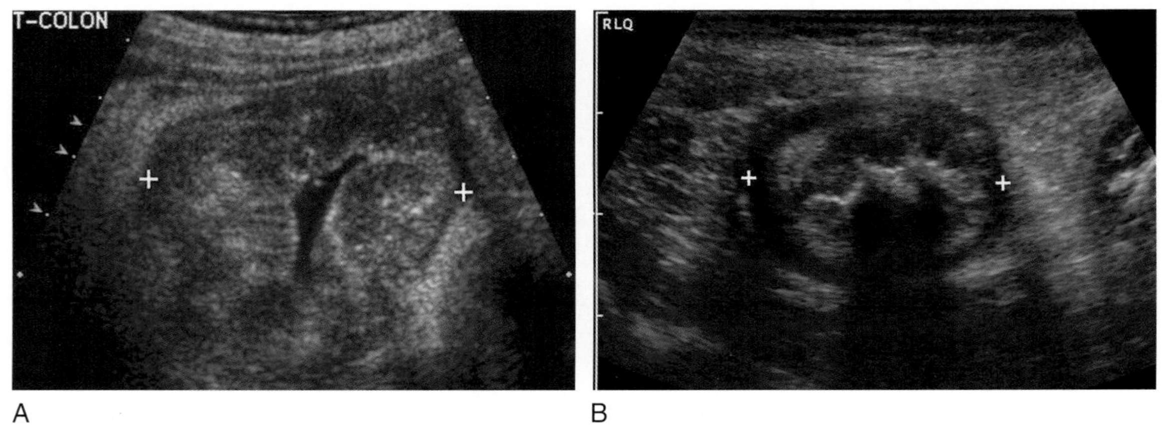

Figure 9-7 Inflammatory thickening of the bowel. **A,** Short-axis view of transverse colon *(cursors)* shows concentric thickening of the colonic wall in a patient with pseudomembranous colitis. **B,** Short-axis view of the terminal ileum *(cursors)* shows concentric wall thickening in a patient with Crohn's disease.

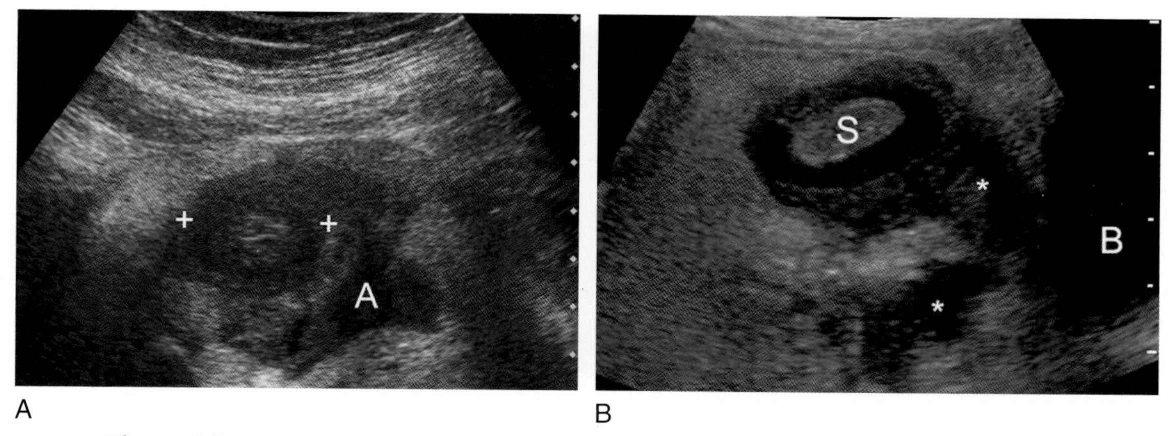

Figure 9-8 Peri-intestinal abscess. **A,** Short-axis view of a small bowel loop *(cursors)* shows concentric thickening of the small bowel with an adjacent irregular fluid collection due to an abscess (A) in a patient with Crohn's disease. **B,** Short-axis view of the sigmoid colon (S) shows concentric colonic wall thickening with extraluminal inflammatory changes and fluid (*) in a patient with diverticulitis. The urinary bladder (B) is seen at the edge of the image.

colitis. Although the sonographic findings are typically nonspecific, the combination of sonographic findings and clinical parameters is often sufficient to suggest the diagnosis. Evaluation of the peri-intestinal structures for extraluminal abscess is also important, especially in patients with Crohn's disease and diverticulitis (Fig. 9-8).

Bowel wall thickening caused by peptic ulcer disease may be eccentric and localized to the region of ulceration (Fig. 9-9A) or concentric from the associated edema. In some cases, peptic ulcers will contain gas within the ulcer crater and produce a ring-down artifact or a dirty shadow (see Fig. 9-9B).

Another condition that can produce bowel thickening is an intussusception. Close inspection will reveal multiple alternating hyperechoic and hypoechoic layers owing to the presence of three overlapping mucosal and muscular layers of the intussuscipiens (distal segment) and the intussusceptum (proximal segment) (Fig. 9-10). Inability to detect blood flow in the intussusception increases the likelihood of necrosis and predicts the need for surgery. Detection of blood flow is reassuring. In adults, approximately 90% are associated with a lead mass of some sort (e.g., polyp, lipoma, stromal tumor, lymphoma, metastasis, cancer). Other causes in adults include Meckel's diverticulum and sprue. With the increased use of CT and ultrasound, transient, idiopathic adult intussusceptions are being diagnosed more often. In children, intussusceptions are usually idiopathic.

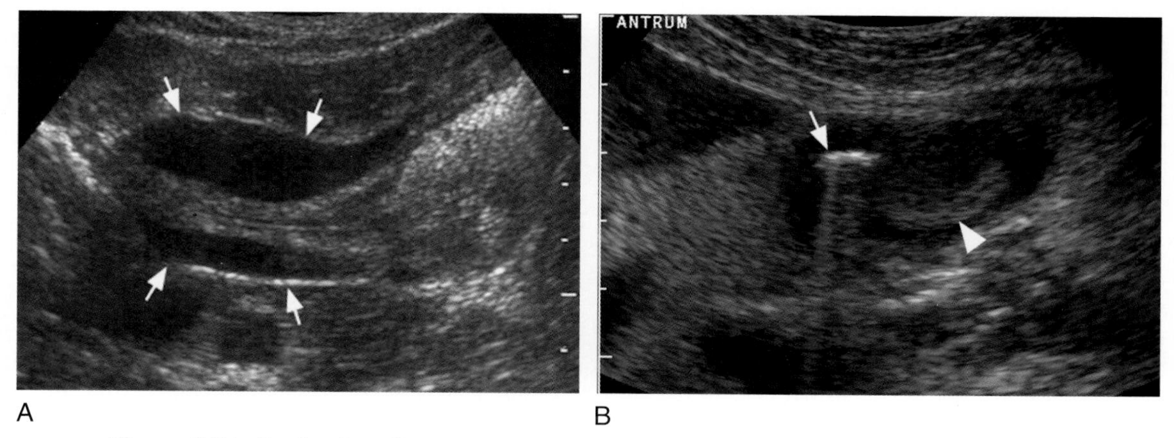

Figure 9-9 Peptic ulcer disease. **A,** Long-axis view of the gastric antrum shows gastric wall thickening *(arrows)* greater along the anterior wall than the posterior wall. **B,** Short-axis view of the gastric antrum in a different patient shows the collapsed lumen and the echogenic mucosa *(arrowhead)*. An ulcer crater containing gas *(arrow)* is seen as a bright intramural reflection within a thickened area of gastric wall. Also note the ring-down artifact posterior to the ulcer.

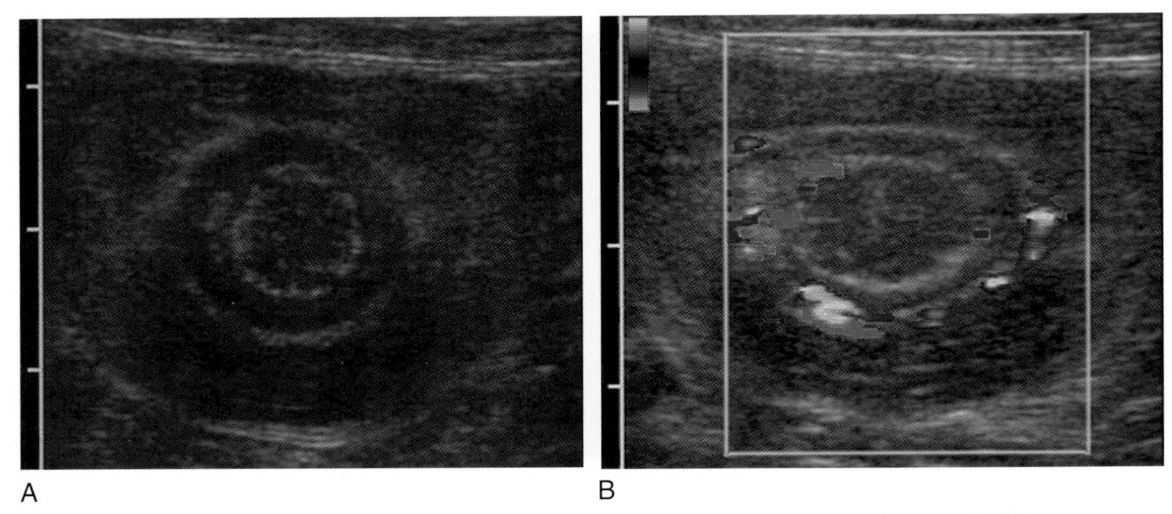

Figure 9-10 Intussusception. **A,** Short-axis view of a loop of small bowel shows multiple concentric rings of increased and decreased echogenicity and thickening of the outer small bowel layer typical of an intussusception. **B,** Color Doppler view shows detectable internal vascularity, which indicates a low likelihood of bowel wall necrosis. A small bowel follow-through study done 1 hour after the ultrasound study showed no detectable intussusception, confirming the sometimes transient nature of this abnormality.

A lesion of the bowel wall that is rarely encountered on sonography is pneumatosis. Nevertheless, because it can indicate bowel ischemia, it is important to recognize when it is encountered. The hallmark on sonography is the presence of echogenic reflectors indicating gas in the dependent wall of the bowel (Fig. 9-11). As elsewhere, ring-down artifacts will sometimes be present and confirm that the reflections are coming from gas.

A common situation in which ultrasound is used as the initial imaging technique is in patients with suspected appendicitis. To be successful, it is important to use a high-resolution probe (usually a linear array or occasionally a curved array operating at least at 5 MHz). To allow for this, graded compression is important to get as close to the appendix as possible. Graded compression also pushes bowel gas out of the way and makes it possible to determine if the appendix compresses. It is also helpful to have the patient localize the region of pain. In many cases, the patient can point to a specific area of pain, and this usually corresponds very precisely to the site of the abnormal appendix. The primary criterion for the diagnosis of appendicitis is an appendiceal diameter greater than 6 mm (Fig. 9-12). In some patients, an intraluminal appendicolith can be detected (see Fig. 9-12C). Other associated findings are inflamed, echogenic periappendiceal fat, loculated periappendiceal fluid collections, and hyperemia on color Doppler imaging (Box 9-2). Localized appendicitis isolated to the tip of the appendix can occur, so it is important to follow the appendix to its blunt tip.

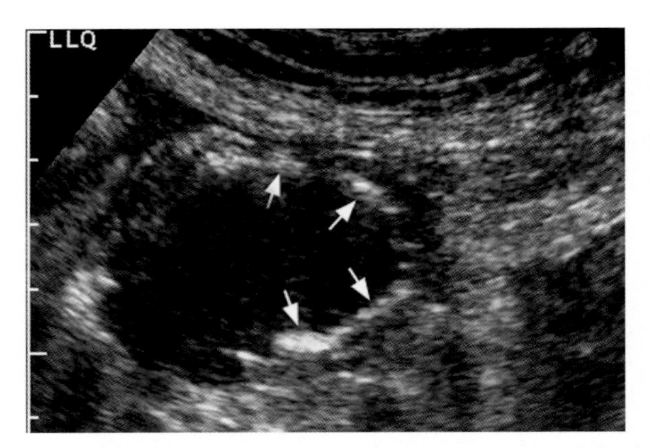

Figure 9-11 Colonic pneumatosis. Short-axis view of the left colon shows bright reflectors along the wall *(arrows)*. Note that some are in the non-dependent portion (as might be seen with intraluminal air), but the presence of reflectors along the dependent portion is difficult to explain and should suggest the diagnosis of pneumatosis. This was subsequently confirmed with an abdominal radiograph.

PERITONEUM

The most common abnormality of the peritoneal cavity is ascites. In addition to transudates and exudates, other less common considerations include urine, blood, pus, cerebrospinal fluid (related to shunts), peritoneal dialysis, and chyle. Sonography is quite sensitive at detecting ascites as well as guiding aspiration of ascites. Small amounts of ascites are seen as anechoic collections

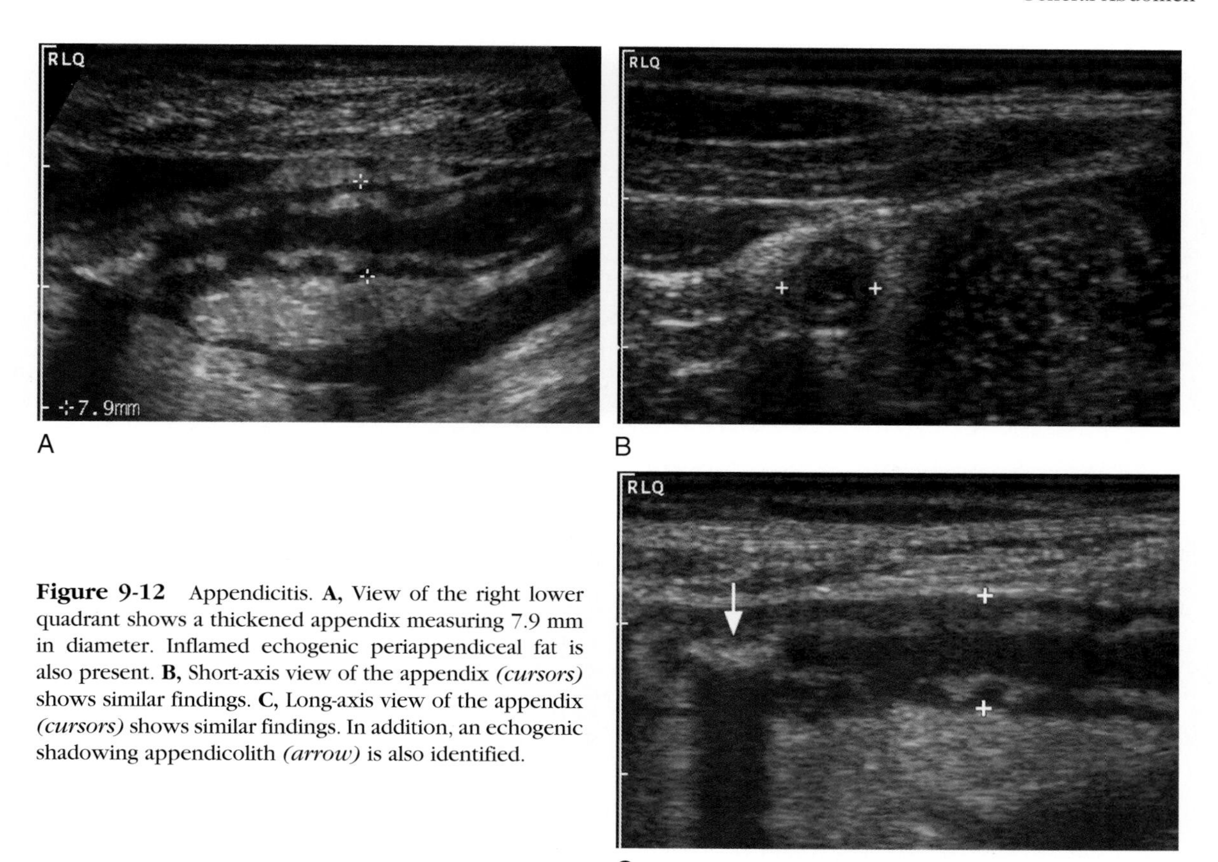

Figure 9-12 Appendicitis. **A,** View of the right lower quadrant shows a thickened appendix measuring 7.9 mm in diameter. Inflamed echogenic periappendiceal fat is also present. **B,** Short-axis view of the appendix *(cursors)* shows similar findings. **C,** Long-axis view of the appendix *(cursors)* shows similar findings. In addition, an echogenic shadowing appendicolith *(arrow)* is also identified.

most often in the pelvic cul-de-sac and in the right upper quadrant (Fig. 9-13A and B) between the liver and the abdominal wall or in the hepatorenal fossa (Morrison's pouch). Larger amounts of ascites will distribute throughout the peritoneal cavity. Uncomplicated ascites lacks internal echoes and although it may displace adjacent structures does not cause significant distortion of adjacent structures (see Fig. 9-13C). On the other hand, complicated ascites may contain internal echoes (due to blood or pus) or may become loculated with multiple septations (see Fig. 9-13D and E).

Box 9-2 Sonographic Signs of Appendicitis

Diameter >6 mm
Lack of compressibility
Inflamed, echogenic periappendiceal fat
Hyperemia
Appendicolith
Adjacent fluid collections

One evolving use of ultrasound is in patients with blunt abdominal trauma. The major role of ultrasound is to identify a hemoperitoneum as a secondary sign of injury to an intra-abdominal organ (Fig. 9-14). In trained hands, sonography is very effective in identifying a hemoperitoneum. Unfortunately, sonography is less effective in identifying the injured organ. On the other hand, contrast medium–enhanced CT is substantially more sensitive in detecting organ injury and is just as sensitive at detecting hemoperitoneum. Therefore, the use of ultrasound in the trauma patient is quite controversial. In the unusual situations in which CT is not readily available or when the patient is too unstable to leave the trauma room, sonography is clearly a valuable tool that can replace the diagnostic peritoneal lavage as a means of detecting a hemoperitoneum. It can also be used as a means of serially following patients who have no abnormalities or have nonsurgical abnormalities detected at initial imaging.

Many primary tumors can metastasize to the peritoneum, but the most common are gynecologic, gastrointestinal, pancreatic, bronchogenic, and breast. Peritoneal metastases are often very small and are not detectable by any imaging technique. When lesions

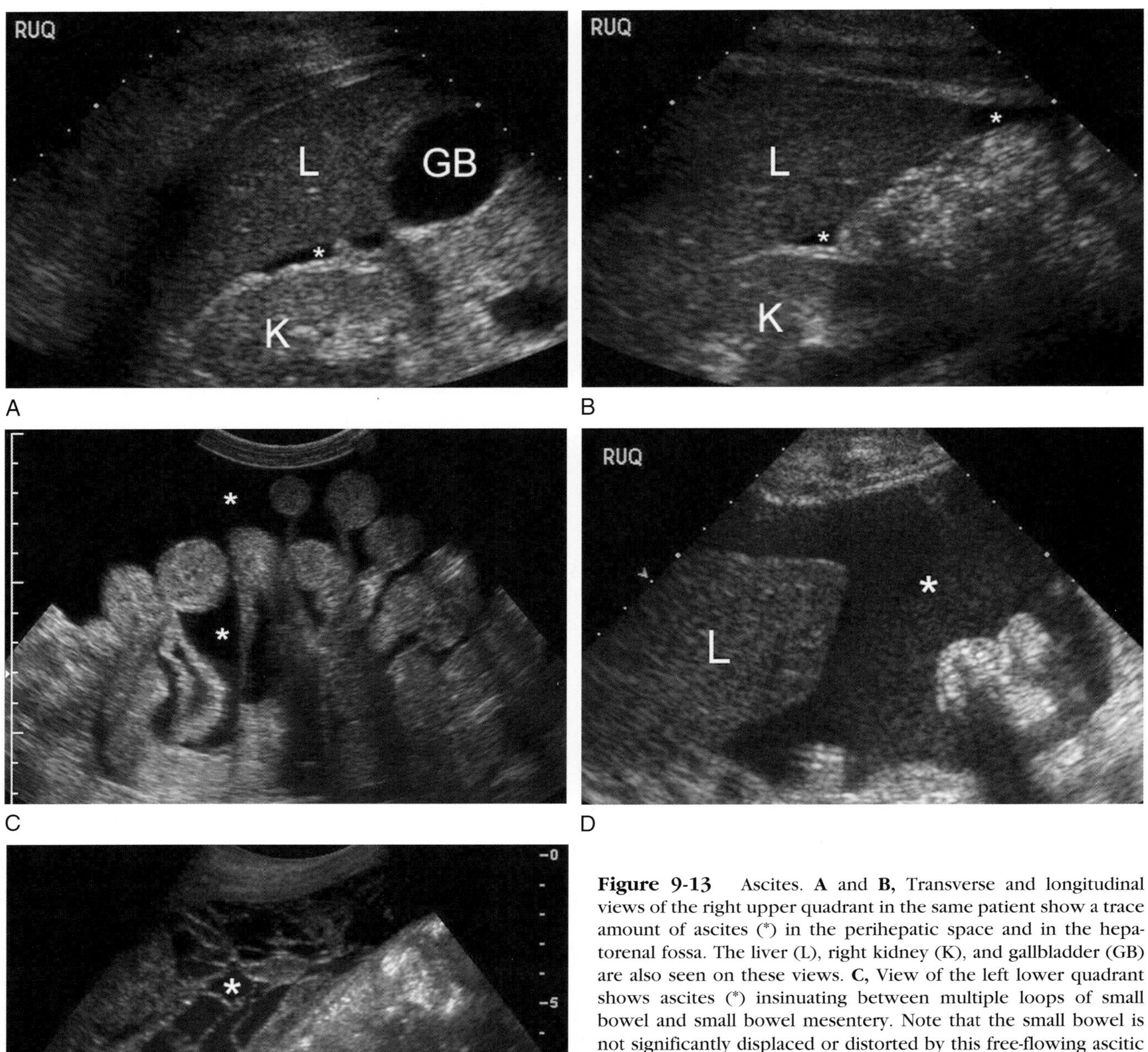

Figure 9-13 Ascites. **A** and **B**, Transverse and longitudinal views of the right upper quadrant in the same patient show a trace amount of ascites (*) in the perihepatic space and in the hepatorenal fossa. The liver (L), right kidney (K), and gallbladder (GB) are also seen on these views. **C**, View of the left lower quadrant shows ascites (*) insinuating between multiple loops of small bowel and small bowel mesentery. Note that the small bowel is not significantly displaced or distorted by this free-flowing ascitic fluid. **D**, Longitudinal view of the right upper quadrant and liver (L) shows complex ascites (*) with diffuse low-level echoes. This is the typical appearance of infected or hemorrhagic fluid. **E**, Transverse view of the right lower quadrant shows a complex multi-septated collection of ascites (*) between the abdominal wall and compressed loops of bowel (B).

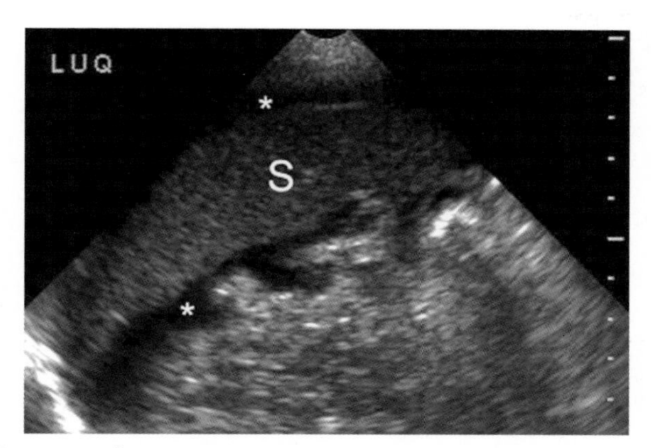

Figure 9-14 Hemoperitoneum secondary to blunt abdominal trauma. Longitudinal view of the left upper quadrant shows the spleen (S) and peritoneal fluid (*) in the perisplenic space. In the setting of trauma, this is assumed to represent a hemoperitoneum and predicts the presence of visceral injury.

reach 1 cm, they can more reliably be detected with sonography and CT. On sonography, they typically appear as hypoechoic soft tissue nodules immediately deep to the abdominal wall (Fig. 9-15A and B). They can be distinguished from adjacent loops of bowel by noting that they are spherical and do not communicate with other loops of bowel. Because they are typically superficial, high-resolution linear arrays or curved arrays can be used and focused at a level just below the deep abdominal fascia. Ascites is often present in patients with peritoneal metastases and can highlight the lesions as soft tissue nodules or sheets of soft tissue lining the peritoneal surfaces (see Fig. 9-15C and D). An unusual type of peritoneal implant is pseudomyxoma peritonei. This consists of mucinous implants and gelatinous peritoneal fluid arising from mucinous tumors of the ovary, gastrointestinal tract (especially the appendix), or rarely other sites. The appearance of pseudomyxoma peritonei is variable, ranging from loculated, anechoic fluid collections that exert mass effect on adjacent structures, to septated collections with or without internal echoes, to more echogenic masses with or without calcification (Fig. 9-16). Mesothelioma, a rare primary malignancy of the peritoneum, can closely mimic peritoneal carcinomatosis (Fig. 9-17), as can tuberculous peritonitis (Box 9-3).

An uncommon cause of a peritoneal mass that can present as an acute abdomen is segmental infarction of the omentum. This is most common in men and most often occurs on the right side. Edematous infiltration of the omentum results in an echogenic mass that may produce marked sound attenuation (Fig. 9-18). This abnormality can be easily overlooked if one is not familiar with its subtle appearance.

Although sonography is not typically used to evaluate a suspected pneumoperitoneum, it is actually a very effective way to make the diagnosis. Free air appears as bright reflectors, usually with dirty shadowing and/or ring-down artifacts, located along the non-dependent aspect of the peritoneal cavity. The reflections are positioned immediately adjacent to the deep abdominal fascia. They will move to the non-dependent portion of the abdomen when the patient changes position and can typically be seen between the liver and the abdominal wall when the patient is in the left lateral decubitus position (Fig. 9-19). They can be distinguished from intraluminal bowel gas by noting lack of peristalsis and lack of motion with inspiration.

ABDOMINAL WALL

Because it is superficial, high-resolution probes can be used to evaluate the abdominal wall with sonography. In some situations, it can be difficult to determine if deep abdominal wall lesions are within the peritoneal cavity or within the abdominal wall. One useful maneuver is to scan in the longitudinal plane and ask the patient to take deep breaths. The respiratory motion of the intra-abdominal structures (bowel, omentum, and mesentery) will help to identify the deep abdominal fascia and confirm that abdominal wall lesions are superficial to this layer.

Masses of the abdominal wall can arise from a number of causes (Box 9-4). Rectus sheath hematomas are one of the more common causes of a palpable or a painful abdominal wall mass. They are most often spontaneous secondary to anticoagulation. They may also occur from direct trauma, forceful contraction of the rectus muscles, or after surgery. The bleeding may involve the rectus muscle itself, the rectus sheath, or both. Above the arcuate line, the hematomas are unilateral. Below the arcuate line they can cross the midline and involve both rectus muscles. They usually appear as complex collections with solid and liquefied areas (Fig. 9-20). Because they are contained in the muscle or the rectus sheath, they usually are lenticular. When rectus sheath hematomas dissect inferior into the suprapubic region, they can enter the prevesical space, assume a more spherical shape, and exert significant mass effect on the bladder (see Fig. 9-20C).

Tumors of the abdominal wall are uncommon. The most frequent are metastases. These can occur in the muscles, in the subcutaneous tissues, or at the site of surgery or percutaneous needle tracts. Metastases usually appear as hypoechoic solid masses or complex solid and cystic masses (Fig. 9-21). The differential diagnosis includes desmoid tumors, endometriomas (Fig. 9-22), lymphomas, lipomas, and complex fluid collections, such as hematomas and abscesses.

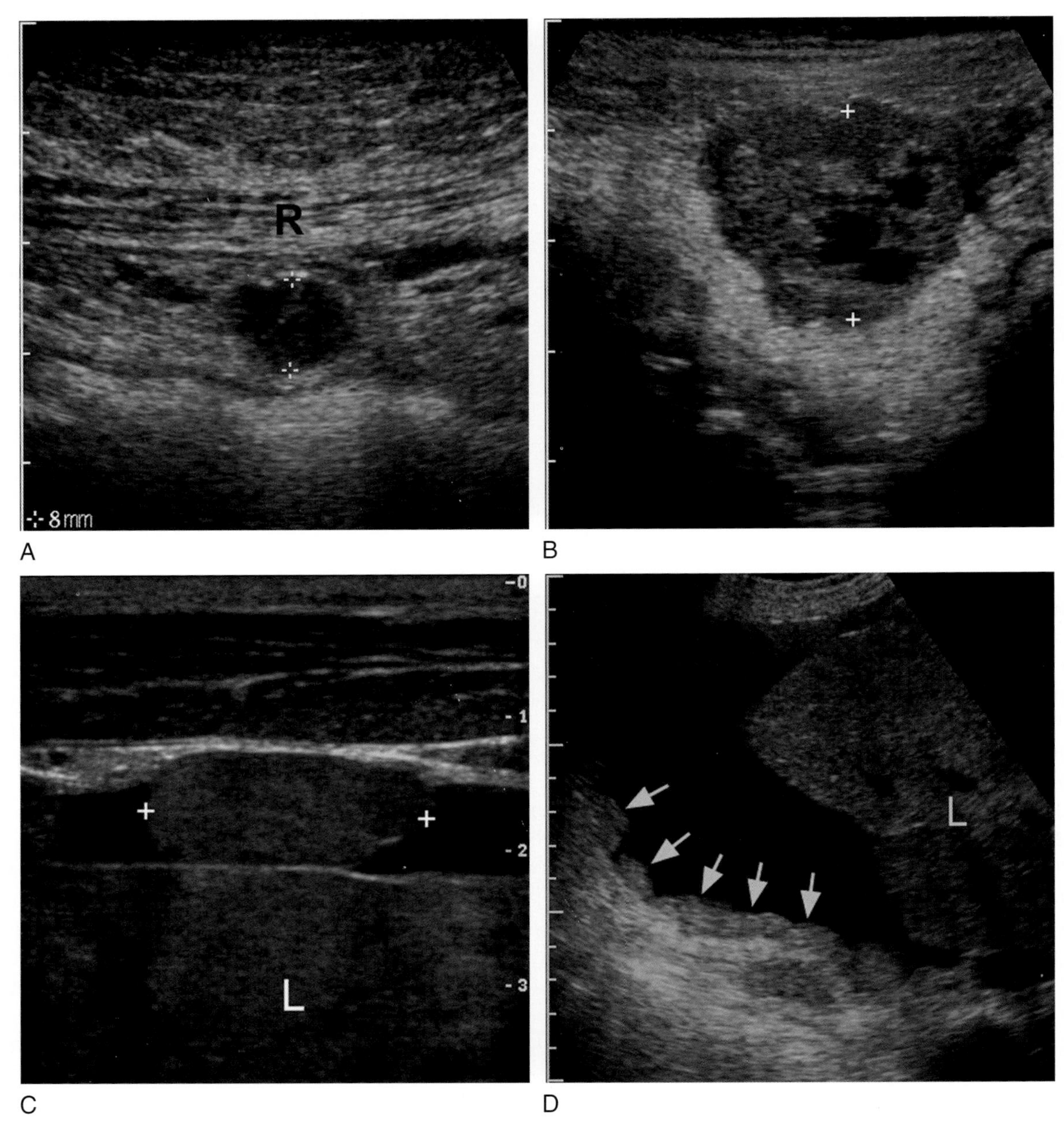

Figure 9-15 Peritoneal metastases. **A,** Longitudinal view of the anterior abdomen shows a hypoechoic solid 8-mm mass *(cursors)* in the peritoneal cavity immediately deep to the rectus muscle (R). This is the typical appearance of a small peritoneal metastasis. **B,** Similar view in a different patient shows a hypoechoic solid 2-cm mass *(cursors)* with small internal cystic components. **C,** Longitudinal view of the right upper quadrant shows a solid mass *(cursors)* surrounded by ascites in the perihepatic space. The liver (L) is seen deep to the mass. **D,** Transverse view of the right upper quadrant shows a nodular sheet of soft tissue implants *(arrows)* along the parietal peritoneum in the perihepatic space. The liver (L) is seen anteriorly.

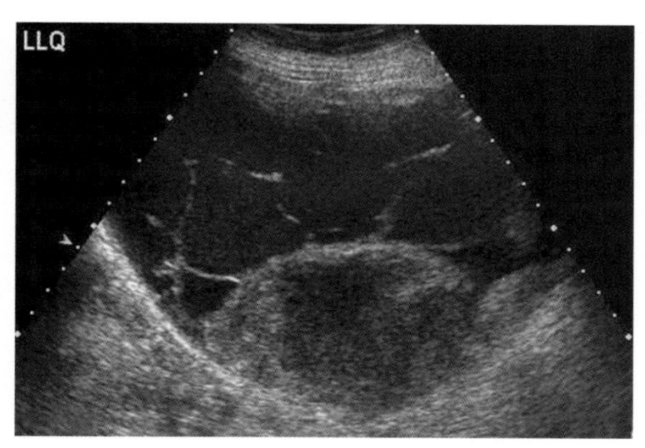

Figure 9-16 Pseudomyxoma peritonei. View of the left lower quadrant shows a complex, multi-septated, loculated-appearing fluid collection with a large solid-appearing nodule posteriorly. Although nonspecific, this appearance is consistent with pseudomyxoma peritonei.

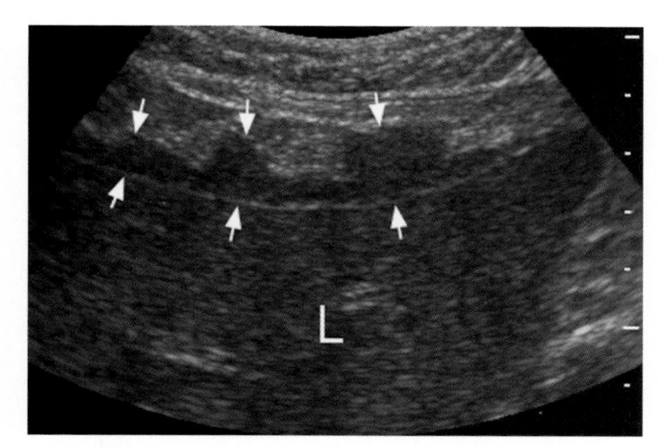

Figure 9-17 Mesothelioma. Longitudinal view of the left lobe of the liver (L) shows nodular hypoechoic soft tissue studding the surface of the liver *(arrows)*. Ultrasound-guided biopsy confirmed mesothelioma.

Box 9-3 Causes of Peritoneal Masses

- Metastases
- Tuberculosis
- Mesothelioma
- Pseudomyxoma peritonei
- Omental infarct

Abdominal hernias occur in areas where the abdominal wall is weak, either naturally weak (i.e., inguinal) or due to surgery (i.e., incisional). Up to 50% of men will develop a hernia during their life. Many hernias can be diagnosed and treated without imaging of any kind. When imaging is necessary, sonography can provide the information necessary for management of the majority of individuals. Incisional hernias are seen as a fascial defect with the hernia contents (bowel, fat, ascites, or a combination of structures) protruding through the defect (Fig. 9-23). Identification of the defect in the fascia is critical in distinguishing hernias that do not contain obvious loops of bowel from complex fluid collections in the abdominal wall. Inguinal hernias originate at the internal inguinal ring, which is immediately adjacent to the inferior epigastric artery. The inferior epigastric artery can be identified in almost all patients as it travels deep to the rectus muscle. When in doubt, the inferior epigastric artery can be followed from its origin off the distal external iliac artery. Direct inguinal hernias arise inferior and medial to the inferior epigastric artery, whereas indirect inguinal hernias arise superior and lateral and travel anterior to the artery. Dynamic maneuvers such as

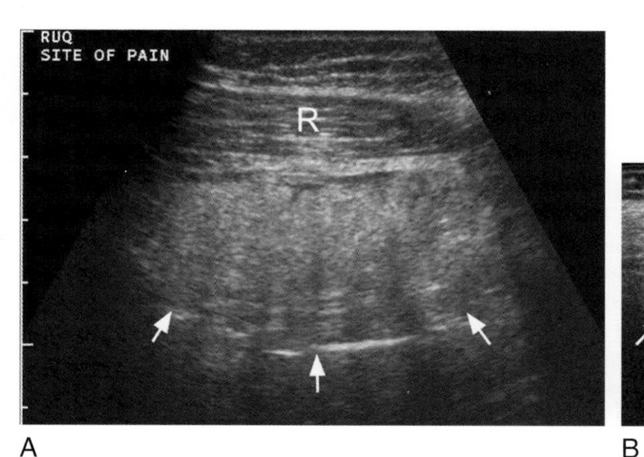

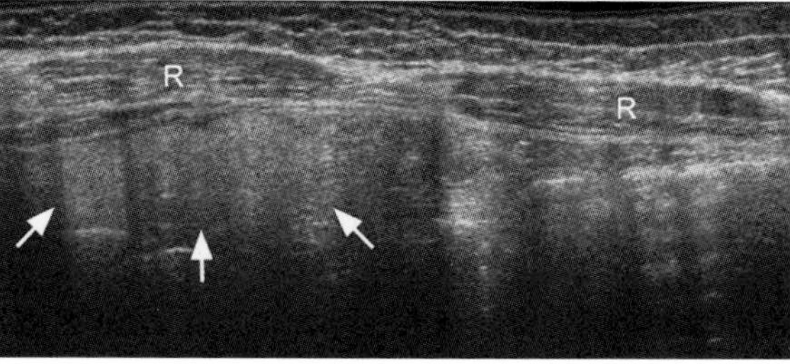

Figure 9-18 Omental infarct. **A,** Transverse view of the right upper quadrant directly over the patient's site of pain shows a very hyperechoic region of omental thickening *(arrows)* immediately deep to the rectus muscle (R). **B,** Transverse extended field of view scan of the upper abdomen shows similar findings and displays the marked asymmetry between the right and left sides. Both rectus muscles (R) are seen.

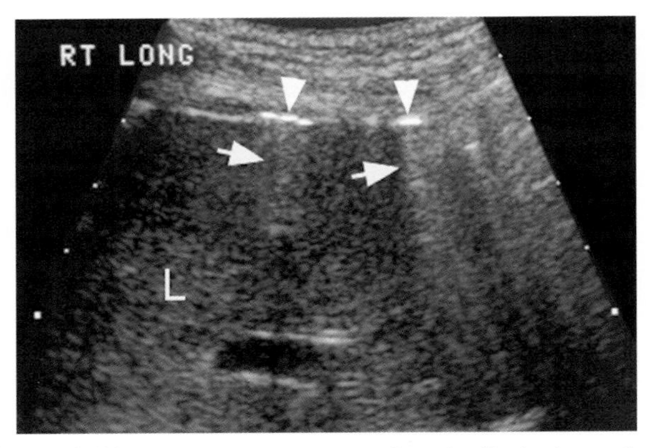

Figure 9-19 Pneumoperitoneum. Longitudinal view of the right upper quadrant shows bright reflectors *(arrowheads)* between the liver (L) and the abdominal wall. Dirty shadows *(arrows)* typical of air are seen posteriorly.

Box 9-4 Causes of Abdominal Wall Masses

Metastases
Lipoma
Hernia
Hematoma
Abscess
Seroma
Desmoid
Endometriosis
Sarcoma
Lymphoma

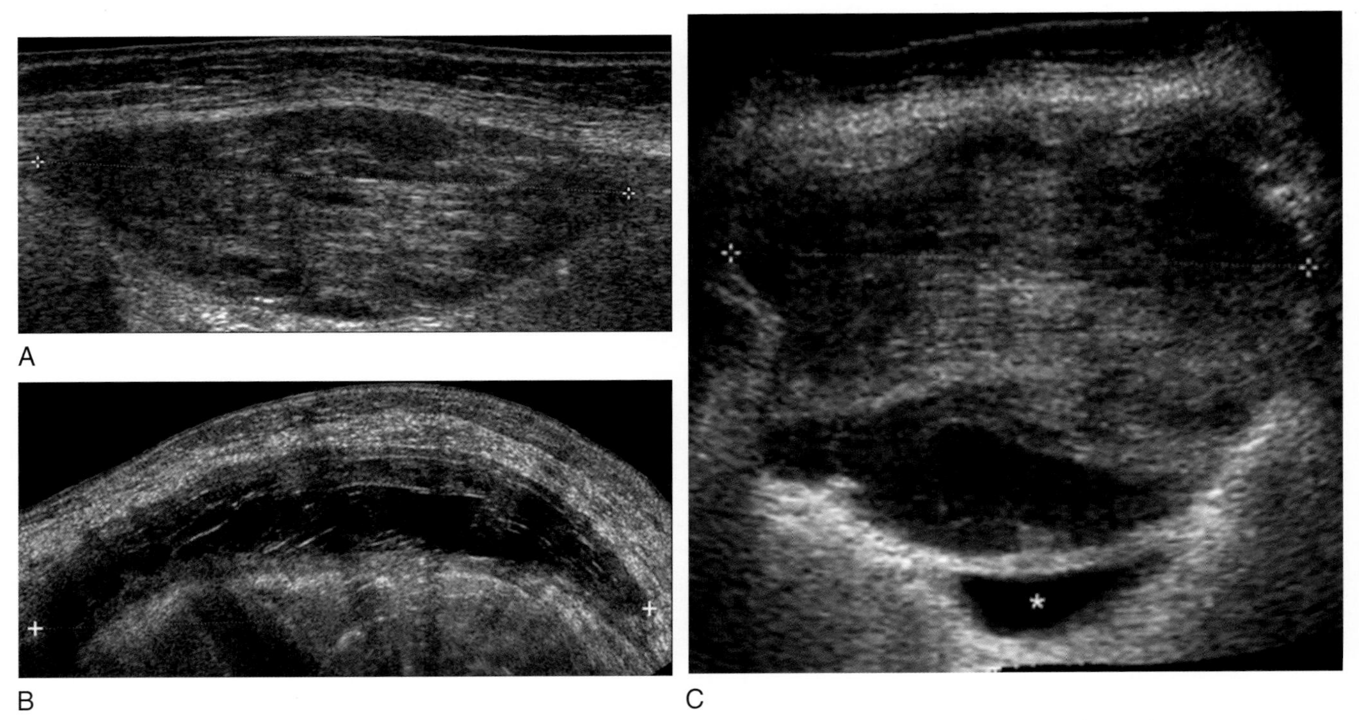

Figure 9-20 Rectus hematoma. **A,** Transverse view of the abdominal wall shows an elliptical, solid-appearing lesion *(cursors)* in the expected location of the rectus muscle. This solid appearance is consistent with a relatively acute hematoma. **B,** Transverse extended field of view scan of another patient shows a complex lenticular multi-septated fluid collection *(cursors)* consistent with a subacute rectus hematoma. **C,** Transverse extended field of view scan of the suprapubic region shows a large rounded mass *(cursors)* with solid elements anteriorly and more liquefied elements posteriorly. Note the compressed and displaced urinary bladder (*) posteriorly. This mass effect on the urinary bladder is typical of rectus hematomas that dissect into the prevesical space.

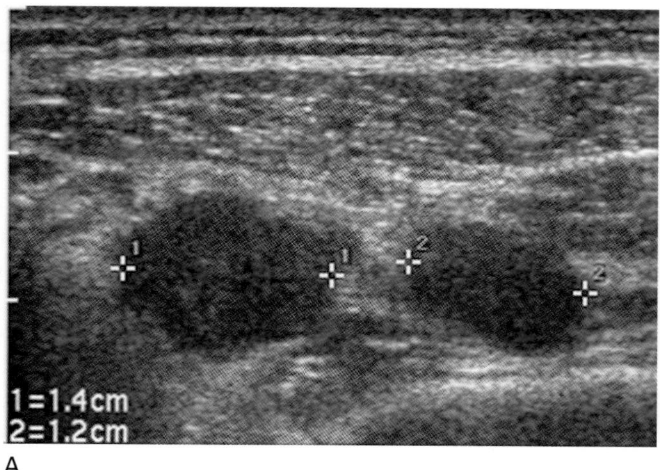

B

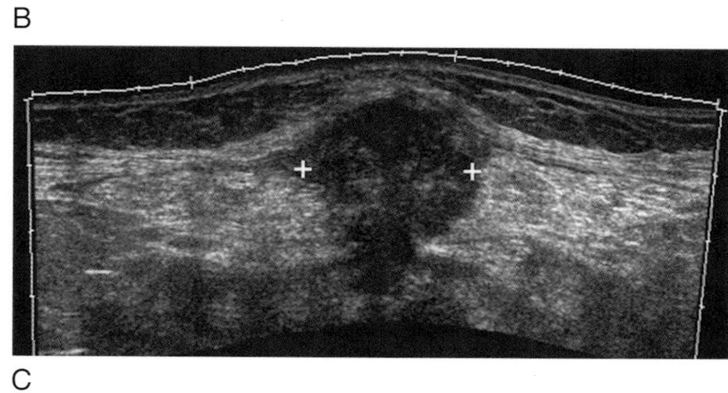

Figure 9-21 Metastases to the abdominal wall. **A,** Transverse view of the right lower quadrant shows two solid hypoechoic masses *(cursors)* within the abdominal musculature in this patient with metastatic bronchogenic carcinoma. **B,** View of the left lower quadrant shows two hypoechoic solid masses *(cursors)* in the subcutaneous fat in a patient with metastatic melanoma. **C,** Transverse extended field of view scan of the lower abdomen shows a solid hypoechoic mass *(cursors)* in the abdominal wall at the site of a prior surgical incision in a patient with metastatic colon cancer.

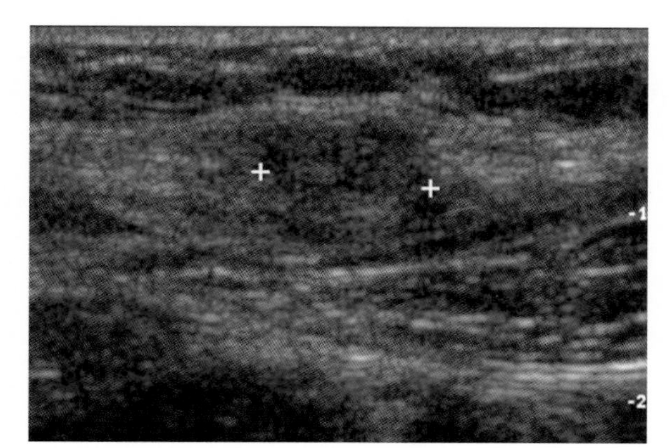

Figure 9-22 Endometrioma. Transverse view of the lower abdomen shows a hypoechoic solid-appearing mass *(cursors)* secondary to endometriosis. This is indistinguishable from abdominal wall neoplasms, and diagnosis was suspected based on the clinical history and confirmed by percutaneous fine-needle aspiration.

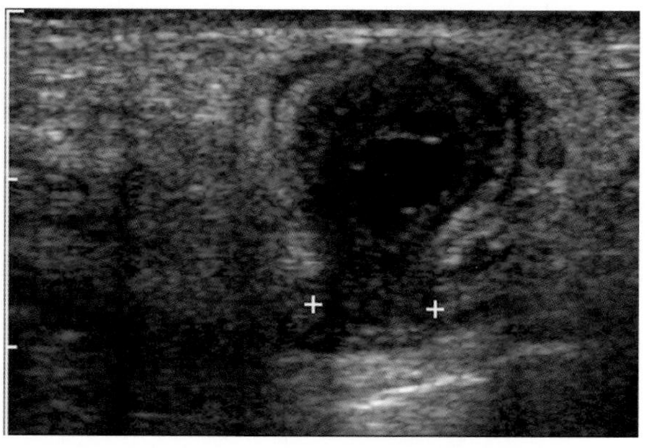

Figure 9-23 Incisional hernia. View of the abdominal wall at the site of a prior surgical incision shows a complex walled-off fluid collection. The diagnosis of a hernia containing complex fluid is made based on the presence of a deep fascial defect *(cursors)*.

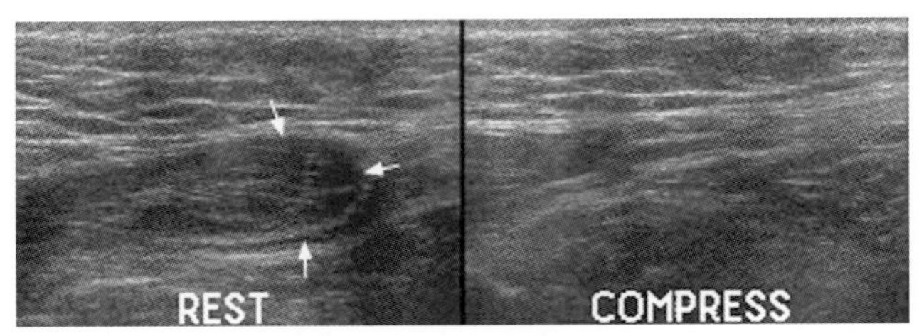

Figure 9-24 Inguinal hernia. Dual longitudinal views of the inguinal canal obtained at rest (left) and with compression (right). Note that at rest there is an elongated hypoechoic sac with a blunt end *(arrows)*. With compression of the inguinal region, the hernia sac was seen to migrate back into the abdominal cavity, leaving an empty inguinal canal.

Valsalva and compression with the transducer should be used to determine if a hernia is incarcerated or reducible (Fig. 9-24).

LYMPHADENOPATHY

Abdominal lymphadenopathy can be due to inflammatory/infectious causes or neoplasms. In most situations, sonography is not capable of determining the cause of the adenopathy, but, in general, the larger the nodes, the more likely they are to be neoplastic. Successful recognition of lymphadenopathy varies, depending on its location and size. Mesenteric lymphadenopathy appears as hypoechoic masses that surround the mesenteric vessels (Fig. 9-25). Small mesenteric nodes must be distinguished from adjacent bowel loops. This is best done during real-time scanning by noting that they are spherical and do not communicate with bowel loops. Extensive mesenteric lymphadenopathy can produce a mantle of concentric tissue that surrounds the vessels. This sometimes simulates the appearance of a kidney and has been called the "pseudokidney sign" (see Fig. 9-25C).

Another common site of lymphadenopathy is around the upper abdominal vessels. Nodes around the celiac axis are often enlarged owing to inflammatory or neoplastic disease of the upper abdominal organs (Fig. 9-26). This is also true of nodes in the porta hepatis and nodes around the head of the pancreas. All of these nodes are usually immediately adjacent to the liver and are usually isoechoic to the liver. Because of this, it is common to overlook them. Careful attention to their

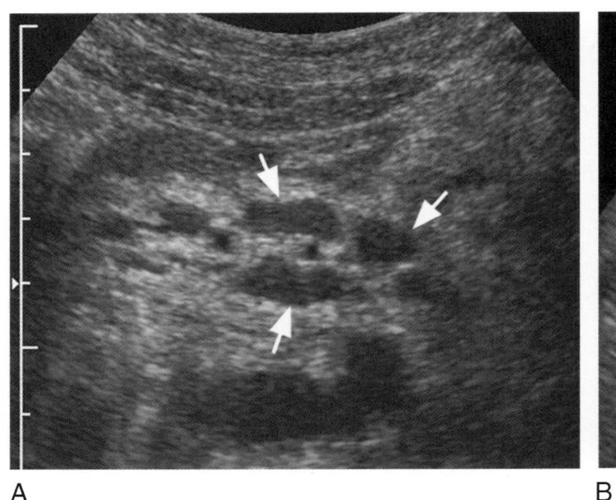

A

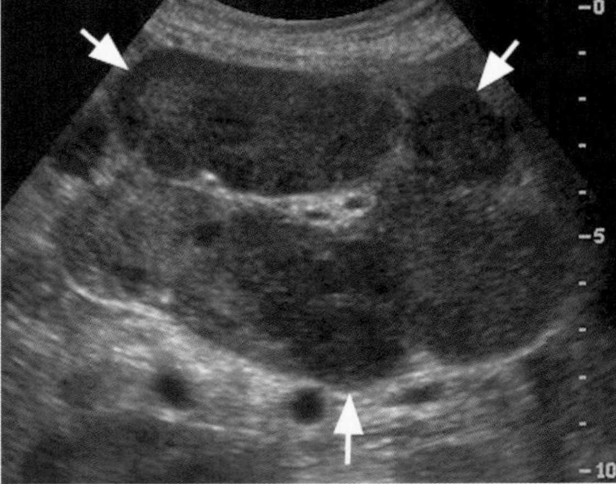

B

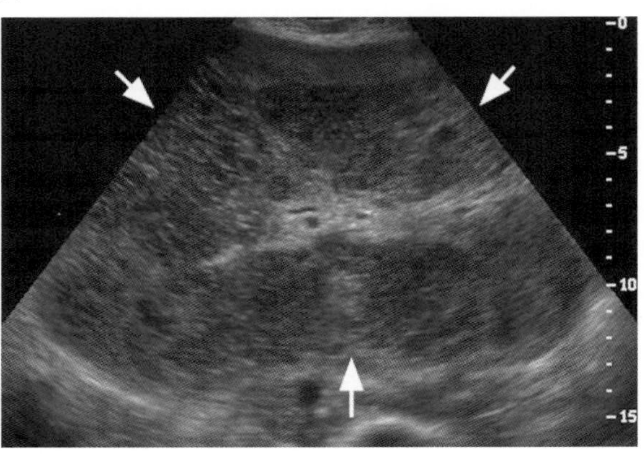

C

Figure 9-25 Mesenteric adenopathy. **A,** Transverse view of the small bowel mesentery shows several small hypoechoic nodes *(arrows)* surrounding the mesenteric vessels. **B,** Transverse view of the mesentery in another patient shows massive confluent hypoechoic adenopathy producing a lobulated-appearing mass *(arrows)* surrounding the mesenteric vessels. **C,** Similar view in a third patient shows a classic "pseudokidney" sign with smooth confluent lymphadenopathy *(arrows)* producing a hypoechoic rind of tissue simulating renal cortex and surrounding the more echogenic mesenteric fat and mesenteric vessels that simulate the renal sinus fat.

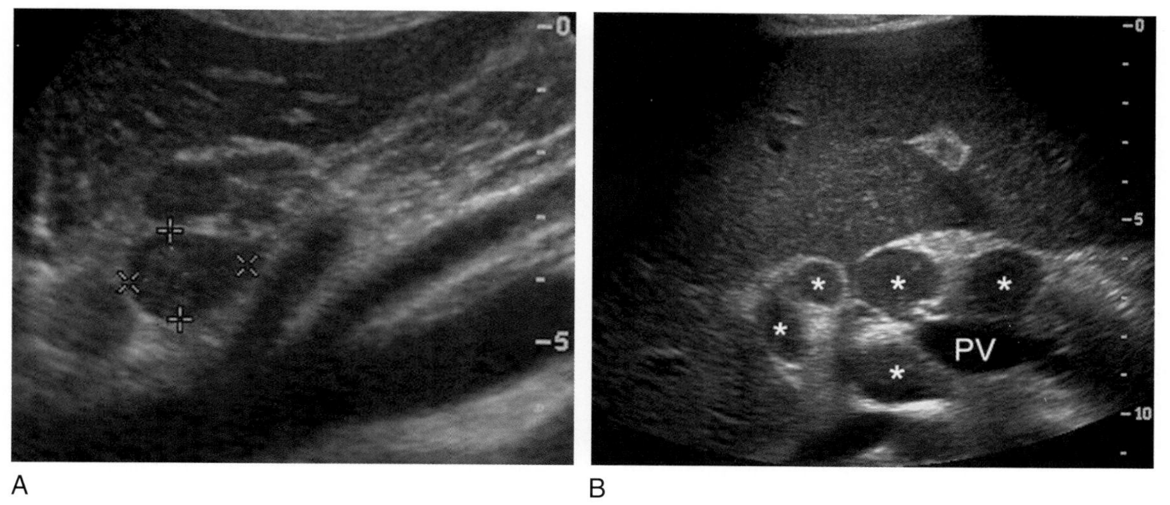

Figure 9-26 Upper abdominal perivascular lymphadenopathy. **A,** Longitudinal view of the upper abdomen shows an enlarged lymph node *(cursors)* immediately superior to the celiac axis. Several other smaller nodes are also present. **B,** Transverse view of the porta hepatis shows multiple enlarged lymph nodes (*) in the porta hepatis surrounding the portal vein (PV).

shape, and familiarity with their typical locations and appearance, allows one to avoid this mistake.

The final common location for adenopathy is the retroperitoneum. These nodes will be intimately related to the aorta and inferior vena cava. Adenopathy that displaces the aorta or cava away from the spine is almost always in the retroperitoneum (Fig. 9-27).

AORTA

Sonography is widely used in the detection and surveillance of abdominal aortic aneurysms. They are common abnormalities and are strongly associated with atherosclerosis. Ninety-five percent occur below the

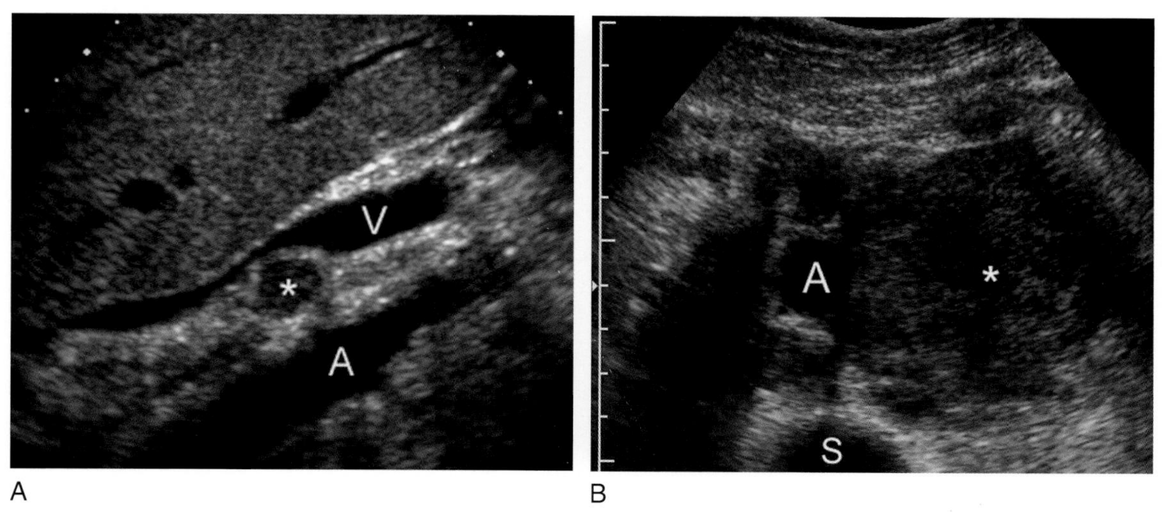

Figure 9-27 Retroperitoneal adenopathy. **A,** Coronal view of the abdomen from a right lateral approach shows an enlarged interaortocaval lymph node (*) in a patient with metastatic esophageal cancer. The inferior vena cava (V) and the aorta (A) are seen on either side of this lymph node. **B,** Transverse view of the abdominal aorta (A) in the mid abdomen shows a large periaortic lymph node (*) with extension into the retroaortic space resulting in displacement of the aorta away from the spine (S). This node was due to metastatic testicular cancer.

level of the renal arteries (Box 9-5). The upper limits of normal for aortic diameter are 2.5 cm at the diaphragm, 2.0 cm in the midabdomen, and 1.8 cm at the bifurcation. An aneurysm is considered to be present when there is a focal dilatation of the aorta that measures 3 cm or more in diameter. Enlarged aortas that are less than 3 cm in diameter are considered ectatic. Surgery should be considered when an aneurysm reaches 5 cm because the cumulative risk of rupture over the next 8 years is 25%. Rapid enlargement of an aortic aneurysm is also an indication for surgery. Different groups use different approaches to the measurement of aortic aneurysms. The most important issue is to use an approach that is reproducible so that comparative measurements over time accurately determine the stability of the aneurysm. It is probably most appropriate to measure the outer wall to the outer wall because this is what surgeons see when they operate. Anteroposterior measurements are obtained from sagittal views, and transverse measurements are obtained from a left coronal view. Measurements in the axial view should be avoided because it is not possible to determine if they are taken perpendicular to the long axis of the aorta and are prone to overestimation (Fig. 9-28). In addition, the lateral borders of the aorta are not well seen on axial views. Mural thrombus is often present, especially in larger aneurysms (see Figs. 9-28 and 9-29). Occasionally, the thrombus will contain crescentic areas of decreased echogenicity that should not be mistaken for dissection, rupture, or impending rupture (see Fig. 9-29). These areas likely are due to liquefied clot. Conventional atherosclerotic aneurysms are usually fusiform. Saccular-shaped aneurysms should raise the suspicion of either a mycotic aneurysm or a pseudoaneurysm (Fig. 9-30).

Box 9-5 Features of Abdominal Aortic Aneurysms

Ninety-five percent are infrarenal.
Vast majority are fusiform.
Mural thrombus is common with large aneurysms.
Surgery considered when >5 cm
Measure anteroposterior diameter on sagittal views.
Measure transverse diameter on coronal views.

Endovascular stent grafts placed from a percutaneous approach are becoming a popular approach for the repair of aortic aneurysms (Fig. 9-31). Perigraft leaks at the attachment sites (type 1) and from patent lumbar and inferior mesenteric arteries (type 2) are potential complications that should be ruled out after graft placement. They are seen on Doppler analysis as areas of blood flow outside the lumen of the graft but within the walls of the aneurysm (Fig. 9-32). Pulsed Doppler analysis of blood flow direction can assist is locating the origin of these leaks.

Sonography is not a primary tool used to evaluate aortic dissections. Nevertheless, patients with dissection may be initially examined with sonography for other reasons. With gray-scale scanning, the intimal flap can be seen well when it is oriented perpendicular to the sound

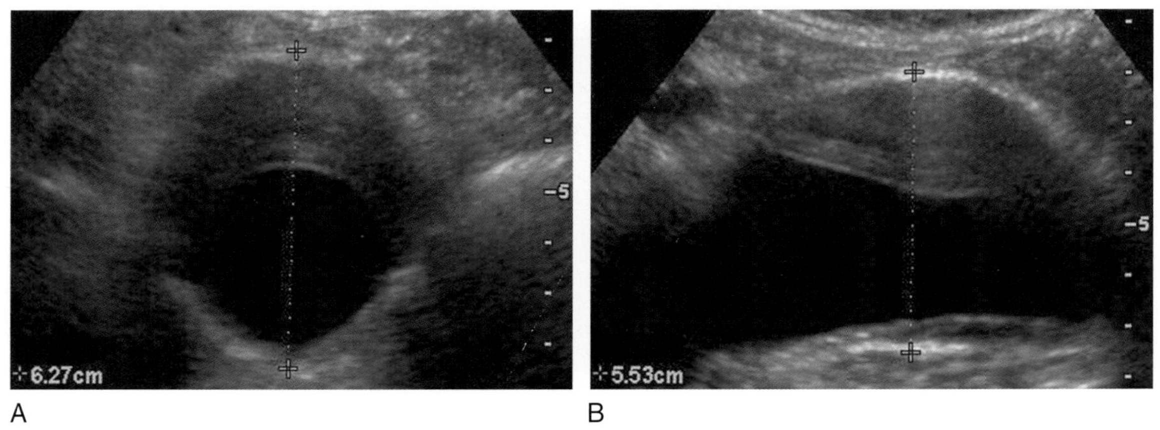

Figure 9-28 Abdominal aortic aneurysm. **A,** Transverse view of the aorta *(cursors)* shows aortic enlargement and eccentric anterior mural thrombus. Note the anteroposterior measurement of 6.27 cm. **B,** Sagittal view of the aorta in the same patient again shows focal aneurysmal dilatation with anterior mural thrombus. On this view, the anteroposterior diameter is more accurately measured at 5.53 cm. The overestimation of the diameter on the transverse view is related to visualization in an oblique plane that is not truly perpendicular to the long axis of the aorta.

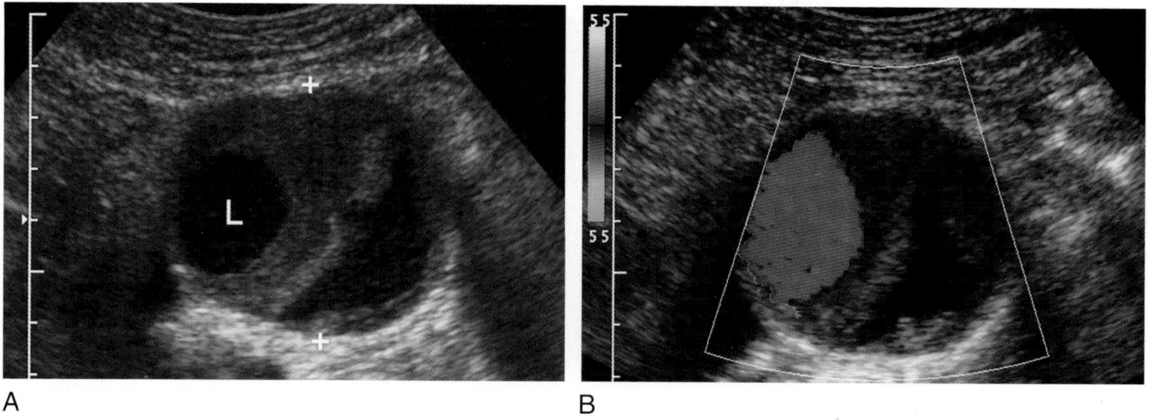

Figure 9-29 Abdominal aortic aneurysm with extensive mural thrombus. **A,** Transverse view of the aorta *(cursors)* shows a large aneurysm with extensive mural thrombus eccentrically surrounding the residual lumen (L). Note the crescentic hypoechoic region within the mural thrombus. **B,** Transverse color Doppler view shows flow within the aneurysm residual lumen but no detectable flow within the mural thrombus. These crescentic areas within large mural thrombi do not imply dissection, rupture, or impending rupture.

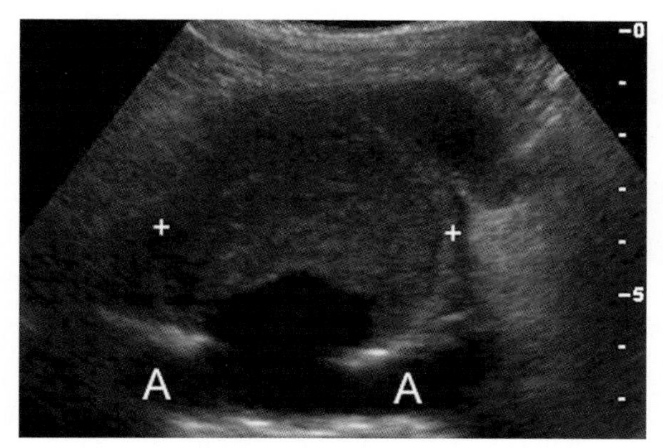

Figure 9-30 Mycotic aneurysm. Coronal view from the left shows the aorta (A) with an eccentric saccular aneurysm *(cursors)* arising from the lateral wall. There is extensive thrombus within this aneurysm. The saccular nature should suggest a pseudoaneurysm or mycotic aneurysm.

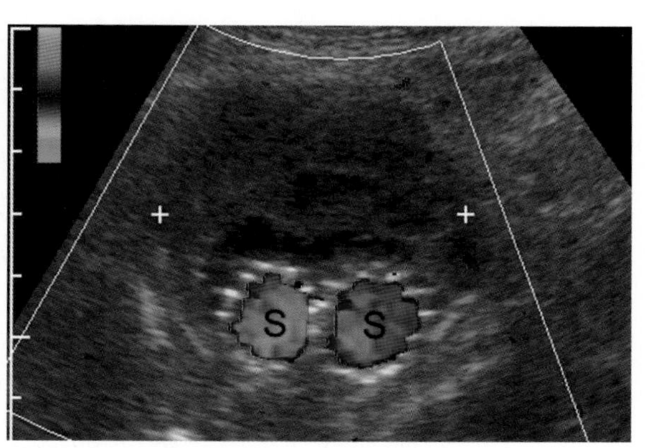

Figure 9-31 Endovascular stent graft. Transverse color Doppler view of an abdominal aortic aneurysm *(cursors)*. The two inferior limbs of an endovascular stent are identified in the posterior aspect of the aneurysm. Note that there is no Doppler signal outside of the stent.

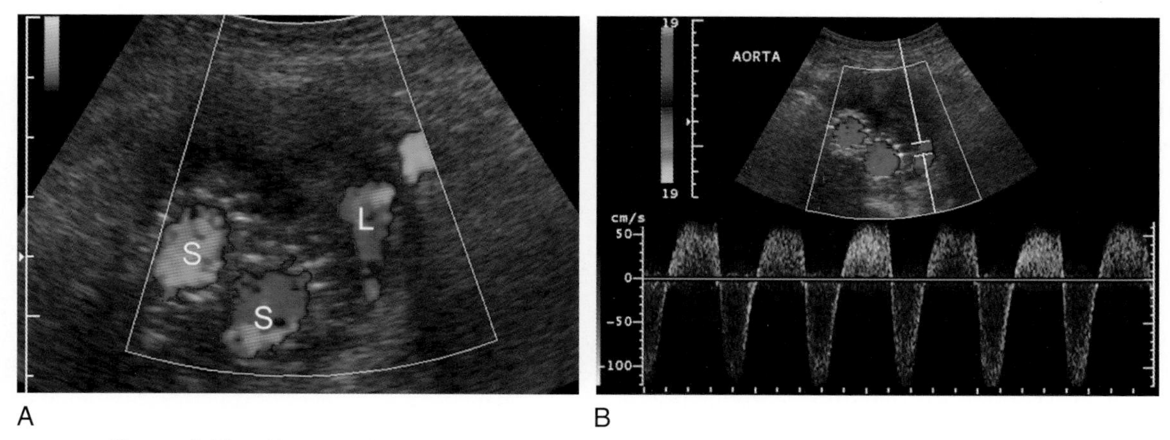

Figure 9-32 Type II endovascular stent graft leak. **A** and **B,** Transverse color, power, and pulsed Doppler views of an aortic aneurysm treated with an endovascular stent show the two limbs of the stent (S) and an area of abnormal color Doppler signal secondary to a leak (L) along the left lateral aspect of the aneurysm. The pulsed Doppler waveform shows that systolic flow is toward the stent, indicating that this is a type 2 leak secondary to back flow from an inferior mesenteric artery.

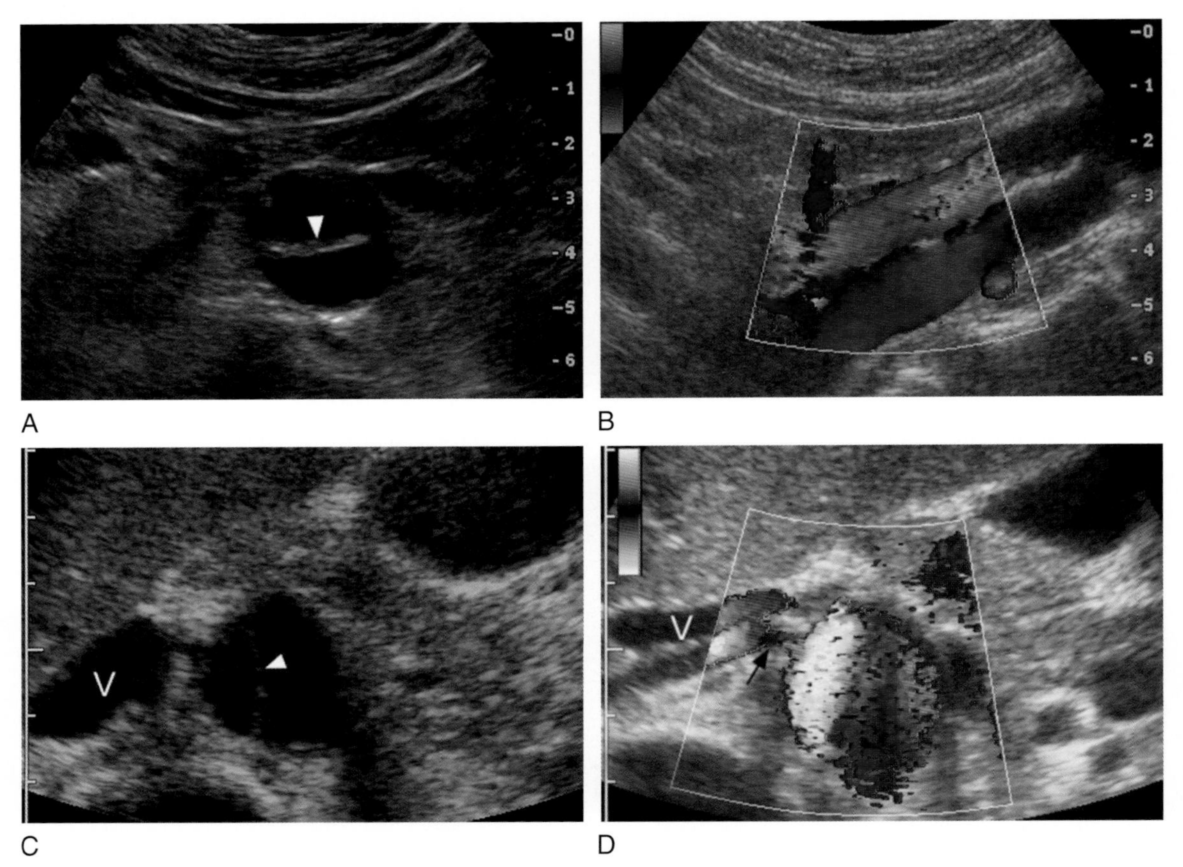

Figure 9-33 Aortic dissection. **A** and **B,** Transverse gray scale view **(A)** and longitudinal color Doppler view **(B)** from the same patient show a readily identifiable intimal flap *(arrowhead)* on the transverse view and differential flow in the anterior and posterior lumen on the color Doppler view. **C** and **D,** Transverse gray scale **(C)** and color Doppler **(D)** views in another patient show an intimal flap *(arrowhead)* that is more difficult to identify on gray scale owing to its orientation. Differential flow is identified on the color Doppler view. The right renal artery *(arrow)* is seen on the color Doppler view. The inferior vena cava (V) is also identified.

beam, but it can be difficult or impossible to see if it is oriented nearly parallel to the sound beam (Fig. 9-33). With color Doppler imaging, differential flow is typically seen in the two lumens.

INFERIOR VENA CAVA

Evaluation of the inferior vena cava (IVC) typically is requested in patients with suspected IVC thrombosis. Detection of caval thrombosis relies on a combination of gray-scale imaging and color Doppler analysis. As in other veins, thrombus appears as abnormal echogenic material within the lumen. When there is focal echogenic thrombus, the diagnosis is relatively easy to make (Fig. 9-34), provided the abnormal segment of the

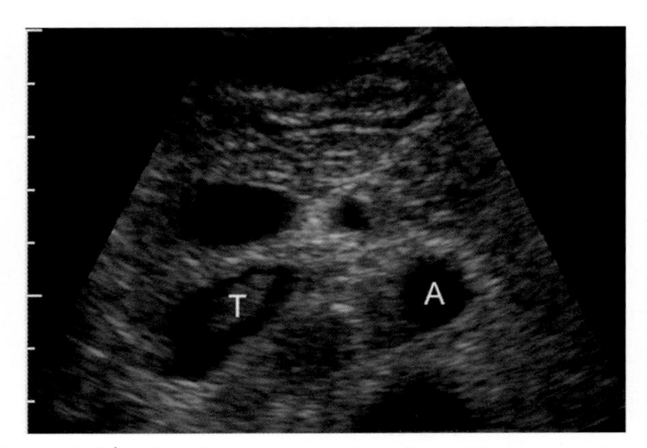

Figure 9-34 Inferior vena cava thrombosis. Transverse view of the abdomen shows a nonobstructive, echogenic thrombus (T) within the lumen of the inferior vena cava. The aorta is also identified (A).

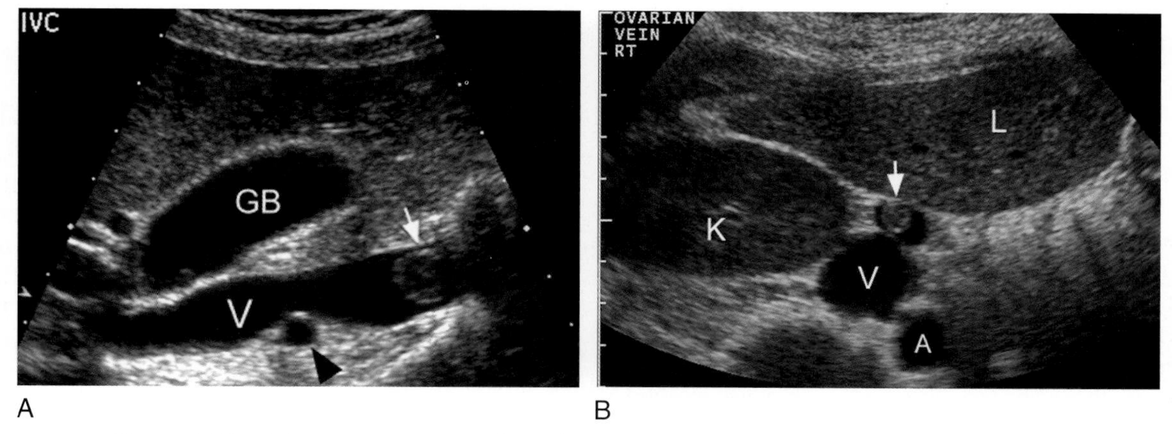

Figure 9-35 Inferior vena cava thrombus related to ovarian vein thrombosis. **A,** Longitudinal view of the inferior vena cava (V) shows a focal thrombus *(arrow)* just inferior to the level of the right renal artery *(arrowhead).* The gallbladder (GB) is also identified. **B,** Transverse view of the inferior vena cava (V) shows a nonobstructed hyperechoic thrombus *(arrow)* within the right ovarian vein immediately anterior to the vena cava. Also seen are the aorta (A), the right kidney (K), and the liver (L).

IVC can be visualized. When the thrombus is more diffuse, the luminal echoes must be differentiated from the low-level artifactual echoes that are frequently present. It also must be distinguished from the echoes arising from slow flowing blood. Detecting flow throughout the lumen on color Doppler sonography can solve the former problem. Noting motion on real-time gray-scale imaging can solve the latter problem.

Primary thrombosis of the IVC occurs but is less common than thrombus that extends from the iliac veins, renal veins, hepatic veins, or gonadal veins. Ovarian vein thrombosis is an unusual postpartum complication that usually occurs on the right and is associated with endometritis. In some cases, the thrombosed vein is directly seen on sonography. However, it is not uncommon for air-filled bowel to obscure the thrombosed ovarian vein. In these instances, the diagnosis can still be made in the majority of cases by noting a small thrombus extending into the IVC from the insertion of the ovarian vein (Fig. 9-35).

Tumor thrombus can extend into the IVC from renal cell cancers, hepatocellular cancers, and primary adrenal cancers. They can usually be diagnosed by identifying the primary tumor. In some instances they differ from bland thrombus by producing expansion of the IVC lumen and by containing internal vascularity that is detectable on color or power Doppler analysis (Fig. 9-36).

Leiomyosarcomas are the most common primary tumor arising from the wall of the IVC. However, all tumors of the IVC are rare. It is much more common for pericaval masses to displace, compress, or encase the IVC.

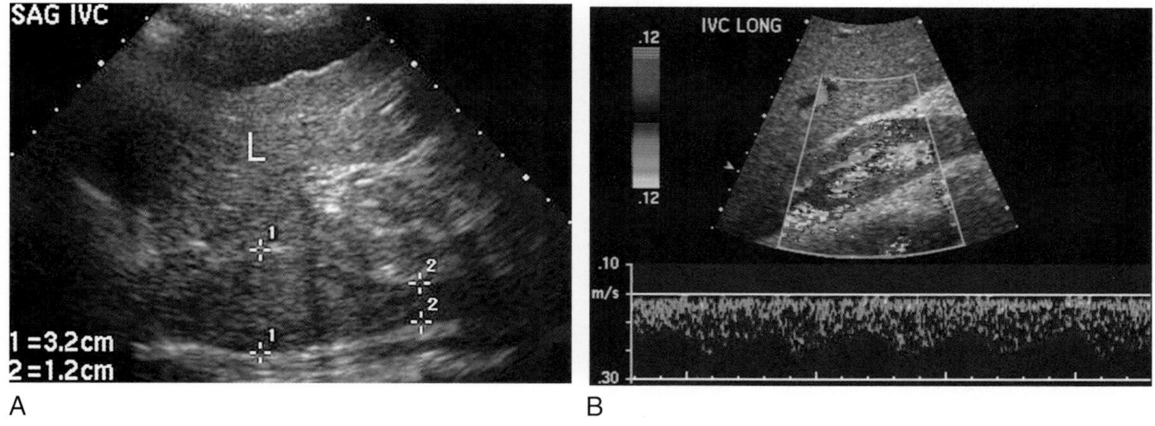

Figure 9-36 Inferior vena cava tumor thrombus. **A,** Longitudinal gray-scale view of the inferior vena cava shows soft tissue *(cursors)* filling and expanding the lumen of the inferior vena cava. The liver (L) is seen anteriorly. **B,** Longitudinal color Doppler and pulsed Doppler view of the inferior vena cava shows identifiable vascularity within tumor thrombus and a low-resistance arterial signal on pulsed Doppler. This pattern is not always seen with tumor thrombus but when present, is diagnostic of tumor thrombus.

ADRENAL

The mainstays of adrenal imaging are CT and MRI because both glands can be reliably identified in almost all patients. With experience, ultrasonography can often identify the normal right adrenal gland. However, sonography generally does not image the normal left adrenal gland and, accordingly, it is not used as a primary imaging method. Nevertheless, ultrasound frequently identifies masses in the right adrenal and occasionally identifies left adrenal masses. Therefore, it is important to recognize these abnormalities when they are encountered. Box 9-6 reviews the most common causes of adrenal masses.

The right adrenal can be imaged from an intercostal or a subcostal approach. By using the liver as a window, the right adrenal appears immediately adjacent to the posterior surface of the liver and lateral and posterior to the IVC. The normal adrenal is a Y- or V-shaped structure. Simultaneous visualization of both limbs is unusual (Fig. 9-37). In most instances, the medial or lateral limb is seen individually as a thin hypoechoic linear structure between the liver and the crus of the diaphragm. The left adrenal is located in a left paraaortic location, medial and anterior to the upper pole of the kidney. It is best identified from an anterior subxiphoid approach or a left coronal intercostal approach using the spleen or kidney as a window.

Adenomas are the most common adrenal mass. Autopsy studies have shown that 1% to 8% of the population have adenomas. They are usually asymptomatic but can produce Cushing's syndrome (excessive glucocortisol) and Conn's syndrome (hyperaldosteronism). They are usually small masses (<3 cm). On CT, they appear as homogeneous low-attenuation lesions because they contain significant amounts of intracytoplasmic

Box 9-6 Common Causes of Adrenal Masses

- Adenoma
- Metastases
- Pheochromocytoma
- Primary carcinoma
- Lymphoma
- Myelolipoma
- Hemorrhage

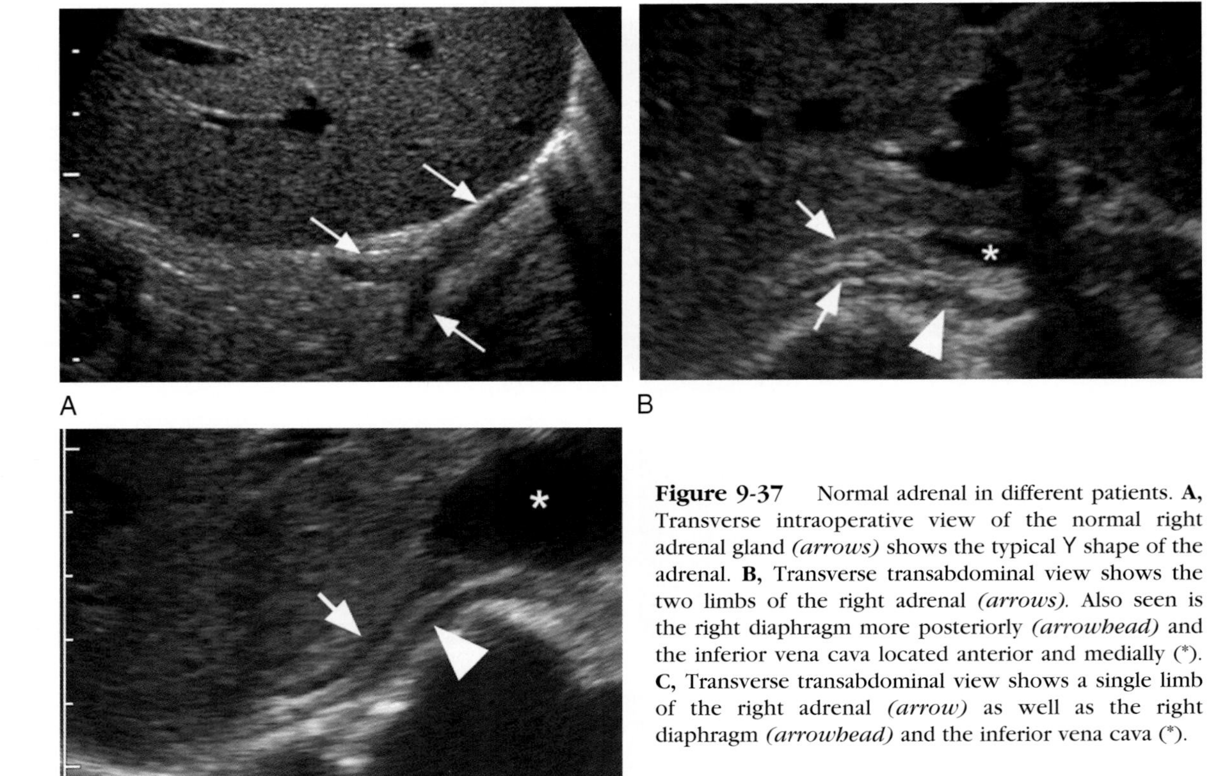

Figure 9-37 Normal adrenal in different patients. **A,** Transverse intraoperative view of the normal right adrenal gland *(arrows)* shows the typical Y shape of the adrenal. **B,** Transverse transabdominal view shows the two limbs of the right adrenal *(arrows)*. Also seen is the right diaphragm more posteriorly *(arrowhead)* and the inferior vena cava located anterior and medially (*). **C,** Transverse transabdominal view shows a single limb of the right adrenal *(arrow)* as well as the right diaphragm *(arrowhead)* and the inferior vena cava (*).

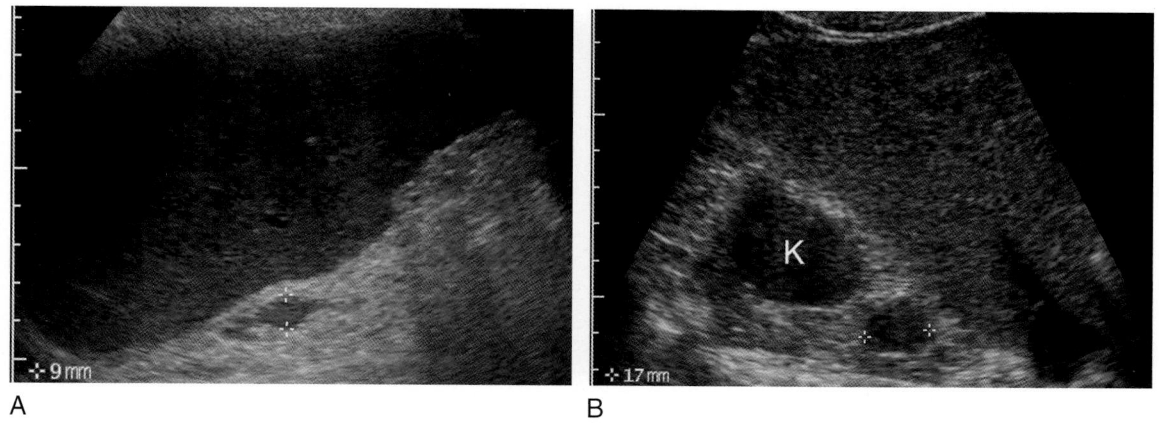

Figure 9-38 Adrenal adenoma in different patients. **A,** Longitudinal view of the right upper quadrant shows a 9-mm adrenal adenoma *(cursors).* **B,** Transverse view of the right upper quadrant shows the upper pole of the right kidney (K) and a 17-mm right adrenal adenoma *(cursors).*

lipid. On MRI, they are characterized by signal dropout on opposed phase chemical shift imaging. On sonography, they appear as homogeneous soft tissue masses that are usually similar in echogenicity to the liver (Fig. 9-38).

Despite their small size, the adrenals are the fourth most common site of metastases. Although many different primary tumors can metastasize to the adrenals, bronchogenic cancer has a particular propensity to spread to the adrenals. Breast cancer and lymphoma also tend to involve the adrenals. On sonography, metastases are often indistinguishable from adenomas, although metastases are usually larger and are often heterogeneous (Fig. 9-39).

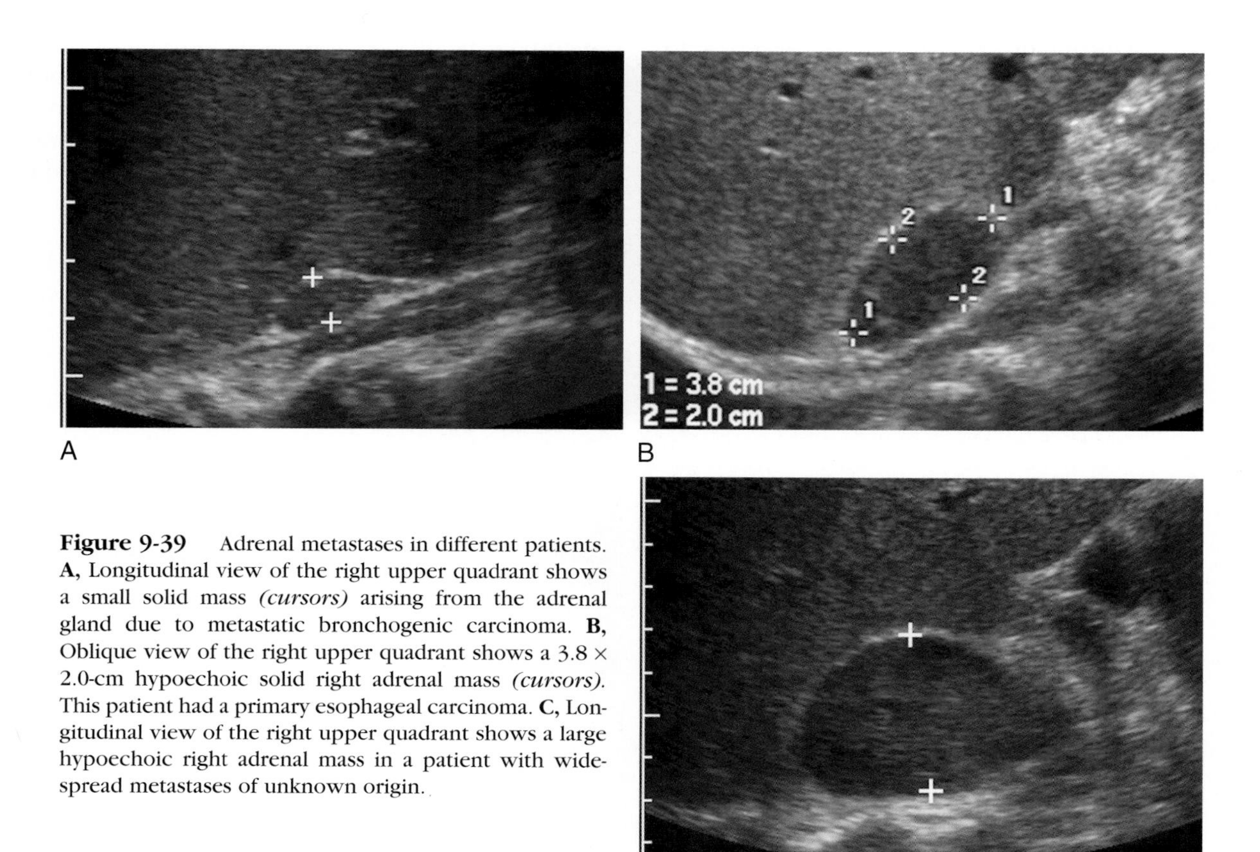

Figure 9-39 Adrenal metastases in different patients. **A,** Longitudinal view of the right upper quadrant shows a small solid mass *(cursors)* arising from the adrenal gland due to metastatic bronchogenic carcinoma. **B,** Oblique view of the right upper quadrant shows a 3.8 × 2.0-cm hypoechoic solid right adrenal mass *(cursors).* This patient had a primary esophageal carcinoma. **C,** Longitudinal view of the right upper quadrant shows a large hypoechoic right adrenal mass in a patient with widespread metastases of unknown origin.

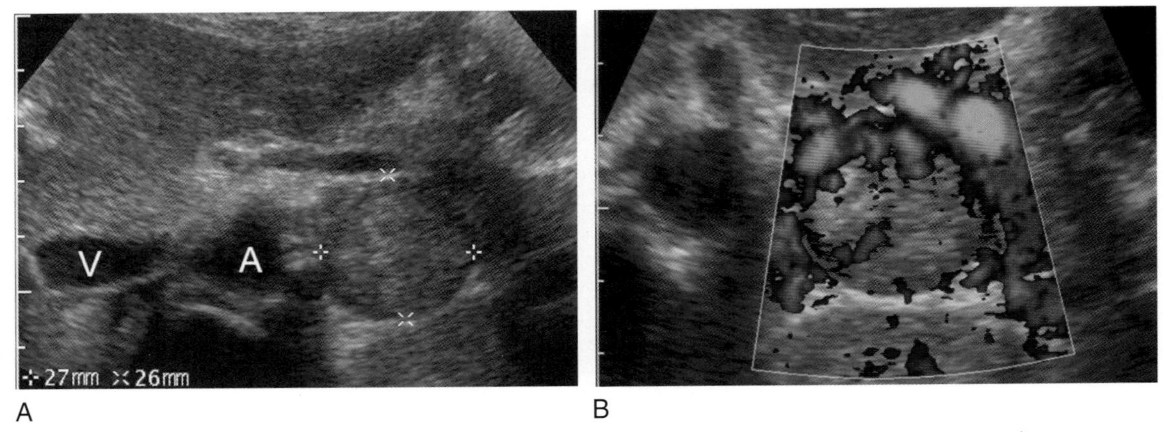

Figure 9-40 Pheochromocytoma. **A,** Transverse view of the upper abdomen shows a 27 × 26-mm solid slightly heterogeneous left adrenal mass *(cursors)* located immediately lateral to the aorta (A). The inferior vena cava (V) is also seen on this image. **B,** Color Doppler view of the same lesion shows readily detectable flow in this vascular lesion. This study was done in a young woman with hypertension. This mass was identified while performing a renal arterial Doppler examination.

Pheochromocytomas are catecholamine-secreting tumors that most often arise from the adrenal medulla. They produce symptoms of hypertension, headache, tachycardia, anxiety, and palpitations. They are referred to as the 10% tumor because 10% are malignant, 10% are extra-adrenal, 10% are bilateral, and 10% are associated with multiple endocrine neoplasia syndromes. Extra-adrenal pheochromocytomas typically occur along the paravertebral sympathetic ganglia from the skull base to the bladder. The vast majority are in the abdomen, in particular in the para-adrenal region and in the organ of Zuckerkandl (para-aortic sympathetic plexus between the inferior mesenteric artery and the aortic bifurcation). The bladder, heart, and mediastinum are well-known but rare sites of pheochromocytomas. Pheochromocytomas are typically large, vascular, heterogeneous tumors (Fig. 9-40). They may rarely be predominantly cystic.

Primary adrenal carcinoma is a very rare tumor. They occur in children and in middle-aged or elderly patients. They are typically very large masses that present as pain or symptoms due to the mass effect. They may be hyperfunctioning in up to 15% of adults, with Cushing's syndrome being the most common clinical manifestation. Necrosis, hemorrhage, and calcification are common. On sonography, they appear as large solid or complex masses. They have a propensity to invade the veins, and tumor thrombus may progress into the vena cava (Fig. 9-41).

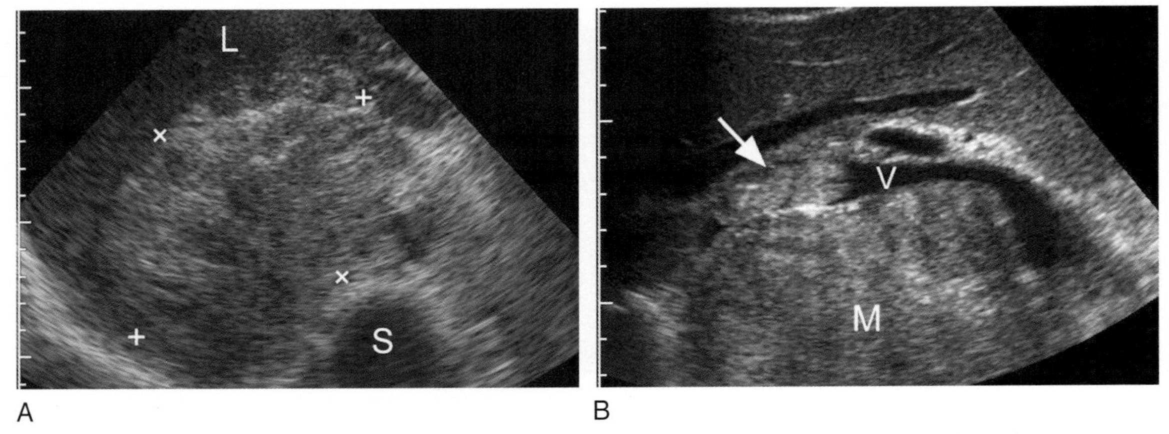

Figure 9-41 Primary adrenal carcinoma. **A,** Transverse view of the right upper quadrant shows a large solid heterogeneous mass *(cursors)* in the expected location of the right adrenal gland. Other views showed this was separate from the kidney. The liver is seen anteriorly (L) and the spine posteriorly (S). **B,** Longitudinal view of the right upper quadrant again identifies the mass (M), which deviates the inferior vena cava (V) anteriorly. A tumor thrombus *(arrow)* is identified within the inferior vena cava.

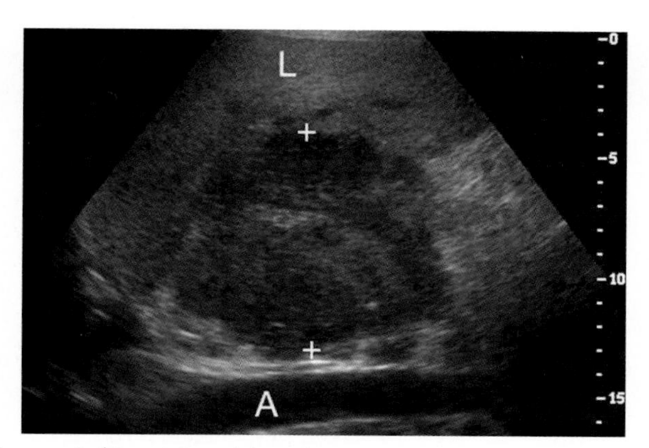

Figure 9-42 Adrenal lymphoma. Coronal view of the right upper quadrant shows a large solid hypoechoic mass in the right adrenal gland *(cursors)*. The liver (L) and the aorta (A) are also identified.

Non-Hodgkin's lymphomatous involvement of the adrenals is not uncommon and usually is caused by direct invasion from retroperitoneal disease. It is bilateral in close to 50% of cases. Primary adrenal lymphoma is very uncommon, but it does occur and should be considered in the differential diagnosis of solid adrenal masses. Like lymphoma elsewhere, adrenal lymphoma is typically a solid, hypoechoic mass (Fig. 9-42).

Myelolipomas are benign tumors that contain hematopoietic and fatty elements. Symptoms are rare, but back pain and hemorrhage may occur. These lesions are typically detected as incidental masses on imaging studies. As expected, the sonographic appearance reflects the amount of fat in the tumor. Thus, they are usually hyperechoic (Fig. 9-43) and they may attenuate the sound and produce partial shadowing. Calcification may also occur.

Adrenal hemorrhage may result from trauma, coagulation dysfunction, sepsis, or iatrogenic from surgery or adrenal venography. Spontaneous hemorrhage may occur with severe stress, hypotension, and tumors. It is unilateral in 80% of cases. On sonography, an adrenal hematoma may appear as a nonspecific mass or it may undergo the typical evolution of a hematoma changing from a hyperechoic lesion, to a complex cystic and solid lesion, to a more purely cystic lesion.

There is significant overlap in the sonographic appearance of various solid adrenal masses. In most cases, sonographic detection of an adrenal mass is followed by CT or MRI for further characterization. In some instances, laboratory studies will suffice to determine the etiology of an adrenal mass.

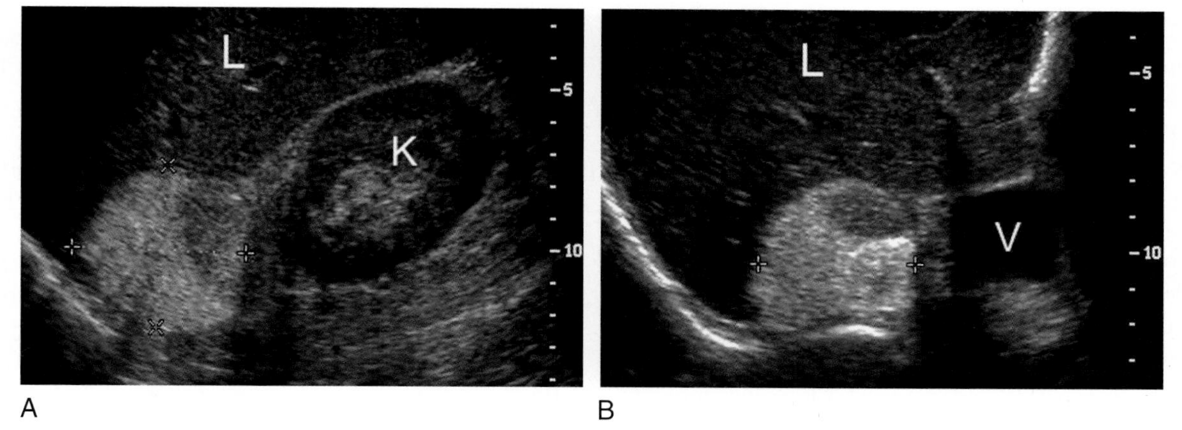

Figure 9-43 Myelolipoma. **A,** Longitudinal view of the right upper quadrant shows a large hyperechoic solid right adrenal mass *(cursors)* located superior to the right kidney (K) and posterior to the liver (L). **B,** Transverse view shows the right adrenal mass *(cursors)* located posterior to the liver and lateral to the inferior vena cava (V).

Key Features

Normal bowel has five layers that are visible on high-resolution sonography. When resolution is limited, as is often the case with routine transabdominal scans, only two layers are visible and the bowel assumes a target appearance.

Bowel wall thickening can be due to neoplasms, inflammatory disease, infections, ischemia, hemorrhage, and edema.

Appendicitis is manifest on sonography as a blunt-ending, noncompressible appendix that is greater than 6 mm in diameter. Associated signs include appendicoliths, inflamed periappendiceal fat, hyperemia, and adjacent fluid collections.

Sonography is very sensitive at diagnosing ascites and guiding paracentesis.

Peritoneal metastatic implants typically appear as solid or complex masses immediately deep to the abdominal wall.

Rectus sheath hematomas are easily detected with sonography and appear as lenticular lesions that initially appear solid and then evolve into more complex collections and ultimately to simple-appearing collections.

Masses and hernias of the abdominal wall can usually be distinguished with sonography.

Sonography is very effective at providing guidance for biopsy of abdominal wall masses that are suspected to be neoplastic.

Extensive mesenteric adenopathy can cause the "pseudokidney" sign.

Abdominal aortic aneurysms can be effectively diagnosed and followed with sonography. So that measurements can be taken perpendicular to the long axis of the aorta, anteroposterior dimensions should be taken from sagittal views and transverse measurements from coronal views.

Primary thrombosis of the inferior vena cava is unusual. Extension from branch vessels is more common.

Tumor thrombus invading the inferior vena cava may expand the lumen and have detectable internal vascularity on color Doppler sonography.

Adrenal masses are easy to detect on the right side but difficult to see on the left side. With the exception of myelolipomas, ultrasound is not capable of characterizing most adrenal masses.

SUGGESTED READINGS

Birnbaum BA, Wilson SR: Appendicitis at the millennium. Radiology 215:337-348, 2000.

Borushok KF, et al: Sonographic diagnosis of perforation in patients with acute appendicitis. AJR Am J Roentgenol 154:275, 1990.

Bru C, Sans M, Defelitto MM, et al: Hydrocolonic sonography for evaluating inflammatory bowel disease. AJR Am J Roentgenol 177:99-105, 2001.

Busch JM, Kruskal JB, Wu B: Malignant peritoneal mesothelioma. Radiographics 22:1511-1515, 2002.

Carson BW, Brown JA, Cooperberg PL: Ultrasonographically guided percutaneous biopsy of gastric, small bowel, and colonic abnormalities: Efficacy and safety. J Ultrasound Med 17:739-742, 1998.

Cobben LPJ, de Mol van Otterloo A, Puylaert JBCM: Spontaneously resolving appendicitis: Frequency and natural history in 60 patients. Radiology 215:349-352, 2000.

Del-Pozo G, Albillos JC, Tejodor D: Intussusception: US findings with pathologic correlation: The crescent in doughnut sign. Radiology 199:688-692, 1996.

Fakuda T, Sakamoto I, Kohzaki S, et al: Spontaneous rectus sheath hematomas: Clinical and radiologic features. Abdom Imaging 21:58-61, 1996.

Fisher AJ, Paulson EK, Sheafor DH, et al: Small lymph nodes of the abdomen, pelvis and retroperitoneum: Usefulness of sonographically guided biopsy. Radiology 205:185-190, 1997.

Greenfield AL, Halpern EJ, Bonn J, et al: Application of duplex US for characterization of endoleaks in abdominal aortic stent-grafts: Report of five cases. Radiology 225: 845-851, 2002.

Haber HP, Stern M: Intestinal ultrasonography in children and young adults: Bowel wall thickness is age dependent. J Ultrasound Med 19:315-321, 2000.

Hadas-Halpern I, Patlas M, Fisher D: Postpartum ovarian vein thrombophlebitis: Sonographic diagnosis. Abdom Imaging 2002 27:93-95.

Hamrick-Turner JE, Chichi MV, Abbitt PL, Ros PR: Neoplastic and inflammatory processes of the peritoneum, omentum, and mesentery: diagnosis with CT. Radiographics 12: 1051-1068, 1992.

Harrison LA, Keesling CA, Martin NL, et al: Abdominal wall hernias: Review of herniography and correlation with cross-sectional imaging. Radiographics 15:315-332, 1995.

Hartman DS, Hayes WS, Choyke PL, Tibbetts GP: Leiomyosarcoma of the retroperitoneum and inferior vena cava: Radiologic-pathologic correlation. Radiographics 12: 1203-1220, 1992.

Jeffrey RB Jr, Jain KA, Nghiem HV: Pictorial essay. Sonographic diagnosis of acute appendicitis: Interpretive pitfalls. AJR Am J Roentgenol 162:55, 1994.

Jeffrey RB Jr, Laing FC, Townsend RR: Acute appendicitis: Sonographic criteria based on 250 cases. Radiology 167:327, 1988.

Jing BS: Diagnostic imaging of abdominal and pelvic lymph nodes in lymphoma. Radiol Clin North Am 28:801-831, 1990.

Korenkov M, Paul A, Troidl H: Color duplex sonography: Diagnostic tool in the differentiation of inguinal hernias. J Ultrasound Med 18:565-568, 1999.

Krebs TL, Wagner BJ: MR imaging of the adrenal gland: Radiologic-pathologic correlation. Radiographics 18:1425-1440, 1998.

Ledermann HP, Borner N, Strunk H, et al: Review: Bowel wall thickening on transabdominal sonography. AJR Am J Roentgenol 174:107-117, 2000.

Mayo-Smith WW, Boland GW, Noto RB, Lee MJ: State-of-the-art adrenal imaging. Radiographics 21:995-1012, 2001.

Muradali D, Wilson S, Burns PN, et al: A specific sign of pneumoperitoneum on sonography: Enhancement of the peritoneal stripe. AJR Am J Roentgenol 173:1257-1262, 1999.

Nevitt MP, Ballard DJ, Hallett JW Jr: Prognosis of abdominal aortic aneurysms: A population-based study. N Engl J Med 321:1009-1014, 1989.

Puylaert JB: Acute appendicitis: US evaluation using graded compression. Radiology 158:355, 1986.

Puylaert JB, et al: A prospective study of ultrasonography in the diagnosis of appendicitis. N Engl J Med 317:666, 1987.

Rao P, Kenney PJ, Wagner BJ, Davidson AJ: Imaging and pathologic features of myelolipoma. Radiographics 17: 1373-1385, 1997.

Rioux M: Sonographic detection of the normal and abnormal appendix. AJR Am J Roentgenol 158:773, 1992.

Rioux N, Michand C: Sonographic detection of peritoneal carcinomatosis: A prospective study of 37 cases. Abdom Imaging 20:47-52, 1995.

Smith C, Kubicka RA, Thomas CR Jr: Non-Hodgkin lymphoma of the gastrointestinal tract. Radiographics 12:887-899, 1992.

Sofia S, Casali A, Bolondi L: Sonographic diagnosis of adult intussusception. Abdom Imaging 26:483-486, 2001.

Sonin AH, Mazer MJ, Powers TA: Obstruction of the inferior vena cava: A multiple-modality demonstration of causes, manifestations, and collateral pathways. Radiographics 12:309-322, 1992.

Spencer JA, Swift SE, Wilkinson N, et al: Peritoneal carcinomatosis: Image-guided peritoneal core biopsy for tumor type and patient care. Radiology 221:173-177, 2001.

Stoupis C, Ros PR, Abbitt PL, et al: Bubbles in the belly: Imaging of cystic mesenteric or omental masses. Radiographics 14:729-737, 1994.

Tudor GR, Rodgers PM, West KP: Bowel lesions: Percutaneous US-guided 18-gauge needle biopsy—preliminary experience. Radiology 121:594-597, 1999.

Turig PS, Cooperberg PL, Madigar SM: The anechoic crescent in abdominal aortic aneurysm: Not a sign of dissection. AJR Am J Roentgenol 1986;146:345-348.

Twickler DM, et al: Imaging of puerperal septic thrombophlebitis: Prospective comparison of MR imaging, CT, and sonography. AJR Am J Roentgenol 169:1039-1043, 1997.

Wilson SR: Gastrointestinal tract sonography. Abdom Imaging 21:1-8, 1996.

Wolf C, Obrist P, Ensinger C: Sonographic features of abdominal wall endometriosis. AJR Am J Roentgenol 169:916, 1997.

Yeh HC: Ultrasonography of peritoneal tumors. Radiology 133:419-424, 1979.

Zhang GQ, Sugiyama M, Hagi H, et al: Groin hernias in adults: Value of color Doppler sonography in their classification. J Clin Ultrasound 29:429-434, 2001.

CHAPTER 10

Neck and Chest

For Key Features summary see p. 275

THYROID

Normal Anatomy

The normal thyroid gland is located in the anterior inferior neck. It is divided into two lobes resting on either side of the trachea. The lobes are connected at their lower third by a thin isthmus that crosses anterior to the trachea (Fig. 10-1). A minority of patients have a thin pyramidal lobe extending superiorly from the isthmus that can be seen in childhood and in conditions that cause generalized enlargement of the thyroid. Immediately anterior to the thyroid are the thin strap muscles (sternohyoid, sternothyroid, and omohyoid). Lateral to the thyroid are the more bulky sternocleidomastoid muscles. The longus colli muscles rest immediately anterior to the vertebrae and posterior to each lobe of the thyroid. The common carotid arteries are located lateral to each thyroid lobe, and the jugular veins are anterior and lateral to the carotids. In most patients the lateral aspect of the esophagus can be seen extending from behind the trachea and the thyroid, more commonly on the left side than on the right side.

In the adult, the thyroid measures 4 to 6 cm in length and 1.3 to 1.8 cm in anteroposterior and transverse diameter. The isthmus measures up to 3 mm in thickness. Thyromegaly is present whenever the transverse or anteroposterior diameter exceeds 2 cm or when parenchyma extends anterior to the carotids (Fig. 10-2). The normal thyroid is very homogeneous and hyperechoic when compared with the adjacent muscles. The amount of internal blood flow seen on color or power Doppler sonography is roughly similar to what is seen in other superficial solid organs, such as the testes. The characteristics of the normal thyroid are reviewed in Box 10-1.

Congenital Anomalies

Congenital abnormalities of the thyroid include ectopia, hypoplasia, and aplasia. Ectopic thyroid tissue is most commonly seen in a midline suprahyoid position between the foramen cecum of the tongue and the epiglottis. This is called a lingual thyroid, and it occurs in approximately 1 in 100,000 healthy individuals. Other sites of ectopic thyroid include sublingual, paralaryngeal, intratracheal, and infrasternal. Ectopic thyroid is generally diagnosed with nuclear medicine scans, and ultrasound plays very little role in most of these patients. On the other hand, hypoplastic and aplastic thyroids are readily evaluated with ultrasound (Fig. 10-3). With unilateral agenesis, contralateral hypertrophy may be seen.

Thyroglossal duct cysts are the most common of the congenital cysts in the neck. During embryogenesis, thyroid anlage migrates from the foramen cecum of the tongue to the lower neck, leaving an epithelial tract

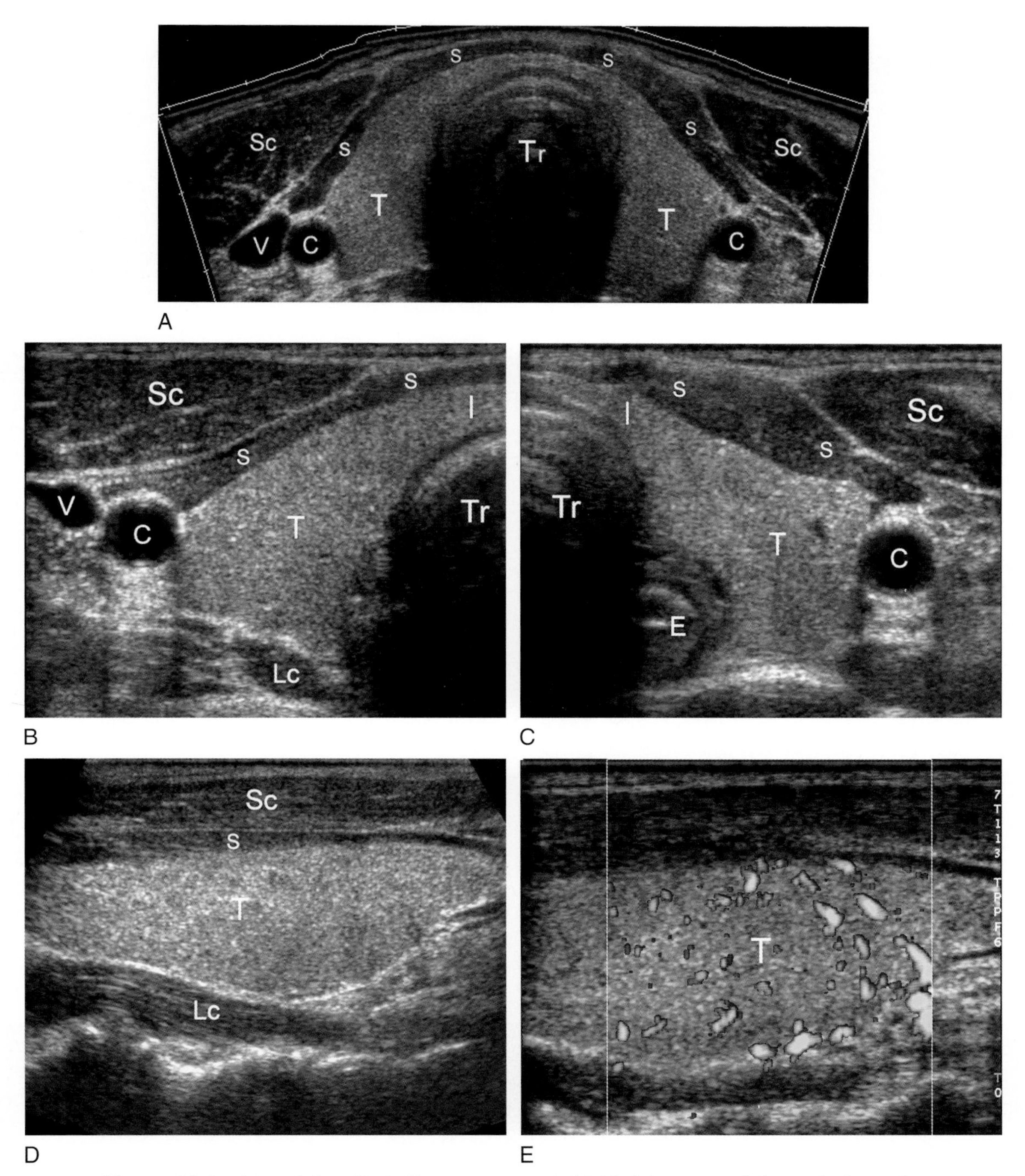

Figure 10-1 Normal thyroid. **A**, Transverse extended-field-of-view scan of the neck shows the normal right and left lobes of the thyroid (T) located on either side of the shadowing produced by the trachea (Tr). The common carotid arteries (C) and the right internal jugular vein (V) are seen lateral to the thyroid. The overlying strap muscles (S) are located immediately anterior to the thyroid, and the sternocleidomastoid muscles (Sc) are seen anterolateral to the thyroid. **B,** Conventional transverse view of the right thyroid lobe shows the thyroid (T) and the trachea (Tr). The isthmus of the thyroid (I) is seen anterior to the trachea. The strap muscles (S) and sternocleidomastoid (Sc) are also seen anteriorly and laterally. The longus colli muscle (Lc) is seen posteriorly. The carotid artery (C) and jugular vein (V) are seen lateral to the thyroid. **C,** Conventional transverse view of the left thyroid lobe shows the same structures as on the right. In addition, the left lateral edge of the esophagus (E) is seen posterior to the trachea. The typical bowel layers are seen in the esophagus. **D,** Longitudinal view of the thyroid (T) shows the lenticular shape of the thyroid and the hyperechoic echogenicity of the thyroid compared with the overlying strap muscles (S) and the sternocleidomastoid (Sc). The longus colli muscle (Lc) is seen posteriorly. **E,** Longitudinal power Doppler view of the thyroid (T) shows the normal expected degree of flow scattered throughout the gland.

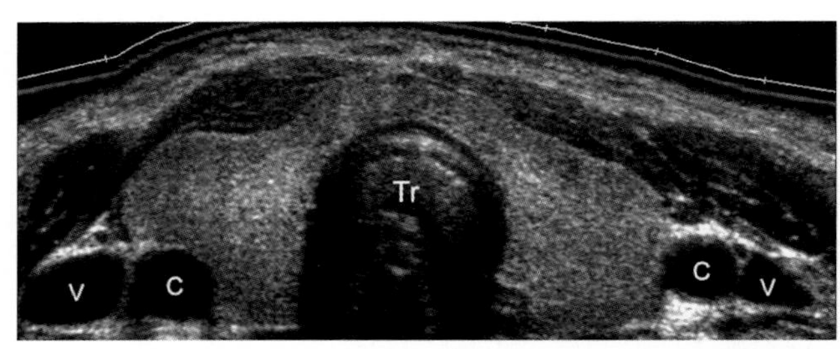

Figure 10-2 Thyromegaly. Transverse extended-field-of-view scan shows that the right lobe of the thyroid has enlarged and extended anterior to the common carotid artery (C). The jugular veins (V) and the trachea (Tr) are also seen.

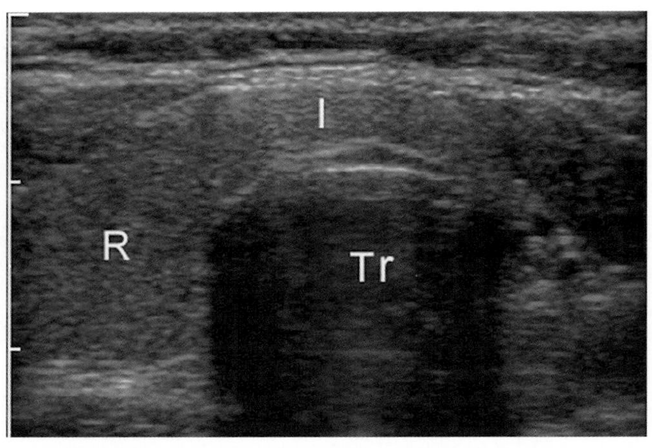

Figure 10-3 Unilateral thyroid agenesis. Transverse view of the thyroid shows a normal right lobe (R) and a normal isthmus (I). No identifiable left lobe is present. The trachea (Tr) is seen centrally.

called the thyroglossal duct. This normally involutes in the eighth week of fetal life. Thyroid cells may remain in the thyroglossal duct in 5% of cases and can potentially give rise to thyroglossal duct cysts. Despite the embryogenesis, thyroid tissue is usually not detected pathologically in resected specimens. They are typically located in the midline between the thyroid gland and the hyoid bone (Fig. 10-4A and B). The more caudad the cyst is located, the more likely it is to be lateral to the midline (see Fig. 10-4C). Only 20% occur above the hyoid. Patients most often present in childhood or young adulthood. Sonographically, thyroglossal duct cysts usually appear as cystic lesions with low-level intraluminal reflectors, presumably due to bleeding or infection. They usually do not appear as simple cysts.

Box 10-1 Characteristics of the Normal Thyroid

Hyperechoic to adjacent muscles
Homogeneous
Scattered readily detectable internal vessels
Lobes less than 2 cm anteroposterior and transverse
Isthmus less than 4 mm

Nodules

Thyroid nodules are extremely common and are the most common indication for thyroid ultrasound. Autopsy studies show that 50% of patients with a clinically normal thyroid have nodules. Sonography detects nodules in approximately 40% of patients who are

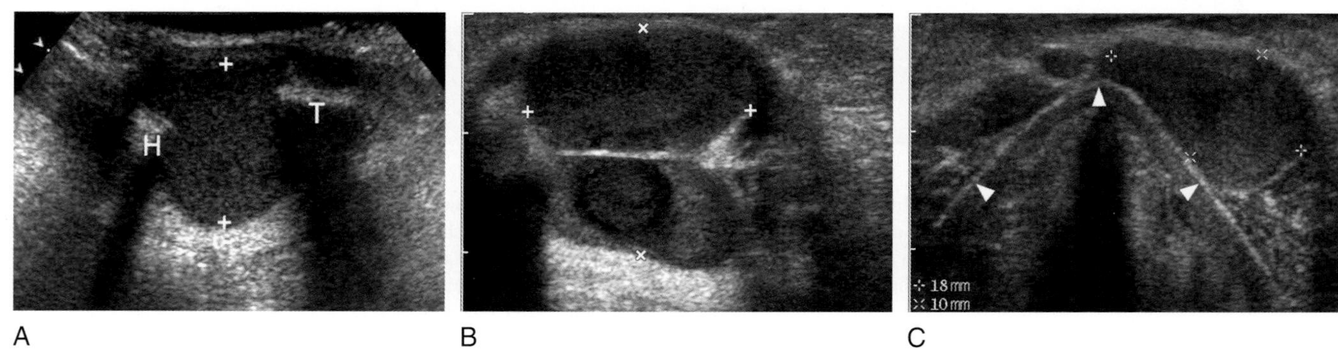

Figure 10-4 Thyroglossal duct cysts in different patients. **A,** Longitudinal view of the midline of the neck in the suprathyroidal region shows the hyoid bone (H) and the thyroid cartilage (T) with their associated shadows. A complex cystic lesion *(cursors)* with diffuse low-level echoes is seen located immediately between these two structures. This is the typical location for a thyroglossal duct cyst. **B,** Transverse view of the midline neck in the suprathyroidal region shows a complex cystic lesion *(cursors)* with low-level echoes and a thin septation. **C,** Transverse view of the neck above the level of the thyroid gland shows the thyroid cartilage *(arrowheads).* Extending from the midline over to the left is a complex cystic lesion *(cursors)* consistent with a thyroglossal cyst.

scanned for other reasons. The prevalence of nodules increases with age, and the percentage of patients with nodules is approximately equal to the age in years minus 10. Despite the high prevalence of thyroid nodules, the percentage of thyroid malignancy is very low (2% to 4%).

In approximately 80% of patients, thyroid hyperplasia is idiopathic, or related to iodine deficiency, familial causes, or medications. An enlarged, hyperplastic gland is called a *goiter*. The male-to-female ratio of thyroid hyperplasia is approximately 1 to 3. When hyperplasia progresses to nodule formation, the pathologic designation of the nodules may be hyperplastic, adenomatous, or colloid. Nodular hyperplasia is the most common cause for thyroid nodules. These types of nodules share some common sonographic appearances (Fig. 10-5). They very frequently have cystic components. When the

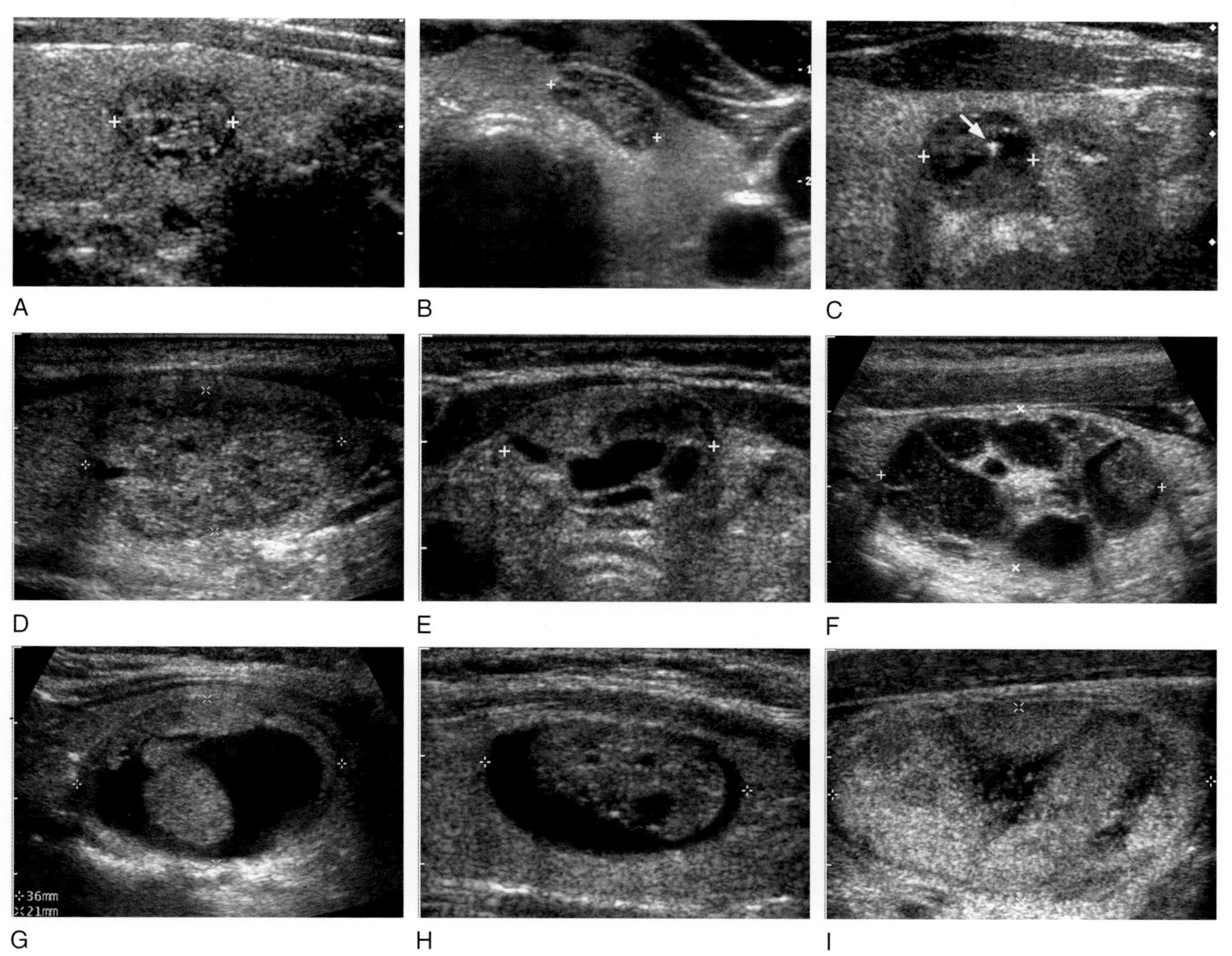

Figure 10-5 Nodular hyperplasia in different patients. **A** and **B**, Hypoechoic nodules *(cursors)* that are predominantly solid with multiple small internal cystic spaces. This is the typical appearance for small lesions. **C**, Nodule similar to those in **A** and **B** with additional finding of inspissated colloid *(arrow)*, which casts a short comet tail artifact. **D**, Larger isoechoic nodule *(cursors)* that is almost entirely solid but contains a few tiny cystic spaces. **E**, Complex nodule *(cursors)* with cystic and solid components. **F**, Predominantly cystic nodule *(cursors)* with thick septations and low-level intraluminal echoes. **G**, Predominantly cystic nodule *(cursors)* with thick wall and a prominent solid mural nodule. **H**, Otherwise simple cyst *(cursors)* with no detectable wall but with a large predominantly solid mural nodule. **I**, Large hyperechoic solid nodule *(cursors)* with minimal internal liquefaction. This nodule simulates a follicular neoplasm.

nodule is small, the cystic components are also very small. As the nodule enlarges, the cystic spaces also may enlarge. When cystic elements are predominant, they are usually associated with multiple internal septations and mural nodules. Bright foci, occasionally with comet-tail artifacts, may be present and indicate inspissated colloid. The echogenicity of nodular hyperplasia is variable and may be hypoechoic, isoechoic, or hyperechoic compared with normal parenchyma.

Benign follicular adenomas account for 5% to 10% of thyroid nodules. A small minority may cause hyperthyroidism owing to autonomous function. They often occur in a gland that has multiple nodules for other reasons. They are typically solid and range from hypoechoic to hyperechoic. Well-defined cystic spaces occur in a minority of these nodules. They are well marginated, and a hypoechoic halo is often present (Fig. 10-6). Follicular adenomas and follicular cancer can be distinguished only on the basis of vascular and capsular invasion. This distinction cannot be made by sonography or by fine-needle aspiration. Therefore, fine-needle aspiration of a follicular lesion should generally be followed by surgical resection.

There are several types of thyroid cancer. Papillary is the most common and accounts for more than 75% of cancers. It is followed in frequency by follicular, medullary, anaplastic, and Hürthle cell cancer.

Papillary cancer is much more common than the other types in patients younger than age 40 years and in women. Lymphatic dissemination is much more common than hematogenous spread, and cervical nodal metastases are often present at the time of diagnosis. The prognosis is excellent, with survival of 90% to 95% at 20 years. In fact, it is not uncommon to find small foci of papillary cancer in the surgical specimens of thyroids removed for other benign nodules. These incidentally detected cancers do not affect the patient's survival. The presence of metastatic cervical nodes also does not affect the good prognosis for papillary cancer. Distant metastases are rare. Papillary cancer is multifocal in 20% of cases, and it grows slowly. Papillary cancer often contains some follicular elements and is then referred to as mixed papillary/follicular or follicular variant. Mixed cancers behave like pure papillary cancers. Microcarcinoma is another variant of papillary cancer. It is a sclerosing carcinoma that is less than 1 cm and presents as

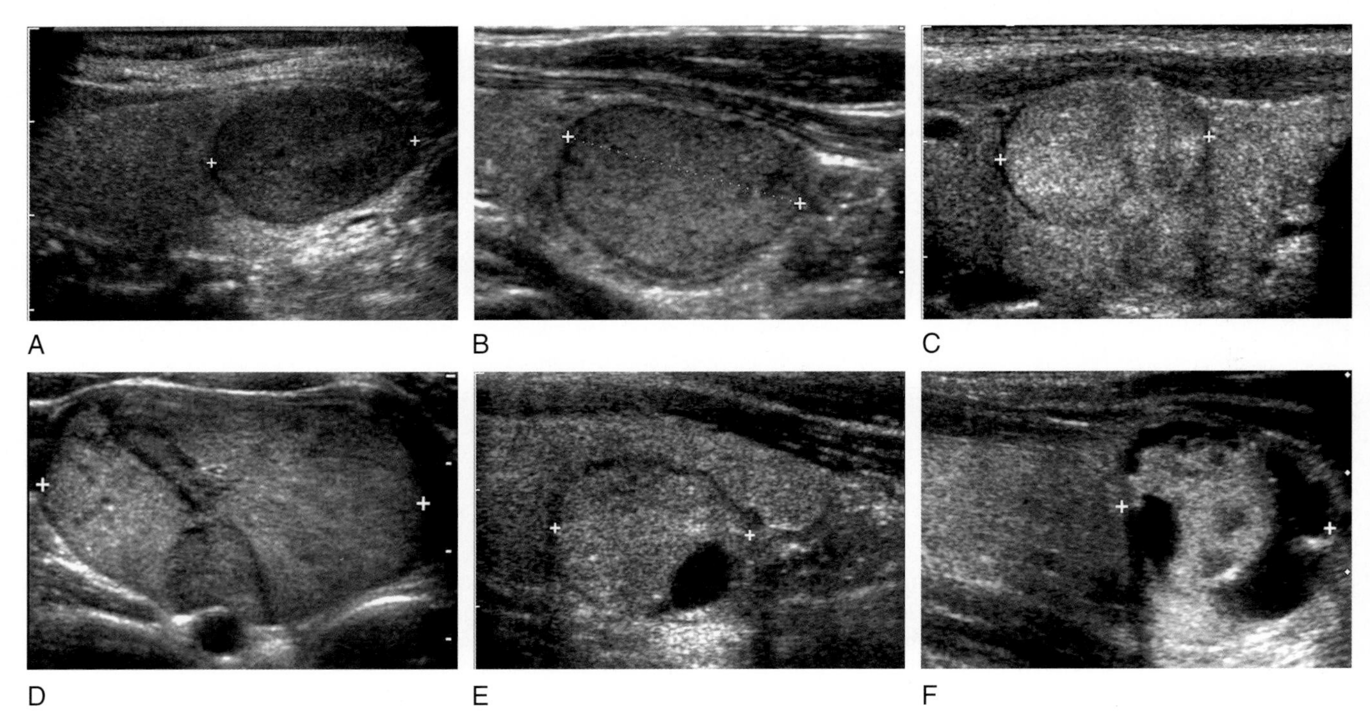

Figure 10-6 Follicular adenomas in different patients. **A,** Solid hypoechoic nodule *(cursors)* with thin peripheral hypoechoic halo. **B,** Solid isoechoic nodule *(cursors)* with peripheral halo. **C,** Solid hyperechoic nodule *(cursors)* with peripheral halo. **D,** Large solid hyperechoic nodule *(cursors)* with scattered internal regions of decreased echogenicity. **E,** Predominantly solid isoechoic nodule *(cursors)* with a peripheral halo and a well-defined internal cyst. **F,** Complex cystic and solid nodule *(cursors)* that simulates nodular hyperplasia.

large metastases to the cervical nodes without clinical evidence of a primary tumor in the thyroid. Papillary cancers are typically hypoechoic and entirely solid (Fig. 10-7). Microcalcifications occur owing to deposition of calcium salts in psammoma bodies and are common in papillary cancer. Although microcalcifications are very uncommon in other thyroid nodules, inspissated crystallinized colloid is very common in nodular hyperplasia and can be confused with microcalcifications. Lymph node metastases are common with papillary cancer, and they may also contain microcalcifications. Cystic degenerative areas in lymph nodes are also very typical of papillary thyroid cancer.

Follicular cancer accounts for approximately 10% of thyroid malignancies and is more common in women in the sixth decade of life. It is divided into minimally and widely invasive forms. Unlike papillary cancer, follicular cancer spreads hematogenously, especially to bone, brain, lung, and liver. Metastases to neck nodes are distinctly rare in follicular cancer. Distant metastases are present in 20% to 40% of the widely invasive variant and 5% to 10% of the minimally invasive variant. Twenty-year mortality for all patients with follicular cancer is approximately 25%. Follicular cancer frequently coexists with multinodular goiters. The microcalcifications and nodal metastases seen with papillary cancer are not present with follicular cancer. As mentioned earlier, follicular cancer overlaps with the appearance of follicular adenomas (Fig. 10-8), and it is not possible to distinguish these lesions on sonography or with fine-needle aspiration.

Medullary cancer is derived from parafollicular cells (also called C cells) that secrete calcitonin, so serum calcitonin can be used as a tumor marker. It accounts for 5% of thyroid malignancies. Ten to 20% of cases of medullary carcinoma are associated with multiple endocrine neoplasia type II. It has a more aggressive behavior than the differentiated carcinomas, and it does not respond to chemotherapy or radiation therapy. On sonography, medullary cancer appears as a hypoechoic, solid mass (Fig. 10-9). Like papillary cancer, microcalcifications are common in both the primary tumor and the nodal metastases.

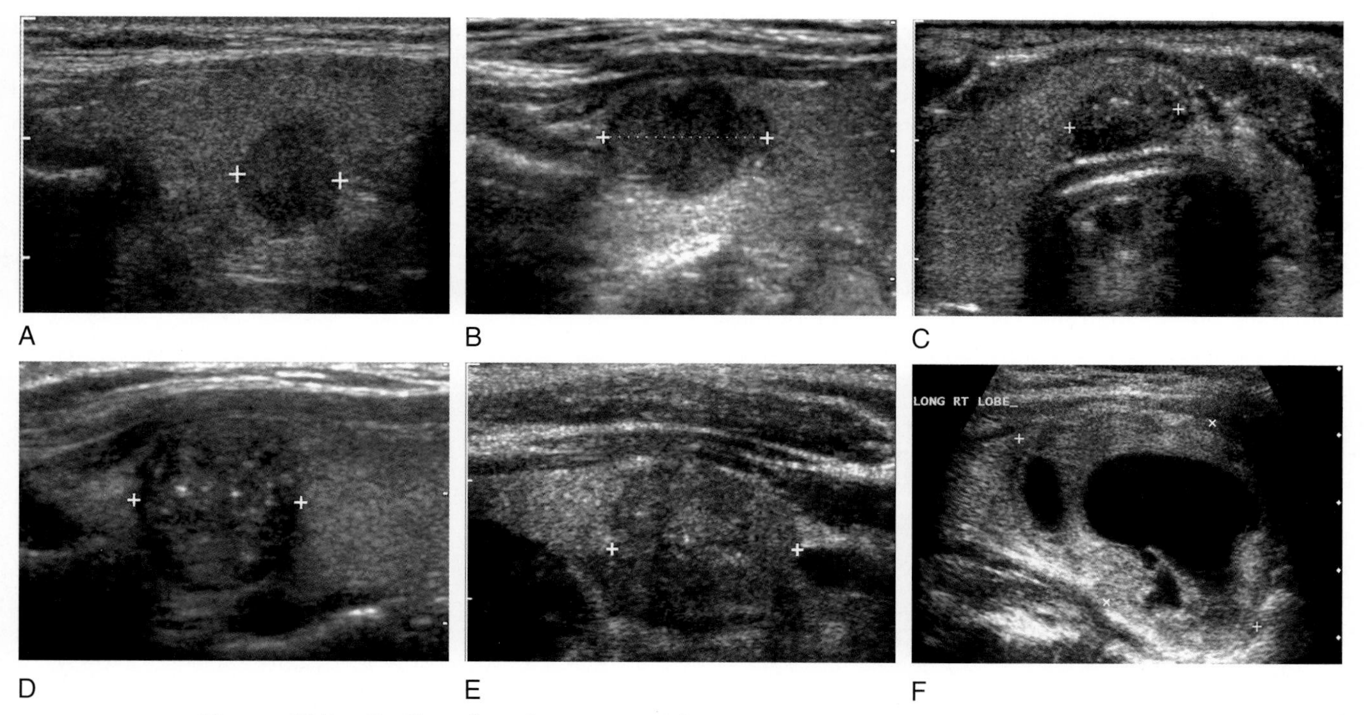

Figure 10-7 Papillary thyroid cancer in different patients. **A,** Longitudinal view shows a hypoechoic homogeneous entirely solid lesion *(cursors)*. **B,** Longitudinal view shows a homogeneous hypoechoic slightly lobulated solid lesion *(cursors)*. **C,** Transverse view shows a hypoechoic solid lesion *(cursors)* that contains a few microcalcifications. **D,** Longitudinal view shows an entirely solid hypoechoic lesion with scattered microcalcifications and an irregular halo. **E,** Longitudinal view shows a solid slightly heterogeneous nodule *(cursors)* containing a few microcalcifications. **F,** Longitudinal view shows a large complex lesion *(cursors)* that is solid but contains large internal cystic components. This is a follicular variant of papillary carcinoma.

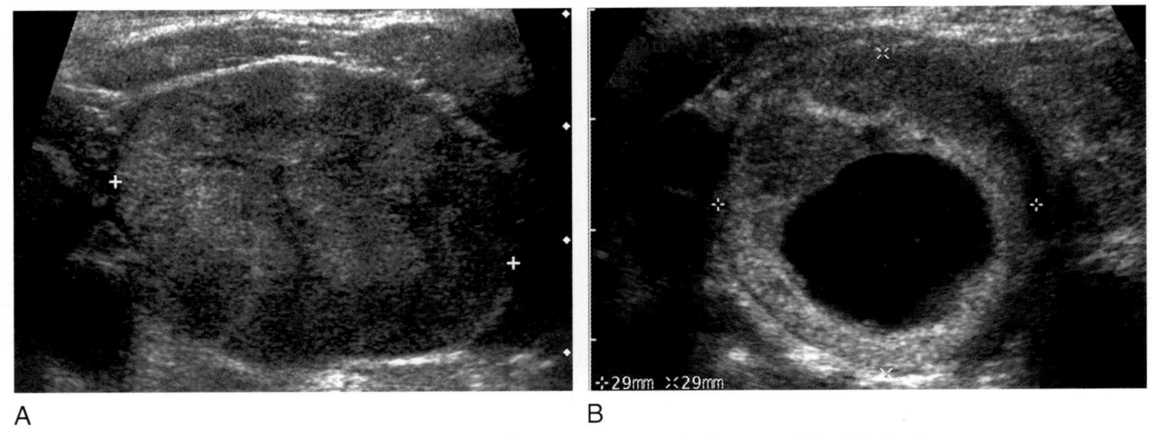

Figure 10-8 Follicular cancer in different patients. **A,** Large solid slightly heterogeneous hypoechoic nodule *(cursors)*. **B,** Predominantly solid, hypoechoic nodule *(cursors)* with a prominent internal cystic component.

Anaplastic cancer accounts for less than 5% of thyroid malignancies. It is rarely seen in patients younger than 60 years old, and it has a dismal prognosis (5-year mortality of greater than 95%). It usually appears as a large, solid, hypoechoic mass (Fig. 10-10). Local invasion of adjacent structures is common at the time of presentation.

Thyroid lymphoma represents less than 5% of thyroid malignancies and can occur as either a manifestation of generalized lymphoma or as a primary abnormality. It is usually of the non-Hodgkin's variety. Women are affected more often than men, and it tends to occur in the elderly. It generally presents as a rapidly growing mass. On sonography, it is usually a large, solid, hypoechoic mass that infiltrates much of the thyroid parenchyma (Fig. 10-11).

Metastases can occur in the thyroid, most commonly from lung, breast, and renal cell cancers. None of these lesions has a characteristic sonographic appearance, but metastatic disease should be considered when a solid thyroid nodule is identified in a patient with a known extrathyroidal malignancy (Fig. 10-12).

When considering nodular thyroid disease, it is important to realize that overlap exists in the sonographic appearance of benign and malignant nodules. Because of this, sonography is not capable of determining with assurance if a nodule is benign or malignant. Nevertheless, based on the description of different thyroid lesions presented previously, it is clear that there are general differences in the appearance of benign and malignant thyroid nodules (Box 10-2). These are worth emphasizing.

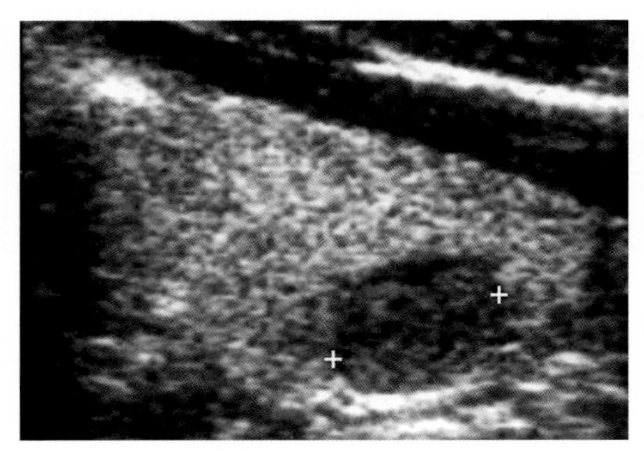

Figure 10-9 Medullary cancer. Longitudinal view shows a solid hypoechoic nodule *(cursors)*. This appearance is very similar to that of papillary cancer.

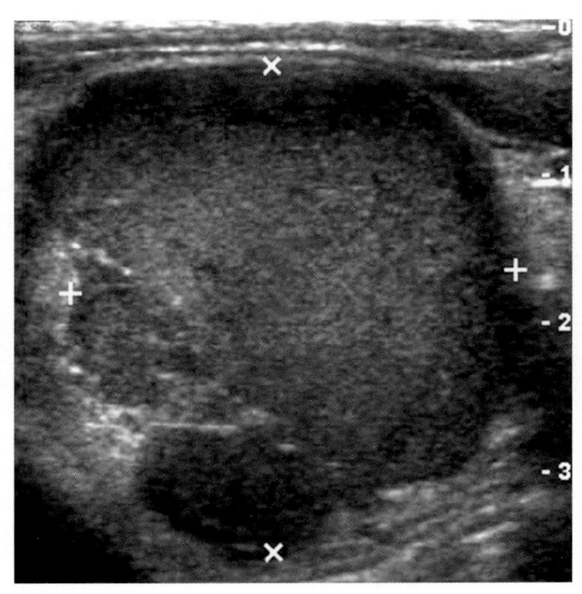

Figure 10-10 Anaplastic cancer. Transverse view shows a large lobulated solid hypoechoic mass *(cursors)* replacing the entire thyroid.

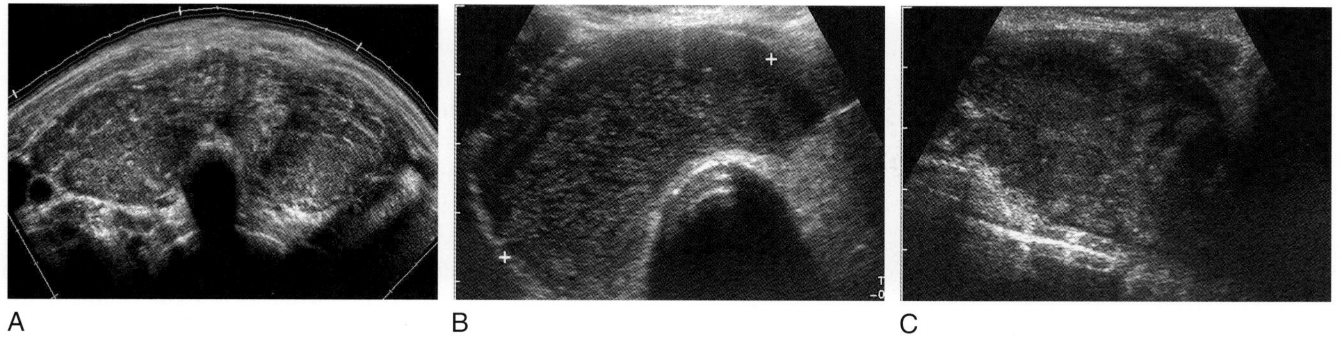

Figure 10-11 Thyroid lymphoma in different patients. **A,** Transverse extended field-of-view scan shows a markedly enlarged slightly heterogeneous hypoechoic thyroid. No discrete masses are seen. **B,** Transverse view shows a solid hypoechoic mass *(cursors)* replacing the entire right lobe and isthmus but sparing the left lobe. **C,** Longitudinal view near the midline shows a hypoechoic heterogeneous solid mass replacing the entire thyroid isthmus.

Sonographic findings that can be used to favor a diagnosis of benign disease include the following:

1. Simple cysts (Fig 10-13). Although these are very uncommon in the thyroid, simple cysts do occur and they are always benign.
2. Significant cystic components. Cystic elements are very common in nodular hyperplasia. They may be very small and require high-resolution probes to detect. Harmonic imaging and real-time compounding help to detect these small cystic spaces. Although there is a cystic form of papillary cancer, it is uncommon.
3. Echogenicity greater than or equal to normal thyroid. Most thyroid malignancies are hypoechoic.
4. Peripheral hypoechoic halo. This is a sign of benign disease when it is thin and regular. However, follicular cancers can also have this appearance.
5. Well-defined margin. This is typical of benign nodules, but there is a great deal of overlap with malignant nodules, and this criterion is not very reliable.
6. Peripheral eggshell calcification (Fig. 10-14). This is occasionally seen in benign nodules and almost never seen in thyroid cancer.
7. Multiplicity. It has traditionally been believed that multiple nodules imply a benign etiology. It is true that most patients with nodular hyperplasia have multiple nodules and some patients with thyroid cancers have solitary nodules. However, approximately 20% of papillary cancer is multifocal and it is not uncommon for thyroid cancer to coexist with nodular hyperplasia. So the presence of multiple nodules on sonography should not decrease the suspicion for a nodule that otherwise has malignant features.

Findings used to favor a malignant nodule include the following:

1. Entirely solid with no cystic elements.
2. Hypoechoic to normal thyroid.
3. Microcalcifications. It should be noted that inspissated colloid may occur in nodular hyperplasia and can be confused with microcalcifications. Crystalinized colloid may have a comet-tail artifact that will distinguish it from microcalcifications.

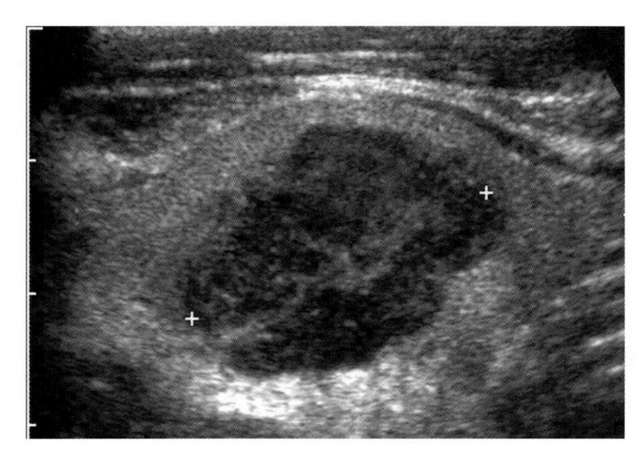

Figure 10-12 Metastatic disease to the thyroid. Longitudinal view of the right lobe of the thyroid shows a slightly lobulated solid predominately hypoechoic nodule *(cursors)*. This patient had a history of melanoma and fine-needle aspiration confirmed metastatic melanoma to the thyroid.

Box 10-2 Differentiation of Thyroid Nodules

BENIGN CHARACTERISTICS	MALIGNANT CHARACTERISTICS
Cystic elements	Entirely solid
Hyper or isoechoic	Hypoechoic
Eggshell calcification	Microcalcifications
Inspissated colloid	Associated cervical adenopathy

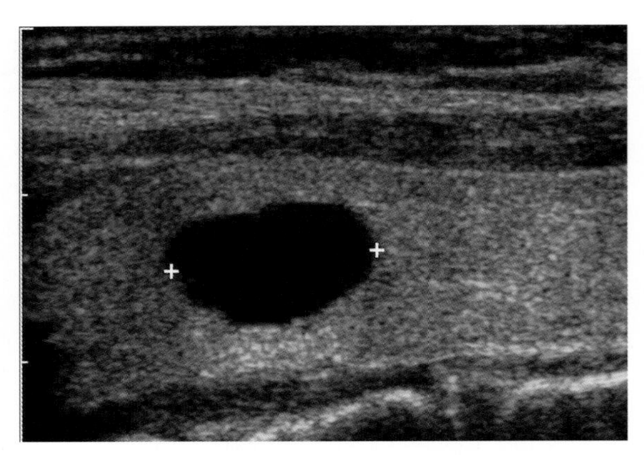

Figure 10-13 Simple thyroid cyst. Longitudinal view shows a simple anechoic cyst *(cursors)* with no solid components.

4. Thick peripheral hypoechoic halo.
5. Associated lymph nodes that appear malignant, especially if the nodes contain microcalcifications or cystic areas of necrosis.

Parenchymal Disease

A number of inflammatory and immune conditions can affect the thyroid. The most common are subacute thyroiditis, Hashimoto's thyroiditis, and Graves' disease. Hashimoto's thyroiditis (also called chronic autoimmune lymphocytic thyroiditis) is believed to be due to autoantibodies to thyroid proteins, especially thyroglobulin. Therefore, the diagnosis is often made serologically. The gland is infiltrated with lymphocytes and plasma cells, and a fibrotic reaction takes place. Patients may be euthyroid initially but generally become hypothyroid owing to replacement of functioning thyroid parenchyma.

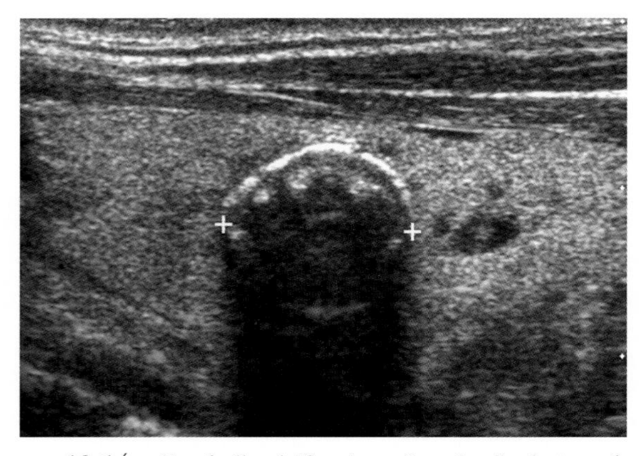

Figure 10-14 Eggshell calcifications. Longitudinal view shows a nodule with a thin peripheral rim of calcification that produces partial shadowing. This appearance is highly suggestive of a benign nodule.

Hashimoto's thyroiditis is the most common cause of hypothyroidism in the United States. It has a peak incidence between the ages of 40 and 60 and is six times more common in women than men. Other autoimmune disorders such as Sjögren's syndrome, lupus, rheumatoid arthritis, fibrosing mediastinitis, sclerosing cholangitis, and pernicious anemia may coexist with Hashimoto's thyroiditis. There is a slight increased risk of thyroid lymphoma in patients with Hashimoto's thyroiditis. On sonography, the gland is normal or enlarged and hypoechoic. Generally, the normal homogeneous echotexture is replaced by a more heterogeneous texture. Thin echogenic fibrous strands may cause a multilobulated or micronodular appearance (Fig. 10-15). Often the gland is extremely hypervascular (see Fig. 10-15F). Hashimoto's thyroiditis can cause nodules (see Fig. 10-15E), and other benign and malignant nodules can coexist with Hashimoto's thyroiditis. In the end stage, the gland becomes atrophic.

Graves' disease is the most common cause of hyperthyroidism. Like Hashimoto's thyroiditis, Graves' disease (also called diffuse toxic goiter) is an autoimmune disorder. Thyroid-stimulating immunoglobulins such as long-acting thyroid stimulator simulate the function of thyroid-stimulating hormone and cause hyperthyroidism. In most cases these can be detected with blood tests. Ultrasound plays a very minor role in the diagnosis and management of Graves' disease. The sonographic findings include gland enlargement, decreased echogenicity, occasional heterogeneity, and hypervascularity ("thyroid inferno") (Fig. 10-16).

Subacute granulomatous thyroiditis (also called de Quervain's thyroiditis) is believed to be caused by a viral infection. It occurs more often in women and produces an enlarged and painful thyroid and often a fever. It is often preceded by an upper respiratory tract infection. The entire gland may be involved, or involvement may be focal. Transient hyperthyroidism may be seen in the initial stages of the disease due to follicular rupture. This may be followed by a transient phase of hypothyroidism. The process is usually diagnosed clinically and responds well to medical treatment. When sonography is performed, it typically shows a poorly marginated area or areas of decreased echogenicity in the involved regions of the thyroid (Fig. 10-17). Blood flow to the area is typically normal or decreased.

PARATHYROID

Normal Anatomy

Most adults have two superior and two inferior parathyroid glands. The superior glands are usually located posterior to the mid portion of the thyroid. The inferior glands are slightly more variable in their

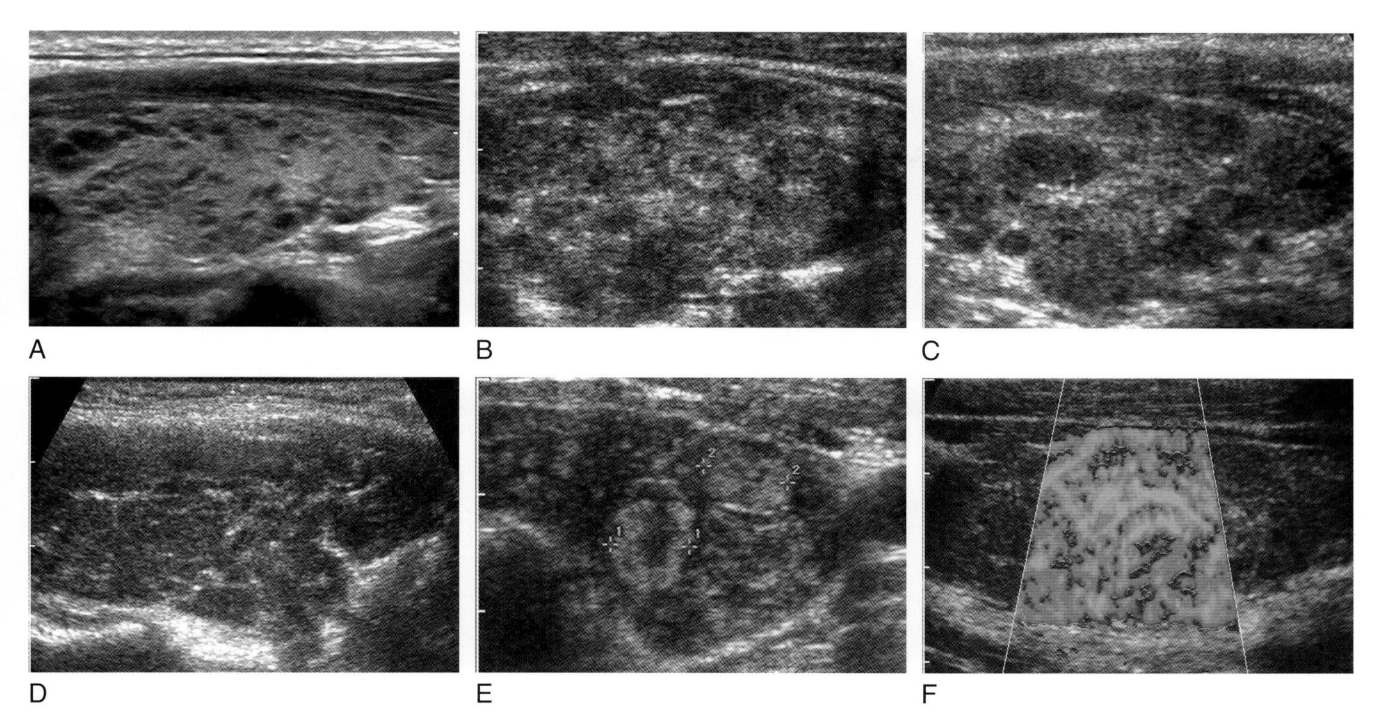

Figure 10-15 Hashimoto's thyroiditis in different patients. **A,** Longitudinal view of the thyroid shows multiple tiny hypoechoic nodules scattered throughout an otherwise normal-appearing thyroid gland. **B,** Longitudinal view shows an enlarged thyroid that is diffusely heterogeneous and more hypoechoic than normal. **C,** Longitudinal view shows a thyroid that is hypoechoic and heterogeneous with several confluent areas of decreased echogenicity. **D,** Longitudinal view shows a thyroid that has decreased echogenicity and several more hyperechoic fibrous strands dispersed in an irregular fashion. **E,** Transverse view of the thyroid shows diffuse heterogeneity and decreased echogenicity with two discrete hyperechoic nodules *(cursors).* Fine-needle aspiration confirmed that these nodules were also due to Hashimoto's thyroiditis. **F,** Longitudinal power Doppler view shows marked hypervascularity throughout the thyroid gland. This can be compared with normal thyroid vascularity shown in Figure 10-1E.

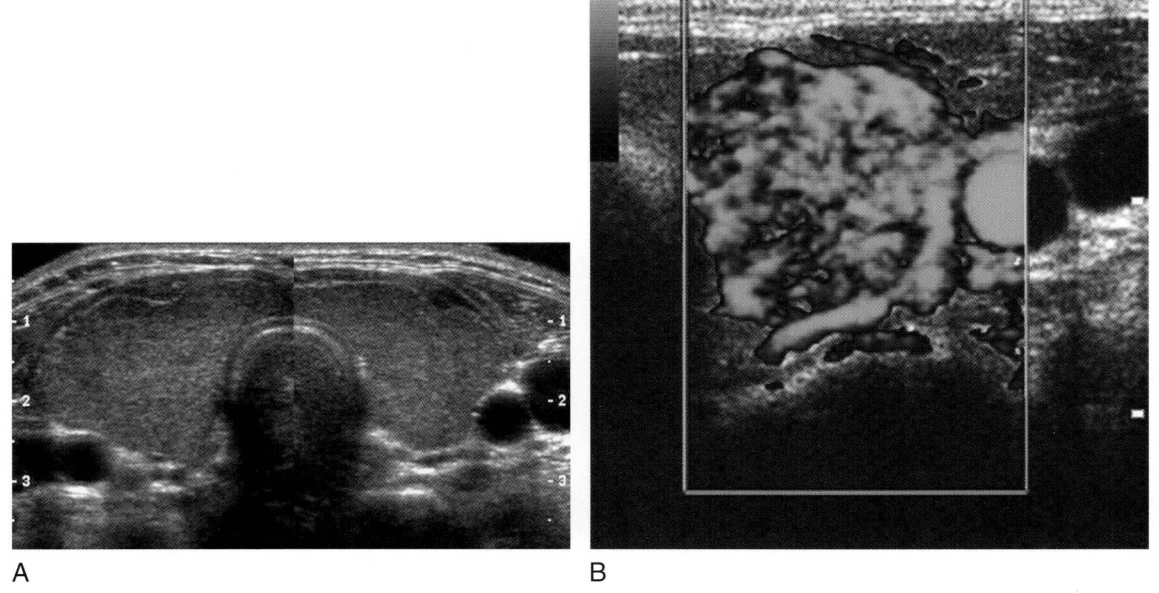

Figure 10-16 Graves' disease. **A,** Dual transverse image of the thyroid shows an enlarged homogeneous but hypoechoic gland without identifiable nodules. **B,** Transverse power Doppler view of the left lobe of the thyroid shows diffuse hypervascularity of the gland.

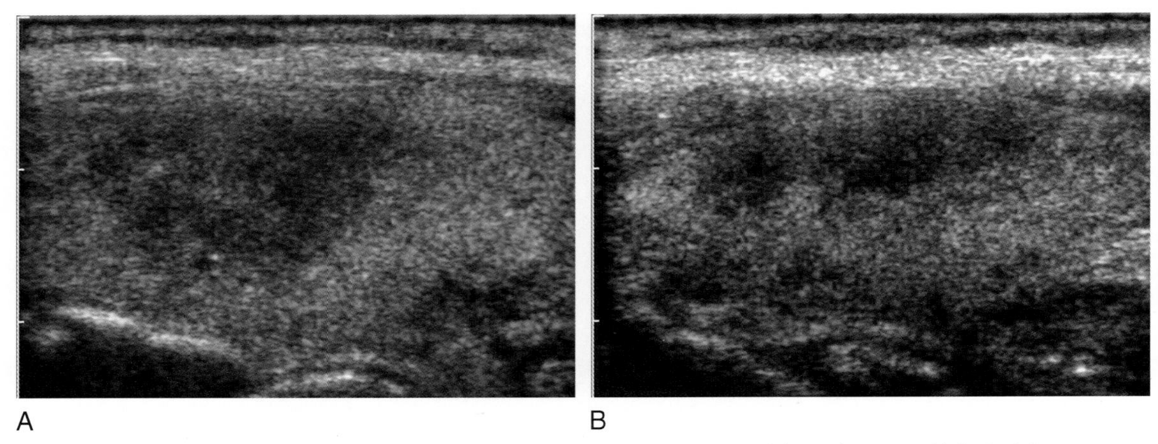

Figure 10-17 Subacute thyroiditis. **A** and **B,** Longitudinal views of the right (**A**) and left (**B**) lobes of the thyroid show poorly marginated regions of decreased echogenicity bilaterally.

location. Approximately 60% are located posterior or just inferior to the lower pole of the thyroid. Another 20% of inferior parathyroids are located within 4 cm of the lower pole of the thyroid. Up to 13% of the population has a fifth parathyroid gland that is often associated with the thymus. Normal parathyroids are oval or almond shaped and measure 1 × 3 × 5 mm. Normal glands are almost never seen with ultrasound.

Hyperparathyroidism

Primary hyperparathyroidism is a relatively common endocrine disorder. The male-to-female ratio is approximately 2.5 to 1. It tends to affect patients between the ages of 40 and 60 years. In 85% of cases it is due to a solitary parathyroid adenoma. In 15% of cases it is caused by multiple gland enlargement. In less than 1% it results from parathyroid cancer. It is characterized clinically by elevated serum calcium levels and inappropriately high levels of parathyroid hormone (PTH) compared with the calcium level. Most cases are detected by routine laboratory tests. Advanced cases of hyperparathyroidism with kidney stones, osteopenia, and subperiosteal resorption are fortunately uncommon. Secondary hyperparathyroidism is usually the result of renal disease and results in variable levels of serum calcium and an elevated PTH value.

On sonography, parathyroid adenomas appear as hypoechoic homogeneous solid masses (Fig. 10-18). In some cases, the lesion is so hypoechoic that it simulates a cyst. Some internal heterogeneity may occur, but true cystic changes are rarely seen. Adenomas are usually oval with the long axis in the craniocaudal direction. Less often they are teardrop shaped or round. Parathyroid adenomas are hypervascular lesions, and this can often be displayed on color Doppler imaging (see Fig. 10-18D and E), although the vascularity of small lesions and deep lesions is often hard to detect with current Doppler equipment (see Fig. 10-18F). The appearance of parathyroid adenomas is summarized in Box 10-3.

Most parathyroid adenomas are located posterior or immediately inferior to the thyroid. Ectopic locations are encountered in approximately 3% of patients (Box 10-4). The retrotracheal region is a common site for ectopic superior adenomas. These can be difficult to visualize sonographically owing to gas shadowing from the trachea. To counteract this, the patient's head should be turned to the opposite side, and scanning should be performed from a lateral location with the transducer angled medially. The caudal aspect of the neck and the superior mediastinum are common locations for ectopic inferior adenomas. When in the mediastinum, they are usually anterior and related to the thymus, although they can occur more posteriorly and as low as the aortopulmonary window. Mediastinal adenomas are difficult to visualize with sonography because high-frequency linear-array transducers that are typically used are often too large to manipulate in the relatively confined region of the suprasternal and supraclavicular regions. This problem can be partially avoided by using curved-array probes with a short radius of curvature. Transvaginal probes are very small and often work very well in looking deep into the lower neck and superior mediastinum (Fig. 10-19A). Ectopic parathyroid adenomas can also be located in the carotid sheath (see Fig. 10-19B and C) or in the thyroid (see Fig. 10-19D). Intrathyroidal adenomas are easy to see sonographically but can be easily confused with thyroid adenomas or other thyroid nodules. They are usually located in the posterior half of

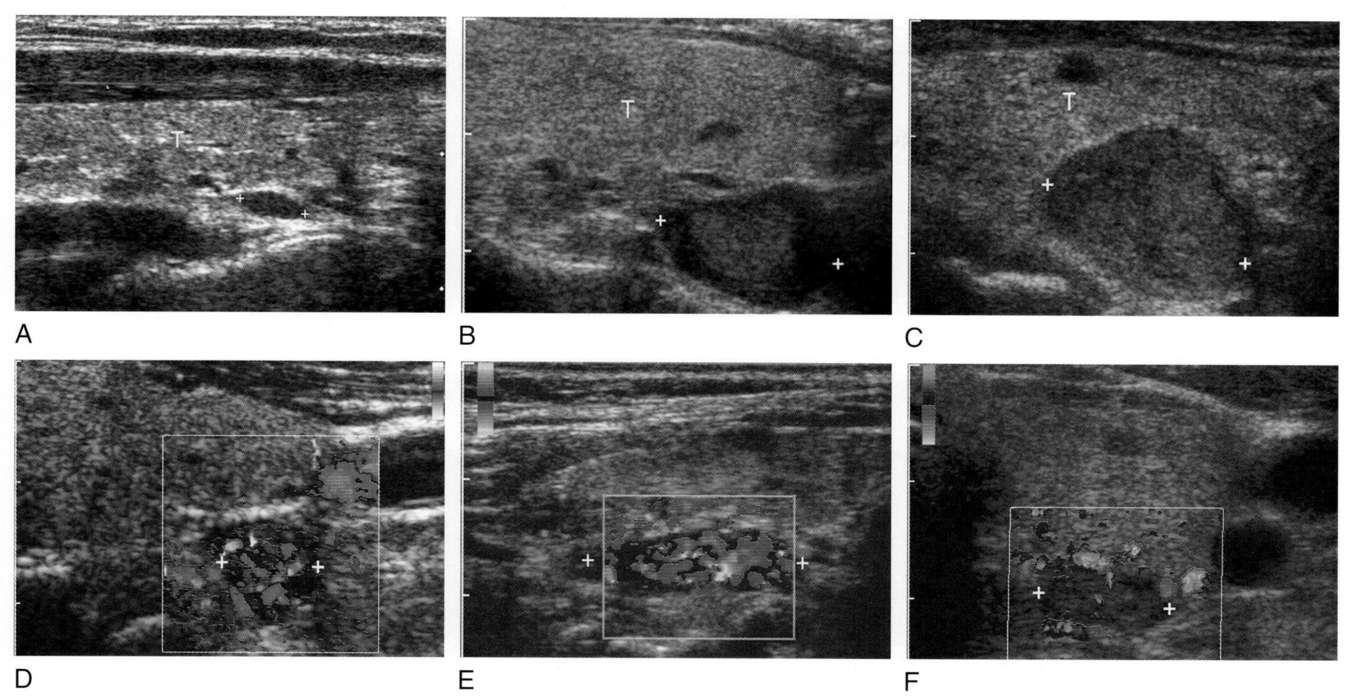

Figure 10-18 Parathyroid adenomas in different patients. **A,** Longitudinal view of the neck shows the thyroid gland (T) and a small hypoechoic solid oval parathyroid adenoma *(cursors).* **B,** Longitudinal view of the neck shows the thyroid gland (T) and a moderate-sized slightly heterogeneous but predominately hypoechoic parathyroid adenoma *(cursors).* **C,** Longitudinal view of the neck shows the thyroid gland (T) and a large solid hypoechoic parathyroid adenoma *(cursors).* **D,** Longitudinal color Doppler view of the neck shows a parathyroid adenoma *(cursors)* with readily detectable internal vascularity. **E,** Longitudinal power Doppler view of the neck shows an ovoid parathyroid adenoma *(cursors)* with marked hypervascularity. **F,** Transverse color Doppler view of the neck shows a parathyroid adenoma *(cursors)* that has very minimal detectable internal blood flow.

the thyroid and have sonographic features similar to other parathyroid adenomas.

The sensitivity of ultrasound in detecting parathyroid adenomas varies greatly. In patients who have not had prior neck surgery, the sensitivity ranges from 34% to 92%, with most studies reporting sensitivities in the 70% to 80% range. Sonographic detection of enlarged parathyroid glands is even harder in patients who present with recurrent or persistent hyperparathyroidism after a previous neck exploration. Nevertheless, sensitivity of 82% and specificity of 86% have been reported even in this difficult group of patients.

Common causes of false-negative scans include small lesions, ectopic lesions (especially mediastinal), and lesions adjacent to an enlarged nodular thyroid gland (Fig. 10-20A). False-positive scans are less of a problem

Box 10-3 Characteristics of Parathyroid Adenomas

Solid
Hypoechoic
Oval shape
Hypervascular (variably detected)
Posterior to thyroid
Medial to carotid

Box 10-4 Locations of Ectopic Parathyroid Adenomas

Low neck
Mediastinum
Retrotracheal/retroesophageal
Carotid sheath
Intrathyroidal

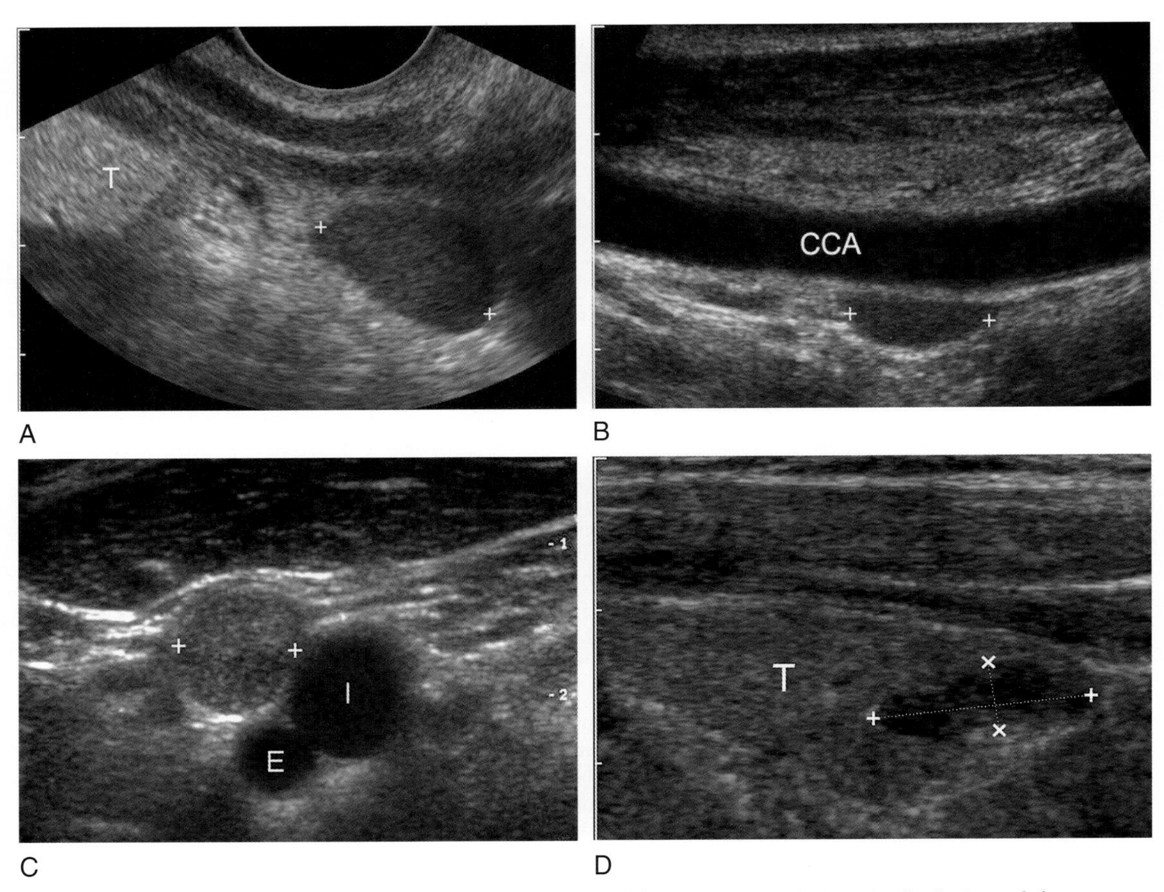

Figure 10-19 Ectopic parathyroid adenomas in different patients. **A,** Longitudinal view of the neck shows the lower pole of the thyroid gland (T). A parathyroid adenoma *(cursors)* is identified significantly below the thyroid in the low neck/superior mediastinum. Note that a tightly curved array typically used for transvaginal scanning was used in this case. **B,** Longitudinal view of the neck shows a parathyroid adenoma *(cursors)* located in the sheath of the common carotid artery (CCA). **C,** Transverse view of the carotid bifurcation shows a parathyroid adenoma *(cursors)* located immediately adjacent to the external (E) and the internal (I) carotid artery. **D,** Longitudinal view of the thyroid (T) shows an intrathyroidal parathyroid adenoma *(cursors)* located in the inferior aspect of the gland.

than false-negative scans. However, structures that can be confused with parathyroid adenomas include posterior thyroid septations (see Fig. 10-20B and C), lymph nodes (see Fig. 10-20D), posterior thyroid nodules, and normal structures posterior to the thyroid, such as veins (see Fig. 10-20E and F), the esophagus, and the longus colli muscle. Lymph nodes often have an echogenic hilum and are typically located lateral in the neck. Parathyroid adenomas are almost always medial to the carotid. Thyroid nodules are generally not homogeneous and hypoechoic, and they lack the linear interface that is typically seen between parathyroid adenomas and the thyroid gland. Veins can be distinguished from parathyroid adenomas with color Doppler imaging. The longus colli muscle and the esophagus can be distinguished from parathyroid adenomas by noting their tubular shape on longitudinal scans. In addition, the linear striations are usually seen in the longus coli muscle, and the target appearance typical of bowel is usually seen in the esophagus.

Alternative methods of localizing enlarged parathyroid glands are scintigraphy using sestamibi, CT scans, MRI, angiography, and venous sampling. All of these methods have strengths and weaknesses. In most practices, scintigraphy is used more than the other techniques. In many practices, a combination of ultrasound and scintigraphy is used and the other modalities are reserved for problem cases, such as when the results of ultrasound and scintigraphy are discordant. When a lesion is seen on sonography but not confirmed on a

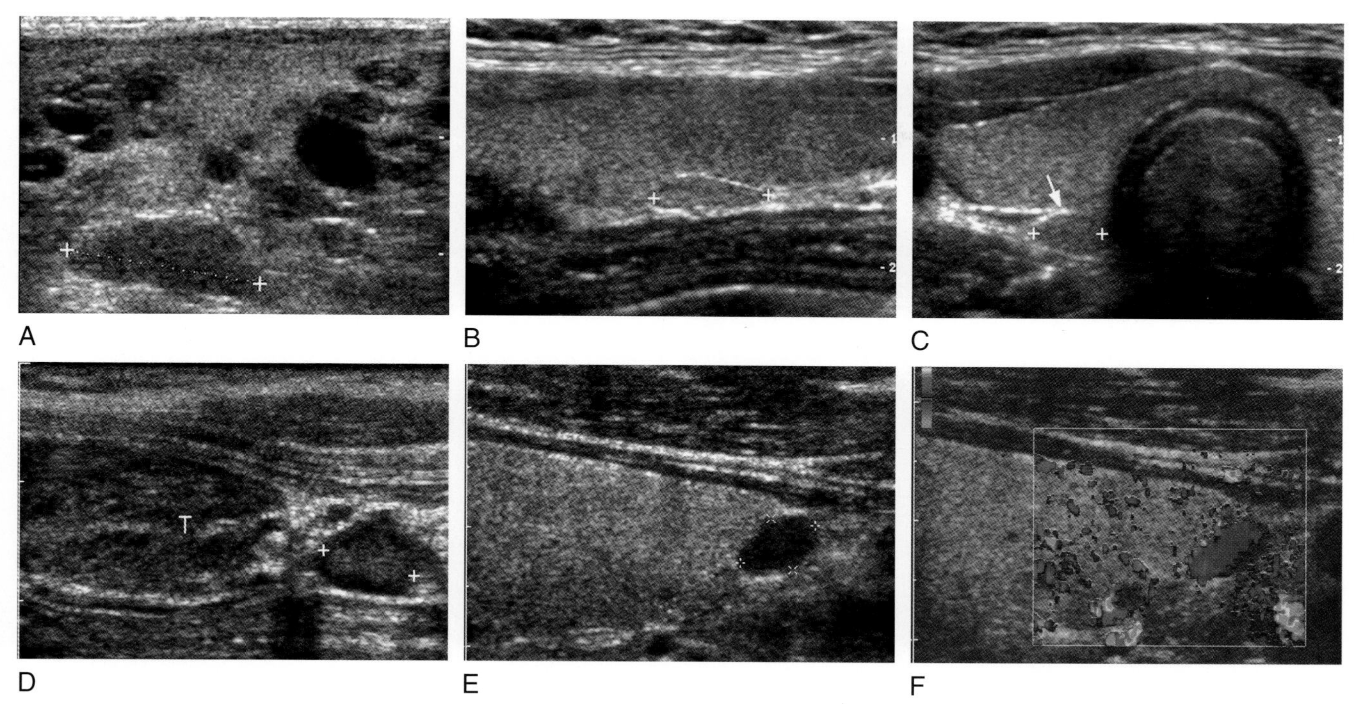

Figure 10-20 Pitfalls in identifying parathyroid adenomas. **A,** Longitudinal view of the neck shows a thyroid gland with multiple nodules. A parathyroid adenoma is present *(cursors)* but is more difficult to identify in the setting of the multinodular thyroid gland. **B** and **C,** Longitudinal (**B**) and transverse (**C**) views of the thyroid show what appears to be an isoechoic nodule *(cursors)* posterior to the thyroid. On the transverse view, it is more apparent that this represents a posterior septation *(arrow)* in the thyroid parenchyma. This is a normal variant that can simulate a parathyroid adenoma. **D,** Longitudinal view of the neck shows a hypoechoic heterogeneous thyroid gland (T) secondary to Hashimoto's thyroiditis. A hypoechoic lesion *(cursors)* is seen inferior to the thyroid that simulates a parathyroid adenoma. This actually represents a lymph node. Lymph nodes are commonly seen in patients with Hashimoto's thyroiditis. **E** and **F,** Longitudinal gray-scale (**E**) and color Doppler (**F**) views of the thyroid show what appears to be a hypoechoic nodule *(cursors)* inferior to the thyroid that simulates a small parathyroid adenoma. On the color Doppler view, it is clear that this represents a prominent vessel adjacent to the thyroid.

sestamibi scan, ultrasound-guided aspiration can be performed and the sample can be sent for chemical analysis of PTH levels.

The treatment of choice for hyperparathyroidism is surgery. In the hands of an experienced head and neck or endocrine surgeon, the success of neck exploration is 95% or higher and the morbidity is low. So preoperative localization is not mandatory. However, it has been shown that unilateral explorations can be performed with similar results to bilateral neck surgery if preoperative localization is obtained. In addition, operating room time is decreased when the correct site of the adenoma is identified preoperatively. Finally, in centers where surgical expertise is limited, preoperative localization can be valuable. In patients who have already had prior neck explorations and have recurrent or persistent hyperparathyroidism, preoperative localization is extremely beneficial. Intraoperative ultrasound can also be helpful in this group of patients.

OTHER NECK ABNORMALITIES

Lymphadenopathy

Normal lymph nodes are frequently identified in the neck, particularly around the carotid artery and jugular vein. Normal nodes are composed of an outer cortex composed of lymphoid follicles and an inner medulla composed of lymphatic sinuses, fat, and vessels. On sonography the nodal cortex appears hypoechoic and the medulla appears as a hyperechoic hilum. Nodes in the neck, especially the nodes in the jugular chain, are

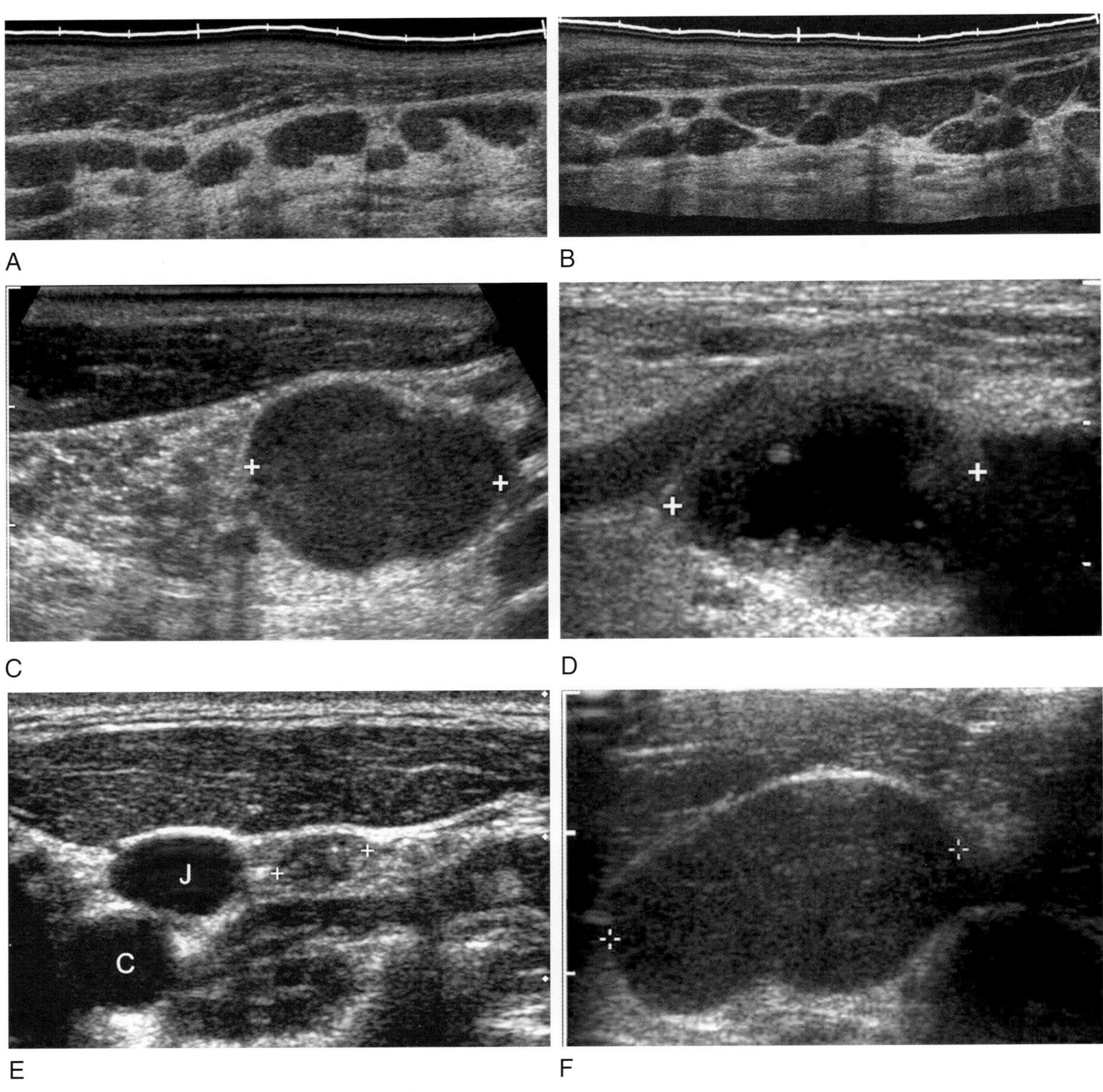

Figure 10-21 Lymphadenopathy. **A,** Longitudinal extended-field-of-view scan of the neck shows multiple predominantly oval nodes deep to the muscle layer. These were reactive nodes that resolved with conservative measures. **B,** Longitudinal extended-field-of-view scan in a patient with lymphoma shows multiple enlarged nodes deep to the muscles. This is similar to the reactive nodes shown in **A**; however, the nodes are more numerous and more crowded together. **C,** Longitudinal view of the neck in a patient with lung cancer shows a metastatic lymph node *(cursors).* Note that the node is rounder than normal with the long-axis dimension less than 1.5 times the short axis dimension. The echogenic hilum has been obliterated. **D,** Longitudinal view of the supraclavicular region in a patient with squamous cell cancer shows a metastatic node *(cursors)* with central liquefaction secondary to necrosis. **E,** Transverse view of the left neck shows a small node *(cursors)* lateral to the jugular vein (J) and common carotid artery (C). There is a small bright reflector in the node owing to microcalcification in this patient with a history of papillary thyroid cancer. **F,** Transverse view of the neck shows a large node *(cursors),* very worrisome for neoplastic involvement. Fine-needle aspiration showed tuberculosis rather than cancer or lymphoma.

normally long in the craniocaudal dimension and short in the axial dimension. In general, the long axis of a node should be 1.5 to 2.0 times the length of the short-axis dimension.

Enlarged nodes can be either reactive or neoplastic, and there are some general differences in their sonographic appearance (Fig. 10-21) (Box 10-5). Neoplastic nodes tend to enlarge asymmetrically, with greater enlargement of the short-axis dimension than the long-axis dimension. When the long- to short-axis ratio is less than 1.5 a malignancy should be considered. In addition, neoplasms will often obliterate or attenuate or displace the echogenic hilum. Metastatic disease from head and neck cancers and papillary thyroid cancer

Box 10-5 Characteristics of Neoplastic Neck Nodes

Obliteration of echogenic hilum
Long-axis to short-axis ratio less than 1.5
Cystic changes
Microcalcifications

often will produce nodal necrosis, and cystic areas will become detectable in the nodes. As mentioned earlier, microcalcifications in nodes can be seen in patients with papillary and medullary thyroid cancers.

Despite these differences, there is enough overlap in the appearance of benign and malignant nodes that biopsy is often necessary. This is easily accomplished in the vast majority of cases using ultrasound guidance.

Salivary Glands

Sonography can be used to image the salivary glands and to guide biopsies. This applies primarily to the parotid and submandibular glands. Indications include imaging of an enlarged gland to determine if it is caused by generalized inflammation, sialolithiasis, or neoplasms.

Tumors of the salivary glands are relatively rare. Most tumors occur in the parotid gland and are benign. Pleomorphic adenomas are benign neoplasms that account for approximately 70% of salivary gland tumors. They are typically solid, hypoechoic, and homogeneous (Fig. 10-22). Warthin's tumors are also benign neoplasms that account for approximately 10% of salivary gland tumors. They are hypoechoic but less homogeneous than the pleomorphic adenoma, and they often have cystic elements (Fig. 10-23).

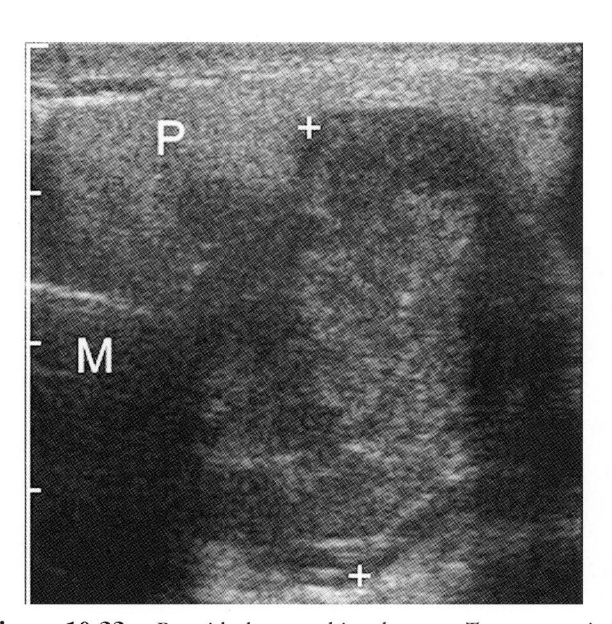

Figure 10-22 Parotid pleomorphic adenoma. Transverse view of the cheek shows the normal parotid gland (P) and the angle of the mandible (M). A large hypoechoic solid slightly heterogeneous mass *(cursors)* is seen arising from the parotid. This is a typical appearance for a pleomorphic adenoma.

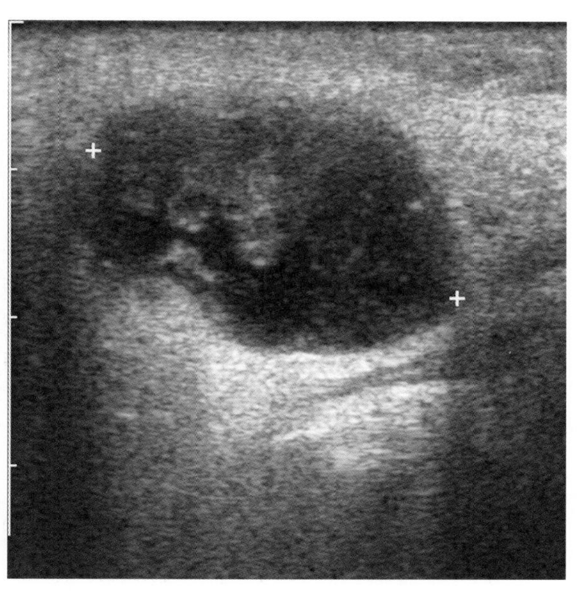

Figure 10-23 Parotid Warthin's tumor. Longitudinal view of the parotid gland shows a complex hypoechoic mass *(cursors)* that contains both solid and cystic components typical of Warthin's tumor.

Stones are more common in the submandibular gland than in the parotid. Sonography is very sensitive and specific in the diagnosis of sialolithiasis. Like stones elsewhere, salivary gland stones appear as echogenic structures that cast an acoustic shadow. Stones can be intraductal (Fig. 10-24) or intraglandular (Fig. 10-25). Intraductal stones are associated with a dilated ductal system.

NECK VESSELS

Carotids

Sonography and Doppler have been used for many years to evaluate the carotid arteries. This was based on the presumption that strokes could be prevented by removing carotid plaques and thus eliminating a source of emboli. Even though there was no definitive scientific proof that they provided clinical benefit, carotid endarterectomies were performed in large numbers. This led to considerable controversy between neurologists, who treated patients medically, and surgeons. Fortunately, this controversy has been largely laid to rest by several large randomized trials performed in the 1980s that compared endarterectomy to medical therapy. Based on these studies, it is now clear that patients with certain degrees of carotid atherosclerosis do benefit from carotid endarterectomy. This was a fortunate result for carotid ultrasound because it is

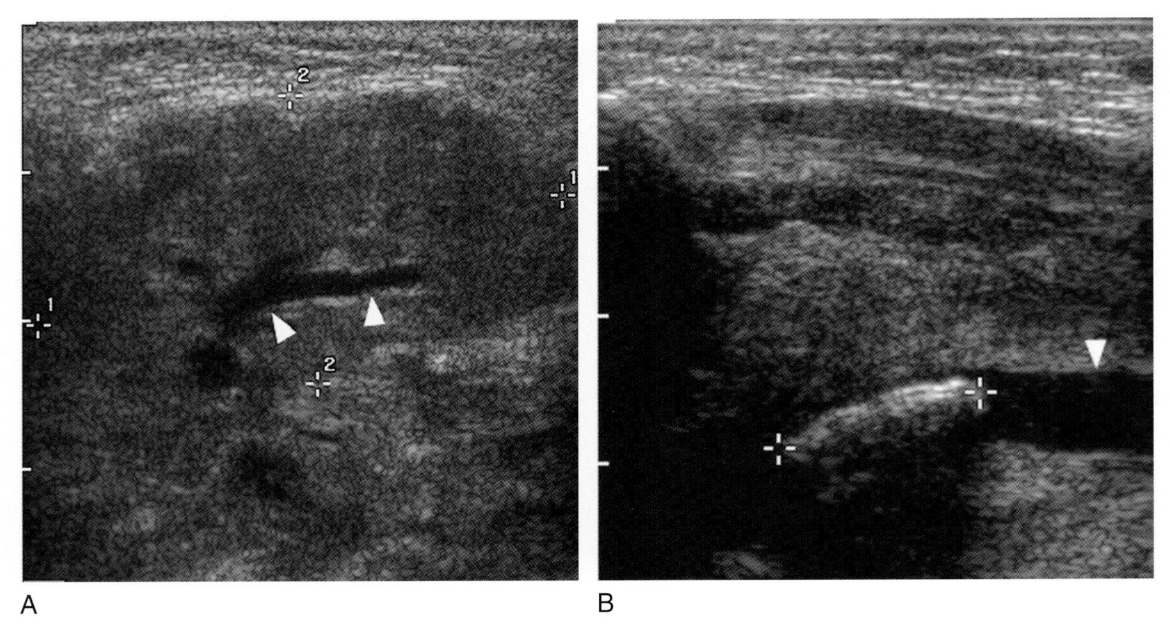

Figure 10-24 Intraductal stone of the submandibular gland. **A,** Oblique view of the submandibular gland *(cursors)* shows a dilated duct *(arrowheads)*. **B,** Oblique view through the submandibular gland shows a more central aspect of the dilated duct *(arrowhead)* and an intraductal stone *(cursors)* with its associated shadow. (Case courtesy of Carol Wilcox, Boston, MA.)

reasonable to look for carotid plaque only if you are going to operate on some of the plaques that are found. Therefore, carotid Doppler has remained an important test in patients with suspected atherosclerosis.

The normal carotid wall appears hypoechoic on gray-scale studies. The reflection from the interface between the intimal surface of the wall and the blood within the lumen produces an inner bright line along the carotid wall. This sonographic morphology of the carotid wall is easily seen in most common carotid arteries (CCA) (Fig. 10-26) but is more difficult to demonstrate in the internal carotid artery (ICA) and external carotid artery (ECA). Normally, the thickness is less than 0.9 mm. As atherosclerosis develops, the carotid artery wall becomes thicker (see Fig. 10-26). In fact, measurements of the wall thickness can categorize a patient's risk of a coronary event or stroke.

When performing carotid Doppler examinations, the ICA must be differentiated from the ECA. Like other parenchymal organs, the brain has a low resistance to arterial inflow; therefore, waveforms from the ICA have broad systolic peaks and well-maintained diastolic flow throughout the cardiac cycle (Fig. 10-27A). The ECA supplies the scalp, muscles, and face, all of which have a high resistance to arterial inflow. This results in a high-resistance arterial waveform with narrower systolic

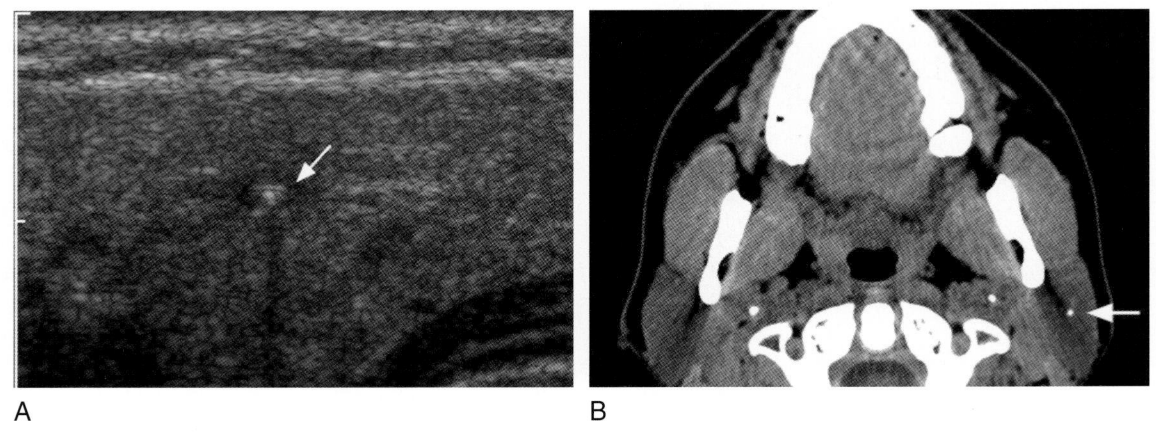

Figure 10-25 Intraglandular stone of the parotid. **A,** Transverse view of the parotid shows a faint hyperechoic structure *(arrow)* with a slight posterior acoustic shadow consistent with an intraglandular stone. **B,** CT scan confirming the presence of an intraglandular stone *(arrow)*. (Case courtesy of Carol Wilcox, Boston, MA.)

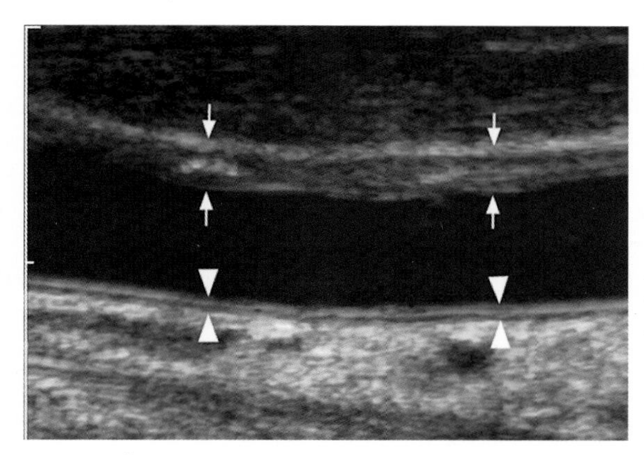

Figure 10-26 Normal carotid artery wall. Longitudinal view of the common carotid shows the normal bilayered appearance to the deep carotid wall *(arrowheads)*. This is in contrast to the appearance of the near carotid wall *(arrows)*, which shows thickening and loss of the normal morphology due to atherosclerotic disease.

peaks and decreased or absent diastolic flow (see Fig. 10-27B). In addition to the differences in the waveforms, the ECA can be distinguished from the ICA on the basis of its more anterior and medial position, its smaller size, and its branch vessels (Fig. 10-28). A maneuver that can also assist in distinguishing these vessels is tapping the superficial temporal artery (located immediately anterior to the ear). Because this vessel is a branch of the ECA, pulsations produced by the tapping are transmitted into the ECA and appear on the waveform (see Fig. 10-27B). It is much less likely for these pulsations to appear in the CCA or ICA waveform. The CCA has characteristics of both the ICA and ECA, but because 70% to 80% of its flow goes to the ICA, the CCA waveform tends to mirror the waveform in the ICA more than the waveform in the ECA. (See Table 10-1 for a summary of the differences between the ICA and ECA.)

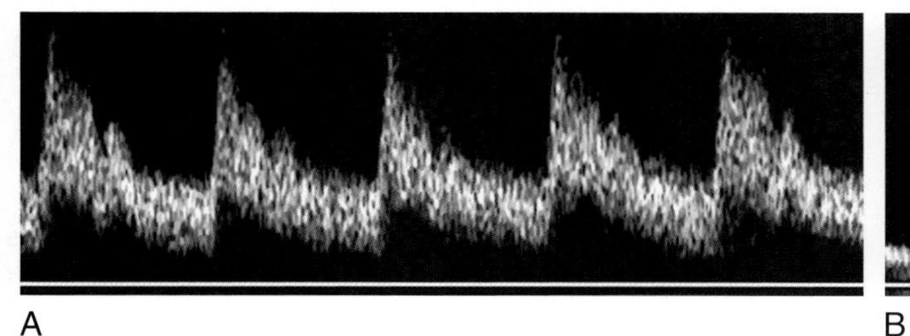

A

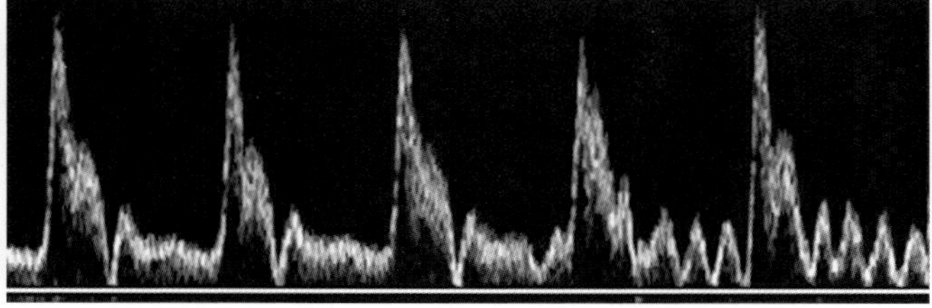

B

Figure 10-27 Normal hemodynamics of the carotid artery. **A,** Internal carotid artery waveform shows a typical low-resistance profile with a broad systolic peak, gradual transition between systole and diastole, and well-maintained diastolic flow throughout the cardiac cycle. **B,** External carotid artery waveform shows a higher resistance pattern with a sharper and narrower systolic peak and lower levels of flow in end diastole. Note the rapid pulsations in the last two cardiac cycles due to the temporal tap maneuver.

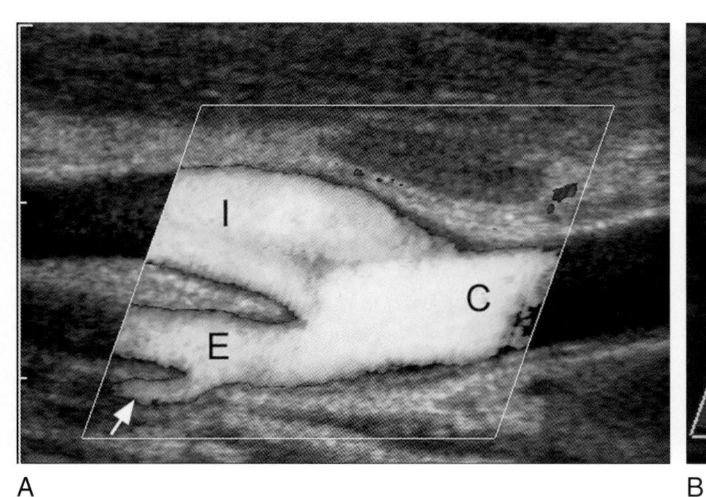

A

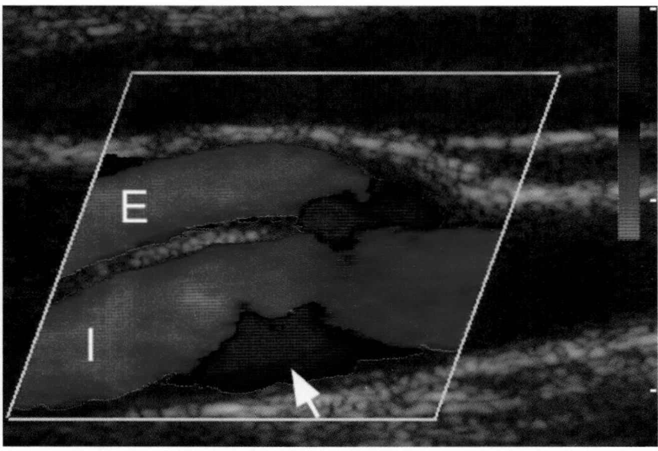

B

Figure 10-28 Normal anatomy of the carotid bifurcation. **A,** Longitudinal power Doppler view of the bifurcation shows the common (C), internal (I), and external (E) carotid arteries. The external is smaller and a branch *(arrow)* is seen posteriorly. **B,** Longitudinal color Doppler view shows the internal (I) and external (E) carotid arteries. A typical region of flow reversal *(arrow)* is seen in the origin of the internal carotid. Note that the internal carotid appears superficial (closer to the surface of the probe) in **A** because the probe was positioned posteriorly. The external carotid appears superficial in **B** because the probe was positioned anteriorly. Also note that the image is oriented with the patient's head to the left and the body to the right. This is the standard convention in carotid sonography.

Table 10-1 Differences between the Internal and External Carotid Arteries

Characteristic	Internal Carotid	External Carotid
Location	Posterior/lateral	Anterior/medial
Size	Larger	Smaller
Branches	No	Yes
Waveform	Low resistance	High resistance
Temporal tap	Negative response	Positive response

A carotid Doppler study should be aimed at identifying atherosclerotic plaques and determining the severity of the plaque. This will determine which patients need to undergo continued follow-up, more extensive tests, or surgery. The North American Symptomatic Carotid Endarterectomy Trial has shown that symptomatic patients who have a stenosis of 70% or greater benefit from carotid endarterectomy. The Asymptomatic Carotid Endarterectomy Study has shown that asymptomatic patients with a stenosis of 60% or greater benefit from endarterectomy.

Determination of carotid stenosis can be potentially accomplished in two ways. Plaque can be identified on gray-scale and color/power Doppler imaging, and measurements of the residual lumen can be made and compared with the normal distal vessel. Unfortunately, plaque is almost always eccentric, so the degree of visible luminal narrowing varies depending on the view. This can lead to both overestimates and underestimates of stenosis (Fig. 10-29). Theoretically, area measurements obtained from transverse views would solve the problem of eccentric plaque. Unfortunately, the margins of plaque are difficult to visualize on transverse gray-scale views and the residual lumen is not accurately displayed on color/power Doppler views. Therefore, direct imaging is usually used in only an ancillary fashion to determine carotid stenosis.

Fortunately, flow velocities increase progressively with the degree of stenosis, and this relationship serves as a basis for estimating the degree of stenosis. Velocity increases are minor for stenosis of less than 50% diameter reduction. So for lesions in this range, visual inspection of gray-scale and color Doppler views (despite the limitations mentioned previously) is the only way to detect and gauge the degree of stenosis (Fig. 10-30). But velocities start to increase rapidly as the stenosis exceeds 50% (Fig. 10-31). A number of parameters have been developed for estimating the degree of carotid stenosis. Those most commonly used include peak systolic flow velocity (PSV), end-diastolic flow velocity (EDV), and the ratio of peak systolic velocity in the ICA (at the site of the stenosis) to the peak systolic velocity in the ipsilateral CCA (usually measured 2 cm proximal to the bifurcation).

The PSV is the simplest and probably the most reliable parameter (Fig. 10-32). However, it has potential limitations. If the baseline carotid velocities are decreased by a second stenosis that is occult (such as at the origin of the CCA), the degree of ICA stenosis may be underestimated. Low cardiac output and aortic valve stenosis can also decrease the baseline velocities. Increased baseline velocities can occur when there is an occlusion or high-grade stenosis in the contralateral ICA or CCA and can lead to overestimation of the ipsilateral

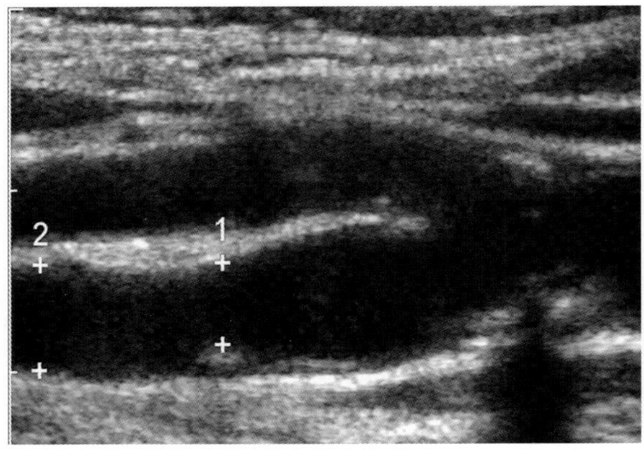

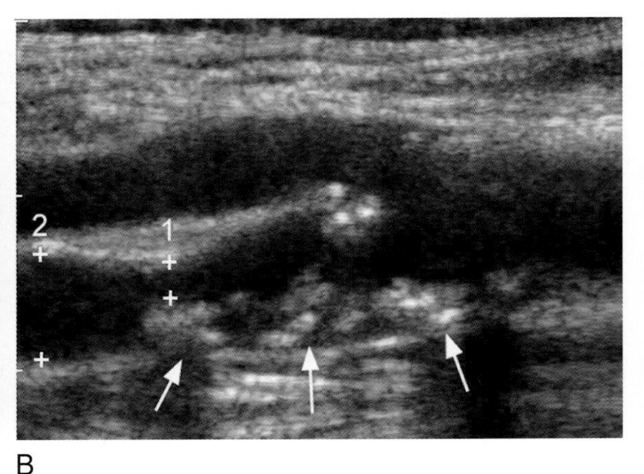

Figure 10-29 Eccentric plaque. **A,** Longitudinal view of the bifurcation shows what appears as minimal plaque in the origin of the internal carotid. Comparison of luminal diameter *(cursors)* at the level of the plaque (1) and the normal distal artery (2) would estimate stenosis at 20%. **B,** Longitudinal view through a slightly different portion of the bifurcations shows what appears to be more extensive plaque *(arrows)*. Estimated stenosis based on this image would be 65%. This discrepancy is due to the eccentric nature of the plaque and emphasizes one of the difficulties with using two-dimensional images to calculate carotid stenosis.

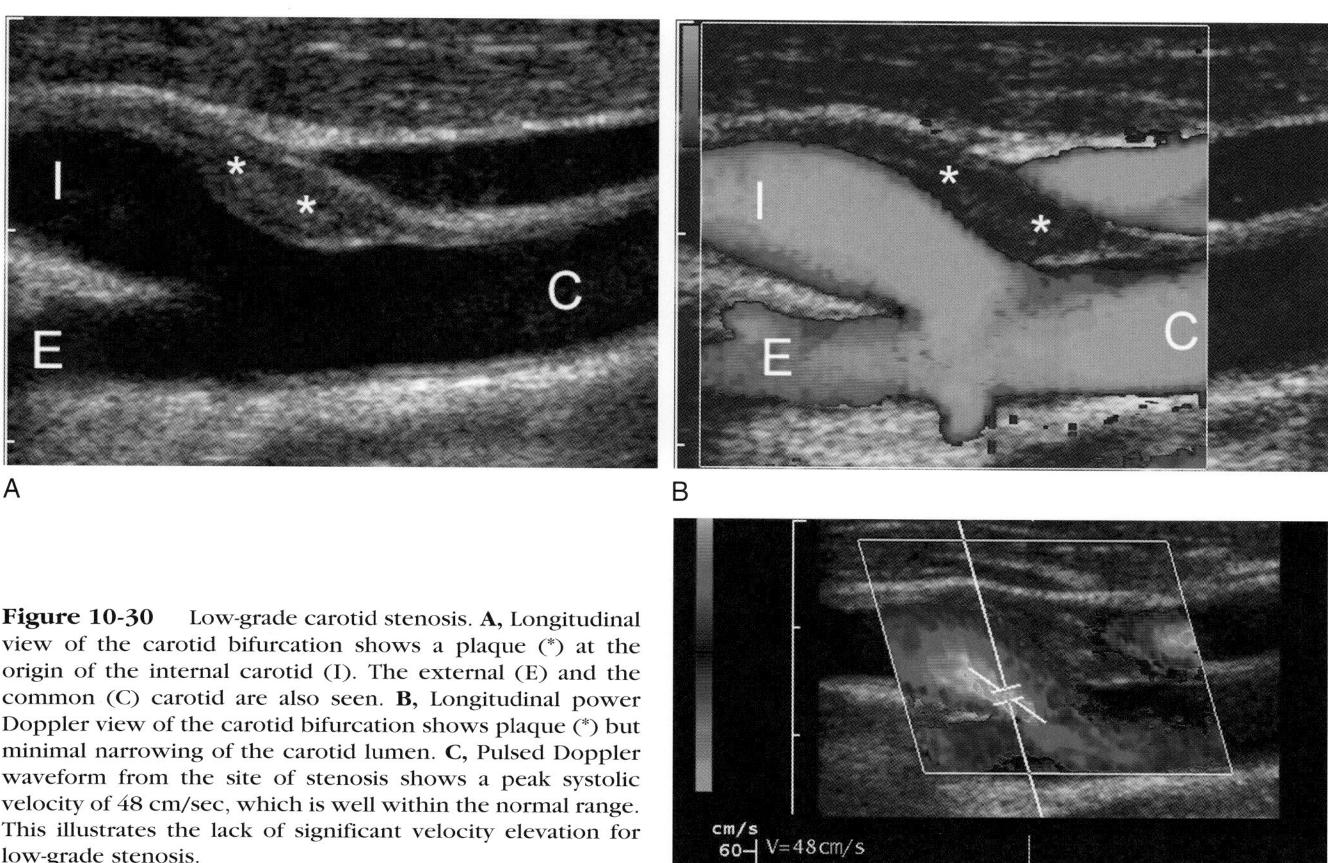

Figure 10-30 Low-grade carotid stenosis. **A,** Longitudinal view of the carotid bifurcation shows a plaque (*) at the origin of the internal carotid (I). The external (E) and the common (C) carotid are also seen. **B,** Longitudinal power Doppler view of the carotid bifurcation shows plaque (*) but minimal narrowing of the carotid lumen. **C,** Pulsed Doppler waveform from the site of stenosis shows a peak systolic velocity of 48 cm/sec, which is well within the normal range. This illustrates the lack of significant velocity elevation for low-grade stenosis.

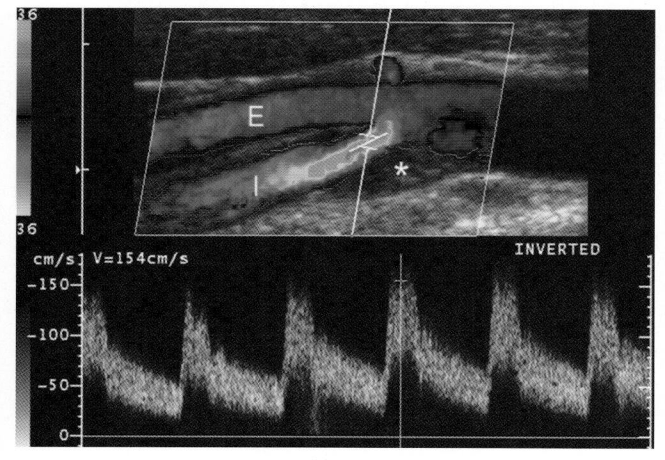

Figure 10-31 Moderate-grade carotid stenosis. Longitudinal color Doppler and pulsed Doppler image shows a plaque (*) at the origin of the internal carotid (I). The external carotid (E) is also seen. Peak systolic velocity is elevated to 154 cm/sec. This predicts a 50% to 70% diameter stenosis.

ICA. The ICA/CCA systolic velocity ratio is theoretically helpful in these situations, because the increases or decreases in baseline velocity are taken into account by using the ipsilateral CCA velocity as a control. Unfortunately, there is unavoidable variability in the measurement of both the ICA and CCA velocities, and these variabilities are multiplied when they are combined in a ratio. Therefore, in practice the ICA/CCA ratio is generally not as reliable as the ICA peak systolic velocity. Nevertheless, the ratio is a valuable parameter that can be especially helpful when the gray-scale or color Doppler image seems discrepant with the PSV. End-diastolic velocity is the third parameter that is commonly used and is particularly valuable when the systolic velocity is so high that it aliases and becomes impossible to measure (Fig. 10-33).

Many different criteria have been proposed to estimate carotid stenosis, and deciding which criteria to use can be a very confusing task. A consensus panel formed

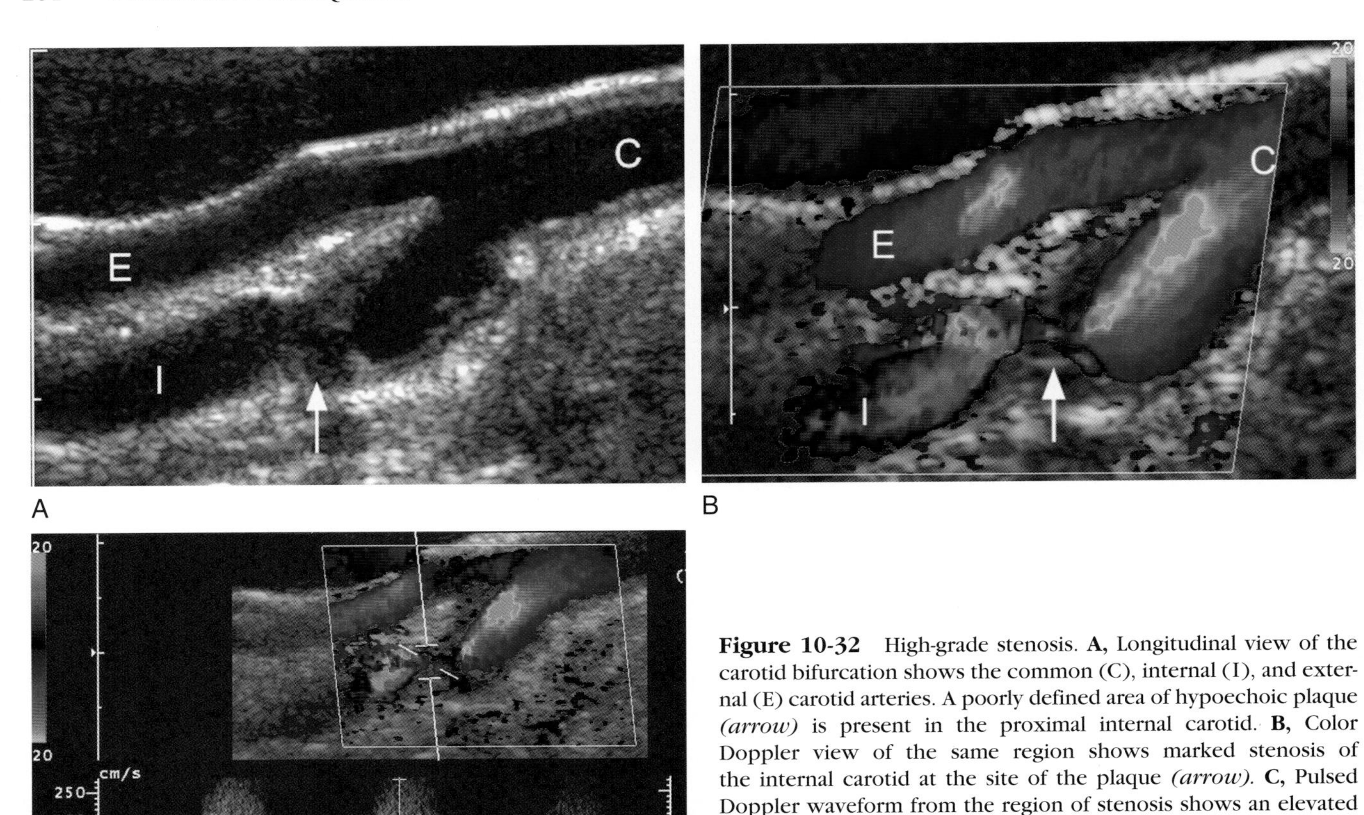

Figure 10-32 High-grade stenosis. **A,** Longitudinal view of the carotid bifurcation shows the common (C), internal (I), and external (E) carotid arteries. A poorly defined area of hypoechoic plaque *(arrow)* is present in the proximal internal carotid. **B,** Color Doppler view of the same region shows marked stenosis of the internal carotid at the site of the plaque *(arrow).* **C,** Pulsed Doppler waveform from the region of stenosis shows an elevated velocity of 271 cm/sec. This predicts a stenosis of greater than 70% diameter narrowing.

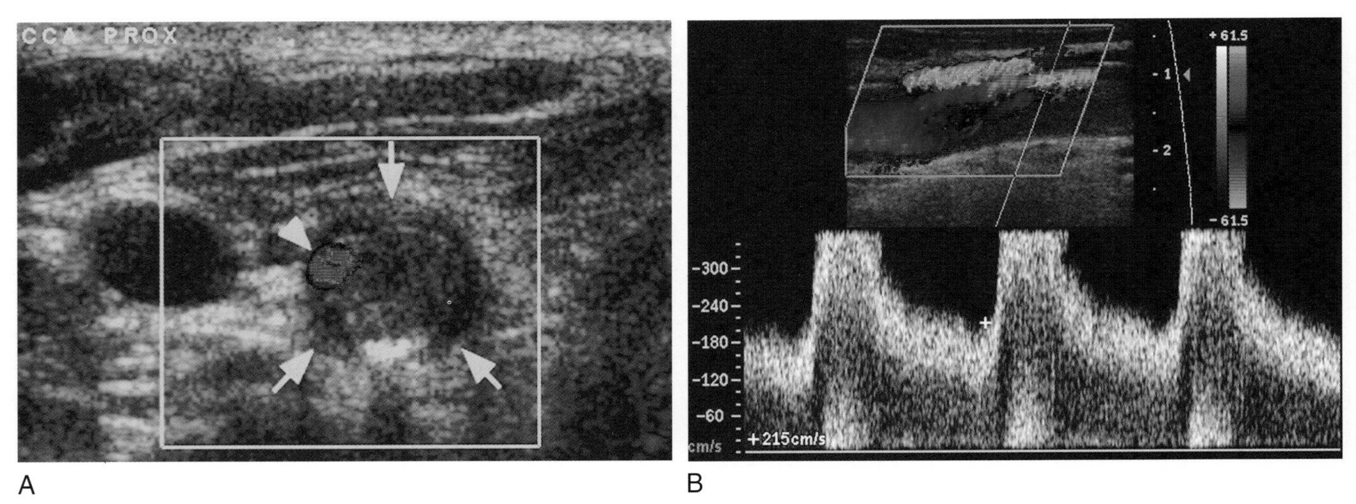

Figure 10-33 High-grade stenosis. **A,** Transverse color Doppler view of the distal common carotid artery *(arrows)* shows an extensive plaque and a very narrow residual lumen *(arrowhead).* **B,** Pulsed Doppler waveform shows velocity elevation so great that the systolic peak is aliased. In cases such as this, the diastolic velocity of 215 cm/sec can be used to estimate a diameter stenosis of greater than 70%.

Table 10-2 Criteria For Estimating Internal Carotid Stenosis

	ICA PSV	ICA/CCA PSV Ratio	ICA EDV	Plaque
Normal	<125 cm/sec	<2.0	<40 cm/sec	None
<50%	<125 cm/sec	<2.0	<40 cm/sec	<50% reduction
50-69%	125-230 cm/sec	2.0-4.0	40-100 cm/sec	>50% reduction
>70%	>230 cm/sec	>4.0	>100 cm/sec	>50% reduction
Near Occlusion	Variable or undetectable	Variable	Variable	Visible
Total Occlusion	No flow	No flow	No flow	Visible

ICA, internal carotid artery; CCA, common carotid artery; PSV, peak systolic flow velocity; EDV, end-diastolic flow velocity.
From: Grant EG, Benson CB, Moneta GL et al: Society of Radiologists in Ultrasound Consensus Conference on Ultrasound and Doppler Diagnosis of Carotid Stenosis. Radiology, Nov 2003 in press.

by the Society of Radiologists in Ultrasound in 2002 specifically studied this issue. The panel was composed of radiologists, vascular surgeons, neurologists, and statisticians. They developed criteria that they believed were most appropriate and recommended that these criteria could be used as a starting point, recognizing that some modification may be necessary on an individual basis based on the results of individual laboratory results. The criteria recommended by this consensus panel are listed in Table 10-2.

As mentioned earlier, the ICA velocities and the ICA/CCA velocity ratio progressively increase as the degree of ICA stenosis worsens. However, when the stenosis becomes so severe that flow volume is close to zero, the velocity starts to drop back down into the normal range. In such cases a high-grade stenosis is generally evident on color Doppler imaging and, despite normal velocities, the pulsed Doppler waveform appears distorted and abnormal. A more common problem is related to the fact that the site of elevated velocity in a high-grade stenosis may be limited to a very small area. Because of this, it may be difficult or impossible to sample the exact site where the velocity is actually elevated (Fig. 10-34). Fortunately, color Doppler sonography will almost always show that the stenosis is severe.

It is important to realize that in most patients it is only possible to see the first 2 to 3 cm of the internal carotid artery. Fortunately, the vast majority of significant stenosis occurs in this region. Stenoses in the more distal internal carotid are generally not visible with ultrasound. When a distal stenosis is severe, the velocities in the proximal internal carotid may be depressed and the waveform may change from the typical low-resistance pattern to a high-resistance pattern (Fig. 10-35).

Total occlusion of the ICA causes a lack of detectable ICA flow on pulsed Doppler and color Doppler studies. When no flow is detected in the ICA, the vessel is very likely occluded (Fig. 10-36). However, it is also possible that an extremely tight stenosis can diminish flow so much that it becomes impossible to detect with Doppler imaging. Because a very tight stenosis represents a surgical lesion, but a complete occlusion does not, angiography of some type (often MRA) is usually performed to further evaluate suspected occlusions. A secondary sign of ICA occlusion is the "externalization" of the CCA waveform. This occurs because all of the CCA flow goes into the ECA.

Occlusion of the CCA can produce interesting collateral pathways to maintain flow in the ICA. The most common involves flow from the contralateral external carotid across the head and neck to supply the ipsilateral external carotid. Retrograde flow in the ipsilateral external carotid then supplies the ipsilateral ICA across the bifurcation (Fig. 10-37).

In addition to using Doppler sonography to detect and quantitate stenosis, there is also potential benefit in using it to evaluate plaque morphology. Studies have suggested that homogeneous plaque tends to be stable over time (Fig. 10-38A). On the other hand, inhomogeneity and hypoechoic defects (see Fig. 10-38B) correlate with the presence of intraplaque hemorrhage. Intraplaque hemorrhage indicates an unstable plaque that is more likely to break down and produce emboli and neurologic symptoms. Despite encouraging results in some studies, the analysis of plaque morphology remains a subjective and controversial method that is only used selectively in some laboratories.

The detection of plaque ulceration is difficult but possible with gray-scale and color-Doppler sonography (Fig. 10-39). Although many ulcers are missed, when a

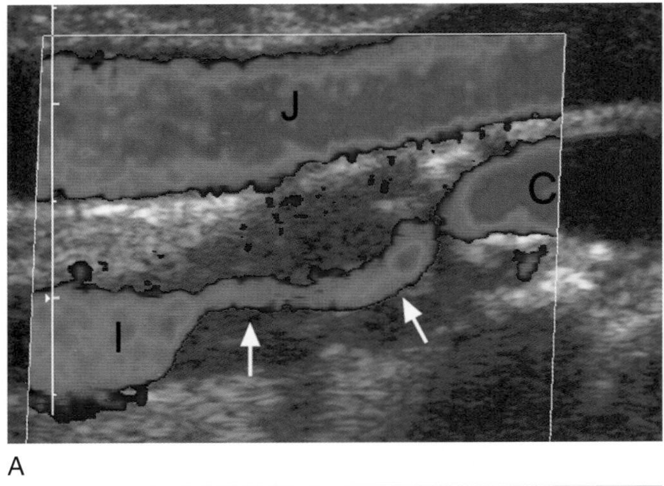

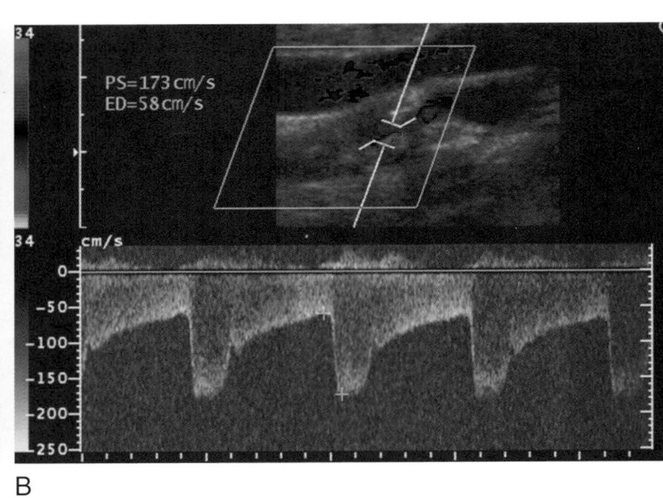

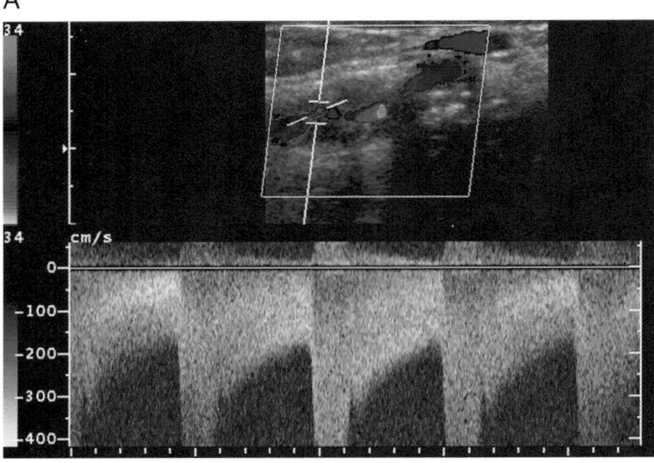

Figure 10-34 High-grade stenosis. **A,** Longitudinal power Doppler view at the junction of the common (C), and internal (I) carotid artery shows a tight stenosis *(arrows)*. The stenosis appears equally severe throughout its course. The jugular vein (J) is seen superficial to the carotid. **B,** Pulsed Doppler waveform from the proximal aspect of the stenosis shows a peak systolic velocity of 173 cm/sec. This velocity would predict a diameter stenosis of 50% to 70%. **C,** Pulsed Doppler waveform from the distal aspect of the stenosis shows a peak systolic velocity that aliases off the scale but exceeds 400 cm/sec. This would predict a diameter stenosis of greater than 70%. This case illustrates that the peak velocity may be limited to a very small region and can potentially be missed. This case also illustrates the need to closely correlate the pulsed Doppler information with the color Doppler image.

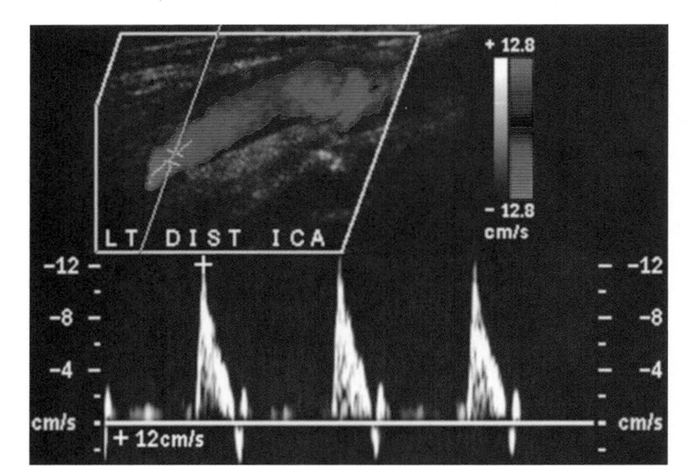

Figure 10-35 Distal internal carotid stenosis. Pulsed Doppler waveform from the internal carotid shows a very high resistance pattern with no diastolic flow. In addition, the systolic velocity of 12 cm/sec is very depressed. This implies a high-grade stenosis in the distal vessel beyond the view of sonography.

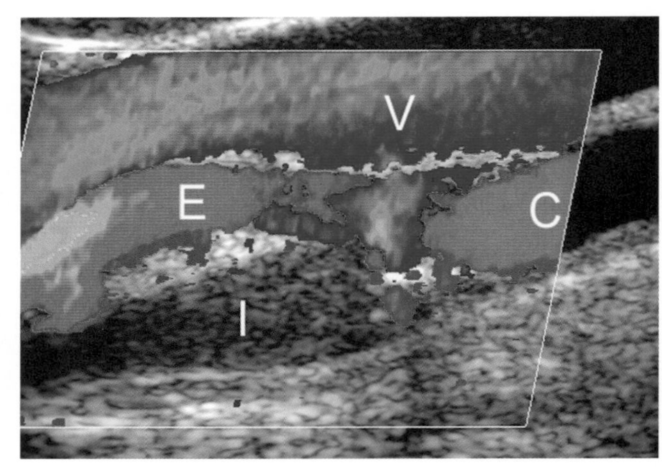

Figure 10-36 Internal carotid occlusion. Longitudinal color Doppler view of the bifurcation shows a patent common (C) and external (E) carotid artery but no detectable flow in the internal carotid (I). The jugular vein (V) is also seen.

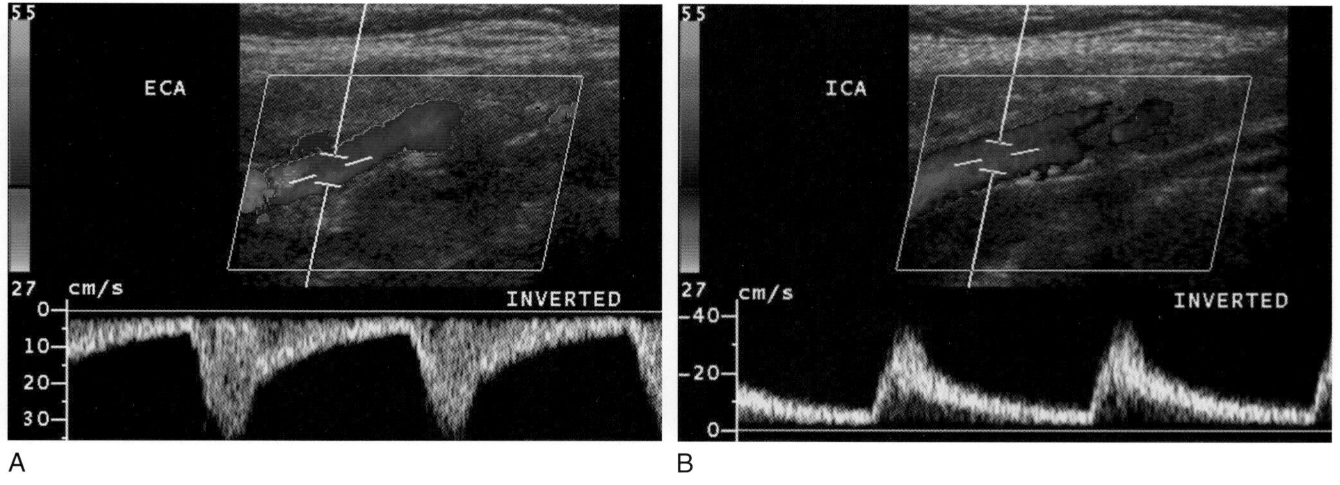

Figure 10-37 Common carotid occlusion. **A,** Longitudinal color Doppler view and pulsed Doppler waveform of the external carotid show reversed blood flow. **B,** Longitudinal color Doppler view and pulsed Doppler waveform of the internal carotid both show antegrade blood flow. Note the similar morphology of the external and internal carotid waveforms.

well-defined crater is detected it should be reported, because this may explain symptoms arising from a hemodynamically insignificant lesion.

Vertebral Arteries

Evaluation of the carotids should always include an evaluation of the vertebral arteries. The vertebral arteries are best seen as they travel between the transverse processes of the cervical spine (Fig. 10-40). In some individuals, the adjacent vertebral vein can be seen, usually located superficial to the artery. Shadowing from the transverse processes results in only segmental visualization of the vertebral arteries, making it difficult to identify stenotic lesions. However, it is possible to determine the patency of the vertebral arteries and the direction of flow in the vertebral arteries. Reversed flow in a vertebral artery indicates a stenosis or occlusion at the origin of the subclavian or innominate artery (Fig. 10-41). In this setting, flow to the ipsilateral upper extremity is maintained by means of antegrade flow in the contralateral carotid and vertebral artery, with cross flow in the basilar artery and circle of Willis allowing for retrograde flow in the ipsilateral vertebral artery. With partial subclavian steal, there is just a dip in the systolic portion of the vertebral artery waveform

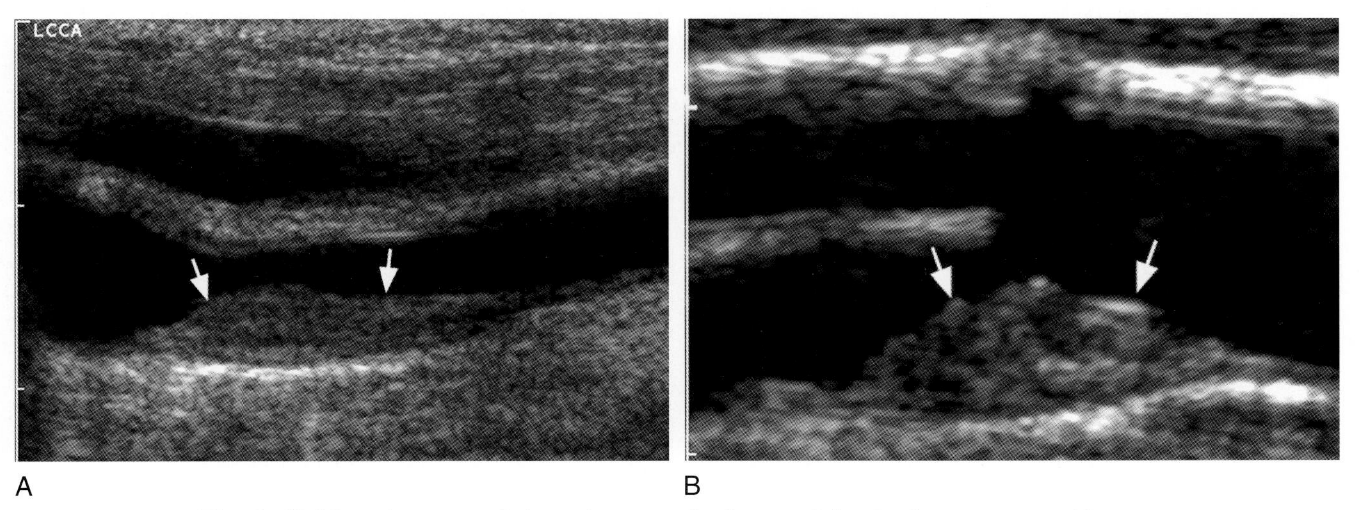

Figure 10-38 Plaque morphology. **A,** Longitudinal view of the distal common carotid artery shows a homogeneous plaque *(arrows)*. **B,** Longitudinal view of the proximal internal carotid shows a heterogeneous plaque with an irregular surface and at least one focal hypoechoic region.

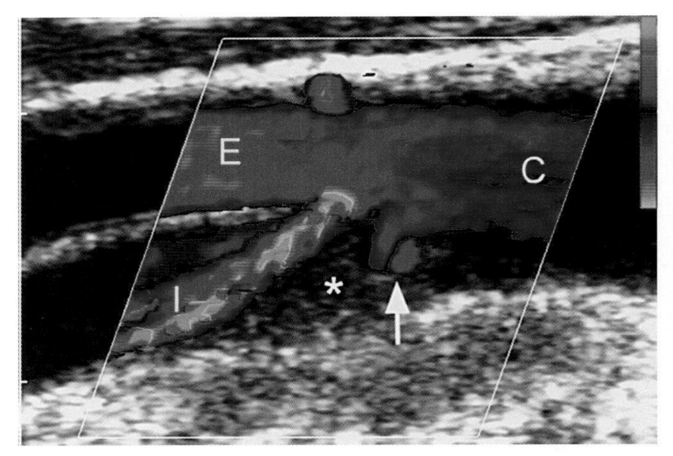

Figure 10-39 Plaque ulceration. Longitudinal color Doppler view of the carotid bifurcation shows a plaque (*) at the origin of the internal carotid (I). A focal rounded area of flow within an ulcer crater *(arrow)* is present within the substance of the plaque. Also seen are the external (E) and the common (C) carotid arteries.

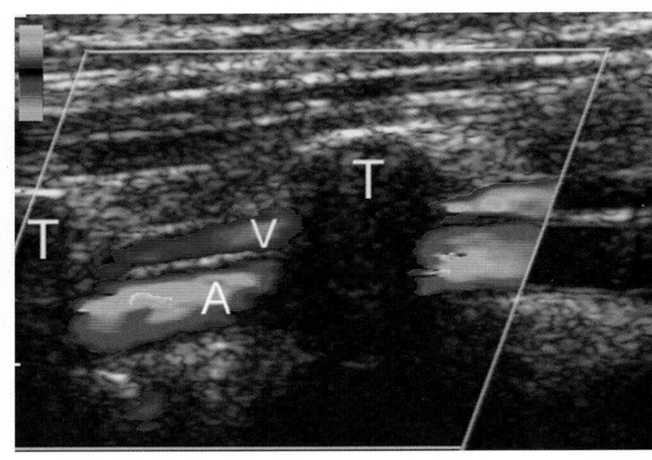

Figure 10-40 Normal vertebral vessels. Longitudinal color Doppler view of the paravertebral region shows two transverse processes (T) and the deep vertebral artery (A) and the more superficial vertebral vein (V). The vertebral vein is not seen in all patients.

(Fig. 10-42). As the subclavian stenosis progresses and the amount of blood flow siphoned from the vertebral artery increases, the systolic peak starts to reverse and, ultimately, there is total reversal of flow. One potential pitfall in the detection of retrograde vertebral arterial flow is the possibility of misconstruing a vertebral vein (which normally has flow directed caudad) to represent a vertebral artery with reversed flow (Fig. 10-43). Doppler waveform analysis of the vessel in question should help to prevent this potential diagnostic error.

Jugular Veins

The internal jugular veins are large vessels located lateral and superficial to the carotid arteries. They are easily seen and evaluated with sonography. Because they are close to the heart, their waveforms are usually pulsatile. Monophasic, flattened flow in the jugular veins should raise suspicion of a more central thrombosis or obstruction, just as it does in the subclavian veins. Thrombosis of the jugular veins themselves is seen most often after placement of central venous catheters. As with venous

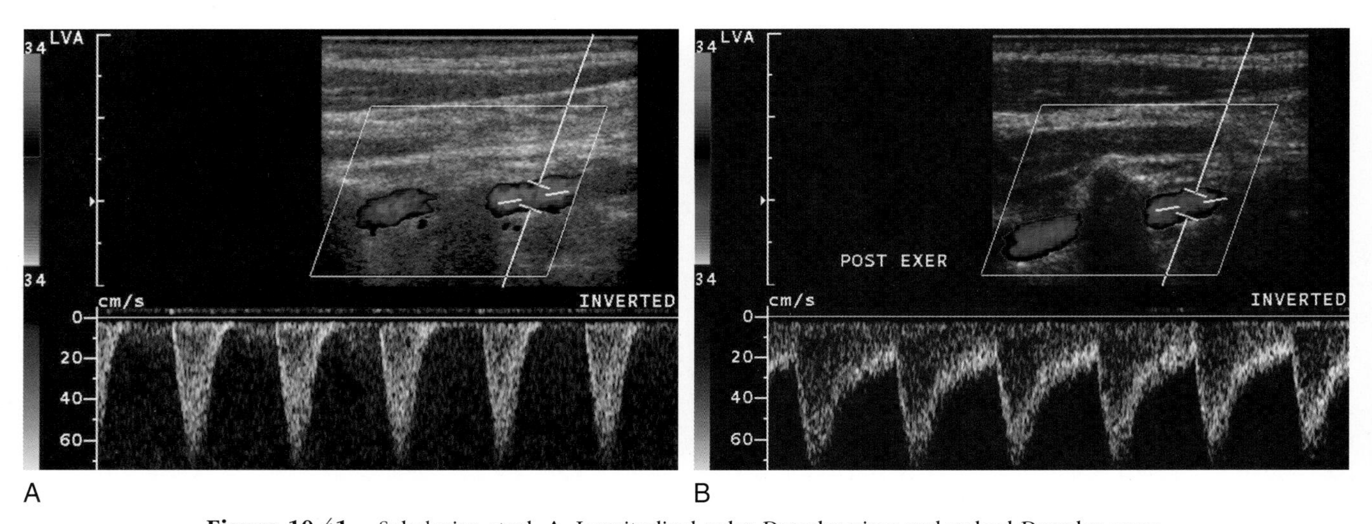

Figure 10-41 Subclavian steal. **A,** Longitudinal color Doppler view and pulsed Doppler waveform of the left vertebral artery obtained with the patient at rest show reversed arterial flow. The waveform is a high resistance pattern typical of an artery supplying an extremity. **B,** After exercise there is increased demand for left upper extremity flow and decreased vascular resistance. This is reflected in increased diastolic flow in the vertebral artery waveform.

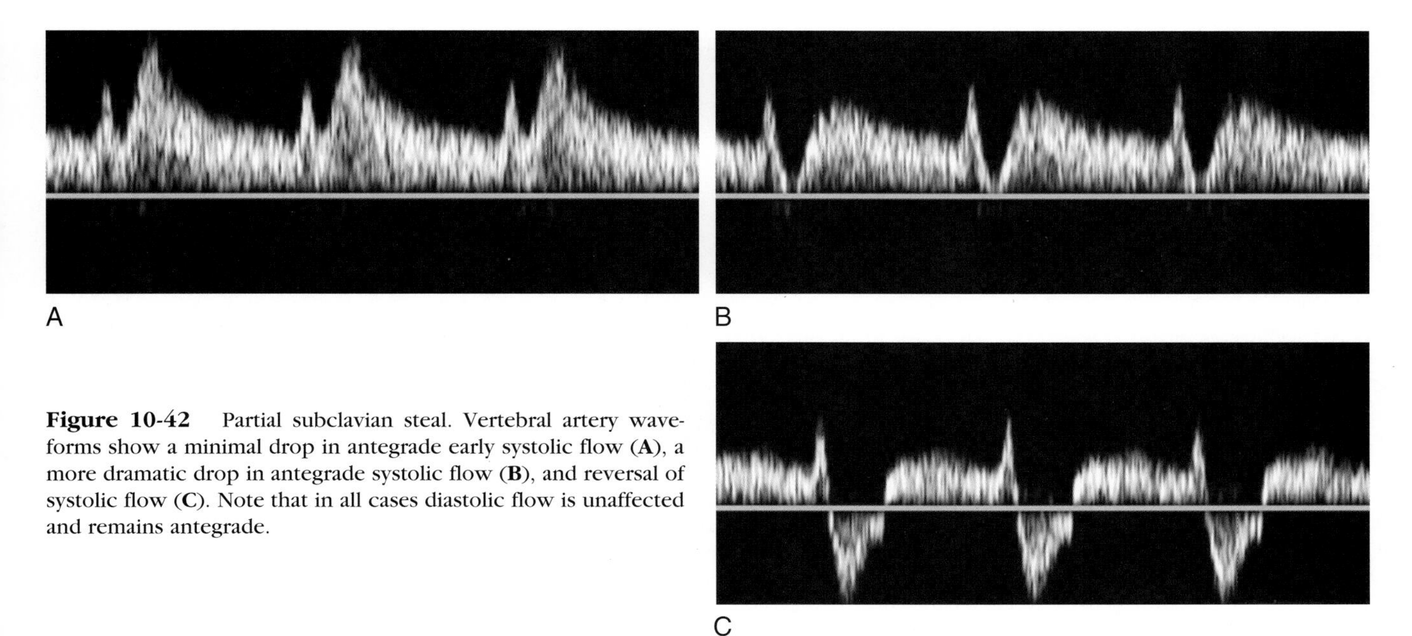

Figure 10-42 Partial subclavian steal. Vertebral artery waveforms show a minimal drop in antegrade early systolic flow (**A**), a more dramatic drop in antegrade systolic flow (**B**), and reversal of systolic flow (**C**). Note that in all cases diastolic flow is unaffected and remains antegrade.

thrombosis elsewhere, jugular vein thrombosis manifests as a lack of compressibility on gray-scale sonography. In general, image quality and resolution is high enough to visualize abnormal intraluminal echoes, indicative of the clot (Fig. 10-44). Low-level echoes due to slow flow can be distinguished from thrombosis by vessel compressibility. In many cases, jugular vein thrombosis is accompanied by an inflammatory reaction resulting in adjacent hyperemia.

CHEST

Because ultrasound cannot penetrate into the substance of aerated lung, it is not a primary modality in evaluating the chest and especially the lung. Nevertheless, there are several situations in which sonography is extremely helpful (Box 10-6). The most common is where guidance is needed to aspirate fluid. Sonography

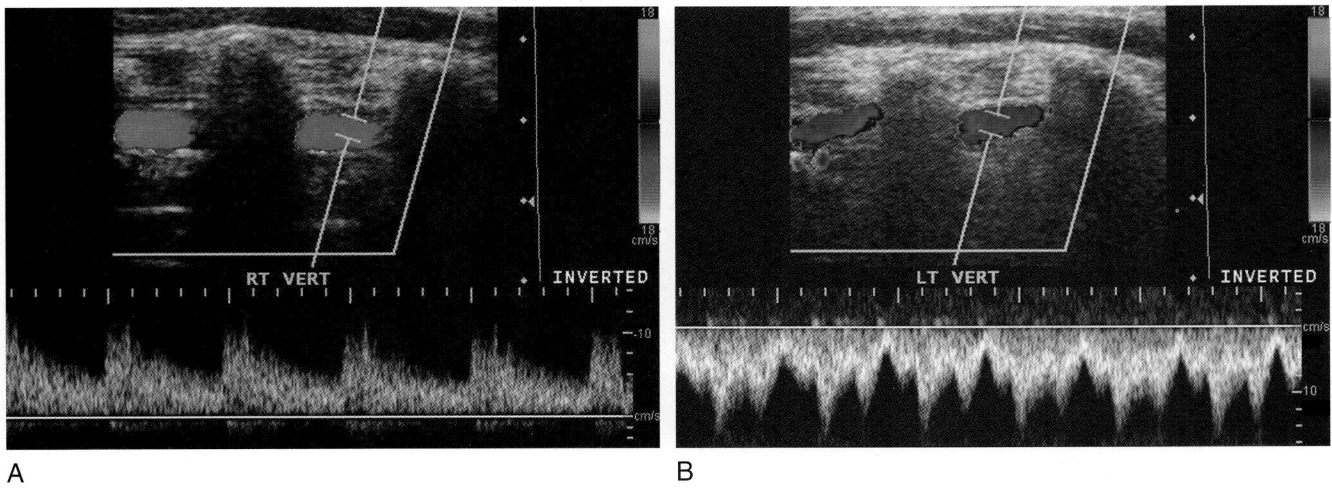

Figure 10-43 Vertebral vein simulating subclavian stenosis. **A,** Longitudinal color Doppler view and pulsed Doppler waveform from the normal right vertebral artery show appropriate direction of flow and a normal-appearing arterial waveform. **B,** Longitudinal color Doppler view and pulsed Doppler waveform from a vessel simulating the left vertebral artery. The color Doppler image shows flow directed from the left to the right, which would indicate a subclavian steal. However, the waveform shows a pulsatile venous signal rather than an arterial signal, indicating that this is a normal vertebral vein. The left vertebral artery could not be identified and was probably hypoplastic or occluded.

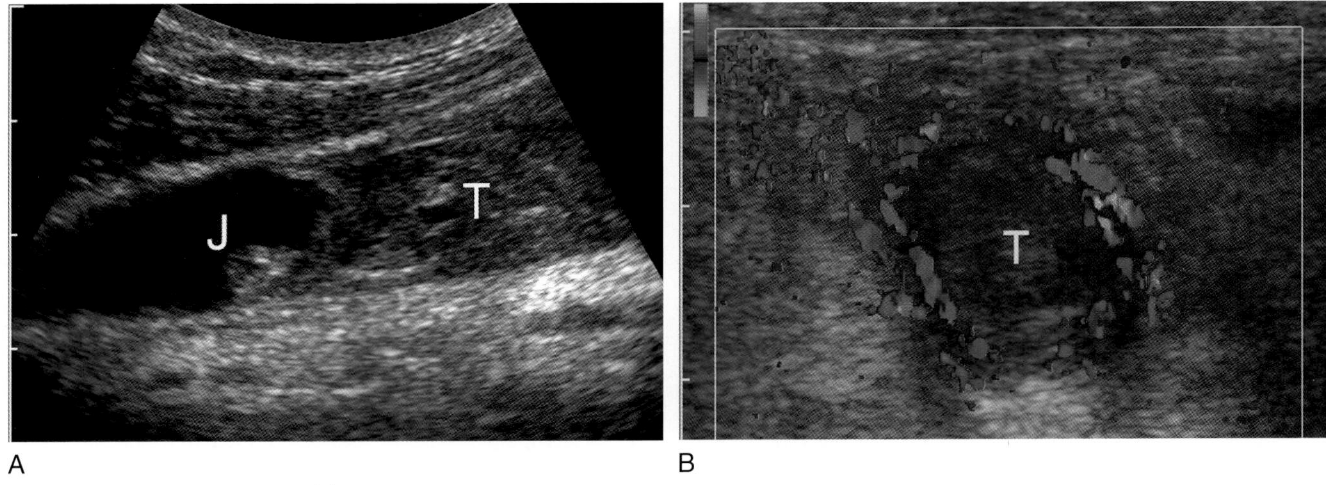

Figure 10-44 Jugular vein thrombosis. **A,** Longitudinal view of the internal jugular vein (J) shows abnormal intraluminal echoes due to thrombus (T) in the inferior aspect of the vein. This was not compressible. **B,** Transverse color Doppler view shows no flow in the thrombosed lumen (T) of the vein. Note the inflammatory hyperemia in the perivascular region.

is capable of detecting as little as 3 mL of fluid in the pleural space. Larger effusions are generally very easy to see with sonography (Fig. 10-45). Once identified, an appropriate site can be localized for thoracentesis. In most cases, an intercostal space associated with the largest volume of fluid is most appropriate. This is usually within one or two interspaces above the diaphragm. Ultrasound guidance may be required when previous attempts guided by physical examination have been unsuccessful, when the effusion is known to be small or loculated, when the patient is frail and tolerance of a potential pneumothorax is low, or when there is a coagulopathy and minimization of trauma is required.

Sonography in general is not capable of determining the etiology of pleural effusions. Both transudates and exudates can be anechoic. However, sonography can identify complex effusions with internal echoes or septations, and these findings are indicative of an exudate in the majority of cases (see Fig. 10-45E and F).

Box 10-6 Uses of Chest Sonography

- Detect pleural effusions
- Provide guidance for thoracentesis
- Characterize chest wall lesions
- Provide guidance for biopsy of peripheral lung/mediastinal lesions
- Localize and analyze paradiaphragmatic lesions
- Detect pneumothorax

When evaluating pleural fluid, it is important to distinguish collapsed or consolidated lung from complex fluid. The presence of air bronchograms can help. These appear as very bright reflectors that often assume a linear configuration and may or may not have detectable shadowing (Fig. 10-46). Color Doppler imaging can also help because pulmonary vessels are often visible in consolidated or atelectatic lung (Fig. 10-47).

Chest wall lesions are amenable to sonographic evaluation in a manner similar to abdominal wall lesions (Fig. 10-48). In most cases the etiology of chest wall masses can be determined based on a combination of clinical factors and sonographic findings. When necessary, ultrasound-guided biopsies or aspirations of chest wall masses can be performed.

Biopsies of mediastinal lesions and apical lung lesions are also possible with sonographic guidance, provided that they make contact with the chest wall without intervening aerated lung. These can be accessed from a parasternal (Fig. 10-49A and B), subclavicular, or supraclavicular (see Fig. 10-49C and D) approach.

Peripheral lung masses that abut the pleura can be visualized by scanning through the adjacent intercostal space. Large masses are readily identified, but even small masses can be seen, especially if prior radiographs or CT scans have already localized the lesion (Fig. 10-50). Once identified, the primary role for sonography is to provide guidance for needle biopsy. Because of the continuous real-time imaging capabilities, it is possible to direct the needle into the lesion during the optimal phase of the

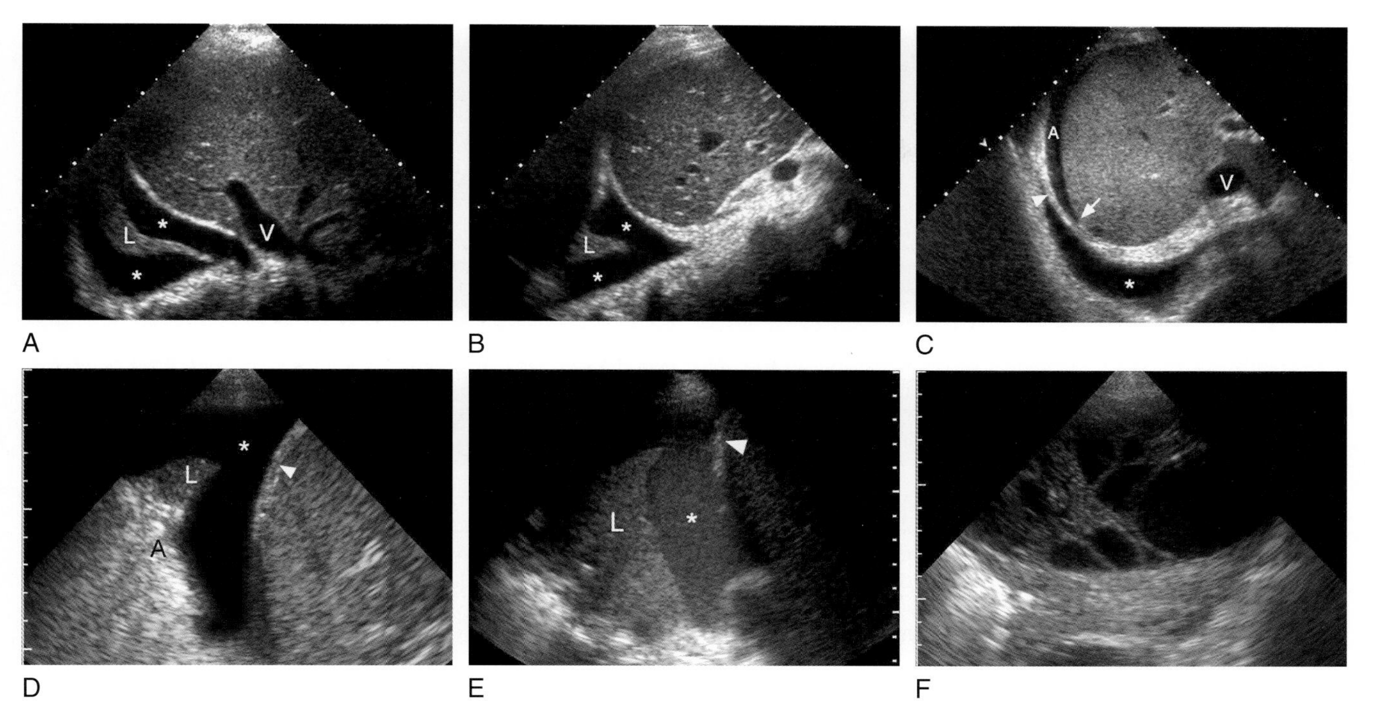

Figure 10-45 Pleural effusions in different patients. Transverse (**A**) and longitudinal (**B**) views of the right upper quadrant and posterior right chest taken from an anterior approach show a moderate pleural effusion (*) and atelectatic lung (L). On the transverse view, note that the effusion is free to pass to the medial aspect of the body and approach the inferior vena cava (V). **C,** Transverse view of the right upper quadrant and posterior chest shows a pleural effusion (*). In this case there is also perihepatic ascites (A) seen below the diaphragm *(arrowhead)*. Note that the ascites is restricted by the bare area of the liver *(arrow)* and cannot flow as far medially as the pleural effusion. The inferior vena cava (V) is also seen. **D,** Longitudinal posterior intercostal view of the chest shows a pleural effusion (*) with adjacent atelectatic lung (L) as well as hyperechoic aerated lung (A). The diaphragm *(arrowhead)* is seen inferiorly. In this case, the location of the probe defines an adequate intercostal site to perform a thoracentesis. **E,** Longitudinal posterior intercostal view of the chest shows a complex pleural effusion (*) with diffuse low-level echoes and adjacent atelectatic lung (L). The diaphragm *(arrowhead)* is located inferiorly. **F,** Transverse posterior intercostal view of the chest shows a complex, loculated, pleural effusion containing multiple internal septations.

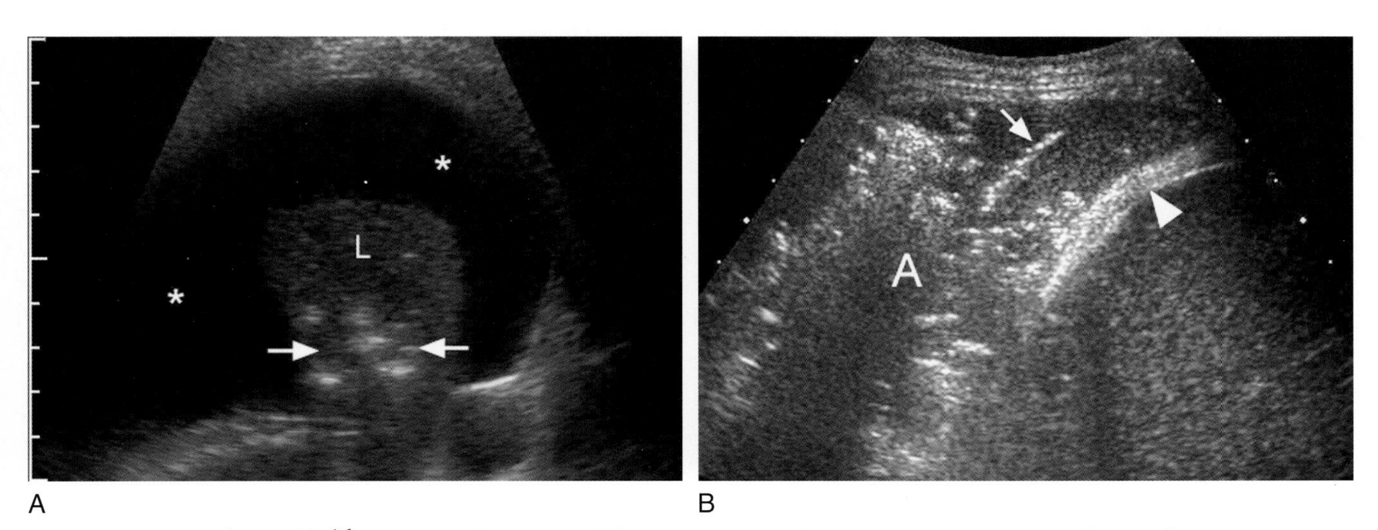

Figure 10-46 Air bronchograms in different patients. **A,** Transverse posterior intercostal view of the chest shows a pleural effusion (*) and atelectatic lung (L). In the deep aspect of the lung there are multiple small bright reflectors *(arrows)* due to residual air in bronchi. **B,** Longitudinal posterior intercostal view of the chest shows an area of atelectatic lung containing a bright linear reflector *(arrow)* due to air in a small peripheral bronchus. There is no separate pleural effusion. Shadowing from more completely aerated lung (A) is seen more centrally, and the diaphragm *(arrowhead)* is seen inferiorly.

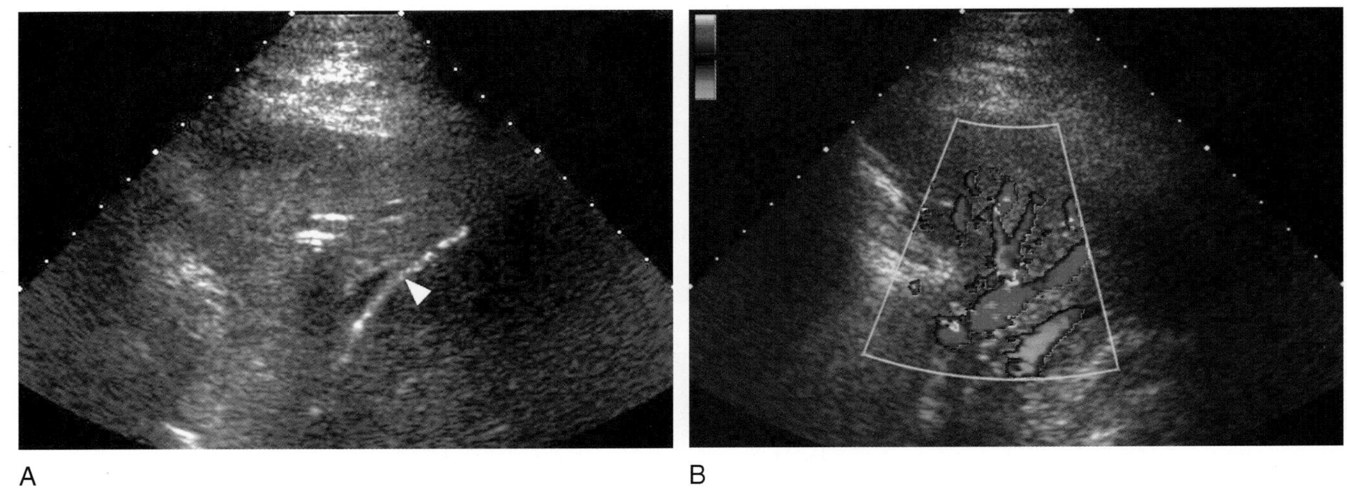

Figure 10-47 Lower lobe collapse. **A,** Longitudinal posterior intercostal view of the chest shows the diaphragm *(arrowhead)* and a hypoechoic structure immediately superior to the diaphragm. From the gray-scale view this most likely represents nonaerated lung, although a complex pleural effusion is also a consideration. **B,** Color Doppler view of the same area shows multiple pulmonary vessels coursing through this region, confirming that this is lung parenchyma rather than a complex effusion.

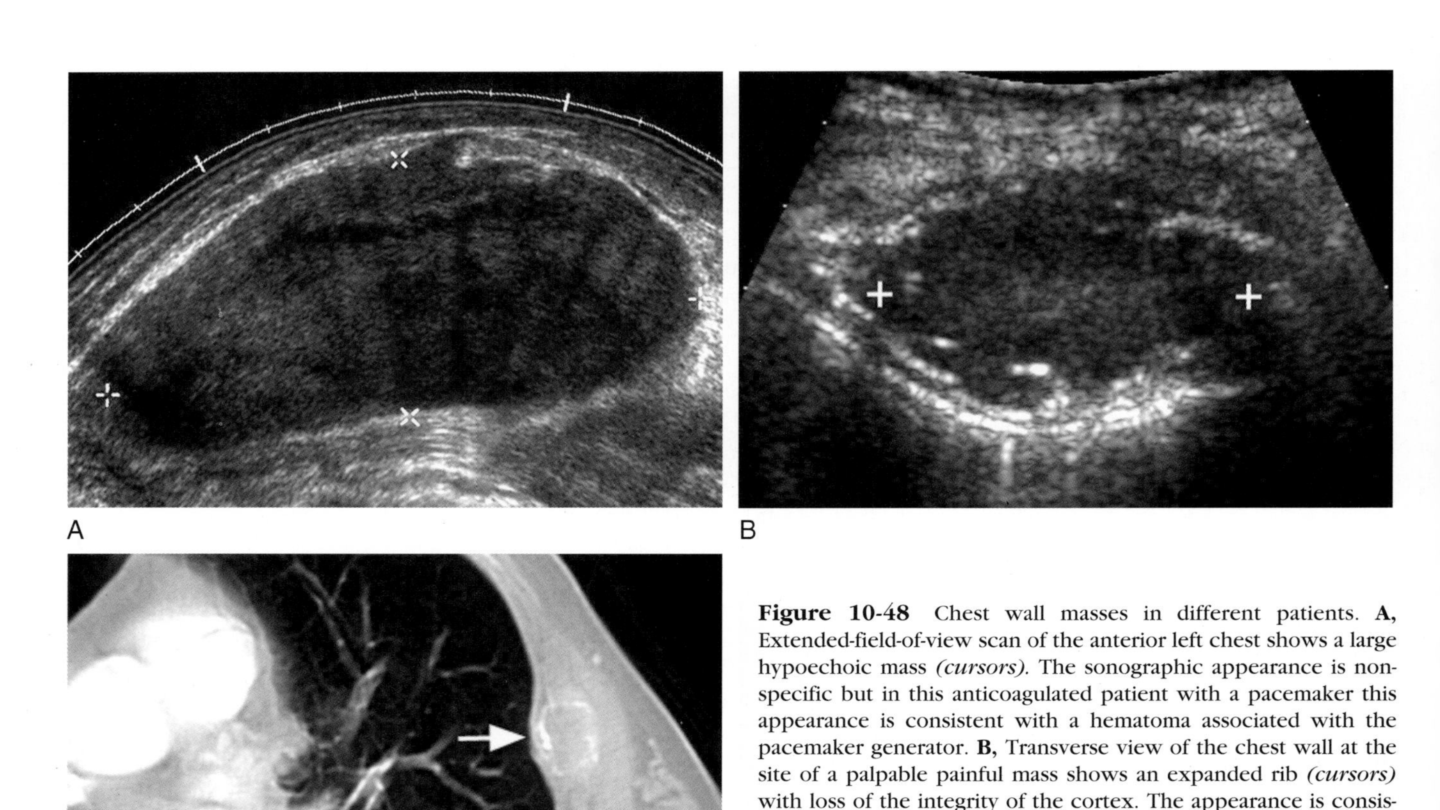

Figure 10-48 Chest wall masses in different patients. **A,** Extended-field-of-view scan of the anterior left chest shows a large hypoechoic mass *(cursors).* The sonographic appearance is nonspecific but in this anticoagulated patient with a pacemaker this appearance is consistent with a hematoma associated with the pacemaker generator. **B,** Transverse view of the chest wall at the site of a palpable painful mass shows an expanded rib *(cursors)* with loss of the integrity of the cortex. The appearance is consistent with a malignant lesion; and in this patient with a history of laryngeal cancer, metastatic disease was considered most likely. **C,** CT scan of the same patient in **B** confirms a destructive lesion of the rib *(arrow).* Subsequent biopsy with ultrasound guidance confirmed metastatic disease.

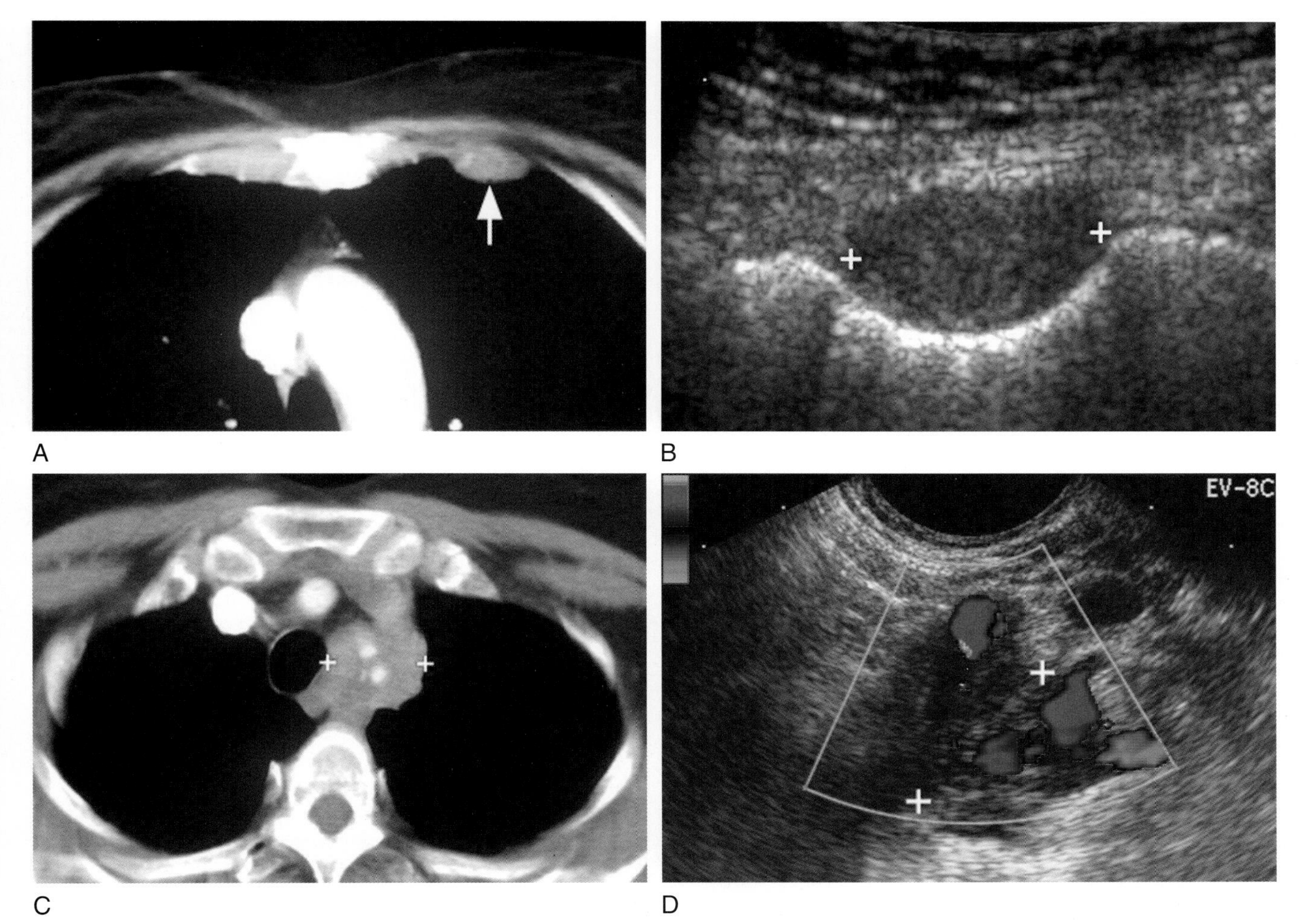

Figure 10-49 Mediastinal masses. **A,** CT of the chest shows an enlarged internal mammary node *(arrow)* in a patient with newly diagnosed pancreatic cancer. **B,** Transverse view of the left anterior chest in the same patient as in **A** confirms an enlarged node *(cursors)*. Ultrasound-guided biopsy showed no evidence of malignancy. **C,** CT scan of the chest shows a superior mediastinal mass *(cursors)* that encases the left common carotid and left subclavian artery origins. **D,** Transverse color Doppler view of the left superior mediastinum obtained from a supraclavicular approach using a transvaginal probe confirms a soft tissue mass *(cursors)* encasing the arteries. Ultrasound-guided biopsy showed a non–small cell cancer.

respiratory cycle. It is also possible to continuously monitor the needle depth to ensure that the aerated lung is not violated.

Although sonography is not frequently used in detecting a pneumothorax, it is actually quite sensitive and can be used in supine patients when radiographs are limited. In normal patients, the visceral surface of the lung can be seen sliding along the parietal pleura during respiratory motion. In patients with a pneumothorax, the extrapulmonary air separates the lung from the parietal pleura, and the sliding motion is lost. In addition, localized comet-tail artifacts are lost in the regions where a pneumothorax is located.

Sonography is also helpful in evaluating paradiaphragmatic lesions. Because sagittal and coronal views are possible, the relationship of lesions to the diaphragm can be determined and the origin of the lesion can often be determined (Fig. 10-51).

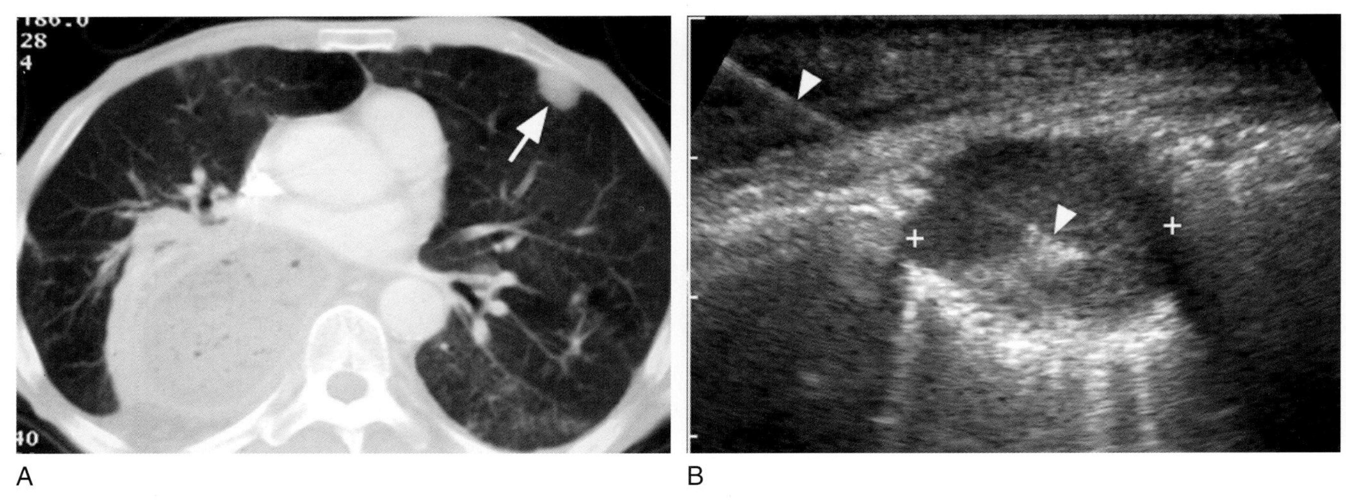

Figure 10-50 Peripheral lung metastasis. **A,** CT scan of the chest in a patient with esophageal cancer shows a small peripheral lung nodule *(arrow)*. This was believed to most likely be a metastasis. **B,** Transverse sonogram of the anterior left chest confirms a small, solid, nodule *(cursors)*. Fine-needle aspiration using a 25-gauge needle *(arrowheads)* proved that this was a metastasis.

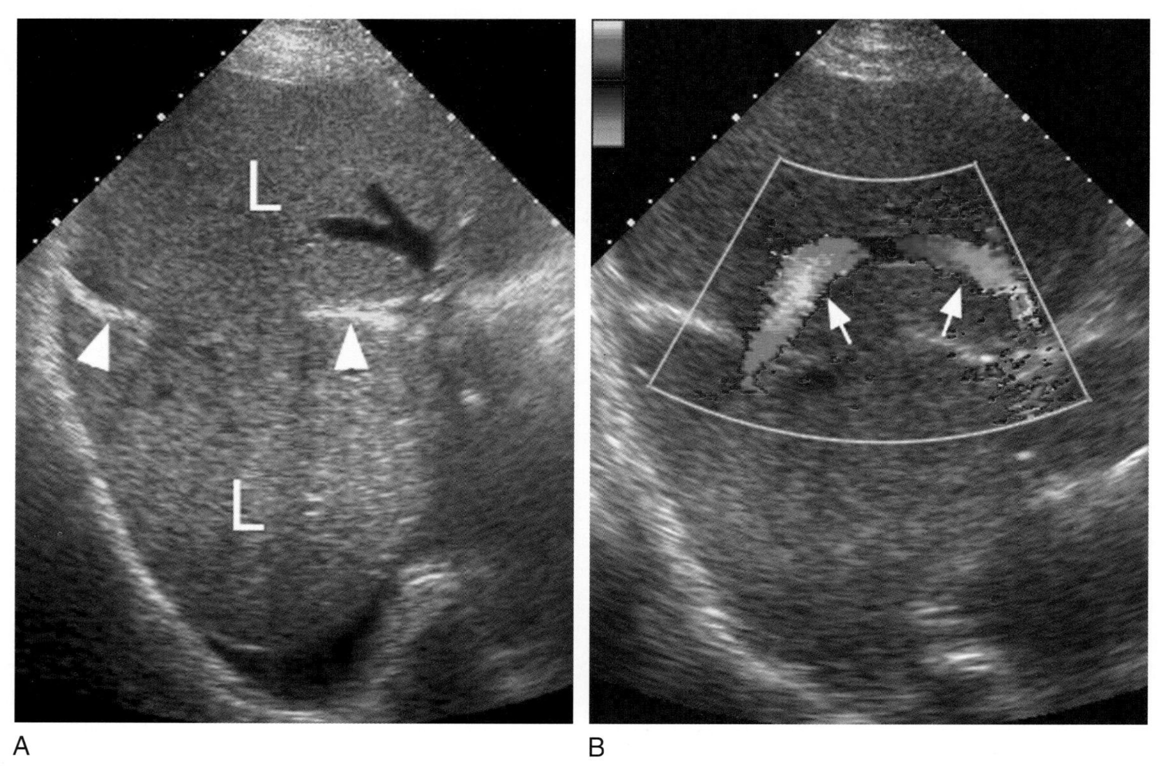

Figure 10-51 Diaphragmatic hernia. **A,** Oblique view of the right upper quadrant in a patient after liver transplantation shows a defect in the diaphragm *(arrowhead)* with herniation of the liver (L) into the lower chest. **B,** Color Doppler view at a slightly different level shows a hepatic vein *(arrows)* passing from the supradiaphragmatic portion of the liver and into the subdiaphragmatic portion of the liver.

Key Features

The normal thyroid is homogeneous and hyperechoic to the adjacent muscles.
Thyroglossal duct cysts are midline lesions that are usually complex and are usually intimately associated with the hyoid bone.
Papillary cancer of the thyroid is typically entirely solid and hypoechoic.
Microcalcifications are tiny, bright, non-shadowing reflectors that are often seen with papillary cancer.
Metastatic neck nodes are common with papillary cancer. They often have microcalcifications and/or cystic changes.
Benign and malignant follicular neoplasms have a range of echogenicities but are usually well defined and often have a hypoechoic halo. They cannot be distinguished with sonography or with fine-needle aspiration.
Medullary cancer has an appearance similar to papillary cancer.
Anaplastic cancer usually presents as a large mass that replaces much of the thyroid and invades adjacent structures.
Thyroid lymphoma is usually a large hypoechoic mass that replaces much of the thyroid.
Benign thyroid nodules usually contain cystic elements and may contain inspissated colloid.
Hashimoto's thyroiditis is the most common cause of hypothyroidism and appears as a diffusely hypoechoic, heterogeneous, hypervascular gland. Focal nodules may coexist.
The most common cause of hyperparathyroidism is a single parathyroid adenoma.
Parathyroid adenomas usually appear as oval, solid, homogeneous, hypoechoic masses posterior and/or slightly inferior to the thyroid.
Parathyroid adenomas are hypervascular; and when they are not too deep, this can be detected with color/power Doppler.
Five percent or less of parathyroid adenomas are ectopic. Sites include the superior mediastinum, the retrotracheal or retroesophageal region, intrathyroidal, or in the carotid sheath.
Malignancy should be considered when lymph nodes in the neck become round (especially those in the jugular chain), when the hilum is obliterated, when cystic changes are seen, or when microcalcifications are present.
Sonography is an excellent means of guiding biopsies and fine-needle aspirations of abnormalities in the thyroid and the remainder of the neck.
Tumors, inflammatory disease, and calculi of the salivary glands are well evaluated with sonography.
The wall of the normal carotid artery appears as a thin inner white line and an outer hypoechoic layer that is less than 0.9 mm thick.
The external carotid can be distinguished from the internal carotid because it is located anterior and medial, it is smaller, it has a high resistance waveform, it has branches, and it responds to the temporal artery tap maneuver.
The most common parameters used to estimate carotid stenosis include peak systolic velocity, end-diastolic velocity, and ICA/CCA peak systolic velocity ratio.
Flow velocities and ratios start to increase when the stenosis exceeds 50% diameter narrowing.
Heterogeneous plaques, especially those with focal hypoechoic regions, tend to be unstable. Homogeneous plaques tend to be stable.
Subclavian steal results in diminished antegrade vertebral blood flow to the brain. As the steal progresses, systolic flow will reverse and, ultimately, diastolic flow will reverse.
Pleural effusions as small as a few milliliters can be detected with sonography.
Chest lesions located adjacent to the pleural surface can be visualized with sonography and can be sampled effectively under ultrasound guidance.

SUGGESTED READINGS

Ahuja AT, Metreweli C: Ultrasound of thyroid nodules. Ultrasound Q 16:111-121, 2000.

Akerstrom G, Malmaeus J, Bergstrom R: Surgical anatomy of human parathyroid glands. Surgery 95:14, 1984.

Bender TM, Ledesma-Medina J, Towbin RB: Pediatric case of the day: Ectopic intrathyroidal parathyroid adenoma. Radiographics 12:1035-1037, 1992.

Bluth EI: Evaluation and characterization of carotid plaque. Semin Ultrasound CT MRI 18:57-65, 1997.

Brander A, et al: Thyroid gland: Ultrasound screening in middle-aged women with no previous thyroid disease. Radiology 173:507, 1989.

Brander AEE, Viikinkoski VP, Kivisaari LM: Importance of thyroid abnormalities detected at US screening: A 5-year follow-up. Radiology 215:801-806, 2000.

DeFeo ML, Colagrande S, Bianini C, et al: Parathyroid glands: Combination of 99m Tc MIBI scintigraphy and US for demonstration of parathyroid glands and nodules. Radiology 214:393-402, 2000.

Dermitzakis I, Minardos I, Kampanarou M, Mitakou D: Color duplex sonography of occlusion of the common carotid artery with reversed flow in the extracranial internal carotid artery. J Clin Ultrasound 30:388-391, 2002.

Frates MC, Benson CB, Doubilet PM, et al: Can color Doppler sonography aid in the prediction of malignancy of thyroid nodules. J Ultrasound Med 22:127-131, 2003.

Gortter M, Niethammer R, Widder B: Differentiating subtotal carotid artery stenoses from occlusion by colour-coded duplex sonography. J Neurol 241:301-305, 1994.

Graif M, et al: Parathyroid sonography: Diagnostic accuracy related to shape, location, and texture of the gland. Br J Radiol 60:439, 1987.

Grant EG, Benson CB, Moneta GL et al: Society of Radiologists in Ultrasound Consensus Conference on Ultrasound and Doppler Diagnosis of Carotid Stenosis. Radiology, Nov 2003, in press.

Grant EG, Duerinckx AJ, El Saden S, et al: Doppler sonographic parameters for detection of carotid stenosis: Is there an optimum method for their selection? AJR Am J Roentgenol 172:1123-1129, 1999.

Grant EG, Duerinckx AJ, Saden SM, et al: Ability to use duplex US to quantify internal carotid arterial stenoses: Fact or fiction? Radiology 214:247-252, 2000.

Gritzmann N, Hollerweger A, Macheiner P, Rettenbacher T: Sonography of soft tissue masses of the neck. J Clin Ultrasound 30:356-373, 2002.

Horrow MM, Stassi J: Sonography of the vertebral arteries: A window to disease of the proximal great vessels. AJR Am J Roentgenol 177:53-59, 2001.

Horrow MM, Stassi J, Shurman A, et al: The limitations of carotid sonography: Interpretive and technology-related errors. AJR Am J Roentgenol 174:189-194, 2000.

Heilo A, Stenwig AE, Solheim OP: Malignant pleural mesothelioma: US-guided histologic core-needle biopsy. Radiology 211:657-659, 1999.

Katz JF, et al: Thyroid nodules: Sonographic-pathologic correlation. Radiology 151:741, 1984.

Kim EK, Park CS, Chung WY, et al: New sonographic criteria for recommending fine-needle aspiration biopsy of nonpalpable solid nodules of the thyroid. AJR Am J Roentgenol 178:687-691, 2002.

Kliewer MA, Hertzberg BS, Kim DH, et al: Vertebral artery Doppler waveform changes indicating subclavian steal physiology. AJR Am J Roentgenol 174:815-819, 2000.

Koeller KK, Alamo L, Adair CF, Smirniotopoulos JG: From the Archives of the AFIP: Congenital cystic masses of the neck: Radiologic-pathologic correlation. Radiographics 19:121-146, 1999.

Langer JE, Khan A, Nisenbaum HL, et al: Sonographic appearance of focal thyroiditis. AJR Am J Roentgenol 176:751-756, 2001.

Lee VS, Hertzberg BS, Kliewer MA, Carroll BA: Assessment of stenosis: Implications of variability of Doppler measurements in normal-appearing carotid arteries. Radiology 212:493-498, 1999.

Lee VS, Hertzberg BS, Workman MJ, et al: Variability of Doppler US Measurements along the common carotid artery: Effects on estimates of internal carotid arterial stenosis in patients with angiographically proved disease. Radiology 214:387-392, 2000.

Lewis BD, Charboneau JW, Reading CC: Ultrasound-guided biopsy and ablation in the neck. Ultrasound Q 18:3-12, 2002.

Miller DL, et al: Localization of parathyroid adenomas in patients who have undergone surgery: I. Noninvasive imaging methods. Radiology 162:133, 1987.

Nicolau C, Gilabert R, Chamorro A, et al: Doppler sonography of the intertransverse segment of the vertebral artery. J Ultrasound Med 19:47-53, 2000.

O'Leary DH, et al: Carotid artery intima and media wall thickness as a risk factor for myocardial infarction and stroke in older adults. N Engl J Med 340:14-22, 1999.

Ralls PW, et al: Color-flow Doppler sonography in Graves' disease: "Thyroid inferno." AJR Am J Roentgenol 150:781, 1988.

Randel SB, et al: Parathyroid variants: Ultrasound evaluation. Radiology 165:191, 1987.

Rao AB, Koeller KK, Adair CF: Paragangliomas of the head and neck: Radiologic-pathologic correlation. Radiographics 19:1605-1632, 1999.

Rausch P, Nowels K, Jeffrey RB Jr: Ultrasonographically guided thyroid biopsy. J Ultrasound Med 20:79-85, 2001.

Reading CC, et al: Postoperative parathyroid high-frequency sonography: Evaluation of persistent or recurrent hyperparathyroidism. AJR Am J Roentgenol 144:399, 1985.

Reeder SB, Desser TS, Weigel RJ, Jeffrey RB: Sonography in primary hyperparathyroidism: Review with emphasis on scanning technique. J Ultrasound Med 21:539-552, 2002.

Rojeski MT, Gharib H: Nodular thyroid disease: Evaluation and management. N Engl J Med 313:428, 1985.

Romero JM, Lev MH, Chan ST, et al: US of neurovascular occlusive disease: Interpretive perils and pitfalls. Radiographics 22:1165-1176, 2002.

Rowan KR, Kirkpatrick AW, Liu D, et al: Traumatic pneumothorax detection with thoracic US: Correlation with chest radiography and CT: Initial experience. Radiology 225:210-214, 2002.

Shawker TH, Avila NA, Premkumar A, et al: Ultrasound evaluation of primary hyperparathyroidism. Ultrasound Q 16:73-87, 2000.

Sheth S, Hamper UM, Stanley DB, et al: US guidance for thoracic biopsy: A valuable alternative to CT. Radiology 210:721-726, 1999.

Soulez G, Therasse E, Robillard P, et al: The value of internal carotid systolic velocity ratio for assessing carotid artery stenosis with Doppler sonography. AJR Am J Roentgenol 172:207-212, 1999.

Stasst J, Cavanaugh BC, Siegal TL, et al: US case of the day: Occlusion of the CCA with segmental reversal of ECA flow and a patent ICA. Radiographics 15:1235-1238, 1995.

Tegos TJ, Sabetai MM, Nicolaides AN, et al: Comparability of the ultrasonic tissue characteristic of carotid plaques. J Ultrasound Med 19:399-407, 2000.

Tessler FN, Tublin ME: Thyroid sonography: Current applications and future directions. AJR Am J Roentgenol 173:437-443, 1999.

van Dalen A, Smit CP, van Vroonhoven TJMV, et al: Minimally invasive surgery for solitary parathyroid adenomas in patients with primary hyperparathyroidism: Role of US with supplemental CT. Radiology 220:631-639, 2001.

Wadsworth DT, Siegel MJ: Thyroglossal duct cysts: Variability of sonographic findings. AJR Am J Roentgenol 163:1475-1477, 1994.

Wernecke K: Pictorial essay: Sonographic features of pleural disease. AJR Am J Roentgenol 168:1061-1066, 1997.

Wiest PW, Hartshorne MF, Inskip PD, et al: Thyroid palpation versus high-resolution thyroid ultrasonography in the detection of nodules. J Ultrasound Med 17:487-496, 1998.

Wunderbaldinger P, Harisinghani MG, Hahn PF, et al: Cystic lymph node metastases in papillary thyroid carcinoma. AJR Am J Roentgenol 178:693-697, 2002.

Yeh HC, Futterweit W, Gilbert P: Micronodulation: Ultrasonographic sign of Hashimoto's thyroiditis. J Ultrasound Med 15:813-819, 1996.

Ying M, Ahuja A, Metreweli C: Diagnostic accuracy of sonographic criteria for evaluation of cervical lymphadenopathy. J Ultrasound Med 17:437-445, 1998.

Yousem DM, Kraut MA, Chalian AA: Major salivary gland imaging. Radiology 216:19-29, 2000.

CHAPTER 11

Extremities

NORMAL ANATOMY

A number of superficial structures in the extremities are well suited for sonographic imaging. This is especially true of tendons. The interfaces between internal tendon fibers produce strong specular reflections when the sound reflects off the tendon at 90 degrees. The result is referred to as a fibrillar pattern and consists of closely spaced, parallel, bright linear reflections (Fig. 11-1). When imaged at less than 90 degrees, the strength of the reflections decrease, tendons become hypoechoic, and the fibrillar pattern is lost (see Fig. 11-1). Variable echogenicity, depending on the relative orientation of the transducer and the structure being scanned, is referred to as anisotropy. Anisotropy is present in many parts of the body but is particularly prominent in tendons. Under most circumstances, tendons should be imaged so that the fibrillar pattern is visible. However, when tendons are surrounded by echogenic tissue, it may be helpful to purposely angle the transducer so that the tendon appears hypoechoic and the contrast between tendon and peritendinous tissues is increased. Additionally, echogenic lesions and abnormal intratendinous interfaces may be best seen when the tendon is purposely made to appear hypoechoic by imaging at less than 90 degrees.

Ligaments in general have a similar sonographic appearance to tendons (Fig. 11-2). However, it is more difficult to image many ligaments at 90 degrees to their long axis; therefore, it is not uncommon for ligaments to appear hypoechoic.

Muscles are composed of many fascicles that are separated by fibrous tissue called the perimysium. Muscle fascicles are very hypoechoic, and this produces an overall appearance of decreased echogenicity to muscles. The perimysium creates interfaces between the fascicles that on longitudinal views appear as linear echogenic reflections and on transverse views appear as diffuse speckles within a hypoechoic background (Fig. 11-3).

Peripheral nerves are composed of multiple internal neuronal fascicles that appear hypoechoic on high-resolution scans (Fig. 11-4). On transverse views, internal nerve fascicles are roughly round and are surrounded by the hyperechoic epineurium, a loose connective tissue composed of collagen and adipose. Peripheral nerves can simulate tendons, but the echogenicity is less than tendons and echoarchitecture of nerves is more fascicular while the architecture of tendons is more fibrillar.

In a number of joints, acoustic access is sufficient to allow for sonographic visualization of articular cartilage. Articular cartilage is very homogeneous and thus produces very few internal echoes. It appears as a thin, smooth hypoechoic to anechoic layer overlying the cortical bone (Fig. 11-5A). Fibrocartilage structures such as the glenoid labrum and the menisci of the knee can also be at least partially visualized with ultrasound. Fibrocartilage has a more complex internal architecture than articular cartilage and appears more echogenic (see Fig. 11-5B).

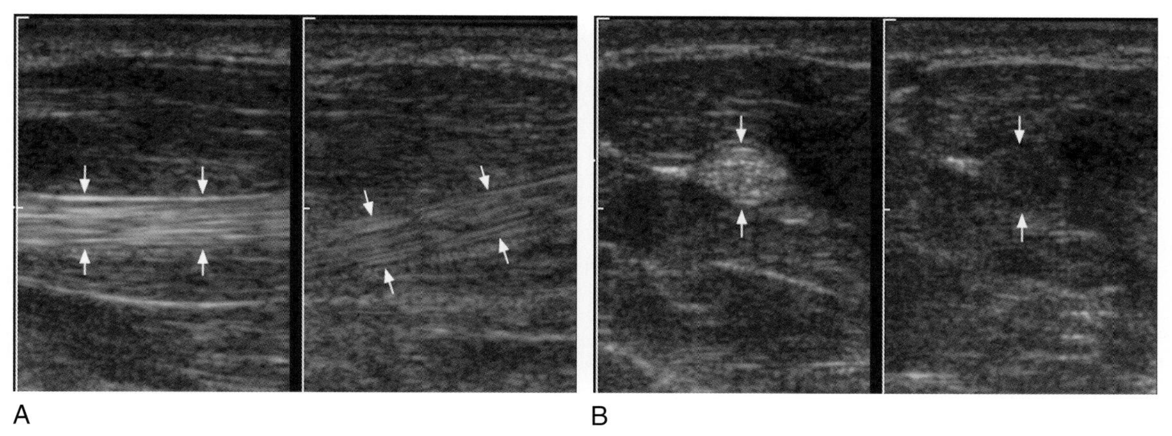

Figure 11-1 Normal tendon. **A,** Longitudinal view of the flexor pollicis longus *(arrows)* shown at 90 degrees to the direction of the sound pulses *(left side)* and at less than 90 degrees *(right side)*. Note the easily identifiable hyperechoic fibrillar echotexture seen on the left but not on the right. **B,** Transverse view of the flexor pollicis longus showing similar findings.

The external cortical surface of superficial bones can be visualized well with sonography as a smooth bright reflection. Therefore, abnormalities that alter the bony surface can be detected sonographically. Although sonography is generally not used as a primary technique for imaging the bones, occult bone lesions are occasionally detected during the evaluation of the overlying soft tissues. Therefore, it is important to observe the bones and recognize abnormalities when they are present.

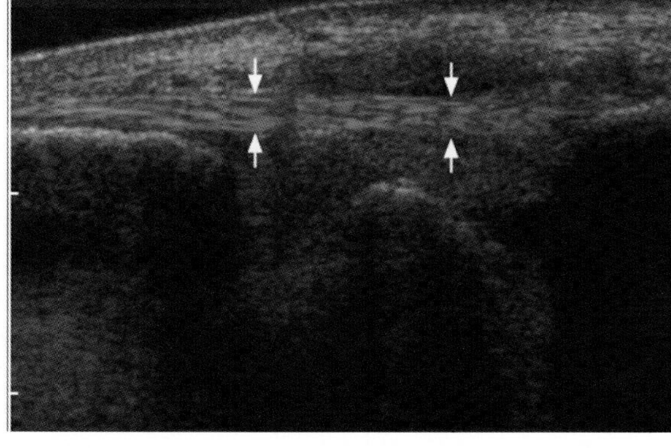

Figure 11-2 Normal ligament. Longitudinal view of the medial ankle shows a normal tibiocalcaneal ligament *(arrows)* displaying characteristics very similar to the normal tendon shown in Figure 11-1.

TENDONS

Probably the most common reason for performing musculoskeletal examinations is to evaluate tendons. Tendon tears are common and are relatively easy to identify and analyze with sonography. Complete tendon tears are associated with a number of sonographic findings (Fig. 11-6). In many cases the end of the retracted proximal tendon will appear blunt on longitudinal views and will appear mass-like on transverse views. In both views there is often shadowing at the site of the torn

Table 11-1 Normal Characteristics of Musculoskeletal Structures

Tendons	Echogenic when imaged at 90% to sound, otherwise hypoechoic Fibrillar architecture
Ligaments	Similar to tendons
Muscles	Hypoechoic
Articular Cartilage	Anechoic to hypoechoic
Fibrocartilage	Hyperechoic
Peripheral Nerves	Hypoechoic Fascicular architecture

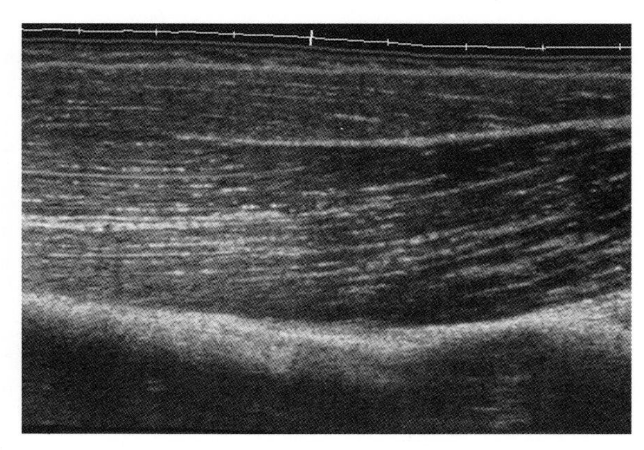

Figure 11-3 Normal muscle. Longitudinal extended field of view scan of the brachioradialis muscle shows the overall hypoechoic appearance of muscle but also shows the multiple linear oriented internal fibrous bands converging to form a central tendon.

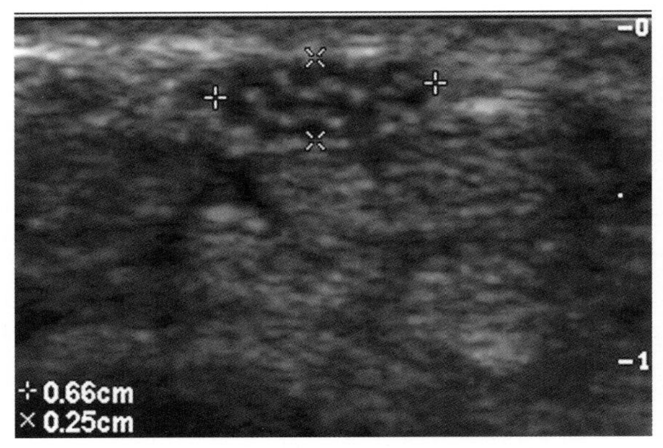

Figure 11-4 Normal nerve. Transverse view of the median nerve *(cursors)* shows the multiple round hypoechoic internal neuronal fascicles.

proximal tendon. In most cases the shadowing is refractive in nature and does not imply underlying calcification or avulsion of bone. Another common finding is loss of the normal fibrillar architecture of the tendon or complete nonvisualization of the tendon. Fluid collections may occur at the site of torn tendons due to a hematoma (especially in the setting of a tear near or at the musculotendinous junction) or a tendon sheath effusion. Partial-thickness tears disrupt the internal fibrillar architecture in a focal region but do not cause tendon retraction (Fig. 11-7).

Tendonitis and tenosynovitis (inflammation of the tendon sheath) can be due to inflammatory processes (rheumatoid arthritis and other synovial based arthritis), infection (either from penetrating trauma or blood borne), crystals (gout), trauma (usually repetitive microtrauma), amyloidosis (chronic hemodialysis), or foreign bodies. Sonographic findings include fluid distending the tendon sheath and/or thickening of the synovial tendon sheath (Fig. 11-8). Synovial thickening may be diffuse and smooth or eccentric and nodular. Infections or hemorrhage may produce fluid with low-level echoes. Hypervascularity is often detectable when there is an active inflammatory process.

Despite the fact that the curved, conjoined tendons of the rotator cuff are more difficult to image than straight tendons, the rotator cuff has received more attention than any other tendon. Perhaps this is because shoulder pain originating from rotator cuff disease is very common and because rotator cuff tears are difficult to diagnose and quantify clinically. Because rotator cuff sonography is among the most commonly performed musculoskeletal examinations, it is important to be familiar with its normal sonographic appearance. All four of the cuff tendons (subscapularis, supraspinatus, infraspinatus, and teres minor) appear as a band of tissue covering the humeral head. The anatomy can be thought of as a series of layers. From deep to superficial, the layers are the echogenic humeral head, the anechoic or hypoechoic articular cartilage, the relatively echogenic rotator cuff, the hypoechoic subdeltoid bursa, the hyperechoic peribursal fat, the hypoechoic deltoid muscle, and, finally, the subcutaneous tissues (Fig. 11-9A). Important normal aspects of the cuff are its outer convex contour (see Fig. 11-9B) and the lack of compressibility with transducer pressure.

Full-thickness rotator cuff tears refer to tears that extend from the deep surface of the cuff to the superficial surface of the cuff. They may be small and only involve a tiny region of a single tendon, or they may be large and involve multiple tendons. The majority of tears originate at the site of insertion of the supraspinatus tendon to the greater tuberosity. From there, they may extend posteriorly to involve the infraspinatus, extend

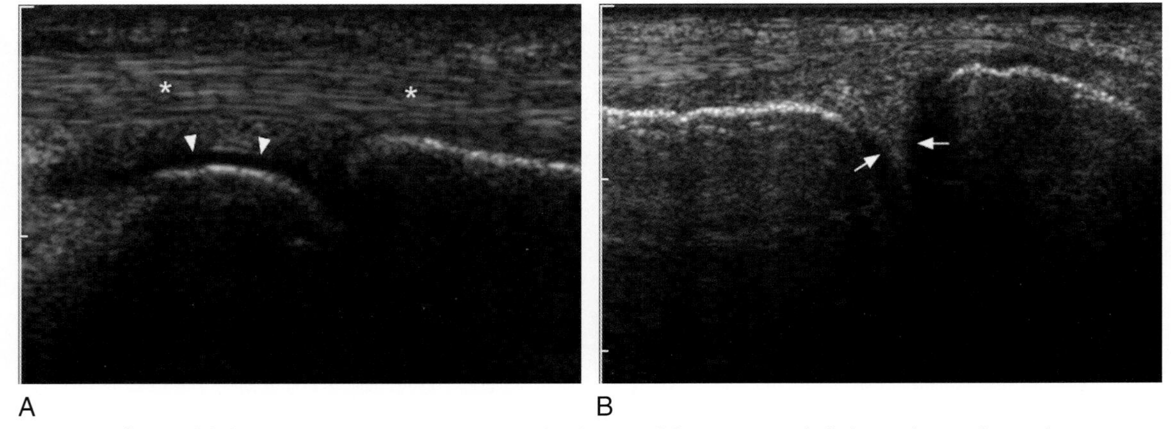

Figure 11-5 Normal cartilage. **A,** Longitudinal view of the metacarpal phalangeal joint shows the articular cartilage of the metacarpal head *(arrowheads)* as a thin anechoic layer overlying the cortical bone. The flexor tendons to this finger are seen superficially (*). **B,** Longitudinal view of the medial meniscus of the knee *(arrows)* shows the hyperechoic appearance of fibrocartilaginous structures.

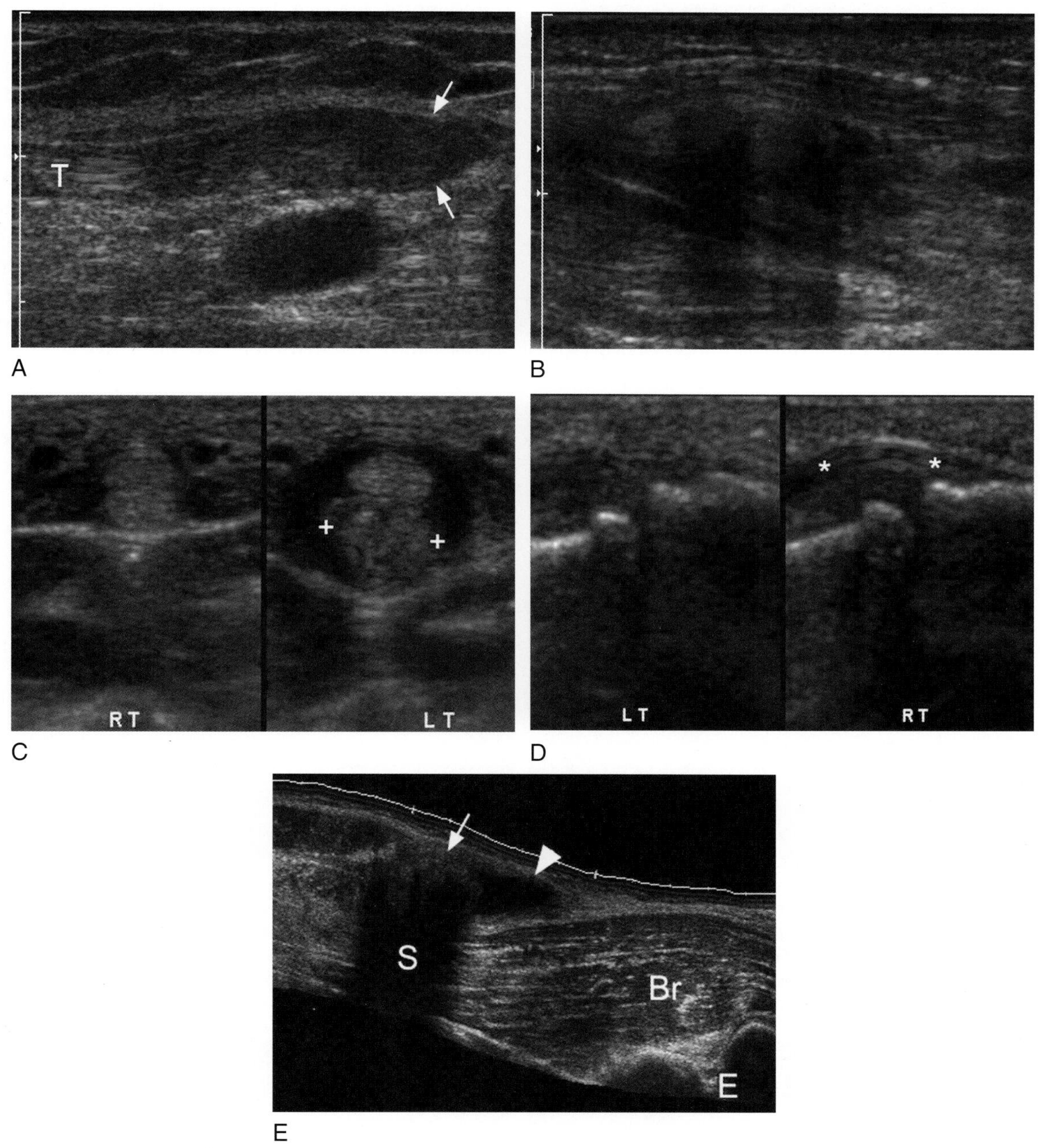

Figure 11-6 Full-thickness tendon tears in different patients. **A,** Torn flexor pollicis longus shows the blunt end of the retracted proximal fragment *(arrows).* Also note the loss of fibrillar architecture in the blunt end as opposed to the more normal proximal tendon (T). **B,** Torn flexor pollicis longus shows classic refractive shadowing at the site of the retracted tendon end. **C,** Dual transverse views of the superficial and deep flexor tendons of the middle finger show the normal tendons on the right side and the tendon sheath effusion and mass effect produced by the torn and retracted deep flexor tendon *(cursors)* on the left side. **D,** Dual longitudinal images of the distal interphalangeal joint of the left and right index finger show a normal intact flexor tendon on the right (*) and no identifiable tendon on the left. **E,** Longitudinal view of the arm shows the level of the elbow joint (E) and the normal overlying brachioradialis muscle (Br). The torn and retracted biceps tendon *(arrow)* casts a distinct refractive shadow (S). An associated fluid collection *(arrowhead)* is seen adjacent to the torn tendon.

Box 11-1 Signs of Complete Tendon Rupture

Blunt tendon tip (longitudinal views)
Mass (transverse views)
Refractive shadowing
Nonvisualization
Loss of fibrillar architecture
Fluid collection

medially to involve the more proximal supraspinatus, or extend in both directions. The subscapularis tendon may also be involved with massive full-thickness rotator cuff tears. However, it is rare to have an isolated tear of the supscapularis tendon in the absence of a prior anterior shoulder dislocation or a dislocated biceps tendon.

The sonographic appearance of full-thickness rotator cuff tears depends on whether there is a significant amount of fluid in the joint (Box 11-2). When fluid is present, the tear appears as a fluid-filled defect (Fig. 11-10A). This type of tear is referred to as a wet tear, and these are generally very easy to identify, and the appearance is easy to understand. With dry tears, the defect created is not filled with fluid and, in most cases, the overlying subdeltoid bursa and peribursal fat drops into the defect. This converts the normal convex interface between the deltoid and the cuff into a concave interface (see Fig. 11-10B and C). In most cases, this concavity is readily visible at rest. If the torn ends of the tendon have not retracted from each other, or if the defect is filled with hypertrophied synovial tissue, a concavity may not be visible at rest. In such a case, compression of the shoulder with the transducer can push the bursa and peribursal fat into the defect at the same time that it

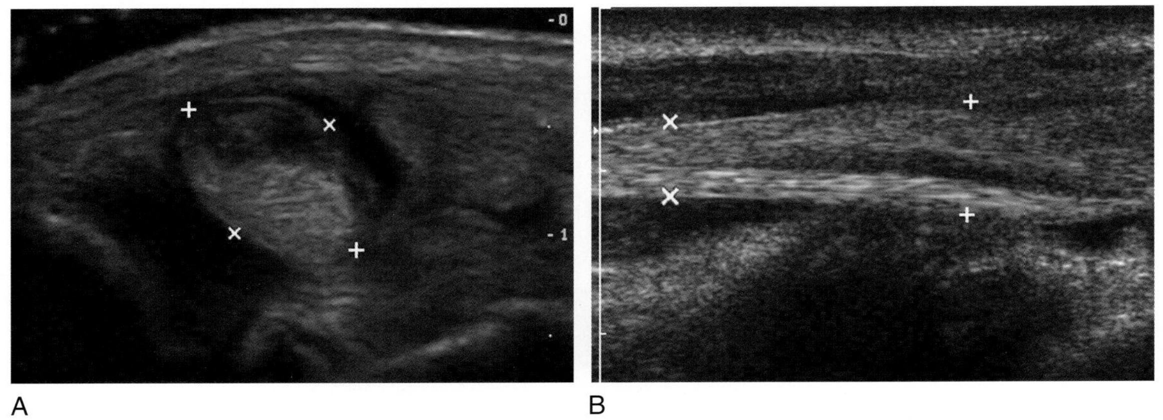

Figure 11-7 Partial-thickness tendon tear in different patients. **A,** Transverse view of the posterior tibial tendon *(cursors)* shows a distinct hypoechoic defect in the superficial aspect of the tendon consistent with a partial tear. **B,** Longitudinal view of the posterior tibial tendon *(cursors)* in another patient shows a distinct linear hypoechoic longitudinally oriented partial tear in the central aspect of the tendon.

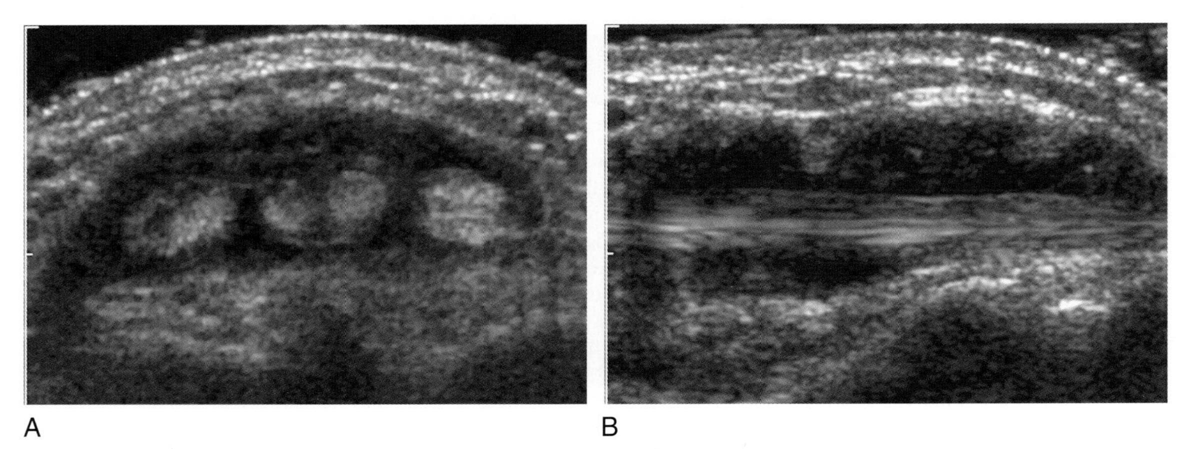

Figure 11-8 Tenosynovitis. **A,** Transverse view of the extensor tendons of the fingers shows fluid in the common tendon sheath as well as proliferative synovium in the tendon sheath. **B,** Longitudinal view of an extensor tendon confirms a tendon sheath effusion as well as irregular thickening of the tendon sheath.

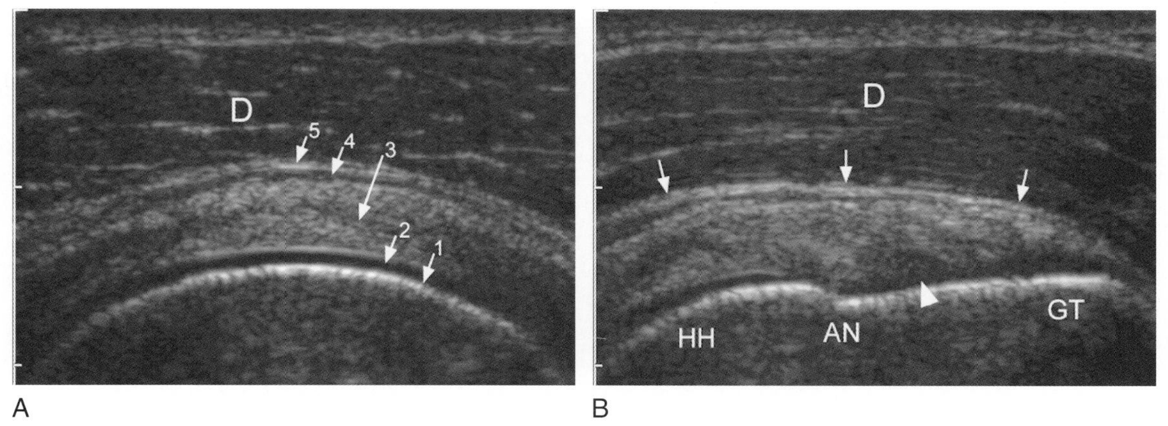

Figure 11-9 Normal rotator cuff. **A,** Transverse view of the shoulder over the region of the rotator cuff shows multiple layers. Layer #1 is the cortical bone of the humeral head. Layer #2 is the articular cartilage of the humeral head. Layer #3 is the thick rotator cuff. Layer #4 is the thin subdeltoid bursa. Layer #5 is the peribursal fat. The hypoechoic deltoid muscle (D) covers all of these structures. Note that the rotator cuff appears echogenic in the middle of the image where it is perpendicular to the direction of sound but becomes hypoechoic on the edges of the image where it loses this orientation. **B,** Longitudinal view of the rotator cuff shows the bright reflection from the bony cortex of the humeral head (HH), anatomic neck (AN), and greater tuberosity (GT). The rotator cuff tapers and assumes a beak-like configuration as it inserts on the greater tuberosity. Note the convex outer contour of the rotator cuff and its adjacent bursa and peribursal fat *(arrows)*. Also note the hypoechoic region of the rotator cuff insertion due to anisotropy *(arrowhead)*.

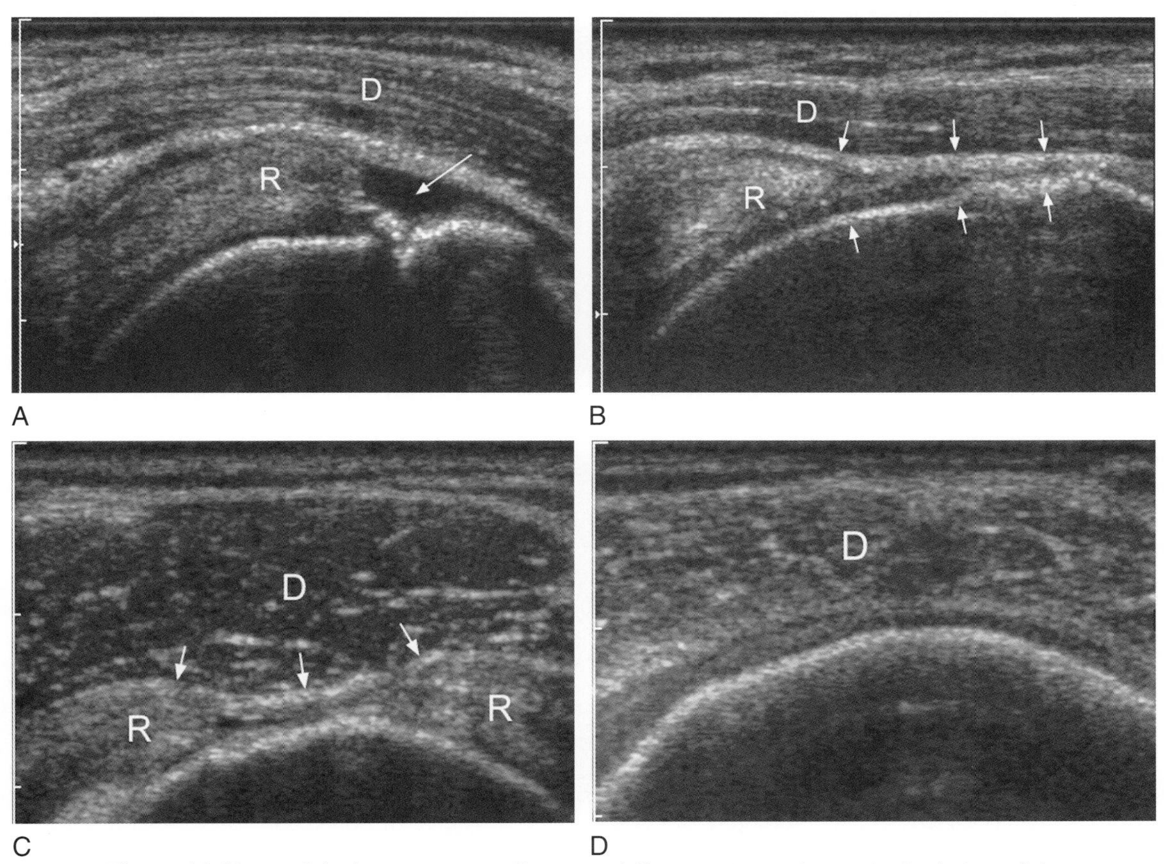

Figure 11-10 Full-thickness rotator cuff tears in different patients. **A,** Longitudinal view of the rotator cuff (R) and deltoid muscle (D) shows a fluid-filled defect *(arrow)* measuring approximately 5 mm located at the insertion of the rotator cuff. **B,** Longitudinal view of the rotator cuff (R) and deltoid muscle (D) shows focal apposition of the peribursal fat and the humeral head and greater tuberosity *(arrows)*. **C,** Transverse view of the rotator cuff (R) and deltoid muscle (D) shows a focal concavity *(arrows)* of the superficial contour at the site of a full-thickness tear. **D,** Deltoid muscle (D) is in close apposition to the humeral head with no identifiable rotator cuff visualized.

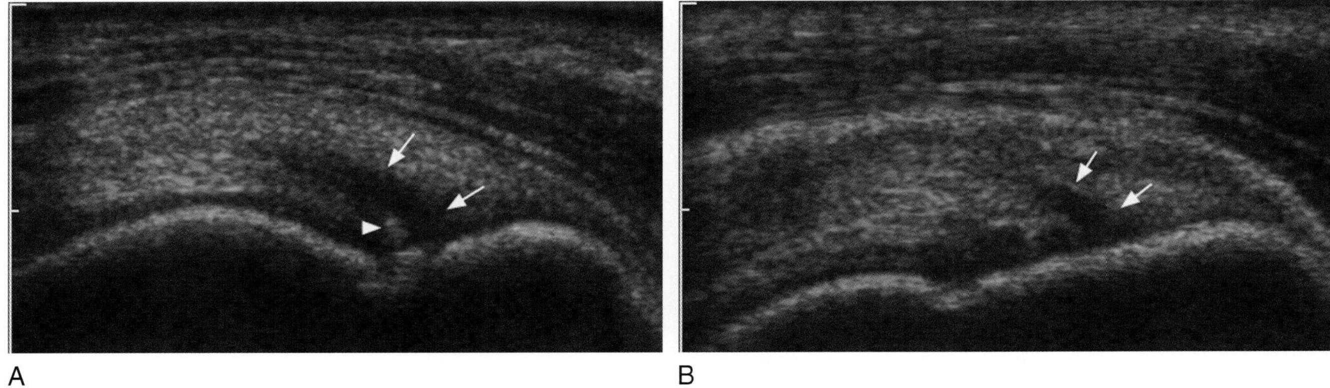

Figure 11-11 Partial-thickness rotator cuff tear in different patients. **A,** Longitudinal view of the rotator cuff shows a relatively well-defined hypoechoic defect *(arrows)* along the deep insertion of the rotator cuff. There is also an associated hyperechoic component *(arrowhead)*. Slight underlying bony pitting is also apparent. **B,** Longitudinal view shows a small well-defined hypoechoic defect along the deep surface of the rotator cuff insertion *(arrows)*. Contrast this better-defined defect with the less well-defined region of anisotropy shown in Figure 11-9B.

produces some separation of the tendon ends. As mentioned earlier, the normal rotator cuff does not compress at all. Massive tears with extensive retraction of the torn tendon produce an uncovered humeral head and no visible cuff on standard images (see Fig. 11-10D). This is referred to as nonvisualization of the cuff.

Once a full-thickness tear has been identified, it is important to determine which tendons are involved. If the tear involves just the first 1.5 cm of cuff behind the biceps tendon, then it is isolated to the supraspinatus. If it extends to involve the cuff more than 1.5 cm behind the biceps, then the infraspinatus is also involved. These measurements are made on the short-axis (transverse) views. The degree of retraction of the cuff from the greater tuberosity is measured on the long-axis (longitudinal) view.

Partial-thickness tears refer to tears that do not extend all the way from the deep to the superficial surface of the cuff. They can involve the deep surface, the superficial surface, or the internal aspect of the cuff. However, the majority arise from the deep surface and involve the supraspinatus tendon insertion. The sonographic appearance of a partial-thickness tear consists of a hypoechoic defect that remains constant despite changes in the orientation of the transducer. In most cases, there is also a bright reflector associated with the hypoechoic area (Fig. 11-11). As with full-thickness tears, the underlying bony cortex is usually irregular. Unlike full-thickness tears, partial-thickness tears are not associated with contour changes and do not compress with transducer pressure. Partial-thickness tears must be distinguished from tendon anisotropy, which normally causes the deep surface of the supraspinatus insertion to appear hypoechoic. Tendon anisotropy usually will become more echogenic when the transducer is angled upward, whereas partial tears will not change. Tendon anisotropy is usually poorly marginated, whereas partial tears are better marginated. Finally, tendon anisotropy is usually entirely hypoechoic, whereas partial tears usually have at least a small hyperechoic component.

The sensitivity of sonography for full-thickness tears is approximately 95%. The sensitivity of sonography for partial-thickness tears is 70% to 90%. A recent

Box 11-2 Signs of Full-Thickness Rotator Cuff Tear

- Anechoic or hypoechoic defect
- Focal superficial contour abnormality
- Compressibility
- Nonvisualization

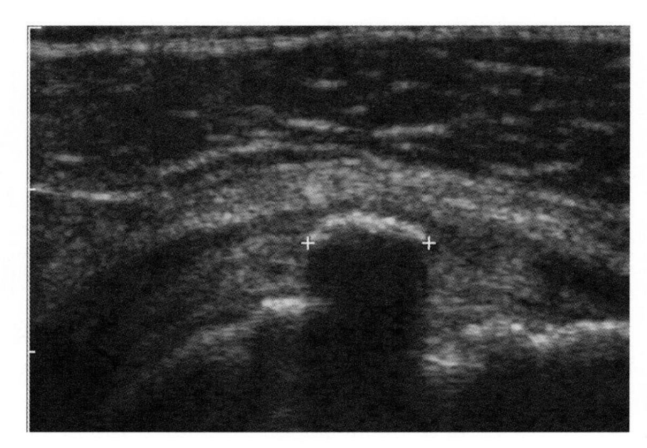

Figure 11-12 Calcific tendinitis. Longitudinal view of the subscapularis tendon shows a shadowing hyperechoic lesion *(cursors)* in the substance of the tendon.

double-blind comparison of ultrasound and MRI using surgery as the gold standard showed similar sensitivity for full- and partial-thickness tears.

In addition to tears, another relatively common painful abnormality of the rotator cuff is calcific tendinitis. Calcium in the rotator cuff produces an area of increased echogenicity and in most cases an associated acoustic shadow (Fig. 11-12). Sonography is the most accurate means of identifying, localizing, and quantifying rotator cuff calcification. It can also be used to guide aspiration of calcific tendonitis. MRI is excellent at detecting most soft tissue abnormalities in the shoulder, but, as elsewhere in the body, it is poor at detecting calcification.

MUSCLES

Muscle injuries can be the result of direct compressive trauma or distraction from sudden forceful muscle contraction. Tears of the muscle are divided into three grades. Grade 1 tears consist of tears of only a limited number of muscle fibers. Grade 2 tears are more extensive partial tears usually associated with some functional weakness. Grade 3 tears are complete disruptions of the entire muscle. On sonography, the severity of the lesion is mirrored by the amount of hematoma. Grade 3 tears are also associated with some degree of muscle retraction, usually at the myotendinous junction. The imaging characteristics of hematomas have been described in previous chapters and are similar in muscles. In the acute stage, they are relatively echogenic and solid (Fig. 11-13A). Over a matter of days they generally start to liquefy and convert to a complex collection (see Fig. 11-13B) and ultimately to a simple-appearing fluid collection (see Fig. 11-13C). When they are close to completely liquefied, they can be aspirated with ultrasound guidance, and this can speed overall recovery time and allow competitive athletes to return to competition earlier. Intramuscular hemorrhage may dissect in between fascicles and not form a discrete collection. This is also known as a contusion and will produce thickening and increased echogenicity of the intermuscular septa.

Intramuscular masses in the absence of trauma should be considered tumors until proven otherwise. Primary sarcomas are often complex, and metastatic tumors are usually solid and homogeneous, but there is considerable overlap in their sonographic appearance (Fig. 11-14). Both lesions should be distinguished from bone lesions with associated soft tissue components. Sonography generally plays little role in the evaluation of

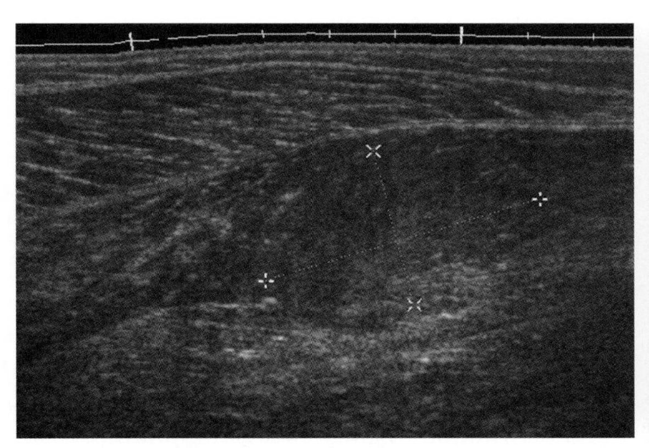

A

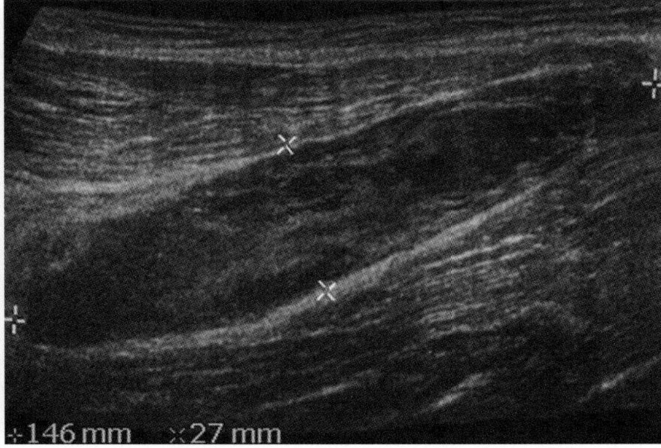

B

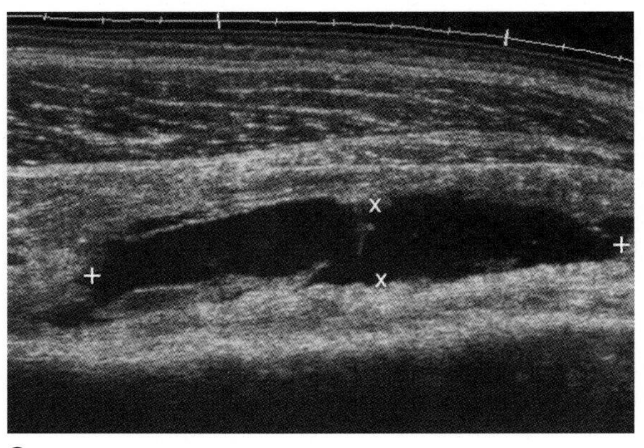

C

Figure 11-13 Muscle hematoma in different patients. **A,** Longitudinal view of the calf shows an isoechoic, solid-appearing acute hematoma *(cursors)* in the soleus muscle. **B,** Longitudinal view of the anterior thigh shows a complex solid and liquefied subacute hematoma *(cursors)* in the quadriceps muscles. **C,** Longitudinal view of the anterior thigh shows an irregularly marginated but completely liquefied hematoma in the quadriceps muscle group.

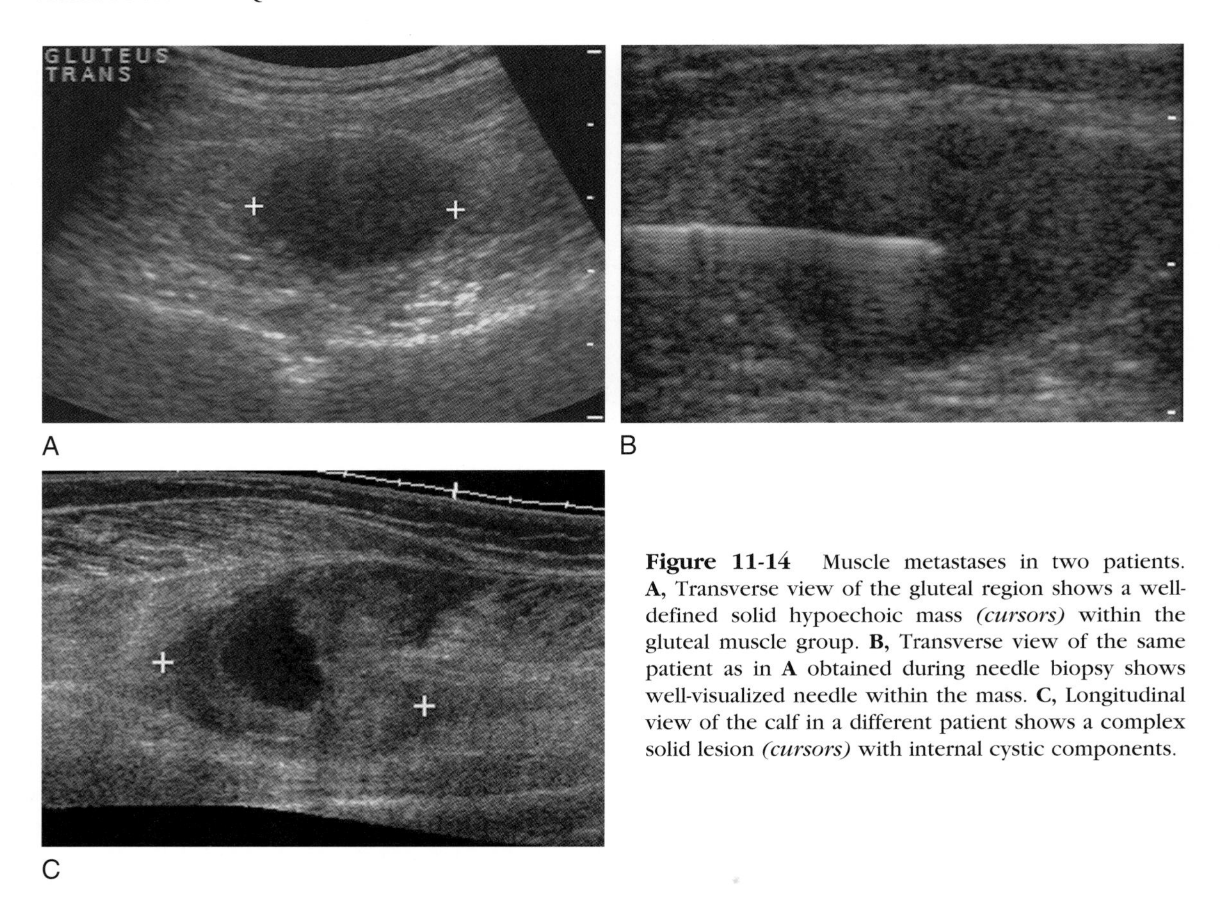

Figure 11-14 Muscle metastases in two patients. **A,** Transverse view of the gluteal region shows a well-defined solid hypoechoic mass *(cursors)* within the gluteal muscle group. **B,** Transverse view of the same patient as in **A** obtained during needle biopsy shows well-visualized needle within the mass. **C,** Longitudinal view of the calf in a different patient shows a complex solid lesion *(cursors)* with internal cystic components.

muscular neoplasms. However, it is an excellent method for providing guidance for biopsy (see Fig. 11-14).

BURSAS

Normal bursas are not visible with sonography. However, abnormal, fluid-filled bursas can be detected around many joints. They are particularly common around the knee. The most common is the bursa between the medial head of the gastrocnemius and the semimembranosus tendon. When distended by fluid, this is referred to as a Baker's cyst. These cysts are best identified by scanning along the medial and superior aspect of the medial head of the gastrocnemius. They may be simple appearing or contain internal septations, thick irregular walls, nodular synovial proliferation, and loose bodies (Fig. 11-15). The neck that extends between the medial gastrocnemius and the semimembranosus tendon produces a beak-like appearance that is a very characteristic feature. Rupture may produce a pointed margin to the inferior aspect of the cyst or fluid tracking into the calf from the inferior aspect of the cyst (see Fig. 11-15D).

Diagnosis of bursitis in other sites depends on a thorough knowledge of the anatomic location of different bursas. This is the only way to distinguish a fluid-filled bursa from other periarticular fluid collections (Fig. 11-16).

MASSES

Sonography of extremity masses should be aimed at determining several specific parameters. The first is whether the mass is cystic, complex, or solid. This can be accomplished with a combination of gray-scale and color Doppler imaging using techniques described in earlier sections. The second is localizing where the mass is located and what structure the mass arises from. The third is determining the relationships of the mass to adjacent structures. The fourth is determining the vascularity of the lesion and whether it is primarily a vascular abnormality. The combination of all this information may not allow for a specific histologic diagnosis, but it will usually provide enough information to guide further management decisions (Fig. 11-17).

There are a number of extremity masses that are commonly encountered. Ganglion cysts are one of the most common causes for palpable masses in the hand and wrist. There are four typical locations. Approximately 70% originate from the scapholunate joint over the

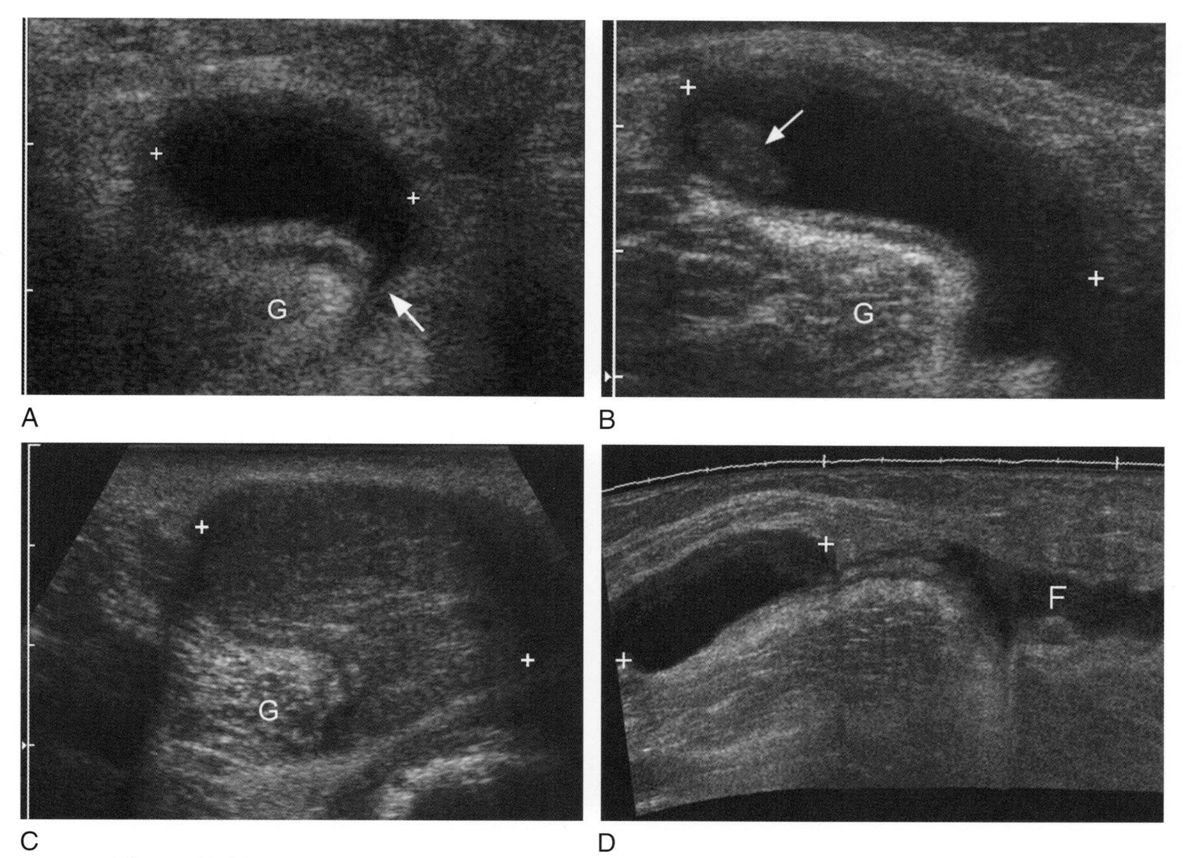

Figure 11-15 Baker's cysts in different patients. **A,** Transverse view of the posterior knee shows a well-defined cystic lesion *(cursors)* adjacent to the medial head of the gastrocnemius muscle (G). Typical beak *(arrow)* that is often seen with Baker's cysts is shown well on this image. **B,** Transverse view shows a Baker's cyst *(cursors)* adjacent to the medial head of the gastrocnemius muscle (G). A small solid nodule *(arrow)* is shown in this image, and similar findings are frequently seen in Baker's cysts. **C,** Transverse view shows a large Baker's cyst *(cursors)* that is filled with diffuse, slightly heterogeneous, but predominately low-level echoes. This appearance is not uncommon with inflammatory arthritis and can represent either proliferative synovium or fibrinous blood clot. **D,** Longitudinal view of the knee and calf shows a Baker's cyst *(cursors)* that has ruptured with fluid (F) dissecting into the calf.

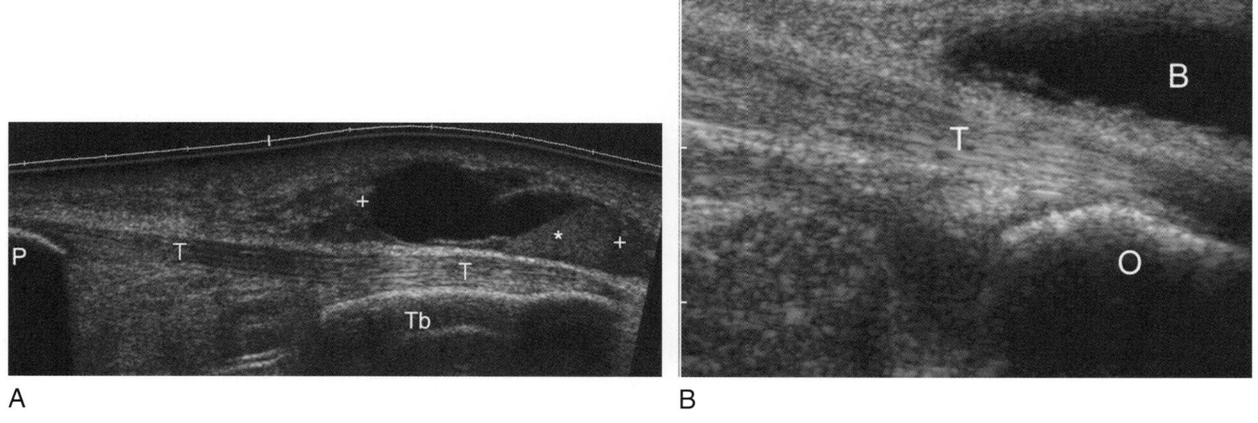

Figure 11-16 Bursitis in two different patients. **A,** Longitudinal view of the knee shows a distended infrapatellar superficial bursa *(cursors)* containing fluid as well as layering blood (*). The patellar tendon (T) is seen immediately posteriorly. Also seen are the patella (P) and the proximal tibia (Tb). **B,** Longitudinal view of the posterior elbow shows fluid distending the olecranon bursa (B). Also seen is the insertion of the triceps tendon (T) into the olecranon process (O).

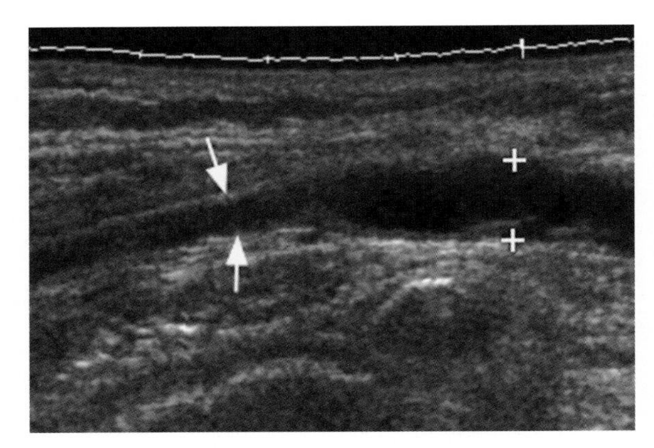

Figure 11-17 Ganglion cyst of the peroneal nerve. Longitudinal view of the posterior knee shows an elongated cystic lesion *(cursors)* that is shown to arise from the peroneal nerve *(arrows)*.

dorsal surface of the wrist (Fig. 11-18A). Approximately 20% arise on the volar side of the wrist around the flexor carpi radialis tendon or the radial artery (see Fig. 11-18B). Approximately 10% of cysts arise along one of the flexor tendon sheaths of the fingers (see Fig. 11-18C). Finally, cysts can arise from the interphalangeal joints, usually owing to underlying degenerative arthritis. Although they are very common in the hand and wrist, they can be seen around many other joints. Although ganglion cysts are filled with thick mucinous fluid, they are still typically anechoic with well-defined walls. Through transmission is usually detectable unless the cyst is small. In some cases, a neck may be seen leading toward the joint of origin. With large ganglia, there are often folds or septations, particularly near the neck.

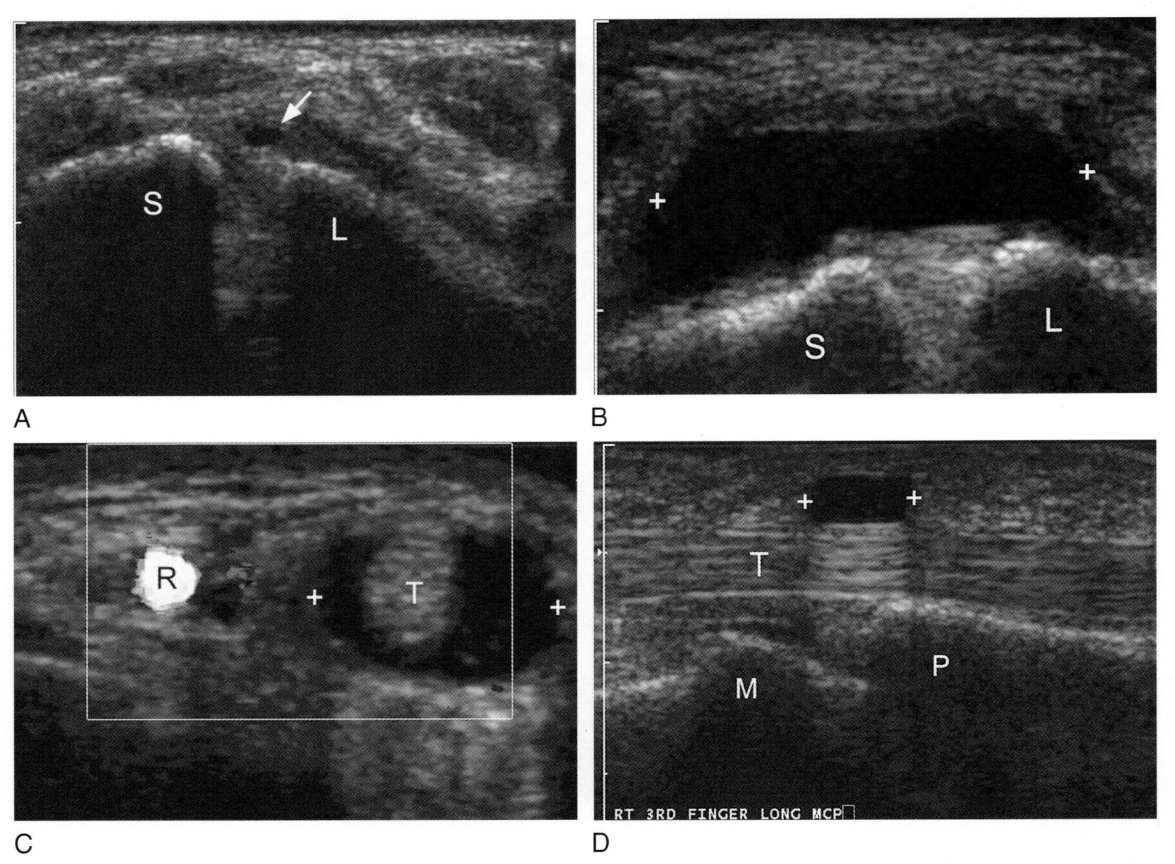

Figure 11-18 Ganglion cysts of the wrist in different patients. **A,** Transverse view of the dorsal surface of the wrist at the level of the joint between the scaphoid (S) and the lunate (L) shows a 2-mm ganglion cyst *(arrow)* immediately over the joint. **B,** Transverse view over the scaphoid (S) and lunate (L) shows a large ganglion cyst *(cursors)* immediately over the joint. **C,** Transverse view over the volar aspect of the wrist shows the radial artery (R) and the extensor carpi radialis tendon (T). A localized ganglion cyst *(cursors)* is seen partially surrounding the tendon. **D,** Longitudinal view of the middle finger shows a ganglion cyst *(cursors)* associated with the flexor tendons (T). The joint between the metacarpal (M) and the proximal phalanx (P) is seen deep to the tendon.

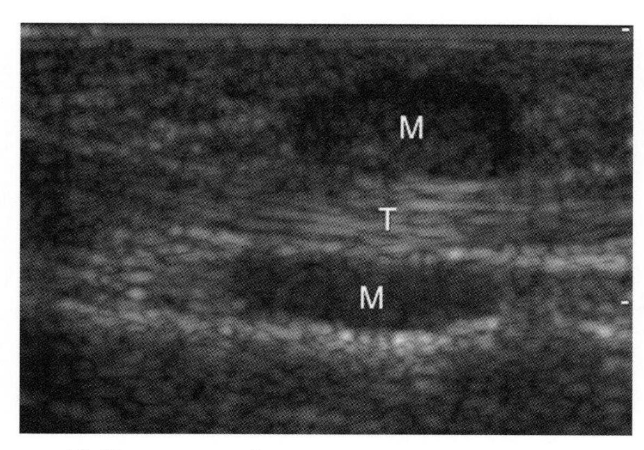

Figure 11-19 Giant cell tumor. Longitudinal view of the thumb shows a solid mass (M) that extends around the superficial and deep aspect of the flexor pollicis longus tendon (T).

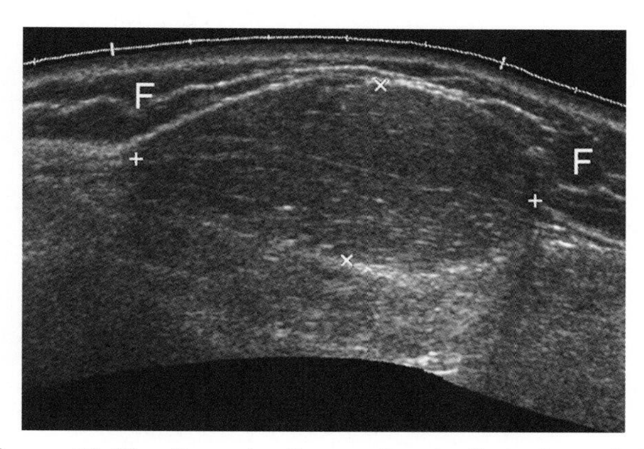

Figure 11-20 Extremity lipoma. Longitudinal view of the shoulder shows an encapsulated soft tissue mass *(cursors)* that is similar in echogenicity to the adjacent subcutaneous fat (F).

Giant cell tumors represent the second most common cause of a mass in the hand. They are benign lesions that are histologically identical to pigmented villonodular synovitis. They are typically slow growing and painless and occur along the volar surface of the fingers. Giant cell tumors are solid, homogeneous, hypoechoic masses that are adjacent to tendons and often partially surround the tendon (Fig. 11-19). However, because they arise from the sheath and not the tendon, they do not move with the tendon when the finger is flexed and extended. High-frequency color Doppler imaging will generally show readily detectable internal blood flow, and the lesions may be quite vascular.

Extremity subcutaneous lipomas are also common. Their echogenicity is variable, and, unlike fatty tumors in most organs, they are often not hyperechoic. They are often isoechoic to subcutaneous fat. They may or may not be encapsulated (Fig. 11-20). As on physical examination, they are usually very compressible with transducer pressure. Color Doppler sonography generally shows little, if any, internal blood flow.

Lymphadenopathy is frequently encountered in the extremities. High-resolution transducers are capable of routinely identifying normal lymph nodes in the axilla and the groin. They are hypoechoic and oval and usually have a detectable central echogenic hilum. As in the neck, there is overlap in the appearance of reactive and neoplastic lymphadenopathy (Fig. 11-21). Neoplasms should be considered when there is a history of lymphoma or a primary malignancy or when the nodes become rounded and the hilum is obliterated.

Masses of the peripheral nerves can occasionally be diagnosed with sonography if they arise from nerves that are big enough to be seen (Fig. 11-22). Tumors in the middle of nerves are usually neurofibromas, and tumors at the periphery are usually schwannomas. Tumors of small nerves are nonspecific and can only be diagnosed with surgical resection. Most nerve tumors are solid, hypoechoic, and vascular. Morton's neuromas are relatively common benign masses of the plantar digital nerves of the foot. The common symptoms are pain and paresthesias. Their location between the metatarsal heads is the key to the diagnosis.

Inflammatory processes can produce localized pain as well as localized swelling. A common clinical scenario is a patient with localized cellulitis and question of underlying abscess. Simple cellulitis produces edema fluid that dissects in the fibrous retinaculum of the subcutaneous fat. This typically results in a marbled appearance without a discrete fluid collection (Fig. 11-23A). On the other hand, cellulitis that results from an underlying abscess will have a discrete collection that usually appears complex (see Fig. 11-23B).

FOREIGN BODIES

Post-traumatic foreign bodies can be a source of chronic pain, swelling, and/or infection. Sonography is an excellent way to detect and localize superficial foreign bodies. Identification is close to 100% for foreign bodies as small as 1 × 4 mm in the palms and just slightly less for objects in the fingers. All foreign bodies appear as a bright reflector (Fig. 11-24A). They may or may not be associated with an adjacent hypoechoic inflammatory process or an adjacent abscess. Acoustic shadowing may be seen if the foreign body is large enough to block a significant amount of the ultrasound beam (see Fig. 11-24B). Glass or metallic objects may show ring-down or comet-tail artifacts. If adjacent inflammation is present, color or power Doppler imaging may demonstrate surrounding hyperemia (see Fig. 11-24C).

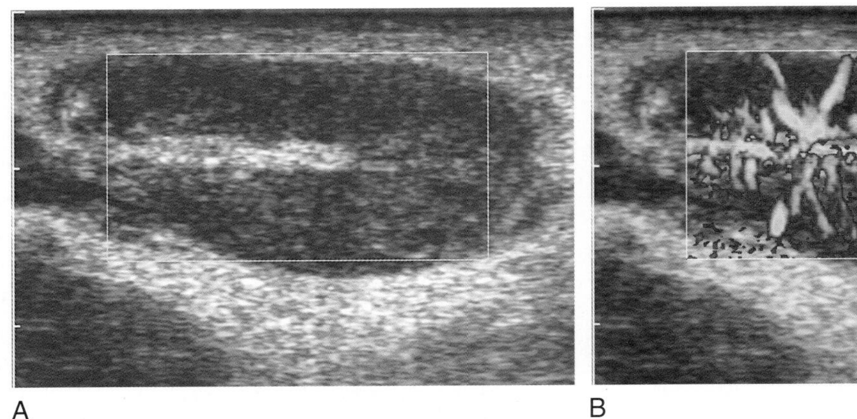

A B

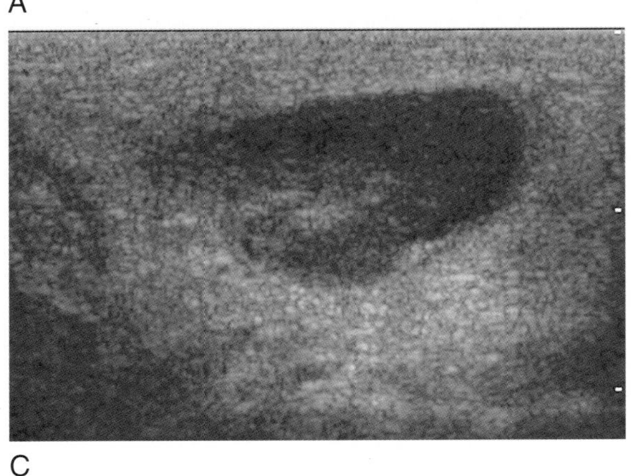

C

Figure 11-21 Lymphadenopathy in different patients. **A** and **B,** Gray-scale (**A**) and power Doppler (**B**) views of the groin show a solid hypoechoic lesion with a linear central echogenic component that extends to the periphery typical of a lymph node with its fatty hilum. Readily detectable hypervascular blood flow in this case is typical of active lymphoma. **C,** View of the groin in a young man with an inguinal abscess shows a reactive lymph node that has features similar to the neoplastic node shown in **A** and **B**.

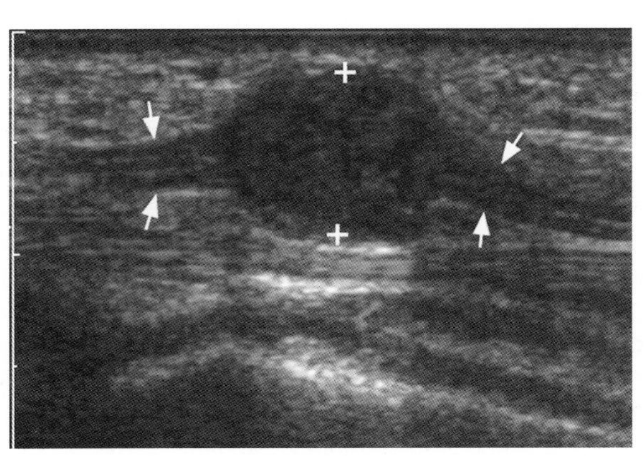

Figure 11-22 Neural tumor. Longitudinal view of the ulnar nerve *(arrows)* shows a solid homogeneous hypoechoic mass *(cursors)* that clearly arises from the nerve. There is increased through transmission that is commonly seen with peripheral nerve tumors.

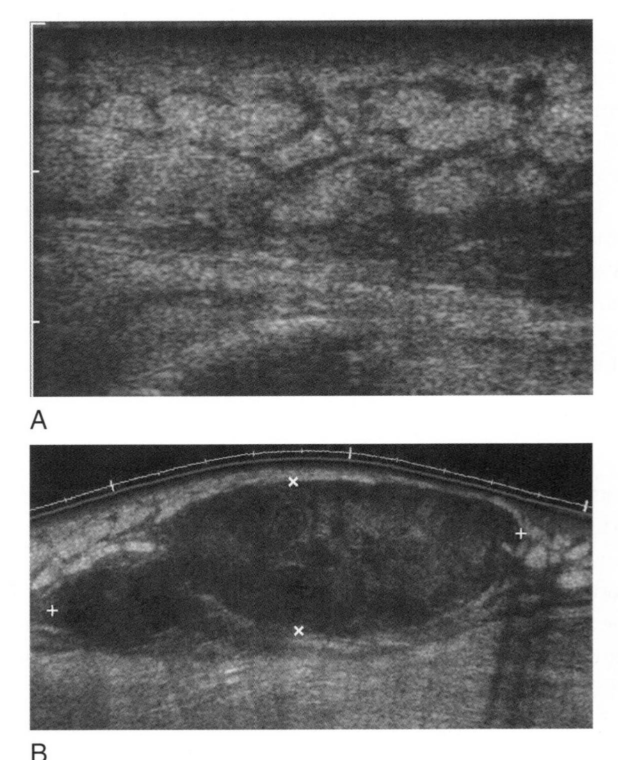

Figure 11-23 Extremity inflammation. **A,** View of the subcutaneous tissues of the thigh in a patient with cellulitis shows the typical marbling pattern in the subcutaneous fat produced by swelling of any type. **B,** Longitudinal view of the subcutaneous tissues of another patient shows a large complex lobulated fluid collection *(cursors)* with adjacent inflammatory changes in the subcutaneous fat due to an abscess.

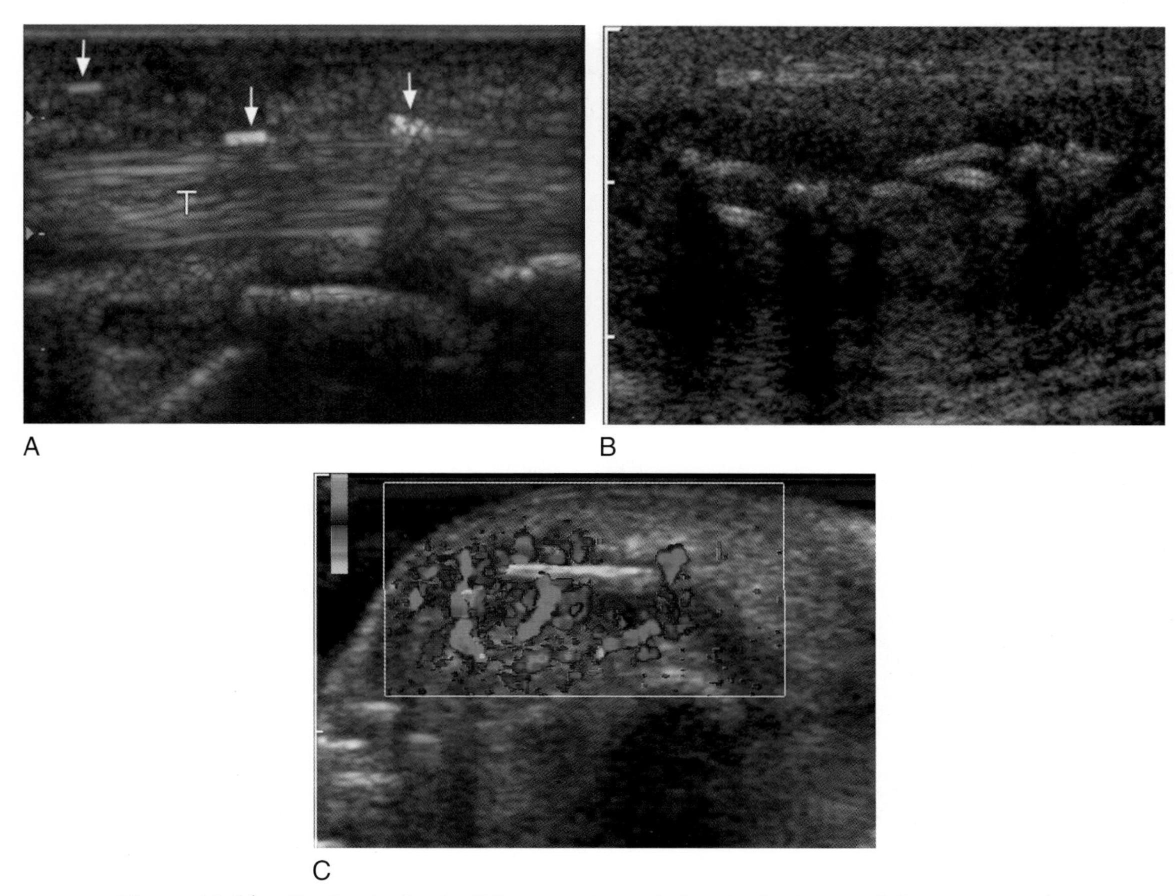

Figure 11-24 Foreign bodies in different patients. **A,** Longitudinal view of the metacarpophalangeal region of the index finger shows three separate hyperechoic linear structures *(arrows),* one of which produces a faint shadow. These were glass fragments from a broken pipette. The flexor tendons (T) are seen deep to the foreign bodies. **B,** Longitudinal view of the region of the Achilles tendon in a patient who is status post repair of a rupture, with subsequent postoperative abscess formation. Multiple hyperechoic linear reflectors are identified, some of which produce shadowing. Note the parallel lines seen within several of these structures. This is typical of suture material that in this case was acting as a foreign body nidus for persistent infection. **C,** Transverse color Doppler view of the base of the third finger shows a linear hyperechoic reflector due to a wooden splinter. There is intense surrounding hyperemia due to the associated inflammatory reaction.

JOINTS

In addition to evaluating the articular and periarticular abnormalities discussed earlier in this chapter, sonography can also be used to detect and guide aspiration of joint effusions. The configuration of joint fluid varies depending on the joint being scanned. The echogenicity of fluid also varies. Most reactive effusions are anechoic or have few internal echoes (Fig. 11-25A). Septic effusions, particularly those in superficial joints, usually have detectable internal echoes (see Fig. 11-25B) and are occasionally hyperechoic. Lipohemarthroses related to trauma can appear as multiple fluid layers (see Fig. 11-25C).

In some patients, synovial diseases will simulate or coexist with effusions. Proliferative synovium can appear diffusely and concentrically thickened, eccentrically thickened, nodular, or complex (Fig. 11-26). Clinical and laboratory correlation is usually required to determine the etiology of synovial proliferation.

BONES

As mentioned earlier, sonography is not a primary means of evaluating the bones because the medullary cavity of bones is not visible. However, sonography is an excellent means of visualizing the surface of bones, and diseases that affect the surface can be evaluated

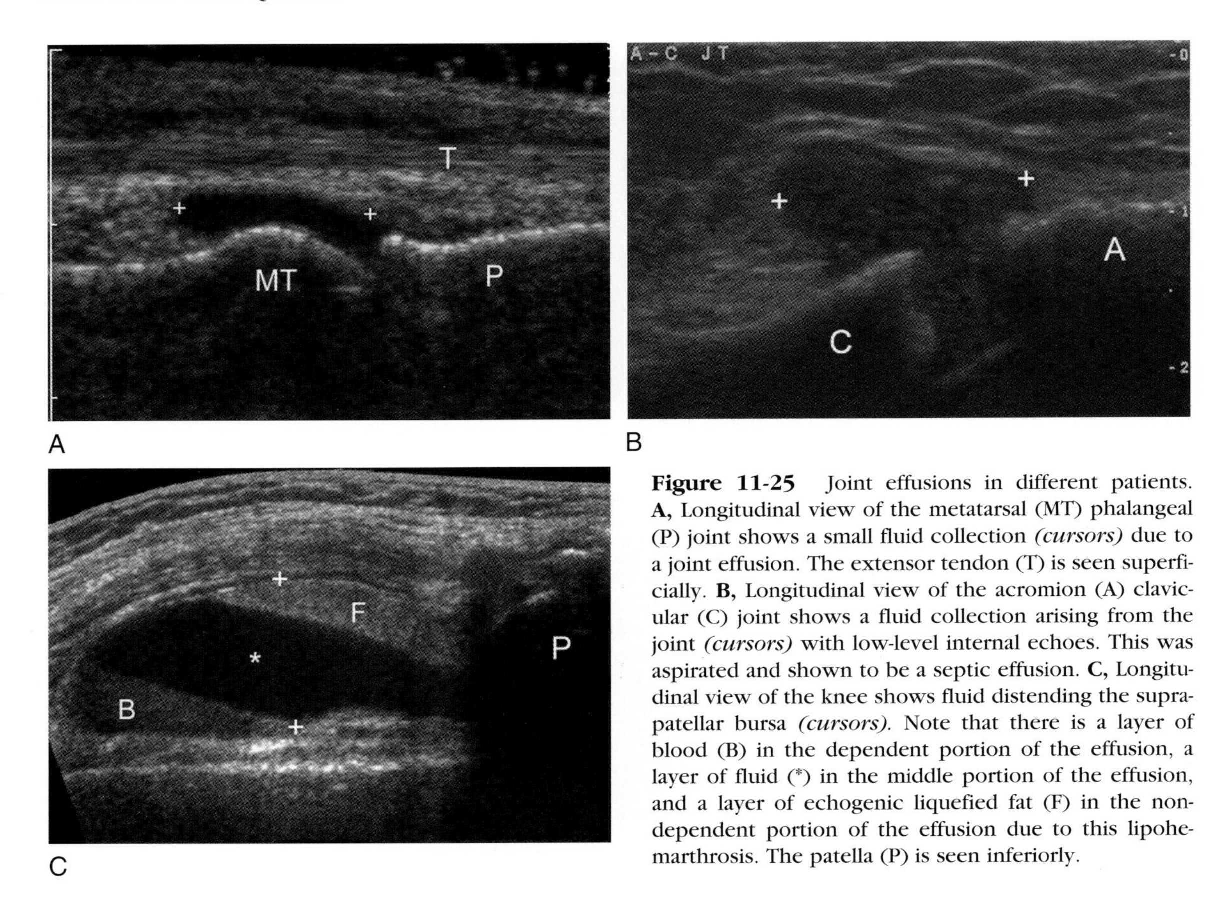

Figure 11-25 Joint effusions in different patients. **A,** Longitudinal view of the metatarsal (MT) phalangeal (P) joint shows a small fluid collection *(cursors)* due to a joint effusion. The extensor tendon (T) is seen superficially. **B,** Longitudinal view of the acromion (A) clavicular (C) joint shows a fluid collection arising from the joint *(cursors)* with low-level internal echoes. This was aspirated and shown to be a septic effusion. **C,** Longitudinal view of the knee shows fluid distending the suprapatellar bursa *(cursors)*. Note that there is a layer of blood (B) in the dependent portion of the effusion, a layer of fluid (*) in the middle portion of the effusion, and a layer of echogenic liquefied fat (F) in the nondependent portion of the effusion due to this lipohemarthrosis. The patella (P) is seen inferiorly.

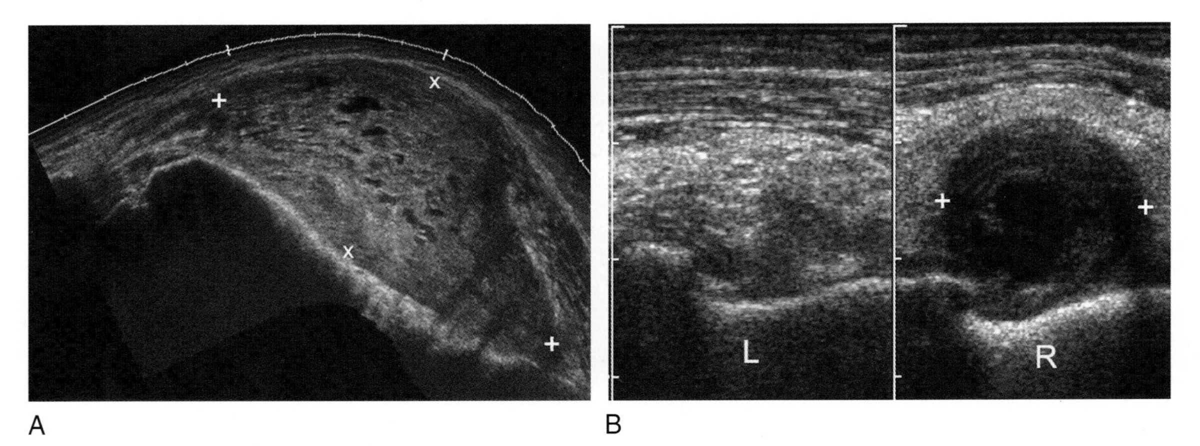

Figure 11-26 Proliferative synovium in different patients with rheumatoid arthritis. **A,** Longitudinal extended field of view scan of the shoulder shows a markedly enlarged subdeltoid bursa filled with solid and cystic proliferative synovium *(cursors)*. **B,** Dual longitudinal views of the elbow joint at the level of the radial head show the normal appearance of the left elbow and a mass anterior to the right elbow due to joint fluid and thickened hypoechoic synovium.

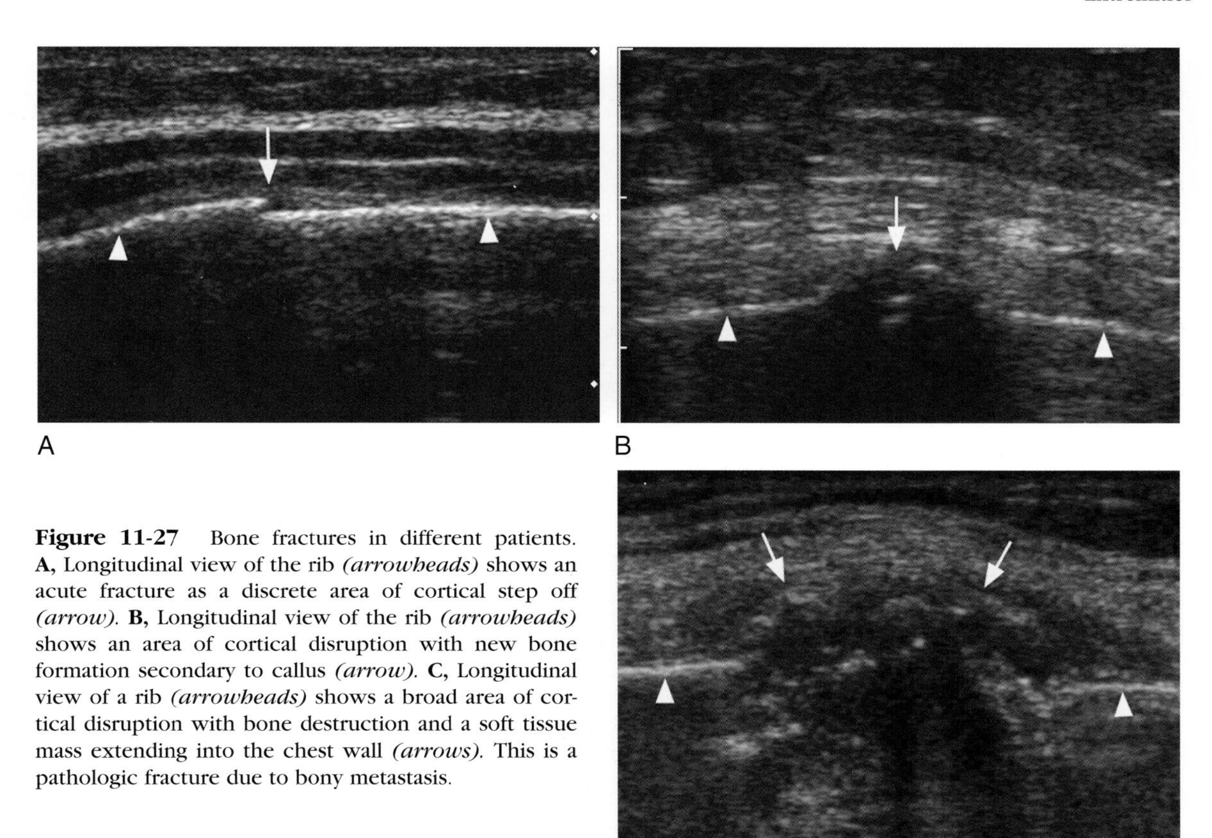

Figure 11-27 Bone fractures in different patients. **A,** Longitudinal view of the rib *(arrowheads)* shows an acute fracture as a discrete area of cortical step off *(arrow)*. **B,** Longitudinal view of the rib *(arrowheads)* shows an area of cortical disruption with new bone formation secondary to callus *(arrow)*. **C,** Longitudinal view of a rib *(arrowheads)* shows a broad area of cortical disruption with bone destruction and a soft tissue mass extending into the chest wall *(arrows)*. This is a pathologic fracture due to bony metastasis.

sonographically. One particular area that has been used in some practices is detection of occult fractures. Nondisplaced fractures can be difficult to detect radiologically, especially in the acute period. On sonography, the area that is painful can be imaged precisely, and disruptions in the surface of the bone can be readily identified (Fig. 11-27A). Over time, callus will form and the surface of the bone will expand and become irregular (see Fig. 11-27B). Pathologic fractures can be distinguished from benign fractures by detecting bone destruction and an associated soft tissue mass (see Fig. 11-27C). Other uses of sonography in bone disease are the early detection of erosions in patients with erosive arthritis, detection of subperiosteal abscess in osteomyelitis, and direction of percutaneous biopsies in patients with suspected metastases and abscesses.

EXTREMITY VESSELS

Normal Hemodynamics

The waveform of normal extremity arteries has a high-resistance profile. There is a sharp, narrow, systolic peak, followed by a short phase of reversed early diastolic flow, followed by another short phase of antegrade flow (Fig. 11-28A). The short period of early diastolic flow reversal is due to elastic recoil of the larger extremity arteries. This waveform appearance is referred to as triphasic and is typical of extremity arteries in a resting individual. After exercise, the waveform will convert to a low-resistance pattern. Extremity venous flow varies depending on location. Veins that are close to the heart will show pulsations related to the cardiac cycle. Veins that are farther away from the heart have much fewer cardiac pulsations but demonstrate gentle phasicity related to the respiratory cycle (see Fig. 11-28B).

Venous Thrombosis

Ultrasound is now the procedure of choice in the evaluation of suspected lower extremity deep vein thrombosis (DVT). In the femoral-popliteal system of symptomatic patients, the sensitivity and specificity exceed 95% and 98%, respectively. The results are more variable in the calf and in asymptomatic patients who are at risk for DVT due to hip and knee surgery.

Normal deep veins are completely compressible (Fig. 11-29). DVT is diagnosed when the veins fail to

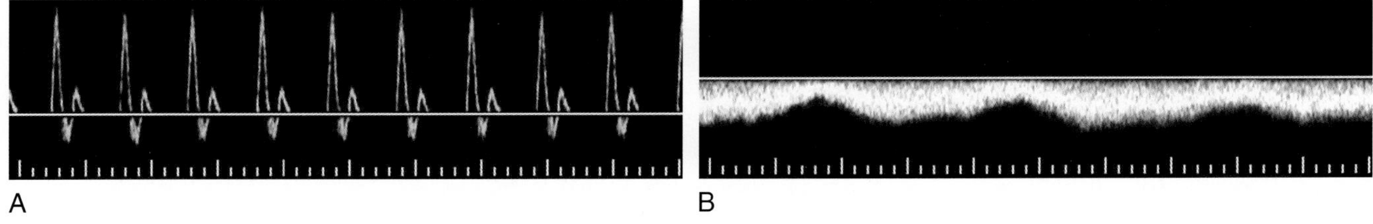

Figure 11-28 Normal extremity hemodynamics. **A,** Ten seconds long waveform from the superficial femoral artery shows the typical triphasic pattern with antegrade flow in systole followed by a transient phase of retrograde flow in early diastole followed by a phase of antegrade flow in mid diastole. No flow is seen in end diastole. **B,** Ten seconds long waveform from the superficial femoral vein shows gentle phasicity related to the respiratory cycle. There are no pulsations related to the cardiac cycle.

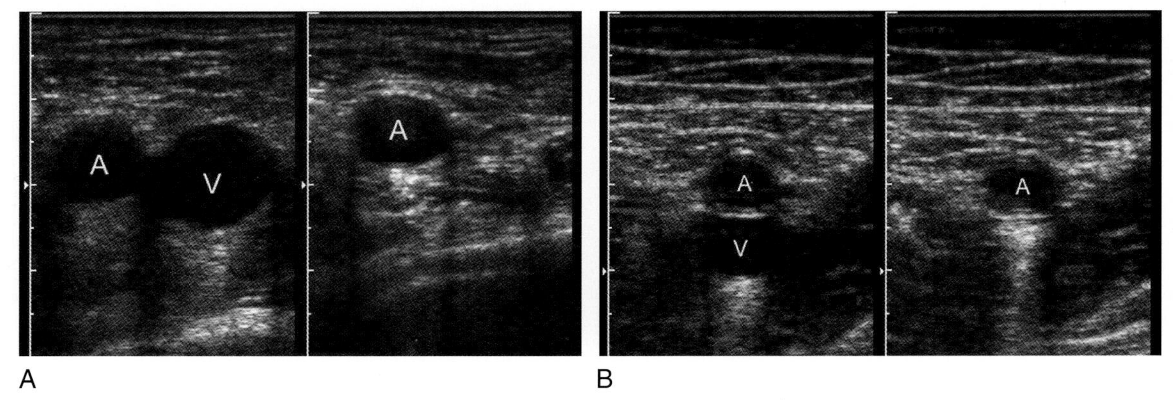

Figure 11-29 Normal extremity venous compressibility. **A,** Transverse dual images of the common femoral artery (A) and vein (V) obtained without *(left side)* and with *(right side)* compression. **B,** Transverse dual images of the superficial femoral artery (A) and vein (V) obtained without compression *(left side)* and with *(right side)* compression. Note the complete compression of the femoral vein during the compression maneuver.

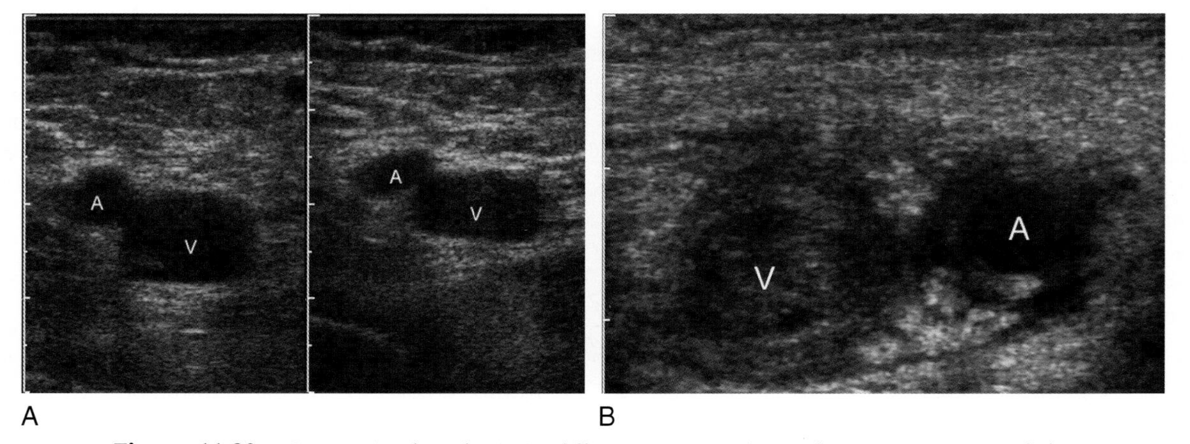

Figure 11-30 Deep vein thrombosis in different patients. **A,** Dual transverse views of the common femoral artery (A) and vein (V) obtained without *(left side)* and with *(right side)* compression. Note the lack of full compressibility of the femoral vein despite enough pressure to produce partial compression of the femoral artery. **B,** Transverse view of the common femoral artery (A) and vein (V) shows echogenic clot filling the lumen of the vein. Also note the inflammatory changes in the tissues around the femoral vein.

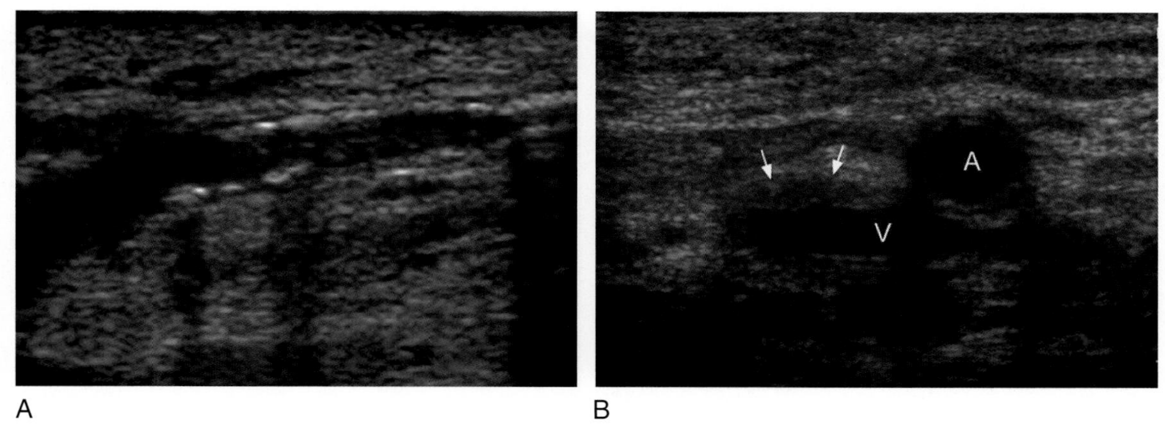

Figure 11-31 Chronic deep vein thrombosis in different patients. **A,** Longitudinal view of the femoral vein shows shadowing calcification along the wall of the vessel. **B,** Transverse view of the femoral artery (A) and vein (V) shows chronic organized clot incorporated into the superficial venous wall producing wall thickening *(arrows)*.

compress completely (Fig. 11-30A). In some cases, thrombus can be seen on gray-scale imaging (Fig. 11-30B). However, the appearance of artifactual intraluminal echoes overlaps with the hypoechoic echoes from clot. Therefore, analysis of echogenicity is not a primary focus of lower extremity venous examinations.

In obese or very edematous persons, gray-scale identification of the femoral and popliteal veins may be very difficult. In these situations, color Doppler imaging may help to localize the vessels. Augmentation of proximal venous flow by compression of the calf or plantar flexion of the foot can accentuate the veins and further assist when color Doppler imaging is required.

After an episode of acute DVT, the vein will either return to a normal appearance and normal function or clot resorption may leave various sequelae that may compromise valvular function and lead to the post-phlebitic syndrome. On sonography, chronic sequelae usually occur and stabilize within 6 months of the initial thrombosis and include focal eccentric thickening of the vein wall, or diffuse thickening of the vein wall, or calcification of the wall, or development of irregular channels within the partially recanalized vein lumen (Fig. 11-31). Because these chronic changes can be difficult to distinguish from acute changes, some experts advocate a repeat ultrasound evaluation after 6 months to establish a new baseline for comparison in case the patient returns with recurrent symptoms and the question of acute versus chronic DVT is raised.

Another result of venous thrombosis or any cause of venous obstruction is alteration of the venous waveform. This occurs because the vein becomes isolated and the normal venous pulsations and phasicity become blunted. It provides a clue to a more central obstruction, especially when the waveforms from the left and right side are asymmetric (Fig. 11-32). This is especially important in diagnosing subclavian vein obstruction because the obstructing process (thrombosis, stenosis, or extrinsic compression) is often hidden in the mediastinum.

Pseudoaneurysms

Postcatheterization pseudoaneurysms are hematomas that maintain an internal area of extravascular blood flow via a patent neck that communicates with the femoral artery. With time, a fibrous capsule will develop around the pseudoaneurysm. Typically, they present as pain, swelling, and ecchymosis in the first 1 or 2 days after the procedure.

On sonography, pseudoaneurysms must be distinguished from simple hematomas (Fig. 11-33A). Both will appear as a complex fluid collection near or adjacent to the artery. If expansion and contraction are seen on real-time imaging, then the two can be distinguished on gray-scale imaging. Sometimes this is difficult to

Box 11-3 Characteristics of Pseudoaneurysms

Complex fluid collection
Single or multiple loculations
Visible pulsations on gray-scale imaging
Internal luminal flow on color Doppler imaging
"To and fro" flow in the neck

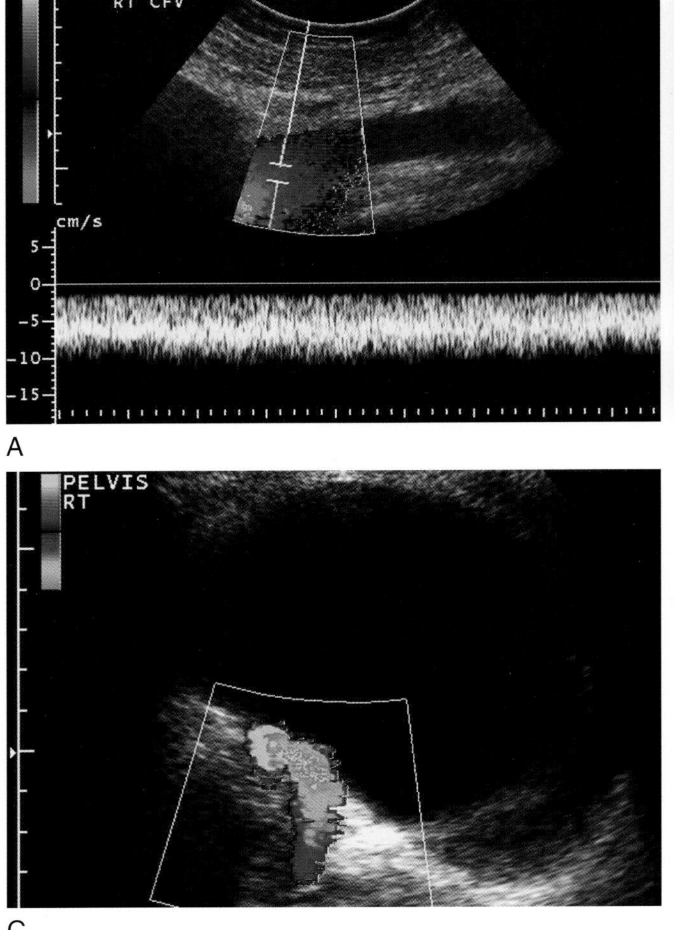

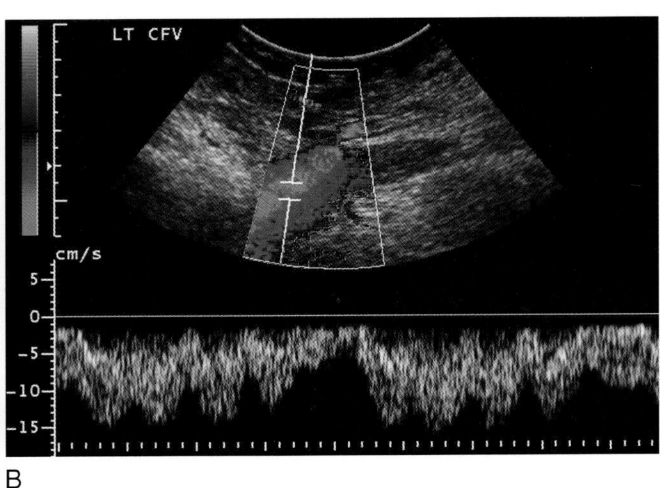

Figure 11-32 Alteration of hemodynamics with venous obstruction. **A,** Longitudinal view of the right common femoral vein with pulsed Doppler waveform shows a flattened waveform with no respiratory phasicity. **B,** Longitudinal view and waveform from the left common femoral vein shows respiratory phasicity as well as transmitted pulsatility from the heart. **C,** View of the right pelvis shows a large lymphocele adjacent to the femoral vessels. This lymphocele produced partial venous obstruction, accounting for the alteration in venous hemodynamics.

distinguish from transmitted pulsations. Solid thrombus is not uncommon in hematomas and at the periphery of pseudoaneurysms.

The key to diagnosing pseudoaneurysms is detecting flowing blood in the lumen with color Doppler. There are many patterns of internal flow depending on the direction of the inflow jet into the aneurysm lumen. The typical pattern is a swirling or "yin-yang" appearance where one half of the lumen is red and the other half is blue. Flow in the neck of the pseudoaneurysm is also unique because systolic flow into the aneurysm and diastolic flow out of the aneurysm occur in sequence in the neck. This produces the "to and fro" waveform on pulsed Doppler with systolic flow above the baseline and pandiastolic flow reversal below the baseline (see Fig. 11-33C). It is not uncommon for there to be multiple loculations connected to each other through narrow tracts (see Fig. 11-33D).

Most pseudoaneurysms can be treated with thrombin injection under ultrasound guidance. Compared with compression repair, this is much faster, almost painless, easier, and more successful and does not require termination of anticoagulation. Techniques vary, but one approach is to fill a 1-mL syringe with saline and 1000 units of thrombin. The amount of thrombin needed varies with the size of the pseudoaneurysm. Usually the aneurysms will thrombose when just a portion of the thrombin solution is injected with a 25-gauge needle (Fig. 11-34). Thrombin injection is contraindicated when the neck to the pseudoaneurysm is wide or when the pseudoaneurysm is part of an arteriovenous fistula. The distal pulses should be checked before the procedure and monitored carefully after the procedure.

Arteriovenous Fistulas

Postcatheterization arteriovenous fistulas (AVF) rarely cause symptoms, unless they are very large, in which case high-output stress on the heart or ischemic symptoms in the lower extremity are possible. They are usually below the bifurcation of the femoral vessels because

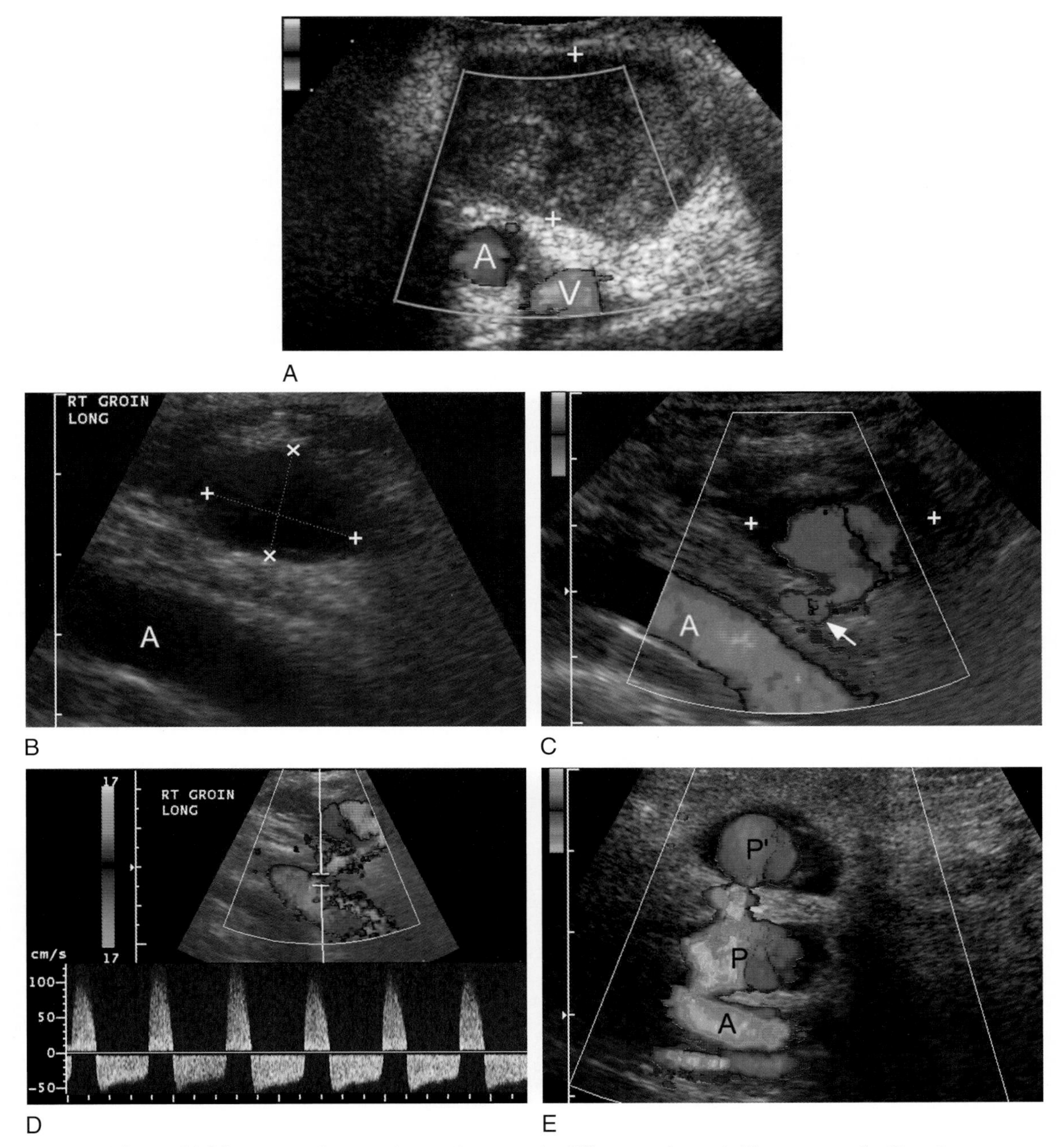

Figure 11-33 Postcatheterization groin masses in different patients. **A,** Transverse color Doppler view of the groin shows a complex fluid collection without internal blood flow *(cursors)* anterior to the femoral artery (A) and vein (V). This is a typical appearance for a hematoma. **B** to **D,** Longitudinal gray-scale (**B**), color Doppler (**C**), and pulsed Doppler (**D**) views of the right groin show a nonspecific fluid collection *(cursors)* anterior to the femoral artery (A) on gray-scale imaging. On color Doppler this fluid collection shows the classic swirling or yin-yang pattern within the pseudoaneurysm lumen and a discrete neck directed toward the femoral artery *(arrow).* Pulsed Doppler waveform from the neck shows a classic to-and-fro pattern with antegrade flow during systole and retrograde flow throughout the diastolic portion of the cardiac cycle. All of these features are typical of a pseudoaneurysm. **E,** Longitudinal color Doppler view of the groin shows a pseudoaneurysm arising from the femoral artery (A) with a deep component (P) and a superficial component (P′).

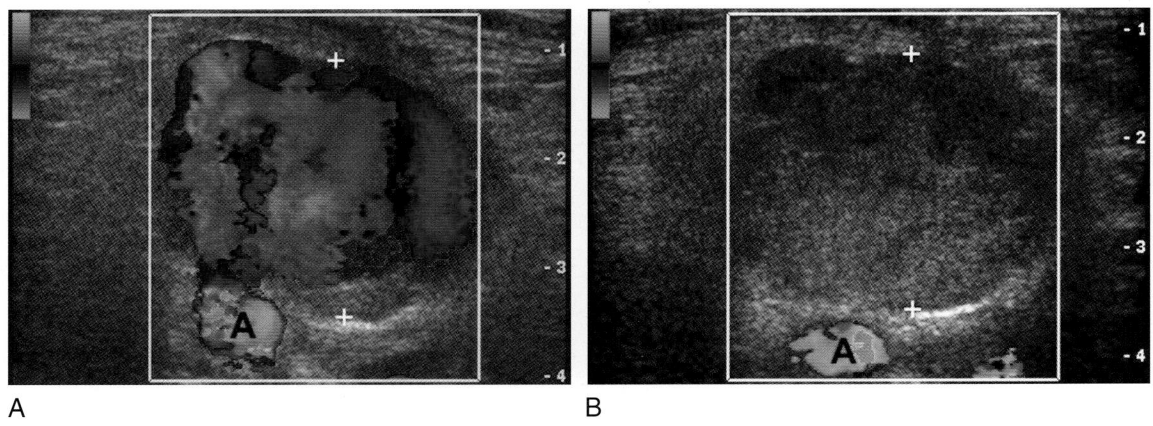

Figure 11-34 Percutaneous treatment of a pseudoaneurysm. **A,** Transverse view of the groin shows a large pseudoaneurysm *(cursors)* anterior to the femoral artery (A). **B,** Similar view immediately after injection of 300 units of thrombin shows low-level echoes throughout the lumen of the aneurysm due to clot and no residual blood flow within the pseudoaneurysm.

the vein starts to travel behind the artery so that it becomes easier to simultaneously puncture both vessels. In addition, a branch of the femoral vein frequently travels between the superficial femoral artery and the profunda artery, and this can be the vein that is involved in the fistula.

Gray-scale changes are rare with AVFs, so it is important to recognize the hemodynamic changes that occur (Fig. 11-35). The low-resistance runoff afforded by the direct arterial communication with the vein causes the arterial waveform to change from the typical high-resistance triphasic pattern to a low-resistance pattern with more diastolic flow. On color Doppler imaging, continuous systolic and diastolic flow is seen in the artery immediately adjacent to the fistula, whereas no flow is seen during diastole in the segments of the artery that are not close to the fistula. On the venous side, the arterial flow entering the compliant vein causes a marked flow disturbance in the vein. This is seen as a haphazard arrangement of intraluminal color and as a distorted and unusually high-velocity venous waveform. In some cases, an arterial pattern can be seen in the venous waveform. The most obvious change seen on color Doppler images is usually perivascular tissue vibration. As discussed in Chapter 1, this is caused by turbulent blood flow and is the color Doppler equivalent of a thrill. It manifests as a mixture of random red and

Box 11-4 Characteristics of Iatrogenic Arteriovenous Fistulas

Usually located below the femoral bifurcation
Perivascular tissue vibration
Low-resistance flow in supplying artery near fistula
High-velocity flow at site of communication
Turbulent and/or arterialized flow in draining vein near fistula

Figure 11-35 Arteriovenous fistula. **A,** Longitudinal view of the femoral bifurcation obtained in systole shows the superficial femoral artery (SF), profunda femoral artery (PF), and the superficial femoral vein (V). **B,** Similar view obtained during end diastole shows cessation of flow in the superficial femoral artery but maintained flow in the proximal profunda femoral artery, suggesting an arteriovenous fistula arising from the profunda femoral artery. **C,** Transverse view through this region shows extensive, random, red and blue color assignment in the tissues around the vessels owing to perivascular soft tissue vibration. **D,** Pulsed Doppler waveform from the superficial femoral artery shows normal high resistance blood flow with early diastolic flow reversal. **E,** Pulsed Doppler waveform from the profunda femoral artery shows abnormal extremity arterial flow with a low resistance pattern and high levels of diastolic flow throughout the cardiac cycle. **F,** Pulsed Doppler waveform from the superficial femoral vein at the site of the fistula shows turbulent flow with an arterialization of the venous waveform. **G,** Pulsed Doppler waveform from the fistula site between the profunda femoral artery and the femoral vein shows extremely high velocity flow with a very low resistance pattern.

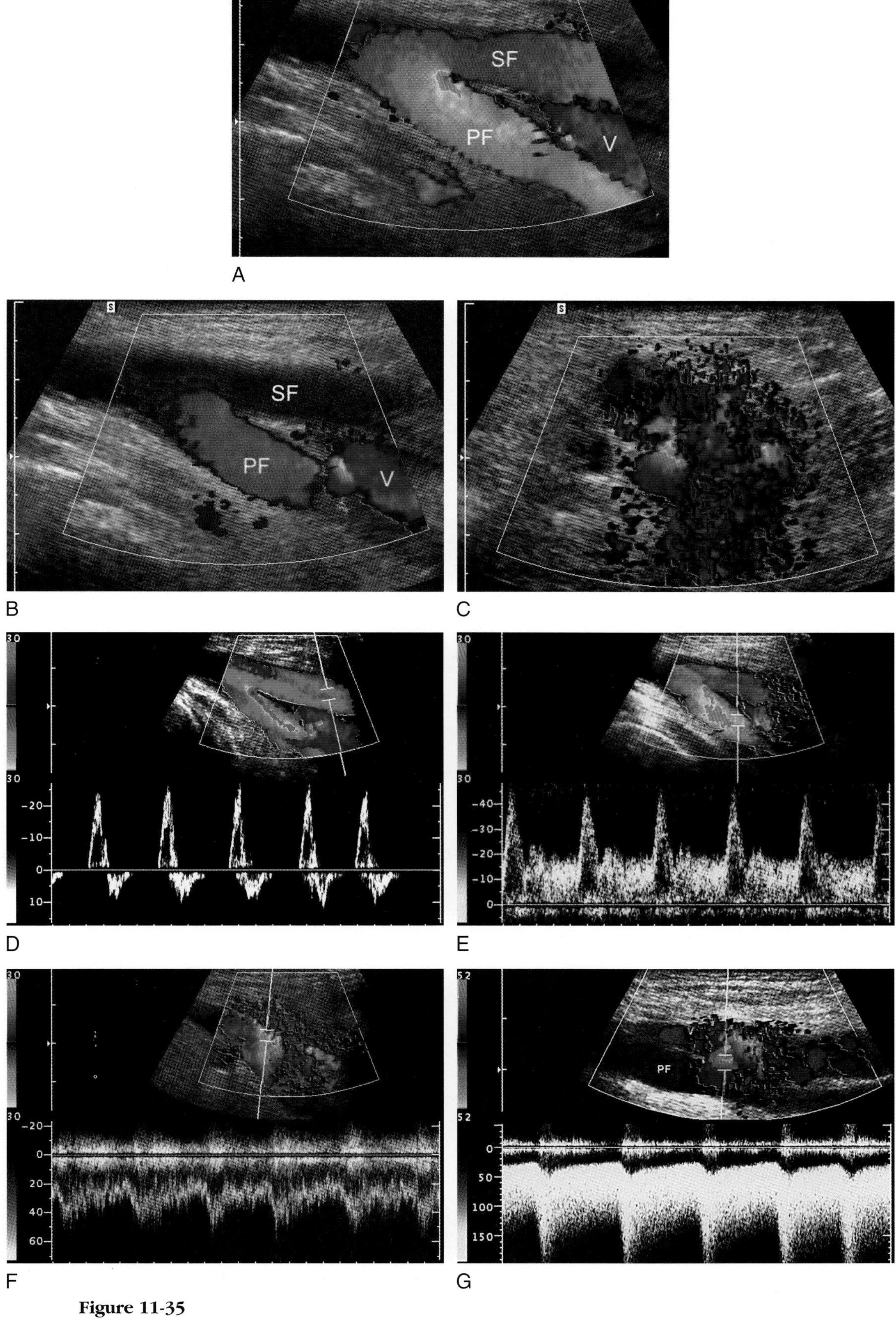

Figure 11-35

blue color assignment in the perivascular soft tissue. The differential diagnosis for tissue vibration includes arterial stenoses and aneurysms, but it is usually much more pronounced with AVFs. Finally, it is sometimes possible to actually visualize the tract that connects the artery and vein on color Doppler imaging. Even when the communication is not seen, the localized hemodynamic changes just described provide convincing evidence that an AVF is present.

SUGGESTED READINGS

Beggs I: Sonographic appearances of nerve tumors. J Clin Ultrasound 27:363-368, 1999.

Belli P, Costantini M, Mirk P, et al: Sonographic diagnosis of distal biceps tendon rupture: A prospective study of 25 cases. J Ultrasound Med 20:587-595, 2001.

Bianchi S, Martinoli C, Abdelwahab IF, et al: Sonographic evaluation of tears of the gastrocnemius medial head ("tennis leg"). J Ultrasound Med 17:157-162, 1998.

Blam O, Bindra R, Middleton W, Gelberman R: The occult dorsal carpal ganglion: Usefulness of magnetic resonance imaging and ultrasound in diagnosis. Am J Orthop 27:107-110, 1998.

Boyse TD, Fessell DP, Jacobson JA, et al: US of soft-tissue foreign bodies and associated complications with surgical correlation. Radiographics 21:1251-1256, 2001.

Bray PW, Mahoney JL, Campbell JP: Sensitivity and specificity of ultrasound in the diagnosis of foreign bodies in the hand. J Hand Surg [Am] 20:661-666, 1995.

Bruneton JN, Rubaltelli L, Solbiati L: Lymph nodes. In Solbiati L, Rizzatto G (eds): Ultrasound of Superficial Structures. Edinburgh, Churchill Livingstone, 1995, pp 279-302.

Bureau NJ, Chhem RK, Cardinal E: Musculoskeletal Infections: US Manifestations. Radiographics 19:1585-1592, 1999.

Cardinal E, Buckwalter KA, Braunstein EM, Mih AD: Occult dorsal carpal ganglion: Comparison of US and MR imaging. Radiology 193:259-262, 1994.

Cardinal E, Chhem RK, Beauregard CG, et al: Plantar fasciitis: Sonographic evaluation. Radiology 201:257-259, 1996.

Cooke KS, Kirpekar M, Abiri MM, Shreefter C: US case of the day: Skeletal metastasis from poorly differentiated carcinoma of unknown origin. Radiographics 17:542-544, 1997.

Craig JG, Jacobson JA, Moed BR: Ultrasound of fracture and bone healing. Radiol Clin North Am 37:737-751, 1999.

Cronan JJ, Leen V: Recurrent deep venous thrombosis: Limitations of US. Radiology 170:739-742, 1989.

Cronin JJ: Controversies in venous ultrasound. Semin Ultrasound CT MR 18:33-38, 1997.

Delgado GJ, Chung CB, Keltrakul N, et al: Tennis leg: Clinical US study of 141 patients and anatomic investigation of four cadavers with MR imaging and US. Radiology 224:112-119, 2002.

Key Features

Tendons are echogenic when they are imaged at 90 degrees to the direction of sound. Otherwise they are hypoechoic. Ligaments have similar characteristics. This property is called anisotropy.

Muscles are normally very hypoechoic and also are anisotropic.

Full-thickness tendon tears are easy to diagnose with sonography. A blunt tendon tip, local mass effect, refractive shadowing, loss of fibrillar pattern, and nonvisualization are all key findings.

Full-thickness rotator cuff tears appear as focal anechoic or hypoechoic defects, focal contour abnormalities, focal compressibility, and nonvisualization.

Important features to determine when imaging an extremity mass are whether it is solid, cystic, or complex, whether it is vascular, what structure it arises from, and what is its relationship to adjacent structures.

Sonography is the most sensitive means of identifying and localizing foreign bodies in the extremities. Foreign bodies almost always are hyperechoic with variable shadowing.

Extremity arteries show high-resistance flow and typically have a triphasic waveform pattern with antegrade flow in systole, reversed flow in early diastole, antegrade flow in mid diastole, and absent flow in end diastole.

Extremity venous flow shows respiratory phasicity and variable cardiac related pulsatility.

Deep venous thrombosis is primarily diagnosed by noting lack of venous compressibility. Altered luminal echogenicity and alterations in flow characteristics are secondary signs.

Pseudoaneurysms are characterized by detectable extravascular blood flow in the lumen and a "to and fro" pattern of flow in the neck.

Pseudoaneurysms can be effectively treated with ultrasound-guided injection of thrombin.

Iatrogenic arteriovenous fistulas typically occur below the femoral bifurcation, display prominent perivascular tissue vibration, and show localized hemodynamic alterations in the supplying artery (low- resistance flow) and the draining vein (turbulence and arterialization).

Erickson SJ: High-resolution imaging of the musculoskeletal system. Radiology 205:593-618, 1997.

Farin PU, Jaroma H: Sonographic findings of rotator cuff calcifications. J Ultrasound Med. 4:7-14, 1995.

Fessell DP, Jacobson JA, Craig J, et al: Using sonography to reveal and aspirate joint effusions. AJR Am J Roentgenol 174:1353-1362, 2000.

Fessell DP, Vanderschueren GM, Jacobson JA, et al: US of the Ankle: Technique, anatomy, and diagnosis of pathologic conditions. Radiographics 18:325-340, 1998.

Fraser JD, Anderson DR: Deep venous thrombosis: Recent advances and optimal investigation with US. Radiology 211: 9-24, 1999.

Griffith JF, Rainer TH, Ching AS, et al: Sonography compared with radiography in revealing acute rib fracture. AJR Am J Roentgenol 173:1603-1609, 1999.

Hartgerink P, Fessell DP, Jacobson JA, van Holsbeeck MT: Full-versus partial-thickness Achilles tendon tears: Sonographic accuracy and characterization in 26 cases with surgical correlation. Radiology 220:406-412, 2001.

Horton LK, Jacobson JA, Powell A, et al: Sonography and radiography of soft-tissue foreign bodies. AJR Am J Roentgenol 176:1155-1159, 2001.

Kruger K, Zahringer M, Sohngen FD, et al: Femoral pseudoaneurysms: Management with percutaneous thrombin injections success rates and effects on systemic coagulation. Radiology 226:452-458, 2003.

Li JC, Cai S, Jiang YX, et al: Diagnostic criteria for locating acquired arteriovenous fistulas with color Doppler sonography. J Clin Ultrasound 30:336-342, 2002.

Lin J, Jacobson JA, Fessell DP, et al: An illustrated tutorial of musculoskeletal sonography: I. Introduction and general principles. AJR Am J Roengtenol 175:637-645, 2000.

Lin J, Jacobson JA, Fessell DP, et al: An illustrated tutorial of musculoskeletal sonography: II. Upper extremity. AJR Am J Roentgenol 175:1071-1079, 2000.

Lin J, Jacobson JA, Fessell DP, et al: An illustrated tutorial of musculoskeletal sonography: III. Lower extremity. AJR Am J Roentgenol 175:1313-1321, 2000.

Lin J, Jacobson JA, Fessell DP, et al: An illustrated tutorial of musculoskeletal sonography: IV. Musculoskeletal masses, sonographically guided interventions, and miscellaneous topics. AJR Am J Roentgenol 175:1711-1719, 2000.

Malghem J, Vande Berg B, Lecouvet R, Maldague B: Costal cartilage fractures as revealed on CT and sonography. AJR Am J Roentgenol 176:429-432, 2001.

Martinoli C, Bianchi S, Derchi LE: Tendon and nerve sonography. Radiol Clin North Am 37:691-711, 1999.

Middleton WD: Duplex and color Doppler sonography of post-catheterization arteriovenous fistulas. Semin Intervent Radiol 7:192-197, 1990.

Middleton WD: Shoulder pain. In Bluth EI, Benson, C, Arger P, et al (eds): The Practice of Ultrasonography. New York, Thieme, 1999.

Middleton WD, Teefey SA, Boyer MI: Hand and wrist sonography. Ultrasound Q 17:21-36, 2001.

Middleton WD, Teefey SA, Yamaguchi K: Sonography of the shoulder. Semin Musculoskeletal Radiol 2:211-221, 1998.

Osterwalder JJ, Widrig R, Stober R, Gachter A: Diagnostic validity of ultrasound in patients with persistent wrist pain and suspected occult ganglion. J Hand Surg [Am] 22:1034-1040, 1997.

Patel MC, Berman LH, Moss HA, McPherson SJ: Subclavian and internal jugular veins at Doppler US: Abnormal cardiac pulsatility and respiratory phasicity as a predictor of complete central occlusion. Radiology 211:579-583, 1999.

Paulson EK, Sheafor DH, Nelson RC, et al: Treatment of iatrogenic femoral arterial pseudoaneurysms: Comparison of US-guided thrombin injection with compression repair. Radiology 215:403-408, 2000.

Peetrons P: Ultrasound of muscles. Eur Radiol 12:35-43, 2002.

Peterson JJ, Bancroft LW, Kransdorf MJ: Wooden foreign bodies: Imaging appearance. AJR Am J Roentgenol 178:557-562, 2002.

Ptasznik R: Ultrasound in acute and chronic knee injury. Radiol Clin North Am. 37:797-830, 1999.

Quinn TJ, Jacobson JA, Craig JG, van Holsbeeck MT: Sonography of Morton's neuromas. AJR Am J Roentgenol 174:1723-1728, 2000.

Rawool NM, Nazarian LN: Ultrasound of the ankle and foot. Semin Ultrasound CT MR 2:275-284, 2000.

Read JW, Conolly WB, Lanzetta M, et al: Diagnostic ultrasound of the hand and wrist. J Hand Surg [Am] 21:1004-1010, 1996.

Rosen MP, McArdle C: Controversies in the use of lower extremity sonography in the diagnosis of acute deep vein thrombosis and a proposal for a unified approach. Semin Ultrasound CT MR 18:362-368, 1997.

Steiner E, Steinbach LS, Schnarkowski P, et al: Ganglia and cysts around joints. Radiol Clin North Am 34:395-425, 1996.

Teefey SA, Hasan SA, Middleton WD, et al: Ultrasonography of the rotator cuff: A comparison of ultrasonography and arthroscopic surgery in one hundred consecutive cases. J Bone Joint Surg Am 82:498-504, 2000.

Teefey SA, Middleton WD, Boyer MI: Sonography of the hand and wrist. Semin Ultrasound CT MR 21:1-14, 2000.

Teefey SA, Middleton WD, Yamaguchi K: Shoulder sonography: State of the art. Radiol Clin North Am 37:767-786, 1999.

VanHolsbeeck MT, Kolowich PA, Eyler WR, et al: US depiction of partial thickness tear of the rotator cuff. Radiology 197:443-446, 1995.

Ward EE, Jacobson JA, Fessell DP, et al: Sonographic detection of Baker's cysts: Comparison with MR imaging. AJR Am J Roentgenol 176:373-380, 2001.

Obstetrics and Gynecology

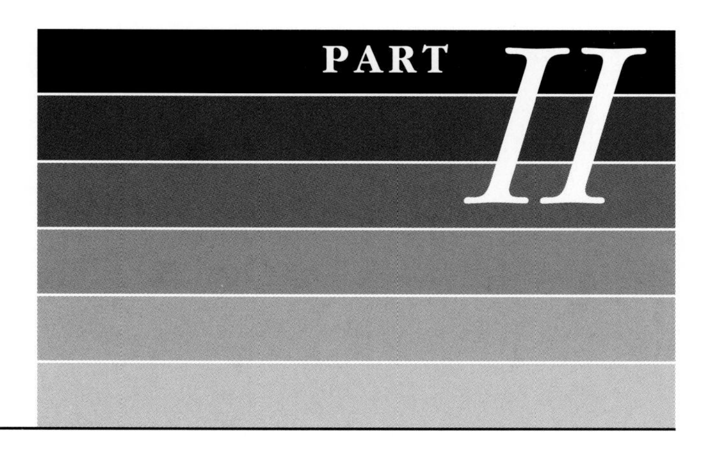

Guidelines to Obstetrical Examination and Appropriate Measurements

Equipment
Documentation
First-Trimester Ultrasound
Second- and Third-Trimester Ultrasound

Ultrasound examinations are performed by sonographers and sonologists with varied experience levels and with equipment of different specifications and image quality. An attempt to standardize all ultrasound studies began in 1985 when the American College of Radiology (ACR) and the American Institute of Ultrasound in Medicine (AIUM) approved the concept of examination guidelines. They created similar but separate antepartum obstetrical ultrasound guidelines. The American College of Obstetricians and Gynecologists (ACOG) was involved in this initial discussion but chose to create an obstetrical ultrasound technical note rather than a guideline. This document was twice updated by the ACR and by the AIUM as a standard. Most recently, in 2003, an updated collaborative antepartum obstetrical ultrasound document, renamed as a practice guideline, was created by a combined effort of the ACR, AIUM, and ACOG. This most recent collaborative guidelines is described below.

Although it is not possible for ultrasound to identify all in utero problems, many significant abnormalities can be detected with a systematic approach. A uniform evaluation is therefore necessary when a pregnant woman needs an ultrasound examination, regardless of clinical history, because most women pregnant with an abnormal fetus will have no predisposing risk factors.

Some examiners originally suggested that the obstetrical ultrasound examination could be divided into two levels of study. Proposed in 1977 in conjunction with maternal serum α-fetoprotein (MSAFP) screening programs, a level 1 sonogram would be performed to detect obstetrical problems, unrelated to structural abnormalities, that could elevate MSAFP levels: most commonly inaccurate menstrual dates but also associated with multiple gestations and fetal demise. Maternal weight can also elevate these levels. If the MSAFP levels are still elevated, in a woman with a living intrauterine pregnancy of appropriate dates, a level 2 sonogram would then be performed to look for fetal anomalies, including open (not skin covered) fetal defects most commonly related to the neural axis and to the abdominal wall. Because it is easier to do a level 1 than a level 2 study, some practitioners interpreted this approach to mean that it might be acceptable to have a level 1 study performed by an examiner with less expertise and equipment; a level 2 study would need more operator experience and better equipment. To make matters more confusing, some practitioners dealing with complex cases declared themselves "level 3" examiners, a designation with no adequate definition. The concept of levels has therefore not been uniformly applied and has consequently lost its validity. A high level of expertise is needed for all ultrasound obstetrical examinations, and it is therefore recommended that this terminology be discarded.

The anteparteum obstetrical ultrasound guideline defines four classifications of examinations: first-trimester, standard second- or third-trimester, limited (to answer a specific question) and specialized (a more detailed anatomic examination). This practice guideline also specifies clinical indications to perform an obstetrical ultrasound. The guideline also defines or references other guidelines that detail expected parameters for physicians performing and interpreting diagnostic examinations, documentation of findings, equipment specifications, and fetal safety. Quality control and improvement, infection control, and patient education concerns are also referenced. Of these, the equipment and fetal safety, documentation, the first-trimester, and the standard second- and third-trimester examinations are discussed below. Direct quotes from the guideline will be shown in bolded type.

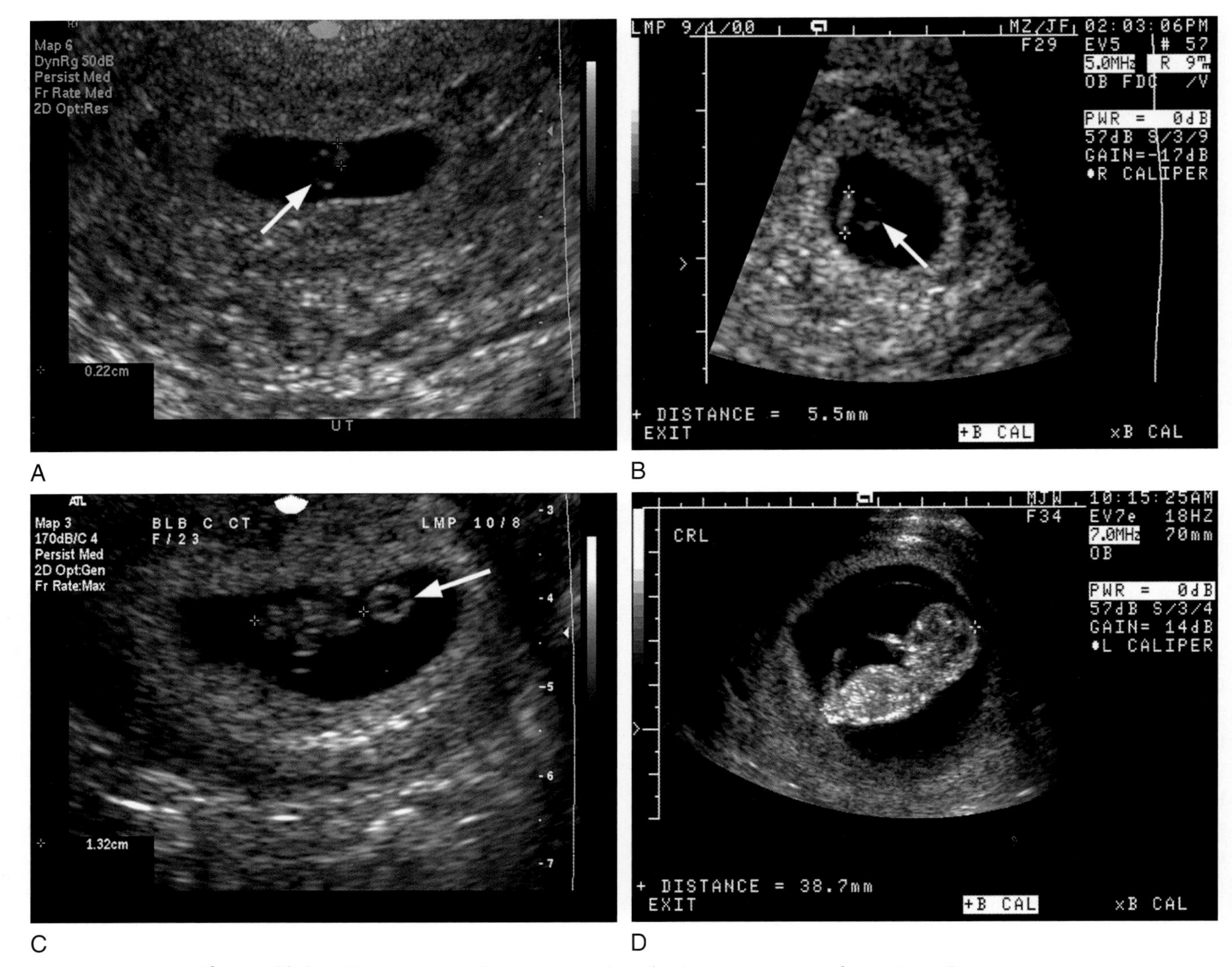

Figure 12-1 Measurement of crown-rump length at various stages of gestation. Crown-rump length is measured from the top of the embryo's head (crown) to the bottom of its torso (rump) *(cursors)*. The yolk sac *(arrows)* should not be included in the measurement. **A,** Crown-rump length of 2.2 mm corresponds to gestational age of 5.7 weeks. **B,** Crown-rump length of 5.5 mm corresponds to gestational age of 6.3 weeks. **C,** Crown-rump length of 13.2 mm corresponds to gestational age of 7.5 weeks. **D,** Crown-rump length of 38.7 mm corresponds to gestational age of 10.8 weeks.

EQUIPMENT

Ultrasound studies should be performed with real-time scanners by the transabdominal (TA) or transvaginal (TV) approach, or both. A transducer of appropriate frequency (≥ 3 MHz for TA examination or ≥ 5 MHz for TV studies) should be used. The choice of frequency is a tradeoff between beam penetration (better at lower frequencies) and resolution (better at higher frequencies). In general, the highest frequency that still affords adequate penetration should be selected. The lowest ultrasound exposure settings should also be used to gain necessary diagnostic information. This has been called the ALARA principle, which means "as low as reasonably achievable."

DOCUMENTATION

Adequate documentation is essential for ensuring appropriate patient care. A permanent record of the ultrasound images is needed, including measurements and anatomic findings. Images should be labeled with the examination date, patient's name, and/or identification number. Image orientation, if important, should be

Table 12-1 Predicted Menstrual Age from CRL Measurements from 5.7 to 12 Weeks

CRL (mm)	Menstrual Age (wk)	Range* (wk)
2	5.7	5.2-6.2
3	5.9	5.4-6.4
4	6.1	5.6-6.6
5	6.2	5.7-6.7
6	6.4	5.8-7.0
7	6.6	6.0-7.2
8	6.7	6.1-7.3
9	6.9	6.3-7.5
10	7.1	6.5-7.7
11	7.2	6.6-7.8
12	7.4	6.8-8.0
13	7.5	6.9-8.1
14	7.7	7.0-8.4
15	7.9	7.2-8.6
16	8.0	7.3-8.5
17	8.1	7.4-8.8
18	8.3	7.6-9.0
19	8.4	7.7-9.1
20	8.6	7.9-9.3
21	8.7	8.0-9.4
22	8.9	8.1-9.7
23	9.0	8.2-9.8
24	9.1	8.3-9.9
25	9.2	8.4-10.0
26	9.4	8.6-10.2
27	9.5	8.7-10.3
28	9.6	8.8-10.4
29	9.7	8.9-10.5
30	9.9	9.1-10.7
31	10.0	9.2-10.8
32	10.1	9.2-10.9
33	10.2	9.3-11.1
34	10.3	9.4-11.2
35	10.4	9.5-11.3
36	10.5	9.6-11.4
37	10.6	9.7-11.5
38	10.7	9.8-11.6
39	10.8	9.9-11.7
40	10.9	10.0-11.8
41	11.0	10.2-11.9
42	11.1	10.2-12.0
43	11.2	10.3-12.1
44	11.2	10.3-12.1
45	11.3	10.3-12.3
46	11.4	10.4-12.4
47	11.5	10.5-12.5
48	11.6	10.6-12.6
49	11.7	10.7-12.7
50	11.7	10.7-12.7
51	11.8	10.8-12.8
52	11.9	10.9-12.9
53	12.0	11.0-13.0
54	12.0	11.0-13.0

*Range is the 95% confidence interval ±8% of the predicted age rounded to farthest 0.1. Only 5.7 to 12.0 weeks are reported.
From Hadlock FP, Shah YP, Kanon DJ, et al: Fetal crown-rump length: Reevaluation of relation to menstrual age (5-18 weeks) with high-resolution real-time US. Radiology 182:501-505, 1992.

labeled. A written report of the ultrasound findings should be prepared and included in the patient's medical record.

FIRST-TRIMESTER ULTRASOUND

Imaging Parameters

Overall Comment

Scanning in the first trimester may be performed either transabdominally or transvaginally. If a transabdominal examination is not definitive, a transvaginal scan or transperineal scan should be performed whenever possible.

a. The uterus should be evaluated for the presence of a gestational sac. If a gestation sac is seen, its location should be documented. The gestational sac should be evaluated for the presence or absence of a yolk sac or embryo, and the crown-rump length should be recorded, when possible.

Comment: The crown-rump length is a more accurate indicator of gestational (menstrual) age than is mean gestational sac diameter. However, the mean gestational sac diameter should be recorded when an embryo is not identified.

Caution should be used in making the presumptive diagnosis of a gestational sac in the absence of definite embryo or yolk sac. Without these findings an intrauterine fluid collection could represent a pseudogestational sac associated with an ectopic pregancy.

In an obstetrical ultrasound examination, the terms *gestational age, embryonic age or fetal age,* and *menstrual age* are used synonymously, all originating from the first day of onset of the woman's last normal menstrual period. The embryo is typically identified by 6 weeks, and the yolk sac is usually seen approximately one-half week earlier. Both are occasionally imaged even earlier by the TV approach. The embryonic or crown-rump length (CRL) is the primary measurement for establishing gestational age during the first trimester, with a precision of ±5 to 7 days. The CRL is measured in the sagittal scan plane from the top of the embryo's head (crown) to the bottom of its torso (rump) (Fig. 12-1). The yolk sac and extremities should not be included in the CRL measurement (Table 12-1). The gestational sac can routinely be identified by 5 weeks' gestation and with TV scanning is occasionally seen earlier. The mean gestational sac diameter or mean sac diameter (MSD) is calculated by averaging three orthogonal measurements of the gestational sac. These measurements of sac diameter are obtained from the inner-to-inner edge of the

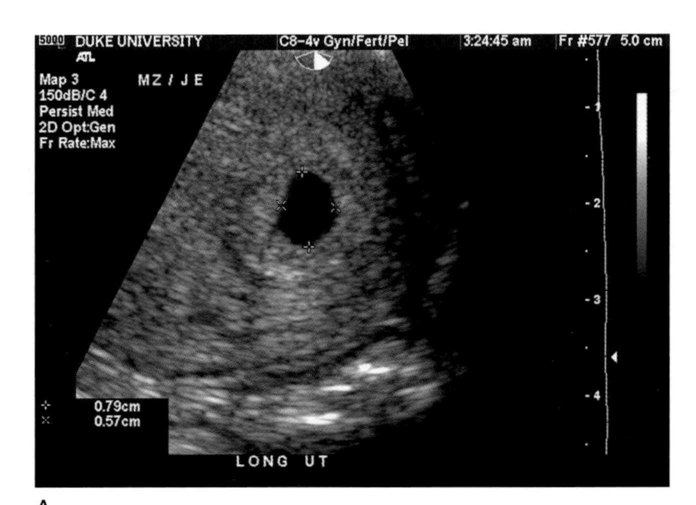

A

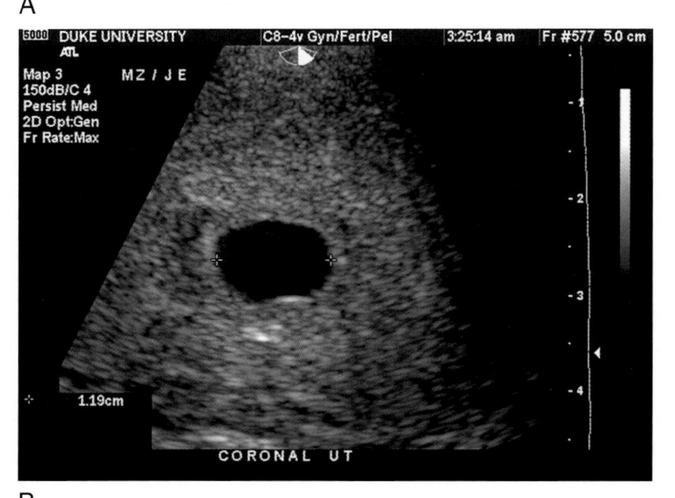

B

Figure 12-2 Transvaginal scans showing measurement of mean sac diameter. **A** and **B,** The mean sac diameter is measured by obtaining three orthogonal diameters of the gestational sac with calipers positioned on the inner edge of the hyperechoic rim. In this case, the average of the three diameters (7.9 mm, 5.7 mm, and 11.9 mm) calculates to a mean sac diameter of 8.2 mm, consistent with a gestational age of 5.7 weeks.

Table 12-2 Mean Diameter of Gestational Sac and Corresponding Estimates of Gestational Age*

Mean Sac Diameter (mm)	Mean	Gestational Age (wk) 95% Prediction Interval (Rounded to Farthest 0.1)
2	5.0	4.5-5.5
3	5.1	4.6-5.6
4	5.2	4.7-5.7
5	5.4	4.8-5.9
6	5.5	5.0-6.0
7	5.6	5.1-6.1
8	5.7	5.2-6.3
9	5.9	5.4-6.4
10	6.0	5.5-6.5
11	6.1	5.6-6.6
12	6.2	5.7-6.8
13	6.4	5.9-6.9
14	6.5	6.0-7.0
15	6.6	6.1-7.1
16	6.7	6.2-7.3
17	6.9	6.4-7.4
18	7.0	6.5-7.5
19	7.1	6.6-7.6
20	7.3	6.7-7.8
21	7.4	6.9-7.9
22	7.5	7.0-8.0
23	7.6	7.1-8.1
24	7.8	7.2-8.3
25	7.9	7.4-8.4
26	8.0	7.5-8.5
27	8.1	7.6-8.7
28	8.3	7.7-8.8
29	8.4	7.9-8.9
30	8.5	8.0-9.0

*The mean gestational age was calculated from a regression equation.
Adapted from Daya S, Woods S, Ward S, et al: Early pregnancy assessment with transvaginal ultrasound scanning. Can Med Assoc J 144:441-445, 1991.

hyperechoic rim, thereby including the fluid in the gestational sac but not the wall of the sac (Fig. 12-2). Like the CRL, the MSD can be used to estimate gestational age with a precision of ±5 to 7 days (Table 12-2), but the primary value of the gestational sac as an age predictor is in the time period before the embryo is visualized, usually between 5 and 6 weeks. Once the embryo can be seen, the CRL, and not the MSD, should be used to assign gestational age. The MSD has not been as extensively studied as the CRL, and there are substantial discrepancies in the MSDs reported in different studies. For example, at 5 weeks, the mean gestational sac sizes reported in the literature range from 2 to 10 mm. Although this may seem a large range, the gestational sac normally grows about 1 mm a day, so that even an 8-mm difference is equivalent to only 1 week.

A note of caution is needed in diagnosing a normal intrauterine pregnancy when only a gestational sac without a yolk sac or embryo is identified. On occasion a pseudogestational sac (fluid within the endometrial canal seen in the setting of an ectopic pregnancy) may exhibit an appearance similar to that of a normal gestational sac.

b. Presence or absence of cardiac activity should be reported.

Embryonic life can be detected by the real-time or color Doppler observation of heart activity. Heart motion should be evident in all embryos with a CRL of at least 5 mm using TV ultrasound (equivalent to an embryonic age of 6.2 weeks) (see Table 12-1) and usually is seen earlier. Heart rate can also be evaluated: at 5 to 6 weeks it should be at least 100 beats per minute, rising to between 140 and 160 beats per minute by 8 weeks.

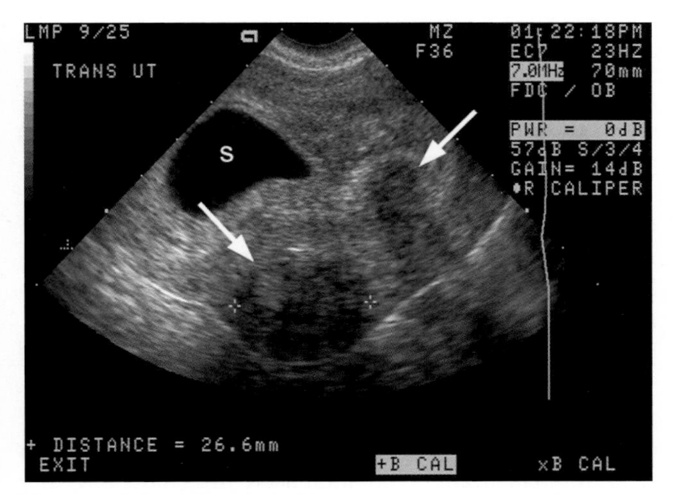

Figure 12-3 Fibroids in first-trimester pregnancy. Transverse endovaginal image of uterus shows two small fibroids *(arrows)* at same level as gestational sac (S).

There is a lower limit of normal for the heart rate: less than 90 beats per minute at 5 to 6 weeks and less than 120 beats per minute by 8 weeks. There is no established upper limit of concern for heart rate. If the rate needs documentation, an M-mode recording can be performed. Pulsed Doppler sonography should be avoided in the first trimester because of its increased power.

c. Fetal number should be reported.

Multiple gestations can be accurately determined by a careful analysis of the number of embryos and the number of gestational sacs. Overestimations of fetal number may occur if fluid in the endometrial cavity, a subchorionic hematoma, or the normal separation of the amnion and chorion is misinterpreted as a gestational sac. Underestimations may also occur, particularly if there are more than two closely situated gestational sacs on transabdominal images. In these cases TV scanning will often be of diagnostic value.

d. Evaluation of the uterus, adnexal structures, and cul-de-sac should be performed.

The size and location of fibroids (Fig. 12-3) need to be noted and monitored, because they tend to enlarge during pregnancy. In the first trimester, fibroids occasionally cause gestational sac malposition and miscarriage.

The most common adnexal mass, the corpus luteal cyst, is usually less than 3 cm in diameter and typically resolves by the mid-second trimester (Fig. 12-4). The amount and echogenicity of cul-de-sac fluid, if present, should be noted. In a normal first-trimester pregnancy, only a small amount of anechoic fluid should be present (Fig. 12-5). Noncystic adnexal and cul-de-sac masses should be evaluated for echogenicity and size. Surgical removal usually in the second trimester, if needed, is related to the mass's size, position, and characteristics that would suggest malignancy (by physical examination, ultrasound, and occasionally MRI).

In the first trimester, the initial ultrasound examination can be performed transabdominally or transvaginally. TA ultrasound allows a more comprehensive overview of the uterus and adnexa, but TV ultrasound provides superior resolution and detail. If TA ultrasound is done first and all normal landmarks are identified, including the gestational sac, the embryo with heart motion, and the ovaries, further evaluation with TV ultrasound is not required. If, however, the gestational sac is not identified, the sac is seen without an embryo,

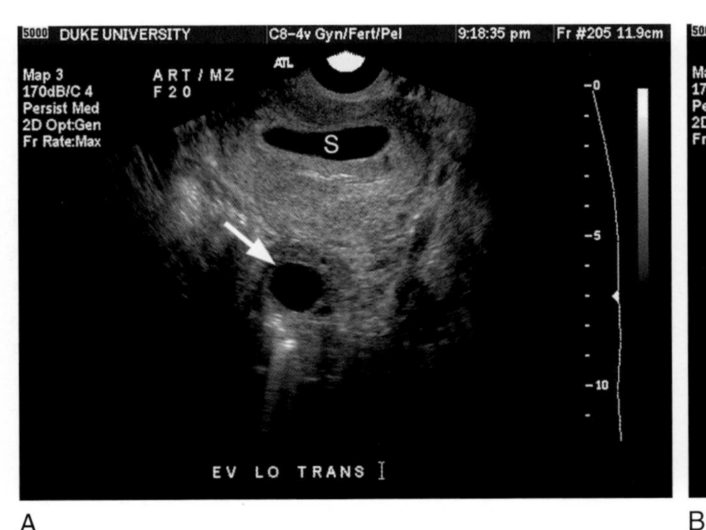

A

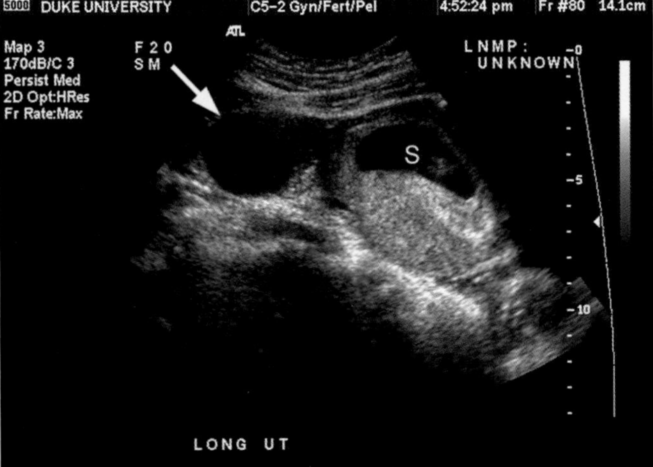

B

Figure 12-4 Examples of corpus luteal cysts during first trimester of pregnancy. **A,** Axial transvaginal image reveals small corpus luteal cyst *(arrow)* in right ovary, immediately posterior to the uterus. **B,** Longitudinal transabdominal image reveals moderate-sized corpus luteal cyst *(arrow)* in an ovary immediately superior to the uterus. S, gestational sac in uterus.

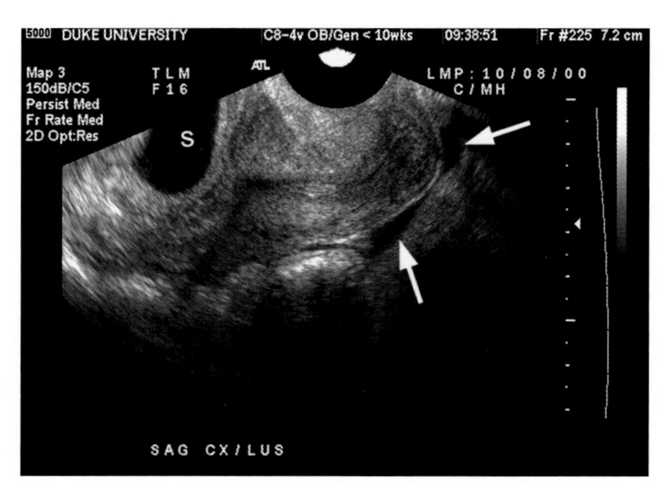

Figure 12-5 Transvaginal ultrasound image during first trimester of pregnancy shows a small, normal amount of anechoic fluid *(arrows)* in the cul-de-sac. S, gestational sac.

or the embryo is identified but no heart motion is detected, a TV study should also be performed. Even in the context of pelvic pain, vaginal bleeding, or cervical pathology, a gentle TV study is almost always indicated when normal pelvic anatomy is not fully identified or an uncertain finding needs further evaluation. Measurements by both the TA and the TV approaches are considered equally accurate, despite the higher frequencies often used transvaginally.

SECOND- AND THIRD-TRIMESTER ULTRASOUND

Imaging Parameters for a Standard Fetal Examination

a. Fetal cardiac activity, number, and presentation should be reported.

Fetal life can be documented by the real-time or color Doppler observation of heart motion. Although an M-mode ultrasound study is not required, an abnormal heart rate or rhythm should be confirmed if possible by M-mode, incorporating a ventricle, atrioventricular valve, and atrium in the tracing. Pulsed Doppler has too much power to be routinely used to document rate but could add information in selected cases. The sustained normal heart rate should be between 140 to 160 beats per minute throughout the second and third trimester, slowing somewhat toward term. For any fetus, a rate of less than 120 or more than 180 beats per minute or an arrhythmia should be considered potentially problematic. However, mild transient episodes of bradycardia are usually normal.

The fetal lie or presentation should be recorded. The most common is cephalic (vertex) and is favored for a normal vaginal delivery. Breech and transverse lies are not uncommon early in pregnancy but at term decrease in incidence to 3% to 4% and 0.25% to 0.5%, respectively. At term the fetal lie can have importance for obstetrical management, including fetal repositioning and mode of delivery.

Fetal number can be reliably documented. The accurate determination of amnionicity and chorionicity of multiple gestations is important information because it helps to assess the inherent potential increased risk to that pregnancy.

b. A qualitative or semi-quantitative estimate of amniotic fluid volume should be reported.

The amount of amniotic fluid is important, because either an increase or decrease is associated with certain fetal anomalies and with increased prenatal morbidity and mortality. This estimate can be accurately performed both qualitatively (subjectively) and quantitatively (by measurement).

c. The placental location, appearance, and relationship to the internal cervical os should be recorded. The umbilical cord should be imaged and the number of vessels in the cord should be evaluated when possible.

The placenta has a uniform echogenicity with a thin hyperechoic chorionic plate abutting on the amniotic fluid. The relationship of the placenta to the internal cervical os should be documented. If the placenta does not extend to the cervix on the initial views, placenta previa is excluded. If, however, the placenta is low-lying or appears to cover the os and the urinary bladder is full or partially distended, the patient should be asked to completely void and the study repeated because a distended bladder could have falsely elongated the lower uterine segment, giving the impression that the placenta covered the internal os. Whereas some examiners prefer the TV approach, a TA study with the bladder empty (imaging through the amniotic fluid) or a translabial examination can often give the same information.

The umbilical cord should be identified and the number of its vessels counted. This is of potential importance because a two-vessel cord (one umbilical artery and one umbilical vein) has a much higher incidence of associated structural abnormalities. Additionally, but not stated in the standard, many examiners believe an attempt should be made to determine the insertion position of the umbilical cord into the placenta because an insertion outside the placental substance can lead to fetal compromise at the time of delivery.

d. Gestational age assessment.

First-trimester crown-rump measurement is the most accurate means for sonographic dating of pregnancy. Beyond this period, a variety of sonographic parameters such as biparietal diameter, abdominal circumference, and femoral diaphysis length can be used to estimate gestational (menstrual) age. The

variability of gestational (menstrual) age estimations, however, increases with advancing pregnancy. Significant discrepancies between gestational (menstrual) age and fetal measurements may suggest the possibility of fetal growth abnormality, intrauterine growth restriction, or macrosomia.

While the crown-rump length (CRL) is an excellent method of establishing gestational age, there is ample evidence in the literature to suggest that the head measurements up to 20 weeks have very good precision, almost equivalent to the CRL, with the femur length considerably less precise (Table 12-3). By the third trimester, while no parameter offers adequate accuracy, the femur length measurement is slightly more precise than the head measurements.

The abdominal measurements are far less precise in both the second and third trimesters and should not be used to establish gestational age (see Table 12-3). Instead, abdominal measurements should be used, along with the head and femur length measurements, to analyze fetal proportionality and growth.

i. **Biparietal diameter is measured at a standard level of the thalami and cavum septi pellucidi. The cerebellar hemispheres should not be visible in this scanning plane. The measurement is taken from the outer edge of the proximal skull to the inner edge of the distal skull. Comment: The head shape may be flattened (dolichocephalic) or rounded (brachycephalic) as a normal variant. Under these circumstances, certain variants of normal fetal head development may make measurement of the head circumference more reliable than biparietal diameter for estimating gestational (menstrual) age.**

ii. **Head circumference is measured at the same level as the biparietal diameter, around the outer perimeter of the calvarium. The measurement is not affected by head shape.**

iii. **Femur diaphysis length can be reliably used after 14th week of gestational (menstrual) age. The long axis of the femur shaft is most accurately measured with the beam of insonation being perpendicular to the shaft, excluding the distal femoral epiphysis.**

iv. **Abdominal circumference should be determined at the skin line on a true transverse view at the level of the junction of the umbilical vein, portal sinus, and fetal stomach when visible. Comment: Abdominal circumference measurement is used with other parameters to estimate fetal weight and may allow detection of intrauterine growth restriction and macrosomia.**

Table 12-3 Gestational Age Interval (Weeks)

Predictor	14-20	20-26	26-32	32-42
BPD	1.4	2.1	3.8	4.1
BPDa	1.2	1.9	3.3	3.8
FL	1.4	2.5	3.1	3.5
HC	1.2	1.9	3.4	3.8
AC	2.1	3.7	3.0	4.5

From Benson CB, Doubilet PM: Sonographic prediction of gestational age: Accuracy of second- and third-trimester fetal measurements. AJR Am J Roentgenol 157:1275-1277, 1991.

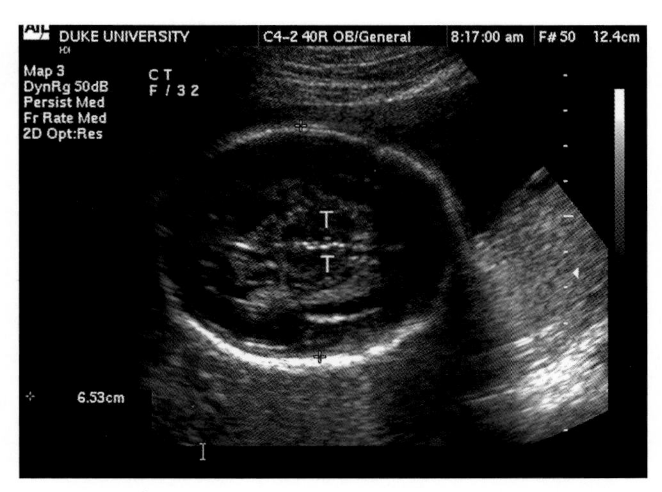

Figure 12-6 Measurement of the biparietal diameter (BPD). The BPD is measured at the level of the thalami (T) or midbrain, from the leading edge to the leading edge (outer to inner) of the calvarium *(cursors)*. In this example, the measured BPD of 65.3 mm corresponds to a gestational age of 25.6 weeks.

The biparietal diameter (BPD) is measured from the leading edge to the leading edge of the temporoparietal bones (Fig. 12-6) and the corresponding gestational age is determined using a standard BPD table (Table 12-4).

The accuracy of the BPD is dependent on a normal head shape. If the fetal head is unusually rounded (brachycephalic) or elongated (dolichocephalic), the BPD measurement will overestimate or underestimate gestational age, respectively. To correct this potential inaccuracy, a second linear measurement is obtained from the same image as the BPD, the fronto-occipital diameter (FOD). Using both measurements, a cephalic index (CI) is calculated by the following formula (Fig. 12-7):

$$CI = (BPD + FOD) \times 2/100.$$

The mean CI is 78.3 with a normal range of 70 to 86 at 2 standard deviations (SD). For the purposes of this correction, both the BPD and FOD should ideally be obtained from outer edge to outer edge. In actuality the BPD is usually not remeasured but is kept as an outer-to-inner-edge measurement.

Table 12-4 Composite Biparietal Diameter

Biparietal Diameter (mm)	Gestational Age (wk) Mean*	Gestational Age (wk) Range 90% Variation†	Biparietal Diameter (mm)	Gestational Age (wk) Mean*	Gestational Age (wk) Range 90% Variation†
20	12.0	12.0	61	24.2	22.6 to 25.8
21	12.0	12.0	62	24.6	23.1 to 26.1
22	12.7	12.2 to 13.2	63	24.9	23.4 to 26.4
23	13.0	12.4 to 13.6	64	25.3	23.8 to 26.8
24	13.2	12.6 to 13.8	65	25.6	24.1 to 27.1
25	13.5	12.9 to 14.1	66	26.0	24.5 to 27.5
26	13.7	13.1 to 14.3	67	26.4	25.0 to 27.8
27	14.0	13.4 to 14.6	68	26.7	25.3 to 28.1
28	14.3	13.6 to 15.0	69	27.1	25.8 to 28.4
29	14.5	13.9 to 15.2	70	27.5	26.3 to 28.7
30	14.8	14.1 to 15.5	71	27.9	26.7 to 29.1
31	15.1	14.3 to 15.9	72	28.3	27.2 to 29.4
32	15.3	14.5 to 16.1	73	28.7	27.6 to 29.8
33	15.6	14.7 to 16.5	74	29.1	28.1 to 30.1
34	15.9	15.0 to 16.8	75	29.5	28.5 to 30.5
35	16.2	15.2 to 17.2	76	30.0	29.0 to 31.0
36	16.4	15.4 to 17.4	77	30.3	29.2 to 31..4
37	16.7	15.6 to 17.8	78	30.8	29.6 to 32.0
38	17.0	15.9 to 18.1	79	31.1	29.9 to 32.5
39	17.3	16.1 to 18.5	80	31.6	30.2 to 33.0
40	17.6	16.4 to 18.8	81	32.1	30.7 to 33.5
41	17.9	16.5 to 19.3	82	32.6	31.2 to 34.0
42	18.1	16.6 to 19.8	83	33.0	31.5 to 34.5
43	18.4	16.8 to 20.2	84	33.4	31.9 to 35.1
44	18.8	16.9 to 20.7	85	34.0	32.3 to 35.7
45	19.1	17.0 to 21.2	86	34.3	32.8 to 36.2
46	19.4	17.4 to 21.4	87	35.0	33.4 to 36.6
47	19.7	17.8 to 21.6	88	35.4	33.9 to 37.1
48	20.0	18.2 to 21.8	89	36.1	34.6 to 37.6
49	20.3	18.6 to 22.0	90	36.6	35.1 to 38.1
50	20.6	19.0 to 22.2	91	37.2	35.9 to 38.5
51	20.9	19.3 to 22.5	92	37.8	36.7 to 38.9
52	21.2	19.5 to 22.9	93	38.8	37.3 to 39.3
53	21.5	19.8 to 23.2	94	39.0	37.9 to 40.1
54	21.9	20.1 to 23.7	95	39.7	38.5 to 40.9
55	22.2	20.4 to 24.0	96	40.6	39.1 to 41.5
56	22.5	20.7 to 24.3	97	41.0	39.9 to 42.1
57	22.8	21.1 to 24.5	98	41.8	40.5 to 43.1
58	23,2	21.5 to 24.9			
59	23.5	21.9 to 25.1			
60	23.8	22.3 to 25.5			

*Weighted least mean square fit equation: BPD (mm) = $-34.5701 + 5.0157GA - 0.00441GA^2$ (GA = mean gestational age).
†For each biparietal diameter, 90% of gestational age data points fell within this range.
From Kurtz AB, Wapner RJ, Kurtz RJ, et al: Analysis of biparietal diameter as an accurate indicator of gestational age. J Clin Ultrasound 8:319-326, 1980.

If the CI computes at or beyond the limits of 70 and 86, one of two approaches can be utilized: (1) an area-corrected BPD (BPDa) to correct the BPD measurement to an ideal head shape at a mean cephalic index of 78 using the formula

$$BPDa = [(BPD \times FOD/1.265)]^{(1/2)}$$

or (2) a head circumference (HC) obtained by tracing the perimeter of the calvarium (Fig. 12-8) or by using the two diameters just described in a formula for the circumference of a circle:

$$\pi(BPD + FOD)/2 = (BPD + FOD) \times 1.57.$$

Both HC techniques have an accuracy to within 2% of the actual measurement. Reference can then be made to any standard HC table to establish gestational age (Table 12-5).

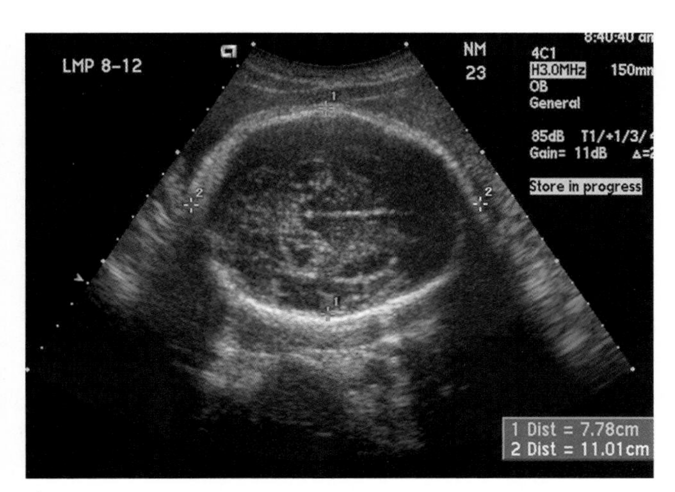

Figure 12-7 Measurement of fronto-occipital diameter (FOD) and calculation of cephalic index. The FOD is measured on the same image as the BPD (cursors labeled 1) by positioning calipers on the outer edge of the frontal and occipital bones in the midline (cursors labeled 2). The cephalic index (CI) is then calculated from the formula: CI = (BPD/FOD) × 100. In this example, the CI of 70.7 is normal (normal range = 70 to 86).

The BPDa and HC measurements in the second trimester (up to 20 and perhaps up to 24 weeks) have a precision of ±1.2 weeks (see Table 12-3), close to that of the first-trimester CRL. By the third trimester, particularly after 26 weeks, the precision of the head measurements decreases to ±3.3 weeks and after 32 weeks it decreases to ±3.8 weeks.

Femur length is used in conjunction with the head measurement to establish gestational age. The femoral diaphysis length (FL) is a linear structure and is measured along its ossified shaft (diaphysis) from one end to

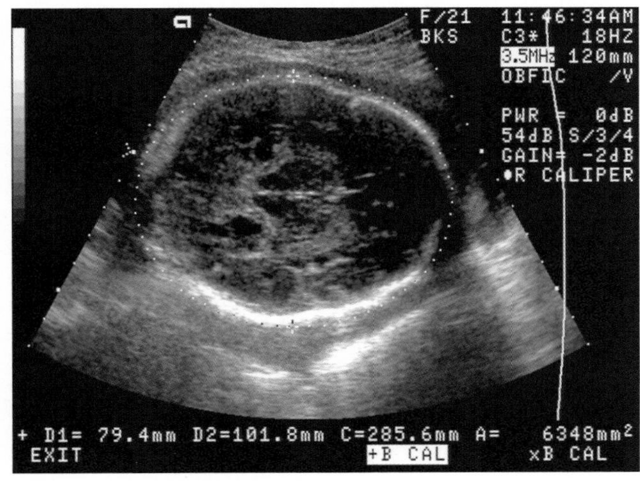

Figure 12-8 Measurement of head circumference (HC). The HC is measured by tracing the perimeter of the calvarium *(dotted line)*, along the outer surface of the calvarium in an axial scan plane at the same level used to measure BPD. In this example, the measured head circumference of 285.6 mm corresponds to a gestational age of 31.4 weeks.

Table 12-5 Head Circumference Measurement

	Gestational Age (wk)	
Head Circumference (mm)	Predicted Mean Values	95% Confidence Limits
80	13.4	12.1 to 14.7
85	13.7	12.4 to 15.0
90	14.0	12.7 to 15.3
95	14.3	13.0 to 15.6
100	14.6	13.3 to 15.9
105	15.0	13.7 to 16.3
110	15.3	14.0 to 16.6
115	15.6	14.3 to 16.9
120	15.9	14.6 to 17.2
125	16.3	15.0 to 17.6
130	16.6	15.3 to 17.9
135	17.0	15.7 to 18.3
140	17.3	16.0 to 18.6
145	17.7	16.4 to 19.0
150	18.1	16 5 to 19.7
155	18.4	16.8 to 20.0
160	18.8	17.2 to 20.4
165	19.2	17.6 to 20.8
170	19.6	18.0 to 21.2
175	20.0	18.4 to 21.6
180	20.4	18.8 to 22.0
185	20.8	19.2 to 22.4
190	21.2	19.8 to 22.8
195	21.6	20.0 to 23.2
200	22.1	20.5 to 23.7
205	22.5	20.9 to 24.1
210	23.0	21.4 to 24.6
215	23.4	21.8 to 25.0
220	23.9	22.3 to 25.5
225	24.4	22.1 to 26.7
230	24.9	22.6 to 27.2
235	25.4	23.1 to 27.7
240	25.9	23.6 to 28.2
245	26.4	24.1 to 28.7
250	26.9	24.6 to 29.2
255	27.5	25.2 to 29.8
260	28.0	25.7 to 30.3
265	28.1	25.8 to 30.4
270	29.2	26.9 to 31.5
275	29.8	27.5 to 32.1
280	30.3	27.6 to 33.0
285	31.0	28.3 to 33.7
290	31.6	28.9 to 34.3
295	32.2	29.5 to 34.8
300	32 8	30.1 to 35 5
305	33.5	30.7 to 36.2
310	34.2	31.5 to 36.9
315	34.9	32.2 to 37.6
320	35.5	32.8 to 38.2
325	36.3	32.9 to 39.7
330	37.0	33.6 to 40.4
335	37.7	34.3 to 41.1
340	38.5	35.1 to 41.9
345	39.2	35.8 to 42.6
350	40.0	36.6 to 43.4
355	40.8	37.4 to 44.2
360	41.6	38.2 to 45.0

From Hadlock FP, Deter RL, Harrist RB, Park SK: Fetal head circumference: Relation to menstrual age. AJR Am J Roentgenol 138:649-653, 1982.

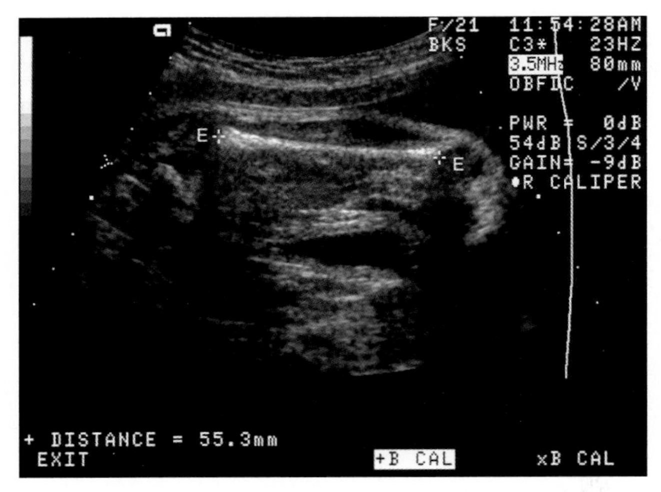

Figure 12-9 Measurement of femur length (FL). The femur length is measured by positioning calipers on the edge of the proximal and distal segments of the diaphysis *(cursors)*. When possible, the femur should be oriented approximately perpendicular to the ultrasound beam. The epiphyseal cartilages (E) should not be included in the measurement. In this example, the femur length of 55.3 mm corresponds to a gestational age of 25.9 weeks.

the other, disregarding the epiphyseal cartilages (Fig. 12-9). The normal diaphysis has a straight lateral and curved medial border. If measured medially, a straight measurement is still obtained disregarding the curvature (Fig. 12-10). The FL is considered slightly more precise in the third trimester (see Table 12-3) and can be used to assign gestational age by itself (Table 12-6) when the BPD and HC are considered unreliable for technical or pathologic reasons. Another use of the FL is to analyze its proportionality to the head, which can detect skeletal dysplasias and growth disturbances (Table 12-7). Whereas the guideline recommends identification and measurement of one femur, with the assumption that the other would also be normal, an attempt to identify and measure the other femur is suggested if the first FL is either too long or short when compared with the BPD.

If more than one study is performed, it is critical that the gestational age *not* be reestablished on each subsequent examination, particularly in the third trimester. Instead, the current fetal age is the initial fetal age (established on the first examination) plus the number of weeks that have elapsed. For example, if a fetus with an initial CRL equivalent to 7 weeks' gestation is restudied 20 weeks later, the gestational age is 27 weeks (7 weeks + 20 weeks = 27 weeks), regardless of the new fetal measurements. A mean gestational age is always given. A range around this mean is sometimes also reported because it gives an assessment of the range of gestational ages likely to correspond to the fetus' actual gestational age.

The fetal abdomen is measured axially at the level of the fetal liver, just below the heart, using the landmark of the umbilical portion of the left portal vein at its junction with the portal sinus and right portal vein (Fig. 12-11). This left portal vein should be imaged entirely within the liver and equidistant from the sides of the abdomen. The abdominal circumference (AC) can be determined either by tracing the perimeter of the abdomen or by averaging two orthogonal abdominal diameters (ADs) and calculating AC from the equation

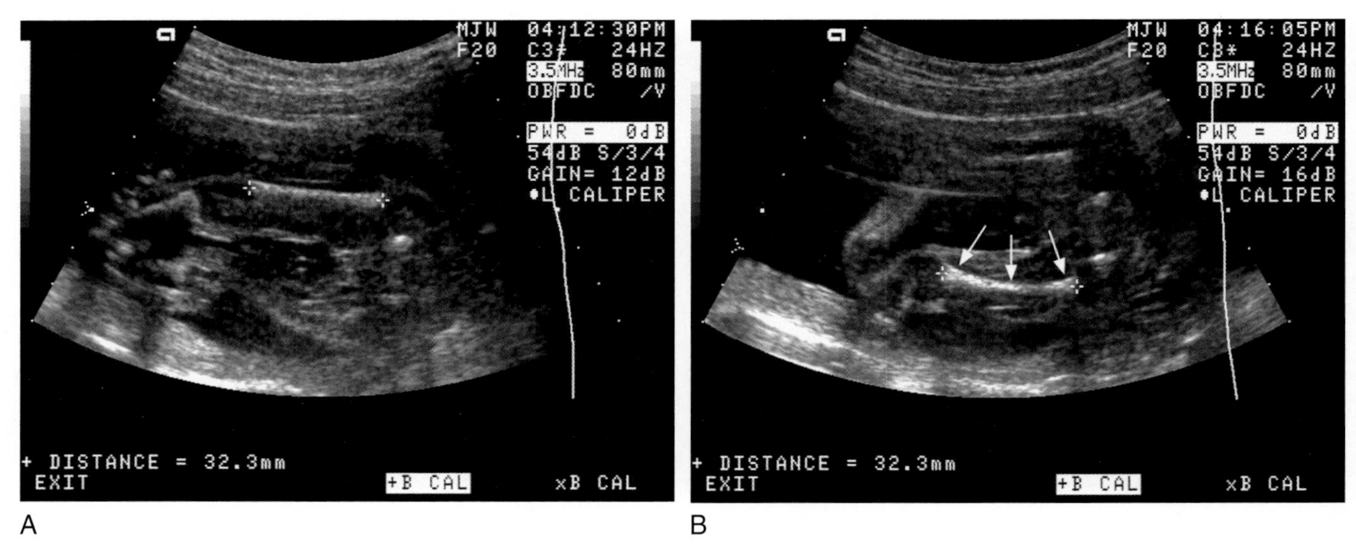

Figure 12-10 Comparison of configuration and length of femur in near and far field. **A,** Femur closest to the transducer. Surface of this femur *(cursors)* appears straight because the lateral surface of the femur is imaged. **B,** Femur farthest from the transducer. Surface of this femur appears to be curved *(cursors, arrows)* because the medial surface of this femur is measured. Despite this, the femur lengths obtained from both femurs are identical (32.3 mm). They correspond to a gestational age of 19.7 weeks.

Table 12-6 Gestational Age (GA) Prediction Based on Femur Length (FL) Measurements

FL (mm)	Predicted GA (wk) Mean	Predicted GA (wk) 2 SD Range*	FL (mm)	Predicted GA (wk) Mean	Predicted GA (wk) 2 SD Range*
10	13.7	12.5 to 14.9	45	24.5	22.6 to 26.4
11	13.9	12.7 to 15.1	46	24.9	23.0 to 26.8
12	14.2	13.0 to 15.4	47	25.3	23.4 to 27.2
13	14.4	13.2 to 15.6	48	25.7	23.8 to 27.6
14	14.6	13.4 to 15.8	49	26.2	23.5 to 28.9
15	14.9	13.7 to 16.1	50	26.6	23.9 to 29.3
16	15.1	13.9 to 16.3	51	27.0	24.3 to 29.7
17	15.4	14.2 to 16.6	52	27.5	24.8 to 30.2
18	15.6	14.4 to 16.8	53	28.0	25.3 to 30.7
19	15.9	14.7 to 17.1	54	28.4	25.7 to 31.1
20	16.2	15.0 to 17.4	55	28.9	26.2 to 31.6
21	16.4	15.2 to 17.6	56	29.4	26.7 to 32.1
22	16.7	15.5 to 17.9	57	29.9	27.2 to 32.6
23	17.0	15.8 to 18.2	58	30.4	27.7 to 33.1
24	17.3	16.1 to 18.5	59	30.9	28.2 to 33.6
25	17.6	16.4 to 18.8	60	31.4	28.7 to 34.1
26	17.9	16.7 to 19.1	61	31.9	29.2 to 34.6
27	18.2	17.0 to 19.4	62	32.5	28.5 to 36.5
28	18.5	17.3 to 19.7	63	33.0	29.0 to 37.0
29	18.8	17.6 to 20.0	64	33.6	29.6 to 37.6
30	19.1	17.9 to 20.3	65	34.1	30.1 to 38.1
31	19.4	18.2 to 20.6	66	34.7	30.7 to 38.7
32	19.7	18.5 to 20.9	67	35.3	31.3 to 39.3
33	20.1	18.2 to 22.0	68	35.9	31.9 to 39.9
34	20.4	18.5 to 22.3	69	36.5	32.5 to 40.5
35	20.7	18.8 to 22.6	70	37.1	33.1 to 41.1
36	21.1	19.2 to 23.0	71	37.7	33.7 to 41.7
37	21.4	19.5 to 23.3	72	38.3	35.1 to 41.5
38	21.8	19.9 to 23.7	73	39.0	35.8 to 42.2
39	22.2	20.3 to 24.1	74	39.6	36.4 to 42.8
40	22.5	20.6 to 24.4	75	40.3	37.1 to 43.5
41	22.9	21.0 to 24.8	76	40.9	37.7 to 44.1
42	23.3	21.4 to 25.2	77	41.6	38.4 to 44.8
43	23.7	21.8 to 25.6	78	42.0	38.8 to 45.2
44	24.1	22.2 to 26.0			

*2 SD = 2 standard deviations.
Adapted from Doubilet PM, Benson CB: Improved prediction of gestational age in the late third trimester. J Ultrasound Med 12:647-653, 1993.

for the circumference of a circle. The ADs should be measured from the outer edge to outer edge of the soft tissues (Fig. 12-12).

Abdominal measurements should not be used to estimate gestational age because they are not as accurate as head and femur measurements for establishing gestational age. Their primary value is instead in the calculation of estimated fetal weight (EFW) and in the determination of normal proportionality with the head so that growth disturbances can be identified by the head-to-abdominal circumference ratio (Table 12-8). Alternatively, the proportionality of the BPD to the AD can be evaluated (Table 12-9). With either method the head is normally larger than the body in the second and early third trimesters, with reversal by term.

A ratio of the FL to the AC has also been proposed. The cut-off ratios separating a normal from a possible large or small abdomen (potential macrosomia and growth restriction) have not been found precise. The ratio is therefore not recommended because too much overlap exists for clinical utility.

e. **Fetal weight estimation. Fetal weight can be estimated by obtaining measurements such as the biparietal diameter, head circumference, abdominal circumference, and femoral diaphysis length. Results from various prediction models can be compared to fetal weight percentiles from published monograms.**

The fetal weight tables are derived from head, body, and femur measurements (Tables 12-10 and 12-11). Their

Table 12-7 Fetal Long Bone Measurements True Mean and Range from 5th to 95th Percentile (mm) (2 SD)

	Biparietal Diameter		Femur		Humerus	
Gestational Age (wk)	True Mean	2 SD	True Mean	2 SD	True Mean	2 SD
13	23	20-26	11	9-13	10	8-12
14	27	24-30	13	11-15	12	10-14
15	30	29-31	15	13-17	14	12-16
16	33	31-35	19	16-22	17	15-19
17	37	34-40	22	19-25	20	16-24
18	42	37-47	25	22-28	23	20-26
19	44	40-48	28	25-31	26	23-29
20	47	43-51	31	28-34	29	26-32
21	50	45-55	35	31-39	32	28-36
22	55	50-60	36	33-39	33	30-36
23	58	53-63	40	36-44	37	34-40
24	61	56-66	42	39-45	38	34-42
25	64	59-69	46	43-49	42	38-46
26	68	63-73	48	44-52	43	40-46
27	70	67-73	49	46-52	45	43-47
28	73	68-78	53	48-58	47	43-51
29	76	71-81	53	48-58	48	44-52
30	77	71-83	56	53-59	50	45-55
31	82	75-89	60	54-66	53	49-57
32	85	79-91	61	55-68	54	50-58
33	86	82-90	64	59-69	56	51-61
34	89	84-94	66	60-72	58	53-63
35	89	82-96	67	61-73	59	53-65
36	91	84-98	70	63-77	60	54-66
37	93	84-102	72	68-76	61	57-65
38	95	89-101	74	68-80	64	61-67
39	95	89-101	76	68-84	65	59-71
40	99	92-107	77	73-81	66	62-70
41	97	91-103	77	73-81	66	62-70
42	100	95-105	78	71-83	68	61-75

From Merz E, Kim-Kern M, Pehl S: Ultrasonic mensuration of fetal limb bones in the second and third trimesters. J Clin Ultrasound 15: 175-183, 1987.

utility is limited by a sizable variation around the mean weight, at least ±17% to 20% for a table using two parameters and ±15% for a table using three parameters. Nevertheless, the mean weight can be of value in determining if the fetus is appropriate in size provided that the fetal age is known from an earlier first- or second-trimester study, when age determination is more precise. Then the calculated weight can be compared with the expected weight of a fetus for that age (Table 12-12). For example, if in Table 12-10, the BPD and AC are 70 and 350 mm, respectively, a weight of 2368 g is obtained. If the fetal age is known to be 35 weeks from a prior ultrasound study, Table 12-12 shows that at 35 weeks a weight of 2368 g is between the 25th and 50th percentile, which is normal. If the weight falls below the 10th percentile the fetus is considered small for gestational age, and if it is above the 90th percentile the fetus is considered large for gestational age.

The guideline recommends that on all follow-up studies the interval growth should be assessed. For this,

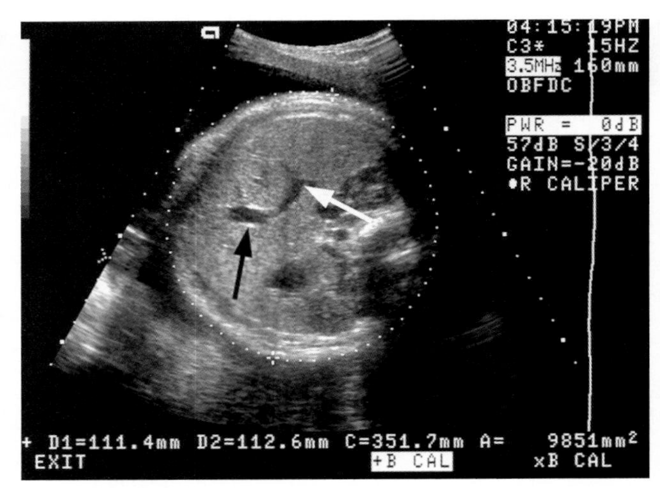

Figure 12-11 Measurement of abdominal circumference (AC). The abdominal circumference is measured on an axial image of the fetal abdomen at the level of the liver, preferably at the confluence of the left *(black arrow)* and right *(white arrow)* portal veins, which assume a C-shaped configuration. The AC should be measured along the outer edge of the soft tissues of the abdomen *(dotted line)*.

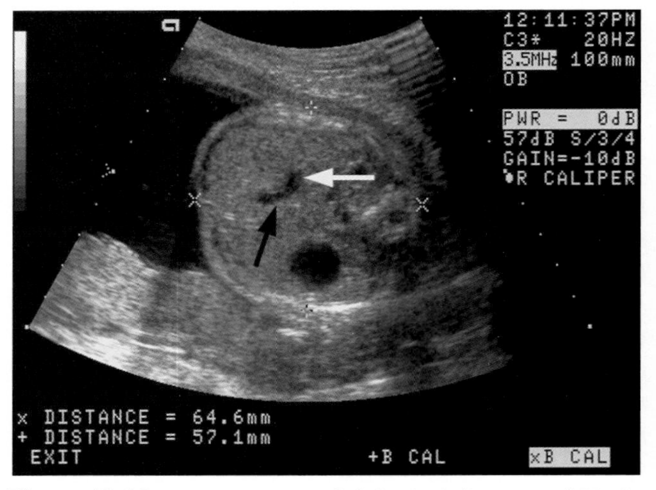

Figure 12-12 Measurement of abdominal diameters (AD). An alternative to directly measuring the abdominal circumference (AC) is to measure two orthogonal abdominal diameters and calculate the AC from the equation for the circumference of a circle. Abdominal diameters are measured at the same level as the AC from the outer edge to the outer edge of the soft tissues *(cursors)*. *Black arrow*, left portal vein; *white arrow*, right portal vein.

Table 12-8 Head to Abdomen Circumference Ratio Table

Gestational Age (wk)	Ratio of Head Circumference/Abdominal Circumference: Mean	Ratio of Head Circumference/Abdominal Circumference: Range from 5th to 95th Percentile
13-14	1.23	1.14-1.31
15-16	1.22	1.05-1.39
17-18	1.18	1.07-1.29
19-20	1.18	1.09-1.39
21-22	1.15	1.06-1.25
23-24	1.13	1.05-1.21
25-26	1.13	1.04-1.22
27-28	1.13	1.05-1.21
29-30	1.10	0.99-1.21.
31-32	1.07	0.96-1.17
33-34	1.04	0.96-1.11
35-36	1.02	0.93-1.11
37-38	0.98	0.92-1.05
39-40	0.97	0.87-1.06
41-42	0.96	0.93-1.00

From Campbell S, Thoms A: Ultrasound measurement of the fetal head to abdomen circumference in the assessment of growth retardation. Br J Obstet Gynaecol 84:165-174, 1977.

Table 12-9 Abdominal Diameter Measurement Table

Gestational Age (wk)	Predicted Mean Biparietal Diameter (mm)	Average Abdominal Diameter (mm): Predicted Mean	Average Abdominal Diameter (mm): Range from 5th to 95th Percentile
13	25.6	22.7	18.2-27.2
14	28.5	26.4	21.7-31.1
15	31.5	30.1	25.3-34.9
16	34.6	33.7	28.6-38.8
17	37.7	37.3	32.0-42.7
18	40.9	40.9	35.4-46.5
19	44.1	44.5	38.7-50.3
20	47.4	48.0	41.9-54.0
21	50.6	51.4	45.2-57.7
22	53.9	54.9	48.3-61.5
23	57.1	58.3	51.4-65.2
24	60.4	61.7	54.5-68.9
25	63.5	65.0	57.5-72.6
26	66.6	68.4	60.5-76.2
27	70.0	71.7	63.4-79.9
28	72.6	74.9	66.3-83.6
29	75.4	78.2	69.1-87.2
30	78.1	81.4	71.9-90.9
31	80.7	84.6	74.6-94.5
32	83.1	87.7	77.2-98.2
33	85.4	90.8	79.8-101.8
34	87.5	93.9	82.4-105.5
35	89.4	97.0	84.8-109.2
36	91.1	100.1	87.3-112.9
37	92.6	103.1	89.5-116.5
38	93.8	106.1	91.9-120.3
39	94.8	109.0	94.1-124.0
40	95.5	112.0	96.2-127.8

From Eriksen PS, Sechor NJ, Weis-Bentzon M: Normal growth of the fetal biparietal diameter and the abdominal diameter in a longitudinal study: An evaluation of the two parameters in predicting fetal weight. Acta Obstet Gynecol Scand 64: 65-70, 1985.

longitudinal growth data should be applied when possible. Most measurement tables use cross-sectional data, which was collected by evaluating multiple fetuses only once. Cross-sectional data permit accurate estimations of gestational age but are not optimal for analysis of interval growth. For evaluation of interval growth, longitudinal growth studies are preferred. Longitudinal growth tables evaluate multiple fetuses multiple times, comparing individual and population growth. Although the mean numbers are approximately the same from cross-sectional and longitudinal studies, the ranges are very different.

There are three main approaches to interval growth analysis. The least precise compares the gestational ages corresponding to fetal measurements from two examinations, sometimes utilizing different gestational age tables. This approach can be used at any time during the pregnancy and is the method most commonly used to assess interval growth between the first and the second trimesters. For example, if the initial ultrasound had detected an embryo of 10 mm, equivalent to mean gestational age of 7.1 weeks (see Table 12-1), 10 weeks later when a second study is performed the assigned gestational age would be 17.1 weeks. If on that second study the BPD measures 36 mm, equivalent to a mean age of 16.4 weeks (see Table 12-4), the measured gestational age by BPD (16.4 weeks) would be within 1 week of the assigned gestational age (17.1 weeks), and it would be assumed that there is likely no problem with head growth. As discrepancies approach or exceed 2 weeks, however, the possibility of a growth disturbance would be raised.

A second method of evaluating interval growth consists of plotting fetal measurements on a graph, which displays a measurement parameter such as EFW or AC on one axis and gestational age on the other axis. Lines delineating the mean and predetermined percentile or standard deviation levels for the parameter are superimposed on the graph to facilitate assessment of whether fetal size is appropriate for gestational age and whether interval growth has been appropriate. A variation of this method uses a table or computer program to report the percentile or standard deviation level of a parameter for the fetus' assigned gestational age. If there is marked

Table 12-10 Estimated Fetal Weight (g) Based on Biparietal Diameter (BPD) and Abdominal Circumference (AC)*

	AC (mm)												
BPD (mm)	**155**	**160**	**165**	**170**	**175**	**180**	**185**	**190**	**195**	**200**	**205**	**210**	**215**
31	224	234	244	255	267	279	291	304	318	332	346	362	378
32	231	241	251	263	274	286	299	312	326	340	355	371	388
33	237	248	259	270	282	294	307	321	335	349	365	381	397
34	244	255	266	278	290	302	316	329	344	359	374	391	408
35	251	262	274	285	298	311	324	338	353	368	384	401	418
36	259	270	281	294	306	319	333	347	362	378	394	411	429
37	266	278	290	302	315	328	342	357	372	388	404	422	440
38	274	286	298	310	324	337	352	366	382	398	415	432	451
39	282	294	306	319	333	347	361	376	392	409	426	444	462
40	290	303	315	328	342	356	371	386	403	419	437	455	474
41	299	311	324	338	352	366	381	397	413	430	448	467	486
42	308	320	333	347	361	376	392	408	424	442	460	479	498
43	317	330	343	357	371	387	402	419	436	453	472	491	511
44	326	339	353	367	382	397	413	430	447	465	484	504	524
45	335	349	363	377	393	408	425	442	459	478	497	517	538
46	345	359	373	386	404	420	436	454	472	490	510	530	551
47	355	369	384	399	415	431	448	466	484	503	524	544	565
48	366	380	395	410	426	443	460	478	497	517	537	558	580
49	376	391	406	422	438	455	473	491	510	530	551	572	594
50	387	402	418	434	451	468	486	505	524	544	565	587	610
51	399	414	430	446	463	481	499	518	538	559	580	602	625
52	410	426	442	459	476	494	513	532	552	573	595	618	641
53	422	438	455	472	489	508	527	547	567	589	611	634	657
54	435	451	468	485	503	522	541	561	582	604	627	650	674
55	447	464	481	499	517	536	556	577	598	620	643	667	691
56	461	477	495	513	532	551	571	592	614	636	660	684	709
57	474	491	509	527	547	566	587	608	630	653	677	701	727
58	488	505	524	542	562	582	603	625	647	670	695	719	745
59	502	520	539	558	578	598	619	642	664	688	713	738	764
60	517	535	554	573	594	615	636	659	682	706	731	757	784
61	532	550	570	590	610	632	654	677	700	725	750	777	804
62	547	566	586	606	627	649	672	695	719	744	770	797	824
63	563	583	603	624	645	667	690	714	738	764	790	817	845
64	580	600	620	641	663	686	709	733	758	784	811	838	867
65	597	617	638	659	682	705	728	753	778	805	832	860	889
66	614	635	656	678	701	724	748	773	799	826	853	882	911
67	632	653	675	697	720	744	769	794	820	848	876	905	935
68	651	672	694	717	740	765	790	816	842	870	898	928	958
69	670	691	714	737	761	786	811	838	865	893	922	952	983
70	689	711	734	758	782	807	833	860	888	916	946	976	1008
71	709	732	755	779	804	830	856	883	912	941	971	1002	1033
72	730	763	777	801	827	853	880	907	936	965	996	1027	1060
73	751	775	799	824	850	876	904	932	961	991	1022	1054	1087
74	773	797	822	847	874	901	928	957	987	1017	1049	1081	1114
75	796	820	845	871	898	925	954	983	1013	1044	1076	1109	1143
76	819	844	870	896	923	951	960	1009	1040	1072	1104	1137	1172
77	843	868	894	921	949	977	1007	1037	1068	1100	1133	1187	1202
78	868	894	920	947	975	1004	1034	1065	1096	1129	1162	1197	1232
79	893	919	946	974	1003	1032	1062	1094	1126	1159	1193	1228	1264
80	919	946	973	1002	1031	1061	1091	1123	1156	1189	1224	1259	1296
81	946	973	1001	1030	1060	1090	1121	1153	1187	1221	1256	1292	1329
82	974	1001	1030	1059	1089	1120	1152	1185	1218	1253	1288	1325	1363
83	1002	1030	1059	1089	1120	1151	1183	1217	1251	1286	1322	1359	1397
84	1032	1060	1090	1120	1151	1163	1216	1249	1284	1320	1356	1394	1433
85	1062	1091	1121	1151	1183	1216	1249	1283	1318	1355	1392	1430	1469
86	1093	1122	1153	1184	1216	1249	1283	1318	1354	1390	1428	1467	1507
87	1125	1155	1186	1218	1250	1284	1318	1353	1390	1427	1465	1505	1545
88	1157	1188	1220	1252	1285	1319	1354	1390	1427	1465	1504	1543	1584
89	1191	1222	1254	1287	1321	1356	1391	1428	1465	1503	1543	1583	1625
90	1226	1258	1290	1324	1358	1393	1429	1456	1504	1543	1583	1624	1666
91	1262	1294	1327	1361	1396	1432	1468	1506	1544	1584	1624	1666	1708
92	1299	1332	1365	1400	1435	1471	1508	1546	1586	1626	1667	1709	1752
93	1337	1370	1404	1439	1475	1512	1550	1588	1628	1668	1710	1753	1796
94	1376	1410	1444	1480	1516	1554	1592	1631	1671	1712	1755	1798	1842
95	1416	1450	1486	1522	1559	1597	1635	1675	1716	1758	1800	1844	1889
96	1457	1492	1528	1565	1602	1641	1680	1720	1762	1804	1847	1892	1937
97	1500	1535	1572	1609	1547	1686	1726	1767	1809	1852	1895	1940	1986
98	1544	1580	1617	1654	1693	1733	1773	1815	1857	1900	1945	1990	2037
99	1589	1625	1663	1701	1740	1781	1822	1864	1907	1951	1996	2042	2089
100	1635	1672	1710	1749	1789	1830	1871	1914	1958	2002	2048	2094	2142

*Estimated fetal weights: Log (birth weight) = −1.7492 + 0.166 (BPD) + 0.046 (AC) −0.00264 (AC × BPD).

From Shepard MJ, Richards VA, Berkowitz RL, et al: An evaluation of two equations for predicting fetal weight by ultrasound. Am J Obstet Gynecol 147:47-54, 1982.

Table 12-10—Cont'd

BPD (mm)	AC (mm) 220	225	230	235	240	245	250	255	260	265	270	275	280
31	395	412	431	450	470	491	513	536	559	584	610	638	666
32	405	423	441	461	481	502	525	548	572	597	624	651	680
33	415	433	452	472	493	514	537	560	585	611	638	666	693
34	425	444	463	483	504	526	549	573	598	624	652	680	710
35	436	455	475	495	517	539	562	587	612	638	666	695	725
36	447	466	486	507	529	552	575	600	626	653	681	710	740
37	458	478	498	519	542	565	589	614	640	667	696	725	756
38	470	490	510	532	554	578	602	628	654	682	711	741	772
39	482	502	523	545	568	592	616	642	669	697	727	757	789
40	494	514	536	558	581	606	631	657	684	713	743	773	806
41	506	527	549	572	595	620	645	672	700	729	759	790	828
42	519	540	562	585	609	634	660	688	716	745	776	807	841
43	532	554	576	600	624	649	676	703	732	762	793	825	859
44	545	567	590	614	639	665	692	719	749	779	810	843	877
45	559	581	605	629	654	680	708	736	765	796	828	861	896
46	573	596	620	644	670	696	724	753	783	814	846	880	915
47	588	611	635	660	686	713	741	770	801	832	865	899	934
48	602	626	650	676	702	730	758	788	819	851	884	919	954
49	617	641	666	692	719	747	776	806	837	870	903	938	975
50	633	657	683	709	736	765	794	824	856	889	923	959	996
51	649	674	699	726	754	783	812	843	876	909	944	980	1017
52	665	690	717	744	772	801	831	863	895	929	964	1001	1039
53	682	708	734	762	790	820	851	883	916	950	986	1023	1061
54	699	725	752	780	809	839	870	903	936	971	1007	1045	1084
55	717	743	771	799	828	859	891	924	958	993	1030	1068	1107
56	735	762	789	818	848	879	911	945	979	1015	1052	1091	1131
57	753	780	809	838	869	900	933	966	1001	1038	1075	1114	1155
58	772	800	829	858	889	921	954	989	1024	1061	1099	1139	1180
59	792	820	849	879	911	943	977	1011	1047	1085	1123	1163	1205
60	811	840	870	900	932	965	999	1035	1071	1109	1148	1189	1231
61	832	861	891	922	955	988	1023	1058	1095	1134	1173	1214	1257
62	853	882	913	945	977	1011	1046	1083	1120	1159	1199	1241	1284
63	874	904	935	967	1001	1035	1071	1107	1145	1185	1226	1268	1311
64	896	927	958	991	1025	1059	1096	1133	1171	1211	1253	1295	1339
65	919	950	982	1015	1049	1084	1121	1159	1198	1238	1280	1323	1368
66	942	973	1006	1039	1074	1110	1147	1185	1225	1266	1308	1352	1397
67	965	997	1030	1065	1100	1136	1174	1213	1253	1294	1337	1381	1427
68	990	1022	1056	1090	1126	1163	1201	1241	1281	1323	1367	1411	1458
69	1015	1048	1082	1117	1153	1190	1229	1269	1310	1353	1397	1442	1489
70	1040	1074	1108	1144	1181	1219	1258	1298	1340	1383	1427	1473	1521
71	1066	1100	1135	1171	1209	1247	1287	1328	1370	1414	1459	1505	1553
72	1093	1128	1163	1200	1238	1277	1317	1358	1401	1445	1491	1538	1586
73	1121	1156	1192	1229	1267	1307	1348	1390	1433	1478	1524	1571	1620
74	1149	1184	1221	1259	1297	1338	1379	1421	1465	1511	1557	1605	1655
75	1178	1214	1251	1289	1328	1369	1411	1454	1499	1544	1592	1640	1690
76	1207	1244	1281	1320	1360	1401	1444	1487	1533	1579	1627	1676	1727
77	1238	1275	1313	1352	1393	1434	1477	1522	1567	1614	1663	1712	1764
78	1269	1306	1345	1385	1426	1468	1512	1557	1603	1650	1699	1749	1801
79	1301	1339	1378	1418	1460	1503	1547	1592	1639	1687	1737	1787	1840
80	1333	1372	1412	1453	1495	1538	1583	1629	1676	1725	1775	1826	1879
81	1367	1406	1446	1488	1531	1575	1620	1666	1714	1763	1814	1866	1919
82	1401	1441	1482	1524	1567	1612	1657	1704	1753	1803	1854	1906	1960
83	1436	1477	1518	1561	1605	1650	1696	1744	1793	1843	1895	1948	2002
84	1473	1513	1555	1599	1643	1689	1735	1784	1833	1884	1936	1990	2045
85	1510	1551	1594	1637	1682	1728	1776	1825	1875	1926	1979	2033	2089
86	1548	1589	1633	1677	1722	1769	1817	1866	1917	1969	2022	2077	2134
87	1586	1629	1673	1717	1764	1811	1859	1909	1960	2013	2067	2122	2179
88	1626	1669	1714	1759	1806	1854	1903	1953	2005	2058	2113	2169	2226
89	1667	1711	1756	1802	1849	1897	1947	1998	2050	2104	2159	2216	2274
90	1709	1753	1799	1845	1893	1942	1992	2044	2097	2151	2207	2264	2322
91	1752	1797	1843	1890	1938	1988	2039	2091	2144	2199	2255	2313	2372
92	1796	1841	1888	1936	1984	2035	2086	2139	2193	2248	2305	2363	2423
93	1841	1887	1934	1982	2032	2083	2135	2188	2242	2298	2356	2414	2475
94	1887	1934	1982	2030	2080	2132	2184	2238	2293	2350	2407	2467	2527
95	1935	1982	2030	2080	2130	2182	2235	2289	2345	2402	2460	2520	2582
96	1984	2031	2080	2130	2181	2233	2287	2342	2398	2456	2515	2575	2637
97	2033	2082	2131	2181	2233	2286	2340	2396	2452	2510	2570	2631	2693
98	2085	2133	2183	2234	2286	2340	2395	2451	2508	2567	2627	2688	2751
99	2137	2186	2237	2288	2341	2395	2450	2507	2565	2624	2684	2746	2810
100	2191	2241	2292	2344	2397	2452	2507	2564	2623	2682	2743	2806	2870

Continued

Table 12-10 Estimated Fetal Weight (g) Based on Biparietal Diameter (BPD) and Abdominal Circumference (AC)*—Cont'd

	AC (mm)												
BPD (mm)	285	290	295	300	305	310	315	320	325	330	335	340	345
31	696	726	759	793	828	865	903	943	985	1029	1075	1123	1173
32	710	742	774	809	844	882	921	961	1004	1048	1094	1143	1193
33	725	757	790	825	861	899	938	979	1022	1067	1114	1163	1214
34	740	773	806	841	878	916	956	998	1041	1087	1134	1183	1235
35	756	789	823	858	896	934	975	1017	1061	1107	1154	1204	1256
35	772	805	840	876	913	953	993	1036	1080	1127	1175	1226	1278
37	788	822	857	893	931	971	1012	1056	1101	1147	1196	1247	1300
38	805	839	874	911	950	990	1032	1076	1121	1168	1218	1269	1323
39	822	856	892	930	969	1009	1052	1096	1142	1190	1240	1292	1346
40	839	874	911	949	988	1029	1072	1117	1163	1212	1262	1315	1369
41	857	892	929	968	1008	1049	1093	1138	1185	1234	1285	1338	1393
42	875	911	948	987	1028	1070	1114	1159	1207	1256	1308	1361	1417
43	893	930	968	1007	1048	1091	1135	1181	1229	1279	1331	1385	1442
44	912	949	987	1027	1069	1112	1157	1204	1252	1303	1355	1410	1467
45	932	969	1008	1048	1090	1134	1179	1226	1275	1326	1380	1435	1492
46	951	989	1028	1069	1112	1156	1202	1249	1299	1351	1404	1406	1518
47	971	1010	1049	1091	1134	1178	1225	1273	1323	1375	1430	1486	1545
48	992	1031	1071	1113	1156	1201	1248	1297	1348	1401	1455	1512	1571
49	1013	1052	1093	1135	1179	1225	1272	1322	1373	1426	1482	1539	1599
50	1034	1074	1115	1158	1203	1249	1297	1347	1399	1452	1508	1566	1626
51	1056	1096	1138	1181	1226	1273	1322	1372	1425	1479	1535	1594	1655
52	1078	1119	1161	1205	1251	1298	1347	1398	1451	1506	1563	1622	1683
53	1101	1142	1185	1229	1276	1323	1373	1425	1478	1533	1591	1651	1713
54	1124	1166	1209	1254	1301	1349	1399	1452	1506	1562	1620	1680	1742
55	1148	1190	1234	1279	1327	1376	1426	1479	1534	1590	1649	1710	1773
56	1172	1215	1259	1305	1353	1402	1454	1507	1562	1619	1678	1740	1803
57	1197	1240	1285	1332	1380	1430	1482	1535	1591	1649	1709	1770	1835
58	1222	1266	1311	1358	1407	1458	1510	1564	1621	1679	1739	1802	1866
59	1248	1292	1338	1386	1435	1486	1539	1594	1651	1710	1770	1834	1899
60	1274	1319	1366	1414	1464	1515	1569	1624	1682	1741	1802	1866	1932
61	1301	1346	1393	1442	1493	1545	1599	1655	1713	1773	1835	1899	1965
62	1328	1374	1422	1471	1522	1575	1630	1686	1745	1805	1868	1932	1999
63	1356	1403	1451	1501	1552	1606	1661	1718	1777	1838	1901	1967	2034
64	1385	1432	1481	1531	1583	1637	1693	1751	1810	1872	1935	2001	2069
65	1414	1462	1511	1562	1615	1669	1725	1784	1844	1906	1970	2037	2105
66	1444	1492	1542	1594	1647	1702	1759	1817	1878	1941	2006	2073	2142
67	1474	1523	1574	1626	1679	1735	1792	1852	1913	1976	2042	2109	2179
68	1505	1555	1606	1658	1713	1769	1827	1887	1949	2012	2078	2147	2217
69	1537	1587	1639	1692	1747	1803	1862	1922	1985	2049	2116	2184	2255
70	1570	1620	1672	1726	1781	1839	1898	1959	2022	2087	2154	2223	2295
71	1603	1654	1706	1761	1817	1875	1934	1996	2059	2125	2193	2262	2334
72	1636	1688	1741	1796	1853	1911	1971	2044	2098	2164	2232	2302	2375
73	1671	1723	1777	1832	1890	1948	2009	2072	2137	2203	2272	2343	2416
74	1706	1759	1813	1869	1927	1987	2048	2111	2176	2244	2313	2384	2458
75	1742	1795	1850	1907	1965	2025	2087	2151	2217	2265	2354	2426	2501
76	1779	1833	1888	1945	2004	2065	2127	2192	2258	2326	2397	2469	2544
77	1816	1871	1927	1985	2044	2105	2168	2233	2300	2369	2440	2513	2588
76	1855	1910	1966	2025	2085	2146	2210	2275	2343	2412	2484	2557	2633
79	1894	1949	2006	2065	2126	2188	2252	2318	2386	2456	2528	2603	2679
80	1934	1990	2048	2107	2168	2231	2296	2362	2431	2501	2574	2649	2725
81	1975	2031	2089	2149	2211	2275	2340	2407	2476	2547	2620	2695	2773
82	2016	2073	2132	2193	2255	2319	2385	2462	2522	2594	2667	2743	2821
83	2059	2116	2176	2237	2300	2364	2431	2499	2569	2641	2715	2791	2870
84	2102	2160	2220	2282	2345	2410	2477	2546	2617	2689	2764	2841	2920
85	2146	2205	2266	2328	2392	2457	2525	2594	2665	2739	2814	2891	2970
86	2192	2251	2312	2375	2439	2505	2573	2643	2715	2789	2864	2942	3022
87	2238	2298	2359	2423	2488	2554	2623	2693	2765	2840	2916	2994	3074
88	2285	2346	2408	2472	2537	2604	2673	2744	2817	2892	2968	3047	3128
89	2333	2394	2457	2521	2587	2655	2725	2796	2869	2944	3021	3101	3182
90	2382	2444	2507	2572	2639	2707	2777	2849	2923	2998	3076	3155	3237
91	2433	2495	2559	2624	2691	2760	2830	2903	2977	3053	3131	3211	3293
92	2484	2547	2611	2677	2744	2814	2885	2958	3032	3109	3187	3268	3350
93	2536	2599	2664	2731	2799	2869	2940	3014	3089	3166	3245	3326	3409
94	2590	2853	2719	2786	2854	2925	2997	3070	3146	3224	3303	3384	3488
95	2644	2709	2774	2842	2911	2982	3054	3129	3205	3283	3362	3444	3528
96	2700	2765	2831	2899	2969	3040	3113	3188	3264	3343	3423	3505	3589
97	2757	2822	2889	2958	3028	3099	3173	3248	3325	3404	3484	3567	3651
98	2815	2881	2948	3017	3088	3160	3234	3309	3387	3466	3547	3630	3715
99	2874	2941	3009	3078	3149	3222	3296	3372	3450	3529	3611	3694	3779
100	2935	3002	3070	3140	3211	3285	3359	3436	3514	3594	3676	3759	3845

*Estimated fetal weights: Log (birth weight) = −1.7492 + 0.166 (BPD) + 0.046 (AC) −0.00264 (AC × BPD).

From Shepard MJ, Richards VA, Berkowitz RL, et al: An evaluation of two equations for predicting fetal weight by ultrasound, Am J Obstet Gynaecol 147:47-54, 1982.

Table 12-10—Cont'd

BPD (mm)	AC (mm) 350	355	360	365	370	375	380	385	390	395	400
31	1225	1279	1336	1396	1458	1523	1591	1661	1735	1812	1893
32	1246	1301	1258	1418	1481	1546	1615	1686	1761	1838	1920
33	1267	1323	1381	1441	1504	1570	1639	1711	1786	1865	1946
34	1289	1345	1403	1464	1528	1595	1664	1737	1812	1891	1973
35	1311	1367	1426	1488	1552	1619	1689	1762	1839	1918	2001
36	1333	1390	1450	1512	1577	1645	1715	1789	1865	1945	2029
37	1356	1413	1474	1536	1602	1670	1741	1815	1893	1973	2057
38	1379	1437	1498	1561	1627	1696	1768	1842	1920	2001	2086
39	1402	1461	1523	1586	1653	1722	1794	1870	1948	2030	2115
40	1426	1486	1548	1612	1679	1749	1822	1898	1977	2059	2145
41	1451	1511	1573	1638	1706	1776	1849	1926	2005	2088	2174
42	1475	1536	1599	1664	1733	1804	1878	1954	2035	2118	2205
43	1500	1562	1625	1691	1760	1832	1906	1984	2064	2148	2236
44	1526	1588	1652	1718	1788	1860	1935	2013	2094	2179	2267
45	1552	1614	1679	1746	1816	1889	1964	2043	2125	2210	2298
46	1579	1641	1706	1774	1845	1918	1994	2073	2156	2241	2330
47	1605	1669	1734	1803	1874	1948	2024	2104	2167	2273	2363
48	1633	1697	1763	1832	1904	1976	2055	2136	2219	2306	2398
49	1661	1725	1792	1861	1934	2009	2086	2187	2251	2339	2429
50	1689	1754	1821	1891	1964	2040	2118	2200	2284	2372	2463
51	1718	1783	1851	1922	1995	2071	2150	2232	2317	2406	2498
52	1747	1813	1882	1953	2027	2103	2183	2266	2351	2440	2532
53	1777	1843	1913	1984	2059	2136	2216	2299	2386	2475	2568
54	1807	1874	1944	2016	2091	2169	2250	2333	2420	2510	2604
55	1838	1906	1976	2049	2124	2203	2284	2368	2456	2546	2640
56	1869	1938	2008	2082	2158	2237	2319	2403	2491	2582	2677
57	1901	1970	2041	2115	2192	2272	2354	2439	2528	2619	2714
58	1934	2003	2075	2150	2227	2307	2390	2475	2564	2657	2752
59	1966	2037	2109	2184	2262	2342	2426	2512	2602	2694	2790
60	2000	2071	2144	2219	2298	2379	2463	2550	2640	2733	2829
61	2034	2105	2179	2255	2334	2416	2500	2588	2678	2772'	2869
62	2069	2140	2215	2291	2371	2453	2538	2626	2717	2811	2909
63	2104	2176	2251	2328	2408	2491	2577	2665	2757	2851	2949
64	2140	2213	2288	2366	2446	2530	2616	2705	2797	2892	2991
65	2176	2250	2328	2404	2485	2569	2656	2745	2838	2933	3032
66	2213	2287	2364	2443	2524	2609	2696	2786	2879	2975	3075
67	2251	2326	2403	2482	2564	2649	2737	2827	2921	3018	3117
68	2290	2365	2442	2522	2605	2690	2778	2869	2964	3061	3161
69	2329	2404	2482	2563	2646	2732	2821	2912	3007	3104	3205
70	2368	2444	2523	2604	2688	2774	2863	2955	3050	3149	3250
71	2409	2485	2564	2846	2730	2817	2907	2999	3095	3193	3295
72	2450	2527	2607	2689	2773	2861	2951	3044	3140	3239	3341
73	2491	2569	2649	2732	2817	2905	2996	3089	3186	3285	3386
74	2534	2612	2693	2776	2862	2950	3041	3135	3232	3332	3435
75	2577	2656	2737	2821	2907	2996	3088	3182	3279	3380	3483
76	2621	2700	2782	2866	2953	3042	3134	3229	3327	3428	3531
77	2666	2746	2828	2912	3000	3090	3128	3277	3376	3477	3581
78	2711	2792	2874	2959	3047	3137	3230	3326	3425	3526	3631
79	2757	2838	2921	3007	3095	3186	3279	3376	3475	3576	3681
80	2804	2886	2969	3056	3144	3235	3329	3426	3525	3627	3733
81	2852	2934	3018	3105	3194	3286	3380	3477	3577	3679	3785
82	2901	2983	3068	3155	3244	3336	3431	3529	3629	3732	3838
83	2950	3033	3118	3206	3296	3388	3483	3581	3682	3785	3891
84	3001	3084	3169	3257	3348	3441	3536	3634	3735	3839	3945
85	3052	3135	3221	3310	3401	3494	3590	3688	3790	3894	4000
86	3104	3188	3274	3363	3454	3548	3644	3743	3845	3949	4056
87	3157	3241	3328	3417	3509	3603	3700	3799	3901	4005	4113
88	3210	3295	3383	3472	3565	3659	3756	3855	3958	4063	4170
89	3265	3351	3438	3528	3621	3716	3813	3913	4015	4120	4228
90	3321	3407	3495	3585	3678	3773	3871	3971	4074	4179	4287
91	3377	3464	3552	3643	3736	3832	3930	4030	4133	4239	4347
92	3435	3522	3611	3702	3795	3891	3989	4090	4193	4299	4408
93	3494	3581	3670	3761	3855	3951	4050	4151	4254	4361	4469
94	3553	3641	3738	3822	3916	4013	4111	4213	4316	4423	4532
95	3614	3701	3791	3884	3978	4075	4174	4275	4379	4486	4595
96	3675	3763	3854	3946	4041	4138	4237	4339	4443	4550	4659
97	3738	3826	3917	4010	4105	4202	4302	4404	4508	4615	4724
98	3802	3890	3981	4074	4170	4267	4367	4469	4573	4680	4790
99	3866	3956	4047	4140	4236	4333	4433	4536	4640	4747	4857
100	3932	4022	4113	4207	4303	4400	4501	4603	4708	4815	4924

Table 12-11 Estimated Fetal Weight (g) Based on Abdominal Circumference and Femur Length*

Femur Length (mm)	Ratio of Head Circumference/Abdominal Circumference																			
	200	205	210	215	220	225	230	235	240	245	250	255	260	265	270	275	280	285	290	295
40	663	691	720	751	783	816	851	887	925	964	1006	1048	1093	1139	1188	1239	1291	1346	1403	1463
41	680	709	738	769	802	836	871	907	946	986	1027	1070	1115	1162	1211	1262	1315	1371	1429	1489
42	697	726	757	788	821	855	891	928	967	1007	1049	1093	1138	1186	1235	1287	1340	1396	1454	1515
43	715	745	776	808	841	875	912	949	988	1029	1071	1116	1162	1209	1259	1311	1365	1422	1480	1541
44	734	764	795	827	861	896	933	971	1010	1051	1094	1139	1185	1234	1284	1336	1391	1448	1509	1568
45	753	783	815	847	882	917	954	993	1033	1074	1118	1163	1210	1259	1309	1362	1417	1474	1534	1596
46	772	803	835	868	903	939	976	1015	1056	1098	1142	1187	1235	1284	1335	1388	1444	1501	1561	1623
47	792	813	856	889	924	961	999	1038	1079	1122	1166	1212	1260	1310	1316	1415	1471	1529	1589	1652
48	812	844	877	911	947	984	1022	1062	1103	1146	1191	1237	1286	1336	1388	1442	1498	1557	1618	1681
49	833	865	899	933	969	1007	1046	1086	1128	1171	1216	1263	1312	1363	1415	1470	1527	1585	1647	1710
50	855	887	921	956	993	1031	1070	1111	1153	1197	1243	1290	1339	1390	1443	1498	1555	1615	1676	1740
51	877	910	944	980	1016	1055	1095	1136	1179	1223	1269	1317	1367	1418	1471	1527	1584	1644	1706	1770
52	899	933	967	1004	1041	1080	1120	1162	1205	1250	1296	1344	1395	1447	1500	1556	1614	1647	1737	1801
53	922	956	992	1028	1066	1105	1146	1188	1232	1277	1324	1373	1423	1476	1530	1586	1645	1705	1768	1833
54	946	981	1016	1053	1091	1131	1172	1215	1259	1305	1352	1401	1452	1505	1560	1617	1675	1736	1799	1865
55	971	1005	1041	1079	1118	1158	1199	1242	1287	1333	1318	1431	1482	1535	1591	1648	1707	1768	1832	1897
56	995	1031	1067	1105	1144	1185	1227	1271	1316	1362	1411	1461	1513	1566	1622	1679	1739	1801	1864	1931
57	1021	1057	1094	1132	1172	1213	1255	1299	1345	1392	1441	1491	1544	1598	1654	1712	1772	1834	1898	1964
58	1047	1084	1121	1160	1200	1242	1285	1329	1375	1422	1472	1533	1575	1630	1686	1744	1805	1867	1932	1999
59	1074	1111	1149	1188	1229	1271	1314	1359	1406	1454	1503	1555	1608	1663	1719	1778	1839	1902	1966	2034
60	1102	1139	1178	1217	1258	1301	1345	1309	1437	1485	1535	1587	1641	1696	1753	1812	1873	1936	2002	2069
61	1130	1168	1207	1247	1289	1331	1376	1421	1469	1518	1568	1620	1674	1730	1788	1847	1908	1972	2038	2105
62	1160	1198	1237	1278	1319	1363	1408	1454	1501	1551	1602	1654	1709	1765	1823	1882	1944	2008	2074	2142
63	1189	1228	1268	1309	1351	1395	1440	1487	1535	1585	1636	1689	1744	1800	1858	1919	1981	2045	2111	2180
64	1220	1259	1299	1341	1384	1428	1473	1520	1569	1619	1671	1724	1779	1836	1895	1956	2018	2082	2149	2218
65	1251	1291	1332	1373	1417	1461	1507	1555	1604	1655	1707	1760	1816	1873	1932	1993	2056	2121	2188	2250
66	1284	1324	1365	1407	1451	1496	1542	1590	1640	1691	1743	1797	1853	1911	1970	2031	2094	2160	2227	2290
67	1317	1357	1399	1441	1486	1531	1578	1626	1676	1728	1780	1835	1891	1949	2009	2070	2134	2199	2267	2330
68	1351	1391	1313	1477	1521	1567	1615	1663	1713	1765	1819	1873	1930	1988	2048	2110	2174	2240	2307	2377
69	1385	1427	1469	1513	1558	1604	1652	1701	1752	1804	1857	1913	1970	2028	2089	2151	2215	2281	2348	2418
70	1421	1463	1506	1550	1595	1642	1690	1740	1791	1843	1897	1953	2010	2069	2130	2192	2256	2322	2391	2461
71	1458	1500	1543	1588	1633	1681	1729	1779	1830	1883	1938	1994	2051	2110	2171	2234	2299	2365	2433	2504
72	1495	1538	1581	1626	1673	1720	1769	1819	1871	1924	1979	2035	2093	2153	2214	2277	2342	2408	2477	2547
73	1534	1577	1621	1666	1713	1761	1810	1861	1913	1966	2021	2078	2136	2196	2258	2321	2386	2453	2521	2592
74	1573	1616	1661	1707	1754	1802	1852	1903	1955	2009	2065	2122	2180	2240	2302	2365	2431	2498	2566	2637
75	1614	1657	1702	1749	1796	1845	1895	1946	1999	2053	2109	2166	2225	2285	2347	2411	2476	2543	2612	2683
76	1655	1699	1745	1791	1839	1888	1939	1990	2043	2098	2154	2211	2270	2331	2393	2457	2523	2590	2659	273[illegible]
77	1698	1742	1788	1835	1883	1933	1983	2035	2089	2144	2200	2258	2317	2378	2440	2504	2570	2638	2707	2778
78	1741	1786	1833	1880	1928	1978	2029	2082	2135	2191	2247	2305	2365	2426	2488	2553	2618	2686	2755	2827
79	1786	1832	1878	1926	1975	2025	2076	2129	2183	2238	2295	2353	2413	2474	2537	2602	2668	2735	2805	2876
80	1832	1878	1925	1973	2022	2073	2124	2177	2232	2287	2344	2403	2463	2524	2587	2652	2718	2785	2855	292[illegible]
81	1879	1926	1973	2021	2071	2121	2173	2227	2281	2337	2394	2453	2513	2575	2638	2702	2769	2837	2906	2977
82	1928	1974	2022	2070	2120	2171	2224	2277	2332	2388	2446	2504	2565	2626	2690	2754	2821	2889	2958	302[illegible]
83	1978	2024	2072	2121	2171	2223	2275	2329	2384	2440	2498	2557	2617	2679	2743	2807	2874	2942	3011	308[illegible]

*Based on regression model: Log_{10} body weight = 1.3598 + 0.051 (abdominal circumference) + 0.1844 (femur length) − 0.0037 (abdominal circumference × femur length).

From Hadlock FP, et al: Sonographic estimation of fetal weight. Radiology 150:535-540, 1984.

Table 12-11—Cont'd

Ratio of Head Circumference/Abdominal Circumference

300	305	310	315	320	325	330	335	340	345	350	355	360	365	370	375	380	385	390	395	400
525	1590	1658	1729	1802	1879	1959	2042	2129	2220	2314	2413	2515	2622	2734	2856	2972	3098	3230	3367	3511
551	1617	1685	1756	1830	1907	1987	2071	2158	2249	2344	2442	2545	2652	2764	2880	3002	3128	3260	3397	3540
578	1644	1712	1783	1858	1935	2016	2100	2187	2279	2373	2472	2575	2683	2794	2911	3032	3159	3290	3427	3570
605	1671	1740	1812	1886	1964	2054	2129	2217	2308	2404	2503	2606	2713	2325	2942	3063	3189	3321	3458	3600
632	1699	1768	1840	1915	1993	2075	2159	2247	2339	2434	2533	2637	2744	2850	2973	3094	3220	3352	3488	3630
660	1727	1797	1869	1944	2023	2105	2189	2278	2370	2465	2565	2668	2776	2888	3004	3125	3251	3383	3519	3661
688	1756	1826	1898	1974	2053	2135	2220	2309	2401	2497	2596	2700	2807	2919	3036	3157	3283	3414	3550	3692
717	1785	1855	1928	2004	2084	2166	2251	2340	2432	2528	2628	2732	2840	2952	3068	3189	3315	3446	3582	3723
746	1814	1885	1959	2035	2115	2197	2283	2372	2464	2560	2660	2764	2872	2984	3100	3221	3347	3478	3613	3754
776	1845	1916	1990	2066	2146	2229	2315	2404	2497	2593	2693	2797	2905	3017	3133	3254	3380	3510	3645	3786
806	1875	1947	2021	2098	2178	2261	2347	2437	2530	2626	2726	2830	2938	3050	3166	3287	3412	3542	3677	3818
837	1906	1978	2053	2130	2210	2294	2380	2470	2563	2659	2760	2864	2972	3084	3200	3320	3445	3575	3710	3850
868	1938	2010	2085	2163	2243	2327	2413	2503	2597	2693	2794	2898	3006	3117	3234	3354	3479	3608	3743	3882
900	1970	2043	2118	2196	2277	2360	2447	2537	2631	2728	2828	2932	3040	3152	3268	3388	3513	3642	3776	3915
933	2003	2076	2151	2229	2311	2395	2482	2572	2665	2762	2963	2967	3075	3176	3302	3422	3547	3676	3809	3948
966	2036	2109	2185	2264	2345	2429	2516	2607	2700	2797	2898	3002	3110	3221	3337	3457	3581	3710	3843	3981
999	2070	2143	2220	2298	2380	2464	2552	2642	2756	2833	2933	3638	3145	3257	3372	3492	3616	3744	3877	4015
33	2104	2178	2254	2333	2415	2500	2587	2678	2772	2869	2970	3074	3181	3293	3404	3572	3651	3779	3911	4048
068	2139	2213	2290	2369	2451	2536	2624	2714	2808	2905	3006	3110	3218	3329	3444	3563	3686	3814	3946	4082
03	2174	2249	2326	2405	2488	2573	2660	2751	2845	2942	3043	3147	3254	3366	3480	3599	3722	3849	3981	4117
39	2211	2286	2363	2442	2525	2610	2698	2789	2883	2980	3080	3184	3292	3403	3517	3636	3758	3885	4016	4151
75	2248	2323	2400	2480	2562	2647	2736	2827	2921	3018	3118	3222	3329	3440	3554	3673	3795	3921	4052	4186
212	2285	2360	2438	2518	2600	2686	2774	2865	2959	3056	3157	3260	3367	3478	3392	3710	3832	3957	4087	4222
250	2323	2398	2476	2556	2639	2725	2813	2904	2998	3095	3195	3299	3406	3516	3630	3747	3869	3994	4124	4257
289	2362	2437	2515	2595	2678	2761	2852	2943	3037	3134	3235	3338	3445	3555	3668	3785	3906	4031	4160	4293
328	2401	2477	2555	2635	2718	2804	2892	2983	3077	3174	3274	3378	3484	3594	3707	3824	3944	4069	4197	4329
367	2441	2517	2595	2675	2759	2844	2933	3024	3118	3215	3315	3418	3524	3633	3746	3863	3983	4106	4234	4366
408	2481	2557	2636	2716	2800	2885	2974	3065	3159	3256	3355	3458	3564	3673	3786	3902	4021	4144	4271	4402
449	2523	2599	2677	2758	2841	2927	3016	3107	3200	3297	3397	3499	3605	3714	3862	3941	4060	4183	4309	4439
490	2564	2641	2719	2800	2884	2969	3058	3149	3242	3339	3438	3541	3646	3754	3866	3981	4100	4222	4347	4477
533	2607	2683	2762	2843	2927	3012	3101	3192	3285	3381	3481	3583	3688	3796	3907	4022	4140	4261	4386	4514
576	2650	2727	2806	2887	2970	3056	3144	3235	3328	3424	3523	3625	3730	3838	3948	4062	4180	4300	4425	4552
620	2694	2771	2850	2931	3014	3100	3188	3279	3372	3468	3567	3668	3772	3880	3990	4104	4220	4340	4464	4591
665	2739	2816	2895	2976	3059	3145	3233	3323	3416	3512	3613	3712	3816	3922	4032	4145	4261	4381	4503	4629
710	2785	2861	2940	3021	3105	3190	3278	3369	3461	3557	3655	3756	3859	3966	4075	4187	4303	4421	4543	4668
756	2831	2908	2987	3065	3151	3236	4324	3414	3507	3602	3700	3800	3903	4009	4118	4230	4344	4462	4583	4708
803	2878	2955	3034	3115	3198	3283	3371	3461	3553	3648	3745	3845	3948	4053	4161	4272	4387	4504	4624	4747
851	2926	3003	3081	3162	3245	3331	3418	3508	3600	4694	3791	3891	3993	4098	4205	4316	4429	4545	4665	4787
899	2974	3051	3130	3211	3294	3379	3466	3555	3647	3741	3838	3937	4039	4143	4250	4360	4472	4588	4706	4827
949	3024	3100	3179	3260	3343	3427	3514	3604	3695	3789	3885	3984	4085	4188	4295	4404	4515	4630	4748	4868
999	3074	3151	3229	3310	3392	3477	3564	3653	3744	3837	3933	4031	4131	4234	4340	4448	4559	4673	4790	4909
50	3125	3202	3280	3360	3443	3527	3614	3702	3793	3886	3981	4079	4179	4281	4386	4493	4604	4716	4832	4950
02	3177	3253	3332	3412	3494	3578	3664	3752	3843	3935	4030	4127	4226	4328	4432	4539	4648	4760	4875	4992
55	3230	3306	3384	2464	3546	3630	3716	3803	3893	3985	4080	4176	4275	4376	4479	4585	4693	4804	4918	5034

Table 12-12 Neonatal Weight Table (Male and Female Subjects Combined)

Gestational Age (wk)*	Weight Percentile (g)						
	5th	10th	25th	50th	75th	90th	95th
25	450	490	564	660	772	889	968
26	523	568	652	760	885	1016	1103
27	609	660	754	875	1015	1160	1257
28	707	765	870	1005	1162	1322	1430
29	820	884	1003	1153	1327	1504	1623
30	947	1020	1151	1319	1511	1706	1836
31	1090	1171	1317	1502	1713	1928	2070
32	1249	1338	1499	1702	1933	2167	2321
33	1422	1519	1696	1918	2169	2421	2587
34	1608	1714	1906	2146	2416	2687	2865
35	1804	1919	2125	2383	2671	2959	3148
36	2006	2129	2349	2622	2927	3230	3428
37	2210	2340	2572	2859	3177	3493	3698
38	2409	2544	2786	3083	3412	3736	3947
39	2595	2735	2984	3288	3622	3952	4164
40	2762	2904	3155	3462	3798	4127	4340
41	2900	3042	3293	3597	3930	4254	4462
42	3002	3142	3388	3685	4008	4322	4523
43	3061	3195	3432	3717	4026	4324	4515

*Age to the nearest week.

From Doubilet PM, Benson CB, Nadel AS, Ringer SA: Improved birth weight table for neonates developed from gestations dated by early sonography. J Ultrasound Med 16:241-249, 1997.

change in this percentile level between studies, a growth disorder is considered. This approach is currently the most widely used for assessing fetal size and growth, but it has the disadvantage that it uses data established from cross-sectional rather than longitudinal studies.

A method of assessing interval growth that is more precise and has the advantage that it uses longitudinal data has been developed and can be used to evaluate growth of the fetal head, abdomen, and femur in the second and third trimesters (Table 12-13). Because this concept may be new to the reader, a detailed discussion and examples follow.

As background, measurement errors cause an inaccuracy of at least 1 mm per study, and this inaccuracy doubles to 2 mm when two studies are compared. As the number of weeks between studies increases, the measurement error decreases in significance. The error is largest when the number of weeks between studies is less than 3 weeks (20% to 30% error) and smallest when there are more than 10 weeks between studies (only 7% to 10% error). Interval growth tables were therefore developed at 4, 6, 8, and greater than or equal to 10 weeks to mathematically correct for this error (see Tables 12-13A to D). The mean measurement numbers in all the tables remain constant, with narrower ranges as the number of weeks between studies increases.

Analysis of interval growth is based on the following principles. The growth of a normal fetus is faster in the early second trimester and decreases until term. Each fetal parameter has a predictable linear or curvilinear growth pattern. The fetus that grows between the 10th and 90th percentile is almost always normal and has little chance of growth disturbance. The fetus with growth *below* the 10th percentile or the fetus that is initially above and then drops below the 10th percentile is *at risk* for growth retardation. Conversely, the fetus that grows above the 90th percentile or is initially below and then rises above the 90th percentile is *at risk* for macrosomia.

Interval growth can be analyzed when there are two fetal studies. The initial and repeat measurements of the head, abdomen, and femur and the time interval between the studies are then known. The rate of change of the measurement parameters is equal to millimeters of growth from the first to the second study divided by the number of interval weeks, or mm/week of growth. This growth rate is then evaluated at the *mean* fetal age *between* the two studies. The growth table to be used depends on the number of weeks *between* studies

Table 12-13A Interval Growth Table (mm/wk): 4 Weeks

Mean Gestational Age (wk)	Biparietal Diameter			Average Abdominal Diameter			Abdominal Circumference			Femur Length		
	Percentiles			Percentiles			Percentiles			Percentiles		
	10%	50%	90%	10%	50%	90%	10%	50%	90%	10%	50%	90%
17	2.5	3.5	4.4	2.3	3.7	5.1	7.2	11.5	15.9	2.1	3.1	4.2
18	2.5	3.4	4.4	2.3	3.7	5.0	7.1	11.5	15.8	2.0	3.0	4.1
19	2.4	3.4	4.4	2.2	3.6	5.0	7.0	11.4	15.7	1.9	2.9	4.0
20	2.4	3.3	4.3	2.2	3.6	5.0	6.9	11.3	15.6	1.8	2.8	3.9
21	2.3	3.3	4.3	2.2	3.5	4.9	6.8	11.1	15.5	1.7	2.7	3.8
22	2.3	3.2	4.2	2.1	3.5	4.9	6.6	11.0	15.4	1.6	2.6	3.7
23	2.2	3.2	4.1	2.1	3.5	4.9	6.5	10.9	15.3	1.5	2.6	3.6
24	2.1	3.1	4.0	2.0	3.4	4.8	6.4	10.7	15.1	1.4	2.5	3.5
25	2.0	3.0	3.9	2.0	3.4	4.8	6.2	10.6	14.9	1.4	2.4	3.4
26	1.9	2.9	3.8	1.9	3.3	4.7	6.0	10.4	14.8	1.3	2.3	3.3
27	1.8	2.8	3.7	1.9	3.3	4.6	5.8	10.2	14.6	1.2	2.2	3.3
28	1.7	2.6	3.6	1.8	3.2	4.6	5.7	10.0	14.4	1.1	2.2	3.2
29	1.5	2.5	3.5	1.7	3.1	4.5	5.5	9.8	14.2	1.1	2.1	3.1
30	1.4	2.4	3.4	1.7	3.1	4.5	5.2	9.6	14.0	1.0	2.0	3.1
31	1.3	2.2	3.2	1.6	3.0	4.4	5.0	9.4	13.8	0.9	2.0	3.0
32	1.1	2.1	3.1	1.5	2.9	4.3	4.8	9.2	13.5	0.9	1.9	3.0
33	0.9	1.9	2.9	1.4	2.8	4.2	4.5	8.9	13.3	0.8	1.9	2.9
34	0.8	1.7	2.7	1.4	2.8	4.2	4.3	8.7	13.0	0.8	1.8	2.9
35	0.6	1.6	2.5	1.3	2.7	4.1	4.0	8.4	12.8	0.7	1.8	2.8
36	0.4	1.4	2.3	1.2	2.6	4.0	3.7	8.1	12.5	0.7	1.7	2.8

The mean growth rates and confidence limits calculated from the regression equations are given at each mean gestational age.
From Nazarian LN, Halpern EJ, Kirtz AB, et al: Normal interval fetal growth rates based on obstetrical ultrasound measurements. J Ultrasound Med 14, 1995.

Table 12-13B Interval Growth Table: 6 Weeks

Mean Gestational Age (wk)	Biparietal Diameter Interval Growth (mm/wk)			Average Abdominal Diameter Interval Growth (mm/wk)			Abdominal Circumference Interval Growth (mm/wk)			Femur Length Interval Growth (mm/wk)		
	Percentiles			Percentiles			Percentiles			Percentiles		
	10%	50%	90%	10%	50%	90%	10%	50%	90%	10%	50%	90%
17	2.8	3.5	4.1	2.7	3.7	4.6	8.6	11.5	14.5	2.4	3.1	3.8
18	2.8	3.4	4.1	2.7	3.7	4.6	8.5	11.5	14.4	2.3	3.0	3.7
19	2.7	3.4	4.0	2.7	3.6	4.6	8.4	11.4	14.3	2.2	2.9	3.6
20	2.7	3.3	4.0	2.7	3.6	4.5	8.3	11.3	14.2	2.1	2.8	3.5
21	2.6	3.3	3.9	2.6	3.5	4.5	8.2	11.1	14.1	2.0	2.7	3.4
22	2.6	3.2	3.9	2.6	3.5	4.4	8.1	11.0	14.0	1.9	2.6	3.3
23	2.5	3.2	3.8	2.5	3.5	4.4	7.9	10.9	13.8	1.9	2.6	3.2
24	2.4	3.1	3.7	2.5	3.4	4.4	7.8	10.7	13.7	1.8	2.5	3.2
25	2.3	3.0	3.6	2.4	3.4	4.3	7.6	10.6	13.5	1.7	2.4	3.1
26	2.2	2.9	3.5	2.4	3.3	4.2	7.5	10.4	13.3	1.6	2.3	3.0
27	2.1	2.8	3.4	2.3	3.3	4.2	7.3	10.2	13.2	1.5	2.2	2.9
28	2.0	2.6	3.3	2.3	3.2	4.1	7.1	10.0	13.0	1.5	2.2	2.9
29	1.9	2.5	3.2	2.2	3.1	4.1	6.9	9.8	12.8	1.4	2.1	2.8
30	1.7	2.4	3.0	2.1	3.1	4.0	6.7	9.6	12.6	1.3	2.0	2.7
31	1.6	2.2	2.9	2.1	3.0	3.9	6.5	9.4	12.3	1.3	2.0	2.7
32	1.4	2.1	2.7	2.0	2.9	3.9	6.2	9.2	12.1	1.2	1.9	2.6
33	1.3	1.9	2.6	1.9	2.8	3.8	6.0	8.9	11.9	1.2	1.9	2.6
34	1.1	1.7	2.4	1.8	2.8	3.7	5.7	8.7	11.6	1.1	1.8	2.5
35	0.9	1.6	2.2	1.7	2.7	3.6	5.5	8.4	11.3	1.1	1.8	2.5
36	0.7	1.4	2.0	1.7	2.6	3.5	5.2	8.1	11.1	1.0	1.7	2.4

The mean growth rates and confidence limits calculated from the regression equations are given at each mean gestational age.
From Nazarian LN, Halpern EJ, Kirtz AB, et al: Normal interval fetal growth rates based on obstetrical ultrasound measurements. J Ultrasound Med 14, 1995.

Table 12-13C Interval Growth Table: 8 Weeks

Mean Gestational Age (wk)	Biparietal Diameter Interval Growth (mm/wk)			Average Abdominal Diameter Interval Growth (mm/wk)			Abdominal Circumference Interval Growth (mm/wk)			Femur Length Interval Growth (mm/wk)		
	Percentiles			Percentiles			Percentiles			Percentiles		
	10%	50%	90%	10%	50%	90%	10%	50%	90%	10%	50%	90%
17	3.0	3.5	4.0	3.0	3.7	4.4	9.3	11.5	13.7	2.6	3.1	3.7
18	2.9	3.4	3.9	2.9	3.7	4.4	9.2	11.5	13.7	2.5	3.0	3.7
19	2.9	3.4	3.9	2.9	3.6	4.3	9.1	11.4	13.6	2.4	2.9	3.4
20	2.9	3.3	3.8	2.9	3.6	4.3	9.0	11.3	13.5	2.3	2.8	3.3
21	2.8	3.3	3.8	2.8	3.5	4.3	8.9	11.1	13.4	2.2	2.7	3.3
22	2.7	3.2	3.7	2.8	3.5	4.2	8.8	11.0	13.2	2.1	2.6	3.2
23	2.7	3.2	3.6	2.8	3.5	4.2	8.7	10.9	13.1	2.0	2.6	3.1
24	2.6	3.1	3.6	2.7	3.4	4.1	8.5	10.7	12.9	1.9	2.5	3.0
25	2.5	3.0	3.5	2.7	3.4	4.1	8.3	10.6	12.8	1.9	2.4	2.9
26	2.4	2.9	3.4	2.6	3.3	4.0	8.2	10.4	12.6	1.8	2.3	2.8
27	2.3	2.8	3.3	2.5	3.3	4.0	8.0	10.2	12.4	1.7	2.2	2.8
28	2.2	2.6	3.1	2.5	3.2	3.9	7.8	10.0	12.2	1.6	2.2	2.7
29	2.0	2.5	3.0	2.4	3.1	3.8	7.6	9.8	12.0	1.6	2.1	2.6
30	1.9	2.4	2.9	2.4	3.1	3.8	7.4	9.6	11.8	1.5	2.0	2.6
31	1.7	2.2	2.7	2.3	3.0	3.7	7.2	9.4	11.6	1.5	2.0	2.5
32	1.6	2.1	2.6	2.2	2.9	3.6	6.9	9.2	11.4	1.4	1.9	2.4
33	1.4	1.9	2.4	2.1	2.8	3.5	6.7	8.9	11.1	1.3	1.9	2.4
34	1.3	1.7	2.2	2.1	2.8	3.5	6.4	8.7	10.9	1.3	1.8	2.3
35	1.1	1.6	2.1	2.0	2.7	3.4	6.2	8.4	10.6	1.3	1.8	2.3
36	0.9	1.4	1.9	1.9	2.6	3.3	5.9	8.1	10.3	1.2	1.7	2.3

The mean growth rates and confidence limits calculated from the regression equations are given at each mean gestational age.
From Nazarian LN, Halpern EJ, Kirtz AB, et al: Normal interval fetal growth rates based on obstetrical ultrasound measurements. J Ultrasound Med 14, 1995.

Table 12-13D Interval Growth Table: ≥10 Weeks

Mean Gestational Age (wk)	Biparietal Diameter Interval Growth (mm/wk)			Average Abdominal Diameter Interval Growth (mm/wk)			Abdominal Circumference Interval Growth (mm/wk)			Femur Length Interval Growth (mm/wk)		
	Percentiles			Percentiles			Percentiles			Percentiles		
	10%	50%	90%	10%	50%	90%	10%	50%	90%	10%	50%	90%
17	3.1	3.5	3.9	3.1	3.7	4.2	9.7	11.6	13.3	2.7	3.1	3.6
18	3.0	3.4	3.8	3.1	3.7	4.2	9.7	11.5	13.3	2.6	3.0	3.5
19	3.0	3.4	3.8	3.0	3.6	4.2	9.6	11.4	13.2	2.5	2.9	3.3
20	3.0	3.3	3.7	3.0	3.6	4.2	9.5	11.3	13.1	2.4	2.8	3.2
21	2.9	3.3	3.7	3.0	3.5	4.1	9.3	11.1	13.0	2.3	2.7	3.2
22	2.8	3.2	3.6	2.9	3.5	4.1	9.2	11.0	12.8	2.2	2.6	3.1
23	2.8	3.2	3.6	2.9	3.5	4.0	9.1	10.9	12.7	2.1	2.6	3.0
24	2.7	3.1	3.5	2.8	3.4	4.0	8.9	10.7	12.5	2.0	2.5	2.9
25	2.6	3.0	3.4	2.8	3.4	3.9	8.8	10.6	12.4	2.0	2.4	2.8
26	2.5	2.9	3.3	2.7	3.3	3.9	8.6	10.4	12.2	1.9	2.3	2.7
27	2.4	2.8	3.2	2.7	3.3	3.8	8.4	10.2	12.0	1.8	2.2	2.7
28	2.3	2.6	3.0	2.6	3.2	3.8	8.2	10.0	11.8	1.7	2.2	2.6
29	2.1	2.5	2.9	2.6	3.1	3.7	8.0	9.8	11.6	1.7	2.1	2.5
30	2.0	2.4	2.8	2.5	3.1	3.6	7.8	9.6	11.4	1.6	2.0	2.5
31	1.8	2.2	2.6	2.4	3.0	3.6	7.6	9.4	11.2	1.6	2.0	2.4
32	1.7	2.1	2.5	2.3	2.9	3.5	7.4	9.2	11.0	1.5	1.9	2.3
33	1.5	1.9	2.3	2.3	2.8	3.4	7.1	8.9	10.7	1.4	1.9	2.3
34	1.4	1.7	2.1	2.2	2.8	3.3	6.9	8.7	10.5	1.4	1.8	2.2
35	1.2	1.6	2.0	2.1	2.7	3.2	6.6	8.4	10.2	1.4	1.8	2.2
36	1.0	1.4	1.8	2.0	2.6	3.2	6.3	8.1	9.9	1.3	1.7	2.2

The mean growth rates and confidence limits calculated from the regression equations are given at each mean gestational age.
From Nazarian LN, Halpern EJ, Kirtz AB, et al: Normal interval fetal growth rates based on obstetrical ultrasound measurements. J Ultrasound Med 14, 1995.

(i.e., 4, 6, 8, or ≥10 weeks). Odd week intervals should be rounded up to the next even number (e.g., for 3 weeks, use the 4-week table). If a clinician wants an interval growth study at less than 3 weeks (particularly in the late third trimester), it should be discouraged because of potentially significant measurement errors.

Two examples of this ultrasound growth analysis are shown. Only the BPD and the AD will be described, although the AC and FL growth are also available (see Appendix I).

In multiple gestations, more commonly twins, gestational age analysis is similar to that of singleton pregnancies and use of the same measurement tables is recommended. In the second and early third trimester, normal growth and weight is the same as in singleton gestations. After that, while these parameters tend to slow down toward the lower 10th percentile, they should not be below the 10th percentile if growth is normal. Because singleton tables are based on many more numbers than multiple gestation tables, it is recommended that the same singleton tables be used.

f. Maternal anatomy—evaluation of the uterus and adnexal structures should be performed.

There should be a careful search for fibroids and adnexal masses. During the second and early third trimester the length and shape of the cervix should be assessed because shortening of the cervix and/or opening of the internal cervical os are important signs of incompetent cervix and preterm labor.

g. Fetal anatomic survey. Fetal anatomy, as described in this document, may adequately be assessed by ultrasound after approximately 18 weeks' gestational (menstrual) age. It may be possible to document normal structures before this time, although some structures can be difficult to visualize due to fetal size, position, movement, abdominal scars, and increased maternal wall thickness.

The following areas of assessment represent the essential elements of a standard examination of fetal anatomy: head (cerebellum, choroid plexus, cisterna magna, lateral cerebral ventricles, midline falx, cavum septi pellucidi), heart (four-chamber view of the heart including its position within the thorax), spine (cervical, thoracic, lumbar, and sacral), abdomen (stomach, kidneys, urinary bladder, and the umbilical cord insertion site into the anterior abdominal wall), extremities (the legs and arms: presence or absence of the legs and arms), and the umbilical cord vessel number. Fetal gender may be obtained when medically indicated.

Whereas these anatomic areas are more completely discussed in the respective chapters, a brief discussion of each anatomic area follows.

In the head, the atria of the lateral ventricles are imaged by tilting the transducer slightly caudad from the standard axial view. The atrial measurement is easily reproducible and essentially constant from 14 to 38 weeks' gestation. The generally accepted upper limit of normal is 10 mm. In addition, the hyperechoic choroid plexus normally fills at least 60% and more often up to 90% of each atrium.

Imaging of the posterior fossa in the axial plane identifies the cerebellum and cisterna magna by tilting the transducer slightly more posteriorly toward the occiput. The cerebellum has a bilobed shape with the midline hyperechoic vermis and larger hypoechoic hemispheres. An axial measurement of the cerebellum can be obtained and compared with the BPD. The normal cisterna magna is always identified as an anechoic space posterior to the vermis and has a normal size range of 2 to 10 mm.

A four-chamber view of the heart is obtained in axial projection. The heart is normally on the left side with the apex pointing toward the left anterior chest wall at an approximately 45-degree angle. The chamber closest to the chest wall is the right ventricle. A four-chamber view can identify both ventricles and their interventricular septa, both atria and their intervening foramina ovalia, and the atrioventricular valves. From 18 weeks to term, a satisfactory view can be obtained in 95% of fetuses. Although the current standard for the obstetric ultrasound examination only requires the four-chamber view of the heart, some observers believe that it should include additional cardiac views and, in particular, images of the ventricular outflow tracts.

Careful analysis of the spine is important to detect neural tube defects. Of the three ossification centers at each vertebral level, the two posterior centers form the neural arches. These arches and the overlying posterior soft tissues are almost always affected by neural defects so that a complete examination requires visualization of all vertebral levels, particularly the lumbosacral region. This can best be accomplished by axial images. If suboptimal, midline sagittal images can visualize the soft tissues and coronal images can visualize the posterior ossification centers.

The fetal stomach is an anechoic structure in the left upper quadrant. It should routinely be identified by 16 weeks. When the stomach is not seen, particularly after 19 weeks with scanning performed for up to 60 minutes, the fetus is likely to be abnormal. When marked oligohydramnios is present, however, the fetus may have no amniotic fluid to fill its stomach.

The kidneys can be identified in their paraspinal location on an axial view just below the level of the liver. The kidneys may be recognized as early as 12 weeks and by 17 weeks may be seen in almost all normal fetuses. In the second trimester, it may be difficult to distinguish the kidneys from the surrounding perinephric tissues; after 26 weeks, the perinephric fat and renal sinus become more hyperechoic and the relatively hypoechoic renal parenchyma is identified more easily. The normal renal sinus is often separated by an anechoic space, corresponding to pyelectasis. Minimal pyelectasis is considered a normal finding. If the subjective impression of the examiner is that there is more than a minimal amount of pyelectasis, the anteroposterior dimension of the renal pelvis should be measured on an axial image. The thresholds reported in the literature for this measurement vary. In the second and early third trimester, pyelectasis can be considered a normal finding if the measurement is less than 4 to 5 mm. Later in the third trimester typically 7 mm (and occasionally up to 10 mm) is considered the upper limit of normal. If caliectasis or ureterectasis is imaged, however, the collecting system dilatation should be considered abnormal regardless of the measurement of the renal pelvis.

The urinary bladder is a round or ovoid anechoic structure in the pelvis. If the normal bladder is not initially identified in the second or third trimester, it will almost always appear if sequential scans are performed at 10- to 15-minute intervals for up to 1 hour. A distended or an absent bladder needs further evaluation, including a careful analysis of the fetal kidneys and the amniotic fluid.

Finally, the insertion site of the umbilical cord into the fetal abdominal wall is an important landmark in the evaluation for a ventral abdominal wall defect. The remainder of the anterior abdominal wall should also be carefully scanned to ensure that no defects are present.

SUGGESTED READINGS

ACR Practice Guidelines for the Performance of Antepartum Obstetrical Ultrasound 2003. Reston, VA, ACR Standards (Res. 19, effective 10/1/03).

Allen LD: A practical approach to fetal heart scanning. Semin Perinatol 24:324, 2000.

American Institute of Ultrasound in Medicine: Guidelines for the Performance of the Antepartum Obstetrical Ultrasound Examination. J Ultrasound Med 15:185, 1996.

Barboza JM, et al: Prenatal diagnosis of congenital cardiac anomalies: A practical approach using two basic views. Radiographics 22:1125, 2002.

Benson CB, Doubilet PM: Sonographic prediction of gestational age: Accuracy of second- and third-trimester fetal measurements. AJR Am J Roentgenol 157:1275, 1991.

Bowie JD, et al: The changing sonographic appearance of fetal kidneys during pregnancy. J Ultrasound Med 2:505, 1983.

Bromley B, et al: Fetal echocardiography: Accuracy and limitations in a population at high and low risk for heart defects. Am J Obstet Gynecol 166:1473, 1992.

Brown DL, et al: Sonography of the fetal heart: Normal variants and pitfalls. AJR Am J Roentgenol 160:1251, 1993.

Budorick NE, et al: Ossification of the fetal spine. Radiology 181:561, 1991.

Budorick NE, Pretorius DH, Nelson TR: Sonography of the fetal spine: Technique, imaging, findings, and clinical implications. AJR Am J Roentgenol 16:421, 1995.

Campbell BA: Utilizing sonography to follow fetal growth. Obstet Gynecol Clin North Am 25:750, 1998.

Cardoza JD, Goldstein BB, Filly RA: Exclusion of fetal ventriculomegaly with a single measurement: The width of the lateral ventricular atrium. Radiology 169:711, 1988.

Chitty LS, Altman DG: Charts of fetal size: Limb bones. BJOG 109:919, 2002.

Clautice-Engle T, Pretorius DH, Budorick NE: Significance of nonvisualization of the fetal urinary bladder. J Ultrasound Med 10:615, 1991.

Copel JA, et al: Fetal echocardiographic screening for congenital heart disease: The importance of the four-chamber view. Am J Obstet Gynecol 157:648, 1987.

Corteville JE, Gray DL, Crane JP: Congenital hydronephrosis: Correlation of fetal ultrasonographic findings with infant outcome. Am J Obstet Gynecol 165:384, 1991.

Doubilet PM, Greenes RA: Improved prediction of gestational age from fetal head measurements. AJR Am J Roentgenol 142:797, 1984.

Farrell TA, et al: Fetal lateral ventricles: Reassessment of normal values for atrial diameter at US. Radiology 193:409, 1994.

Filly RA: Level 1, level 2, level 3 obstetric sonography: I'll see your level and raise you one. Radiology 172:312, 1989.

Frates MC: Sonography of the normal fetal heart: A practical approach. AJR Am J Roentgenol 173:1363, 1999.

Goldstein RB, Filly RA: Sonographic estimation of amniotic fluid volume: Subjective assessment versus pocket measurements. J Ultrasound Med 7:363, 1988.

Gotoh H, Masuzaki H, Fukuda H, et al: Detection and assessment of pyelectasis in the fetus: Relationship to postnatal renal function. Obstet Gynecol 92:226, 1998.

Grumbach K, et al: Twin and singleton growth patterns compared using ultrasound. Radiology 158:237, 1986.

Hadlock FP, et al: Estimating fetal age: Effect of head shape on BPD. AJR Am J Roentgenol 137:83, 1981.

Hadlock FP, et al: Fetal abdominal circumference as a predictor of menstrual age. AJR Am J Roentgenol 139:369, 1982.

Heiserman J, Filly RA, Goldstein RB: Effect of measurement errors on sonographic evaluation of ventriculomegaly. J Ultrasound Med 10:121, 1991.

Hertzberg BS, et al: Diagnosis of placenta previa during the third trimester: Role of transperineal sonography. AJR Am J Roentgenol 159:83, 1992.

Hertzberg BS, et al: Sonographic evaluation of fetal CNS: Technical and interpretive pitfalls. AJR Am J Roentgenol 172: 253, 1999.

Hilpert PL, Hall BE, Kurtz AB: The atria of the fetal lateral ventricles: A prospective study of normal size and choroids plexus filling. AJR Am J Roentgenol 164:731, 1995.

Kurtz AB, et al: Twin pregnancies: Accuracy of first-trimester abdominal US in predicting chorionicity and amnionicity. Radiology 185:759, 1992.

Levi CS, et al: Endovaginal US: Demonstration of cardiac activity in embryos of less than 5.0 mm in crown-rump length. Radiology 176:71, 1990.

Mahony BS, Filly RA, Callen PW: Amnionicity and chorionicity in twin pregnancies: Prediction using ultrasound. Radiology 155:205, 1985.

McGahan JP: Sonography of the fetal heart: Findings on the four-chamber view. AJR Am J Roentgenol 156:547, 1991.

McKenna KM, Goldstein RB, Stringer MD: Small or absent fetal stomach: Prognostic significance. Radiology 197:729, 1995.

Millener PB, Anderson NG, Chisholm RJ: Prognostic significance of nonvisualization of the fetal stomach by sonography. AJR Am J Roentgenol 160:827, 1993.

Monteagudo A, et al: Early and simple determination of chorionic and amniotic type in multifetal gestations in the first fourteen weeks by high-frequency transvaginal ultrasonography. Am J Obstet Gynecol 170:824, 1994.

Pennell RG, et al: Prospective comparison of vaginal and abdominal sonography in normal early pregnancy. J Ultrasound Med 10:63, 1991.

Perez CG, Goldstein RB: Sonographic borderlands in the fetal abdomen. Semin Ultrasound CT MR 19:336, 1998.

Persutte WH, Hussey M, Chyu J, et al: Striking findings concerning the variability in the measurement of the fetal renal collecting system. Ultrasound Obstet Gynecol 15:186, 2000.

Persutte WH, Klyle M, Lenke RR, et al: Mild pyelectasis ascertained with prenatal sonography is pediatrically significant. Ultrasound Obstet Gynecol 10:12, 1997.

Pilu G, Reece EA, Goldstein I, et al: Sonographic evaluation of the normal developmental anatomy of the fetal cerebral ventricles: II. The atria. Obstet Gynecol 783:250, 1989.

Pretorius DH, et al: Sonographic evaluation of the fetal stomach: Significance of non-visualization. AJR Am J Roentgenol 151:987, 1988.

Scardo JA, et al: Prospective determination of chorionicity, amnionicity, and zygosity in twin gestations. Am J Obstet Gynecol 173:1376, 1995.

Seeds JW: Borderline genitourinary tract abnormalities. Semin Ultrasound CT MR 19:347, 1998.

Wilcox DT, Chitty LS: Non-visualization of the fetal bladder: Aetiology and management. Prenat Diagn 21:977, 2001.

Appendix I

Example 1: The first study is performed at 20 weeks' gestation, and the second study is done at 30 weeks' gestation. The *mean* fetal age is 25 weeks' gestation. There are 10 weeks between studies so Table 12-13D (interval growth = 10 weeks) is used. At 20 weeks the biparietal diameter (BPD) and abdominal diameter (AD) measurements are both 45 mm. At 30 weeks, the BPD and AD measurements have increased to 79 mm and 81 mm, respectively. The interval growth rate for the BPD is 79 mm – 45 mm/10 weeks = 3.4 mm/week. The interval growth rate for the AD is 81 mm – 45 mm/10 weeks = 3.6 mm/week. Table 12-13D shows that, at a mean of 25 weeks, both parameters are growing normally, between the 10th and the 90th percentiles.

Example 2: The first study is performed at 32 weeks' gestation, and the second study is done at 36 weeks' gestation. The *mean* gestational age is 34 weeks. There are 4 weeks between studies, and Table 12-13A (interval growth of 4 weeks) is used. The BPD and AD at 32 weeks are 81 mm and 79 mm, respectively, and at 36 weeks have increased to 89 mm and 84 mm, respectively. The interval growth rate for the BPD is 89 mm – 81 mm/4 weeks = 2.0 mm/week, equivalent to growth between the 50th and 90th percentiles. The interval growth rate for the AD is 84 mm – 79 mm/4 weeks = 1.25 mm/week, a growth *below* the 10th percentile. The abdomen is growing too slowly, relative to the BPD, and the fetus is at risk for asymmetric growth restriction.

Fetal Growth and Well-Being

For Key Features summary see p. 340

Improved equipment and increased ultrasound sophistication have permitted the examiner to go beyond a routine evaluation of the fetal structure. Particularly in the third trimester, fetal function and measurements, separately or in combination with the clinical findings, have been used to analyze fetal well-being. These findings have helped in the prediction of fetuses that are either too small or too large, allowing increased accuracy in the detection of the compromised fetus and, in some cases, in the timing of delivery.

INTRAUTERINE GROWTH RESTRICTION

Intrauterine growth restriction (IUGR) is a complex problem not always detected in utero. By definition, a child with a low birth weight is deemed small for gestational age (SGA). There are two main types of SGA infants: the constitutionally small infant is small but otherwise normal, whereas the infant with IUGR is pathologically smaller than its expected gestational age.

The overall incidence of growth restriction varies in different studies but is usually between 3% and 10% of all births. On average, 1 in every 20 infants (5%) is growth restricted, approaching 1 in 10 infants (10%) in certain high-risk groups. Most studies use a weight cutoff for SGA infants of less than the lower 10th percentile. The specificity of detection of IUGR infants increases with even lower weights, at the lower 5th and 2.5th percentile, for example.

Two characteristics, age and weight (size), are needed to evaluate infants and also fetuses for growth restriction. In utero, the weight of the fetus for its gestational age can predict size appropriateness. Unfortunately, in utero determination of age and weight are not precise. By using 2 standard deviations (2 SD or 95%) in a large group of women, an optimal menstrual history can only predict fetal age to within ±2.5 weeks. With uncertain dates, this precision decreases to ±4 weeks or more. Using ultrasound, the first-trimester crown-rump length and second-trimester head measurements are accurate to ±1 to 1.2 weeks with the third-trimester precision decreased to ± 3 to 4 weeks. Fetal weight is even less precise, with an accuracy of at best ±15% when three parameter tables (head, abdomen, and femur) are used. A 3000-g fetus for example would have a weight range of 900 g, from 2550 to 3450 g.

To further complicate this analysis, there are two types of growth restriction and numerous risk factors that can be separated into maternal, fetal, and placental, with some overlap. The maternal risk factors range from a young maternal age to chronic hypoxia and include systemic hypertension, collagen vascular diseases, insulin-dependent diabetes, smoking, and certain drugs (including alcohol and cocaine). Fetal risk factors include a previously growth-restricted fetus, structural abnormalities, chromosomal abnormalities, and in utero infections such as the TORCH viruses of toxoplasmosis, rubella, cytomegalovirus, and herpes simplex. Placental problems include infarction, abnormal umbilical cord insertion, placenta previa, and abruption. Premature placental aging (dysmaturity), vascular problems (anticardiolipin antibodies and hypercoagulable states), and placental tumors also adversely affect the fetus.

Although not fully understood, women with persistently elevated α-fetoprotein levels (without structural fetal causes) suggest increased placental permeability and have a higher incidence of growth-restricted fetuses later in the pregnancy.

Abnormally low growth stems from two distinct mechanisms: fetal malnutrition and diminished cellular growth. These manifest themselves as the two types of IUGR: asymmetric and symmetric. There is significant overlap between the asymmetric and symmetric forms of IUGR. Asymmetric IUGR (malnutrition) constitutes the majority (up to 90%) of the cases. It is uncommonly detected earlier than the third trimester. Placental and maternal problems predominate, with the fetus receiving a less-than-adequate blood supply and nourishment. Because asymmetric IUGR is a form of starvation, there is an initial loss of subcutaneous tissue and liver glycogen stores, and thus a decrease in abdominal size. Head and femur measurements (part of the fetal skeleton) are also affected, but to a lesser extent. As starvation persists, however, the entire fetus becomes equally affected. The fetus then assumes a "symmetric" appearance that signifies severe growth restriction.

Asymmetric IUGR creates chronic stress on the fetus and is not infrequently accompanied by oligohydramnios (Fig. 13-1). The differentiation in the third trimester between this severe form of asymmetric growth and the truly symmetric growth restriction (described in the next paragraph) must often rely on history and, if present, on the finding of decreased amniotic fluid. Because asymmetric IUGR is a late onset in utero problem, not affecting organ development, the prognosis depends on the severity of the perinatal and immediate neonatal problems. If successfully treated, this type of child will experience normal development.

The symmetric type of IUGR (diminished cellular growth) comprises the remaining cases of pathologic IUGR. It occurs early in pregnancy, usually in the first trimester, as a result of an insult to the fetus or its mother. Chromosomal abnormalities, drug toxicities, and in utero infections are among the causes of this form of IUGR. The fetus is stunted. The head and body (and femur) are equally affected, and the fetus is symmetrically small. The volume of amniotic fluid is usually normal. Because it occurs early, it can adversely affect organ development, particularly in the central nervous system, and thus manifest as slow development after birth.

Ultrasound

Fetal Structures and Measurements

Because fetal anomalies either may be the cause of or be associated with growth restriction, the fetus should be carefully evaluated to determine structural normalcy. Even when the fetus appears grossly normal, however, chromosomal anomalies and/or in utero infections may still adversely affect fetal growth and development. Measurement of fetal parts, in particular the head, body, and femur, are therefore important on both the first and on any follow-up examination. Amniotic fluid, occasional Doppler evaluation, and, very infrequently, placental appearance may be of value. Additionally, there are internal fetal structures that will be discussed that have been suggested, but not as yet proven, to be useful in the diagnosis of IUGR.

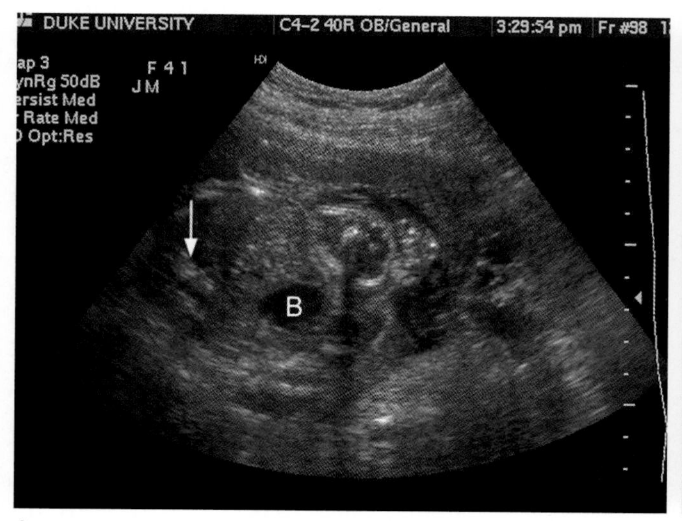

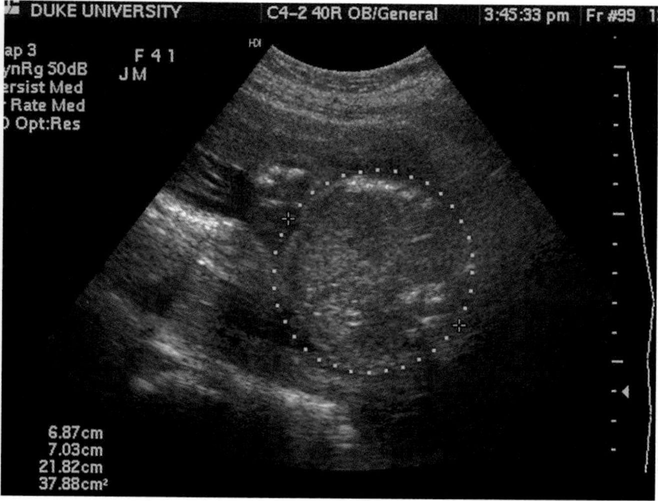

Figure 13-1 Oligohydramnios associated with IUGR. **A,** Axial image of lower abdomen of a 29-week fetus shows severe oligohydramnios. B, bladder; *arrow*, spine. **B,** Abdominal circumference measurement on same fetus as in **A**. Value of 21.8 cm is less than the 2.5th percentile for 29 weeks (see Table 13-1). Likewise, the estimated fetal weight of 716 g is less than the 10th percentile.

All standard ultrasound measurements are performed according to the antepartum obstetric ultrasound standard (see Chapter 12). The gestational age is ideally established within the first 20 to 24 weeks by either a first-trimester crown-rump length or second-trimester head and femur length measurement (see Tables 12-1, 12-3, and 12-4). If follow-up examinations are performed, the fetal age is the initial ultrasound age plus the number of intervening weeks. The fetal body measurement (usually obtained as a circumference rather than an average diameter) is of value in the determination of fetal size and growth. Its use in the weight formulas has been well established.

The overall ultrasound detection rate for IUGR is 70%. Asymmetric growth restriction is more commonly detected. When combined with the clinical assessment of a fetus into low and high risk for IUGR, ultrasound can be used to accomplish different tasks: to suggest that a low-risk fetus is smaller than expected, to confirm that a fetus at high risk is too small, to find out if the ultrasound findings are compatible with the clinical impression of a small fetus, and to monitor the pregnancy when the diagnosis of a small fetus is made.

The accuracy of ultrasound in detecting IUGR is different in these different circumstances. A small fetal abdomen detected during an examination performed solely to establish fetal age is less likely to be caused by IUGR than a small fetal abdomen found in a woman with hypertension. In a "screening" group, there is a larger proportion of constitutionally small fetuses and consequently higher false-positive and lower positive predictive values for diagnosing IUGR than in a group of higher-risk women. If only abnormal fetal measurements are found, suggesting a small fetus, it is more prudent to initially call the fetus SGA rather than IUGR and to request a follow-up study.

The calculated fetal weight uses a combination of measurements of the head, body, and femur (see Tables 12-10 and 12-11). Similarly, the abdominal circumference (AC) can help predict if there is a small fetal body (Table 13-1). Percentile tables are available for both, using the lower 10th percentile as the cut-off limit to separate normal for gestational age fetuses from SGA fetuses. To make this determination, however, a comparison of the calculated fetal weight (or the AC) to the anticipated fetal weight (or the AC) for the assigned fetal age is needed (see Table 12-12). This expected age is ideally established earlier in the pregnancy; in a late-registrant woman the fetal age may be uncertain. And when uncertain, the calculated weight (or AC) is of limited value.

For example, if the fetal biparietal diameter and AC are 80 and 340 mm, respectively, the fetal weight would be 2649 g (Table 12-10). If the fetal age is known to be 36 weeks from an earlier study, this weight would be normal, between the 50th and 75th percentiles (see Table 12-12). However, if the fetal age were uncertain and believed to be as advanced as 39 weeks, this same weight would be below the 10th percentile, and a SGA fetus with possible growth restriction would be more likely.

A comparison of the fetal head and body can predict the presence of asymmetric IUGR if fetal age is known. Because the abdomen is initially affected more severely than either the head or femur, a ratio of its head-to-abdominal circumferences has a high degree of sensitivity. A table of the circumference ratios from 13 to 42 weeks' gestation shows the head to be normally larger than the abdomen in the second trimester (ratio of >1), with reversal near term (ratio of <1) (see Table 12-8). Because the ratio is not constant but changes with gestational age, precise gestational age is important. This ratio can create uncertainty if the age is not known in a late registrant woman. A comparison of the BPD to the average body diameter yields comparable results without its dependence on gestational age (see Table 12-9). Both methods suggest that a normal proportion of the head to abdomen likely diagnoses a normal fetus except in the situations of advanced malnutrition (starvation) in which the head and body are both adversely affected. In symmetric IUGR all fetal parts are affected equally, and this comparison is not of diagnostic value.

Ratios of other fetal parameters have not shown predictive advantages in asymmetric IUGR but nevertheless deserve mentioning. The initially promising femur length-to-abdominal circumference ratio is an age-independent ratio from 22 weeks to term. Although this ratio is elevated in asymmetric IUGR (small body) and decreased in macrosomia (large body), subsequent studies have shown poor sensitivities and poor positive predictive value for both conditions. In symmetric IUGR this ratio is not of diagnostic value. The head to femur ratio may have value in certain skeletal disproportions but does not appear to be of diagnostic value in either symmetric or asymmetric IUGR. Although some case reports have suggested that the femur may be shorter than normal in asymmetric IUGR, this has not been borne out in larger studies.

Normal growth of the fetal parameters (head, body, and femur) is usually linear or mildly curvilinear, faster in the second trimester, and then progressively slower until term. In asymmetric IUGR the fetus typically grows normally into the third trimester, with decreased growth (which can be marked) in the third trimester. In symmetric IUGR the fetus grows slowly from the time of the initial early insult. Regardless of the types of IUGR, the small fetus with IUGR grows slower than a normal fetus of similar size.

Interval change in fetal weight or abdominal size can be evaluated and even plotted on a graph. Interval

Table 13-1 Fetal Abdominal Circumference (mm)

Weeks of Gestation	Percentile								
	2.5	5	10	25	50	75	80	95	97.5
18	98	103	109	119	131	142	145	159	164
19	111	116	123	133	144	156	159	172	178
20	121	126	133	143	154	166	169	182	188
21	137	142	148	159	170	181	184	198	203
22	147	152	158	169	180	191	194	208	213
23	160	165	171	182	193	204	207	221	226
24	172	177	183	194	205	216	219	233	238
25	180	185	191	202	213	224	227	241	246
26	188	193	199	210	221	232	235	249	254
27	204	209	215	226	237	248	251	265	270
28	220	225	231	242	253	264	267	281	286
29	236	241	247	258	269	280	283	297	302
30	241	246	252	263	274	285	288	302	307
31	247	252	258	269	280	291	294	308	313
32	254	259	265	276	287	298	301	315	320
33	257	262	268	279	290	301	304	318	323
34	268	273	279	290	301	312	315	329	334
35	289	294	300	311	322	333	336	350	355
36	300	305	311	322	333	344	347	361	366
37	311	316	322	333	344	355	358	372	377
38	324	329	335	346	357	368	371	385	390
39	326	331	337	348	359	370	373	387	392
40	328	333	339	350	361	372	375	389	394
41	338	343	349	360	371	382	385	399	404

From Tamura RK, Sabbagha RE: Percentile ranks of fetal sonar abdominal circumference measurements. Am J Obstet Gynecol 138:475, 1980.

growth of fetal parameters is, however, the best method for identifying both types of growth restriction. A discussion and examples of this approach using the head (biparietal diameter), abdominal (diameter and circumference), and femur length measurements were given in Chapter 12 and its Appendix 1 using Table 12-13.

It is anticipated that normal fetal growth should be above the 10th percentile. Although 10% of normal fetuses will grow slower (SGA fetuses), so will almost all fetuses with IUGR. It is also expected that most fetuses will maintain predetermined growth percentiles throughout fetal life so that a fetus growing at the 10th or 50th percentile early in pregnancy, for example, will typically remain at a similar percentile until term. Using this, four types of growth patterns have been described. Growth consistently above the 10th percentile and growth spurts from below to above the 10th percentile should be considered normal. Continued slow growth (below the 10th percentile) or a growth slowdown, particularly if from above to below the 10th percentile is likely to be abnormal.

Amniotic Fluid

The uterine cavity should be scanned to determine the amount of amniotic fluid. Amniotic fluid volume can be analyzed either qualitatively (subjectively) or quantitatively (by measurement). When the results of measurement techniques are compared with the findings from the subjective analysis of amniotic fluid, the subjective impression is as accurate as the objective (quantitative) approach, with excellent intraobserver and interobserver agreement.

Nevertheless, quantitative analysis can at times be helpful. Although different measurement techniques have been proposed, the most widely used in a singleton pregnancy is a four-quadrant analysis called the amniotic fluid index (AFI). Taking the largest anteroposterior (AP) fluid pocket in each quadrant (either in a sagittal or axial projection), the four measurements are totaled (Fig. 13-2). There is a lack of consensus regarding the optimal technique for measuring the AFI. Some groups only include fluid pockets that are free of fetal parts or umbilical cord, whereas others use fluid pockets that contain umbilical cord or an extremity, provided the pocket is predominantly fluid filled. Although there are week-to-week fluctuations, the AFI is usually normal when between 7 and 25 cm (Table 13-2). The AFI should be performed with the patient supine, and each measurement should be obtained strictly perpendicular even if a larger pocket of fluid can be imaged in an oblique scan plane.

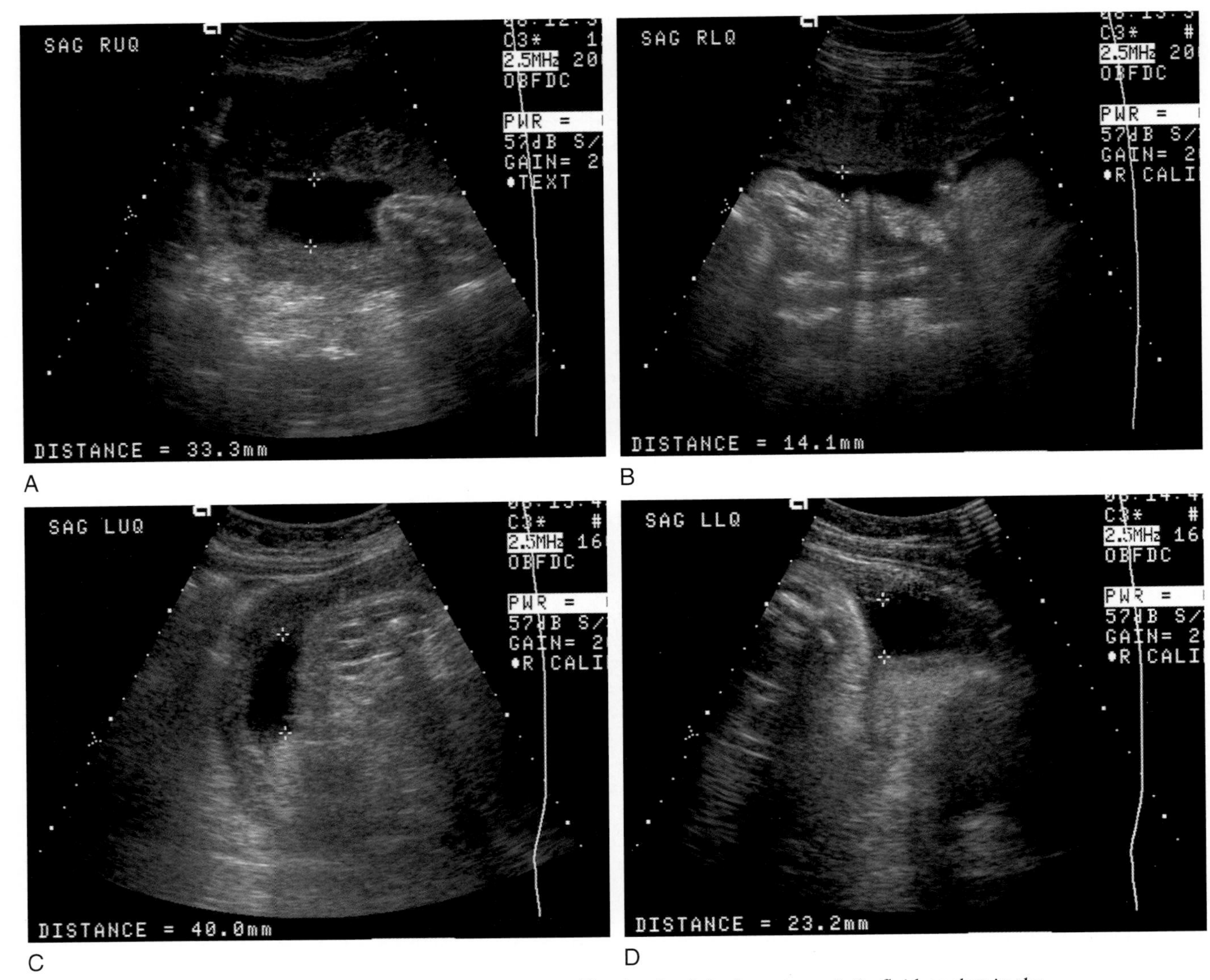

Figure 13-2 Amniotic fluid index (AFI). The depth of the largest amniotic fluid pocket in the right upper (**A**), right lower (**B**), left upper (**C**), and left lower (**D**) quadrants has been measured with electronic calipers *(cursors)*. The sum of the corresponding four values, 11.1 cm, is a normal AFI for the fetus' gestational age of 36 weeks.

The subjective analysis of the amniotic fluid volume is of particular importance in borderline high and low fluid. In these cases, especially when there is a discrepancy between the subjective analysis and the AFI, it is recommended that the subjective determination be favored. If, for example, the AFI calculates in the low normal range but subjectively the fluid appears decreased in volume, the examiner should consider favoring the subjective interpretation and diagnosing oligohydramnios.

The Placenta

Asymmetric IUGR is caused by a placenta that does not supply adequate blood and nutrition to the fetus. Although there are no absolute criteria for identifying a dysfunctioning placenta, three placental properties have been analyzed: its thickness and its echogenicity (discussed in Chapter 20) and Doppler waveforms of the umbilical artery (described later in this chapter).

As the placenta ages, it begins to thin and in the third trimester may calcify. These changes are variable, but in approximately 15% of cases the calcifications extend completely through the substance of the placenta, completely outlining the cotyledons (see Fig. 20-5D). These are termed grade 3 changes and should not occur before 34 weeks. Although data from prospective studies are not available, a composite of data from case reports has shown that the incidence of asymmetric IUGR approaches 50% in fetuses younger than 34 weeks' gestation with grade 3 changes. Conclusive work on

Table 13-2 Amniotic Fluid Index Values (cm) in Normal Pregnancy

Week	Amniotic Fluid Index Percentile Values		
	5th	50th	95th
16	7.9	12.1	18.5
17	8.3	12.7	19.4
18	8.7	13.3	20.2
19	9.0	13.7	20.7
20	9.3	14.1	21.2
21	9.5	14.3	21.4
22	9.7	14.5	21.6
23	9.8	14.6	21.8
24	9.8	14.7	21.9
25	9.7	14.7	22.1
26	9.7	14.7	22.3
27	9.5	14.6	22.6
28	9.4	14.6	22.8
29	9.2	14.5	23.1
30	9.0	14.5	23.4
31	8.8	14.4	23.8
32	8.6	14.4	24.2
33	8.3	14.3	24.5
34	8.1	14.2	24.8
35	7.9	14.0	24.9
36	7.7	13.8	24.9
37	7.5	13.5	24.4
38	7.3	13.2	23.9
39	7.2	12.7	22.6
40	7.1	12.3	21.4
41	7.0	11.6	19.4
42	6.9	11.0	17.5

From Moore TR, Cayle JE: The amniotic fluid index in normal human pregnancy. Am J Obstet Gynecol 162:1168, 1990.

placental thickness in evaluating for IUGR is not available. Therefore, although of theoretical importance, early appearance of these findings cannot at present be considered definite risk factors for IUGR.

Other Fetal Parameters

Two internal fetal parameters may be of value in diagnosing IUGR: the length of the liver and the epiphyseal centers around the knee.

The liver is a major store of glycogen in utero and a source of extramedullary hematopoiesis. In starvation states, in particular asymmetric IUGR, the liver would be expected to decrease in size and may be the major reason for the decrease in the size of the abdomen. The length of the right lobe of the liver and its potential value is discussed in Chapter 17 (see Table 17-1). Certain epiphyseal centers are expected to develop at specific fetal ages (see Fig. 19-2C). The distal femoral epiphysis has been shown to be larger than 5 mm in longest length by 32 weeks, with the proximal tibial epiphysis growing to more than 5 mm by 36 weeks. If these are detected and yet the fetus is otherwise too small (by at least 2 weeks), this might suggest growth retardation. Although both need further evaluation in large prospective studies, they hold promise in the detection of growth restriction.

Umbilical Artery Doppler Velocity Waveform Analysis

Placental circulation is composed of two parallel low-resistance, high-flow circulations. From the maternal side, approximately 100 spiral arteries feed the placenta through the uterine artery. From the fetal side, usually two but sometimes one umbilical artery flows to and one umbilical vein flows away from the placenta. The capillary vessels are long, tortuous, and dilated. These create slow flow and a large surface area so that a maximum exchange of nutrients and waste products can take place. The low resistance ensures continuous blood flow throughout the fetal and maternal cardiac cycles.

Obstetric Doppler evaluates the velocity waveform in the umbilical artery. It is important to remember that this is not a measurement of true flow volume. To obtain true flow, an accurate blood vessel cross-sectional area and vessel angle would have to be computed simultaneously with the Doppler shift. These cannot be performed on routine ultrasound machines, and currently true flow has an error of 30% to 100%. Instead, the arterial velocity waveform is analyzed by comparing peak systole (A) to end diastole (B) in the same cycle as an A/B ratio, thereby providing an assessment of resistance to blood flow in the placenta (Fig. 13-3). The A/B ratio has also been termed an S/D (systolic/diastolic) ratio. For maximum consistency, sampling should be repeated from at least three different waveforms and averaged. If variations in the ratio exist, some observers have suggested averaging as many as six consecutive A/B ratios. Because this is a comparison of the height of systole to end diastole, the angle of insonation is not important unless an adequate signal cannot be obtained.

The A/B ratio of the umbilical artery normally decreases throughout the second and third trimesters, from mean values of 4.25 at 16 weeks to 2.51 by term, with an abnormal ratio set at greater than the 90th percentile (Table 13-3). The ratio decreases because of increasing diastolic flow, a representation of less placental resistance, and more perfusion as the fetus matures. But because the ratio changes, knowledge of the fetal age is important. A top normal A/B ratio at 28 weeks, for example, would be above the 90th percentile (abnormal) at 34 weeks' gestation.

Decreased blood flow to the fetus is usually caused by increased vascular resistance within the placental

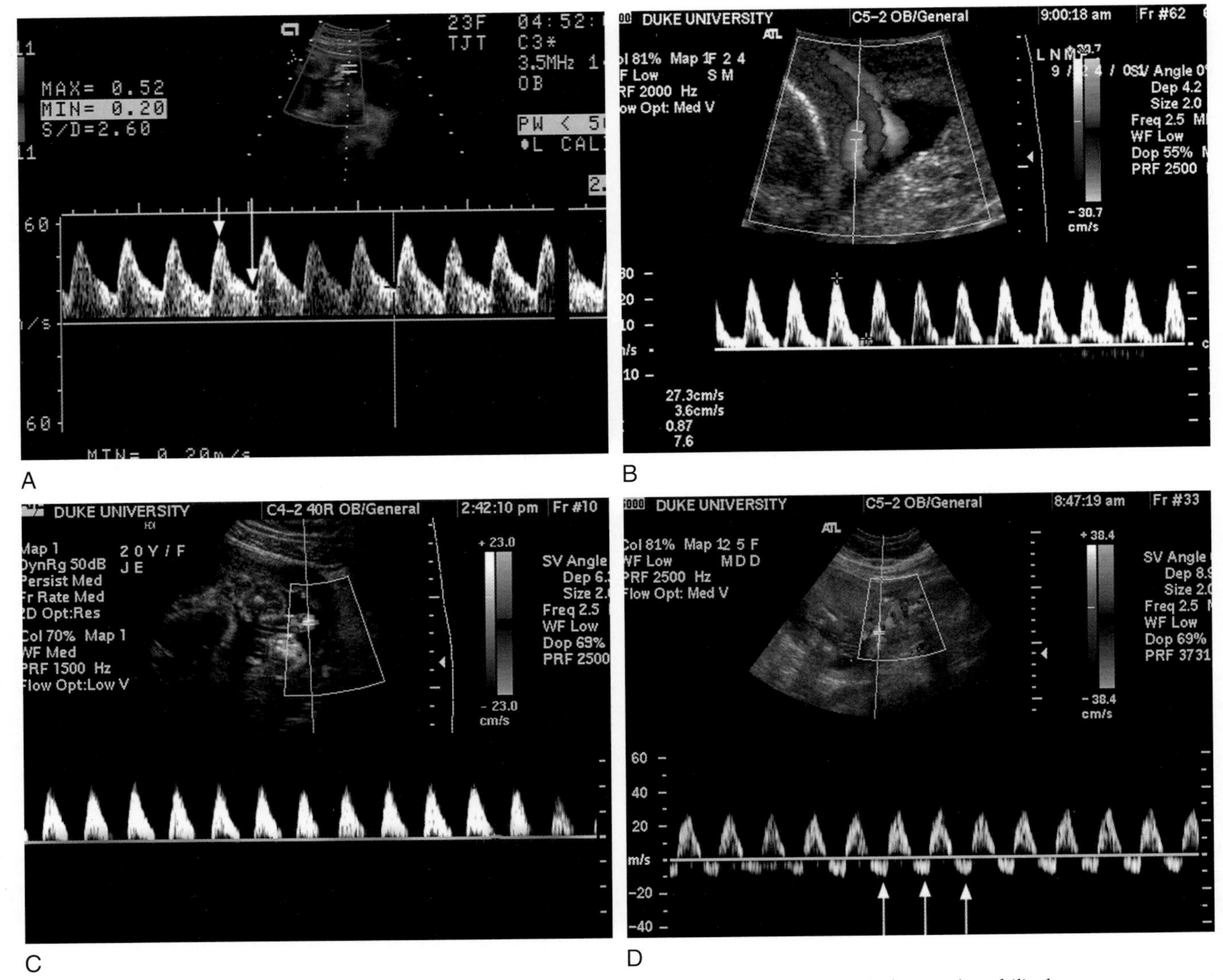

Figure 13-3 Umbilical artery Doppler imaging. Examples of normal and abnormal umbilical artery Doppler waveforms. **A,** Normal waveform. Spectral Doppler tracing obtained from umbilical artery in the mid cord at 36 weeks shows a normal waveform with good diastolic flow. The A/B ratio of .52/.20 is 2.6, which is normal for 36 weeks (see Table 13-3). *Short arrow,* peak systole; *long arrow,* end diastole. **B,** Decreased diastolic flow. Umbilical artery spectral Doppler tracing at 31 weeks shows decreased diastolic flow resulting in a markedly elevated A/B ratio of 7.6 (see Table 13.3). The fetus also was small for gestational age. Electronic calipers *(cursors)* indicate peak systole and end diastole. **C,** Absent diastolic flow. Spectral Doppler tracing from umbilical artery at 29 weeks shows a markedly abnormal waveform, with no diastolic flow. **D,** Reversed diastolic flow. Spectral Doppler waveform from umbilical artery of a 26-week fetus with severe growth restriction is markedly abnormal, with reversed diastolic flow *(arrows).*

vascular bed, in the vessels supplying the placenta, or from the fetus. Less commonly, it stems from maternal cardiovascular problems. As the resistance increases in any of these conditions, the diastolic component decreases initially toward the baseline value (see Fig. 13-3B). This elevates the A/B ratio above the 90th percentile. As the resistance further increases, end diastole can become nonexistent (see Fig. 13-3C) and even reverse (see Fig. 13-3D) in more severe cases. Further increase in resistance can cause the systolic component to become blunted and decreased in height.

An abnormal Doppler ratio indicates an underlying problem that is adversely affecting fetal circulation. A normal Doppler ratio is more difficult to interpret. If there are clinical and/or other ultrasound findings of IUGR, then a normal ratio tells the examiner little. It might be that the fetus will not exhibit an abnormal signal (not all fetuses with IUGR have abnormal ratios)

Table 13-3 Umbilical Artery Peak Systolic–to–End-Diastolic Ratio

Gestational Age	Percentile		
	10th	50th	90th
16	3.01	4.25	6.07
20	3.16	4.04	5.24
24	2.70	3.50	4.75
28	2.41	3.02	3.97
30	2.43	3.04	3.80
32	2.27	2.73	3.57
34	2.08	2.52	3.41
36	1.96	2.35	3.15
38	1.89	2.24	3.10
40	1.88	2.22	2.68
41	1.93	2.21	2.55
42	1.91	2.51	3.21

From Fogarty P, et al: Continuous wave Doppler flow velocity waveforms from the umbilical artery in normal pregnancy. J Perinat Med 18:51, 1990.

or that the fetus is not as yet severely affected. A differentiation of these two possibilities may be very difficult or impossible.

Furthermore, when an abnormal signal is detected that suggests fetal compromise, can the abnormal ratio be equated with the extent of that compromise (distress or demise)? The answer to this question is at present unfortunately "no." Although the abnormal Doppler signal, particularly when other variables such as fetal biometric measurements are abnormal, elevates the fetus to an increased risk level, there is no definitive correlation with the extent of the fetal compromise. In most pregnancies, if diastolic flow is still seen, close observation without intervention is considered the correct approach unless the fetus is mature enough to be delivered. Absent or reversed diastolic flow is of more concern and is often an indicator of severe fetal compromise, but even these markedly abnormal spectral waveform patterns sometimes improve on follow-up examinations. As a general rule, however, the earlier an abnormal ratio is detected, the worse the prognosis.

It is not recommended that all fetuses have a routine Doppler examination, even in the third trimester. Umbilical artery Doppler should be considered an adjunctive test and the indications for performing Doppler ultrasound should be limited to the selected cases that are likely to have IUGR and more specifically to those likely to be malnourished (asymmetric IUGR).

More recently there has been an attempt to directly analyze the fetus' internal circulation (the descending thoracic aorta or kidneys) and cranial circulation (the carotid or middle cerebral arteries (Fig. 13-4). By convention this is usually performed with another Doppler index, the pulsatility index (PI), which is a ratio of peak systole minus end diastole divided by the area under the curve of one waveform. In fetuses with asymmetric IUGR, there is evidence that blood flow to the head will initially remain stable at the expense of blood flow to the remainder of the body. As the fetus further fails, however, the cerebral PI will rise as the diastolic component of the waveform elevates. This indicates that the fetus has now lost its ability to autoregulate its blood flow and has increasing distress. Although this analysis added to the umbilical artery Doppler is being used more often in suspected fetal compromise, its clinical significance and its predictive value in fetal distress have not been worked out. At present, at most institutions, the A/B ratio of the umbilical artery is performed first, and if it is normal, the Doppler examination is stopped. Only when the ratio is abnormal, or when there are additional clinical or ultrasound concerns for an abnormal fetus, is the cerebral PI performed.

Biophysical Profile

Perinatal mortality is of clinical concern in the late third trimester. Deaths in premature deliveries are to a large extent caused by the prematurity itself (46%). In term deliveries, deaths are usually secondary to gross fetal anomalies (57%). In both settings, however, 17% of perinatal mortality (one out of every six fetuses) is caused by hypoxia. Can hypoxia be detected?

The biophysical profile (BPP) is an extensively studied in utero evaluation that can help in the prediction and management of fetuses with hypoxia. Five tests are combined in the BPP: four are of the fetus (assessing acute hypoxia) evaluating cardiac function, breathing,

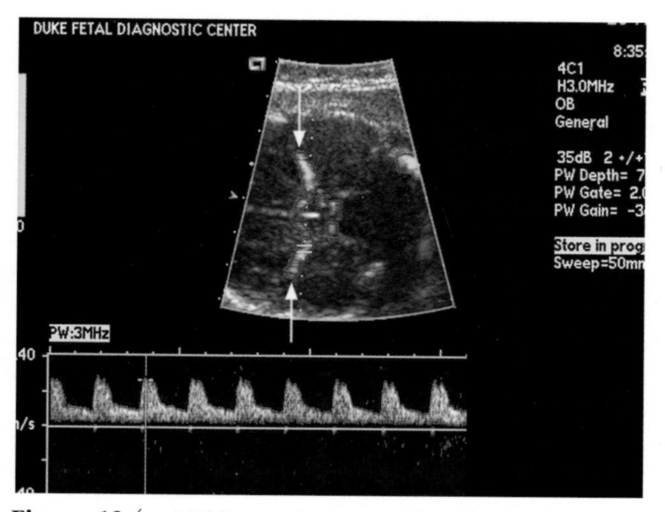

Figure 13-4 Middle cerebral artery Doppler imaging. Axial color Doppler image of fetal head at 26 weeks shows the right and left middle cerebral arteries *(arrows)*. A spectral tracing has been obtained from the middle cerebral artery.

gross body movement, and overall tone, and one is of the amniotic fluid (assessing chronic hypoxia). Of these, the heart rate study (the nonstress test [NST]) uses an external monitor to analyze passive normal episodes of cardiac accelerations whereas the other four (breathing, gross body movements, tone, and amniotic fluid) are evaluated by ultrasound.

The BPP uses a binomial grading system, with each variable assigned a 2 if that characteristic is present (normal) or 0 if absent (abnormal), for a maximum score of 10 and a minimum score of 0. The four fetal characteristics develop from different central nervous system centers. During embryogenesis the earliest developing center involves fetal tone, followed by development of the areas associated with fetal movement, then fetal breathing movements, and lastly fetal heart rate. Hypoxia appears to affect these centers in reverse order. Therefore, it is possible to evaluate the degree of acute hypoxia by observing how many fetal characteristics are involved. These centers, and in particular the cardiac center, are not fully developed until 26 to 28 weeks' gestation so that the BPP is a third-trimester evaluation.

A normal fetus goes through sleep-wake cycles lasting 20 to 40 minutes. An important assumption of the BPP is that a fetus cannot be spontaneously awakened. When it is asleep, the normal fetus will resemble a compromised (hypoxic) fetus. However, the sleeping fetus will eventually awaken and start to move, whereas the compromised fetus will not. The BPP is scheduled to last 30 minutes. During that time the examiner is looking for four parameters. If the fetus is normally responsive the study can be completed within 10 minutes. If the fetus is not moving, however, it is necessary to continuously observe the fetus for the full 30 minutes. If still unresponsive, the fetus is probably compromised.

Definitions have been given to each of the variables. Since the initial studies, only the definition of gross body movements has remained unchanged; the definitions of the other four have been modified, and this is described by Finberg and coworkers. It has been suggested that fetal tone too closely mirrors gross body movements and that fine body movements such as those of the hands should be used instead. Another group has suggested giving the fetus a "partial credit" of 1 (instead of 2) for any response that is somewhere between a full response and no response. Still others have recommended using the contraction stimulation test, an active cardiac test requiring nipple stimulation or the administration of oxytocin, either in addition to or instead of the NST. Lastly, evaluation of the amniotic fluid has undergone changes from a single pocket measurement, with most examiners now using the AFI.

These variations notwithstanding, there is a high degree of correlation between the BPP and perinatal morbidity (fetal distress) and mortality (fetal demise). Fetal distress has a linear relationship to the BPP: there is almost no likelihood of fetal distress (<3%) associated with a BPP of 10, with this likelihood increasing steadily to 100% with a BPP of 0. A score of 0 or 2, meaning that every characteristic is abnormal or that only one characteristic is normal, is highly associated with impending demise. For a BPP score of 8 or 10, the negative predictive accuracy for a normal live outcome within 1 week of the test is 99.224%. Certain groups of high-risk mothers, particularly insulin-dependent diabetics, may need to be reexamined more than once a week. The meaning of the intervening scores of 4 to 7, unfortunately, has not been resolved.

It would be tempting to assume that all growth-restricted fetuses should have their BPP assessed. However, a number of fetuses with IUGR are not hypoxic and a number of hypoxic fetuses are not growth restricted. Therefore, although there is overlap in the characteristics of both, and many IUGR fetuses may be studied with the BPP, these two groups should not be considered the same.

A full BPP may not be needed in most cases, because the cardiac portion (NST), representing acute hypoxia, and the amniotic fluid assessment, representing chronic hypoxia, may be representative of the entire BPP. In particular, when comparing the BPP against the NST, the positive predictive value for an abnormal BPP score is much greater than that for an abnormal NST result (56.6% vs. 13.1%), but the negative predictive value for a normal BPP score is virtually identical to a normal NST result (98.8% vs. 98.0%). As a result, it may be reasonable to perform the NST first and obtain a BPP only when the NST result is abnormal.

There is a distinct difference between the indications for a full ultrasound obstetrical antenatal examination and a BPP. The ultrasound examination is performed any time in pregnancy to establish fetal age and to evaluate for anomalies and amniotic fluid; the BPP is performed to evaluate fetal function in the late second trimester and third trimester.

Summary Of IUGR

When the gestational age is known, weight and abdominal circumference are helpful predictors of SGA fetuses with the lower 10th percentile picked as the cutoff. The lower the weight or abdominal circumference, the greater likelihood that IUGR is present. When the gestational age is not known or uncertain, the only consistently useful characteristic for the analysis of symmetric growth restriction is slow interval growth. Multiple additional characteristics are potentially available for determining asymmetric growth retardation: an abnormal head-to-body proportion, slow interval growth, decreased volume of amniotic fluid, and abnormal

Doppler velocity waveforms. Each case of asymmetric IUGR differs in its presentation and in its abnormal characteristics.

The BPP is a valuable test for predicting both normal (nonhypoxic) fetuses and impending fetal demise. However, there is need for uniform definitions of the characteristics and the scoring system needs to be standardized.

MACROSOMIA

The terms *large for gestational age* (LGA) and *macrosomia* are often used interchangeably to describe a newborn above the 90th percentile by weight or one who weighs more than either 4000 or 4500 g. However, if strictly defined, the terms are not synonymous. LGA fetuses are symmetrically large with fat distributed evenly over the entire body. In contradistinction, macrosomic fetuses are asymmetrically enlarged with fat distributed more to the shoulders and body, so macrosomic fetuses are at greatest risk for shoulder dystocia during vaginal delivery; that is, the head can be delivered without difficulty but the shoulders may impact. If excessive traction on the neck is required to disengage the shoulders, injury to the newborn, most commonly Erb's palsy (neurologic damage to the brachial plexus), can result. At times, despite the use of all aggressive obstetrical maneuvers, the results of delivery may be disastrous. Macrosomia is commonly associated with maternal gestational diabetes and mild insulin-dependent diabetes (Fig. 13-5).

Estimated fetal weight alone cannot predict the disproportionality of the shoulders and body and therefore does not optimally predict the potential for shoulder dystocia. In addition, because there is a minimum of a 15% error in the calculation of the fetal weight, the fetus would have to have a mean weight of at least 4600 g to confidently predict a weight of more than 4000 g.

There have been attempts to measure the head, the head-to-body ratio, and shoulder length (from the neck to the edge of the shoulder) for the prediction of dystocia. This work is incomplete and has not been consistent in predicting potential problems at time of delivery. At present, therefore, macrosomia can only be inferred from the estimated fetal weight and clinical suspicion.

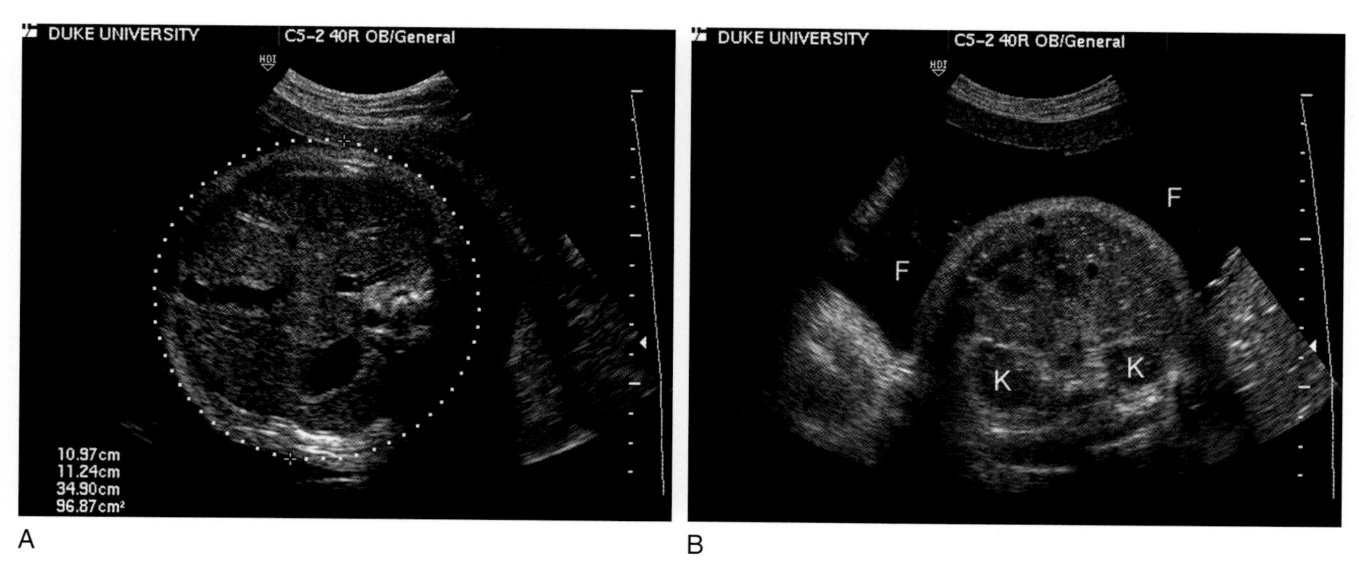

Figure 13-5 Macrosomia associated with gestational diabetes. **A,** AC measurement of 34.9 cm in this 34-week pregnancy complicated by gestational diabetes is above the 97.5th percentile for gestational age (see Table 13-1). The EFW was at the 99th percentile. **B,** Axial image of abdomen of same fetus obtained at the level of the kidneys (K) shows polyhydramnios, also due to gestational diabetes. F, amniotic fluid.

Key Features

- Neonates with small birth weights, usually defined as below the 10th percentile, are considered small for gestational age (SGA). These SGA children can be either constitutionally small or growth restricted.
- Intrauterine growth restriction (IUGR) varies in incidence. On average, it affects 5% of the general population. In a high-risk population, this rate can rise to 10% of fetuses.
- There are two types of IUGR: diminished cellular growth leading to a symmetrically small fetus (usually occurring in the first or early second trimester) and fetal malnutrition leading to an asymmetrically small fetus (usually occurring in the third trimester). If the malnutrition is extreme, however, the asymmetric fetus may appear symmetric.
- If an accurate fetal age is known, either from an early ultrasound examination or accurate menstrual dates, or both, then the measured abdominal circumference and calculated fetal weight can be used to determine if the fetal size and weight are appropriate.
- When an accurate age is not known, additional less sensitive and less specific characteristics for identifying IUGR are needed. They are interval growth, the head-to-body ratio, the amniotic fluid volume, and the Doppler velocity waveform. Of these, only interval growth can be used to assess both types of IUGR.
- Structural anomalies may be either the cause of or associated with IUGR.
- The ability of ultrasound to detect IUGR is different in different clinical risk groups. A slightly small fetus or a fetus growing at the lower 10th percentile is often less of a clinical concern if the woman is in a low-risk rather than in a high-risk group.
- The volume of amniotic fluid can be evaluated either subjectively by scanning the entire uterine content or by a four-quadrant measurement (the amniotic fluid index [AFI]). Subjective analysis is as accurate as the AFI and is of particular value in borderline cases.
- Doppler evaluation makes use of a ratio of peak systole and end diastole from the arterial waveform in the umbilical artery. With decreasing diastole (higher vascular resistance), the ratio increases and the fetus is then at greater risk for circulatory problems. More recently, the fetal cerebral circulation has been studied but no specific conclusions as to its predictive accuracy have yet been made.
- It is not recommended that Doppler sonography be performed in all pregnancies. When there is a suggestion of a compromised fetus, however, the umbilical artery Doppler study is performed. Only if the study is abnormal does the fetal cerebral circulation need to be studied.
- The biophysical profile (BPP) can predict perinatal mortality by detecting in utero hypoxia (17% of all fetuses).
- The BPP consists of five tests, four fetal for identifying acute hypoxia and one of the amniotic fluid for identifying chronic hypoxia. Each characteristic is rated as 2 if normal and 0 if absent, for a total score of from 0 to 10.
- The fetus with a BPP score of 7 or more can be considered "safe" in most cases for up to a week but is at risk for impending demise if the score is less than 4. Intervening numbers indicate risk but usually not the danger of sudden demise.
- The two most sensitive BPP tests are the cardiac test for acute hypoxia (the nonstress test [NST]) and amniotic fluid assessment for chronic hypoxia.
- The terms *large for gestational age* (LGA) and *macrosomia* have been used interchangeably. There are three definitions: a weight exceeding 4000 g, a weight exceeding 4500 g, or ultrasound findings that suggest that the fetus is larger than the 90th percentile.
- There are no problems with a macrosomic fetus in utero. At delivery, particularly if asymmetrically large with fat distributed more in the shoulders and body, the fetus is at risk for shoulder dystocia.

SUGGESTED READINGS

Baschat AA, Harman CR: Antenatal assessment of the growth restricted fetus. Curr Opin Obstet Gynecol 13:161, 2001.

Benson CB, et al: Intrauterine growth retardation: Diagnosis based on multiple parameters: A prospective study. Radiology 177:499, 1990.

Campbell BA: Utilizing sonography to follow fetal growth. Obstet Gynecol Clin North Am 25:750, 1998.

Craigo SD: The role of ultrasound in the diagnosis and management of intrauterine growth retardation. Semin Perinatol 18:292, 1994.

Doubilet PM, Benson CB: Sonographic evaluation of intrauterine growth retardation. AJR Am J Roentgenol 164:709, 1995.

Finberg HJ, et al: The biophysical profile: A literature review and reassessment of its usefulness in the evaluation of fetal well-being. J Ultrasound Med 9:583, 1990.

Fong KW, Ohlsson A, Hannah ME, et al: Prediction of perinatal outcome in fetuses suspected to have intrauterine growth restriction: Doppler US study of fetal cerebral, renal, and umbilical arteries. Radiology 213:681, 1999.

Galan HL, Ferrazzi E, Hobbins JC: Intrauterine growth restriction (IUGR): Biometric and Doppler assessment. Prenat Diagn 22:331, 2002.

Goldstein RB, Filly RA: Sonographic estimation of amniotic fluid volume: Subjective assessment versus pocket measurements. J Ultrasound Med 7:363, 1988.

Hershkovitz R, Kingdom JC, Geary M, et al: Fetal cerebral blood flow redistribution in late gestation: Identification of compromise in small fetuses with normal umbilical artery Doppler. Ultrasound Obstet Gynecol 15:209, 2000.

Landon MB: Prenatal diagnosis of macrosomia in pregnancy complicated by diabetes mellitus. J Matern Fetal Med 9:52, 2000.

Manning FA: Fetal biophysical profile. Obstet Gynecol Clin North Am 26:557, 1999.

Manning FA, Platt LD, Sipos L: Antepartum fetal evaluation: Development of a fetal biophysical profile. Am J Obstet Gynecol 136:787, 1980.

Marsal K: Intrauterine growth restriction. Curr Opin Obstet Gynecol 14:127, 2002.

Pollack RN, Divon MY: Intrauterine growth retardation and etiology. Clin Obstet Gynecol 35:99, 1992.

Resnick R: Intrauterine growth restriction. Obstet Gynecol 99:490, 2002.

Rochelson B, et al: The significance of absent end-diastolic velocity in umbilical artery velocity waveforms. Am J Obstet Gynecol 156:1213, 1987.

Rochelson BL, et al: The clinical significance of Doppler umbilical artery velocimetry in the small for gestational age fetus. Am J Obstet Gynecol 156:1223, 1987.

Sacks DA, Chen W: Estimating fetal weight in the management of macrosomia. Obstet Gynecol Surv 55:229, 2000.

Sholl JS, et al: Intrauterine growth retardation risk detection for fetuses of unknown gestational age. Am J Obstet Gynecol 144:709, 1982.

Trudinger BJ, et al: Fetal umbilical artery velocity waveforms and subsequent neonatal outcome. Br J Obstet Gynaecol 98:378, 1991.

Vintzileos AM, et al: The fetal biophysical profile and its predictive value. Obstet Gynecol 62:271, 1983.

The First Trimester and Ectopic Pregnancy

For Key Features summary see p. 371

The obstetrical literature fails to give a precise definition to the first trimester. For convenience, it is simplest to describe the early pregnancy as the first 12 weeks from the beginning of the last normal menstrual period (LMP) to the end of the first 3 months. The embryo is defined as the time from conception to 8 weeks (10 weeks from LMP) when organ development begins; after that the conceptus is termed a fetus. From an ultrasound standpoint, the most useful definition for both the first trimester and for the embryo is the first 12 weeks, because in a normal pregnancy this is the junction between analysis of the embryo and evaluation of fetal structures.

This first trimester, the early pregnancy, is a critical diagnostic interval in the pregnancy. The ultimate proof of a normal intrauterine pregnancy (IUP) is awaiting the detection of a living embryo. However, miscarriages (spontaneous incomplete or complete abortions), ectopic pregnancies, hydatidiform moles, and even unrelated pelvic pathologic conditions such as pelvic inflammatory disease and endometriosis may confuse this analysis.

The two most important diagnostic studies of an early pregnancy are the pregnancy test (urine and/or serum) and the ultrasound examination. The pregnancy test is an immunoassay of the β subunit of human chorionic gonadotropin (βhCG). This hormone is produced by the placenta, differs from other pituitary glycoprotein hormones, and is therefore highly specific for identifying a pregnancy. False-positive diagnoses are extremely rare. The only false-negative diagnoses are when the hCG levels are too low for detection. The serum test can be analyzed qualitatively and quantified to levels as low as 5 IU/L, equivalent to less than a 1-week pregnancy (<3 weeks from the LMP). These quantitative serum levels of hCG correlate in the first trimester with embryonic age. The urine levels, qualitative only, approach the lowest serum levels when tested in a concentrated first-morning sample.

Ultrasound is an important diagnostic test in the early pregnancy. It is best used in conjunction with the knowledge of the pregnancy test because specific pelvic processes are anticipated and others are excluded by the knowledge of a positive pregnancy test. The study can be performed by a combination of transabdominal (TA) and transvaginal (TV) techniques. The TA approach permits evaluation of the overall pelvic structures whereas the TV technique can aid in the identification of landmarks not appreciated transabdominally and can reanalyze structures not completely appreciated by the TA approach.

All pregnancies are defined as the age of the conceptus from the first day of the LMP. The LMP is not a precise method for establishing gestational age. Menstrual dates assume a regular 28-day cycle. A woman who has a regular but different cycle will have an error; for example a woman with a 35-day cycle will have a 7-day error. In addition, as many as 20% of women are uncertain of their menstrual dates, primarily because of irregular periods, oligomenorrhea, or failure to accurately recall their LMP. Therefore, although the LMP can be precise in any individual patient, its overall precision in the population is no better than ±2.5 weeks at the 95% confidence level (2 SD). First- and second-trimester ultrasound, up to at least 20 weeks and perhaps to 24 weeks, can determine gestational age to ±1 to 1.2 week at 2 SD. Therefore, one of the primary uses for an initial ultrasound study in the first 24 weeks is to establish gestational age. Comparison of this age to the LMP has limited value because a sizeable discrepancy (often more than 3 to 4 weeks in either direction) may require a follow-up study of fetal interval growth to rule out growth restriction or macrosomia.

THE GESTATIONAL SAC AND ITS MEASUREMENT

Both TA and TV scanning can be used to identify the gestational sac. The TA technique often requires a distended urinary bladder, with scans performed suprapubically to identify the uterus and the sac. As the uterus enlarges, the gestational sac is often identified above the urinary bladder, with the bladder still used to identify the lower uterine segment. The TV study in contradistinction is performed with the bladder empty.

The gestational sac can be routinely identified by both TA and TV scanning but often earlier transvaginally at 5 gestational weeks (3 weeks from conception). There is often a delay between the identification of the gestational sac and the identification of the embryo, which is usually not seen until almost 6 weeks transvaginally. The yolk sac is often identified in between, at 5.5 weeks. In some cases, these structures can be identified earlier.

Analysis of the gestational sac is of primary importance before embryonic visualization. The gestational sac is an anechoic space surrounded by a hyperechoic rim of trophoblastic tissue. Only the anechoic space is measured. The mean gestational sac diameter (MGSD) is obtained by averaging three orthogonal (perpendicular) measurements. Although this can be performed in any two perpendicular projections, the most useful method is to take measurements from the long-axis (usually sagittal) and the perpendicular short-axis (usually axial) images of the uterus. The maximal long-axis and maximal anteroposterior diameters are obtained from the long-axis images and the maximal widest measurement from the short-axis images (Fig. 14-1).

The gestational sac (using the MGSD) grows in a linear fashion. From the earliest ultrasound studies, some dating from the late 1960s, a 10-mm sac was equivalent to a 5-week gestation, increasing to 60 mm by 12.2 weeks. More recently, the early first-trimester measurements have been reevaluated, with the smallest measurable sac of 2 mm equivalent to a 5-week gestation. The difference between 2 and 10 mm MGSD for a 5-week gestation cannot be explained because both the TA and TV techniques are similarly accurate. This difference is unlikely to be of clinical significance, however, because the sac normally grows 1.2 mm/day and the difference of 8 mm

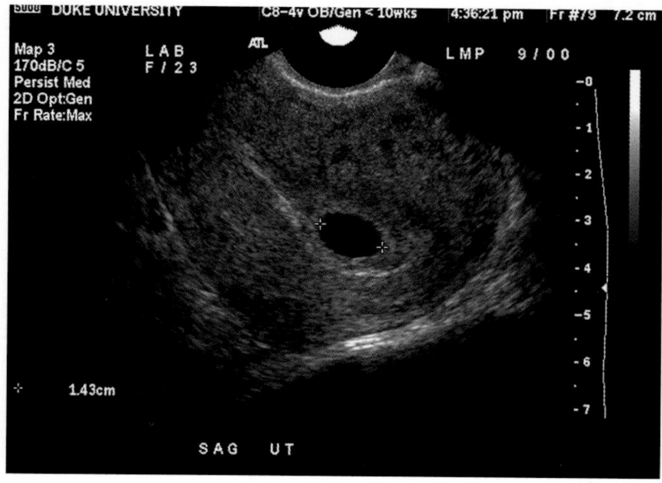

A

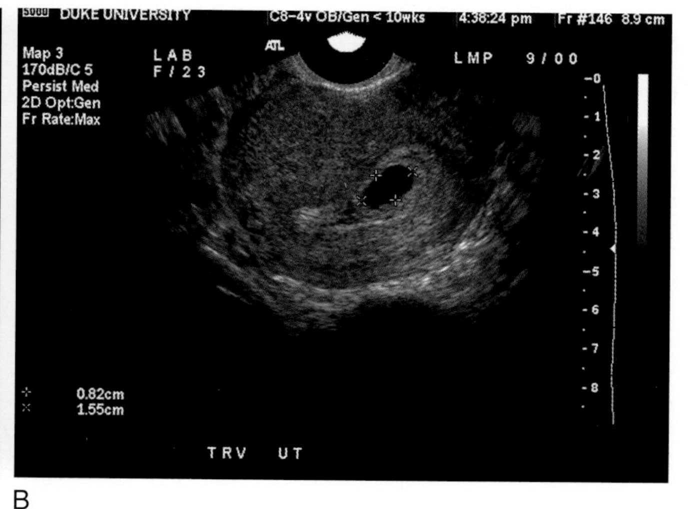

B

Figure 14-1 Measurement of mean gestational sac diameter (MGSD). **A** and **B**, The gestational sac is measured by positioning calipers on the inner edge of the hyperechoic rim of decidua *(cursors)* in three orthogonal planes. In this example, diameters of 14.3, 8.2, and 15.5 mm calculate to a mean of 12.7 mm. This corresponds to 6.3 weeks.

is only a variance of slightly less than 1 week. Because the range of precision for a first-trimester parameter (primarily from work performed on crown-rump length [CRL] measurements) is ±1 week (2 SD), this discrepancy would be within acceptable limits. However, we have arbitrarily picked a table that defines a 2-mm gestational sac as equivalent to 5 gestational weeks, performed in a TV study by Daya and coworkers (see Chapter 12, Table 12-2). This table continues up to 8.5 weeks (30 mm) and not to the end of the first trimester because gestational age established by the MGSD is of little value once the embryo is identified.

THE EMBRYO AND ITS MEASUREMENT

The embryo can be routinely identified by 6 weeks and, not infrequently, earlier by the TV approach. In most cases, heart motion can be detected when the embryo is seen. This is definitive for proving a living IUP. It is not often necessary to use an M-mode tracing to document heart motion. Rather, observation with real-time ultrasound or color Doppler imaging will suffice. Because of its increased power levels, pulsed Doppler imaging is not recommended in the early pregnancy.

The embryo grows progressively from 6 to 12 weeks, slowly at first with faster growth after 9 weeks. Its measurement, the embryonic or CRL, is performed along the embryo's longest observed axis. It should be possible to obtain an accurate and consistent CRL at any time in the first trimester. When the embryo is visualized at 6 to 7 weeks, it is difficult to identify the embryonic anatomy or even to differentiate the crown from the rump; by 8 to 9 weeks, the head and body can be identified (Fig. 14-2).

Early studies on the precision of the CRL had suggested an accuracy of ±3 days in 95% of the pregnant population. More recent studies have revealed a more realistic precision of ±5 to 7 days (2 SD). The CRL is less accurate after 12 weeks because the fetus can flex

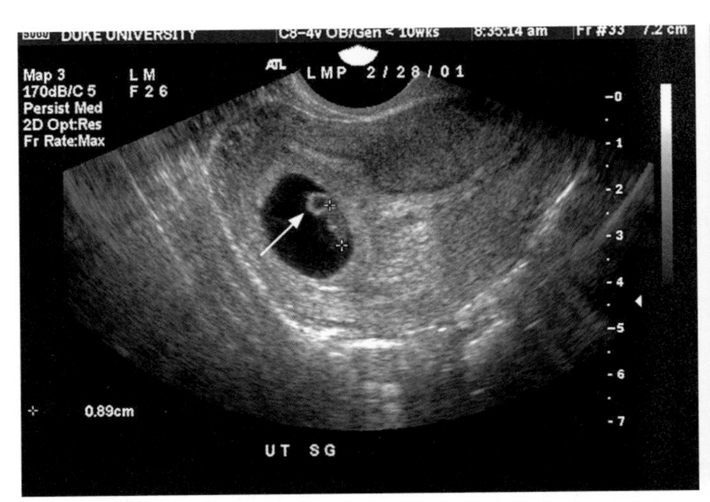

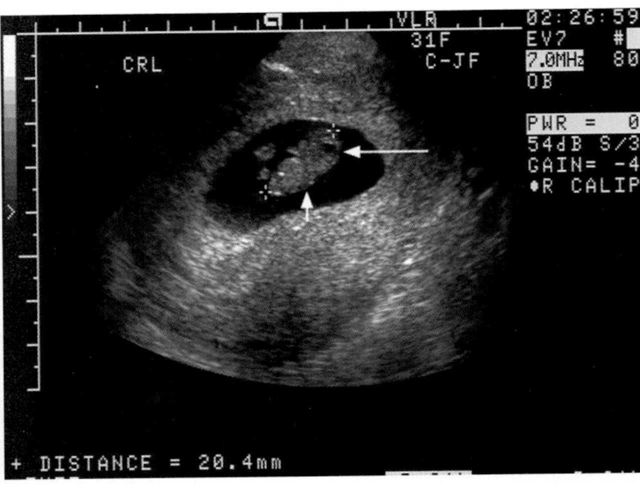

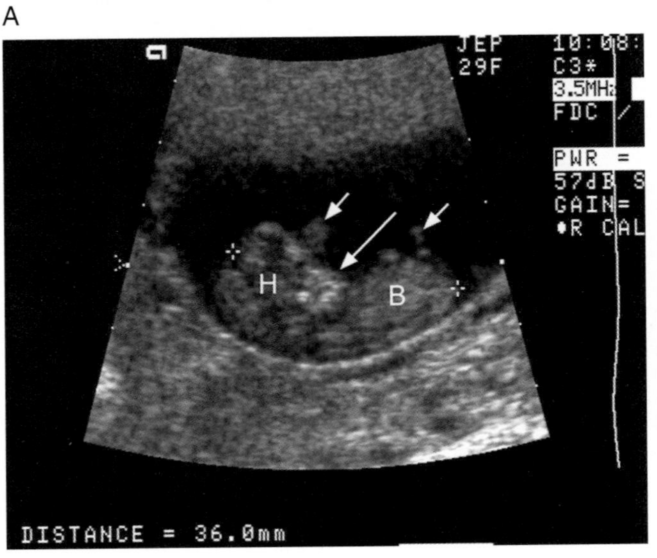

Figure 14-2 Growth and development of the embryo. **A,** Endovaginal scan of embryo *(cursors)* with a CRL of 8.9 mm, consistent with 6.8 weeks. At this early stage it is difficult to distinguish embryonic head from body. *Arrow,* yolk sac. **B,** By 8 to 9 weeks the head *(long arrow)* and body *(short arrow)* can be distinguished. In this example, the CRL of 20.4 mm corresponds to 8.6 weeks. **C,** Limb buds *(short arrows)* and ossification in mandible and maxilla *(long arrow)* are seen in this 10.5-week embryo (CRL, 36 mm). H, head; B, body.

and extend, thus causing measurement variability. The head measurements (biparietal diameter and head circumference), on the other hand, are routinely imaged in the second trimester, are less variable, and have approximately the same precision as the CRL, up to 20 and possibly to 24 weeks at ±1 to 1.2 weeks (2 SD). It is therefore recommended that the CRL be used until 12 weeks and a head measurement be used thereafter to determine gestational age.

In one of the earliest and best-regarded studies, the smallest routinely measured CRL of 6.7 mm was equivalent to 6.3 weeks using TA ultrasound. This work has been reevaluated using both TA and TV ultrasound. Unlike the MGSD, no significant measurement differences from previous studies have been found. A newer table by Hadlock and coworkers, however, assigns a gestational age to an embryo as small as 2 mm, equivalent to 5.7 weeks, thus permitting earlier determination of the embryonic age by approximately half a week (see Chapter 12, Table 12-1).

COMPARISON OF GESTATIONAL SAC AND EMBRYO

There is potential value in comparing the size of the gestational sac (MGSD) to the embryonic length (CRL), a concept roughly equivalent in the second and third trimesters to a comparison of amniotic fluid volume to fetal size. However, because the MGSD and CRL measurements come from different and unrelated populations, their analysis is restricted to comparing gestational ages from different tables. A more direct comparison of the two has been found in a formula subtracting the CRL (mm) from the MGSD (mm). A value greater than 5 mm is normal. When the value is less than 5 mm, almost all (94%) aborted spontaneously. This has been termed "first-trimester oligohydramnios." In all of the abnormal cases, the amount of fluid surrounding the embryo was obviously decreased (Fig. 14-3). A larger study is needed before the clinical value of this method can be determined.

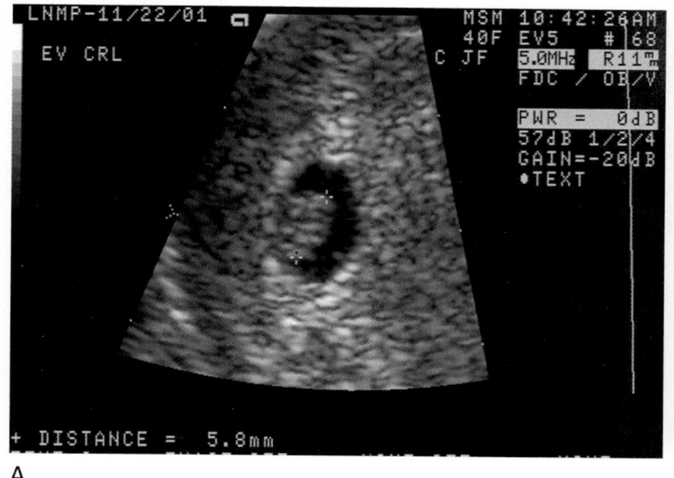

A

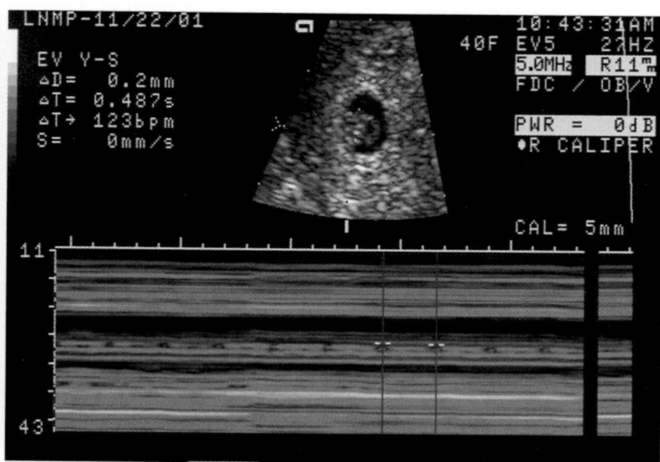

B

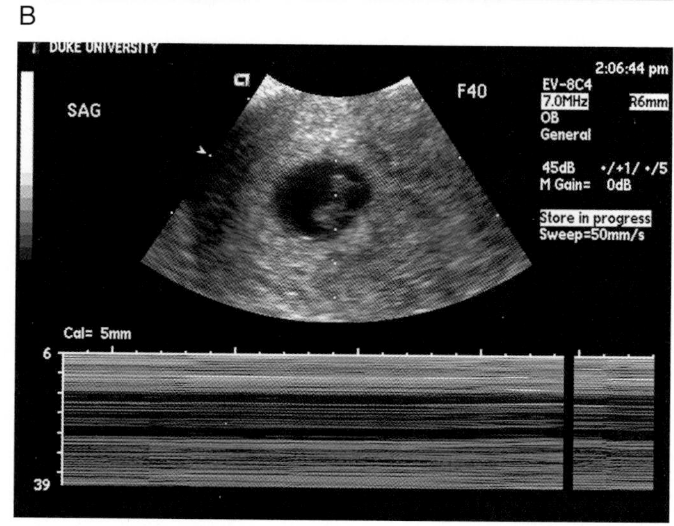

C

Figure 14-3 First-trimester oligohydramnios: a poor prognostic finding. **A,** Endovaginal ultrasound image reveals an early embryo *(cursors)*. Subjectively, the amount of fluid surrounding the embryo appears decreased. The MGSD of 8 mm minus crown-rump length of 5.8 mm = 2.2 mm, considerably less than the normal threshold of 5 mm. **B,** M-mode tracing obtained on the same day as image in **A** reveals cardiac activity, with a normal rate of 123 beats per minute. **C,** M-mode tracing obtained 2 weeks after the images in **A** and **B** reveals absence of cardiac activity, consistent with interval embryonic death.

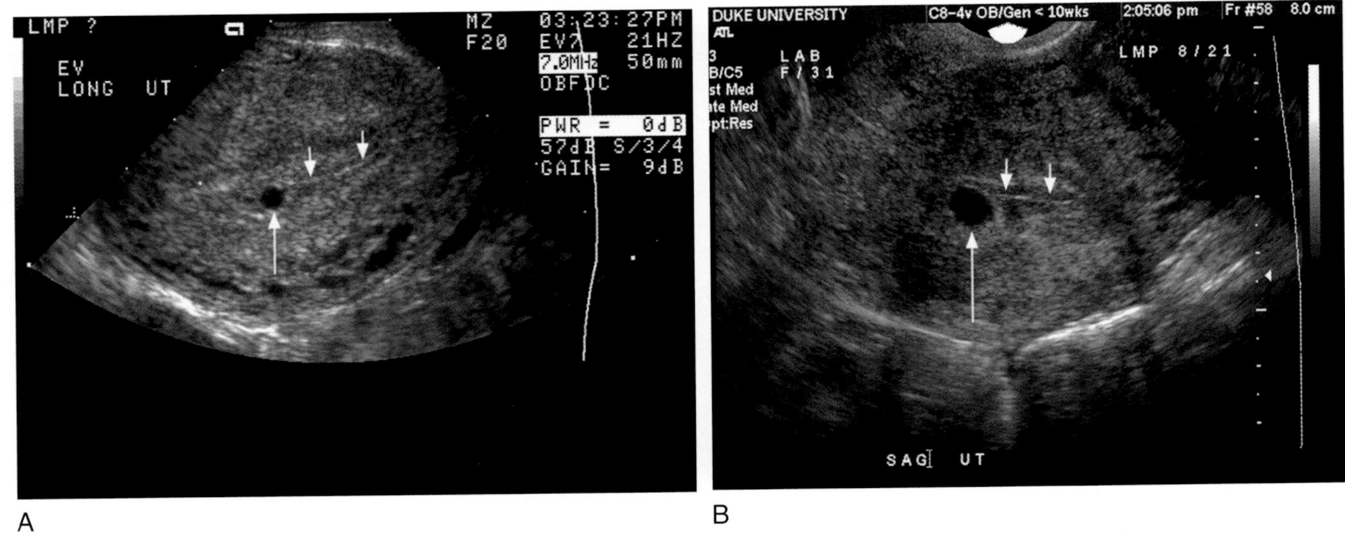

Figure 14-4 Two examples of the intradecidual sign. **A** and **B,** The early gestational sac *(long arrow)* is seen as a small anechoic space within the decidua, adjacent to but separate from the endometrial cavity *(short arrows).*

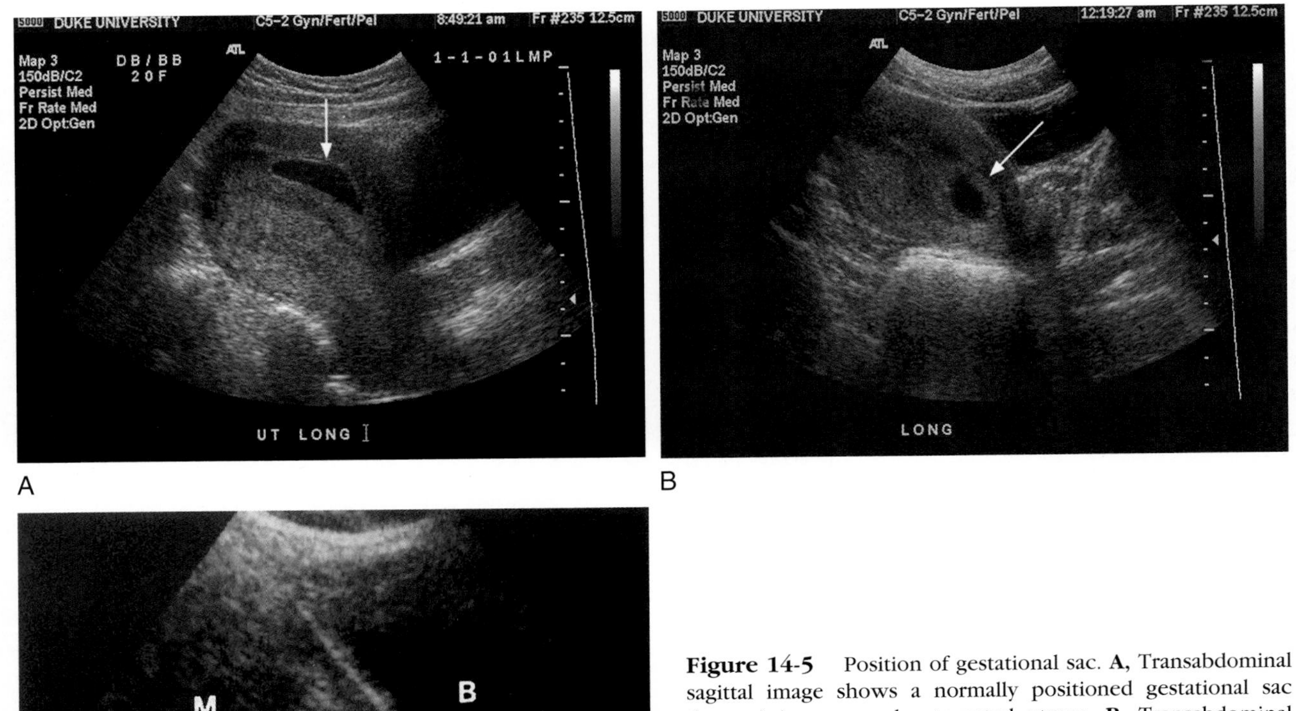

Figure 14-5 Position of gestational sac. **A,** Transabdominal sagittal image shows a normally positioned gestational sac *(arrow)* in a normal anteverted uterus. **B,** Transabdominal sagittal image of a different patient shows a gestational sac *(arrow)* implanted lower than expected in the uterus. The patient subsequently had a miscarriage. **C,** Transabdominal sagittal image of a 6.6-week pregnancy shows a fundal fibroid (M) displacing the gestational sac *(arrowheads)* downward into the lower part of the uterine body. e, embryo; B, urinary bladder.

THE NORMAL AND ABNORMAL APPEARANCE OF THE GESTATIONAL SAC

Before identification of the embryo, even before visualization of the gestational sac, the hyperechoic endometrial thickness may be a helpful but nonspecific sign in separating normally developing IUPs from abnormal IUPs and ectopic pregnancies. Using a cut-off thickness of 8 mm (97% of cases), normal IUPs were significantly thicker, averaging 13 mm, compared with an endometrial thickness in ectopic pregnancies of 6 mm. The initial identification of the gestational sac is a small anechoic sac within the thickened decidua, adjacent to but separate from the uterine cavity. This has been termed the *intradecidual sign.* It is seen at or before 5 weeks when the sac is still too small to indent the endometrial canal and too small to exhibit the other features of a larger gestational sac (Fig. 14-4).

The position of the gestational sac is important. In a normal anteverted uterus, the sac should be situated in the upper uterine body, in a midposition between the uterine walls (Fig. 14-5A). A lower-lying gestational sac may be normal but is more suggestive of a miscarriage (either an impending spontaneous pregnancy loss or one in progress) (see Fig. 14-5B), a cervical ectopic pregnancy (to be discussed later in the chapter), or the presence of fundal and/or uterine body fibroids displacing the sac downward (see Fig. 14-5C). If the uterus is either retroverted or retroflexed, a less common uterine position, it assumes (for unexplained reasons) a more globular shape. The position of the gestational sac tends to be more asymmetric in position, often posterolateral, and sometimes within 10 mm of the uterine margin.

As it grows, the gestational sac can be evaluated for a number of normal characteristics: double decidual sac (DDS), continuous hyperechoic rim of at least 2 mm in thickness, spherical or ovoid shape without marked angulation, and growth of more than 1.2 mm/day. To evaluate growth, at any time in the pregnancy, a measurement error of 1 mm on a single study and 2 mm on any two studies needs to be taken into account. To minimize this error, at least 6 mm of actual growth (at least 5 days for the CRL) should separate the two studies.

The DDS sign is an important feature. As the embryo implants into the uterine wall, it causes a hyperechoic trophoblastic reaction around the sac and a secondary endometrial hyperechoic decidual reaction around the endometrial cavity (Fig. 14-6). As the sac grows, it impinges on and causes the hypoechoic endometrial canal to close, and the hyperechoic rim is then interrupted around a part of the sac by a hypoechoic line that corresponds to the still unopposed endometrial cavity (Fig. 14-7). It is a very useful sign and when it is

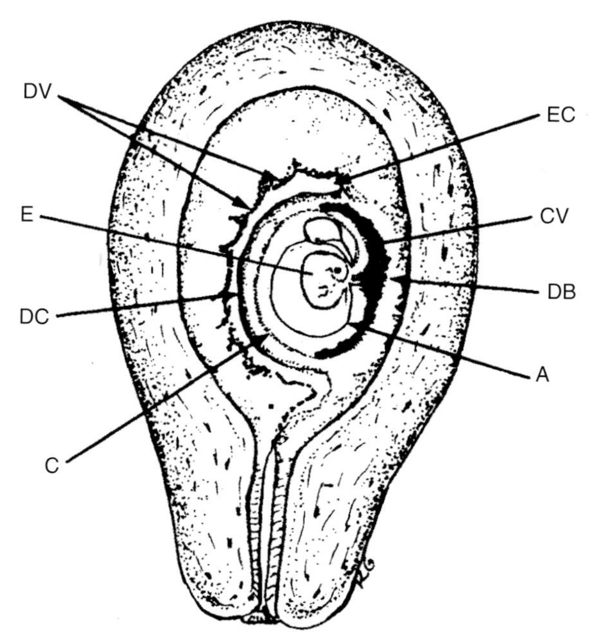

Figure 14-6 The uterus in the first trimester. The embryo (E) is developing within the amniotic sac (A). The chorionic sac (C), containing the yolk sac, surrounds the amniotic sac. The chorionic villi (CV) and the decidua basalis (DB) will form the placenta. On the opposite side of the chorionic sac, the decidua capsularis (DC) is greatly thinned. Between it and the opposite decidua, the decidua vera (DV), is the endometrial canal (EC). The potential uterine normal spaces are the endometrial canal and the separation of the amnion from the chorion.

specifically sought can be seen in the majority of normal early IUPs. Conversely, a hyperechoic rim without a DDS is more likely to be present in an abnormal IUP (a spontaneous incomplete abortion) (Fig. 14-8A) or a pseudogestational sac (see Fig. 14-8B) of fluid within the endometrial canal secondary to an ectopic pregnancy. The finding of a DDS confirms a normal IUP; its absence does not rule out an IUP (see Fig. 14-8C), but inability to demonstrate the DDS sign after a concerted effort to demonstrates it suggests the existence of an abnormality.

Identification of the embryo can be appreciated by certain MGSD sizes. By the TV approach, the embryo can be routinely identified earlier than by the TA approach. Transvaginally, the embryo is often first seen when the gestational sac has an MGSD of approximately 12 mm, equivalent to a mean gestational age of 6.2 weeks. Transabdominally, the MGSD routinely needs to be at least 27 mm or 8.1 weeks. If the embryo is not seen at these lower limits, waiting an extra week before declaring the pregnancy abnormal is appropriate because in some normal pregnancies the embryo will not be seen at these sac diameters. Transvaginally, the embryo is almost always seen by an MGSD of 16 mm; by

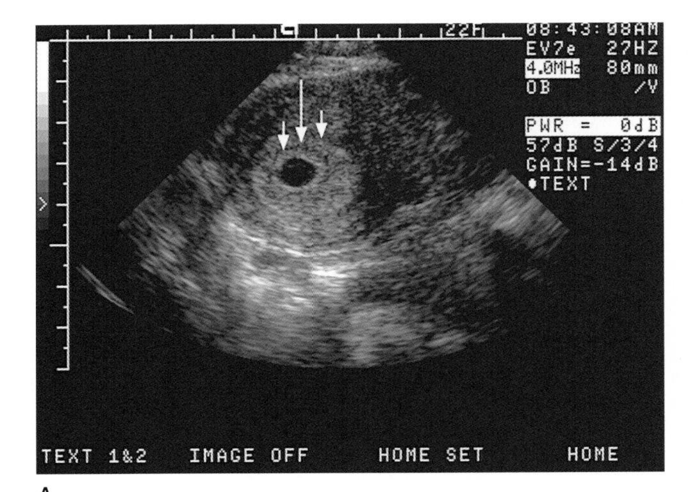

A

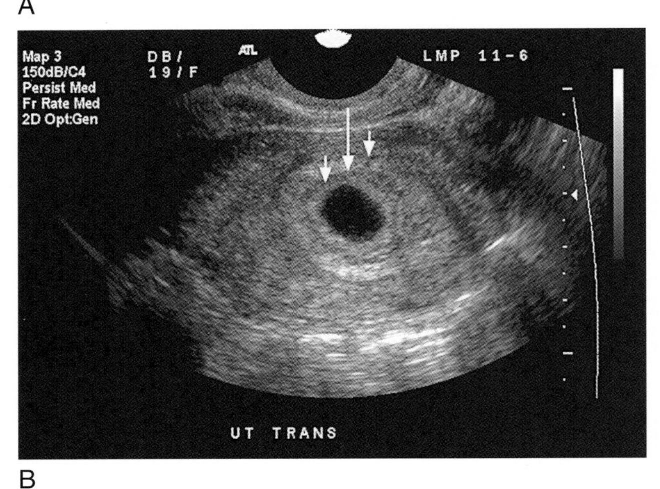

B

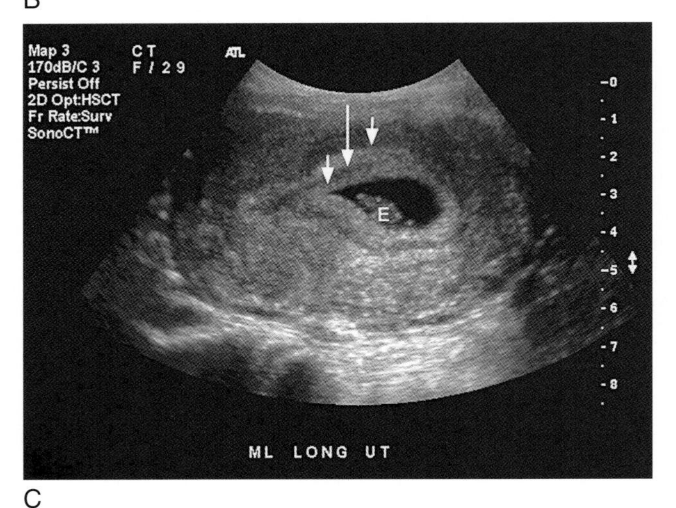

C

Figure 14-7 Double decidual sac sign. Examples of the double decidual sac sign in three patients (**A**—transvaginal scan; **B** and **C**—transabdominal scans) with normal early intrauterine pregnancies. Three discrete layers of echogenicity surround the gestational sac: the outer and inner echogenic layers *(short arrows)* correspond to decidua surrounding the gestational sac along both sides of the uterine cavity. The hypoechoic middle layer *(long arrows)* corresponds to the uterine cavity. E, embryo.

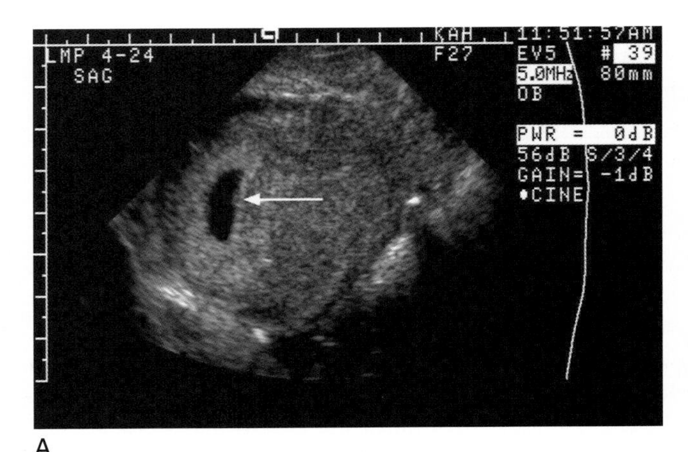

A

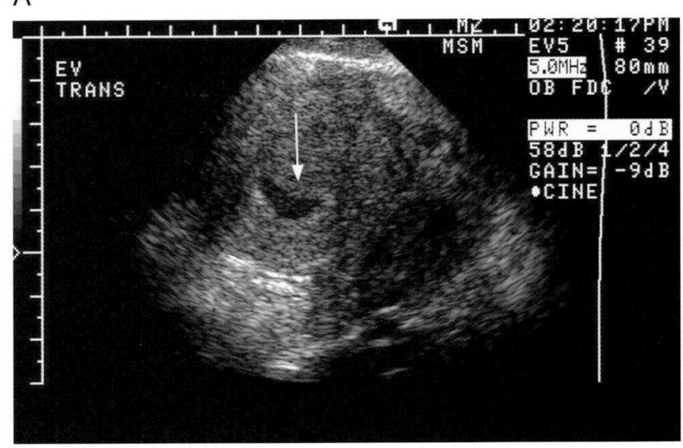

B

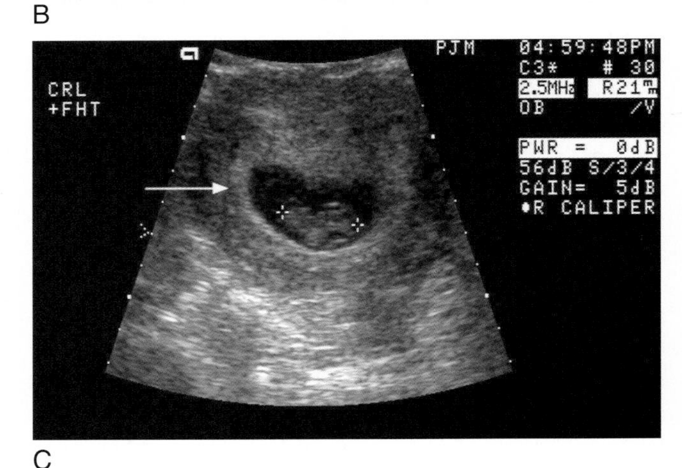

C

Figure 14-8 Absence of double decidual sac sign: etiology. **A,** Failed intrauterine pregnancy: the gestational sac *(arrow)* is surrounded by a hyperechoic rim of decidual reaction, but there is no double decidual sac sign. Additionally, there was no evidence of an embryo or yolk sac. Patient subsequently had a spontaneous miscarriage. **B,** Pseudogestational sac associated with ectopic pregnancy: a fluid collection surrounded by a hyperechoic rim of decidual reaction *(arrow)* is seen in the uterine cavity of this patient with an ectopic pregnancy. Note the absence of a double decidual sac sign surrounding this pseudogestational sac. **C,** Normal intrauterine pregnancy: although no double decidual sac sign is seen, there is a live embryo *(cursors)* in the gestational sac *(arrow)*. The pregnancy progressed normally, and a normal infant was delivered at term. The double decidual sac sign is not always seen in normal pregnancies and may require a concerted effort to demonstrate it.

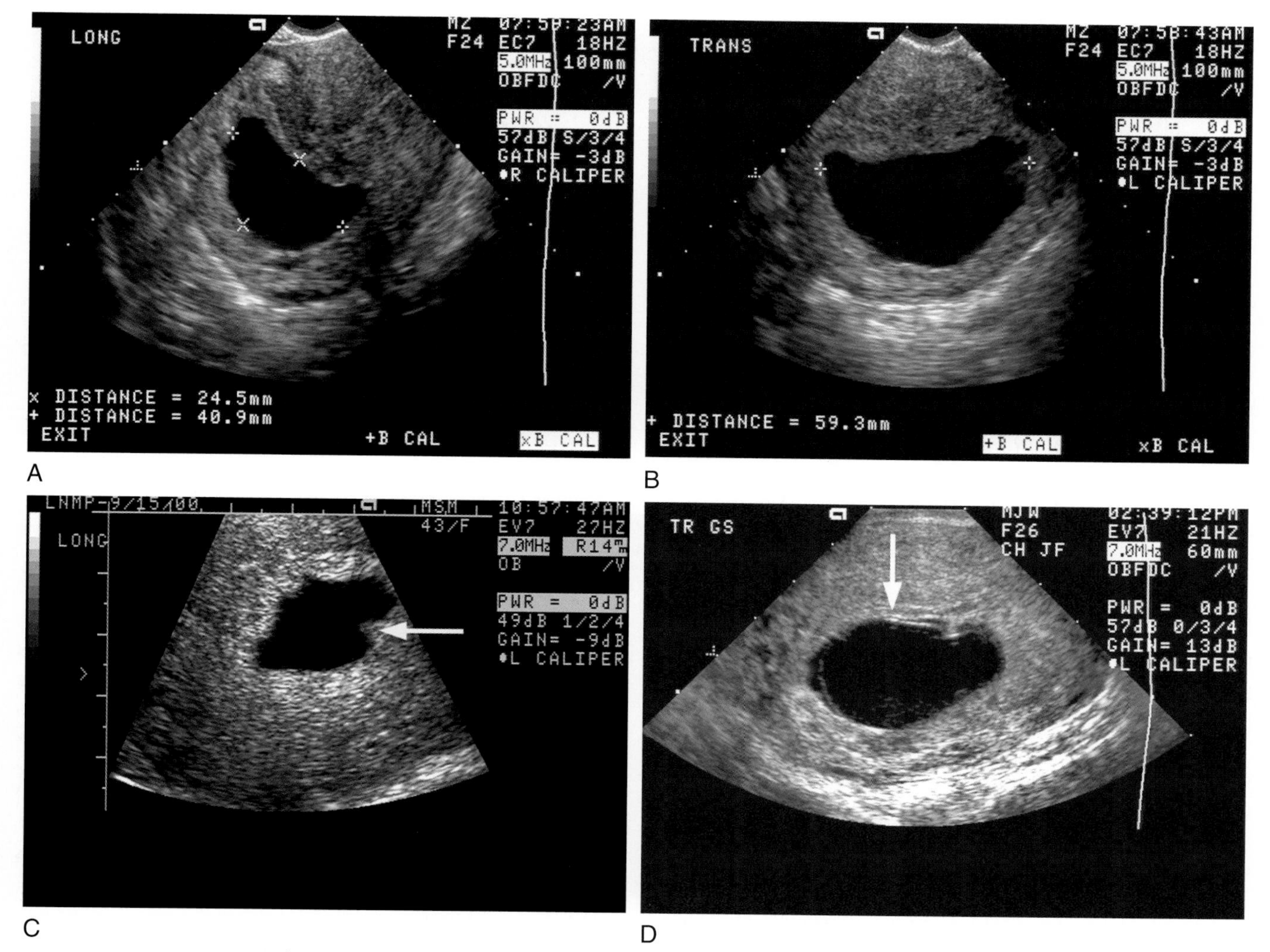

Figure 14-9 Gestational sac: findings in abnormal intrauterine pregnancies. **A** and **B,** Longitudinal (**A**) and axial (**B**) transvaginal scans reveal a mean gestational sac diameter of 41.6 mm (based on three orthogonal measurements of 24.5, 40.9, and 59.3 mm) with failure to depict an embryo or yolk sac. This is diagnostic of a failed intrauterine pregnancy. **C,** Distorted, irregular contour of gestational sac *(arrow).* Patient subsequently had a spontaneous miscarriage. **D,** A thin, weakly hyperechoic rim surrounds the gestational sac *(arrow)* of this nonliving intrauterine pregnancy.

the time the gestational sac has increased to greater than 25 mm, the embryo can be identified or the pregnancy should be considered abnormal (Fig. 14-9A and B). The yolk sac is usually seen by an MGSD of 8 mm at TV ultrasound, but failure to identify the yolk sac by this MGSD is not considered sufficient evidence that a pregnancy is abnormal. In addition, certain gestational sac characteristics suggest an abnormal pregnancy: distorted contour, thin decidual (<2 mm) hyperechoic rim, a weakly hyperechoic rim, and a low gestational sac position (see Fig. 14-9C and D; see also Fig. 14-5B). When in doubt as to whether a pregnancy is abnormal, it is recommended that the pregnancy be given the benefit of the doubt and a follow-up ultrasound should be suggested.

POTENTIAL UTERINE SPACES OR COLLECTIONS

In the early pregnancy, intrauterine findings other than a normal gestational sac can sometimes be seen: fluid within the endometrial canal, a normal chorioamniotic separation, a "vanishing twin," an implantation bleed, and a necrotic fibroid. The endometrial canal is a potential space, apposed but patent throughout the first trimester, surrounded by the hyperechoic decidual reaction (see Fig. 14-7). Any fluid, usually blood, can cause the endometrial canal to distend and can outline the free unembedded margin of the gestational sac. A variety of terms, including subchorionic hematoma, implantation

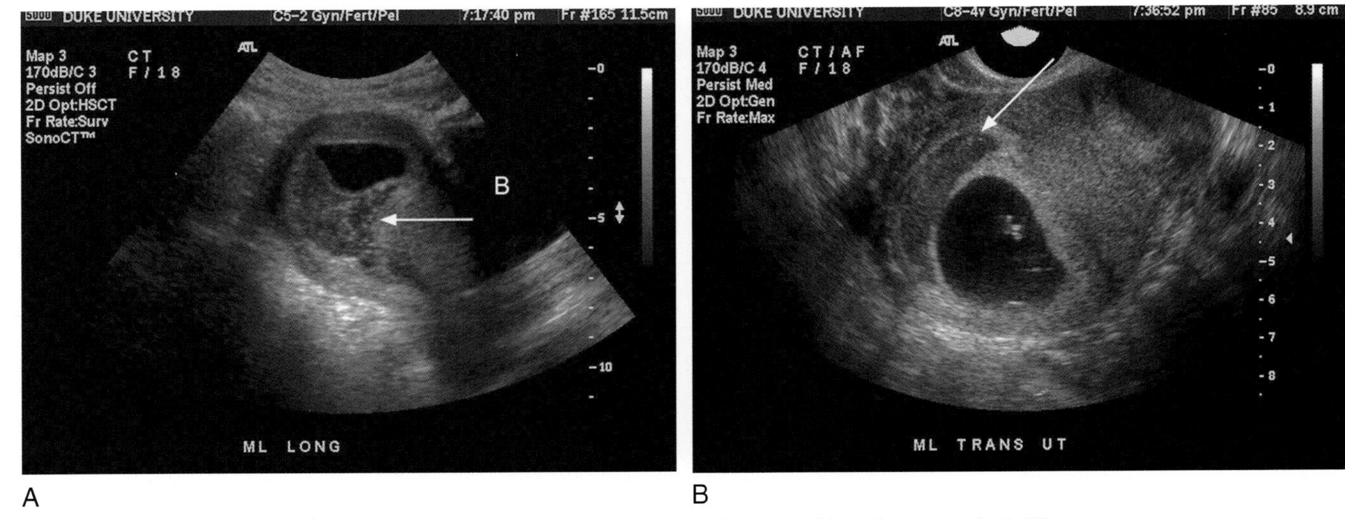

Figure 14-10 Subchorionic hematoma. Transabdominal (**A**) and transvaginal (**B**) scans performed for vaginal bleeding in an 8-week pregnancy show a hypoechoic collection of blood *(arrow)* adjacent to the gestational sac. The blood distends the endometrial cavity and outlines the outer surface of the chorionic sac. B, urinary bladder.

bleed, perigestational hematoma, and intrauterine hematoma, have been used to describe a collection of blood in this region (Fig. 14-10).

The gestational sac can also be called the chorionic sac because the chorion lines the inner surface of the hyperechoic rim. Within this sac, the embryo develops within a smaller amniotic sac. Ultimately, the amnion expands to the chorion and the two fuse, as late as at 16 weeks. These two spaces can be likened to a balloon within a balloon, the smaller inner balloon the amniotic sac and the larger outer balloon the chorionic sac (Fig. 14-11). The normal amnion is a thin membrane (<1 mm). Some observers believe that the amnion is abnormal if it is unusually thick or "lumpy" or if the amniotic sac is unusually large or both. More work is needed to more fully evaluate these findings, although the observations appear correct. The secondary yolk sac develops within the chorionic space on a stalk and subsequently detaches from the embryo (see Fig. 14-11).

The "vanishing twin," an implantation bleed, and a necrotic fibroid can cause problems in interpretation. The "vanishing twin" is an abnormal anechoic space, previously the second twin, now appearing next to but separate from the normal gestational sac (see Fig. 21-7).

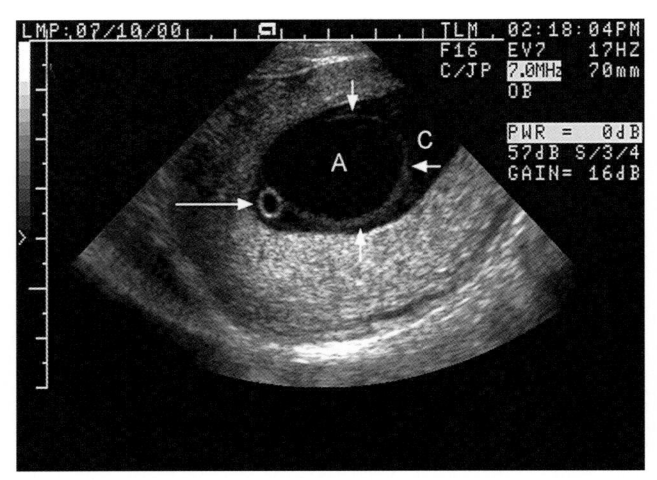

Figure 14-11 Amniotic and chorionic sacs. Transvaginal ultrasound of a normal 6-week pregnancy shows the amniotic sac (A) within the chorionic sac (C). The yolk sac *(long arrow)* is located immediately outside the amnion, within the chorionic sac. The embryo was seen in a different scan plane, in the amniotic sac, adjacent to the yolk sac. *Short arrows*, amnion.

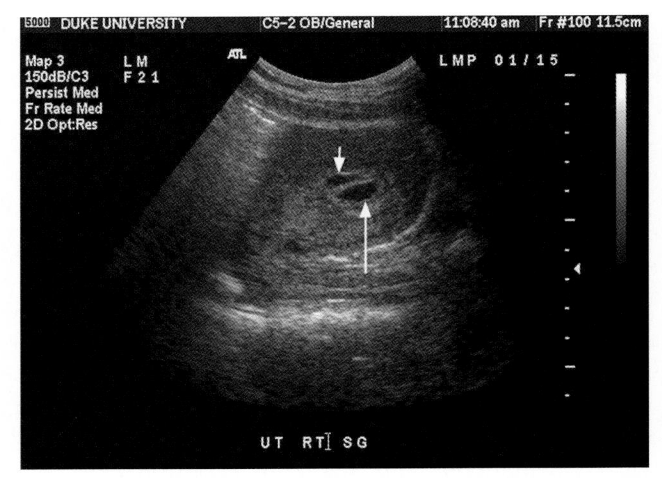

Figure 14-12 Implantation hemorrhage. Transabdominal sagittal scan of an early intrauterine pregnancy shows a small hypoechoic collection of blood *(short arrow)* immediately adjacent to the gestational sac *(long arrow)*. The collection of blood is caused by bleeding at the site of chorionic attachment and has also been termed a *subchorionic hematoma.*

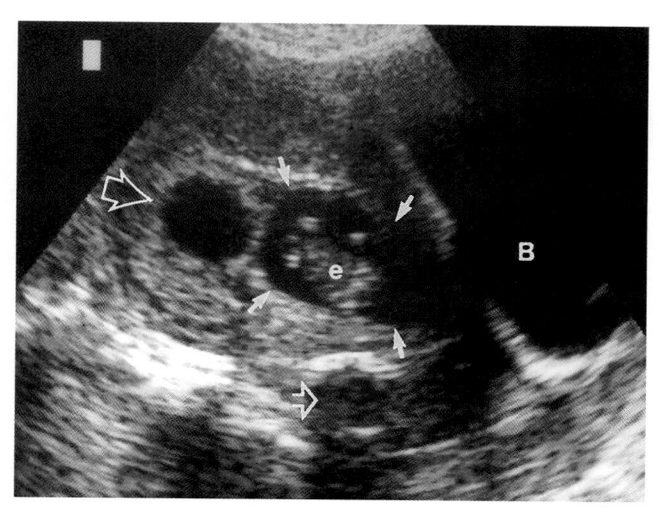

Figure 14-13 First-trimester pregnancy with a necrotic fibroid. This transabdominal sagittal image of an 8-week pregnancy shows a well-defined gestational sac *(arrows)* in the lower part of the uterus with a normal embryo (e). More superiorly a fibroid *(open large arrow)* is seen as a solid mass with a hypoechoic center that exhibits no distal acoustic enhancement. This mass is responsible for causing the unusually low gestational sac position. A second smaller fibroid with a hyperechoic rim of calcification *(small open arrow)* is seen posterior to the gestational sac. B, urinary bladder.

Unlike the normal sac, its contour is often distorted, ovoid or curvilinear, and without an embryo. A definitive diagnosis can only be made if an earlier examination had shown a twin pregnancy or if the βhCG levels were above that for a normal singleton pregnancy. It is called "vanishing" because this sac will almost always resolve by the second trimester. An implantation bleed is bleeding within the uterus where the chorionic insertions attach into the endometrium (Fig. 14-12). It has been given many names, including subchorionic hematoma, perigestational hematoma, and intrauterine hematoma. Bleeding can assume any degree of echogenicity, ranging from anechoic to hyperechoic, and is similar in concept to an abruptio placentae seen later in pregnancy. However, unlike an abruption, these implantation bleeds are often only incidental findings and, when small, of little clinical concern. Once detected, however, they should be followed to rule out propagation. Infrequently, a necrotic fibroid may resemble a twin gestational sac and can even enlarge as the pregnancy progresses (Fig. 14-13). Fibroids are discussed later in this chapter.

TRANSVAGINAL SCANNING IN EARLY PREGNANCY

TV scanning has had a significant impact on the evaluation of early pregnancies. After the probe is sterilized and placed into a latex sheath (usually a condom), it is inserted approximately halfway into the vagina. It does not routinely touch the cervix unless intentionally inserted farther. Its use is therefore not contraindicated in the first trimester, even in problem pregnancies. Although a careful TV examination can be performed without undue concern, the obstetrician should be notified before the start of the examination if there is doubt about its appropriateness or if the patient expresses undue concern. After its use, the probe should again be appropriately sterilized.

TV sonography is a valuable and accepted technique for three primary reasons. The study is performed with an empty or near-empty bladder, and any inconvenience from the use of a probe outweighs the discomfort of a distended urinary bladder. The TV study uses a high-frequency short-focused transducer, which is capable of achieving better detail to a depth of approximately 8 to 10 cm. Landmarks can be evaluated in different projections, including the coronal plane.

The TV technique, however, has pitfalls. Because the probe is intracavitary (within the vagina), its positioning is limited. A long-axis view of the uterus is sometimes the only consistently definable landmark. Any structure or mass that is more than 8 to 10 cm from the transducer face either cannot be identified or its full extent cannot be appreciated. Depending on the probe, the ultrasound beam may be angled anteriorly as it exits the TV probe. Although this angulation is useful for the long-axis examination of an anteverted uterus, a retroverted uterus may be imaged incompletely. It may be necessary to turn the transducer 180 degrees (then reverse the image on the ultrasound machine) so that posterior areas can be defined more clearly. Similarly, the probe may have to be turned 180 degrees when evaluating the adnexal regions so that both sides are identified fully. Transducer angulation cannot be appreciated so the examiner must keep this limitation in mind when full visualization is not achieved.

VALUE OF TRANSVAGINAL VS. TRANSABDOMINAL STUDIES IN INTRAUTERINE PREGNANCIES

In a few very early IUPs, between 4 to 5 weeks, an additional sign within the gestational sac, the double-bleb sign, can sometimes be seen. A very early gestational sac, when detected, can often only be evaluated by the TV approach. By scanning the margins of the gestational sac (the chorionic sac), two cystic structures can sometimes be identified: the smaller amniotic sac (closer to the wall) and the larger secondary yolk sac (farther away) before its stalk elongates (Fig. 14-14). Between the two, the prochordal plate of the developing embryo can be seen as a 2- to 4-mm linear hyperechoic

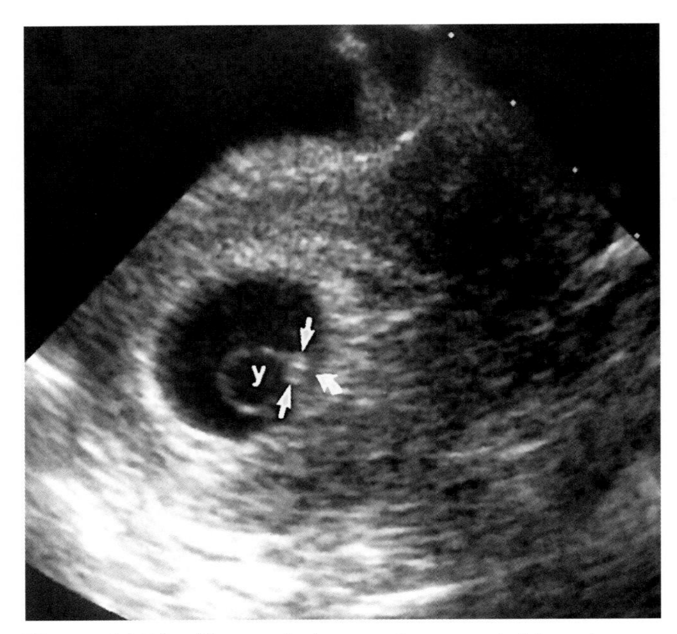

Figure 14-14 Transvaginal scan of a normal 4.5-week pregnancy shows a well-defined gestational (chorionic) sac with a hyperechoic rim. Along one of its walls is a combination of three findings, termed the *double-bleb sign,* and these consist of two cystic spaces, the larger the secondary yolk sac (y) and the smaller *(curved arrow)* amniotic sac, with a small 3-mm hyperechoic prochordal plate *(arrows)* of the developing embryo in between. Heart motion could already be identified.

disc, occasionally even with detectable heart motion. This double-bleb sign is only rarely detected. When it is, its position serves as a reminder that the initial development of the embryo takes place along the gestational sac wall.

The primary or primitive yolk sac develops and resolves early in the pregnancy (by 2 weeks of implantation) and is not detected by ultrasound. The secondary yolk sac then develops, and it can be imaged as early as 4.5 weeks as a 0.4-mm cystic structure. The secondary yolk sac exhibits slight curvilinear growth, increasing in average diameter to 4 mm by 10 weeks; after 11 weeks it begins to involute (Fig. 14-15A and B). As stated earlier, it can be identified about half a week before the normal embryo is seen. In one study, the embryo was seen transvaginally at an MGSD of 16 mm whereas the yolk sac was identified earlier at 8 mm. An upper limit of normal has been established at 5 to 6 mm in diameter. A yolk sac that is too large or is calcified is considered a poor prognostic sign (see Fig. 14-15C and D).

The identification of the yolk sac within the gestational sac is a valuable sign that an IUP is developing. It would also rule out that the gestational sac could instead be a pseudogestational sac of an ectopic pregnancy. However, the literature is mixed about the overall diagnostic value of identifying a yolk sac because in a normal pregnancy within less than 1 week the embryo will be seen. Conversely, whereas some of the literature states that failure to see the yolk sac at its expected time before identifying an embryo is a poor prognostic sign, this is not always the case. It is therefore believed that the determination of a normal or abnormal pregnancy should await identification of the embryo and its cardiac motion, although the prior identification of the yolk sac is an encouraging initial sign.

Comparison studies of the TA and TV techniques have shown the value of TV scanning when the TA study is suboptimal. It is particularly helpful in large women in whom the distance from the anterior abdominal wall to the uterus is more than 10 cm (Fig. 14-16). The TV approach commonly sees the gestational sac, yolk sac, and embryo at least half a week earlier.

The TV study has also been shown to be superior in the early detection of heart motion by more than half a week. Transabdominally, heart motion is detected in all embryos with a CRL larger than 9 mm (6.9 weeks). Transvaginally, heart motion is detected in all normal embryos larger than 5 mm (6.2 weeks). In most cases it can be detected even earlier.

Despite the earlier detection of first-trimester parameters by the TV approach, the TA examination should not be abandoned. Instead, it should be performed first. If it shows a normal intrauterine embryo with normal heart motion, a TV study is not required. If there are uncertain findings for a definitive normal IUP, TV imaging should be performed to identify a gestational sac, to look for an embryo when only a gestational sac is detected, or to identify heart motion when an embryo without heart motion is seen.

In the early pregnancy, at approximately 5 weeks from the LMP, heart motion can be identified even before the heart is fully formed. Its rate is commonly more than 100 beats per minute. By 8 weeks, and from then until near term, the rate averages 140 beats per minute, with a range of 120 to 180 beats per minute. A slow heart rate of less than 90 beats per minute at 5 weeks and less than 120 beats per minute from 8 weeks should be closely observed because a number of these pregnancies are lost. Faster heart rates are rare and not shown to be of pathologic significance in the first trimester.

Because there is a known background of 20% to 25% spontaneous loss rate in the first trimester, does the early detection of cardiac activity imply a "safe" ongoing pregnancy? A study by Levi and coworkers of embryos less than 5 mm (<6.2 weeks) revealed that even when cardiac activity was detected there was still a 24% miscarriage rate. When vaginal bleeding was present, spontaneous loss increased to 33%. Therefore, although it may be tempting to say that an embryo less than 5 mm with heart motion is "normal" and that it will progress normally to term, this determination should await embryos that exceeds at least 10 mm (>7.1 weeks).

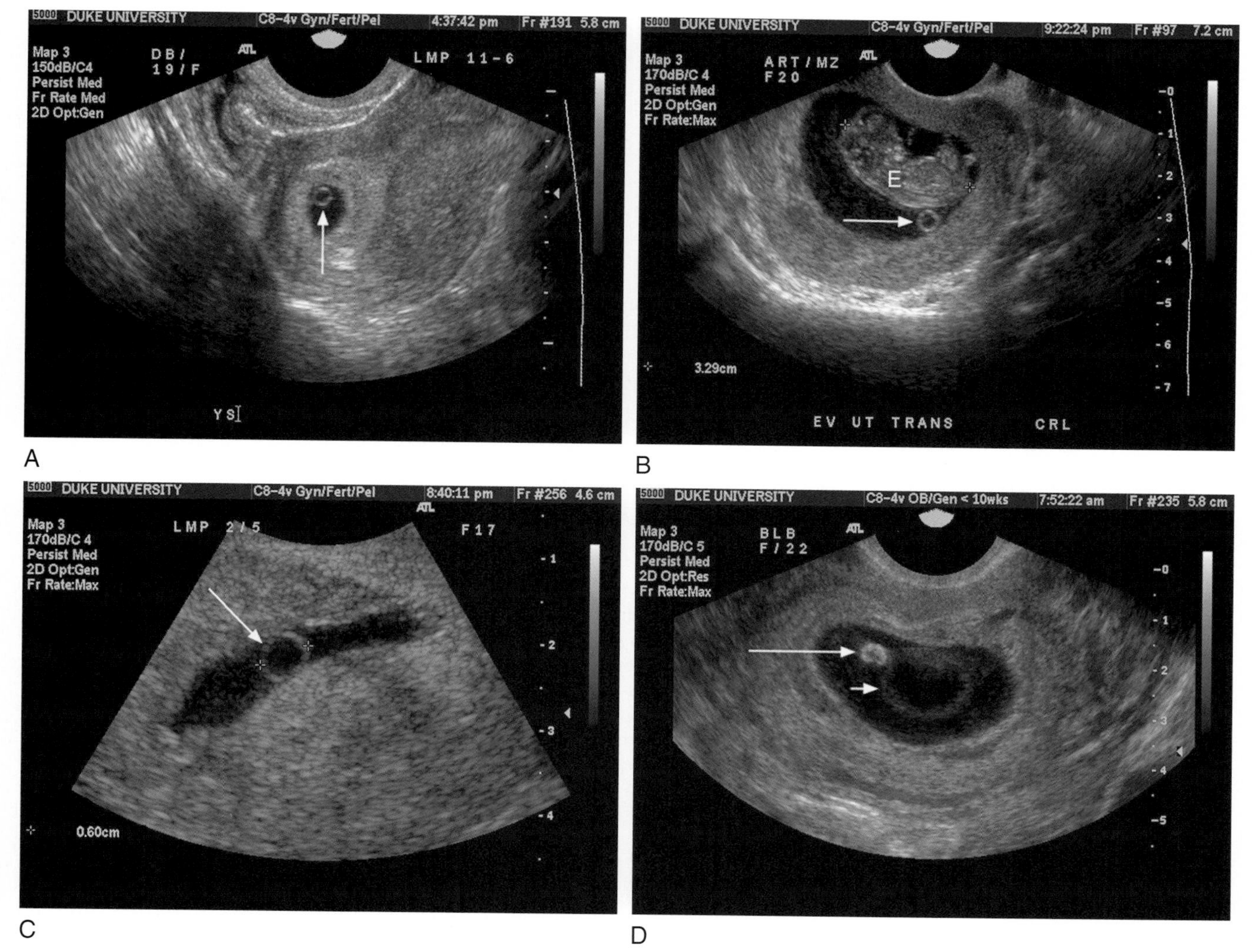

Figure 14-15 Examples of normal and abnormal yolk sacs. **A,** Endovaginal scan of normal yolk sac *(arrow)* in a 6-week pregnancy. **B,** Endovaginal scan of 10.2-week pregnancy shows normal yolk sac *(arrow)* posterior to embryo (E). **C,** Enlarged yolk sac *(arrow)* measuring 6 mm. This is considered a poor prognostic finding, although some pregnancies with enlarged yolk sacs have normal outcomes. The pregnancy in this example subsequently was shown to be nonviable. **D,** Calcified yolk sac *(long arrow)* in a nonviable pregnancy. *Short arrow,* amnion.

There is still a smaller 1% to 2% loss rate that continues into the early second trimester. Conversely, some of the initial embryos smaller than 5 mm had no initially detectable cardiac activity but progressed normally to term. The presence or absence of heart motion in the small, less than 5-mm embryo should therefore be used cautiously in predicting the outcome of that pregnancy.

Comparison of the TV ultrasound findings and quantitative serum βhCG levels in early pregnancy has been studied. A variety of different assays have been used to quantitate βhCG levels. Currently, the 3rd International Reference Preparation (World Health Organization ([WHO] [3rd IRP WHO]) is most commonly employed. Using this standard, TV ultrasound has been found to identify the gestational sac in most normal pregnancies when the βhCG exceeded 1800 to 2000 IU/L (<5 weeks), although it is frequently seen earlier, by 1000 IU/L. This level of 1800 to 2000 IU/L has been termed by some the discriminatory zone because theoretically it discriminates normal pregnancies from abnormal and ectopic pregnancies. That is, if the gestational sac is not seen at a βhCG level above the discriminatory zone, a normal IUP is unlikely, thereby raising the likelihood of an ectopic pregnancy. However, as an isolated finding, a single βhCG above the discriminatory zone is not sufficient evidence of an ectopic or abnormal pregnancy: occasionally, the gestational sac will not be seen by this βhCG level in a normal pregnancy.

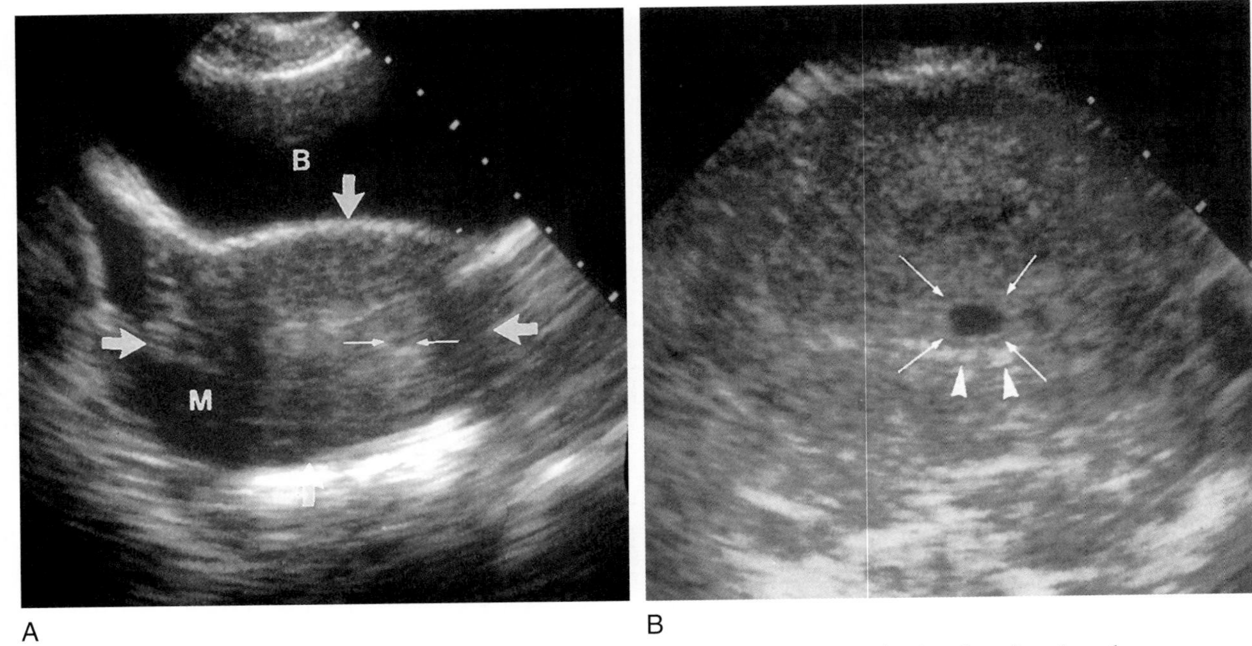

Figure 14-16 Comparison of the transabdominal and transvaginal studies in a less than 5-week pregnancy. **A,** The transabdominal transaxial view shows a large bulky uterus *(arrows)*, with at least one hypoechoic solid mass, a fibroid (M), identified on the right posterolaterally. A possible early intrauterine pregnancy is noted on the left *(small arrows)*. B, urinary bladder. **B,** The intradecidual sign. This transvaginal study in the transaxial-coronal projection shows a well-defined gestational sac with a normal hyperechoic rim *(small arrows)* embedded within the endometrium, adjacent to the apposed hyperechoic endometrial canal *(arrowheads)*. An embryo could not yet be identified.

FETAL ANATOMY

The ability of TA ultrasound to detect normal early embryonic anatomic characteristics is limited. Only the embryo, its heart motion, and the differentiation of the head from the body can be consistently identified by 8 to 9 weeks. With TV imaging, embryonic anatomic detail is seen earlier and more completely. The embryonic head can be distinguished from the body by 7 to 8 weeks, with additional intraembryonic structures possible by 8 weeks: the forebrain (prosencephalon) and hindbrain (rhombencephalon) as two hypoechoic intracranial structures (Fig. 14-17). On occasion, the heart chambers and great vessels can be seen by 9 to 10 weeks. Between 9 to 12 weeks, a hyperechoic fullness can be identified at the base of the umbilical cord, owing to normal midgut herniation (Fig. 14-18A and B). Although an excess of soft tissue in this region has been correctly diagnosed as an omphalocele, this diagnosis must be made cautiously because the soft tissue protrusion is normal when less than 7 mm in diameter or less than one third the diameter of the adjacent abdomen. By 11 weeks the spine and extremities can be routinely identified.

Because of the increased detection capabilities of TV imaging, one might consider performing a TV study to search for fetal anomalies during all late first-trimester pregnancies. Although this is tempting, at present there has been no study that has shown an increased ability to diagnose anomalies compared with second-trimester ultrasound.

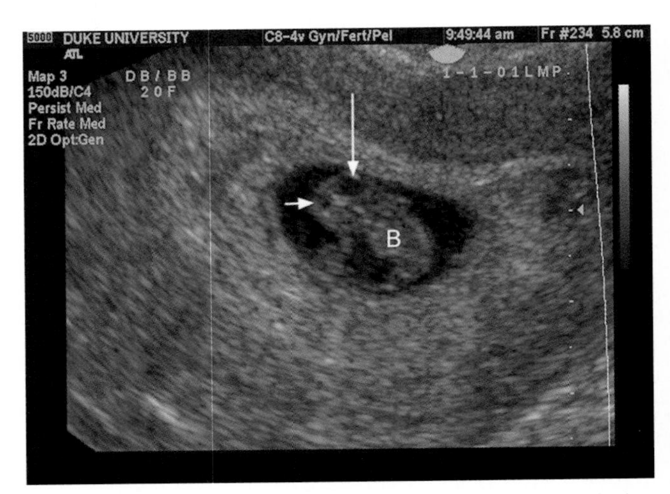

Figure 14-17 Embryonic head at 8 weeks. Endovaginal ultrasound image of normal embryo shows two well-defined hypoechoic structures in the head, corresponding to the normal forebrain *(short arrow)* and hindbrain *(long arrow)*. The hindbrain, or rhombencephalon, is the more prominent structure and should not be mistaken for a pathologic process. B, body of embryo.

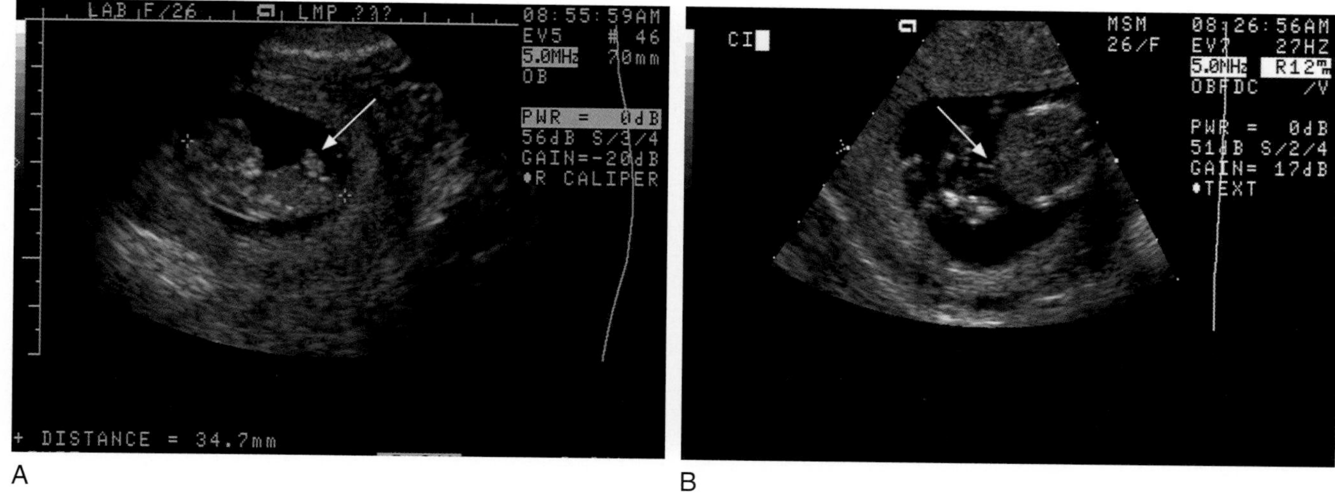

Figure 14-18 Normal midgut herniation into umbilical cord. **A,** Sagittal endovaginal scan of embryo at 10 weeks 3 days shows a focal bulge in contour of abdomen *(arrow)* due to physiologic herniation of bowel into base of umbilical cord. This normal process should not be mistaken for an omphalocele or gastroschisis. The bowel returns to the abdominal cavity by 12 weeks in the normal fetus. **B,** Axial image of abdomen obtained during follow-up ultrasound at 14 weeks shows normal abdominal cord insertion *(arrow),* with no evidence of an abdominal wall defect.

MULTIPLE GESTATIONS

The TA evaluation of multiple gestations in early pregnancy often suffices to determine the number of gestations, cardiac activity of each gestation, and the type of separating membranes. The type of separating membrane is of particular importance, and this can be best determined in the first trimester. Unless the TA study detects a thick, hyperechoic, at least 2-mm membrane, diagnostic for a dichorionic-diamniotic twinning, a TV study should be performed to determine if a membrane is present and its thickness. In addition, if there is any doubt about the number of gestational sacs or spaces within the uterus, a TV study can be of value. This is discussed more completely in Chapter 21.

HYDATIDIFORM MOLES AND FIBROIDS

When the pregnancy test is positive and ultrasound detects multiple hypoechoic and hyperechoic spaces filling and distending the endometrial canal (without a well-defined embryo), a hydatidiform mole is likely (Fig. 14-19). The classic clinical triad for a hydatidiform mole is an enlarged uterus, hyperemesis, and a markedly elevated βhCG level (often > 100,000 mIU/L). However, these findings may not be present or may be due to other causes. In particular, the βhCG levels can be greater than 100,000 mIU/L in normal gestation at more than 8 weeks or in a late first- or early second-trimester spontaneous incomplete abortion. Both a hydatidiform mole and a miscarriage can further overlap because both could present after vaginal expulsion of material.

The differential diagnosis should also include a partial mole with hydropic placental changes, which is of lower malignant potential than a complete mole. A partial mole (Fig. 14-20A) is usually triploid and can result in significant maternal complications. Additionally, hydropic change in retained placenta after spontaneous miscarriage should be considered but is not a form of gestational trophoblastic disease and will have much lower βhCG levels (see Fig. 14-20B). Of these, a hydatidiform mole is of the most concern because of its malignant possibility in a small percentage of cases, invasion into the wall (choradenoma destruens), or metastatic choriocarcinoma. In up to 50% of cases, hydatidiform moles are accompanied by multiseptated cystic ovarian masses (theca lutein cysts), which are bilateral (see Fig. 14-20C). Theca lutein cysts typically do not occur in patients with hydropic change in the placenta but no gestational trophoblastic disease because βhCG levels are relatively low in these patients.

Fibroids may markedly distort and enlarge the uterus. In the pregnant uterus, fibroids often continue to enlarge and can become necrotic as the pregnancy progresses (Fig. 14-21). If a fibroid contains an unusual necrotic cystic space, it can potentially be misdiagnosed as a second sac (see Fig. 14-13). More commonly,

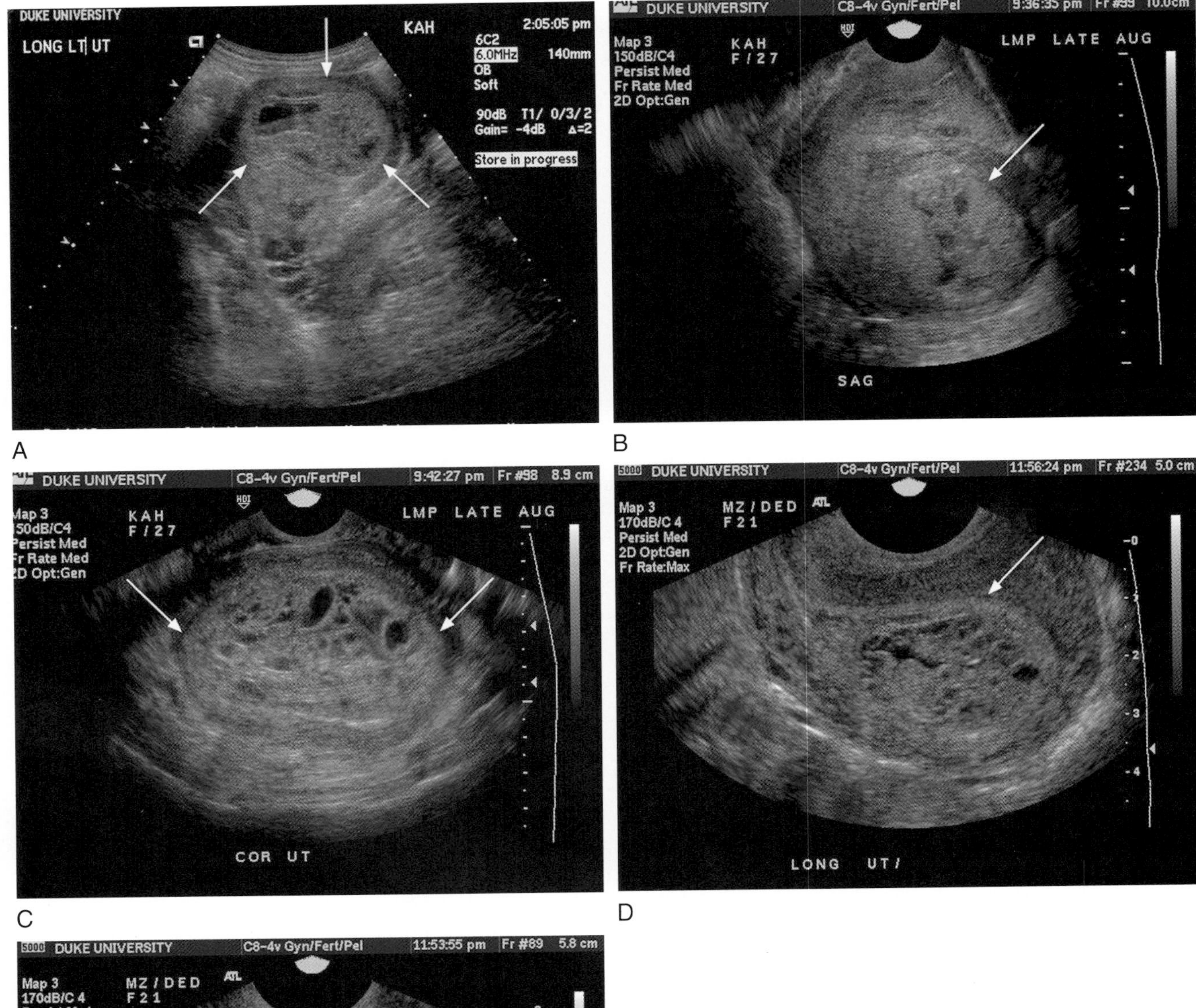

Figure 14-19 Hydatidiform mole: Examples in three patients. **A,** Transabdominal sagittal scan shows echogenic mass *(arrows)* with cystic spaces expanding the uterine cavity. **B** and **C,** Longitudinal (**B**) and axial (**C**) transvaginal scans of a different patient with a complete mole show echogenic mass *(arrows)* with innumerable well-defined cystic spaces in uterine cavity. **D** and **E,** Longitudinal (**D**) and axial (**E**) transvaginal scans of a third patient with a complete mole show echogenic mass *(arrows)* with small cystic spaces in uterine cavity.

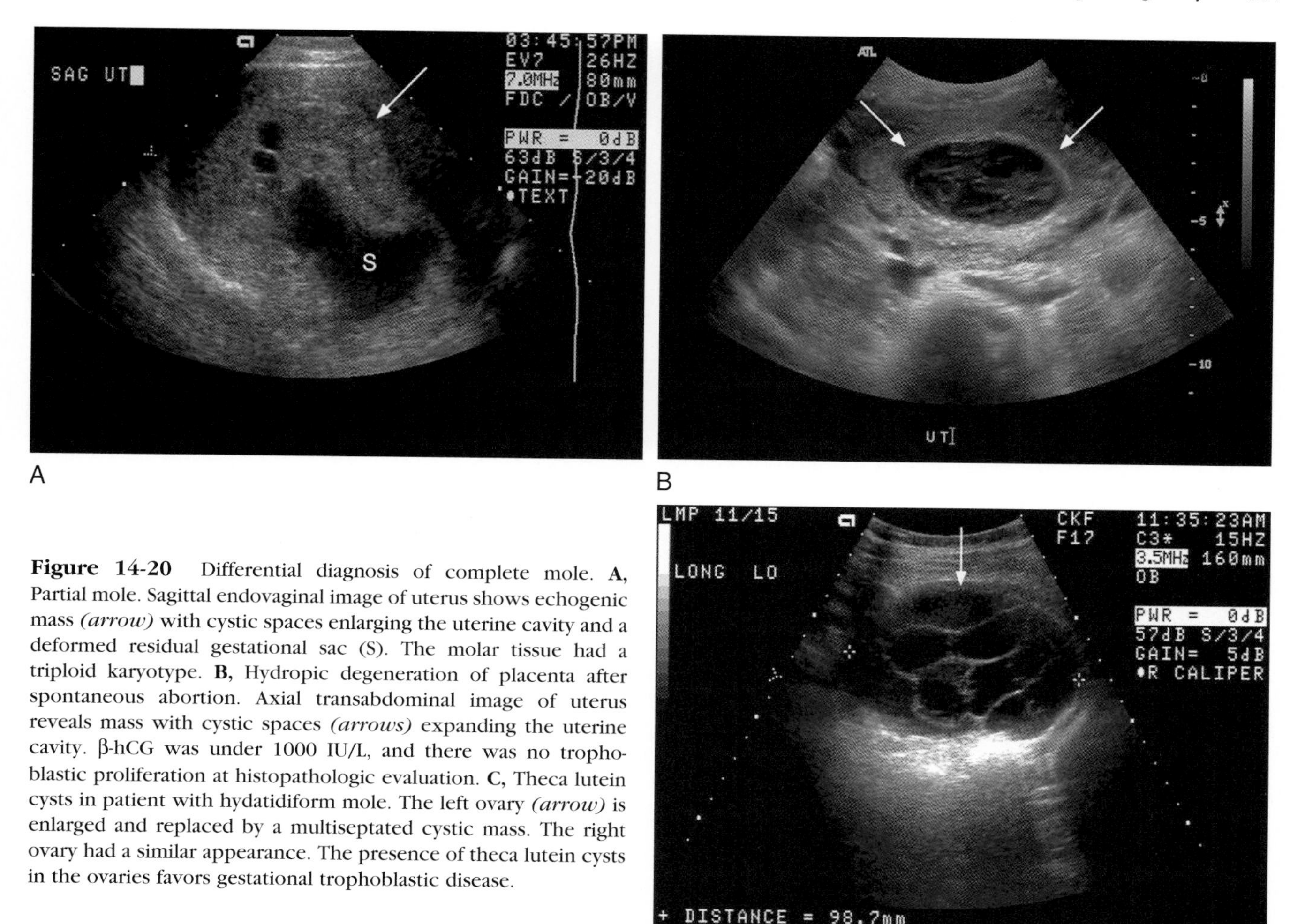

Figure 14-20 Differential diagnosis of complete mole. **A,** Partial mole. Sagittal endovaginal image of uterus shows echogenic mass *(arrow)* with cystic spaces enlarging the uterine cavity and a deformed residual gestational sac (S). The molar tissue had a triploid karyotype. **B,** Hydropic degeneration of placenta after spontaneous abortion. Axial transabdominal image of uterus reveals mass with cystic spaces *(arrows)* expanding the uterine cavity. β-hCG was under 1000 IU/L, and there was no trophoblastic proliferation at histopathologic evaluation. **C,** Theca lutein cysts in patient with hydatidiform mole. The left ovary *(arrow)* is enlarged and replaced by a multiseptated cystic mass. The right ovary had a similar appearance. The presence of theca lutein cysts in the ovaries favors gestational trophoblastic disease.

multiple fibroids can greatly distort the position of the gestational sac (see Fig. 14-5C), sometimes making it appear to be in an extrauterine (ectopic) position. If extensive, fibroids can precipitate a miscarriage.

ECTOPIC PREGNANCY

Overview

The incidence of ectopic pregnancies has risen considerably in the United States from 17,800 in 1970 to more than 70,000 in 1986. It now appears to be leveling off. Fortunately, the death rate, mostly related to blood loss, has substantially decreased during this same interval, from 3.6 per 1000 ectopic pregnancies in 1970 to 0.5 per 1000 in 1986. The improved death rate is most likely due to better earlier detection and increased awareness.

The typical presenting signs and symptoms of an ectopic pregnancy are not always present. For example, only 60% of women have a history of a missed menstrual period. The classic triad of irregular menstrual bleeding, abdominal or pelvic pain, and a palpated tender adnexal mass are not always present. However, certain groups of women are at particularly high risk: (1) those with abnormal fallopian tubes as the result of previous infection (salpingitis), developmental defects, or prior tubal reconstructive surgery; (2) those with normal fallopian tubes but who have an intrauterine device, who are taking ovulation-inducing agents, who are treated by in vitro fertilization–embryo transfer, or who suffer from delayed ovulation or tubal transport; and (3) those who have a history of prior ectopic pregnancies.

The βhCG serum and urine blood tests are very sensitive, without false-positive diagnoses and only false-negative results when levels are too low to be detected. Combining a positive test, first qualitative to know that a pregnancy exists and then quantitative to expect certain intrauterine findings in a normal IUP, with the use of ultrasound, in particular the TV method, has allowed

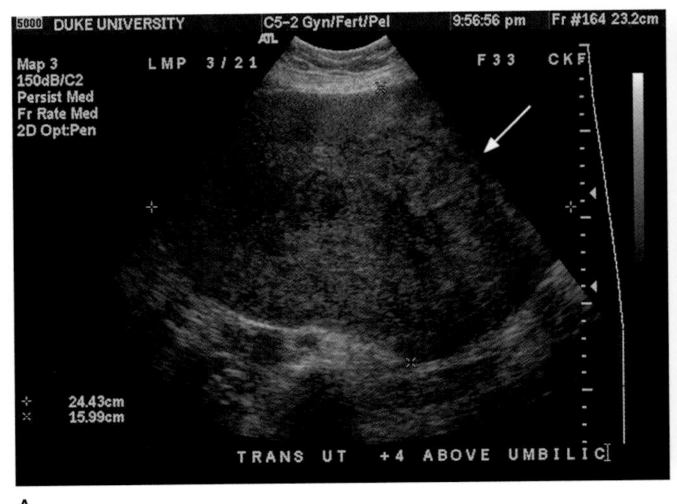

A

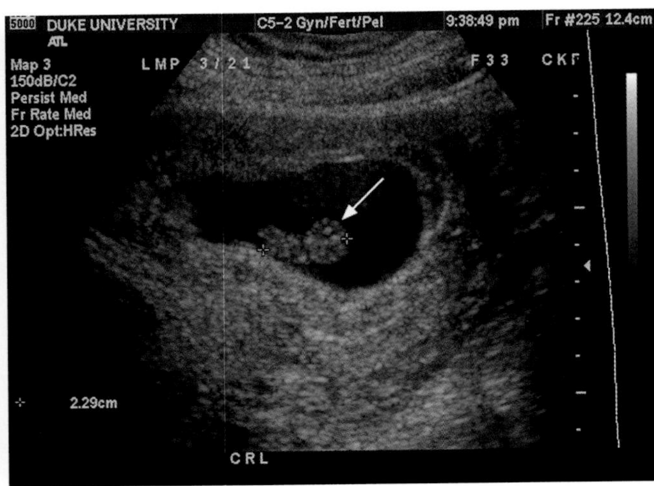

B

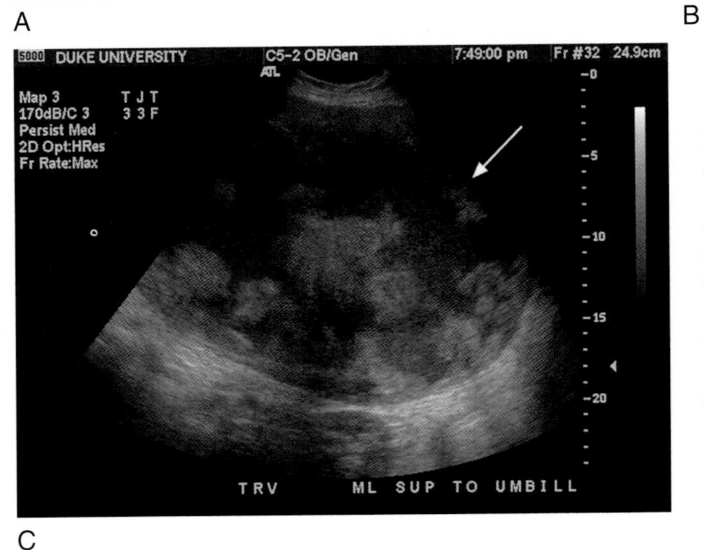

C

Figure 14-21 Interval infarction and necrosis of a large fibroid during pregnancy. **A,** Large solid fibroid *(arrow)* was seen at 09 weeks of pregnancy. **B,** Image obtained the same day as **A.** A live intrauterine embryo *(arrow)* was also identified. **C,** Scan performed 7 weeks later at 16 weeks of pregnancy shows dramatic interval change in appearance of the previously seen fibroid *(arrow)* which has become complex in appearance owing to infarction and necrosis. The fibroid is now predominantly cystic but contains numerous irregular solid regions. The patient had presented with acute onset of abdominal pain. Fetus was alive and had grown appropriately.

much more precise and earlier diagnoses. By using the 3rd IRP, a quantitative serum βhCG level of more than 2000 IU/L is expected to yield a detectable intrauterine gestational sac in most, but not all, normal pregnancies. In early pregnancy, βhCG levels normally double every 2 days, slightly faster at 1.4 days before 7 weeks.

The differential diagnosis of a positive pregnancy test includes a normal early IUP, an abnormal IUP, and an ectopic pregnancy. As a general rule, a woman with a positive pregnancy test and without a definite IUP is at higher risk for an ectopic pregnancy, although in some instances an early normal IUP (before the gestational sac can be detected) or a miscarriage (spontaneous complete or incomplete abortion) is still possible.

Because of the expected doubling time of the βhCG, not only a single value but also serial quantitative βhCG values can be used in conjunction with the ultrasound examination. If there is a normal doubling time, a normal IUP is highly likely. If the change is either too slow or slightly declining, an abnormal IUP or an ectopic pregnancy is likely. Rapidly decreasing βhCG levels are more typical of a miscarriage.

Definitions

An ectopic pregnancy is defined as the implantation of a fertilized ovum outside the endometrial lining of the uterus. Ectopic pregnancies are most common in the fallopian tubes (95% to 97%), usually in the ampullary or isthmus regions. However, ectopic implantation can occur anywhere in the tube, from the fimbriated end (near the ovary) to the interstitial portion (as it enters the muscular wall of the uterus). Adnexal ectopic pregnancies sometimes occur outside the fallopian tube: within the ovary (<1%), between the leaves of the broad ligament, and on the intraperitoneal surface (approximately 0.03%), which is the rarest form and called an abdominal pregnancy. It is often not possible to predict the exact anatomic position of an adnexal pregnancy before surgery.

Within the uterus, ectopic pregnancies can occur in the cornual region of the uterine fundus (<5%) and in the cervix (0.1%). Cervical pregnancies are very low uterine implantations located in the endocervical canal at or below the internal cervical os. They have increased in frequency because of the use of in vitro fertilization, with transcervical insertion of fertilized ova.

Because of the small diameter of most of the fallopian tube, particularly the isthmus and interstitial regions, these ectopic pregnancies frequently cause early signs and symptoms. Conversely, pregnancies outside the tube, particularly in the expandable muscular cornual portion of the uterus and in the abdomen, may present later, even in the second and rarely in the third trimester. The onset of symptoms can vary in women with cervical pregnancies.

A heterotopic pregnancy is a concomitant intrauterine and extrauterine pregnancy. Although it was initially rare, with an incidence of 1 in 30,000 births, it has become more common: it now occurs in 1 in 7,000 pregnancies with an approximate range of 1 in 4,000 to 1 in 8,000 pregnancies. This increased incidence appears to be related to the presence of partially damaged fallopian tubes (a causative factor for many ectopic pregnancies), often owing to partially treated pelvic inflammatory disease and to the use of assisted reproductive techniques.

Intrauterine Findings

When the pregnancy test is positive, the primary value of ultrasound is its ability to identify an IUP, specifically the intrauterine identification of an embryo with heart motion. When only a gestational sac is identified, the signs of a normal-appearing sac are often reassuring that an early IUP is present. Certainly the identification of a yolk sac within the gestational sac confirms that the pregnancy is intrauterine. An intrauterine collection surrounded by a hyperechoic rim but without the DDS sign could represent an early intrauterine gestational sac, an abnormal gestational sac, or a pseudogestational sac of an ectopic pregnancy (see Fig. 14-8).

The uterine cavity can exhibit a range of appearances in patients with an ectopic pregnancy. The endometrial stripe can appear normal, thickened, or heterogeneous or contain decidual cysts or a pseudogestational sac (Fig. 14-22). A pseudogestational sac is a collection of either fluid or hyperechoic material (termed a *decidual cast*) that distends the endometrial canal. It occurs in approximately 5% of ectopic pregnancies. A pseudogestational sac cannot always be differentiated from an IUP. Occasionally, it can even contain a small collection of debris or cells that simulates the appearance of an early embryo (see Fig. 14-22G). However, an abnormal IUP sac is more likely round or oval, whereas a pseudogestational sac is more likely elongated because it conforms to the endometrial canal. Lastly, decidual cysts, simple cysts seen in the periphery of the hyperechoic endometrium (see Fig. 14-22H), in a woman with a positive pregnancy test and no IUP have been found to be associated with a higher risk for an ectopic pregnancy and have occasionally been the first sign that an ectopic pregnancy was present. A decidual cyst, however, can be difficult, if not impossible, to distinguish from an early intrauterine gestational sac.

On occasion, the hyperechoic material blends with the hyperechoic rim. It then looks like (and probably is) a thickened endometrium. If less than 8 mm in thickness (as stated earlier in this chapter), this hyperechoic endometrium is more likely related to an extrauterine pregnancy (averaging 6 mm), although an abnormal IUP (averaging 9 mm) cannot be excluded.

Some ectopic pregnancies may initially (and falsely) look like normal IUPs. The ectopic pregnancies within the cornual portion of the uterine fundus and within the cervix are both easily identified as pregnancies but may be difficult to appreciate as being ectopic in location. An interstitial (cornual) pregnancy refers to implantation of the ectopic gestation in the interstitial portion of the fallopian tube, that is, in the segment of tube that traverses the uterine wall. An interstitial ectopic pregnancy is eccentrically positioned within the most lateral portion of the uterine fundus (Fig. 14-23). A careful examination can often reveal the absence or marked thinning of myometrium surrounding a portion of the gestational sac. This can be apparent if the sac abuts on the distended urinary bladder. However, a thickened rim of trophoblastic tissue of more than 10 mm in an ectopic interstitial pregnancy may not be able to be differentiated from an eccentrically placed IUP surrounded by 10 mm of myometrium. This can be particularly difficult in a retroverted or retroflexed uterus, which is normally more globular, whereas a typical IUP is eccentrically placed, usually posterolateral and close to the uterine margin. Fibroids, too, can displace a normal IUP into a position that appears ectopic. In these cases, if no definitive diagnosis can be made, close clinical and sonographic follow-up may be necessary.

A suggestive sign of an interstitial pregnancy is the interstitial line sign. Ackerman and coworkers have found that the hyperechoic endometrial canal could be followed as a line into the uterine fundus. When an interstitial ectopic pregnancy is present, the line abuts on the midportion of the sac or mass rather than goes around it. They found this sign to be more sensitive than the eccentric placement of the gestational sac or myometrial thinning in predicting a cornual ectopic. Although an intriguing observation, the fundal portion of a retroverted or retroflexed uterus can be difficult to image and further work on its predictive value is needed.

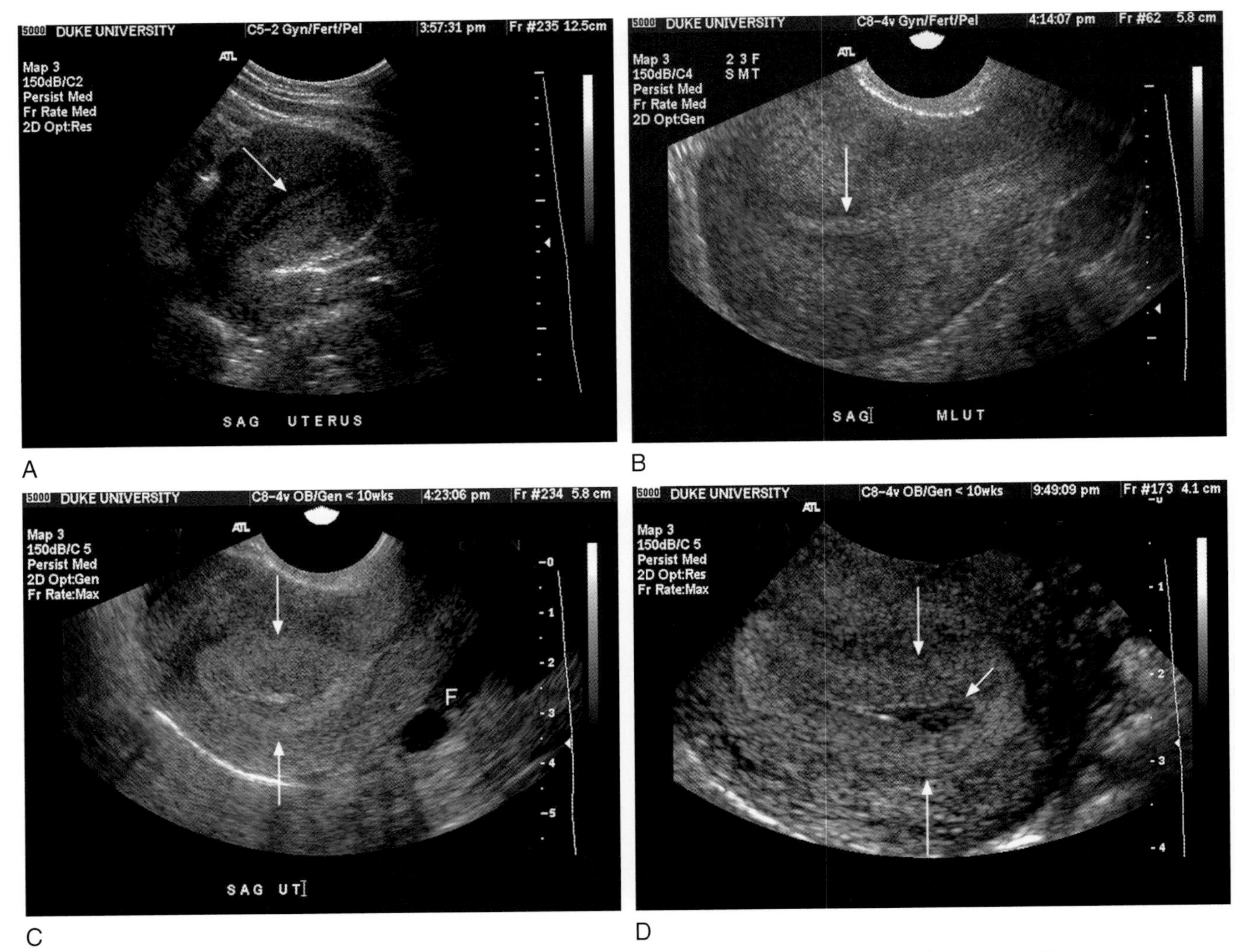

Figure 14-22 Range of appearances of uterine cavity: images of the uterus in eight patients with proven ectopic pregnancies. **A,** Normal thin endometrium *(arrow)* evident on transabdominal ultrasound evaluation. **B,** Normal thin endometrium *(arrow)* in a different patient at endovaginal ultrasound evaluation. **C,** Thick uterine stripe *(arrows)* at endovaginal ultrasound. Free fluid (F) is also seen in the cul-de-sac. **D,** Thick uterine stripe *(long arrows)* with a small amount of fluid *(short arrow)* on endovaginal ultrasound evaluation.

Continued

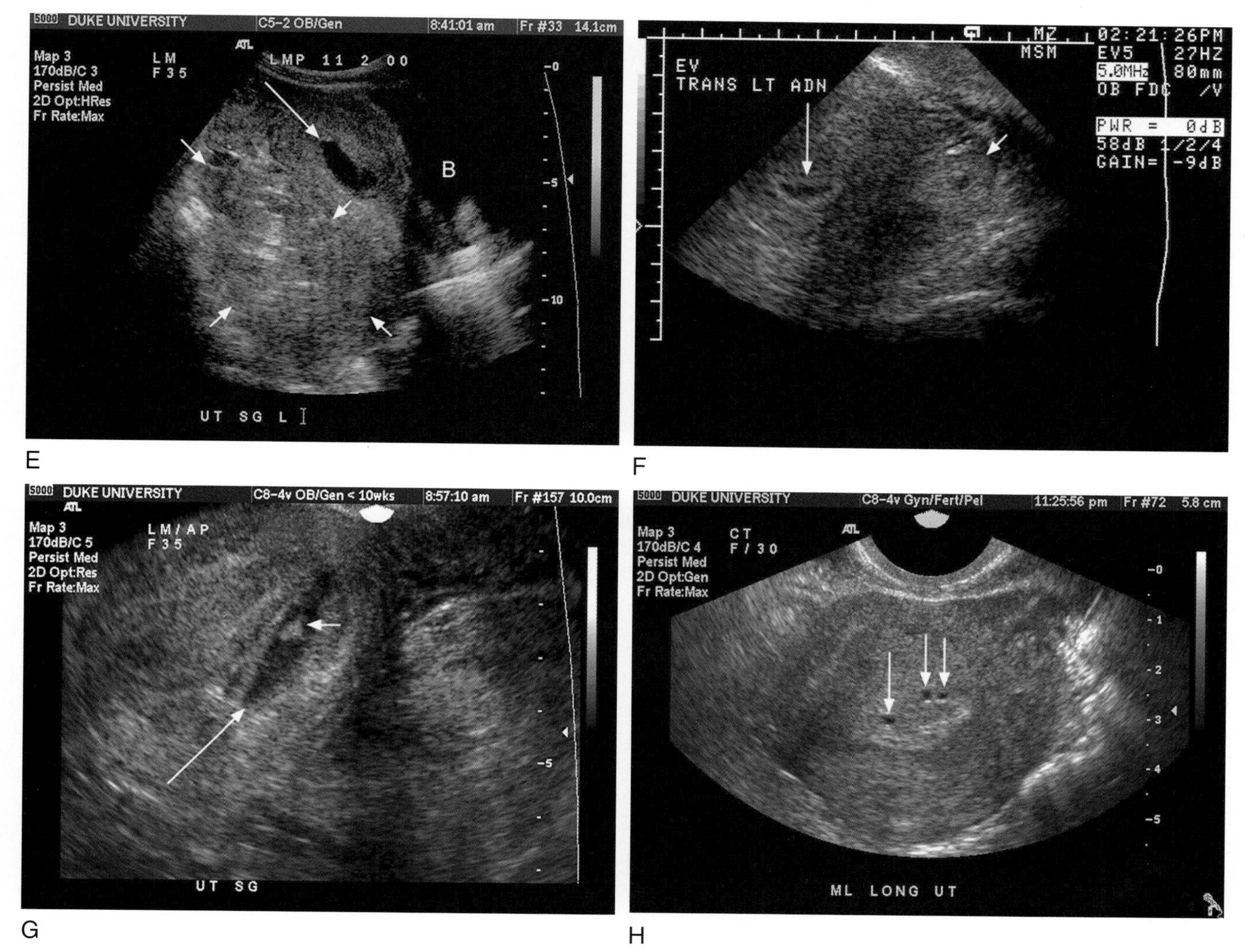

Figure 14-22, cont'd **E,** Large fluid collection *(long arrow)* in uterine cavity consistent with a pseudogestational sac at transabdominal ultrasound. A large pelvic hemoperitoneum *(short arrows)* is also seen posterior to the uterus. B, urinary bladder. **F,** Small fluid collection *(long arrow)* in uterine cavity consistent with a pseudogestational sac on axial transvaginal scan. The ectopic gestation *(short arrow)* is located to the left of the uterus. **G,** Moderate fluid collection consistent with a pseudogestational sac *(long arrow)* in uterine cavity on longitudinal endovaginal scan. Note the focal collection of echoes *(short arrow)* due to blood and debris in the pseudogestational sac. Although superficially this collection of echoes may resemble an embryo, it did not exhibit cardiac activity and was not associated with a yolk sac. It is important not to mistake a pseudogestational sac containing a focal collection of echoes for an early intrauterine gestational sac with an embryo. **H,** Three small decidual cysts *(arrows)* in endometrium on transvaginal scan. When only a single decidual cyst is seen it can be indistinguishable from a very early intrauterine gestational sac.

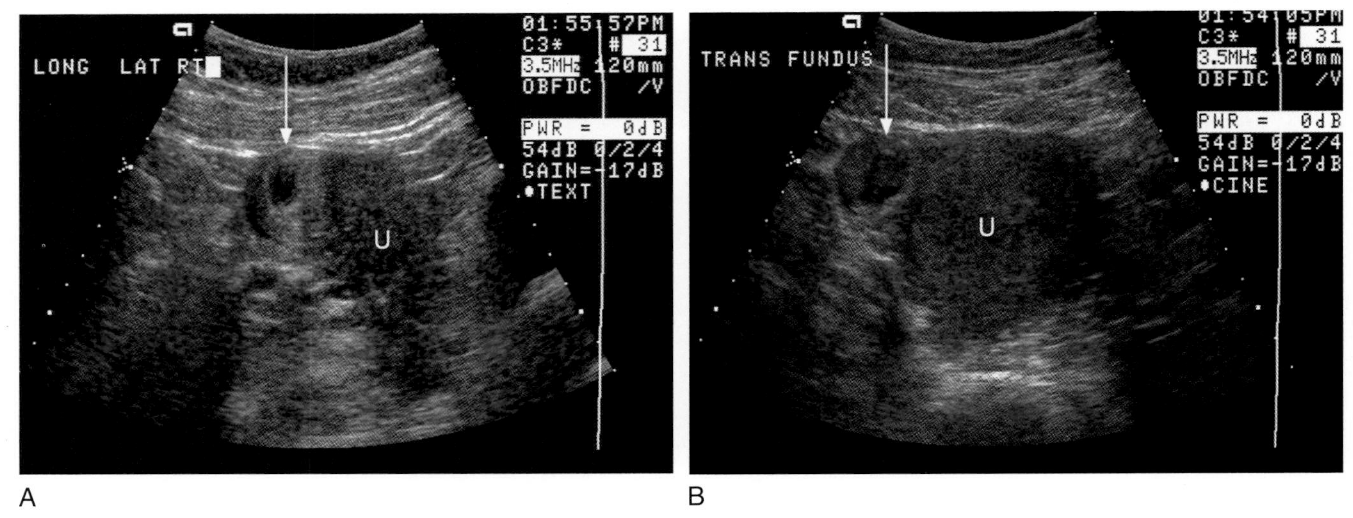

Figure 14-23 Interstitial (cornual) ectopic pregnancy. **A** and **B,** Transabdominal longitudinal image through right lateral surface of uterus (**A**) and axial image obtained high in uterine fundus (**B**) reveal the ectopic gestational sac *(arrow)* along the most superior, right lateral surface of the uterus (U). Note the marked thinning of the myometrium around the sac.

A cervical ectopic pregnancy needs to be differentiated from a low but normal IUP (see Fig. 14-5B) and from a spontaneous abortion in progress. Although in the first trimester the internal cervical os may be difficult to identify, insertion of the uterine arteries into the lateral margin of the uterus can define this region. A pregnancy below this insertion should be considered too low. Pregnancies (cervical and normal) are highly vascular; a miscarriage typically is not. The differentiation of a cervical ectopic pregnancy may therefore be possible with the use of color Doppler imaging, but further investigation is needed to further assess the specificity of this finding. Identification of a live embryo in a sac in the cervix favors a cervical ectopic pregnancy, whereas the presence of severe pain and cramping favors a spontaneous abortion in progress (Fig. 14-24).

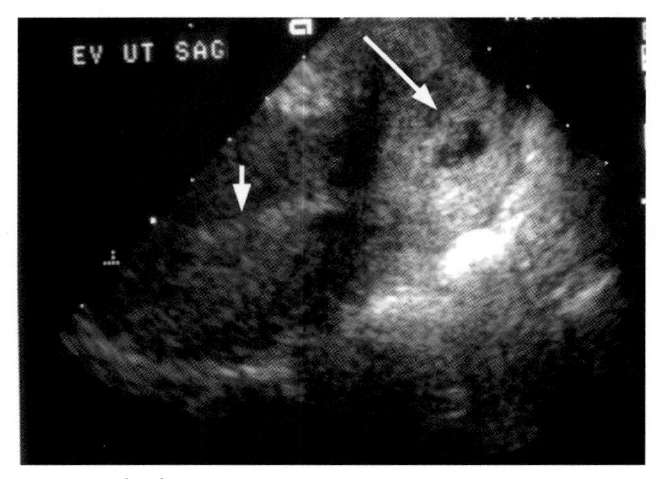

Figure 14-24 Spontaneous abortion in progress. Sagittal endovaginal scan of uterus shows a gestational sac *(long arrow)* in the cervix. The uterine stripe *(short arrow)* is normal with no evidence of a pregnancy in the body of the uterus. Patient was experiencing pain and cramping at the time of the study and miscarried shortly thereafter.

Extrauterine Findings

Most ectopic pregnancies are tubal. Although the examiner would expect extrauterine findings, in 10% to 20% of cases the ultrasound examination is either nonspecific or normal, even when a TV study is performed. Therefore, when the pregnancy test is positive, the only finding that rules out the presence of an ectopic pregnancy is the detection of an IUP, except in the rare instance of a heterotopic pregnancy. If an IUP is not detected by either TV or TA scanning, the likelihood of an ectopic pregnancy is therefore increased.

But when extrauterine findings are detected, the diagnosis of an ectopic pregnancy is usually definitive. TV scanning is often better at detecting subtle abnormalities than is TA scanning (Fig. 14-25). However, TA scanning is important for giving an initial overview of the pelvis and abdomen and should be performed even when the urinary bladder is empty (Fig. 14-26). If the TA study clearly identifies a live IUP and normal adnexa or if the TA study detects a live ectopic pregnancy, the study can usually be stopped. The TA study is also important to look for findings outside of the pelvis, in particular abdominal ascites (Fig. 14-27).

When the pregnancy test is positive and there is no evidence of an IUP, any adnexal finding other than an intraovarian cyst should be considered an ectopic

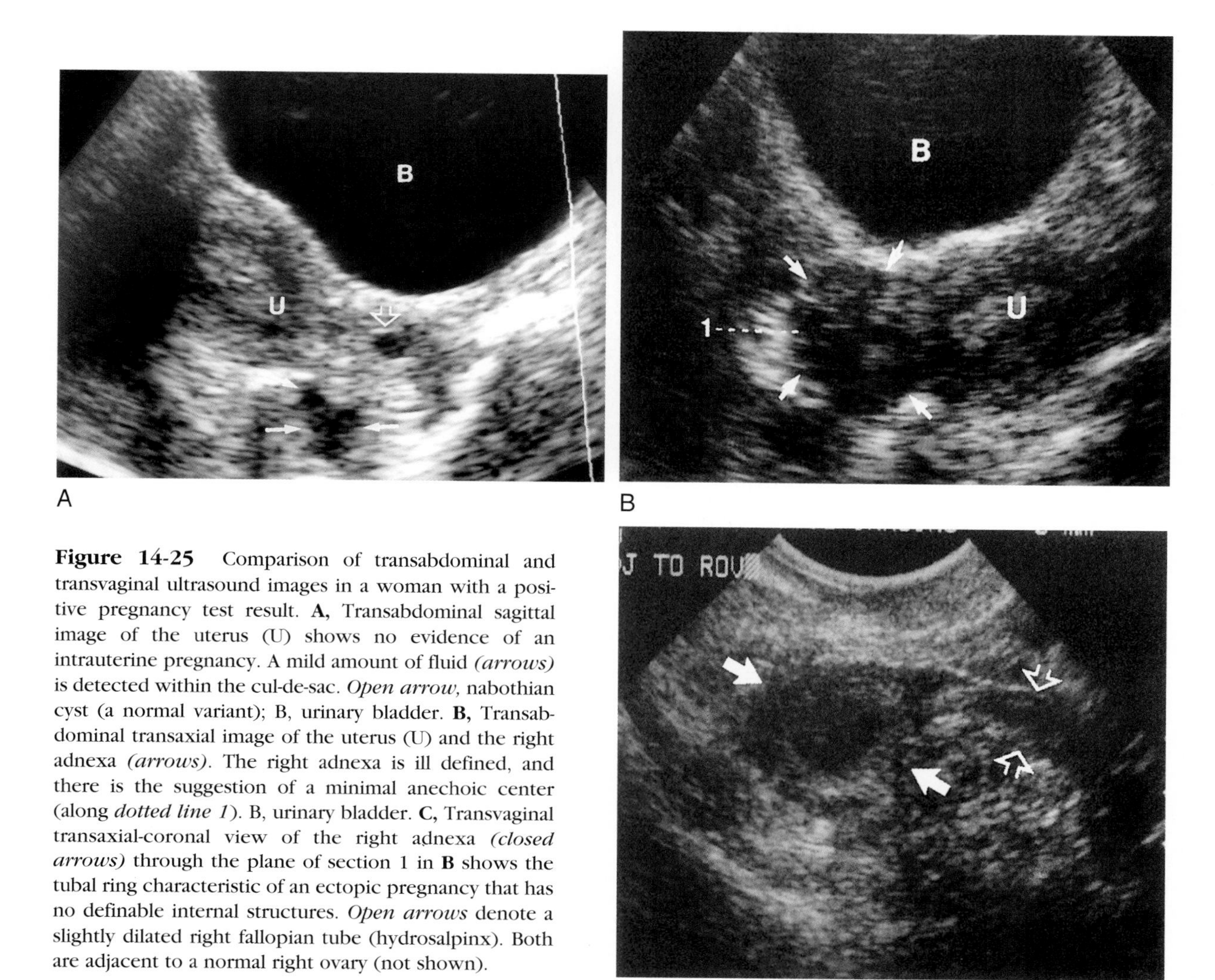

Figure 14-25 Comparison of transabdominal and transvaginal ultrasound images in a woman with a positive pregnancy test result. **A,** Transabdominal sagittal image of the uterus (U) shows no evidence of an intrauterine pregnancy. A mild amount of fluid *(arrows)* is detected within the cul-de-sac. *Open arrow,* nabothian cyst (a normal variant); B, urinary bladder. **B,** Transabdominal transaxial image of the uterus (U) and the right adnexa *(arrows)*. The right adnexa is ill defined, and there is the suggestion of a minimal anechoic center (along *dotted line 1*). B, urinary bladder. **C,** Transvaginal transaxial-coronal view of the right adnexa *(closed arrows)* through the plane of section 1 in **B** shows the tubal ring characteristic of an ectopic pregnancy that has no definable internal structures. *Open arrows* denote a slightly dilated right fallopian tube (hydrosalpinx). Both are adjacent to a normal right ovary (not shown).

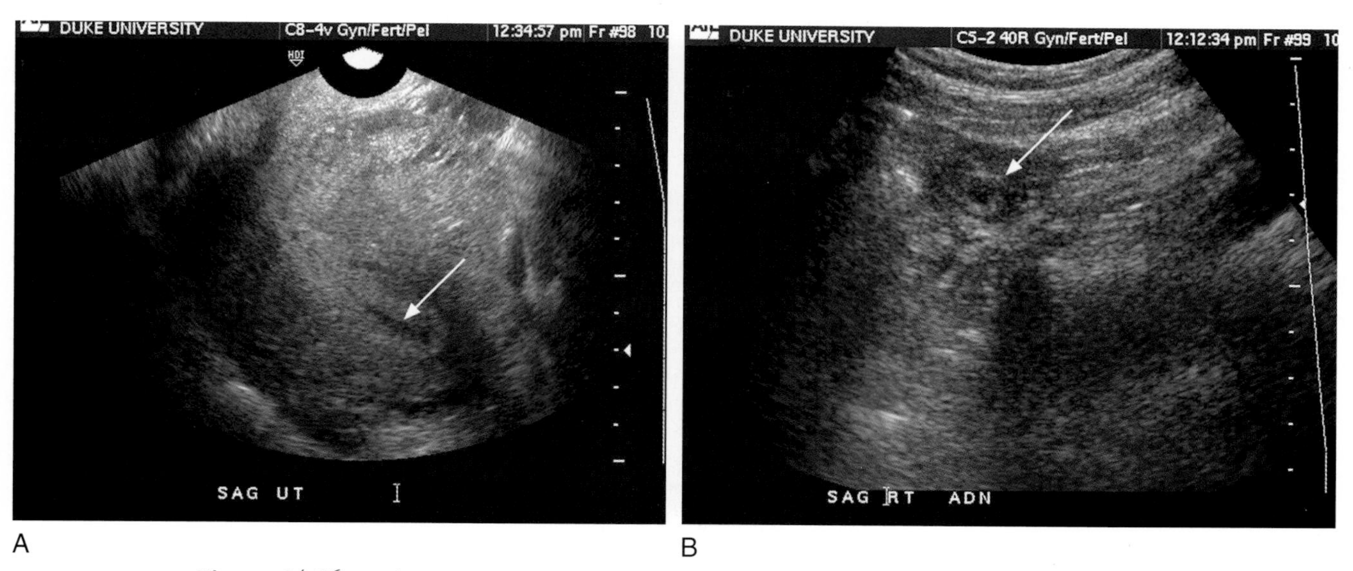

Figure 14-26 Value of transabdominal examination: ectopic pregnancy seen only at transabdominal ultrasound. **A,** Transvaginal image of uterus in sagittal plane shows a small amount of fluid in the endometrial cavity *(arrow)* but no intrauterine pregnancy. An ectopic gestation was not seen at transvaginal ultrasound evaluation. **B,** Transabdominal image obtained high in the pelvis with the urinary bladder empty shows an ectopic gestational sac *(arrow)*. The ectopic sac would have been missed if only transvaginal ultrasound analysis had been performed.

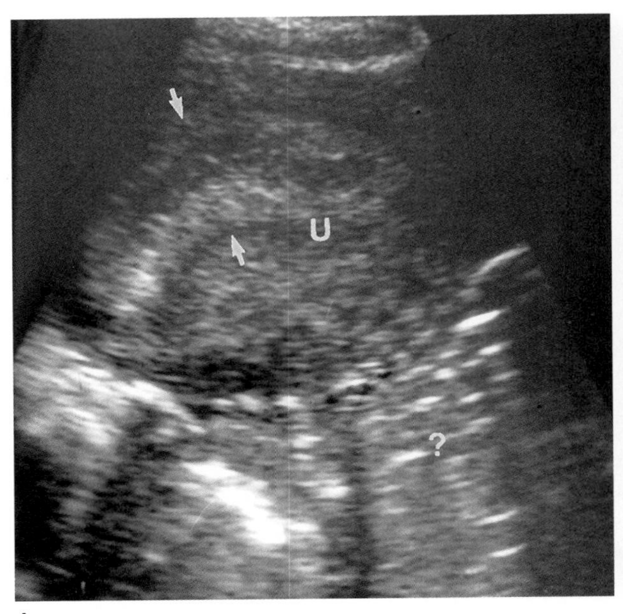

A

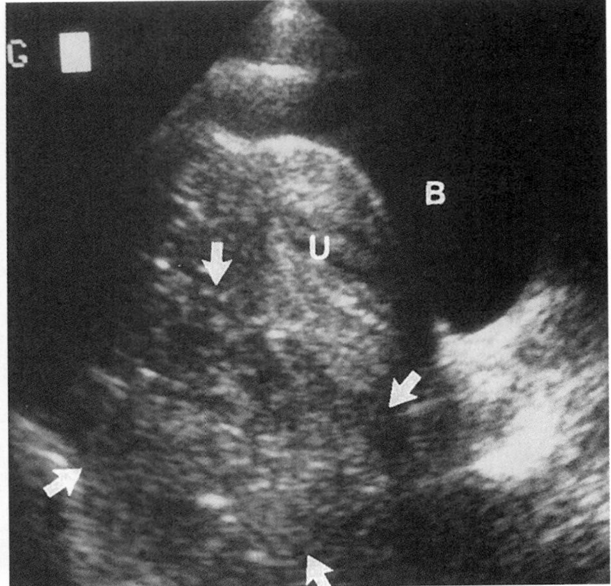

B

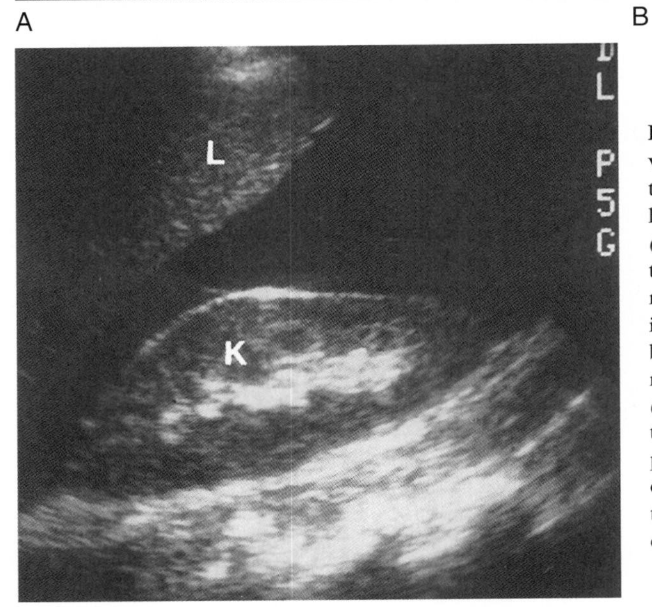

C

Figure 14-27 The value of the transabdominal study in a woman with a positive pregnancy test result. **A,** This initial transvaginal sagittal study of the uterus (U) shows a markedly hyperechoic, thickened decidual cast or endometrium *(arrows)*. No intrauterine pregnancy is detected. Posterior to the uterus is an ill-defined area (?) that was thought to be normal nonperistalsing bowel. **B,** Transabdominal midline image of the uterus (U), scanned through a distended urinary bladder (B), confirms the absence of an intrauterine pregnancy. The large hyperechoic area posterior to the uterus *(arrows)* is pushing the uterus anteriorly. It is trophoblastic tissue and hemorrhage stemming from a ruptured ectopic pregnancy. **C,** Transabdominal sagittal scan of the right upper quadrant shows anechoic fluid (hemoperitoneum) between the liver (L) and right kidney (K) secondary to the ruptured ectopic pregnancy.

Table 14-1 Diagnosis of Ectopic Pregnancies Based on Ultrasound Adnexal Findings*

Positive Ultrasound Findings	Predictive Value
Extrauterine embryo with positive heart motion	100%
Adnexal mass containing a yolk sac or nonliving embryo	100%
"Tubal" or "adnexal" ring surrounding a fluid collection	95%
Complex or solid adnexal mass (no embryo, yolk sac, or tubal ring)	92%

*All patients had a positive pregnancy test result and no evidence of an intrauterine pregnancy.

Adapted from Brown DL, Doubilet PM: Transvaginal sonography for diagnosing ectopic pregnancy: Positivity criteria and performance characteristics. J Ultrasound Med 13:259, 1994.

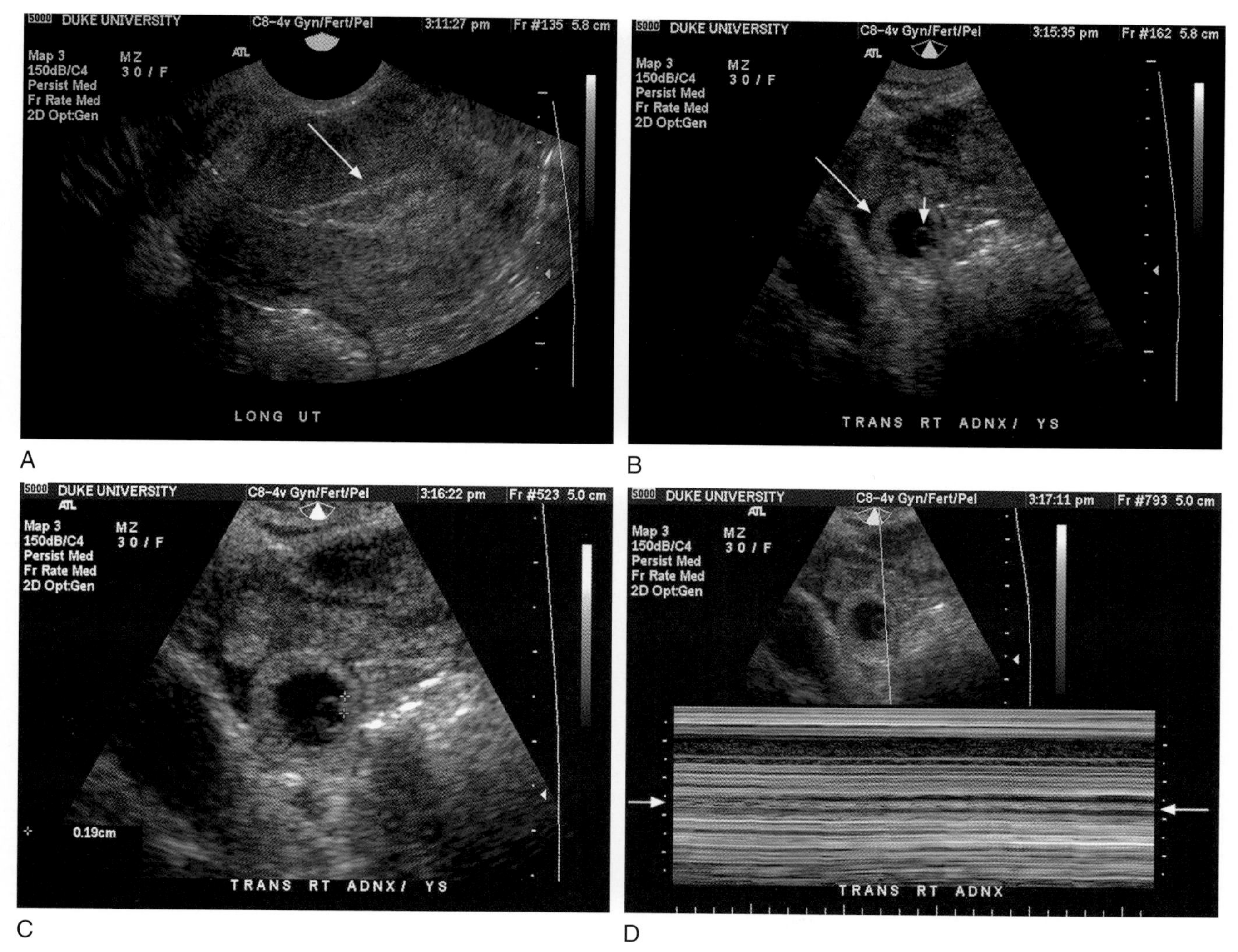

Figure 14-28 Live ectopic pregnancy at transvaginal ultrasound evaluation. **A,** Longitudinal scan of uterus reveals no evidence of an intrauterine pregnancy. *Arrow,* endometrial stripe. **B,** Axial image of right adnexa shows adnexal ring *(long arrow)* containing a yolk sac *(short arrow).* **C,** High resolution image of the adnexal ring in **B** shows a 1.9-mm embryo *(cursors)* adjacent to the yolk sac. **D,** M-mode tracing reveals the ectopic embryo has cardiac activity *(arrows).* Cardiac activity was also observed at real-time evaluation.

pregnancy until proven otherwise. The adnexal abnormalities can be divided into four categories (Table 14-1). A living embryo with heart motion in an extrauterine gestational sac can be detected in up to 15% of TA and in up to 20% to 30% of TV studies (Fig. 14-28). Its positive predictive value (PPV) is 100% in diagnosing an ectopic pregnancy. The PPV of an adnexal mass (not a well-defined gestational sac) with a positive pregnancy test containing either a yolk sac or nonliving embryo also approaches 100% (Fig. 14-29).

Less sensitive, but with PPVs of 92% and 95%, respectively, are the ultrasound findings of a tubal ring and an adnexal mass. The tubal ring (also called an adnexal ring, bagel sign, and donut sign) is a mass with a hyperechoic rim of trophoblastic tissue surrounding extrauterine fluid (Fig. 14-30). An adnexal mass can be complex or solid and of any shape from round to ovoid to irregular. If the ectopic pregnancy has ruptured, the mass can be very irregular because it conforms to the available space (Fig. 14-31).

An additional important finding in a woman with a suspected ectopic pregnancy is the detection of intraperitoneal fluid, particularly if it contains internal echoes (hemorrhage) (Fig. 14-32). A small amount or "sliver" of intraperitoneal fluid in the cul-de-sac can be seen in normal pregnancies (see Fig. 12-5). A larger amount of intraperitoneal fluid, especially if it extends into the flanks and upper abdomen, must be considered

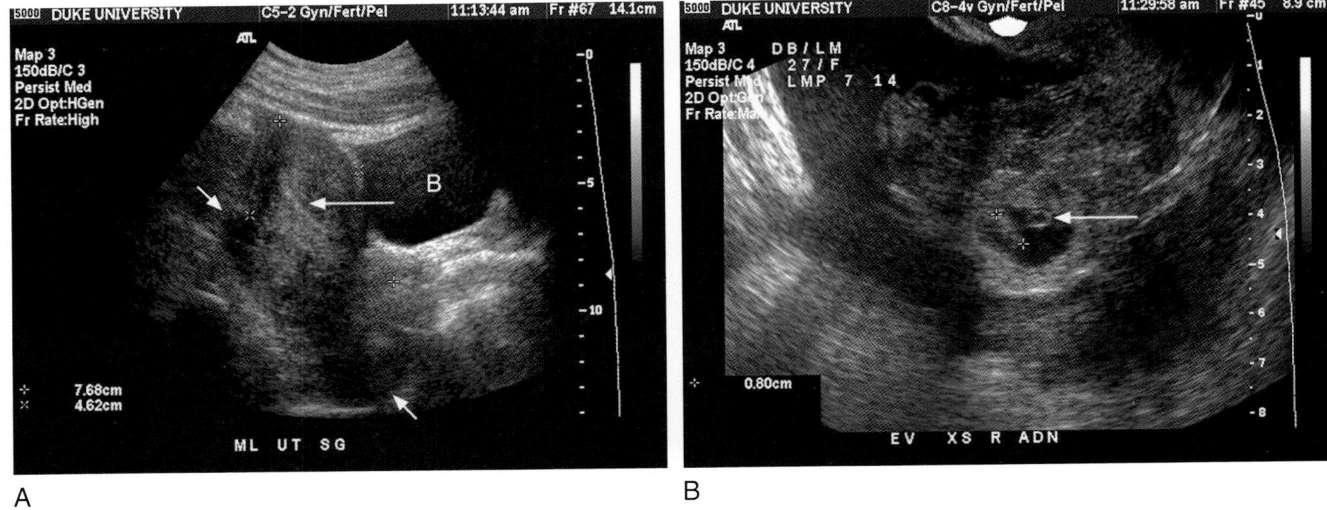

Figure 14-29 Ectopic pregnancy: diagnosis based on adnexal mass containing yolk sac and non-living embryo. **A,** Transabdominal ultrasound shows a normal uterine stripe *(long arrow)* with no evidence of intrauterine pregnancy. A large pelvic hemoperitoneum *(short arrows)* is also seen posterior to the uterus. B, urinary bladder. **B,** Transvaginal scan of right adnexal mass demonstrates a yolk sac *(arrow)* and an embryo *(cursors)*. Even though no cardiac activity was observed, this combination of findings is virtually diagnostic of ectopic pregnancy.

abnormal. Although there is no quantitative amount, if the volume of fluid is judged subjectively to be anything more than mild, the likelihood of an ectopic pregnancy is considerably increased when the pregnancy test is positive and no IUP is present.

A combination of these extrauterine findings further increases the likelihood of an ectopic pregnancy. A noncystic extraovarian adnexal mass with a moderate to large amount of amniotic fluid has been found to be highly specific for an ectopic pregnancy. Even if there is a normal IUP, if any of these adnexal findings are observed, the probability of a concomitant extrauterine pregnancy is greatly increased (Fig. 14-33).

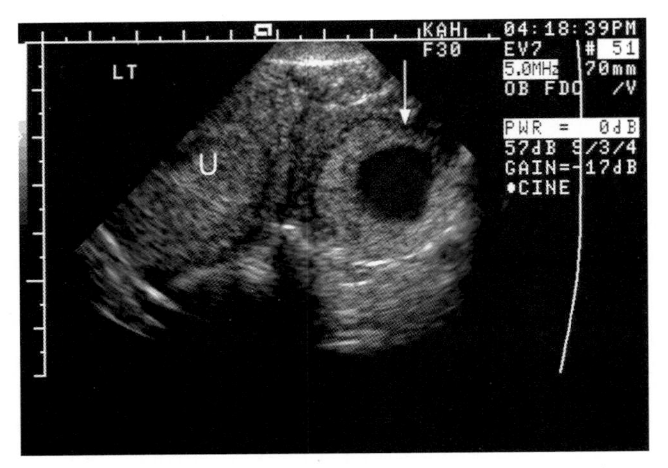

Figure 14-30 Tubal (adnexal) ring sign. Axial transvaginal scan reveals a highly echogenic ring *(arrow)* corresponding to trophoblastic tissue surrounding fluid in the ectopic gestational sac. The left ovary was seen in a different scan plane, separate from the tubal ring. U, uterus.

The separation of a corpus luteum cyst of pregnancy from an ectopic pregnancy can be difficult. When the luteal cyst is simple, it can be accurately diagnosed. When complex and especially with a thick rim, its appearance can overlap a non-cyst adnexal ectopic pregnancy. It has recently been suggested that the echogenicity of the ectopic rim is more often increased when compared with the ovary than the echogenicity of the corpus luteum cyst, but this finding does not always hold true. Assessment of the relationship of an adnexal ring to the ovary in a patient with a positive βhCG value is critical (Fig. 14-34). If the ring can be shown to be separate from the ovaries, it is not a corpus luteal cyst and can therefore be presumed to be an ectopic pregnancy. If instead it is located within the ovary and does not contain a yolk sac or embryo, it is likely a corpus luteal cyst (because a true intraovarian ectopic pregnancy is a rare phenomenon).

All of the sonographic findings characteristic of an ectopic pregnancy, aside from the identification of an extrauterine embryo with heart motion, can occur with other abnormalities. When the pregnancy test is negative, endometriomas, pelvic inflammatory disease without or with abscess formation, hydrosalpinx or pyosalpinx, and even dermoids on occasion exhibit some of the appearances described earlier (Fig. 14-35). For this reason, knowledge of the βhCG is critical in establishing the diagnosis of an ectopic pregnancy.

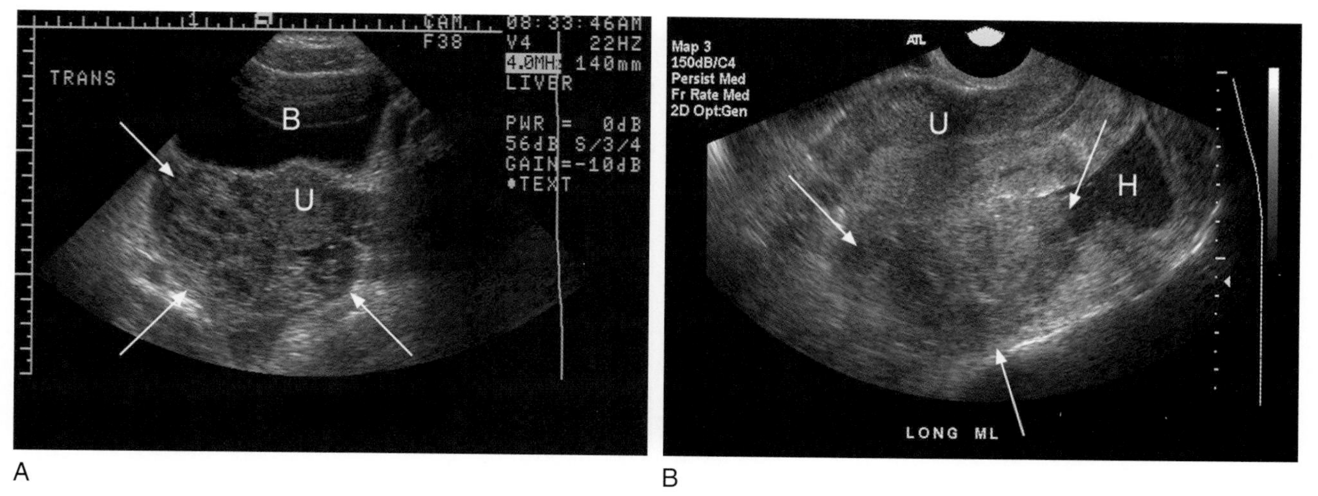

Figure 14-31 Examples of irregularly shaped adnexal masses due to pelvic hematomas after rupture of ectopic pregnancy. **A,** Axial transabdominal image shows large heterogeneous right adnexal mass *(arrows)* extending posterior to the uterus (U). B, urinary bladder. **B,** Longitudinal transvaginal image of a different patient shows an irregular heterogeneous mass *(arrows)* posterior to the uterus (U). Hemoperitoneum (H) is seen immediately caudad to the mass.

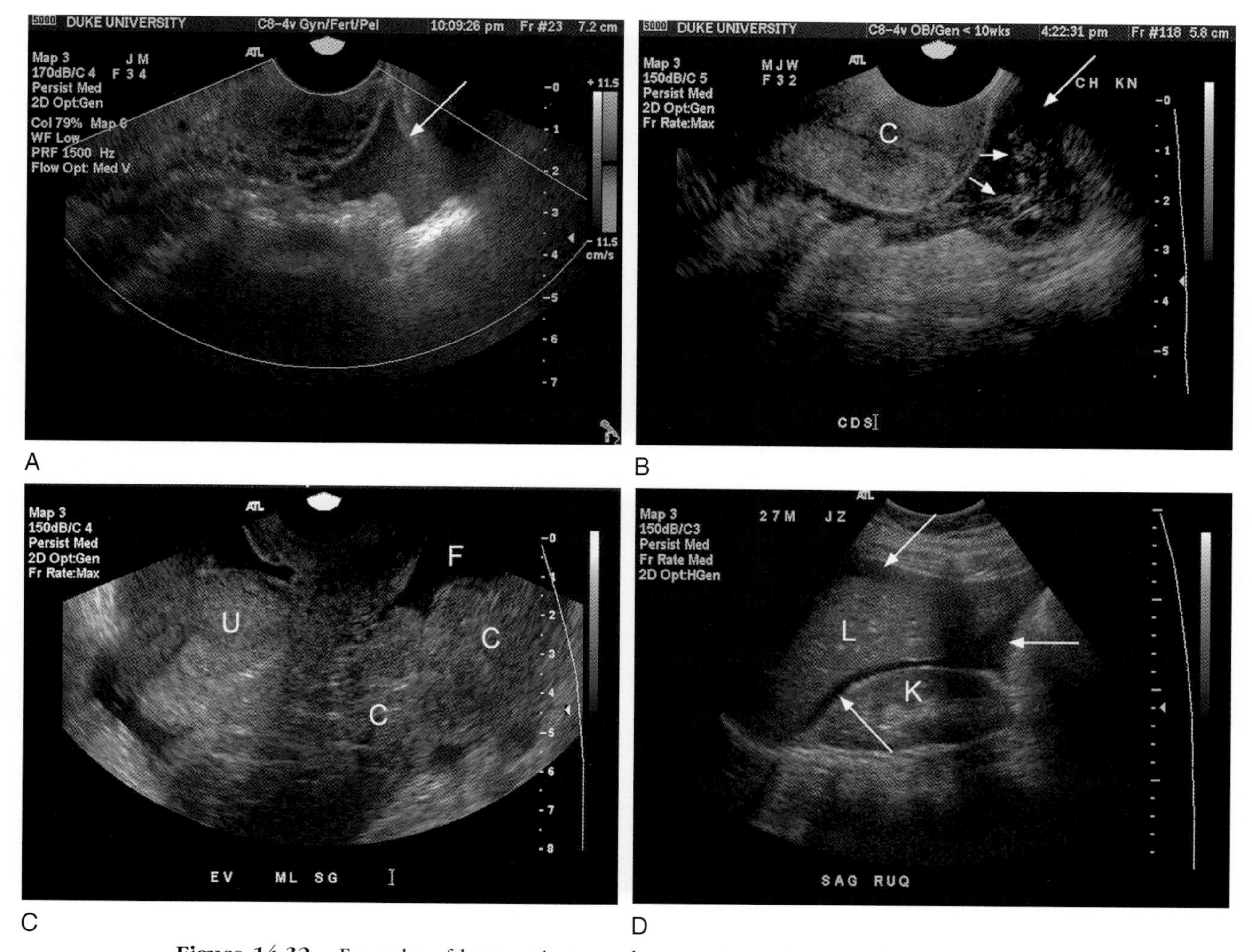

Figure 14-32 Examples of hemoperitoneum due to ectopic pregnancy. **A,** Endovaginal image shows fluid-containing echoes *(arrow)* due to hemoperitoneum in cul-de-sac. **B,** Longitudinal endovaginal image shows fluid *(long arrow)* containing irregular strands and blood clots *(short arrows)* in cul-de-sac. C, cervix. **C,** Longitudinal endovaginal scan of uterus (U) shows anechoic fluid (F) containing large blood clots (C). **D,** Longitudinal transabdominal image of right upper quadrant shows anechoic fluid *(arrows)* surrounding the liver (L) corresponding to hemoperitoneum from a ruptured ectopic pregnancy. K, kidney.

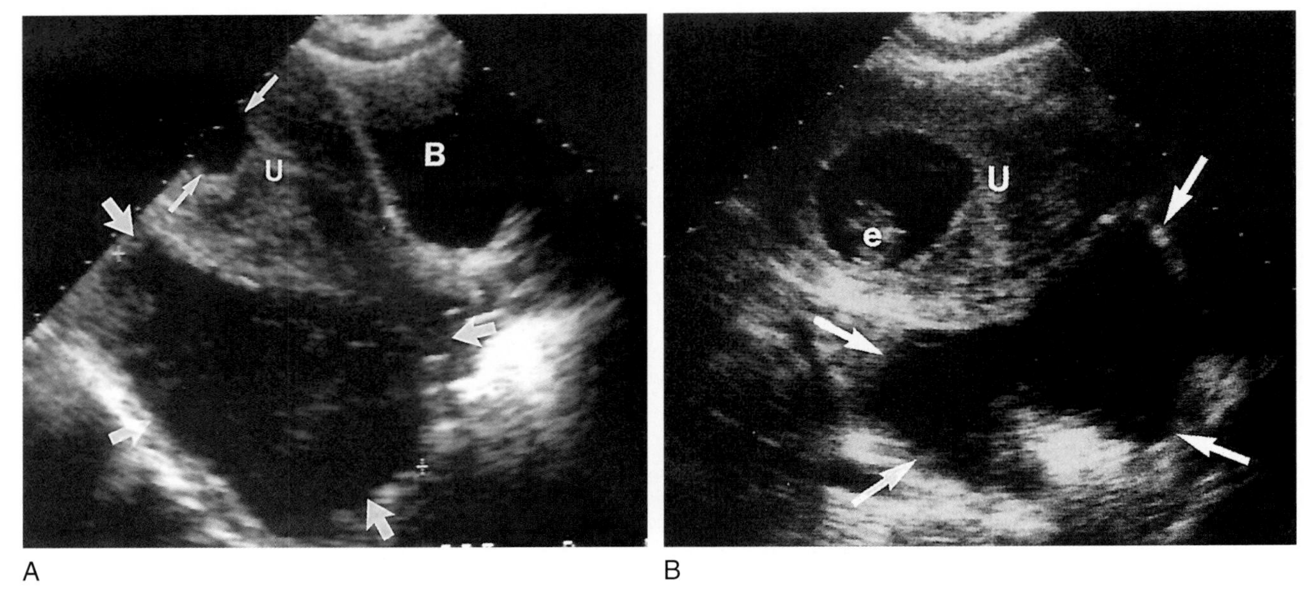

Figure 14-33 Heterotopic pregnancy, a concomitant intrauterine and extrauterine pregnancy. **A,** Transabdominal sagittal midline view of the uterus (U) shows part of a normal intrauterine gestational sac *(small arrows)*. A large, irregular, primarily anechoic fluid collection is identified within the cul-de-sac, which shows multiple small hyperechoic internal echoes *(large arrows)*. B, urinary bladder. **B,** Transabdominal transaxial image through the upper part of the uterus (U) shows a normal intrauterine gestational sac with a well-defined living embryo (e). Posteriorly, within the cul-de-sac, is the same large complex fluid collection *(arrows)*.

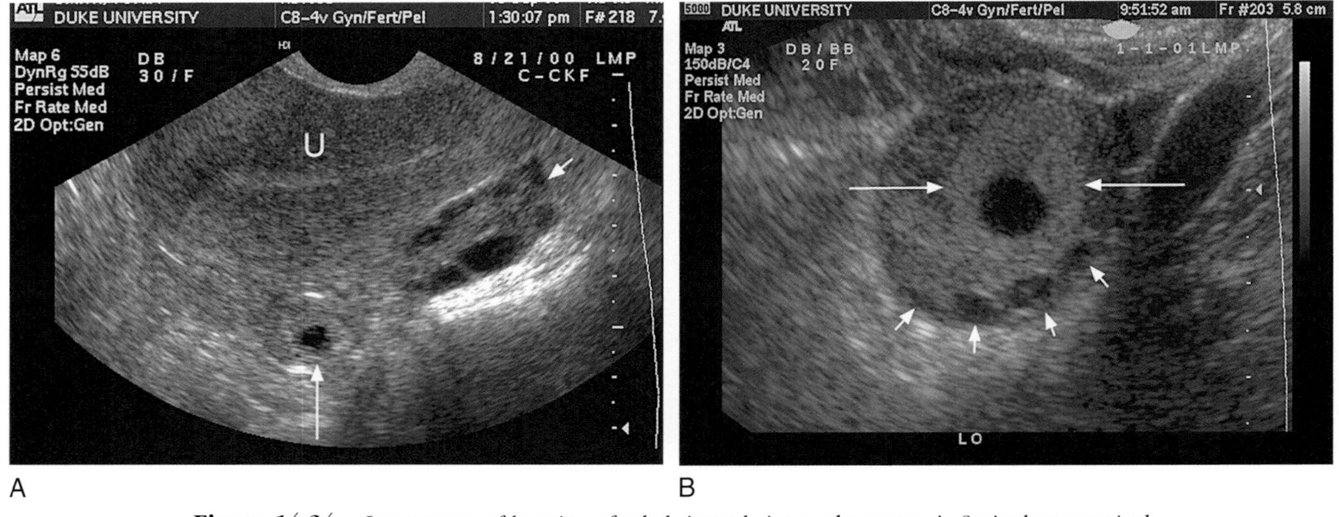

Figure 14-34 Importance of location of tubal ring relative to the ovary. **A,** Sagittal transvaginal scan shows tubal ring *(long arrow)* is separate from the ovary *(short arrow),* consistent with ectopic pregnancy. U, uterus. **B,** Axial image of left adnexa reveals a ring of increased echogenicity *(long arrows)* surrounding a round fluid collection, suggestive of a tubal ring sign. However, peripheral follicles *(short arrows)* are seen, indicating the ring is contained within the ovary and does not contain an embryo or yolk sac, so it is most consistent with a corpus luteal cyst. A true intraovarian ectopic pregnancy is a rare phenomenon.

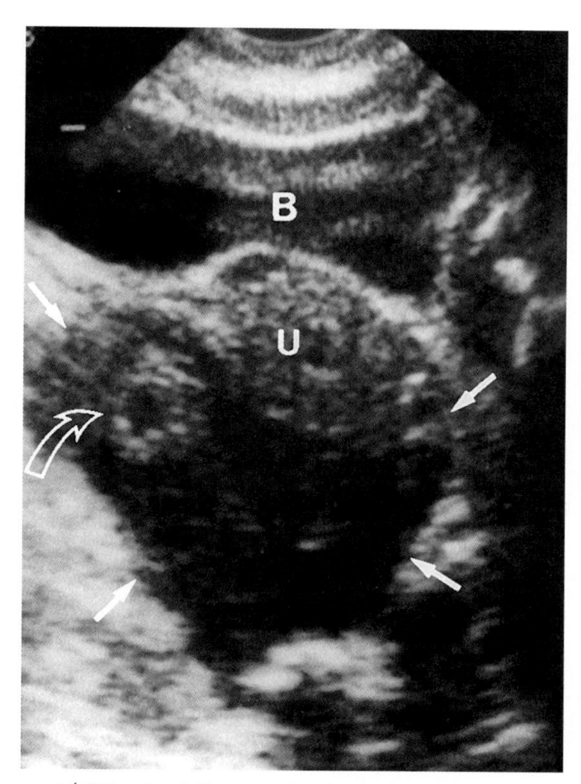

Figure 14-35 Partially treated pelvic inflammatory disease in a woman with a negative pregnancy test result. This transabdominal transaxial view shows a grossly normal uterus (U). Behind the uterus is an ill-defined complex collection *(straight arrows)* that fills the cul-de-sac and extends into the right adnexa where there is the suggestion of a tubal ring *(open curved arrow)* characteristic of an ectopic pregnancy. However, the pregnancy test result was negative, and this area proved to be part of a large abscess. B, urinary bladder.

If abnormal fallopian tubes are found or there is a known clinical history of pelvic inflammatory disease, the level of suspicion for an ectopic pregnancy also increases.

The Use of Doppler Imaging

Both color and pulsed Doppler analysis have been attempted in ectopic pregnancies. Color Doppler imaging can survey a large amount of tissue and find arterial signals; pulsed Doppler sonography can then obtain an arterial waveform. The trophoblastic tissue that surrounds a pregnancy, whether intrauterine or extrauterine, commonly has a low-resistance (high-diastolic) arterial waveform (Fig. 14-36). This waveform is suggestive but not diagnostic for trophoblastic tissue and has been seen in certain cancers (malignant neovascularity), endocrine-active tumors, and inflammation.

It has been suggested that in an ectopic pregnancy, this high-diastolic arterial pattern of trophoblastic tissue in the adnexa can be of value in identifying the trophoblastic tissue of an ectopic pregnancy. However, the Doppler waveform is nonspecific because there are multiple arteries (both uterine and ovarian) under the influence of a woman's menstrual cycles and in pregnancy. This low-resistance, high-diastolic arterial pattern may be detected in normal ovaries and in the walls of a corpus luteum cyst of pregnancy. Additionally, certain masses (e.g., endometriomas, abscesses, and dermoid cysts) unrelated to an ectopic pregnancy may have arterial waveforms with elevated diastolic flow. Likewise, the absence of this waveform pattern does not exclude an ectopic pregnancy: if ultrasound findings are typical of ectopic pregnancy, an ectopic gestation should be diagnosed even in the absence of the high diastolic arterial pattern.

The intrauterine trophoblastic reaction of the gestational sac (its hyperechoic rim) in an IUP can also have the same arterial waveform. This finding should in theory differentiate an IUP from the pseudogestational sac of an ectopic pregnancy. But it is only of diagnostic value in cases in which only the gestational sac (not with a yolk sac and embryo) is identified. The specificity of this sign is not known, particularly in the context of an abnormal IUP. Because of the increased power needed for pulsed Doppler, it is not recommended that pulsed Doppler be used except in cases of diagnostic necessity.

The Importance of Diagnosing an Ectopic Pregnancy

There is an important subset of women with ectopic pregnancy in whom, if the diagnosis is not quickly established, there can be rapid deterioration and possible death. Many of these women present with severe pelvic pain and hypotension. However, these are the minority of ectopic pregnancy cases.

Instead, most women with ectopic pregnancies present with vague symptomatology and are clinically stable. They should obviously be treated cautiously but not necessarily as emergencies, particularly if their presentation (by clinical examination, serum hCG levels, and ultrasound) still includes the consideration of an early normal IUP. In this setting, it is important for the examiner to give all the options for that pregnancy and, if possible, the most favored diagnosis. Close follow-up without compromise to the patient can often be performed until the diagnosis has been established. To rush into the diagnosis of an ectopic pregnancy, particularly if treatment of an ectopic pregnancy with methotrexate is considered, may result in the loss of the normal IUP.

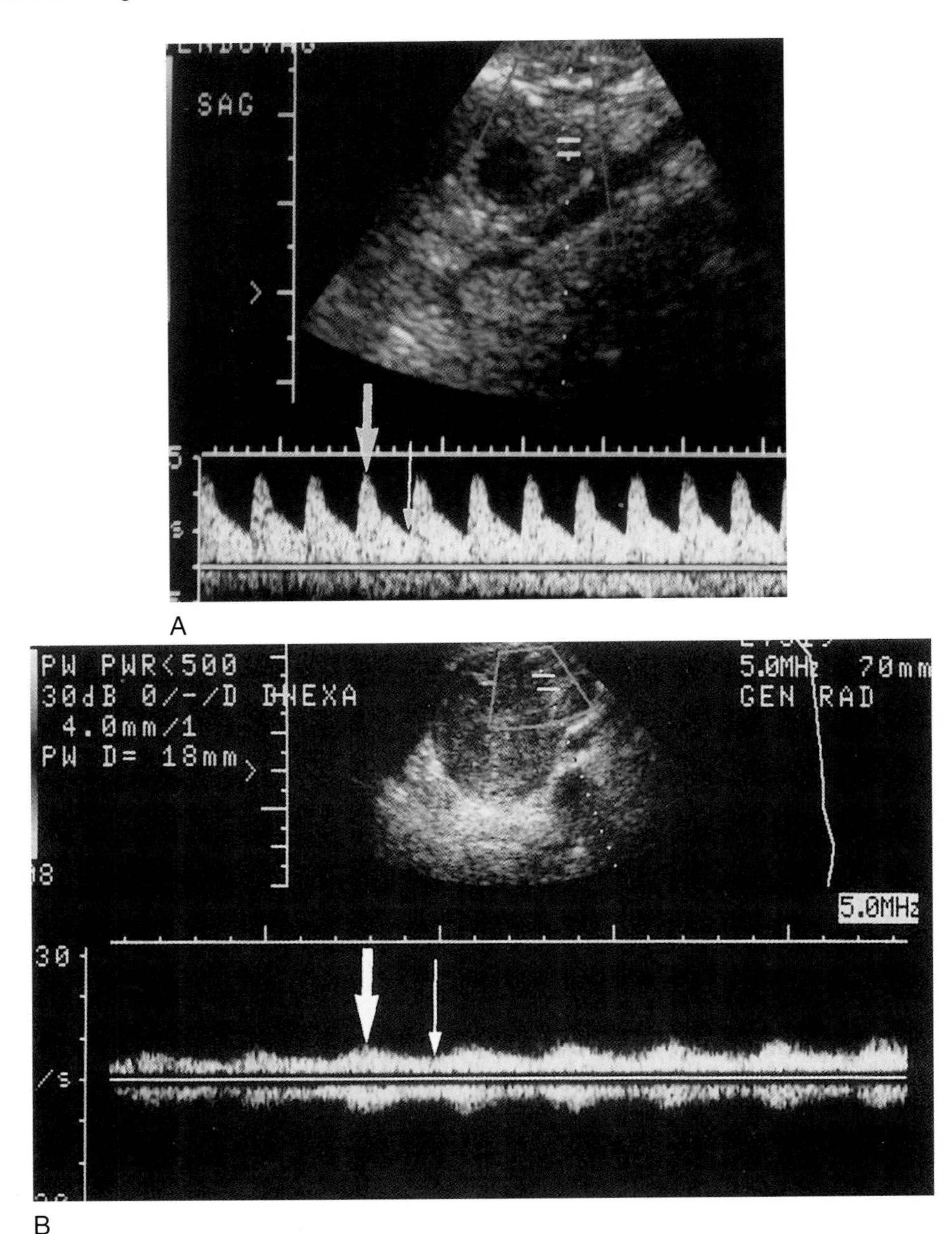

Figure 14-36 Doppler arterial spectral waveforms in two cases of ectopic pregnancy. **A,** Split image showing the transvaginal image of an adnexal tubal ring at the top. The Doppler sample is taken from the edge of the tubal ring. On the bottom, the Doppler arterial waveform shows a relatively small amount of diastolic flow (end-diastole is denoted by a *long thin arrow*) compared with the systolic flow (peak systole is denoted by a *large thick arrow*). This waveform is nonspecific. **B,** Split image showing the transvaginal image of a large hyperechoic adnexal mass at the top with the Doppler sample taken from its edge. On the bottom the Doppler arterial waveform is seen to have a relatively large amount of diastolic flow (end-diastole is denoted by a *long thin arrow*) compared with the systolic flow (peak systole is denoted by a *large thick arrow*). This pattern is more typical for trophoblastic tissue but can be seen in other conditions.

Key Features

In the first trimester the two most important diagnostic tests are the pregnancy test (urine and/or serum) and the ultrasound examination.

The age of a pregnancy is defined as the age of the conceptus from the first day of the last normal menstrual period.

The early pregnancy can be evaluated by two ultrasound techniques: the transabdominal (TA) and the transvaginal (TV) examinations.

The TV ultrasound examination allows earlier assessment of the gestational sac, yolk sac, and embryo. The gestational sac can be routinely identified at 5 weeks, with the yolk sac and embryo seen by 5.5 and 6 weeks, respectively.

Measurements obtained by the TV and TA methods are both accurate.

Analysis of the gestational sac is of primary importance before embryonic visualization. Identification of the yolk sac confirms the presence of a developing intrauterine pregnancy (IUP), even before the embryo is identified.

The first-trimester crown-rump length (CRL) and second-trimester biparietal diameter are both accurate (±1 week) in predicting gestational age. Both are more accurate than menstrual history, which is ±2.5 weeks in the general population.

The normal gestational sac typically has the following characteristics: correct positioning within the uterus, a double decidual sac (DDS) sign, a continuous hyperechoic rim of 2 mm in thickness or greater, a grossly spherical or ovoid shape, and growth of more than 1.2 mm/day.

The finding of the DDS (two hyperechoic lines surrounding a hypoechoic closed endometrial canal) is highly predictive of an IUP. Its absence is more suggestive of an ectopic pregnancy or a miscarriage but does not exclude a normal IUP.

Potential uterine findings that can cause confusion in the first trimester include fluid within the endometrial canal, chorioamniotic separation, a "vanishing twin," implantation bleed, and a necrotic fibroid.

The definitive diagnosis of a normal and abnormal IUP may need to await the detection of an embryo with a CRL of 5 mm, when heart motion is expected.

The embryonic heart rate is important. By 5 weeks the rate is commonly greater than 100 beats per minute. After 8 weeks, it is anticipated to be between 120 and 180 beats per minute.

Fetal anatomy is more completely identified by TV scanning. Currently this has not caused more precise first-trimester diagnosis of anomalies.

TV scanning should be performed in multiple gestations whenever there is an uncertainly about the number of gestations and type of twinning.

Hydatidiform moles may present in the first trimester, occasionally mimicking a spontaneous incomplete abortion.

The incidence of ectopic pregnancies has risen in the United States. Although the death rate has fallen, ectopic pregnancy should still be considered a significant health risk.

The detection of a pregnancy using the β subunit of the human chorionic gonadotropin (βhCG) in urine and serum is highly accurate. Using the 3rd International Reference Preparation, at a quantitative serum βhCG level of 2000 IU/L transvaginal ultrasound will usually detect a normal intrauterine gestational sac.

In the early pregnancy, the quantitative serum βhCG level normally doubles every 2 days.

The differential diagnosis of a positive pregnancy test is a normal IUP, a miscarriage, and an ectopic pregnancy.

The presentation of ectopic pregnancy is variable. High-risk women have a history of abnormal fallopian tubes, a history of ectopic pregnancies or an intrauterine device, are on fertility medication, or are undergoing in vitro fertilization.

The βhCG level in a woman with an ectopic pregnancy often increases more slowly than in a normal intrauterine pregnancy.

An ectopic pregnancy is defined as the implantation of a fertilized ovum outside the endometrial lining. Most are in the fallopian tubes.

Ectopic pregnancies within the uterus can occur in the cornual portion of the fundus and the cervix.

A heterotopic pregnancy, a concomitant intrauterine and extrauterine pregnancy, now occurs in approximately 1 in 7000 pregnancies, with an even higher incidence in patients who have undergone ovulation induction for infertility.

When an IUP is identified and there are adnexal findings other than an ovarian cyst or a small amount of simple cul-de-sac fluid, a heterotopic pregnancy should be considered.

Pseudogestational sacs occur in approximately 5% of ectopic pregnancies. These are caused by a collection of fluid or a decidual cast within the endometrial canal or a thickened endometrium.

In a retroverted uterus or in a uterus with multiple fibroids, an intrauterine sac may be displaced to the margin of the uterus and falsely appear in an ectopic position. If myometrium can be shown to encompass the sac, the pregnancy is intrauterine.

With a positive pregnancy test, there are five adnexal findings that have high positive predictive values in diagnosing an ectopic pregnancy: (1) a gestational sac in an ectopic location, (2) an adnexal mass containing either a yolk sac or an embryo, (3) a tubal ring appearing as an empty gestational sac, (4) a complex or solid adnexal mass, and (5) a moderate to a large amount of intraperitoneal fluid, particularly with internal echoes.

Doppler waveform analysis is of limited value in the evaluation of most intrauterine and extrauterine pregnancies.

SUGGESTED READINGS

Ackerman TE, Levi CS, Dashefsky SM, et al: Interstitial line: Sonographic finding in interstitial (cornual) ectopic pregnancy. Radiology 189:83, 1993.

Ackerman TE, Levi CS, Lyons EA, et al: Decidual cyst: Endovaginal sonographic sign of ectopic pregnancy. Radiology 189:727, 1993.

Atri M, Leduc C, Gillett P, et al: Role of endovaginal sonography in the diagnosis and management of ectopic pregnancy. Radiographics 16:755, 1996.

Bar-Hava I, Aschkenazi S, Orvieto R, et al: Spectrum of normal intrauterine cavity sonographic findings after first-trimester abortion. J Ultrasound Med 20:1277, 2001.

Barnhart KT, Simhan H, Kamelle SA: Diagnostic accuracy of ultrasound above and below the beta-hCG discriminatory zone. Obstet Gynecol 94:583, 1999.

Bennett GL, Bromley B, Lieberman E, et al: Subchorionic hemorrhage in first-trimester pregnancies: Prediction of pregnancy outcome with sonography. Radiology 200:803, 1996.

Benson CB, Chow JS, Chang-Lee W, et al: Outcome of pregnancies in women with uterine leiomyomas identified by sonography in the first trimester. J Clin Ultrasound 29:261, 2001.

Benson CB, Doubilet PM: Slow embryonic heart rate in early first trimester: Indicator of poor pregnancy outcome. Radiology 192:343, 1994.

Benson CB, Doubilet PM: Sonographic prediction of gestational age: Accuracy of second- and third-trimester fetal measurements. AJR Am J Roentgenol 157:1275, 1991.

Benson CB, Genest DR, Bernstein MR, et al: Sonographic appearance of first trimester complete hydatidiform moles. Ultrasound Obstet Gynecol 16:188, 2000.

Bowerman RA: Sonography of fetal midgut herniation: Normal size criteria and correlation with crown-rump length. J Ultrasound Med 5:251, 1993.

Brown DL, Doubilet PM: Transvaginal sonography for diagnosing ectopic pregnancy: Positivity criteria and performance characteristics. J Ultrasound Med 13:259, 1994.

Bromley B, et al: Small sac size in the first trimester: A predictor of poor fetal outcome. Radiology 178:375, 1991.

Chen PC, Sickler GK, Dubinsky TJ, et al: Sonographic detection of echogenic fluid and correlation with culdocentesis in the evaluation of ectopic pregnancy. AJR Am J Roentgenol 170:1299, 1998.

Dillon EH, et al: Endovaginal US and Doppler findings after first-trimester abortion. Radiology 186:87, 1993.

Dillon EH, Feyock AL, Taylor KJW: Pseudogestational sacs: Doppler US differentiation from normal or abnormal intrauterine pregnancies. Radiology 176:359, 1990.

Doubilet PM, Benson CB: Embryonic heart rate in the early first trimester: What rate is normal? J Ultrasound Med 14:431-434, 1995.

Doubilet PM, Benson CB: Long term prognosis of pregnancies complicated by slow embryonic heart rates in the early first trimester. J Ultrasound Med 18:818, 1999.

Frates MC, et al: Cervical ectopic pregnancy: Results of conservative treatment. Radiology 191:773, 1994.

Frates MC, et al: Tubal rupture in patients with ectopic pregnancy: Diagnosis with transvaginal US. Radiology 191:769, 1994.

Frates MC, Laing FC: Sonographic evaluation of ectopic pregnancy: An update. AJR Am J Roentgenol 165:251, 1995.

Frates MC, Visweswaran A, Laing FC: Comparison of tubal ring and corpus luteum echogenicities: A useful differentiating characteristic. J Ultrasound Med 20:27, 2001.

Fylstra DL: Tubal pregnancy: A review of current diagnosis and treatment. Obstet Gynecol Surv 53:320, 1998.

Goldstein SR: Embryonic death in early pregnancy: A new look at the first trimester. Obstet Gynecol 84:294, 1994.

Gracia CR, Barnhart KT: Diagnosing ectopic pregnancy: Decision analysis comparing six strategies. Gynecol Obstet 97:464, 2001.

Gun M, Mavrogiogis M: Cervical ectopic pregnancy: A case report and literature review. Ultrasound Obstet Gynecol 19:297, 2002.

Hadlock FP, et al: Fetal crown-rump length: Reevaluation of relation to menstrual age (5-18 weeks) with high-resolution real-time US. Radiology 182:501, 1992.

Hertzberg BS, Kliewer MA: Ectopic pregnancy: Ultrasound diagnosis and interpretive pitfalls. S Med J 88:1191, 1995.

Hertzberg BS, Kliewer MA, Bowie JD: Sonographic evaluation for ectopic pregnancy: Transabdominal scanning of patients with nondistended urinary bladders as a complement to endovaginal sonography. AJR Am J Roentgenol 173:773, 1999.

Hertzberg BS, Kliewer MA, Bowie JD: Adnexal ring sign and hemoperitoneum caused by hemorrhagic ovarian cyst: Pitfall in the sonographic diagnosis of ectopic pregnancy. AJR Am J Roentgenol 173:1301, 1999.

Kopta MM, May RR, Crane JP: A comparison of the reliability of the estimated date of confinement predicted by crown-rump length and biparietal diameter. Am J Obstet Gynecol 145:562, 1983.

Kucuk T, Duru NK, Yenen MC, et al: Yolk sac size and shape as predictors of poor pregnancy outcome. J Perinatol Med 27:316, 1999.

Kurtz AB, et al: Can detection of the yolk sac in the first trimester be used to predict the outcome of pregnancy? A prospective sonographic study. AJR Am J Roentgenol 158:843, 1992.

Laing FC, Brown DL, Price JF, et al: Intradecidual sign: Is it effective in diagnosis of an early intrauterine pregnancy? Radiology 204:655, 1997.

Lemus JF: Ectopic pregnancy: An update. Obstet Gynecol 12:369, 2000.

Levi CS, Lyons EA, Lindsay DJ: Early diagnosis of nonviable pregnancy with endovaginal US. Radiology 167:383, 1988.

Levi CS, et al: Endovaginal US: Demonstration of cardiac activity in embryos of less than 5.0 mm in crown-rump length. Radiology 176:71, 1990.

Lindsay DJ, et al: Yolk sac diameter and shape at endovaginal US: Predictors of pregnancy outcome in the first trimester. Radiology 183:115, 1992.

Mahony BS, Filly RA, Nyberg DA, Callen PW: Sonographic evaluation of ectopic pregnancy. J Ultrasound Med 4:221, 1985.

Marks WM, Filly RA, Callen PW, Laing FC: The decidual cast of ectopic pregnancy: A confusing ultrasonographic appearance. Radiology 133:451, 1979.

McKenna KM, Feldstein VA, Goldstein RB, et al: The "empty amnion": A sign of early pregnancy failure. J Ultrasound Med 14:117, 1995.

Mehta TS, Levine D, Beckwith B: Treatment of ectopic pregnancy: Is a human chorionic gonadotropic level of 2,000 mIU/mL a reasonable threshold? Radiology 205:569, 1997.

Mehta TS, Levine D, McArdle CR: Lack of sensitivity of endometrial thickness in predicting the presence of an ectopic pregnancy. J Ultrasound Med 18:117, 1999.

Moore KL: The Developing Human: Clinically Oriented Embryology. Philadelphia, WB Saunders, 1982.

Nyberg DA, et al: Extrauterine findings of ectopic pregnancy at transvaginal US: Importance of echogenic fluid. Radiology 178:823, 1991.

Nyberg DA, et al: Endovaginal sonographic evaluation of ectopic pregnancy: A prospective study. AJR Am J Roentgenol 149:1181, 1987.

Nyberg DA, Laing FC, Filly RA: Threatened abortion: Sonographic distinction of normal and abnormal gestation sacs. Radiology 158:397, 1986.

Nyberg DA, et al: Ultrasonographic differentiation of the gestational sac of early intrauterine pregnancy from the pseudogestational sac of ectopic pregnancy. Radiology 146:755, 1983.

Nyberg DA, et al: Distinguishing normal from abnormal gestational sac growth in early pregnancy. J Ultrasound Med 6:23,1987.

Parvey HR, Maklad N: Pitfalls in the transvaginal sonographic diagnosis of ectopic pregnancy. J Ultrasound Med 3:139, 1993.

Pennell RG, et al: Complicated first-trimester pregnancies: Evaluation with endovaginal US versus transabdominal technique. Radiology 165:79, 1987.

Pennell RG, et al: Prospective comparison of vaginal and abdominal sonography in normal early pregnancy. J Ultrasound Med 10:63, 1991.

Pittaway DE, Reish RL, Wentz AC: Doubling times of human chorionic gonadotropin increase in early viable intrauterine pregnancies. Am J Obstet Gynecol 152:299, 1985.

Robinson HP, Fleming JEE: A critical evaluation of sonar "crown-rump length" measurements. Br J Obstet Gynaecol 82:702, 1975.

Rowling SE, Langer JE, Coleman BS, et al: Sonography during early pregnancy: Dependence of threshold and discriminatory values on transvaginal transducer frequency. AJR Am J Roentgenol 172:983, 1999.

Russell SA, Filly RA, Damato N: Sonographic diagnosis of ectopic pregnancy with endovaginal probes: What really has changed? J Ultrasound Med 3:145, 1993.

Sohaey R, Woodward P, Zweibel WJ: First-trimester ultrasound: The essentials. Semin Ultrasound CT MR 17:2, 1996.

Spandorfer SD, Barnhart KT: Endometrial stripe thickness as a predictor of ectopic pregnancy. Fertil Steril 66:474, 1996.

Stampone C, Nicotra M, Muttinelli C, et al: Transvaginal sonography of the yolk sac in normal and abnormal pregnancy. J Clin Ultrasound 24:3, 1996.

Wachsberg RH, Levine CD: Echogenic peritoneal fluid as an isolated sonographic finding: Significance in patients at risk of ectopic pregnancy. Clin Radiol 53:520, 1998.

Zinn HL, Cohen HL, Zinn DL: Ultrasonographic diagnosis of ectopic pregnancy: Importance of transabdominal imaging. J Ultrasound Med 16:603, 1997.

Fetal Central Nervous System: Head and Spine

For Key Features summary see p. 410

The overall frequency of congenital anomalies is 1:500 to 1:600 births. Central nervous system (CNS) abnormalities constitute the majority and include anencephaly and spina bifida, both with an incidence of 1:1000 births, and cephalocele, with an incidence of 1:4000 births. If a woman has had a previous child with a CNS defect, the risk for another CNS anomaly (of any type) in a subsequent child increases to greater than 1 in 50 (2%). If she has had two previous children with CNS defects, the risk then exceeds 1 in 10 (10%)!

Many CNS anomalies are large and obvious. However, small subtle defects may also occur. Because any abnormality can lead to a clinically significant deficit, a careful sequential evaluation of the head and spine is warranted in all pregnancies.

ANENCEPHALY

Anencephaly is a lethal anomaly caused by lack of development of the fetal brain. It is one of the easiest CNS anomalies to recognize. By the beginning of the second trimester, at 12 to 14 weeks, the normal fetal head with its bright calvarium and its intracranial structures, in particular the lateral ventricles with choroid plexus, are routinely identified (Fig. 15-1). Using transvaginal (TV) scanning, it is likely that these structures can be identified earlier, perhaps as early as at 9 to 10 weeks. For now, however, it is still prudent to delay the definitive diagnosis of this and any other structural abnormality until the early second trimester.

Inability to identify the normal calvarium and intracranial structures should prompt a consideration for anencephaly. If it proves difficult to find the calvarium, scanning from the spine to the skull base should identify a normal head. If not, anencephaly should be considered. Ultrasound of the fetus with anencephaly reveals the absence of normal brain tissue and calvarium above the level of the orbits, producing a cranial appearance that has been called "frog-like" (Fig. 15-2A). On occasion, hyperechoic ill-defined soft tissue can be identified (without the normal surrounding calvarium) above the facial structures (see Fig. 15-2B). This appearance is most commonly seen when an anencephalic fetus is imaged early in the second trimester. It is termed *angiomatous stroma* or *area cerebrovasculosa* and represents the residuum of dysmorphic brain.

Infrequently, anencephaly may be difficult to image owing to maternal body habitus or fetal position or because the fetus is not studied until late in pregnancy. If the calvarium and intracranial structures are difficult to identify, particularly if the head is either in an unusually high breech position under the mother's ribs or in a deep vertex presentation below the pubic symphysis, the examiner may be tempted to deem the head technically difficult to image rather than diagnose anencephaly. Instead, failure to identify the calvarium, regardless of fetal position, should make the examiner strongly suspect anencephaly. If transabdominal images are not definitive, this diagnosis can be confirmed by

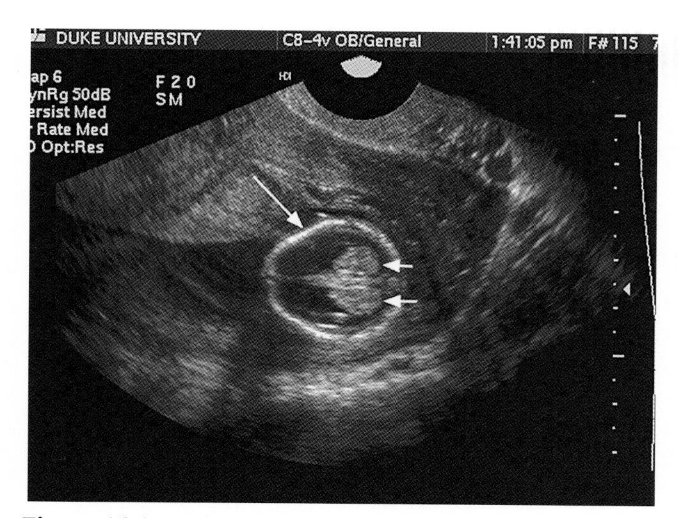

Figure 15-1 Normal fetal head at 13 weeks. Axial transvaginal sonogram of fetal head shows normal appearance of choroid plexus *(short arrows)* filling the atria of the lateral ventricles. *Long arrow,* calvarium.

a TV study if the fetal head is in the vertex presentation (Fig. 15-3).

Polyhydramnios is frequently a secondary finding in cases of anencephaly. It can be accurately diagnosed and graded as mild, moderate, or severe by the subjective observation of increased amniotic fluid volume. Measurement of either a single anteroposterior fluid pocket (>8 cm) or the amniotic fluid index (AFI) can also be used to diagnose polyhydramnios, although a measurement is not necessary to make the diagnosis. The AFI is obtained by calculating the sum of the anteroposterior diameters of the deepest fluid pocket in each of the four quadrants (left upper, left lower, right upper, and right lower) of the uterus (Fig. 15-4). Some ultrasound practices only include fluid pockets that do not contain fetal parts or umbilical cord, whereas in other practices fluid pockets with umbilical cord or an extremity are included, provided the pocket is predominantly fluid. The upper limit for the AFI varies with gestational age (see Table 13-2). If polyhydramnios is very severe, the placenta can appear thin, owing to uterine distention (Fig. 15-5).

Polyhydramnios has many causes (Table 15-1). Approximately one third of cases are idiopathic (not associated with anomalies), and the polyhydramnios is then usually mild. In the remaining two thirds, maternal or fetal problems (or both) are present. Women with diabetes mellitus may have polyhydramnios, which is usually only mildly increased. The overall amount of amniotic fluid in multiple gestations is normally increased because of the composite fluid from each gestation. Although this increase is often mild to moderate, polyhydramnios may be marked in the settings of complicated monochorionic pregnancies (e.g., twin-twin transfusions) and monoamniotic pregnancies.

The remaining cases of polyhydramnios are associated with the fetus and include structural anomalies and fetal hydrops. Structural anomalies appear to cause polyhydramnios by failure of either normal swallowing or of normal intestinal absorption: severe CNS abnormalities, obstruction of the upper and sometimes lower

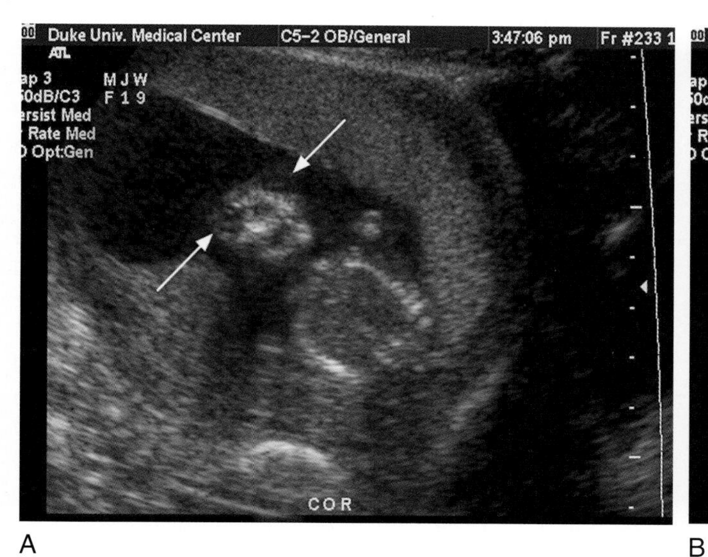

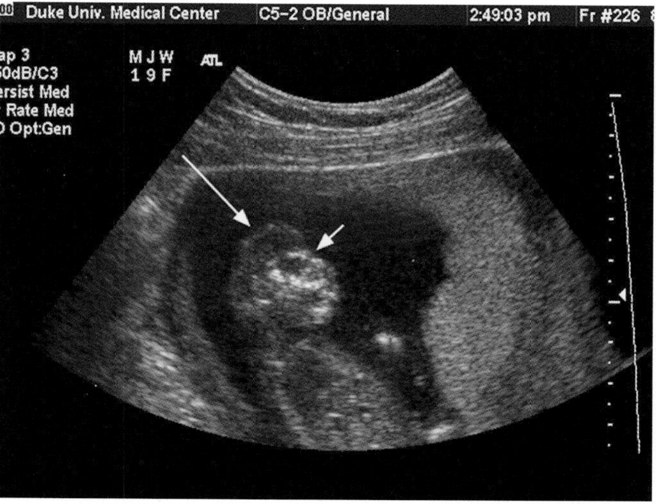

Figure 15-2 Anencephaly. **A,** Coronal view of the head of a 15-week fetus with anencephaly shows absence of calvarium and lack of normal brain tissue above level of orbits *(arrows),* resulting in a "frog-like" appearance of the craniofacial structures. **B,** Sagittal view of same fetus confirms absence of calvarium above level of orbit *(short arrow)* and shows dysmorphic brain tissue *(long arrow)* corresponding to angiomatous stroma above the level of the facial structures.

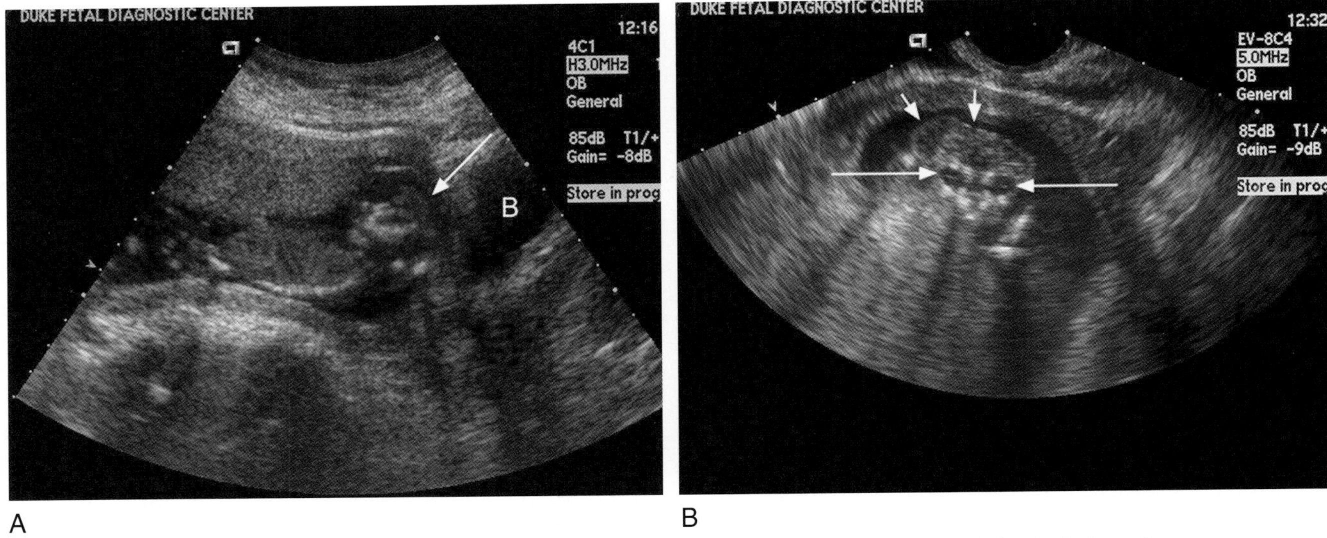

A B

Figure 15-3 Anencephaly: value of transvaginal ultrasound. **A,** Sagittal transabdominal view of fetal head *(arrow)* is suboptimal because of unfavorable position abutting uterine wall. Because normal calvarium was not seen, anencephaly was suspected and transvaginal ultrasound was performed to confirm the diagnosis. B, maternal bladder. **B,** Transvaginal coronal image of fetal head confirms absence of calvarium and normal brain tissue above level of orbits *(long arrows)*. Dysmorphic tissue *(short arrows)* corresponding to angiomatous stroma is seen.

gastrointestinal tract, marked chest narrowing, large chest or neck masses, and congenital severe muscular hypotonia or dystrophy. In general, the increase in amniotic fluid due to polyhydramnios is a slow process and may not manifest itself until after 24 weeks and rarely not even by term. On the other hand, the more severe the polyhydramnios the more likely it is that a fetal problem exists, and a careful search for a structural abnormality is indicated once maternal causes have been ruled out. Hydrops is discussed later in this chapter and in Chapter 16.

NORMAL ANATOMY OF THE HEAD

Normal structures can be identified outside the calvarium. They are subcutaneous tissue, skin, hair, and ears (Fig. 15-6). All are inconstantly seen and should not be confused with pathologic conditions.

Axial images of the head, identifying the midline hypoechoic paired thalami and occasionally the slightly more caudad hypoechoic heart-shaped midbrain, are common starting points for analysis of intracranial structures (Fig. 15-7). At the level of the thalami, the normal cavum septi pellucidi is frequently seen as a cystic structure immediately anterior to the thalami. It should not be confused with the normal slit-like (<2 mm) third ventricle, which is situated posterior to the cavum septi pellucidi, between the two thalami.

An accurate measurement of the head can be obtained with either the thalami or midbrain identified in the midline. Standard measurement tables allow for comparison of the biparietal diameter (BPD) and head circumference (HC) to the gestational age. To ensure that the BPD measurement is technically correct, the head shape can be evaluated by calculating the cephalic index (see Fig. 12-7). If the head is too round (brachiocephalic) or elongated (dolichocephalic), so that the cephalic index approaches or exceeds 2 SD from the norm, the BPD can be corrected by calculating an area-corrected BPD (BPDa) or the head circumference can be used. This is discussed more completely in Chapter 12. Up to 20 weeks (and most likely up to 24 weeks), the precision of the BPD and HC is ±1.2 weeks, similar to that of the first-trimester embryonic (crown-rump) length. After that, the precision decreases and by the late third trimester is only ±3.8 weeks.

The antepartum ultrasound standard also recommends evaluation of the lateral ventricles. The lateral ventricles are formed from the prosencephalon in the first trimester and once formed remain relatively constant in size throughout gestation. Subsequent head growth is caused by growth of the brain parenchyma around these ventricles. The lateral ventricles should be measured on an axial image demonstrating the choroid plexus at the level of the atrium immediately anterior to the junction of the body and occipital horns (Fig. 15-8). This measurement was chosen because the ventricular atrium is most sensitive to the development of early hydrocephalus and because the lateral ventricle farther from the transducer is usually easy to identify in this scan plane. The measurement should be obtained on an

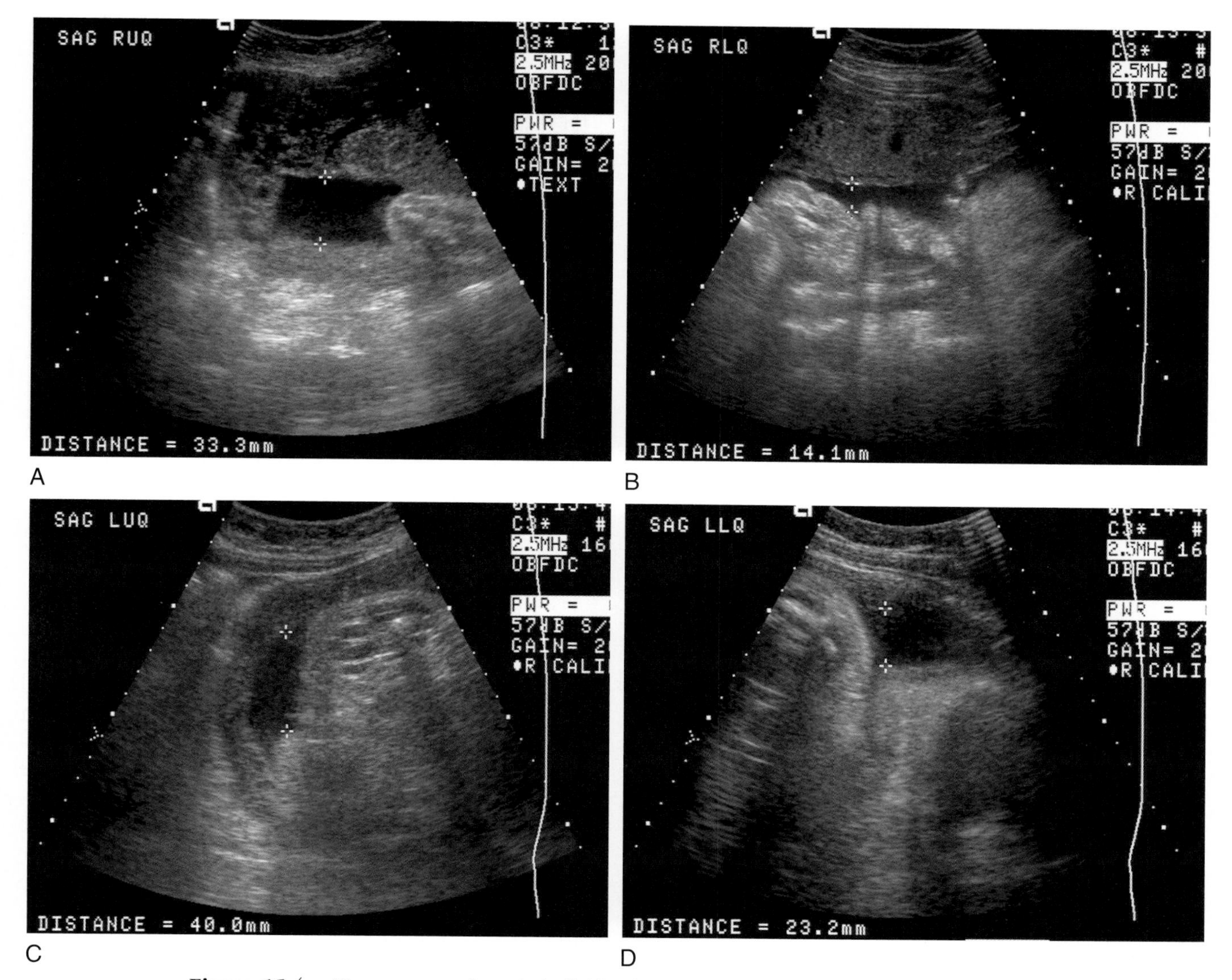

Figure 15-4 Measurement of amniotic fluid index (AFI). The AFI is calculated by adding the depths of the largest fluid pocket *(cursors)* in the right upper quadrant (**A**), right lower quadrant (**B**), left upper quadrant (**C**), and left lower quadrant (**D**). The AFI of 11.0 is normal for a 36-week pregnancy (see Table 13-2).

image that demonstrates a substantial length of choroid plexus superior to the level of the thalami. To obtain this view, particularly during the third and late second trimesters, it may be necessary to angle the posterior portion of the scan plane inferiorly.

Each atrium is measured perpendicular to its walls. Care should be taken not to measure off-axis because this can spuriously increase the measurement. The generally accepted upper limit of normal for the width of the atrium is 10 mm. Measurements between 10 and 12 mm are termed *minimal or mild ventriculomegaly*. Fetal outcome may be normal in fetuses with isolated minimal ventriculomegaly, but even in the setting of only minimal ventriculomegaly a detailed anatomic search and follow-up examinations should be performed to assess for other fetal abnormalities and rule out progressive ventricular enlargement. Fetuses with mild ventriculomegaly also are at increased risk for aneuploidy, and many practices offer fetal karyotyping in this setting.

Another helpful sign in identifying fetuses with dilated lateral ventricles is the relative amount of hyperechoic choroid plexus filling the lateral ventricles. In normal fetuses the choroid plexus should fill more than 60% to 90% of the width of the atria. If true ventricular enlargement is present, the choroid plexus typically decreases in size (relative to the atria) and may "dangle" downward toward the gravity-dependent wall of the ventricle in the enlarged atrium (Fig. 15-9). This has been called the "dangling choroid plexus sign."

It is important for the examiner to be aware of the potential problem of identifying only one normal atrium, usually the one in the far field. Although the assumption

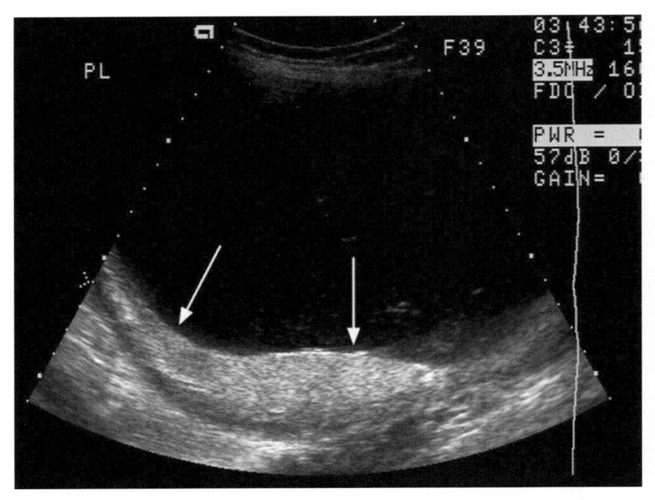

Figure 15-5 Thin placenta due to severe polyhydramnios. Longitudinal transabdominal scan of a 32-week pregnancy shows thinning of the placenta *(arrows)* due to severe polyhydramnios.

Table 15-1 Causes of Polyhydramnios

Cause	Approximate Percentage
Idiopathic	33
Maternal: diabetes mellitus	25
Multiple gestations	10
Fetal	
Anomalies*	20
Hydrops	12

*Central nervous system, gastrointestinal, thoracic, skeletal, chromosomal, cardiac.

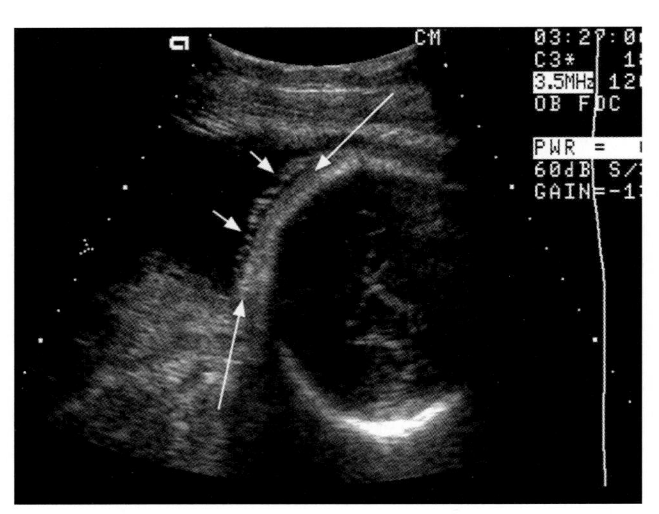

Figure 15-6 Normal fetal hair. Oblique image of fetal head at 34 weeks shows normal scalp *(long arrows)* and hair *(short arrows)*.

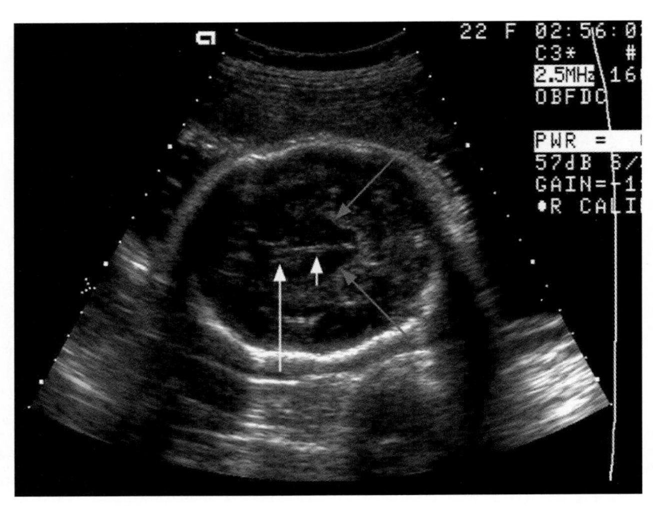

Figure 15-7 Normal intracranial anatomy at level of thalami. Axial image of fetal head at 29 weeks shows third ventricle *(short white arrow)* between the thalami *(long gray arrows)*. The cavum septum pellucidum *(long white arrow)* is located anterior to the thalami and third ventricle.

is often correct that both atria are the same size, there are cases of asymmetric lateral ventricular enlargement (Fig. 15-10). The inability to visualize the near-field atrium is primarily caused by reverberation artifact from the near-field calvarium obscuring the atrium. This difficulty can be partially overcome by turning or tilting the transducer to image through the lambdoid or sometimes through the coronal suture. At least partial identification of the near-field atrium is then possible (Fig. 15-11). Therefore, although it is not standard practice to image both atria, when possible an attempt should be made to do so, particularly if one ventricle is dilated.

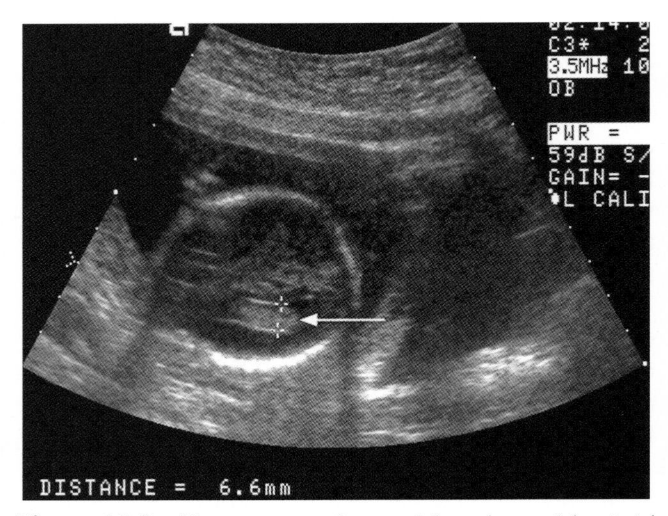

Figure 15-8 Measurement of normal lateral ventricle. Axial scan of fetal head at 19 weeks shows choroid plexus filling atrium of lateral ventricle *(arrow)*. The ventricle is measured perpendicular to its walls *(cursors)* at the level of the atrium. The measurement of 6.6 mm is normal.

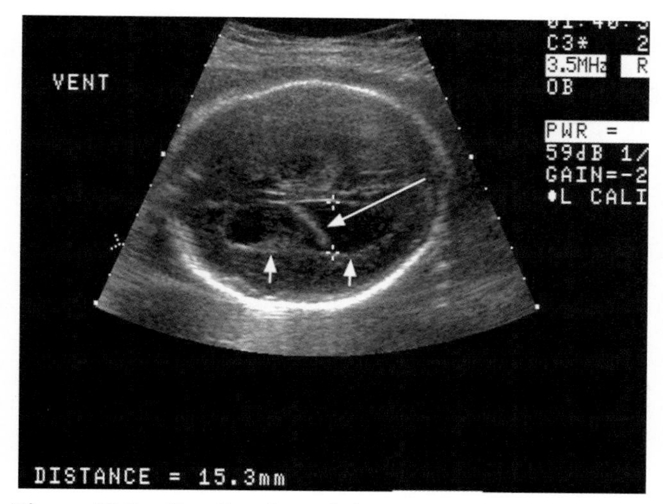

Figure 15-9 Dangling choroid plexus. Axial image of fetal head shows a dilated lateral ventricle *(short arrows)* measuring 15.3 mm in width. The choroid plexus *(long arrow)* is decreased in thickness and dangles toward the gravity-dependent lateral ventricular wall.

HYDROCEPHALUS AND HYDRANENCEPHALY

Ventriculomegaly (enlarged lateral ventricles) is caused by either increased intraventricular pressure or an ex vacuo phenomenon in which the ventricles expand to "fill in" the space previously occupied by brain parenchyma. The condition of enlarged ventricles due to increased pressure is called hydrocephalus, whereas enlarged ventricles without increased pressure suggests brain parenchymal underdevelopment, dysgenesis, or destruction. In the latter conditions, the atria of the lateral ventricles are often affected first. With more marked ventriculomegaly, the entire lateral ventricular system becomes enlarged (Fig. 15-12).

Sonographically, hydrocephalus (increased pressure) can be diagnosed if, in addition to ventricular enlargement, the head is enlarged, the lesion (e.g., a mass)

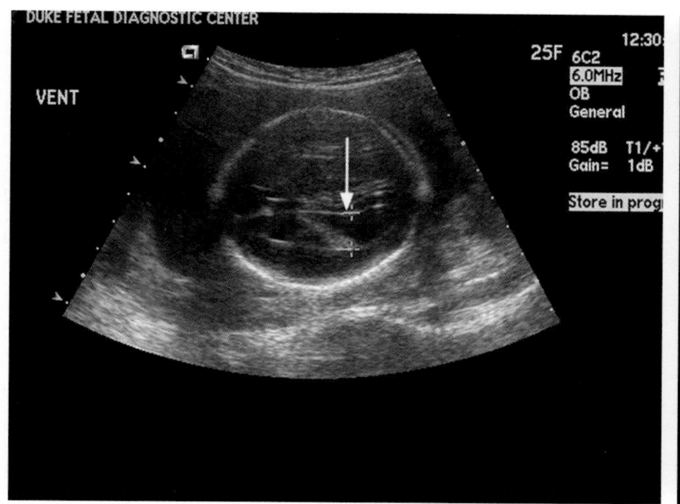

A

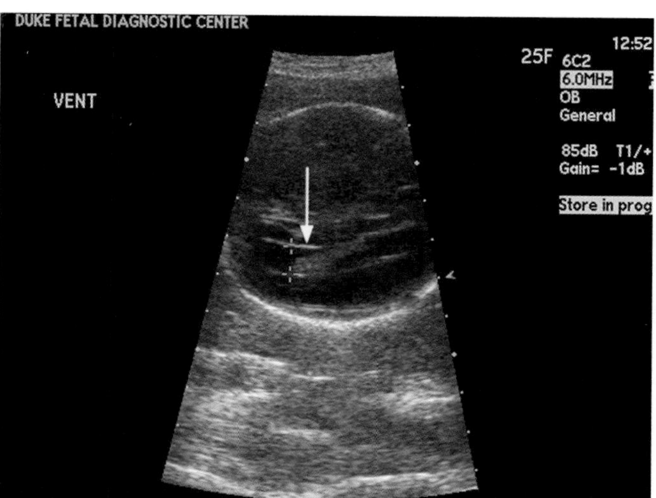

B

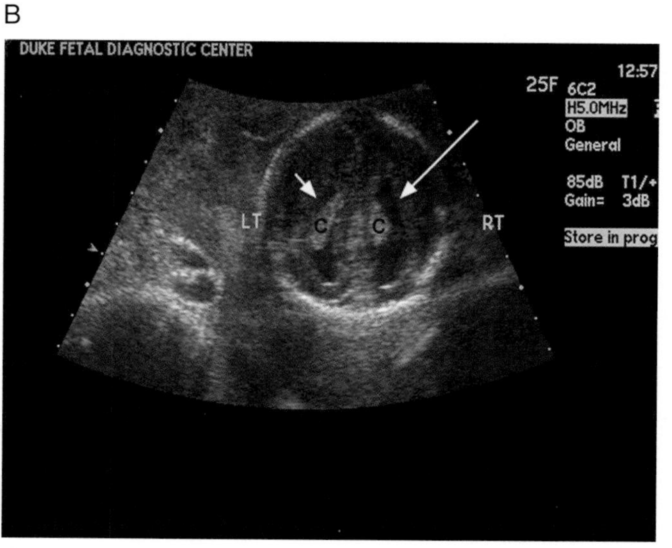

C

Figure 15-10 Unilateral mild ventriculomegaly. **A,** Axial image of fetal head during the second trimester shows mild ventriculomegaly *(arrow)* with a dangling choroid plexus. The atrium of the lateral ventricle measured 11.6 mm in width. **B,** Axial image of same fetus as in **A**, obtained after the fetus changed position, shows the contralateral ventricle *(arrow)* is not dilated. The atrium of the lateral ventricle measured 7.2 mm in width. **C,** Coronal image of head confirms the presence of unilateral ventriculomegaly. The left lateral ventricle *(short arrow)* is normal in appearance but there is mild dilatation of the right lateral ventricle *(long arrow)*. C, choroid plexus.

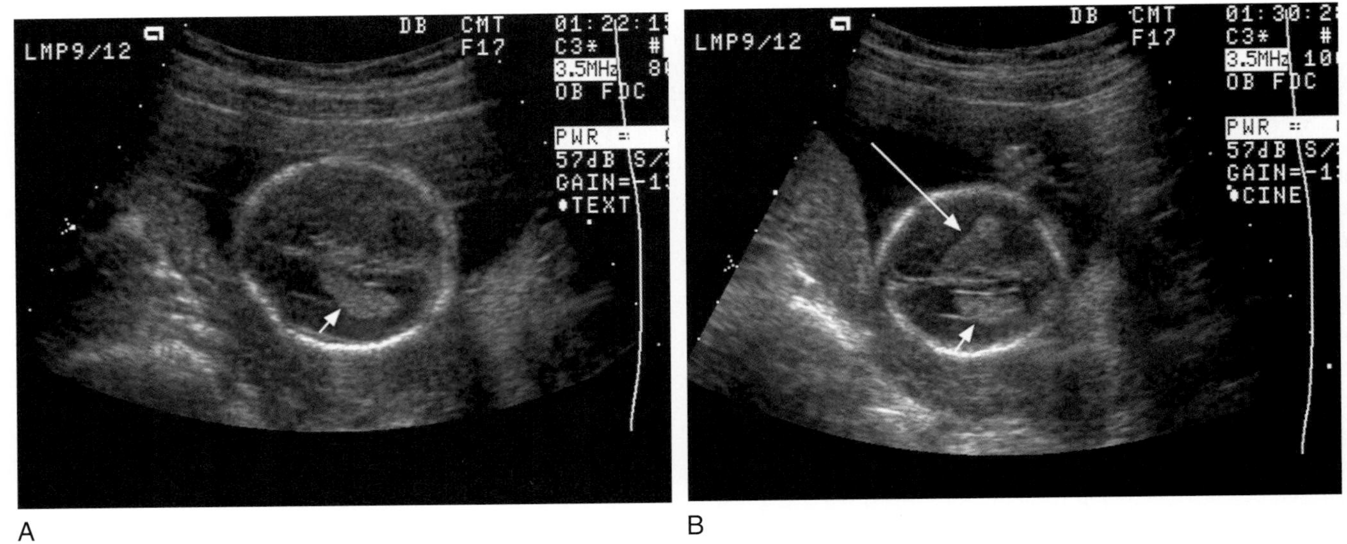

Figure 15-11 Visualization of near-field lateral ventricle. **A,** Axial scan of fetal head at 17 weeks fails to depict the near-field lateral ventricle due to reverberation artifact. The far-field lateral ventricle *(arrow)* is seen. **B,** Adjustment of the scan plane used in **A** facilitates visualization of the choroid plexus in the near-field lateral ventricle *(long arrow)*. The far-field lateral ventricle *(short arrow)* is again seen.

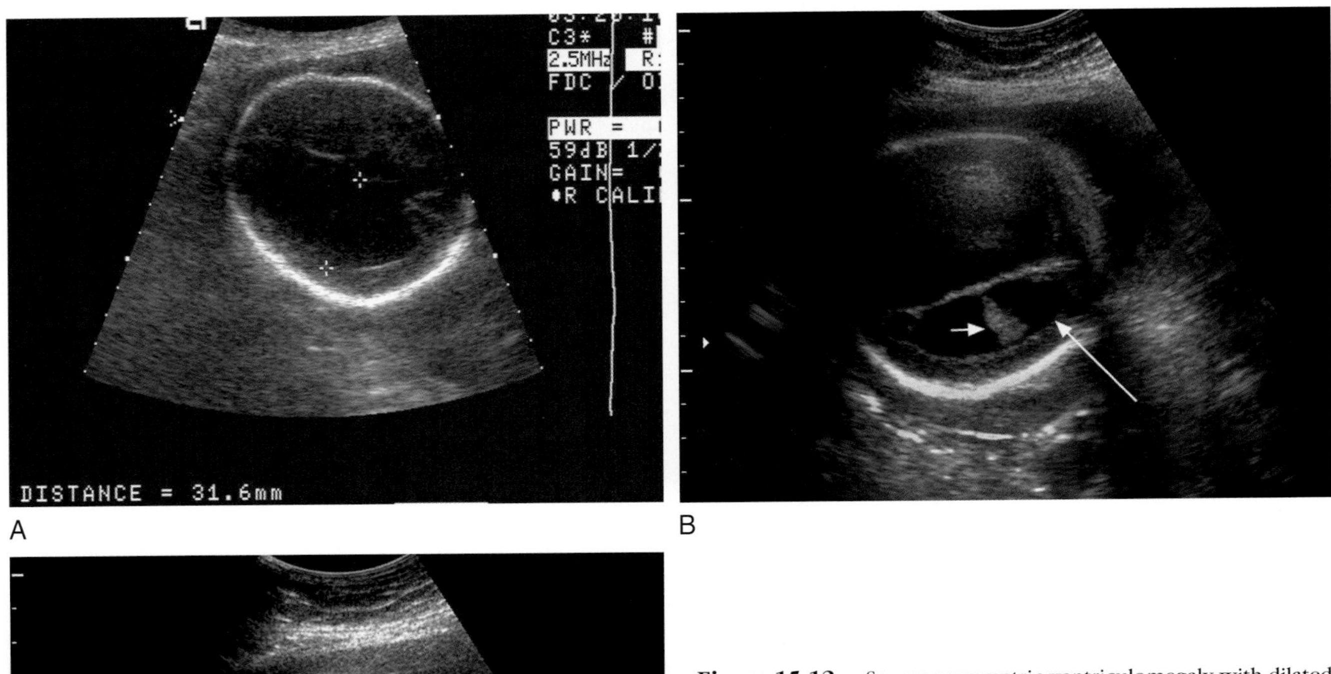

F
F
C

Figure 15-12 Severe asymmetric ventriculomegaly with dilated frontal horns and third ventricle. **A,** Axial image of fetal head at 25 weeks shows severe dilatation of atrium of lateral ventricle (cursors), which measured 31.6 mm in width. **B,** Axial scan of head performed 2 weeks after **A** with the fetus in a different position shows the contralateral ventricle *(long arrow)* is also dilated, with a dangling choroid plexus *(short arrow)*. This ventricle is less dilated than the ventricle in **A**. **C,** Coronal image of head of same fetus shows dilatation of the frontal horns (F) and the third ventricle *(long arrow)*. The dilated third ventricle extends between the thalami *(short arrows)* and splays the thalami apart.

causing the obstruction is seen, certain types of posterior fossa abnormalities are identified, or the falx echo is disrupted. On occasion, a dilated third ventricle can also be seen, although this may be misleading when there is an enlarged high-riding third ventricle in such developmental conditions as agenesis of the corpus callosum.

Head enlargement is only occasionally present. In most cases, unless the hydrocephalus is pronounced, the fetal head size remains normal and in proportion to the fetal body. Enlargement of any body part is somewhat arbitrarily defined but is usually considered increased when 2 SD or more above the norm. In obstetrical ultrasound, on average, each 1 SD is equivalent to 3 mm with 2 SD = 6 mm. Therefore, for the fetal head to be considered enlarged, the area-corrected BPD (BPDa) would need to be more than 6 mm larger than the average abdominal diameter (assuming a normal body size). A circumference measurement uses the equation for a circumference of a circle = diameter × π. At 2 SD the head circumference would need to be more than 18 mm (6 mm × π) larger than the abdominal circumference (again assuming a normal body size). Another approach is to use gestational age. If the true fetal age is known, the head would need to be larger than its expected size by at least 2 weeks.

A dilated third ventricle would be rounded or triangular and exceed 3 mm in diameter (Fig. 15-13; see also Fig. 15-12C). Posterior fossa abnormalities that suggest ventricular enlargement are due to increased pressure (hydrocephalus) and include an abnormally enlarged cisterna magna, seen as a component of a Dandy-Walker malformation, or a small or obliterated cisterna magna with abnormal cerebellar shape, due to an Arnold-Chiari type II malformation (see later discussion). Lastly, a disrupted falx midline echo, imaged as a wavy line within the dilated ventricles, is very suggestive of marked hydrocephalus (Fig. 15-14A).

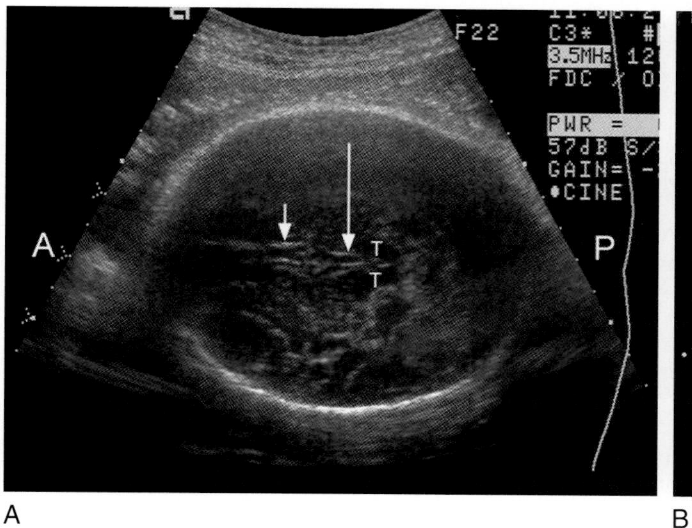

A

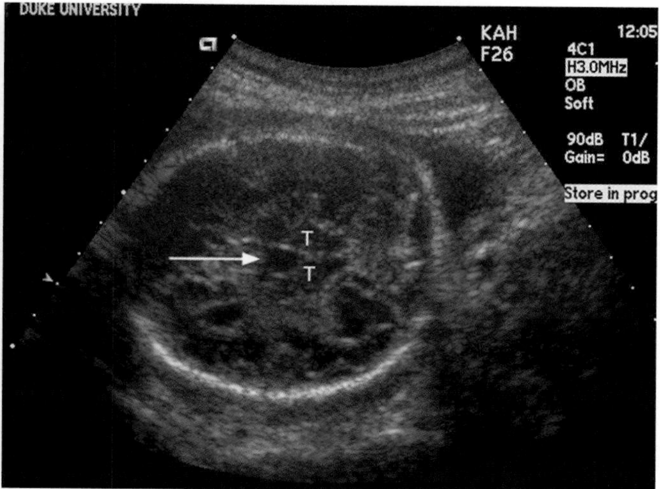

B

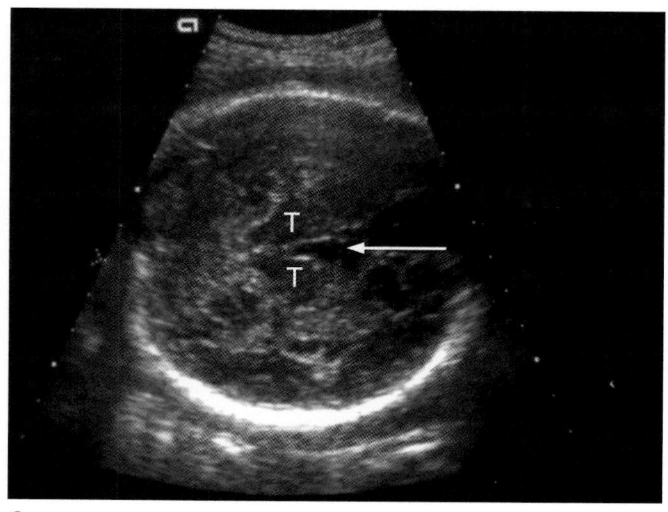

C

Figure 15-13 Examples of normal and enlarged third ventricles. **A,** Axial image of fetal head at 37 weeks shows normal third ventricle *(long arrow)* between the thalami (T). The cavum septum pellucidum *(short arrow)* is located anterior to the third ventricle. A, anterior; P, posterior. **B,** Axial image of fetal head at 26 weeks shows dilated third ventricle *(arrow)* as a rounded fluid-filled structure between the thalami (T). **C,** Axial image of fetal head at 27 weeks shows dilated third ventricle *(arrow)* as a triangular fluid-filled structure between the thalami (T).

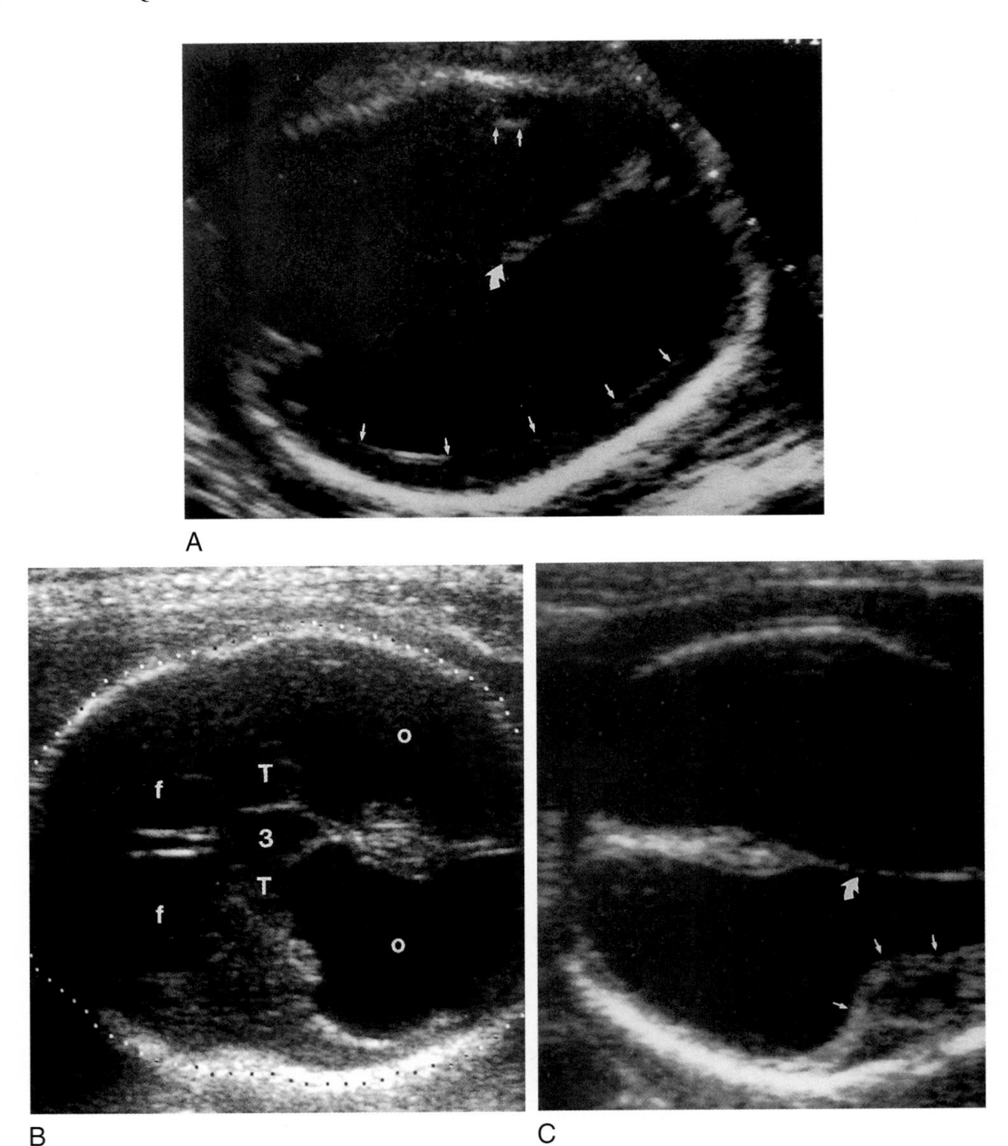

Figure 15-14 Comparison of marked hydrocephalus to hydranencephaly in three third-trimester fetuses. **A,** Hydrocephalus. A disrupted falx midline echo is detected, with the edge denoted by a *curved arrow.* Despite the marked ventriculomegaly, a thin mantle of parenchyma can still be identified *(small arrows)*, and this is better seen on the far side of the head. **B,** Hydrocephalus. Transaxial image of the head shows marked spreading of the thalami (T) caused by a markedly dilated third ventricle (3). The occipital horns (o) and the frontal horns (f) of the lateral ventricles are also markedly dilated. The enlarged head (compared with the body) is outlined by a *dotted line.* **C,** Hydranencephaly. There is an intact falx echo *(curved arrow)*. Although a small amount of residual tissue *(small arrows)* still remains in the occipital region, the frontal and parietal regions on both the near and far side of the head do not have a mantle of cortical tissue. This is consistent with brain parenchymal destruction. The head is larger than the body.

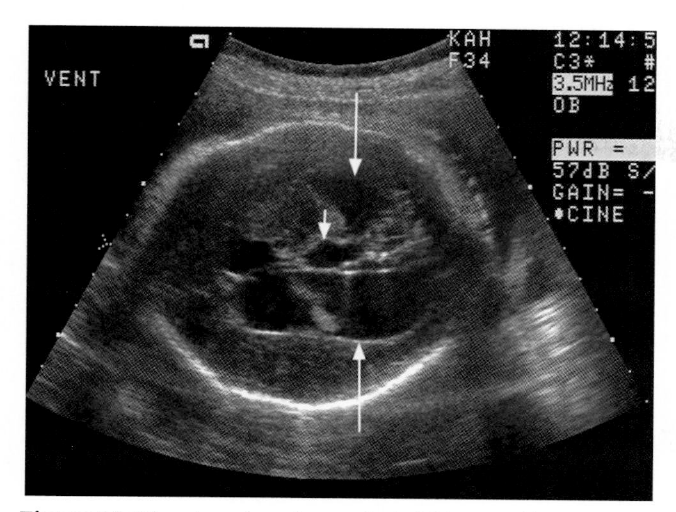

Figure 15-15 Aqueductal stenosis. Axial image of head of third-trimester fetus with aqueductal stenosis shows dilated lateral *(long arrows)* and third ventricles *(short arrow)*. The fourth ventricle (not shown) was not dilated.

Although hydrocephalus can be diagnosed accurately, the precise level of obstruction cannot always be identified. As a rule of thumb, the level of obstruction is never higher than the lowest dilated structure, but it may be lower. The sonographic finding of only lateral ventricular dilatation, for example, is rarely an obstruction at the foramen of Monro; the obstruction is usually lower. If the lateral and third ventricles are dilated, in the absence of other intracranial abnormalities, the hydrocephalus may be at the aqueduct of Sylvius (Fig. 15-15) but may be at the level of the fourth ventricle or even part of a communicating hydrocephalus.

In all cases of hydrocephalus, regardless of severity, there is always a residual rim or mantle of brain parenchyma (see Fig. 15-14A and B). This is in contradistinction to a condition called hydranencephaly, or "water head" (see Fig. 15-14C). Hydranencephaly results from destruction of the brain parenchyma in the frontal, temporal, and parietal regions, with the lateral ventricles expanding to fill in the space left by the destroyed brain (the ex vacuo phenomenon). It is most commonly caused by thrombosis of both middle cerebral arteries or an in utero infection. The occipital lobes, posterior fossa, and brain stem regions are typically normal because the posterior cerebral circulation has not been disrupted. Unlike the more common hydrocephalus, with its variable long-term prognosis (even on occasion normal), hydranencephaly is a lethal condition.

The sonographic appearance of the fetal brain in hydranencephaly varies from the visualization of irregular areas (if the destruction is ongoing) to a complete absence of brain in the frontal and temporoparietal areas. No cortical mantle is visible. The head is typically enlarged and even continues to grow as the fetus matures. Although the reason for this enlargement is not known, the continued production of cerebrospinal fluid from the intact choroid plexuses with impaired resorption appears to cause increased pressure and continued enlargement. The falx midline echo is usually maintained but may be disrupted, owing to the increased intraventricular pressure. Severe hydrocephalus with marked cortical thinning may be difficult to differentiate from advanced hydranencephaly by either ultrasound or MRI.

MICROCEPHALY

Microcephaly (small brain) has many causes. Among the most common are some of the TORCH infections (rubella, cytomegalovirus, and herpes simplex), developmental abnormalities (particularly holoprosencephaly), and genetic conditions (especially trisomies) (Fig. 15-16). Toxoplasmosis (the "T" in TORCH) is an in utero infection that can affect the fetal brain but is not typically associated with microcephaly. Less commonly, pollutants such as radiation, toxins, and heavy metals can be causative agents.

The incidence of microcephaly is known from mental institution statistics to range from 1:6000 to 1:8500 births. However, not infrequently, affected fetuses die in utero or in infancy and are not counted. The true incidence is undoubtedly higher. Microcephaly must take into account a clinically significant small head, with the likelihood of concomitant small brain and mental retardation. Microcephaly has been found to be clinically significant when the BPD or HC is more than 3 SD below the norm. If the BPD or HC is smaller but by only 1 or 2 SD, with no other anomaly, the prognosis is variable and often normal.

For microcephaly to be sonographically diagnosed, the head must measure smaller than expected by 3 SD. Based on the same concept that 1 SD = 3 mm (discussed earlier), at 3 SD *below* the norm the BPDa would be expected to be less than 9 mm smaller than the abdominal diameter and the head circumference less than 27 mm smaller than the abdominal circumference (both assuming a normal body). Alternatively, some investigators have suggested the size of the head should lag behind that of the body by 3 or more gestational weeks.

If the lateral ventricles are seen to be dilated in conjunction with a small head, this suggests loss of brain parenchyma with the ex vacuo enlargement of the lateral ventricles expanding to fill the void. Concomitant intracranial calcifications, both periventricular and parenchymal, suggest the presence of cytomegalovirus infection (Fig. 15-17). If calcifications are seen in a normal-sized head, however, toxoplasmosis may instead be the causative infection. These hyperechoic areas do not always shadow. In the appropriate clinical setting

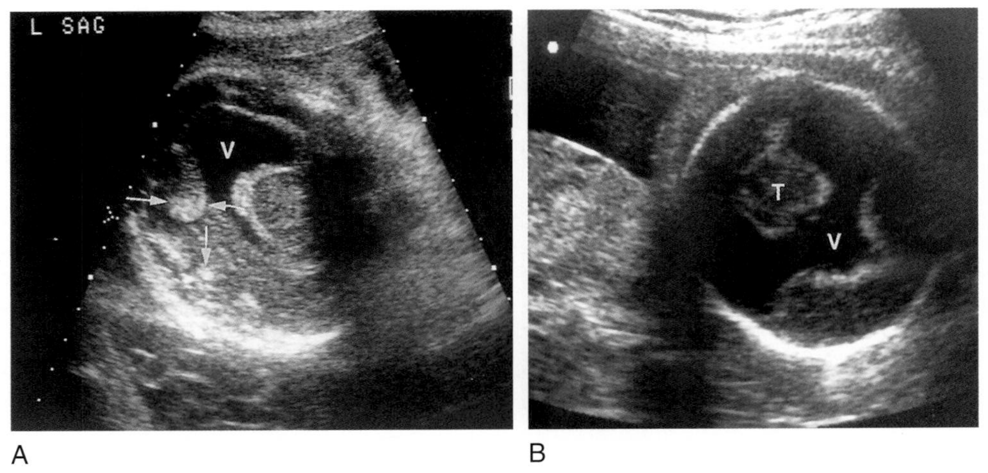

Figure 15-16 Two cases of microcephaly. **A,** Cytomegalovirus infection at 22 weeks. The parasagittal image through the left lateral ventricle (V) shows a dilated ventricle and both periventricular and intraparenchymal hyperechoic calcifications *(arrows)* in a small head. Note that there is no distal acoustic shadowing. **B,** Alobar holoprosencephaly at 17 weeks. This coronal image shows fused thalami (T) and a single ventricle, or monoventricle (V). Some ill-defined occipital tissue has formed superior to the ventricle. Hypotelorism (not shown) is also detected.

these areas may instead represent the tubers of tuberous sclerosis. If further differentiation is needed, an in utero MRI or a neonatal CT or MRI could be of value.

Holoprosencephaly is a midline developmental anomaly that comprises a spectrum of malformations affecting the brain and face, owing to failure of cleavage of brain parenchyma during forebrain development in the first trimester. Its reported incidence varies widely in the literature, from 1:2,000 to 1:16,000 births. Holoprosencephaly is frequently associated with chromosomal abnormalities, most commonly trisomy 13 (Fig. 15-18), but also with 18P syndrome, 13Q syndrome,

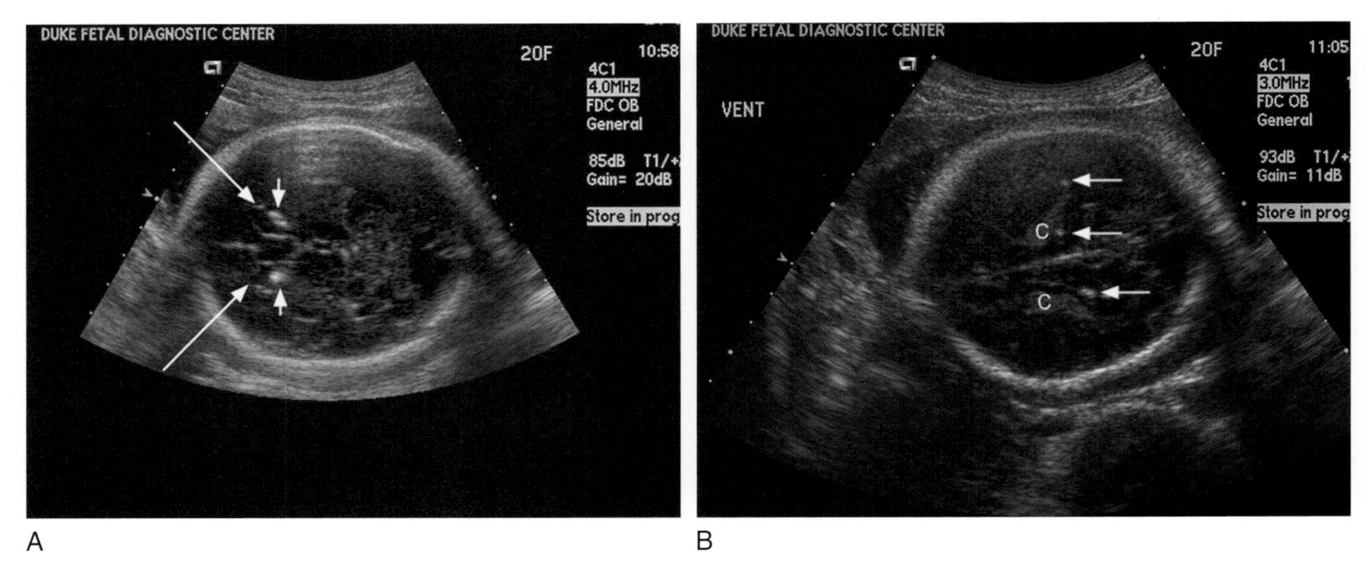

Figure 15-17 Intracranial calcifications due to cytomegalovirus infection. **A,** Axial image of head of second-trimester fetus shows prominence of the frontal horns *(long arrows)* of the lateral ventricles with adjacent periventricular calcifications *(short arrows)*. **B,** Calcifications *(short arrows)* are also seen adjacent to the atria of the lateral ventricles. C, choroid plexus.

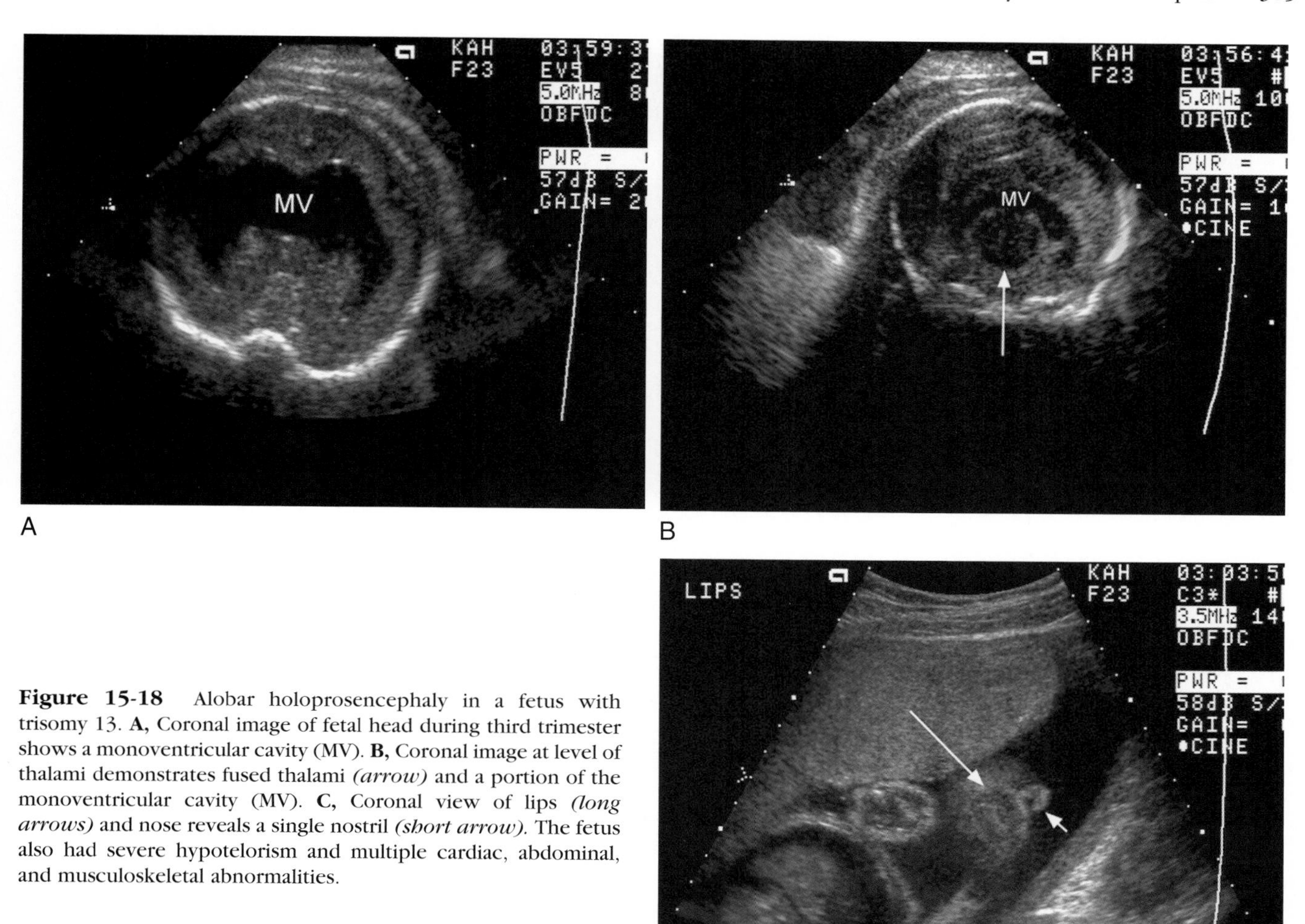

Figure 15-18 Alobar holoprosencephaly in a fetus with trisomy 13. **A,** Coronal image of fetal head during third trimester shows a monoventricular cavity (MV). **B,** Coronal image at level of thalami demonstrates fused thalami *(arrow)* and a portion of the monoventricular cavity (MV). **C,** Coronal view of lips *(long arrows)* and nose reveals a single nostril *(short arrow)*. The fetus also had severe hypotelorism and multiple cardiac, abdominal, and musculoskeletal abnormalities.

and triploidy. It is classified into three main forms termed *alobar, semilobar,* and *lobar holoprosencephaly* (from most to least severe).

In the alobar form there is a single monoventricular cavity in association with fused thalami, absence of midline structures such as the falx cerebri and cavum, and facial abnormalities. The monoventricular cavity may communicate with a dorsal cyst, replacing the usual configuration of the ventricular system (Fig. 15-19A). Brain tissue surrounds the monoventricular cavity, forming an anterior wedge of tissue resembling a boomerang. A wide range of midline facial abnormalities such as cyclopia, proboscis, severe hypotelorism, and cleft lip/palate are seen. Overall head size can be normal, macrocephalic, or microcephalic (see Fig. 15-16). The semilobar form is of intermediate severity and consists of partial development and separation of the lateral ventricles with a monoventricular cavity anteriorly that communicates with partially formed lateral ventricles posteriorly. The thalami and basal ganglia are typically fused and, as in the alobar form, facial anomalies are common and the head can be small, large, or of normal size. The least severe form is lobar holoprosencephaly, in which the head is normal in size with absence of the frontal horns of the lateral ventricles and cavum septi pellucidi.

The alobar form can be sonographically diagnosed by the early second trimester because of its obvious intracranial and frequently additional abnormalities: midline defects of the face (>80% of cases) (see Figs. 15-18 and 15-19), heart, and abdomen. The semilobar form with its partially developed lateral ventricles and falx can often be detected by the mid-second trimester. The lobar form is most difficult to diagnose. Its ultrasound findings resemble those of agenesis of the corpus callosum, and the two disorders can be indistinguishable at antenatal sonography. Although examiners are not asked to routinely identify the frontal horns during a routine fetal

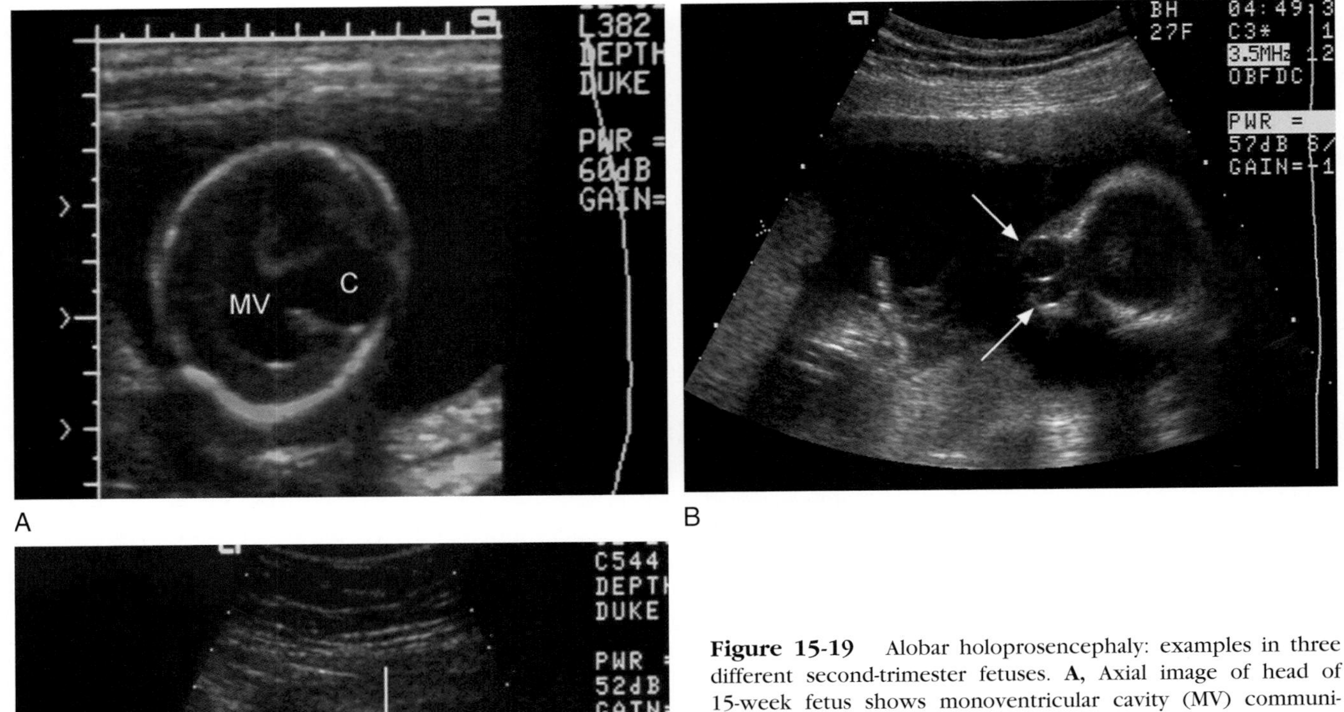

Figure 15-19 Alobar holoprosencephaly: examples in three different second-trimester fetuses. **A,** Axial image of head of 15-week fetus shows monoventricular cavity (MV) communicating with a dorsal cyst (C) posteriorly. Note that the wedge of brain tissue anterior to the monoventricular cavity has a configuration resembling a boomerang. **B,** Coronal image of head of 18-week fetus with holoprosencephaly shows malformed orbits *(arrows)* and severe hypotelorism. **C,** Coronal image of head and cervicothoracic spine of a 16-week fetus with holoprosencephaly shows monoventricular cavity (MV), fused thalami *(arrow)*, and microcephaly.

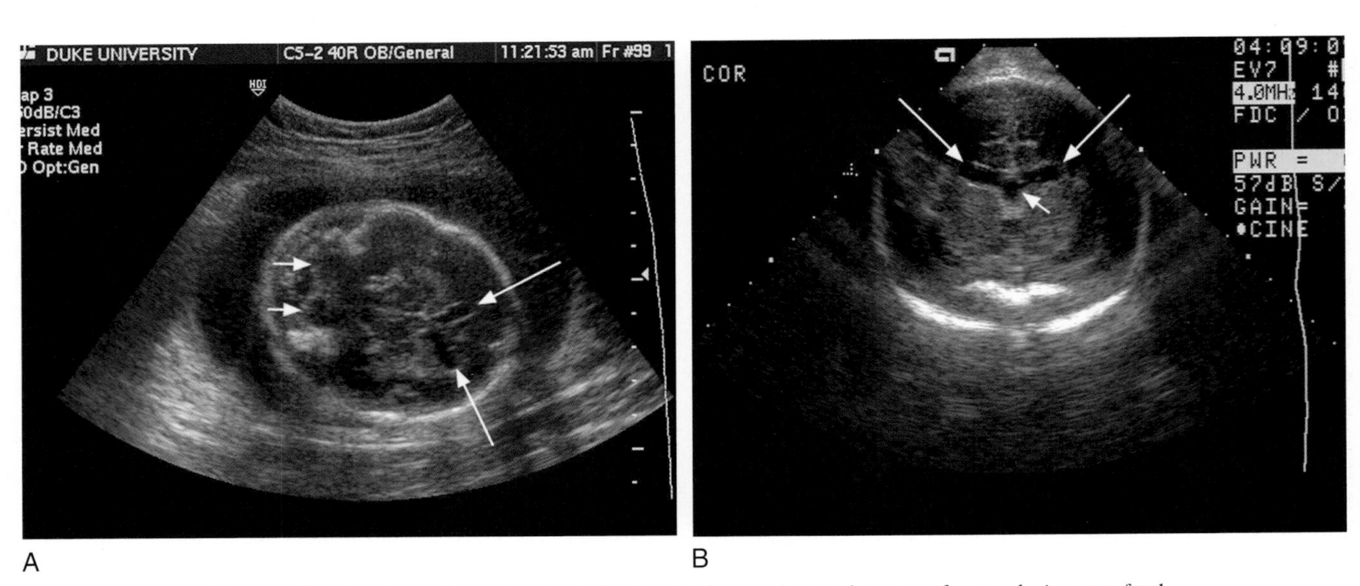

Figure 15-20 Scan planes for depicting frontal horns. **A,** Axial image of second-trimester fetal head with scan plane tilted superiorly toward frontal bone shows cerebellar hemispheres *(short arrows)* in the posteroinferior portion of head and mildly dilated frontal horns *(long arrows)* anteriorly. **B,** Coronal image through anterior portion of a different fetus with dilated ventricles shows dilated frontal horns *(long arrows)* on either side of the cavum septum pellucidum *(short arrow)*.

examination, these can be seen in an axial image of the head or one tilted superiorly toward the frontal bone (similar in angulation to that used to identify the posterior fossa inferiorly) or in a coronal scan plane obtained through the anterior portion of the head (Fig. 15-20).

FACIAL STRUCTURES

Facial anomalies can be isolated or associated with more complex anomalies and/or karyotype abnormalities. Although analysis of the face is not considered a part of the routine antepartum ultrasound evaluation, a number of normal facial structures can be identified.

Cleft lips and cleft palates are the most common congenital facial anomalies. A solitary cleft lip deformity occurs in 1:800 births; a combined cleft lip and palate occurs in 1:1300 births. Clefts vary in severity from involvement of only the soft tissues of the upper lip to posterior extension into the hard and even into the soft palate. Occasionally, the palate can be affected without involvement of the soft tissues. If only an isolated palate abnormality is present, it is usually not appreciated in utero.

Cleft defects can be single (central or eccentric) or bilateral. Eccentric and bilateral clefts are more deforming and more likely to be associated with additional abnormalities, including trisomies and holoprosencephaly. By scanning through the face in either the coronal or axial plane, depending on fetal position, or using 3-D ultrasound, the normal soft tissues of the lips can be identified (Fig. 15-21) and facial clefts can be seen (Fig. 15-22). The axial projection is preferred for confirming extension of abnormalities into the palate. As might be expected, the larger defects are easier to detect.

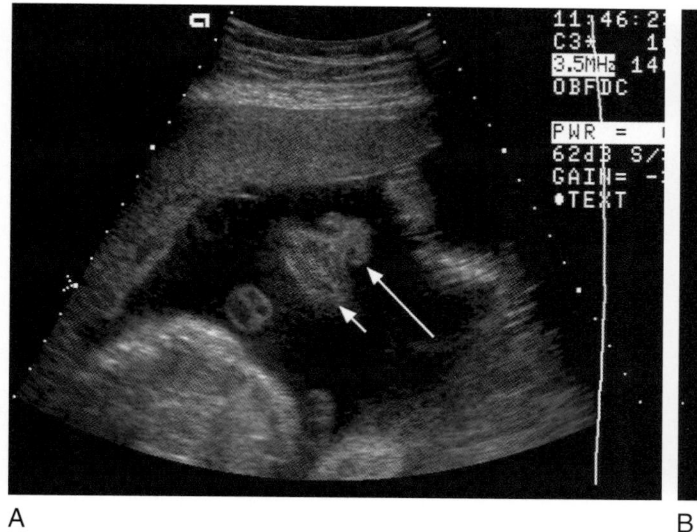
A

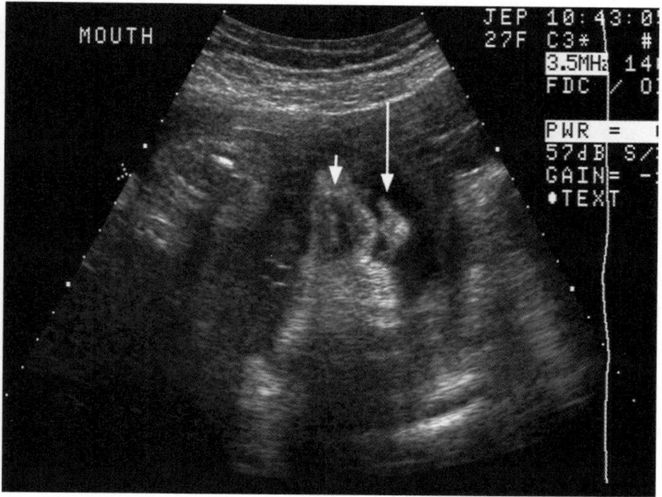

B

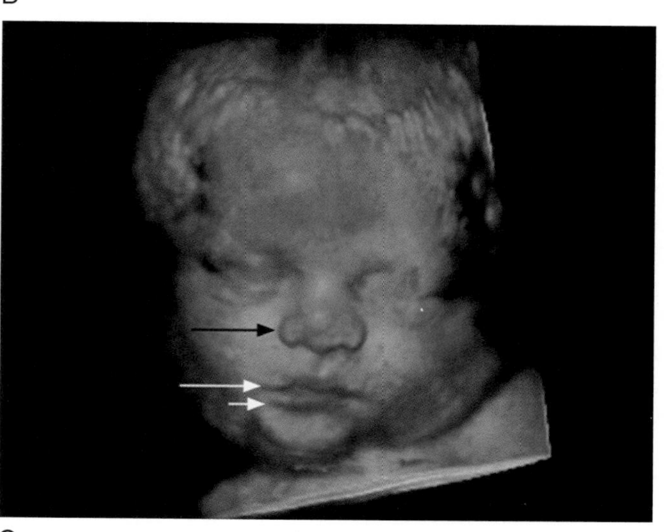
C

Figure 15-21 Nose and lips: examples in normal fetuses. **A,** Coronal image of anterior portion of face at 26 weeks shows normal appearance of nose *(long arrow)* and lips *(short arrow).* **B,** Coronal image of a 35-week fetus shows normal nose *(long arrow)* and lips *(short arrow).* **C,** Surface-rendered 3D image of 34-week fetal face shows normal nose *(black arrow)* and lips. *Long white arrow,* upper lip; *short white arrow,* lower lip.

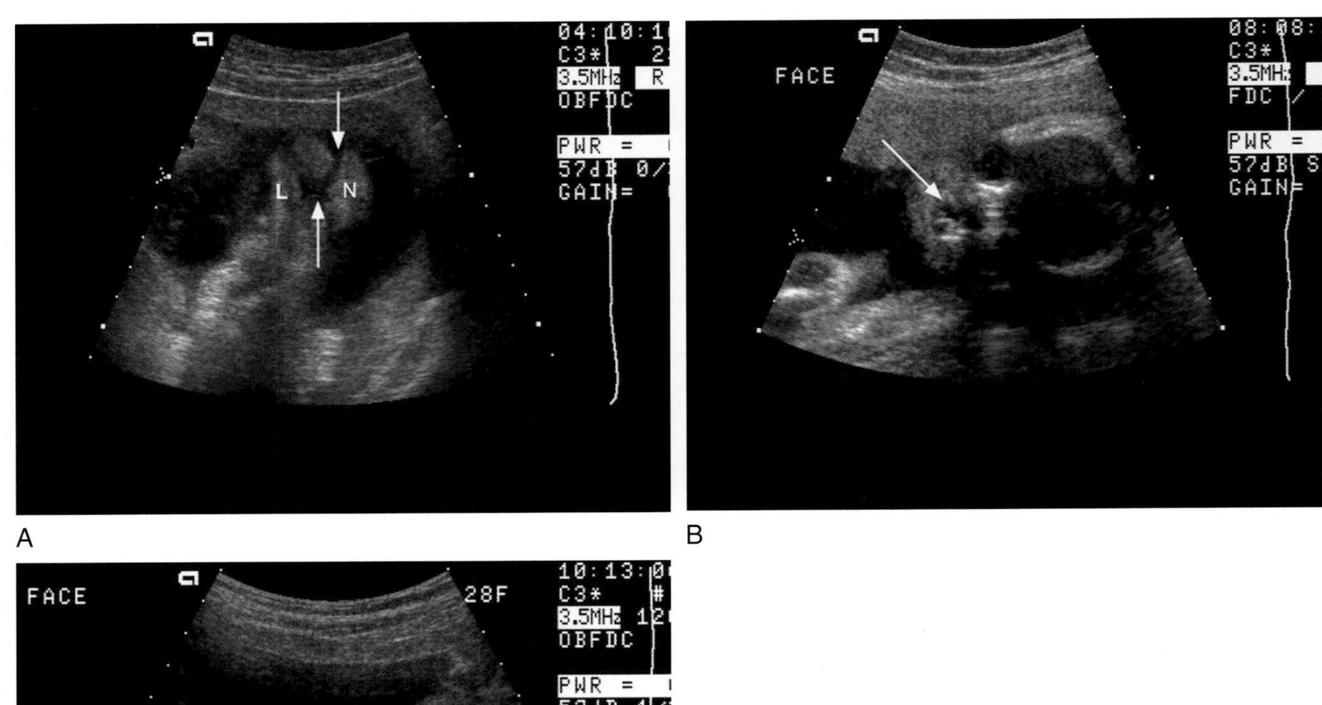

Figure 15-22 Cleft lip and palate. **A,** Coronal image of nose and lips of 34-week fetus shows large cleft *(arrows)* extending from upper lip into nose. L, lower lip; N, nose. **B,** Coronal image of face of third-trimester fetus with large cleft lip and palate shows gap in fetal face *(arrow).* **C,** Axial image of face of third-trimester fetus obtained at level of upper lip reveals cleft lip *(arrow).*

Interorbital distance can be determined by scanning either axially or coronally. An outer-to-outer diameter (OOD) can be measured and shows proportionate growth to the BPD and to the gestational age (Fig. 15-23). Inaccuracies of this measurement occur because the outer margins of the orbits are difficult to define, and errors of at least 2 to 3 mm are not uncommon. Nevertheless, hypotelorism (Fig. 15-24A) and hypertelorism (see Fig. 15-24B) can be confirmed by measurement of the OOD.

Detection of a small chin (micrognathia), a finding associated with trisomy 13, trisomy 18, triploidy, and a variety of other syndromes, is possible. Care must be taken in rendering this diagnosis. A true midline sagittal view of the face is necessary. Because the mandible normally tends to be small (relatively underdeveloped) in utero, only flattening should be interpreted as abnormal (Fig. 15-25).

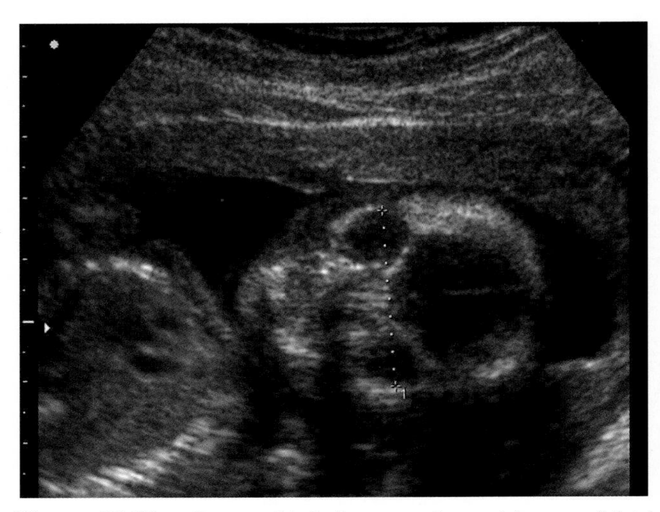

Figure 15-23 Outer orbital diameter. Coronal image of fetal face at 18 weeks shows measurement of outer orbital diameter *(cursors and dotted line)* from the outer edges of the bony orbits.

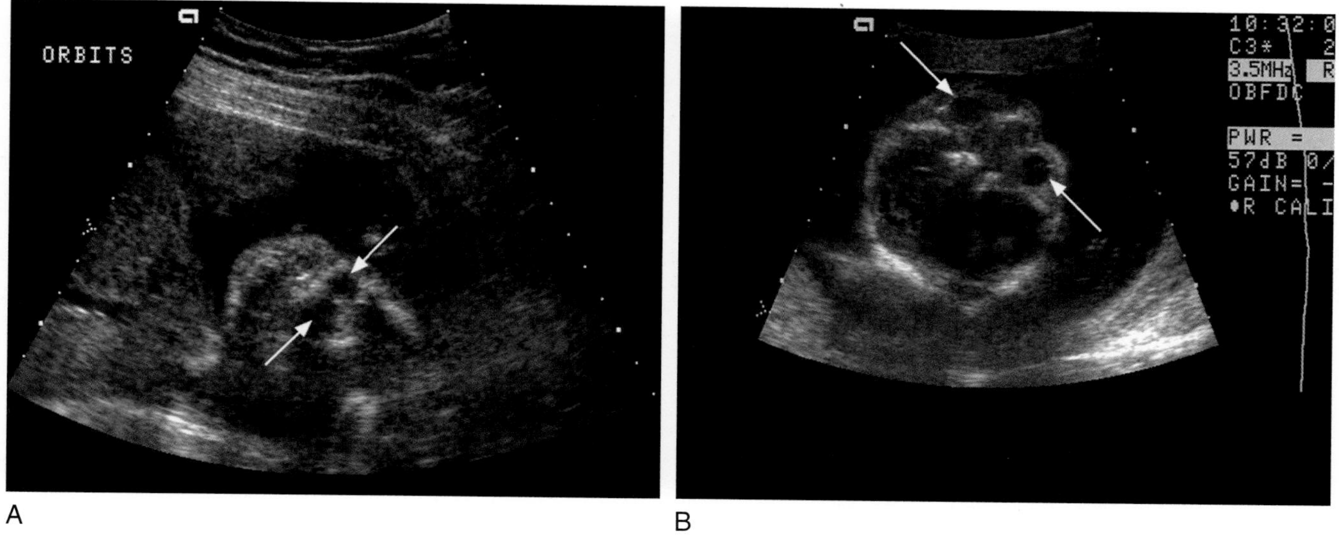

Figure 15-24 Hypotelorism and hypertelorism. **A,** Hypotelorism in a second-trimester fetus with holoprosencephaly. Coronal view of face shows the orbits *(arrows)* are too close together. **B,** Hypertelorism in a second-trimester fetus with multiple congenital anomalies. Axial view of head shows the orbits *(arrows)* are widely separated.

Facial tumors have also been sonographically identified. They are primarily isolated anomalies and yet can still be quite deforming and extensive. Hemangiomas are common; they are usually hyperechoic and somewhat compressible. Typically, no Doppler signal is detected because their blood flow is too slow. Teratomas are solid tumors, sometimes with cystic components, either confined to the face or extending into the neck and even to the thoracic outlet (Fig. 15-26). Concomitant polyhydramnios may be present, caused by an inability of normal swallowing. If large, teratomas can obstruct the airway and lead to serious respiratory compromise at the time of delivery. Some teratomas are very vascular, and color Doppler evaluation may be of value to analyze the extent of the tumor.

CEPHALOCELE

A cephalocele is a protrusion of intracranial structures through a calvarial defect. Cephaloceles fall into two categories: cranial meningoceles contain only

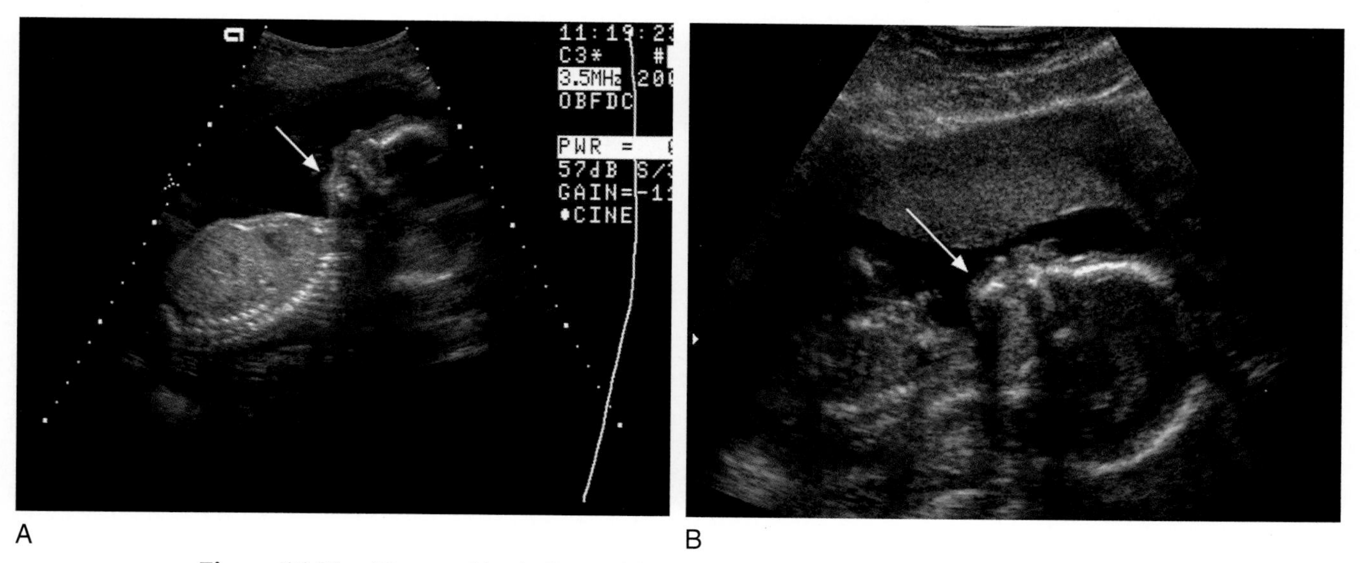

Figure 15-25 Micrognathia. **A,** View of face of second-trimester fetus with micrognathia and multiple other anomalies shows small recessed chin *(arrow)*. Compare with profile of normal fetus in **B**. **B,** Normal chin. Midline sagittal view of face of normal second-trimester fetus shows normal configuration of fetal chin *(arrow)*.

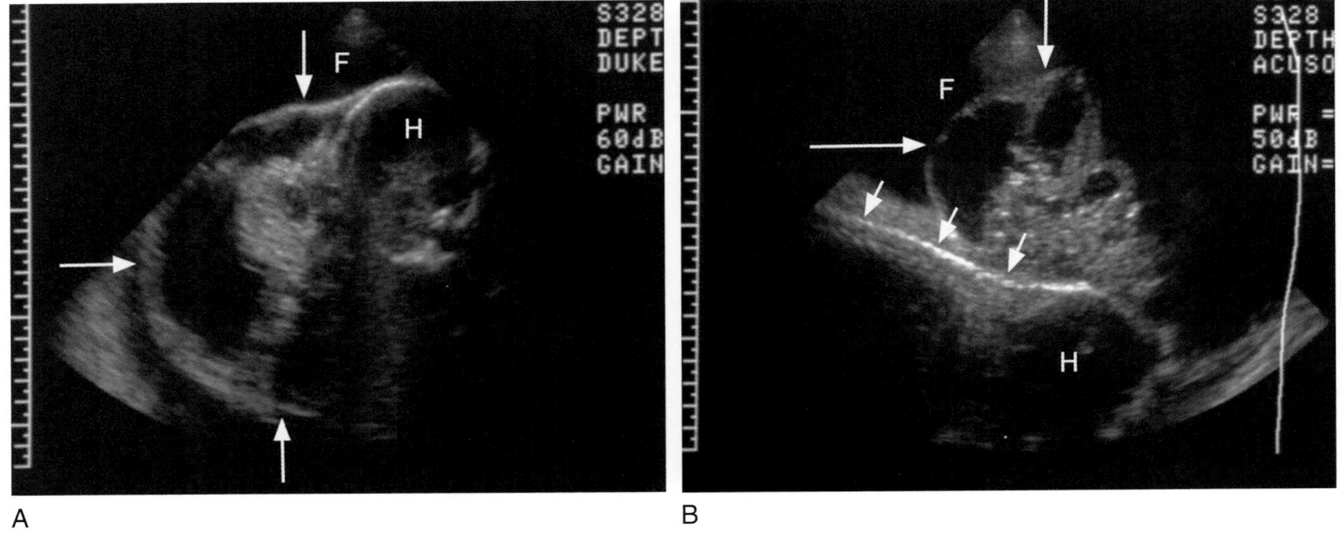

Figure 15-26 Facial and cervical teratoma. **A,** Oblique image of fetal head (H) during third trimester shows large complex tumor *(arrows)* with cystic and solid components extending laterally into amniotic fluid (F). **B,** Sagittal image of fetal head (H) and cervicothoracic spine *(short arrows)* shows the mass *(long arrows)* in **A** extends into the soft tissues of the posterior portion of the neck. Punctate foci of increased echogenicity in the mass corresponded to calcifications at histopathologic evaluation. F, amniotic fluid.

meninges, and encephaloceles contain brain tissue. Severity and prognosis are primarily related to the amount of brain within the defect. Because exposed brain is often dysmorphic, there is often a significant CNS deficit even if the brain can be surgically repaired. In addition, the incidence of additional associated CNS, extra-CNS, and chromosomal abnormalities is high.

Encephaloceles range in size from a small bubble of meninges that extends through the calvarium to nearly the entire brain (and meninges) located outside a collapsed calvarium (Fig. 15-27). In the latter, identification of the collapsed calvarium may be difficult and scanning up the spine to the skull base may be needed. Identification of the calvarial defect is critical in distinguishing encephaloceles from other diagnostic possibilities such as teratomas and cystic hygromas.

In the United States, particularly in the non-Asian population, at least 80% of the cephaloceles are posterior, extending through a defect in the occipital bone. With the exception of very small defects, occipital cephaloceles are relatively easy to detect, commonly identified on the routine axial head images. However, a cephalocele can occur anywhere along the midline, including at the top of the head and anteriorly within the ethmoidal sinus region. A cephalocele in the ethmoidal region may be very subtle, and because the facial structures are not routinely imaged during the fetal ultrasound evaluation, these defects may not be appreciated in utero.

THE POSTERIOR FOSSA AND NUCHAL SKIN

The posterior fossa is imaged starting with the standard axial view, at the level of the thalami or midbrain, with the transducer then tilted inferiorly toward the occiput. The bilobed cerebellum is identified by its two prominent hypoechoic lateral hemispheres and its smaller midline hyperechoic vermis (Fig. 15-28A). More posteriorly, the cisterna magna is imaged between the cerebellum and the occiput. The cisterna magna is the largest cistern of the head and contains anechoic cerebrospinal fluid, sometimes with additional normal hyperechoic strands thought to represent arachnoid septa.

The cerebellum and cisterna magna have expected sizes. The cerebellum is measured in the axial projection from the outer edges of its hemispheres. It grows steadily as the head grows and its size correlates with the BPD and gestational age. The cisterna magna, measured from the posterior margin of the cerebellar vermis to the inside of the occipital bone, is normally between 2 and 10 mm (see Fig. 15-28B).

The fourth ventricle can be seen anteriorly in the posterior fossa in up to 75% of normal fetuses during the second and third trimesters if specifically sought (see Fig. 15-28). The normal fourth ventricle increases in size with gestational age, both in anteroposterior and width dimensions, measuring up to 8 mm in width by term.

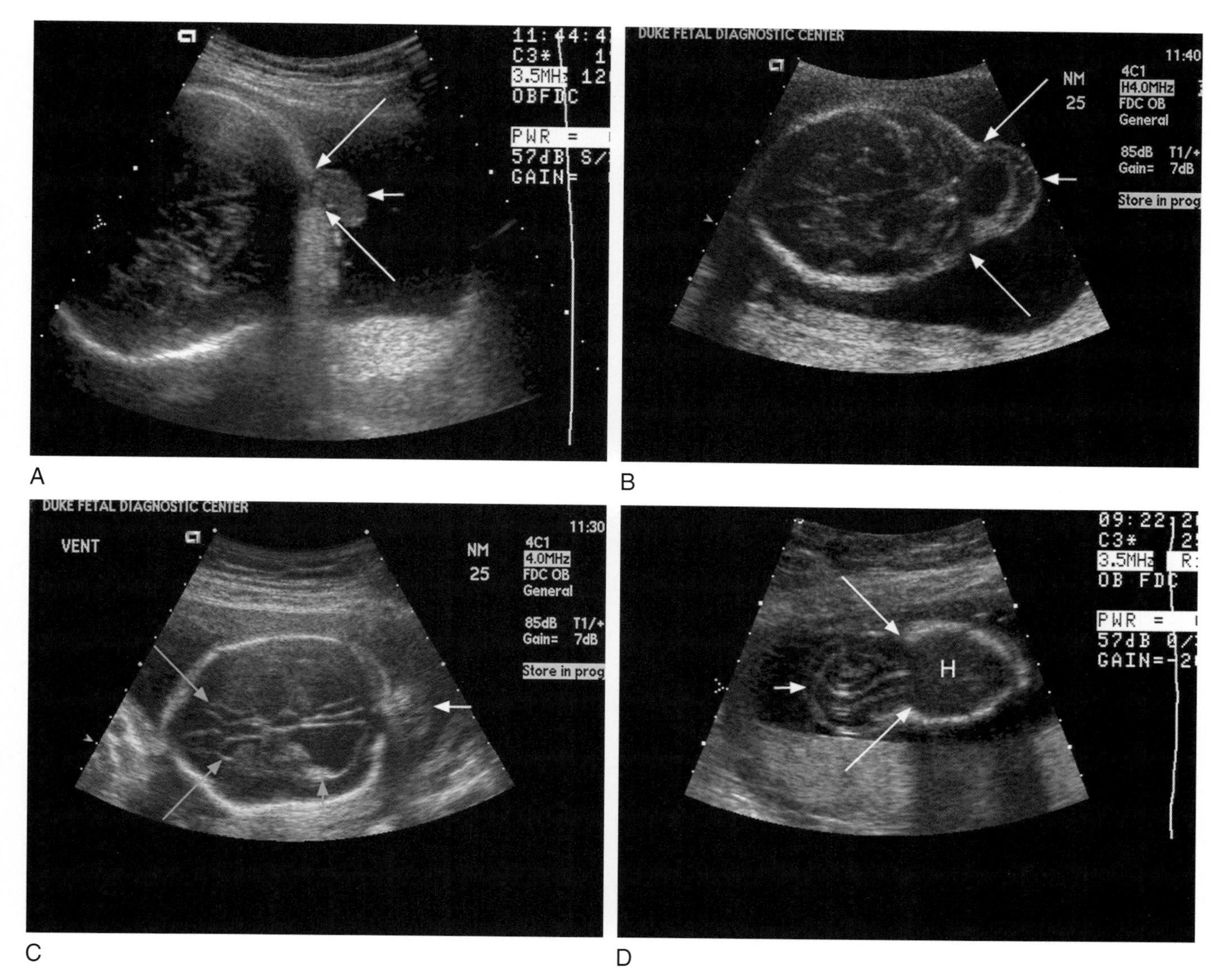

Figure 15-27 Encephalocele. Images of encephaloceles in three different fetuses depict a wide range of size and echo pattern. **A,** Oblique image of fetal head at 34 weeks shows a small occipital encephalocele *(short arrow)* protruding through a small calvarial defect *(long arrows).* **B,** Axial image of 24-week fetal head shows a predominantly cystic occipital encephalocele *(short arrow)* protruding through a large calvarial defect *(long arrows).* **C,** Axial image of same fetus as in **B** obtained cephalad to image in **B** shows solid component of the encephalocele *(short white arrow)* and hydrocephalus. *Long gray arrows,* dilated frontal horns; *short gray arrow,* dilated atrium of lateral ventricle. **D,** Axial image of head of a different fetus shows a large encephalocele *(short arrow)* protruding through a large calvarial defect *(long arrows).* The encephalocele is similar in size to the remainder of the head (H).

Its shape can be slit-like, triangular, or ovoid, or it can resemble a "boomerang" in configuration .

The cisterna magna can be abnormally small or large. An obliterated cisterna magna is caused by an Arnold-Chiari type II malformation, owing to downward displacement of the medulla oblongata and cerebellar structures into or through the foramen magnum. When the cisterna magna is obliterated, a neural tube defect is almost always the causative factor (see the section on neural tube defects). In contrast, when the cisterna magna is enlarged and the cerebellar hemispheres are splayed apart, the diagnosis is a Dandy-Walker malformation or Dandy-Walker variant. In Dandy-Walker anomalies a posterior fossa "cyst" communicates with the fourth ventricle (often referred to as "cystic dilatation of the fourth ventricle" due to vermian agenesis or hypoplasia) through a defect in the cerebellar vermis (Fig. 15-29). Dilatation of the lateral ventricles is often an associated finding.

The Dandy-Walker variant has ultrasound findings that are similar to but less severe than those of the Dandy-Walker malformation. In the variant, the posterior

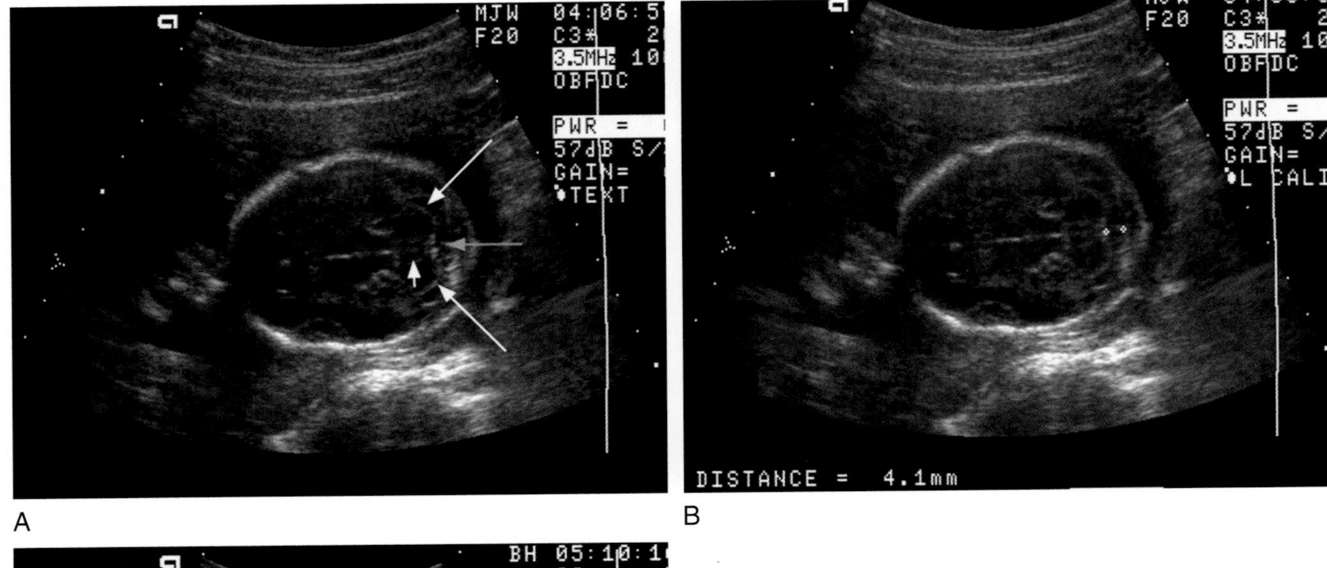

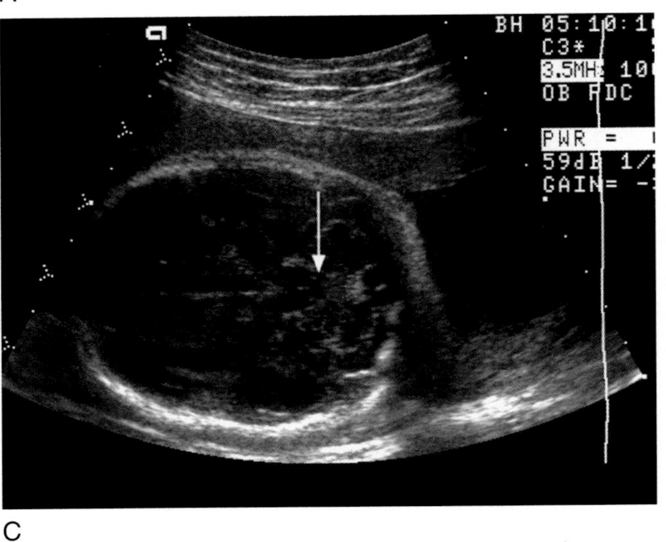

Figure 15-28 Posterior fossa and fourth ventricle. **A,** Axial image of normal 20-week fetal head at level of thalami, with transducer tilted inferiorly toward occiput demonstrates normal appearance of posterior fossa. Cerebellar hemispheres *(long white arrows),* cerebellar vermis *(short white arrow),* and cisterna magna *(gray arrow)* are seen. **B,** Image of same fetus as in **A** shows measurement of cisterna magna *(cursors).* The cisterna magna is measured from the posterior margin of the cerebellar vermis to the inside of the occipital bone. **C,** Axial image of head of a different fetus at 28 weeks shows normal fourth ventricle *(arrow)* in the anterior portion of the posterior fossa.

fossa cyst is smaller and does not enlarge the posterior fossa, vermian hypoplasia is milder, and the likelihood of ventricular dilatation is lower.

Dandy-Walker abnormalities are frequently associated with additional fetal anomalies (often midline), which include CNS malformations such as agenesis of the corpus callosum, cephalocele, and meningocele; extra-CNS abnormalities involving the cardiac, genitourinary, gastrointestinal, and musculoskeletal systems; and chromosomal aneuploidies. The CNS anomalies may be subtle, and in the more difficult cases a TV ultrasound study (if the fetal head is the presenting part) or a fetal MRI may be of value.

There are technical and developmental issues to be considered when assessing the axial view of the posterior fossa. The standard axial view of the cerebellum and the cisterna magna depicts the mid to upper part of the cerebellum, so a subtle abnormality of the inferior (lower) portion of the vermis may not be appreciated. On the other hand, too steep an angulation during scanning, into a semicoronal view angled toward the cervical spine, should also be avoided because it can create a false impression of an enlarged cisterna magna (Fig. 15-30). Ultrasound clues that suggest the scan plane has been angled too sharply include visualization of the posterior fossa and the cervical spine on the same image, apparent thickening of the soft tissues of the neck, and round head shape. Developmentally, the cerebellum is not completely formed until 16 to 18 weeks so a cleft can be seen between the cerebellar hemispheres in the expected position of the vermis as a normal embryologic event in some fetuses early in the second trimester. As a result, the diagnosis of Dandy-Walker variant should not be based solely on identification of a small vermian cleft in the absence of additional features before 18 weeks.

An enlarged cisterna magna, measuring more than 10 mm in anteroposterior diameter may, on occasion, be

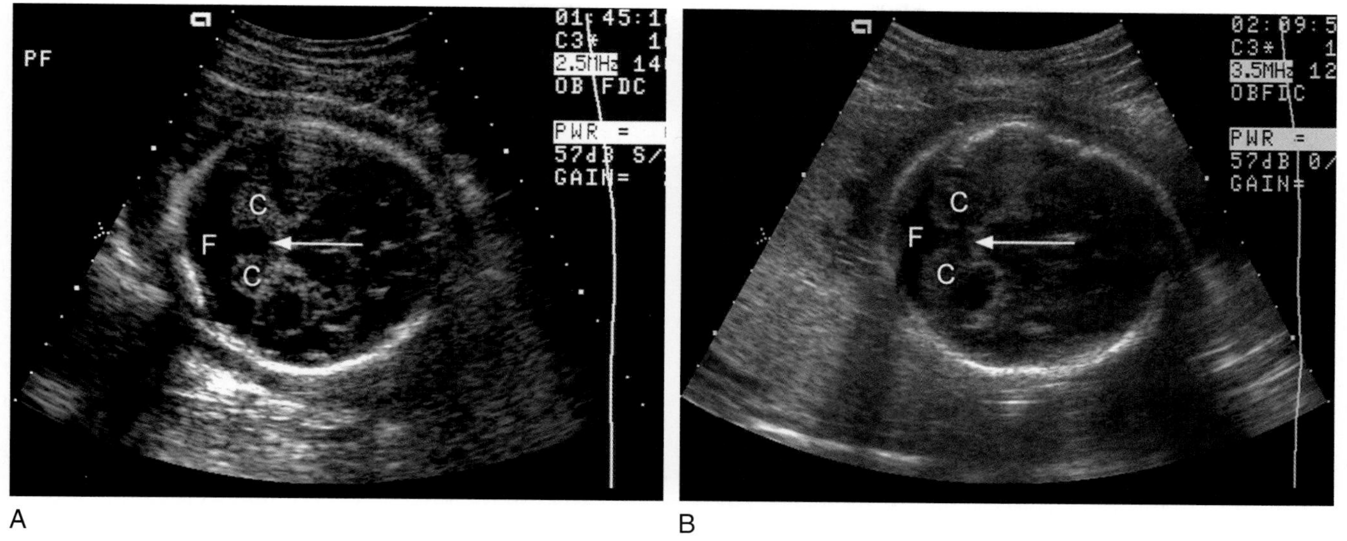

Figure 15-29 Dandy-Walker abnormality: examples in two fetuses. **A,** Axial image of head of second-trimester fetus with Dandy-Walker malformation shows large fluid collection (F) in posterior fossa, communicating with fourth ventricle *(arrow)* due to absence of cerebellar vermis. The cerebellar hemispheres (C) are splayed apart. **B,** Axial image of second-trimester fetus with Dandy-Walker variant and mild ventriculomegaly shows fluid (F) in posterior fossa communicating with fourth ventricle *(arrow)* across defect due to absence of cerebellar vermis. C, cerebellar hemispheres.

identified during routine posterior fossa imaging in an otherwise normal fetus (Fig. 15-31). If the vermis and fourth ventricle appear normal and a detailed fetal anatomic survey reveals no structural anomalies or technical issues, this is most likely a normal variant that is termed *megacisterna magna.*

A posterior fossa arachnoid cyst can also be the source of an abnormal fluid collection in the posterior fossa. Sonographic features that favor a posterior fossa arachnoid cyst include asymmetric location of the fluid, rounded cyst margins (Dandy-Walker cysts tend to be more triangular), and either normal cerebellar anatomy

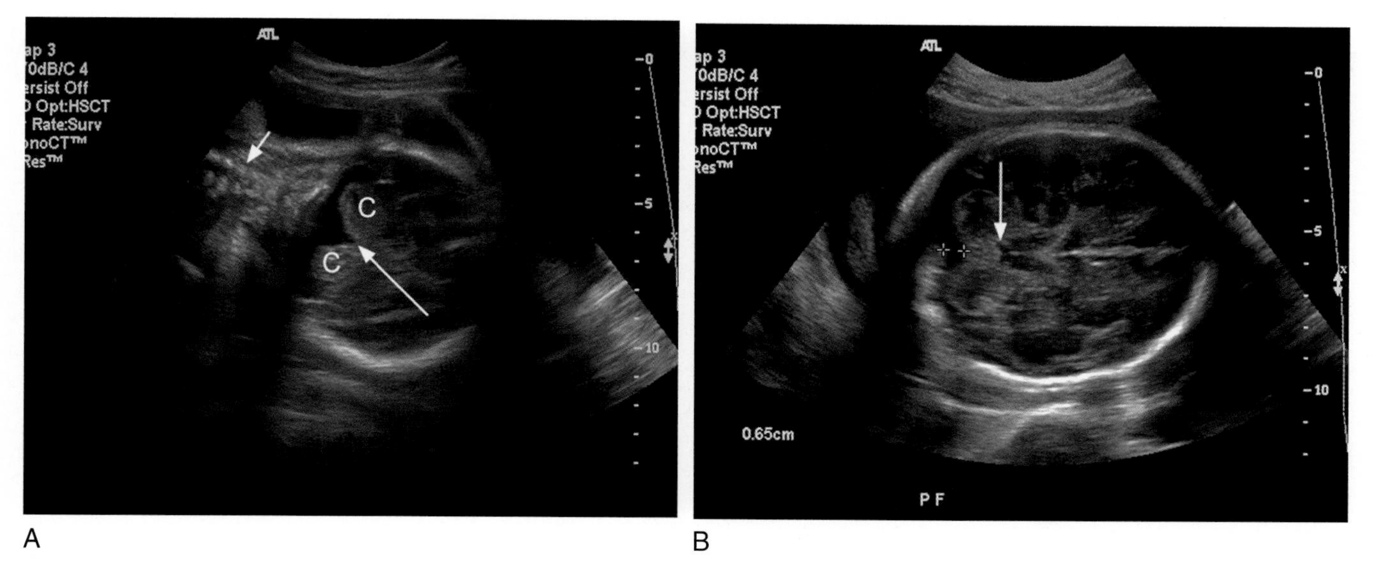

Figure 15-30 Spurious appearance of Dandy-Walker abnormality due to incorrect scan plane in a normal fetus. **A,** Image of posterior fossa in coronal scan plane shows apparent enlargement of cisterna magna *(long arrow)* suggesting a Dandy-Walker abnormality. Identification of cervical spine *(short arrow)* on same image as posterior fossa and rounded contour of fetal head suggest the scan plane is coronal rather than axial. C, cerebellar hemispheres. **B,** Image of same fetus in axial scan plane reveals normal posterior fossa. Cisterna magna measurement (cursors) of 6.5 mm is normal, and a normal fourth ventricle *(arrow)* is seen.

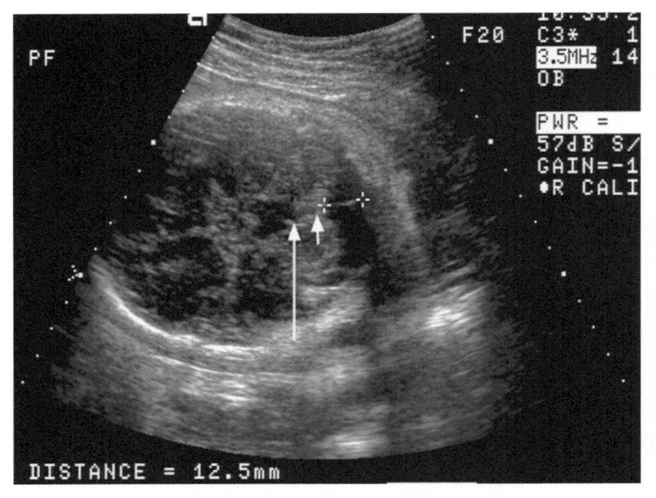

Figure 15-31 Megacisterna magna. Axial image of fetus, tilted inferiorly toward the occiput, shows enlarged cisterna magna *(cursors)*, which measures 12.5 mm. The cerebellar vermis *(short arrow)* and fourth ventricle *(long arrow)* are intact, distinguishing this example of megacisterna magna from a Dandy-Walker abnormality.

or en bloc displacement and compression of the cerebellar hemispheres in the absence of splaying or a vermian defect.

The nuchal fold refers to the layer of soft tissue identified immediately posterior to the occipital bone in the same scan plane as that used to identify the cerebellum and cisterna magna (Fig. 15-32). The anteroposterior diameter of the nuchal fold is measured in the midline in fetuses between 15 and 21 weeks and is considered abnormal if it is 6 mm or greater. The 6-mm threshold does not apply later in pregnancy because the nuchal skin often becomes redundant and thicker with advancing gestation. Some investigators use a slightly lower threshold of 5 mm before 18 weeks. Care must be taken not to angle too steeply toward the cervical spine, because this can falsely increase the nuchal fold measurement. A true increase in nuchal skin thickness (see Fig. 15-32B) is considered the most sensitive and specific single ultrasound marker for trisomy 21 (Down syndrome) during the mid-second trimester and is thought to detect approximately one third of fetuses with Down syndrome. Fetal karyotyping should be offered in the setting of a thick nuchal fold.

Earlier in the pregnancy, the nuchal region is also the site of a more recently described marker for aneuploidy. This is termed *nuchal translucency* and refers to the hypoechoic region along the posterior portion of the fetal neck. Nuchal translucency is measured earlier in pregnancy than the nuchal fold, from 11 to 14 weeks. An abnormally thickened nuchal translucency is highly correlated with aneuploidy, but it can also be seen with other conditions, including fetal cardiac abnormalities, diaphragmatic hernia, abdominal wall defects, skeletal dysplasias, and other fetal syndromes in the absence of aneuploidy. Trisomy 21 is the most commonly associated aneuploidy, although a variety of other abnormal karyotypes such as Turner's syndrome, trisomies 13 and 18, and triploidy have also been reported. Thickened

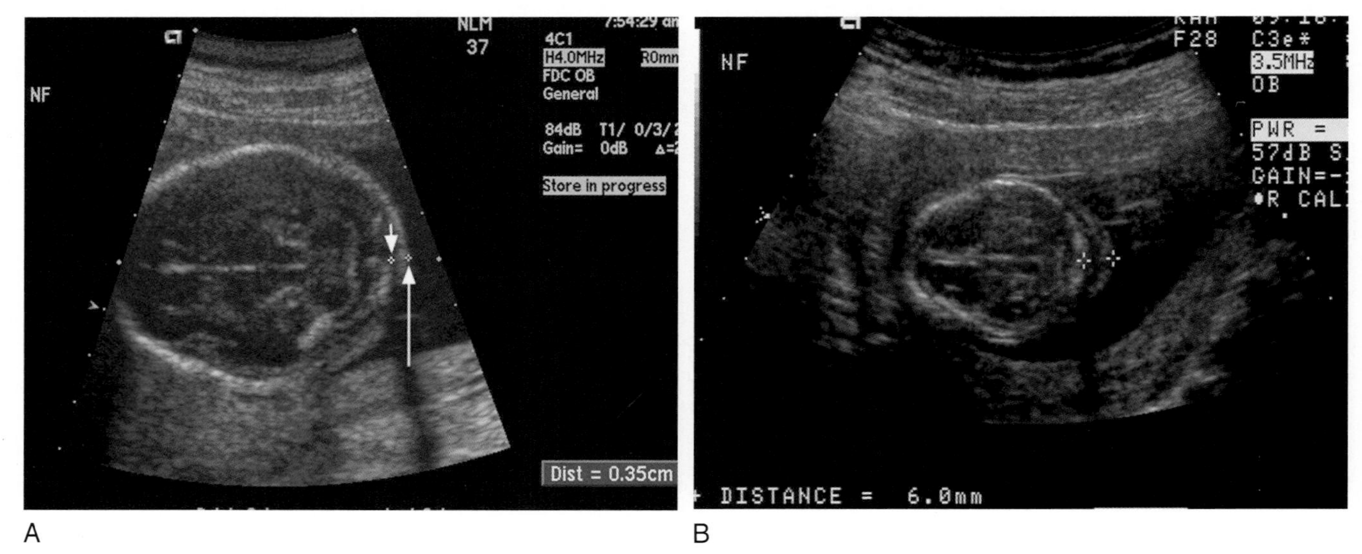

Figure 15-32 Measurement of nuchal fold: normal and abnormal. **A,** Normal nuchal fold. Axial image of fetal head at 18 weeks angled posteriorly toward occiput shows measurement of nuchal fold. Calipers are positioned on the outer margin of the occipital bone *(short arrow)* and outer margin of the nuchal skin *(long arrow)*. The measurement of 3 mm is normal. **B,** Thickened nuchal fold in fetus with trisomy 21. Axial image of fetal head at 16 weeks, angled posteriorly toward occiput shows thick nuchal fold *(cursors)*. The measurement of 6 mm is elevated.

nuchal translucency can resolve after 14 weeks, so it is thought to be from a different etiology than the nuchal thickening seen during the mid-second trimester. Because this thickness can resolve, there are those who argue that all fetuses, especially those at high risk, should be examined during this time period.

The measurement of nuchal translucency should be obtained at the level of the neck on a sagittal image of the fetus, rather than in the axial projection used to measure the nuchal fold during the mid-second trimester. Electronic calipers should be positioned on the inner margins of the lines delineating the lucency so that only the lucent area, and not the specular reflector from the adjacent spine or skin surface, is measured (inner to inner measurement) (Fig. 15-33). A nuchal translucency measurement of greater than 3 mm is always considered abnormal from 11 to 14 weeks. The normal nuchal translucency thickens with increasing gestational age, however, so the sensitivity of the measurement can be improved if the threshold selected is likewise adjusted for gestational age. The 95th percentile (which increases from 2.2 mm at a crown-rump length [CRL] of 38 mm to 2.8 mm at a CRL of 84 mm) is therefore often used to define the upper limit of normal. Further improvements in the prediction of aneuploidy using the nuchal translucency can be obtained by adding maternal age and first-trimester biochemical markers (free βhCG and protein-associated plasma protein) to the analysis. Currently, a large multicenter trial is underway assessing the use of nuchal translucency and first-trimester biochemical markers.

Because measurement differences on the order of only tenths of a millimeter determine the difference between a normal and abnormal value, meticulous technique is critical when measuring the nuchal translucency. To decrease measurement error, the image should be adjusted so that the fetus occupies the majority of the image and so that a movement of the cursor produces less than a 0.1-mm change in the measurement. The scans can be performed either transabdominally or transvaginally, but care must be taken so that the unfused amnion (which may not completely fuse with the chorion of the normal gestational sac until approximately 16 weeks) is not mistaken for the fetal skin line, potentially leading to overestimation of the nuchal translucency (see Fig. 15-33).

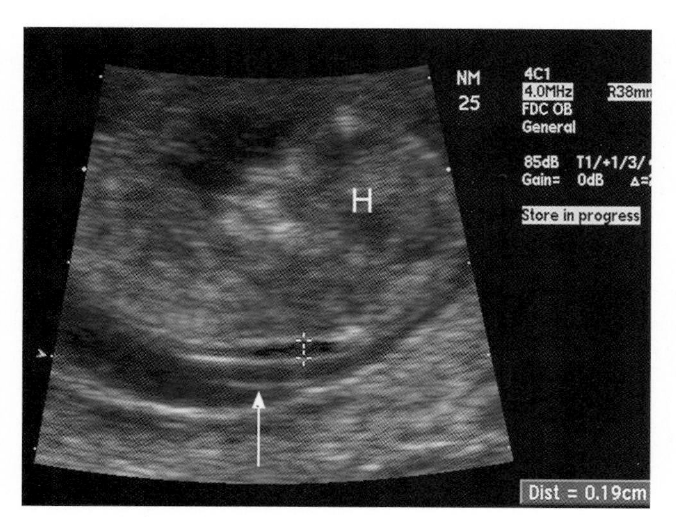

Figure 15-33 Measurement of nuchal translucency. Sagittal image of head (H) and neck of 12-week fetus shows measurement of normal nuchal translucency *(cursors)*. The amnion *(arrow)* is also seen and should not be mistaken for the fetal skin line.

THE CHOROID PLEXUS

The choroid plexus is easily compressible. A decrease in choroid plexus size is usually caused by raised intraventricular pressure (hydrocephalus). However, the choroid plexuses are also a source of energy (glycogen) and may be important in the early developmental stages of the brain. Therefore, if hydrocephalus is not present, a decrease in size might suggest impaired brain development.

There has been intense interest in choroid plexus cysts, particularly in the second trimester. Initial observations had suggested that these were normal variants, occurring in 1.8% to 3.6% of the normal population. However, choroid plexus cysts were subsequently found to be disproportionately associated with chromosomal abnormalities, in particular trisomy 18.

Trisomy 18 is usually associated with other structural anomalies, which can include a wide range of lesions such as heart defects, abnormal feet (clubfeet or rocker-bottom deformity), clenched hands with overlapping digits, facial clefts, neural tube defects, radial ray abnormalities, and two-vessel umbilical cord. Because of the association of trisomy 18 with choroid plexus cysts and structural abnormalities, it is generally agreed that chromosomal analysis should be offered when a fetus has both a choroid plexus cyst and additional structural anomalies. Therefore, when a choroid plexus cyst is identified, in addition to the routine anatomic survey, a targeted search for structural abnormalities frequently associated with trisomy 18 should be performed. This should include detailed evaluation of the heart, images of the face and feet, and an attempt to image the open fetal hand (Fig. 15-34). Some observers consider the configuration of the fingers particularly helpful. A normal fetus intermittently opens and closes its hands and extends its fingers, whereas the majority of fetuses with trisomy 18 have a clenched fist with overlapping index or third and fourth fingers (Fig. 15-35). A serum triple screen of α-fetoprotein, human chorionic gonadotropin (hCG), and unconjugated estriols, with

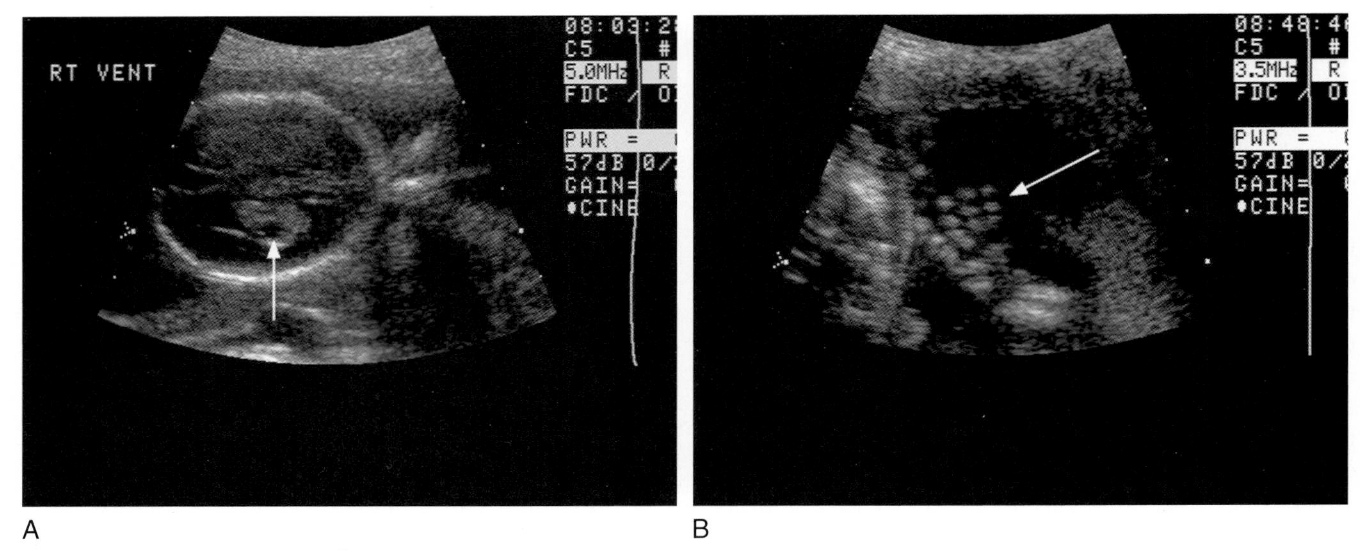

Figure 15-34 Choroid plexus cyst in an otherwise normal 18-week fetus. **A,** Axial image of fetal head at level of lateral ventricles shows a choroid plexus cyst *(arrow)*. **B,** Image of open hand *(arrow)* is normal. The hand was seen to open and close normally at real-time evaluation.

maternal age adjustment, has been found helpful in detecting trisomy 18 and 21 (Down syndrome) and can help determine if karyotyping should be offered in the setting of an isolated choroid plexus cyst. In trisomy 21 the α-fetoprotein and unconjugated estriol levels are low and that of hCG is high, whereas in trisomy 18, all three levels are low. The triple screen can detect 65% to 70% of fetuses with Down syndrome but has a significant false-positive rate. The interplay of ultrasound and the serum triple screen is important. If an age-adjusted triple screen assigns an increased risk for trisomy 18 or 21, a normal ultrasound leaves that risk unchanged or decreased while an abnormal ultrasound further increases that risk. The definitive test for a chromosomal abnormality is the amniocentesis. Unfortunately, amniocentesis is not without complications. A second-trimester amniocentesis is associated with an average estimated pregnancy loss rate of 1:200 to 1:300 and needs to be balanced between the potential loss of a normal pregnancy and the benefit of detecting a chromosomally abnormal fetus. If the serum triple screen is positive for trisomy 18 and an isolated choroid plexus

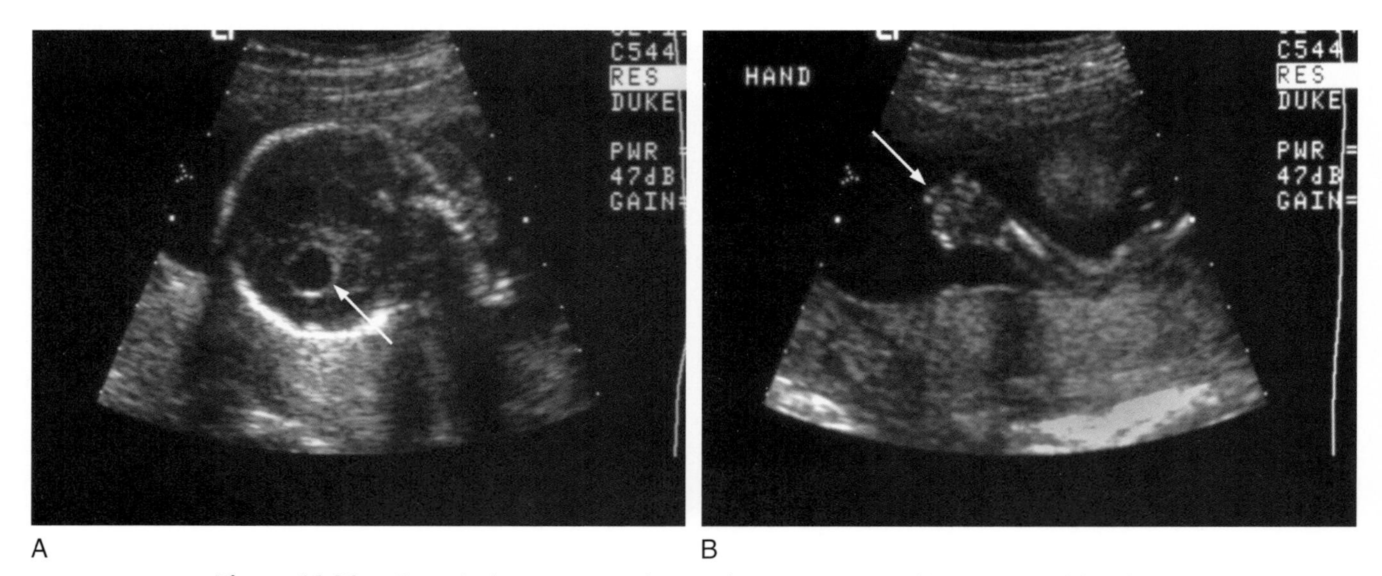

Figure 15-35 Choroid plexus cyst in a fetus with trisomy 18. **A,** Oblique image of fetal head shows a choroid plexus cyst *(arrow)*. **B,** Image of hand shows clenched fist and overlapping digit *(arrow)*. At real-time evaluation, the hand was fixed in this position and did not open.

cyst is seen, many practices will offer amniocentesis. The question that remains is when the fetal ultrasound reveals a choroid plexus cyst but a detailed targeted ultrasound and a triple screen are normal, what is the risk of having a fetus with trisomy 18? It is the belief of most observers that a fetus with isolated choroid plexus cyst(s), a normal serum triple screen, and a normal targeted ultrasound examination in which all relevant anatomy was well seen is highly likely to be normal and that in most cases amniocentesis need not be offered.

A pitfall in the identification of choroid plexus cysts can occur if the atria of the lateral ventricle are imaged in an oblique/coronal rather than a true axial plane. Ovoid hypoechoic structures may be seen to project into the choroid plexuses on their lateral margins from the adjacent corpus striatum. Although superficially resembling cysts, these hypoechoic regions become oblong when the transducer is turned 90 degrees. Because of this observation, it has been suggested that the overall incidence of choroid plexus cysts may be overstated.

OTHER HEAD ABNORMALITIES

Isolated CNS abnormalities can be detected sonographically. Agenesis of the corpus callosum (AGCC) can be an isolated anomaly, or it can be seen in association with chromosomal abnormalities, CNS abnormalities (such as Dandy-Walker malformation, holoprosencephaly, and Arnold-Chiari type II malformation), and a wide variety of other congenital anomaly syndromes. AGCC can be partial or complete. When it is partial, the posterior portion of the corpus callosum is missing and there is little to suggest the abnormality at antenatal ultrasound evaluation unless a midline sagittal image or multiple coronal images of the fetal head through the expected location of the entire corpus callosum can be obtained.

Antenatal ultrasound diagnosis of complete agenesis of the corpus callosum can also be difficult. Ventriculomegaly is common and may dominate the sonographic picture. Because the ventricular enlargement is not due to obstruction, it does not improve with shunting. In some fetuses, the ventriculomegaly is recognized but the specific diagnosis of AGCC is not made antenatally. Despite this, there are a number of ultrasound features that can suggest this diagnosis. Because the ventriculomegaly is caused by the secondary effects of absence of the callosal tracts on the adjacent ventricular system, the lateral ventricles tend to be located farther laterally and oriented more parallel to one another than usual. The callosal tract superior to the ventricles is absent, so the third ventricle extends cephalad and can herniate between the cerebral hemispheres, resulting in a midline interhemispheric cyst (Fig. 15-36). The third ventricle is often enlarged. Colpocephaly (disproportionate enlargement of the posterior portion of the lateral ventricles) is another common finding and can result in a "teardrop" configuration to the lateral ventricles in axial scan planes. Additionally, the cavum septum pellucidum is absent and a radiating pattern of gyri can be seen extending peripherally from the interhemispheric fissure. TV ultrasound evaluation (if the head is in vertex presentation) and/or an MRI study of the fetal head may prove of value in making the diagnosis.

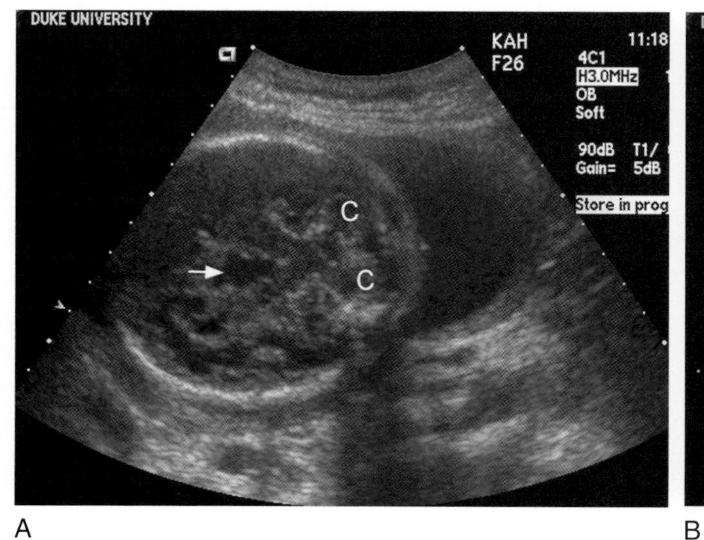

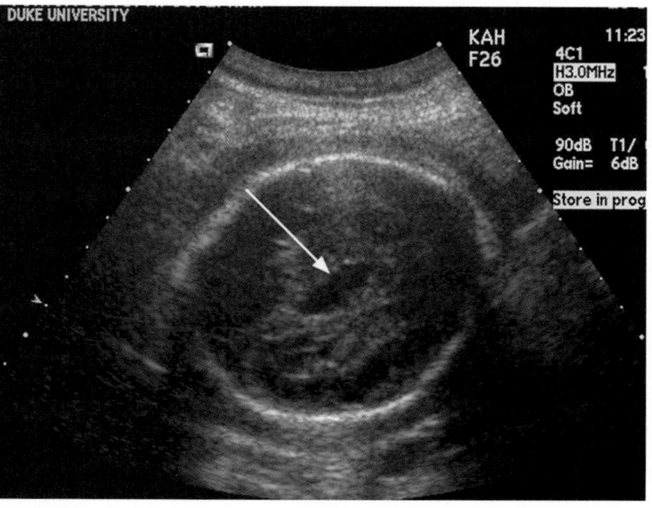

Figure 15-36 Agenesis of corpus callosum. **A** and **B**, Axial views of head of 27-week fetus with agenesis of corpus callosum shows dilated third ventricle (*short arrow*, **A**) with midline interhemispheric cyst (*long arrow*, **B**). C, cerebellar hemispheres.

A cystic structure identified posterior to the thalami or brain stem has the differential diagnoses of a Dandy-Walker malformation or variant, megacisterna magna, an enlarged fourth ventricle, a posterior fossa arachnoid cyst, or a vein of Galen aneurysm.

The term *vein of Galen aneurysm* is a misnomer. The vein of Galen aneurysm is not a true aneurysm but instead corresponds to marked dilatation of the vein of Galen due to increased blood flow through a communication between major branches of the carotid and/or vertebrobasilar system and the venous plexus in the region of the vein of Galen. On gray-scale ultrasound analysis, a rounded or ovoid fluid collection is seen in the midline, posterosuperior to the third ventricle and thalamus (Fig. 15-37). The collection elongates posteriorly into a more tubular configuration in sagittal and posteroinferiorly angled axial scan planes, because the vein extends posteriorly to drain into the sagittal sinus. The vein of Galen aneurysm opacifies on color Doppler evaluation, and spectral analysis reveals high-velocity turbulent flow. Color Doppler analysis should be considered an important component of the ultrasound examination whenever an abnormal cystic midline structure is identified in the fetal head, because of the possibility of a vein of Galen aneurysm. Increased flow from a vein of Galen aneurysm can cause high-output failure, so additional ultrasound findings that are frequently seen include cardiomegaly and fetal hydrops. Obstruction of the aqueduct of Sylvius by the dilated vein can cause hydrocephalus.

Intracranial masses are occasionally detected. Teratomas with cystic and solid components are rare tumors that can occupy most of the midline and severely distort the intracranial anatomy. These tumors are often very large and therefore of severe consequence to the fetus (Fig. 15-38). They may be very vascular at Doppler examination.

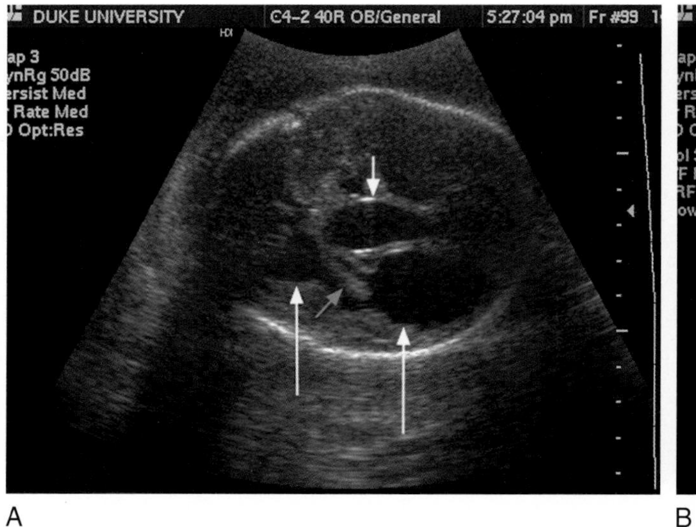

A

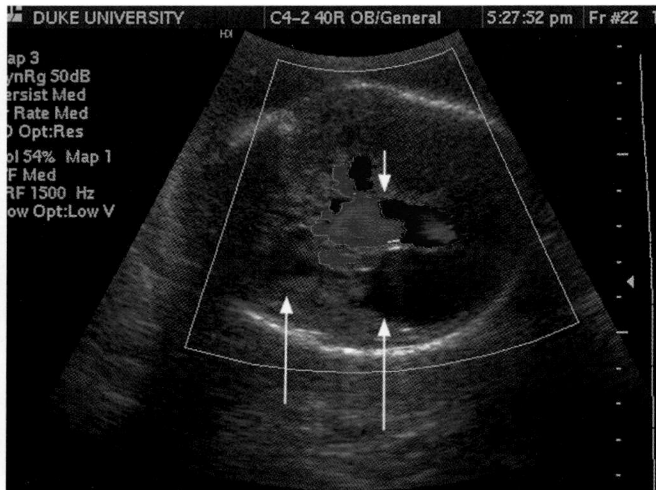

B

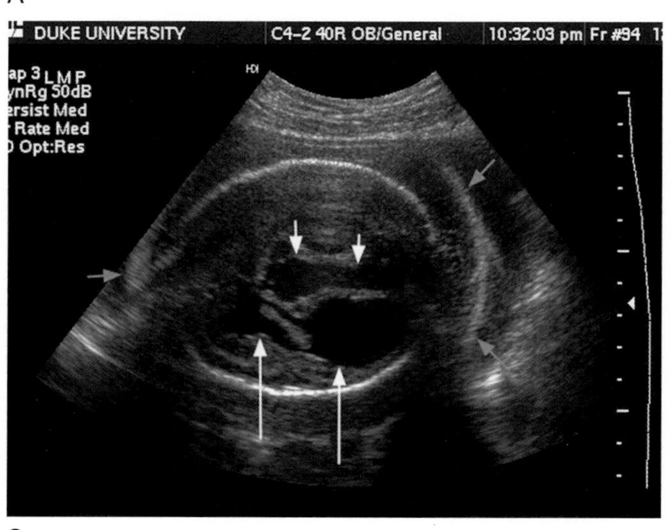

C

Figure 15-37 Vein of Galen aneurysm. **A,** Axial image of head of third-trimester fetus shows midline ovoid fluid collection *(short white arrow),* ventriculomegaly *(long white arrows),* and a dangling choroid plexus *(short gray arrow).* **B,** Color Doppler image corresponding to **A** shows the midline fluid collection is vascular *(short arrow),* consistent with a vein of Galen aneurysm. *Long arrows,* dilated lateral ventricle. **C,** Axial image angled posteroinferiorly demonstrates the vein of Galen aneurysm *(short white arrows)* elongates posteriorly as it extends toward the sagittal sinus. The fetus also had hydrops. Marked scalp edema *(short gray arrows)* is seen. *Long white arrows,* dilated lateral ventricle.

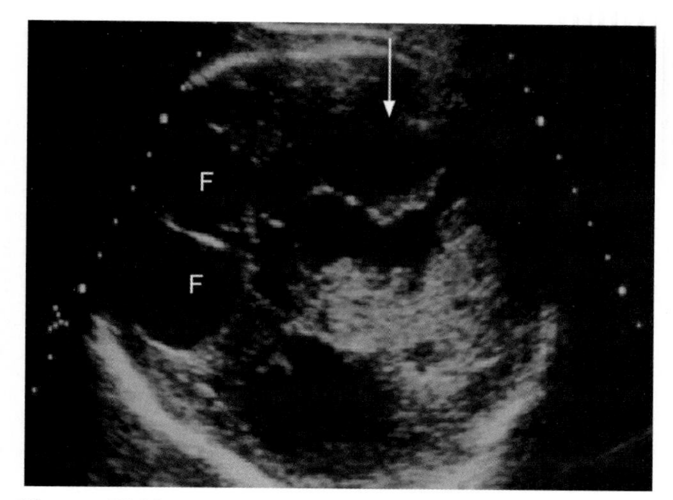

Figure 15-38 Intracranial teratoma. Axial image of head of third-trimester fetus shows a large echogenic mass with cystic and solid components *(arrow)* causing hydrocephalus. F, dilated frontal horns of lateral ventricles.

Intracranial hyperechoic areas can also be detected. As discussed under microcephaly, calcifications secondary to an in utero infection (see Fig. 15-17) or the tubers in tuberous sclerosis can sometimes be seen. When hyperechoic areas without acoustic shadowing are identified either in the germinal matrix region or within the lateral ventricles, they are more likely areas of hemorrhage. Hyperechoic areas due to hemorrhage can occasionally have a sonographic appearance similar to that of an intracranial tumor. Initially, intracranial hemorrhage was considered possible in utero only in cases of direct trauma near term, when there was less amniotic fluid to protect the fetus. However, cases of spontaneous bleeding have now been reported in the late second trimester and in the third trimester, and when detected the intracranial hemorrhage grading system for neonates can be used: grade 1 hemorrhage is within the germinal matrix; grade 2 has intraventricular bleeding; grade 3 also is associated with hydrocephalus; and grade 4 includes an intraparenchymal bleed. When intraventricular, the hemorrhage can blend with and assume the appearance of an enlarged choroid plexus (Fig. 15-39). As with neonates, the higher the grade of hemorrhage, the worse the prognosis.

Porencephalic cysts can also be detected in utero. Although their etiology is uncertain, porencephaly is generally assumed to be secondary to a vascular accident because brain parenchymal loss is typically in a vascular distribution (Fig. 15-40). The "cystic" area of destroyed brain often communicates with and/or enlarges part of a ventricle (an ex vacuo enlargement). The porencephalic cyst can vary in size and not infrequently enlarges with advancing gestation, presumably caused by the continued production (without resorption) of cerebrospinal fluid. On occasion, the enlarging area can impinge on normal brain structures, cause a midline shift, and even protrude through the suture lines and be seen outside the calvarium.

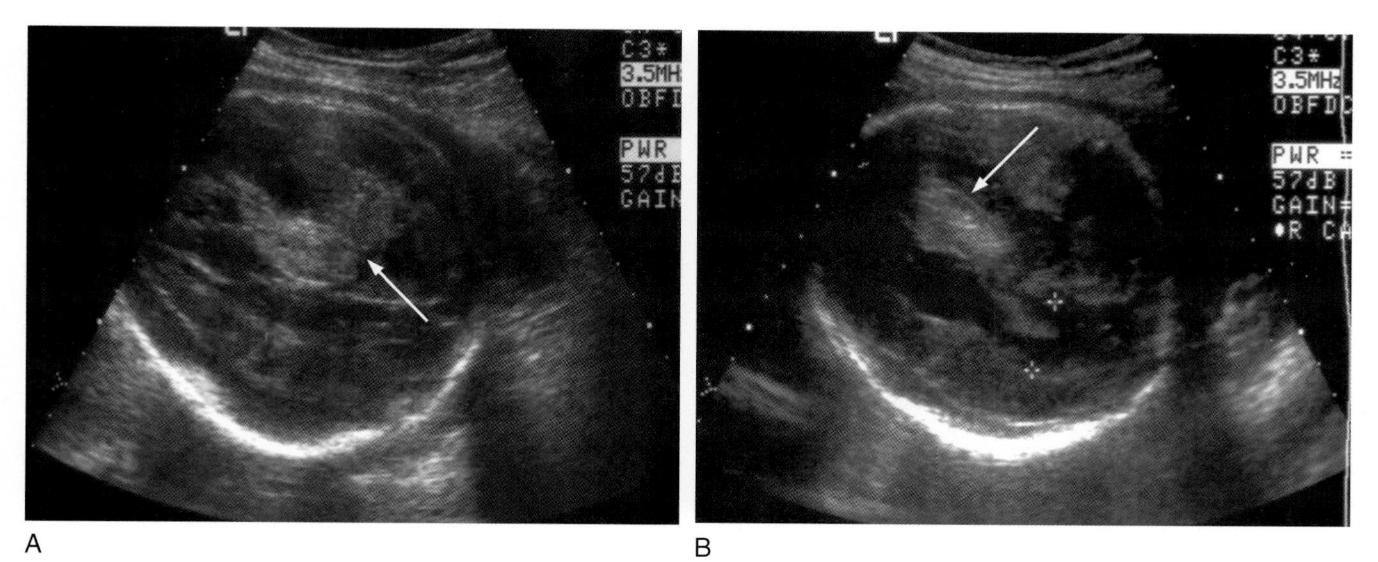

Figure 15-39 Intracranial hemorrhage. **A,** Oblique view of third-trimester fetal head shows irregularly shaped heterogeneous material *(arrow)* in near-field lateral ventricle, owing to a combination of choroid plexus and hematoma. **B,** Axial view of head shows the hemorrhage *(arrow)* has extended into the brain parenchyma and caused dilatation of the contralateral lateral ventricle *(cursors).*

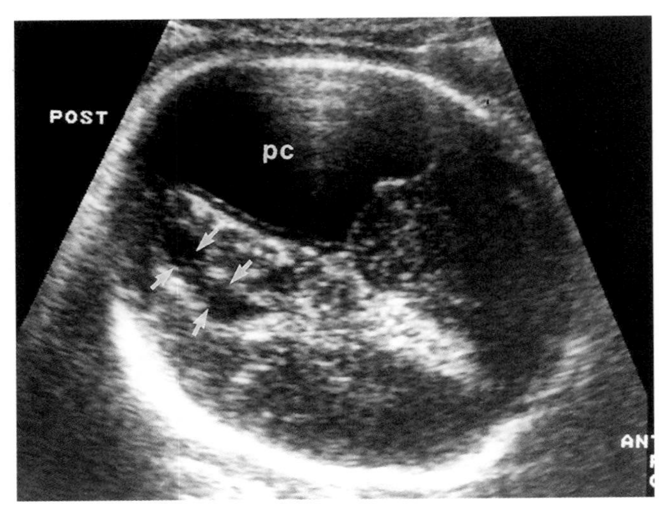

Figure 15-40 Large porencephalic cyst (pc) in the left parieto-occipital region in the distribution of the posterior cerebral artery. The occipital horn on the left is not identified because the "cyst" actually represents the enlarged ventricle filling the space of the destroyed brain. The normal right occipital horn is noted *(small arrows)*. There is some evidence of a mass effect from the porencephalic area, with slight bulging of the midline toward the right.

THE FETAL SPINE

Serum α-fetoprotein (AFP) measurements have assumed considerable importance in screening pregnant women in the second trimester for the presence of open (not skin-covered) fetal anomalies. AFP is a normal fetal protein that is synthesized throughout fetal life, first in the yolk sac and then by the liver. Because it is excreted by the fetal kidneys, it can be identified in the amniotic fluid, with a normal fetal-to-amniotic fluid ratio of 1000:1. It is highest in concentration in the first trimester and decreases as the pregnancy progresses. AFP can also be detected in the maternal serum (MSAFP), caused by a transplacental diffusion gradient, also at a ratio of 1000:1. The level of MSAFP increases as placental permeability increases and is normally highest, in the second trimester.

There are bell-shaped distribution curves for the expected normal AFP levels in both the maternal serum and amniotic fluid, both adjusted for the age of the pregnancy. When there is an open fetal defect, these AFP levels elevate. By using an arbitrary upper limit of normal, different in different laboratories, but commonly 2.5 multiples of the median adjusted for obesity and multiple gestations, the abnormal cases have higher levels. These anomalies are usually neural (e.g., anencephaly, encephalocele, and spinal defects). However, any open fetal defect, for example an anterior abdominal wall defect, can elevate the AFP levels. Nevertheless, there is some overlap between the normal and the abnormal groups. Of interest, used in the serum triple screen, a low (rather than elevated) MSAFP level is a marker after maternal age adjustment for Down syndrome.

In the analysis of MSAFP, false-negative results are very uncommon and almost always occur in the setting of closed (skin-covered) fetal defects. False-positive results (elevated levels but not caused by fetal anomalies) are much more frequent and have been estimated to constitute upward of 50% of the cases. The errors are mostly the result of inaccurate gestational dates, so fetal age-adjustment is frequently all that is necessary to ensure normalcy. When elevated MSAFP levels are still present after adjustment for fetal age, two additional tests should be considered: (1) a thorough fetal ultrasound evaluation and (2) amniocentesis to obtain amniotic fluid for AFP and acetylcholinesterase levels (the latter specific for neural tube defects). Pregnant women who do not have structural abnormalities but have persistently elevated AFP levels tend as a group to have placental problems and have a poorer prognosis, particularly in the third trimester, than the general population (discussed more completely in Chapter 20).

An abnormal neural axis is one of the primary causes of elevated MSAFP levels. To perform a complete examination of the spine, every vertebral level from the cervical to the sacral region should be examined, and images should be obtained at representative levels. In the axial scan plane, there are three hyperechoic bony structures (the anterior centrum and two posterior elements) at each vertebral level (Fig. 15-41). Optimally, axial images of the spine should be performed with the spine located immediately under the transducer, that is, in the 12 o'clock position. In this orientation, the two posterior ossification centers should converge posteriorly, pointing toward each other (see Fig. 15-41A to D). When axial images are obtained with the spine in other orientations, the normal convergence of the posterior ossification centers may not be apparent. For example, with the spine pointing toward the side in the 3 or 9 o'clock position, the posterior elements may appear to be parallel in a normal fetus. The spine should also be imaged in longitudinal projection (sagittal and/or coronal). In longitudinal scan planes the bony elements should taper caudad in the sacrococcygeal region (see Fig. 15-41E). It is also important to attempt to demonstrate that the soft tissues posterior to the spine are intact.

The majority of the spine can be identified in most pregnancies by 16 weeks. By that time, the fifth lumbar vertebra is the most caudad level to be ossified. Thereafter, the sacral spine ossifies sequentially every 2 to 3 weeks, so that S2 will normally ossify by 22 weeks, with S3 through S5 ossifying even later. This observation would suggest that, at least in theory, abnormalities of the sacrum may not be diagnosed before the late second

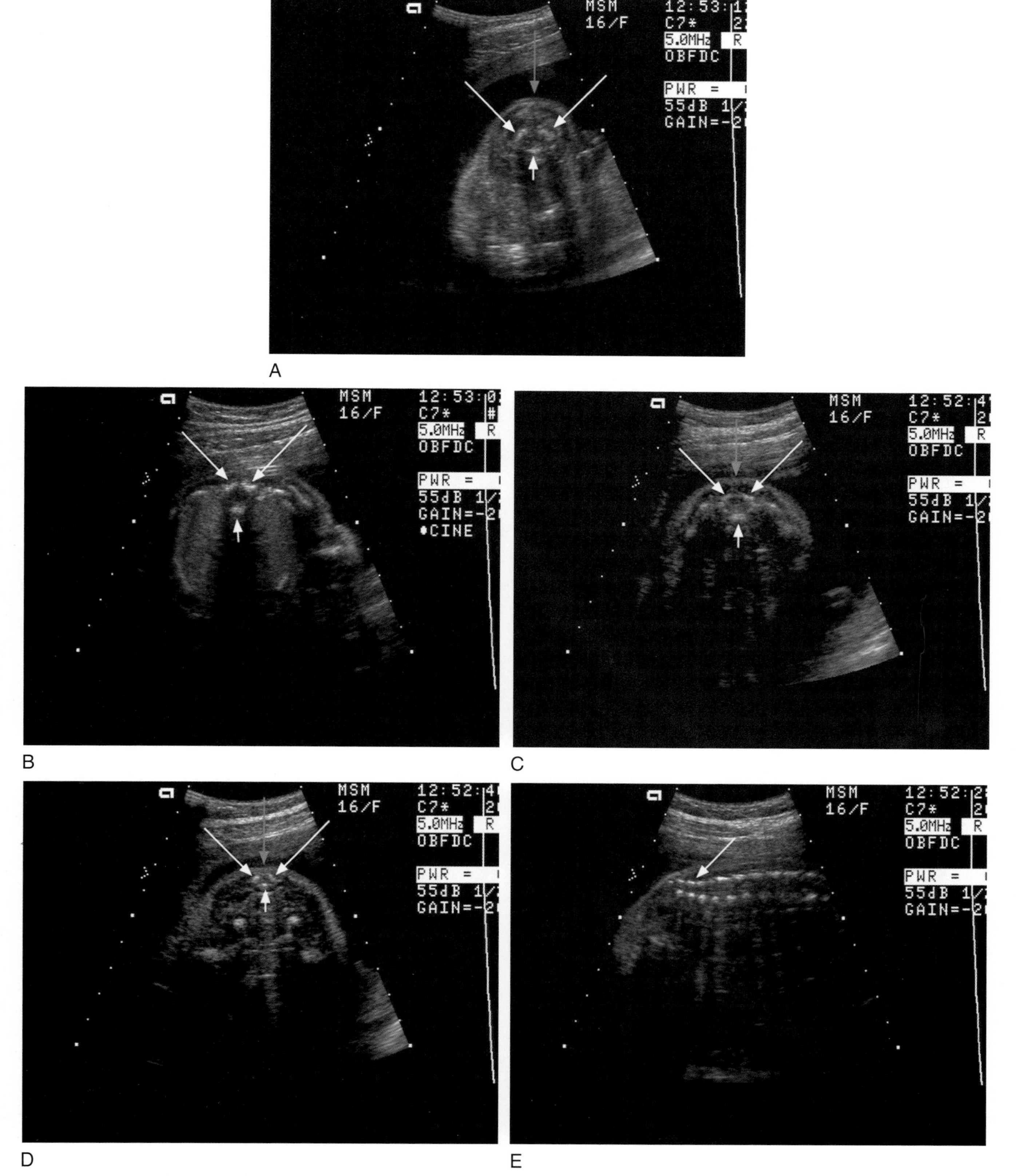

Figure 15-41 Normal fetal spine at 24 weeks. **A** to **D**, Axial images of spine at representative levels including cervical spine (**A**), thoracic spine (**B**), lumbar spine (**C**), and sacral spine (**D**) show a normal configuration with posterior ossification centers *(long white arrows)* pointing toward each other and a vertebral body *(short white arrow)*. The soft tissues posterior to the spine *(long gray arrow)* are intact. **E**, Sagittal image of distal spine shows normal tapering *(arrow)* of the sacrococcygeal spine.

trimester. In practice, if fetal position is favorable, most defects can be identified accurately after 18 weeks. Spine defects are almost always associated with the Chiari II malformation (described later), and the cranial abnormalities of the Chiari II malformation may be more apparent than the spine defect itself. Indeed, cranial findings may be the first to alert the examiner to the presence of a spine defect and occasionally are the only abnormalities seen even after a targeted evaluation of the fetal spine.

NEURAL TUBE DEFECTS (MENINGOCELES AND MENINGOMYELOCELES)

Neural tube defects are most common in the lumbosacral region. They are called meningoceles (if they contain only meninges) and meningomyeloceles (if they also have neural elements). Sonographic features of the spine defect include splaying of the posterior elements,

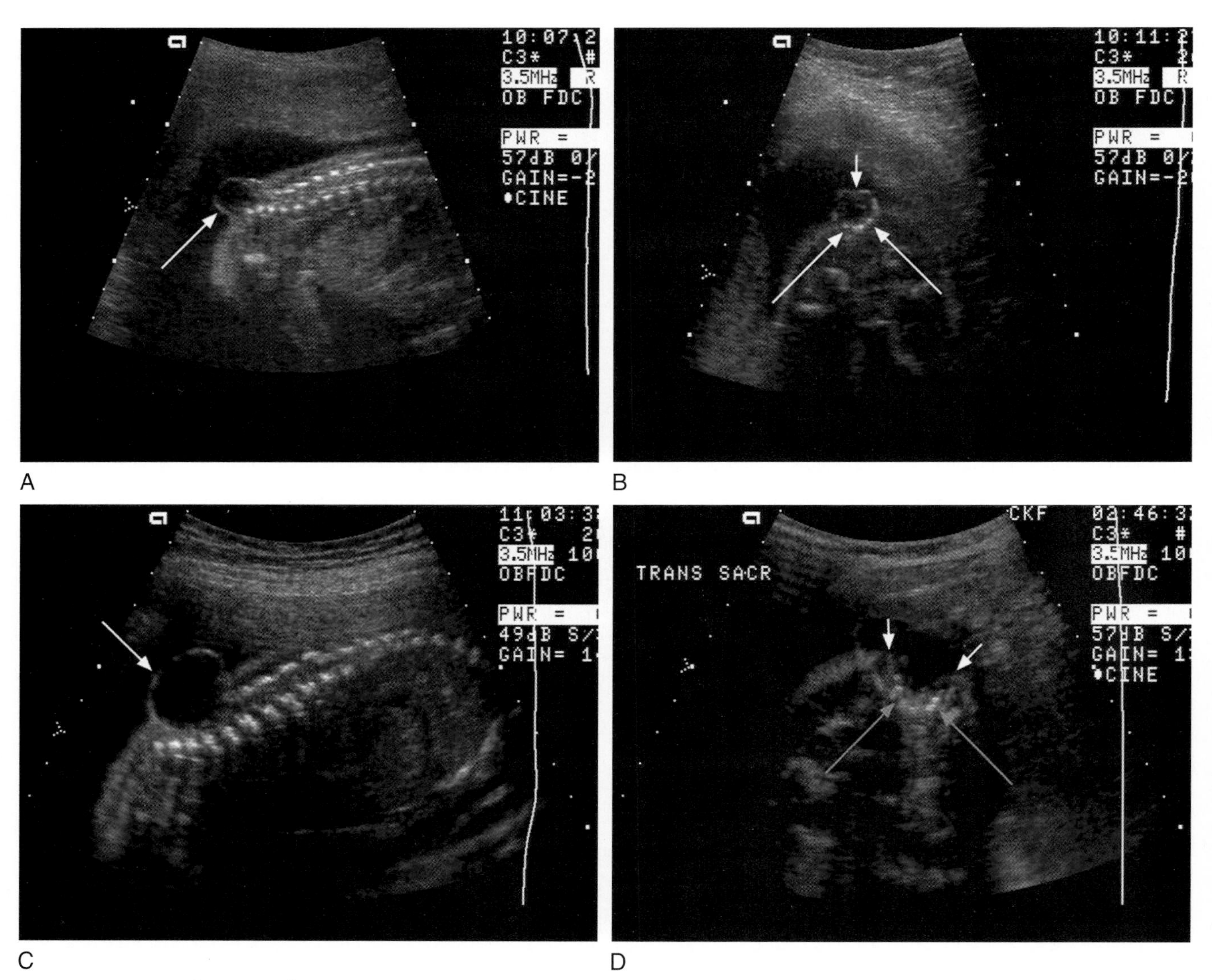

Figure 15-42 Myelomeningocele: examples in two fetuses. **A,** Midline longitudinal image of distal spine of a second-trimester fetus depicts myelomeningocele sac as a cystic mass *(arrow)* extending from posterior aspect of distal spine. **B,** Axial image of distal spine of same fetus as in **A**, at level of the myelomeningocele sac *(short arrow)* shows splaying of the posterior ossification centers *(long arrows)*. **C,** Midline longitudinal image of distal spine of third-trimester fetus shows disruption of the spine by a large myelomeningocele sac *(arrow)*. **D,** Axial image of distal spine of same fetus as in **C** shows a large defect in the soft tissues *(short white arrows)* and splaying of the posterior ossification centers *(long gray arrows)*.

a defect in the overlying soft tissues, and identification of the meningocele sac as a cystic or complex mass extending off the posterior aspect of the spine (Fig. 15-42). The sac can be identified on either a midline sagittal or an axial scan and may be relatively easy to identify if it is surrounded by amniotic fluid and the fetus is in a favorable position. In contrast, the sac may be more difficult to identify and may not be appreciated at all if the fetal back is against the uterine wall obscuring soft tissue visualization, the fetus is in a face-up presentation with the back away from the transducer (Fig. 15-43), or oligohydramnios is present. In these situations, identification of the posterior (bony) elements and of intracranial findings assumes an even greater importance. Splaying of the posterior elements, best evaluated in axial and coronal views, is diagnostic for a neural defect. If the cystic sac is filled with thin hyperechoic strands, nerve roots (myeloid elements) are most likely present (although arachnoid bands could give a similar appearance). If instead the cystic sac is completely anechoic, the sac could correspond to a meningocele without neural elements or it could be a myelomeningocele in which the neural elements are present but not seen.

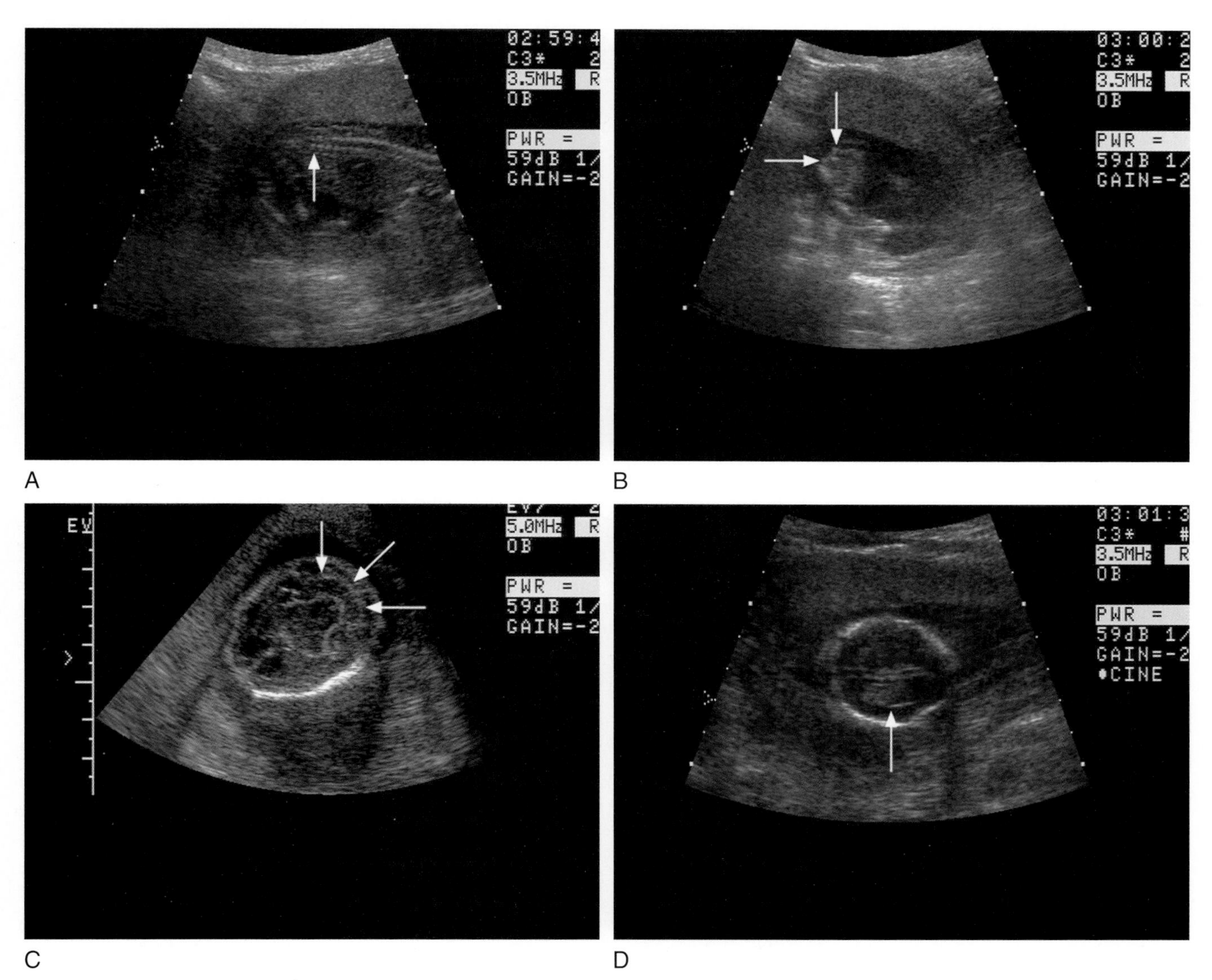

Figure 15-43 Value of axial images of spine and of "banana sign" when myelomeningocele is difficult to identify. **A,** Midline sagittal image of distal spine *(arrow)* of a 15-week fetus with a myelomeningocele fails to identify the myelomeningocele sac because fetal back abuts uterine wall, obscuring skin surface. **B,** Axial image of distal spine of same fetus reveals splaying of the posterior elements *(arrows)* consistent with a neural tube defect. **C,** Axial transvaginal image of fetal head shows obliteration of the cisterna magna and distortion of the shape of the cerebellar hemispheres ("banana sign") *(arrows),* further confirming a neural tube defect and Chiari II malformation. **D,** Despite the presence of a Chiari II malformation, the ventricles are normal in size, with no hydrocephalus. *Arrow,* lateral ventricle.

The extent of the defect is also important because the number of involved vertebral bodies can help predict the severity of a neural tube defect. If only the lower sacral vertebrae are abnormal, the neurologic consequences will be less than if the defect extends into the lumbar region. Because early in fetal life the neural tube occupies the entire length of the vertebral column and is tethered by the neural defect, a long sacral or lumbosacral defect affects many more neural levels than an abnormality in the same area acquired after birth (when the cord ends at L3). Ideally, the affected vertebrae should be counted if possible and the potential level for the neurologic deficit predicted. An intraspinal hypoechoic to hyperechoic fatty tumor (lipoma) or a hyperechoic bony spur with shadowing (diastematomyelia) is occasionally associated with a myelomeningocele (Fig. 15-44). When the defect is severe, there may be an additional sharp angulation or deformity of the spine in the region of the abnormality (Fig. 15-45).

Whenever a neural tube abnormality is detected, the fetal head should be carefully evaluated for evidence of an Arnold-Chiari type II malformation. Ultrasound features of the Chiari II malformation include obliteration of the cisterna magna, decrease in size and distorted shape of posterior fossa structures (particularly the cerebellum), altered head shape, and hydrocephalus.

The names "banana sign" and "lemon sign" have been coined to describe the cranial features of the Chiari II malformation. The "lemon" sign refers to flattening or concavity of the bilateral frontal bones, resulting in a calvarial shape that resembles the shape of a lemon. (Figs. 15-46 and 15-47). Although its etiology is not known, the sign is present before 24 weeks in 98% of the fetuses with open spinal defects; after 24 weeks, the sign is inexplicably present in only 13% of the affected fetuses. The lemon sign is helpful in corroborating the diagnosis of Chiari II malformation in fetuses with other typical ultrasound features, but it is nonspecific because it can be associated with other structural abnormalities, some not even related to the neural axis (e.g., omphalocele). Moreover, some normal fetuses may have a milder, less indented, lemon configuration (1% to 2% of normal fetuses before 24 weeks). Additionally, the lemon sign can resemble an abnormal skull shape seen in some fetuses with trisomy 18, referred to as the "strawberry sign." The strawberry sign describes flattening of the occiput due to hypoplasia of the hindbrain, in conjunction with flattening of the frontal bones due to hypoplasia of the frontal lobes (Fig. 15-48).

The "banana sign" refers to an abnormal curved shape of the cerebellum. The banana configuration is the direct pathologic consequence of an Arnold-Chiari type II malformation. The cerebellum and medulla oblongata are pulled downward and posteriorly by the tethered cord, resulting in obliteration of the cisterna magna and loss of the normal shape of the cerebellum with anterior curving of the cerebellar hemispheres. On ultrasound,

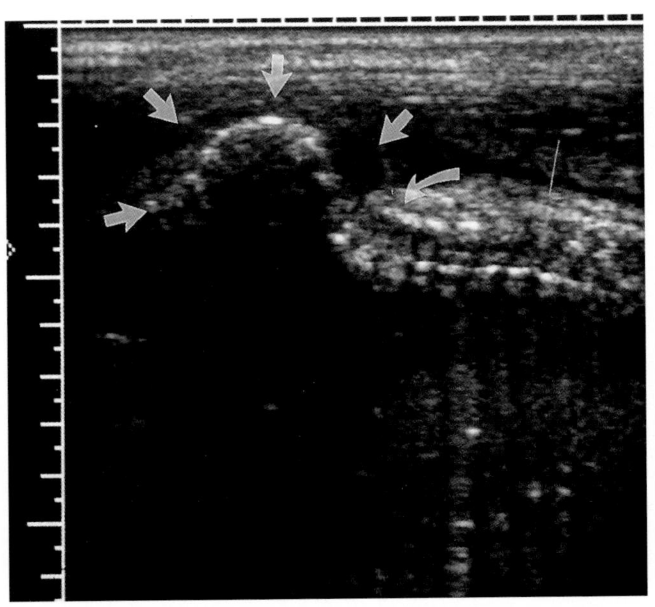

Figure 15-45 Abrupt spine curvature associated with myelomeningocele. Sagittal view of spine with fetal head toward the reader's right shows normal soft tissues and posterior elements down to the *curved arrow* at the L3 level. Below this, there is marked spine curvature with an overlying cystic area *(arrows)*.

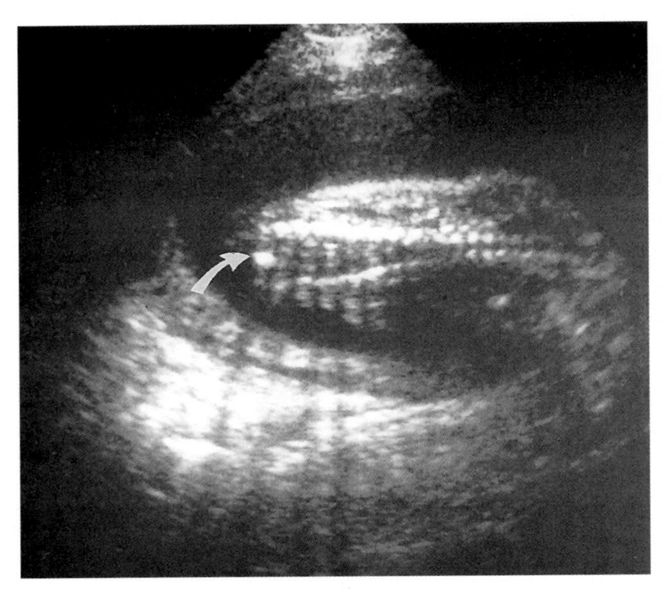

Figure 15-44 Diastematomyelia associated with myelomeningocele. Coronal view of spine with fetal head toward the reader's right shows significant spreading of the posterior elements and a well-defined hyperechoic ossification *(curved arrow)* within the canal at the L5 level.

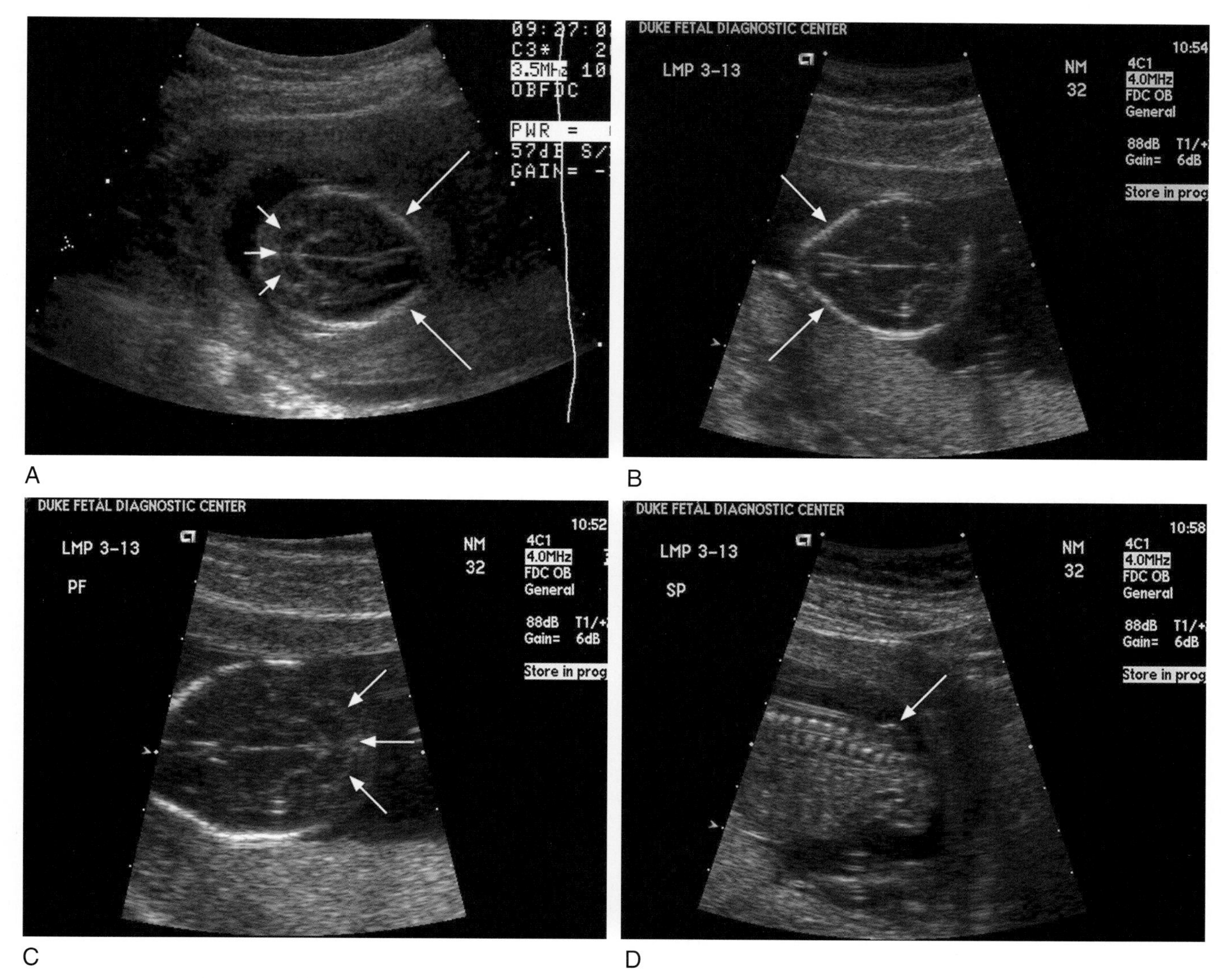

Figure 15-46 Lemon and banana signs. **A,** Axial image of head of 16-week fetus demonstrates banana sign, with "C"-shaped curvature of the cerebellar hemispheres *(short arrows)* and obliteration of cisterna magna. Flattening of the frontal bones *(long arrows)* corresponds to the lemon sign. Fetus also had a myelomeningocele (not shown). **B,** Axial image of head of a different 16-week fetus shows lemon sign, with flattening of frontal bones *(arrows).* **C,** Image of posterior fossa of same fetus as in **B** shows banana sign with "C"-shaped curvature of the cerebellum *(arrows),* resembling the shape of a banana. **D,** Midline sagittal image of distal spine of same fetus as in **B** and **C** confirms the presence of a myelomeningocele *(arrow).*

the cerebellum is changed in shape from bilobed to a downward-curved "C" (see Fig. 15-46). The banana sign represents a permanent intrinsic deformity of posterior fossa structures and consequently is more specific than the lemon sign. With today's ultrasound equipment, the abnormal configuration of the cerebellum should be identified in the majority of fetuses with a Chiari II malformation. The likelihood of detection of a banana sign depends partly on the severity of the posterior fossa malformation: if the downward displacement of the posterior fossa structures is very severe, the cerebellum may be displaced so far caudad that it is not imaged on views of the head. A true banana sign will then not be appreciated, but the key diagnostic feature, obliteration of the cisterna magna, will still be present. Conversely, the Chiari malformation is sometimes relatively mild and then cannot be appreciated with ultrasound.

Hydrocephalus is seen in many, but not all, fetuses (see Figs. 15-43 and 15-47) with the Chiari II malformation and is presumably caused by obstruction at the outlet of the fourth ventricle. It is more common later in gestation and when the posterior fossa malformation is severe. There is no definite direct correlation, however, between the extent of the spinal defect and the severity of the hydrocephalus.

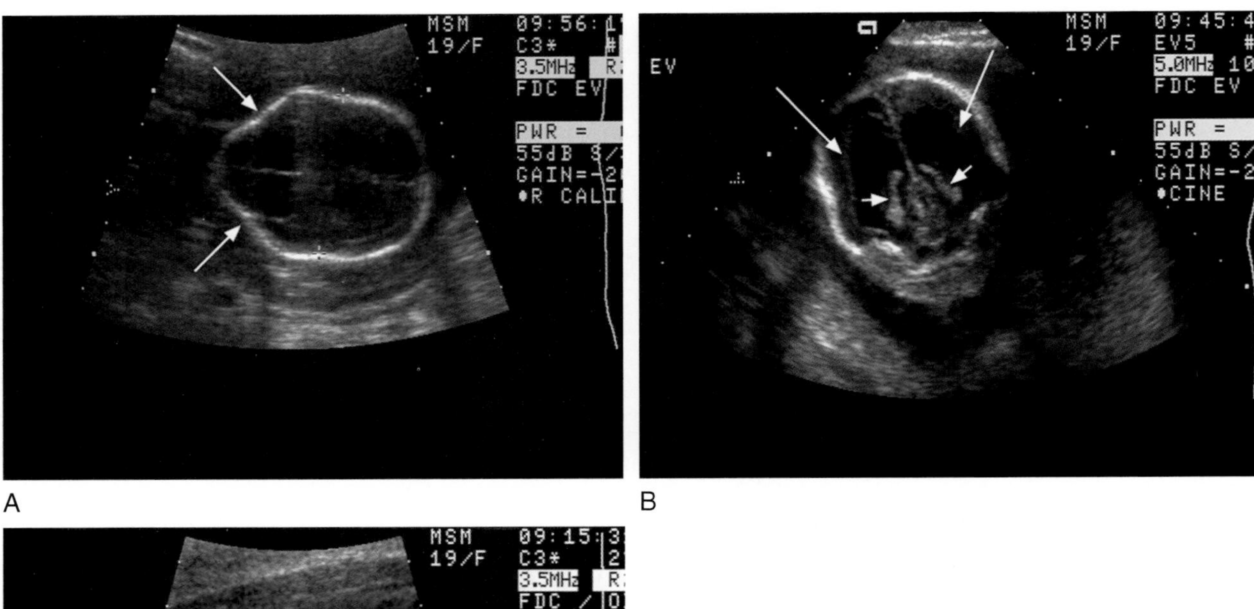

Figure 15-47 Lemon sign and hydrocephalus in fetus with Chiari II malformation. **A,** Axial image of fetal head at 19 weeks shows prominent lemon sign, with concavity of the frontal bones *(arrows)*. **B,** Coronal transvaginal image of head shows dilated lateral ventricles *(long arrows)* and small choroid plexus *(short arrows)* due to hydrocephalus. **C,** Midline sagittal image of distal spine confirms presence of a myelomeningocele *(arrow)*.

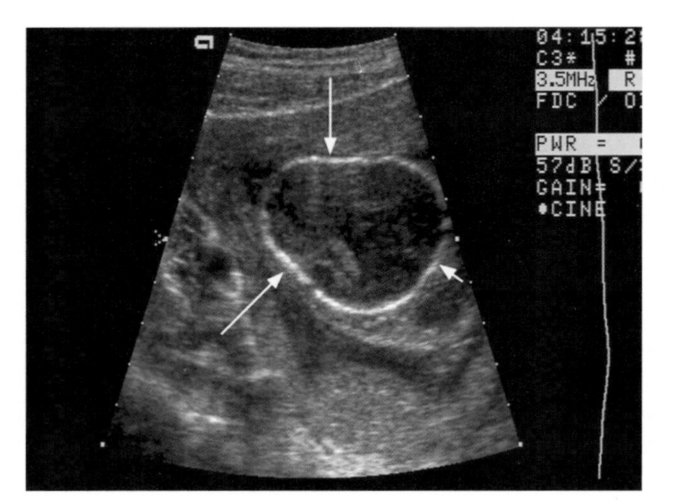

Figure 15-48 Strawberry sign in trisomy 18. Axial image of head of second-trimester fetus with trisomy 18 demonstrates the strawberry sign. There is flattening of the frontal bones *(long arrows)* due to hypoplasia of the frontal lobes and flattening of the occiput *(short arrow)* due to hypoplasia of the hindbrain. Overall shape of head resembles that of a strawberry, even though the frontal bones have a configuration resembling the lemon sign seen with Chiari II malformations.

There are instances when the fetal spine may appear normal and yet the "banana" sign with or without hydrocephalus is present. A more careful evaluation of the spine, particularly the lumbosacral area, is then needed to search for a subtle spinal defect (see Fig. 15-43). It can be argued that a spinal defect must exist if the "banana" sign is detected so that if it is still not identified, a TV ultrasound should be considered (if the fetus is in breech presentation); or, alternatively, an MRI may be performed.

PARASPINAL ANOMALIES

Additional pathologic conditions may be detected in the paraspinal regions. A spoked-wheel–shaped cystic structure can be identified posterior and lateral in the soft tissues of the neck, with the underlying cervical spine normal. This pattern is characteristic for a lymphocele and in this location is diagnostic of a cystic hygroma (Fig. 15-49). Although cystic hygromas can be

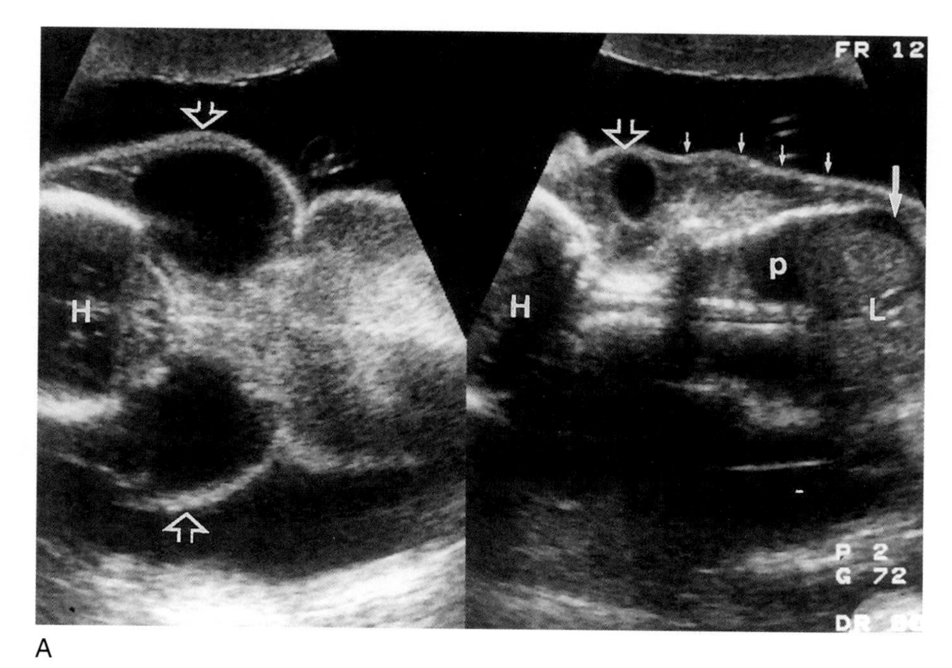

A

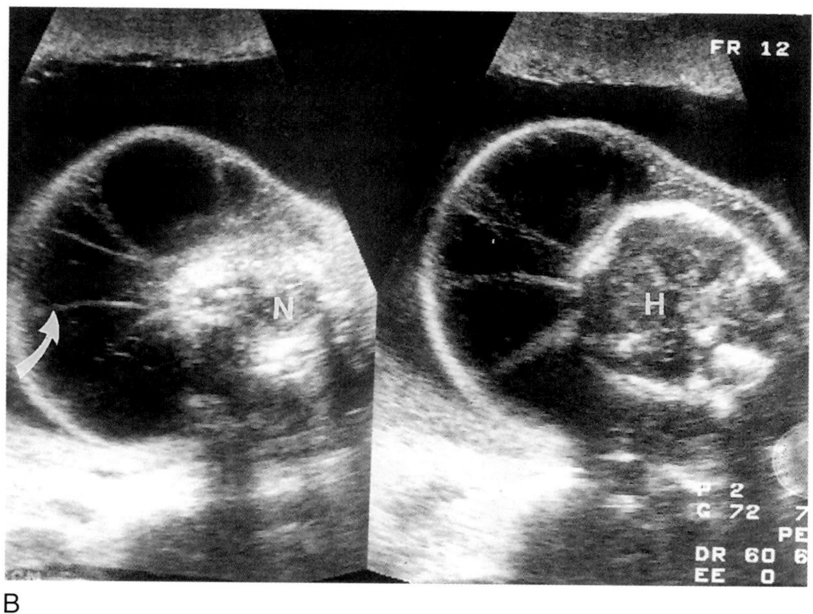

B

Figure 15-49 Cystic hygroma with diffuse hydropic changes in a fetus with Turner's syndrome at 28 weeks. Two long-axis coronal views with the head (H) toward the reader's left and body toward the right. **A,** In the left image, a defect in the soft tissues of the neck represents a large cystic mass *(open arrows)* characteristic of cystic hygroma. In the right image, the liver (L) is surrounded by ascites *(arrow)*. Anechoic spaces in the thoracic cavity are consistent with pleural effusions (p). One of the cystic areas of the hygroma is seen in the neck *(open arrow)*. Continued soft tissue thickness extends downward into the abdominal wall *(small arrows)*; these are findings consistent with diffuse edema. **B,** Two transaxial views of the head (H) and neck (N) region. The large cystic mass exhibiting a characteristic "spoke wheel" pattern extends posteriorly, with one of the septations denoted by a *curved arrow*.

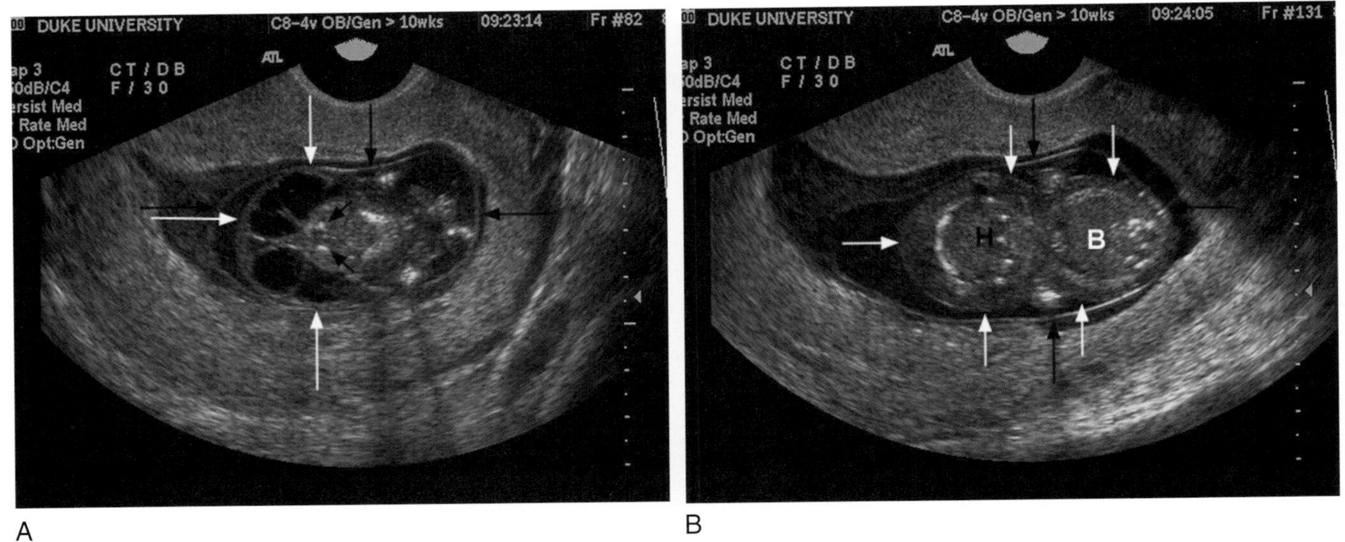

Figure 15-50 First-trimester cystic hygroma with diffuse skin thickening. **A,** Axial transvaginal image of neck of an 11-week embryo shows a large cystic mass *(white arrows)* with a spoke wheel pattern of septations posterior and lateral to the neck. *Short black arrows,* spine ossification centers; *long black arrows,* amnion. **B,** Longitudinal transvaginal image of same fetus as in **A** shows marked diffuse skin thickening *(white arrows)* due to lymphatic obstruction. H, head; B, abdomen; *black arrows*, amnion.

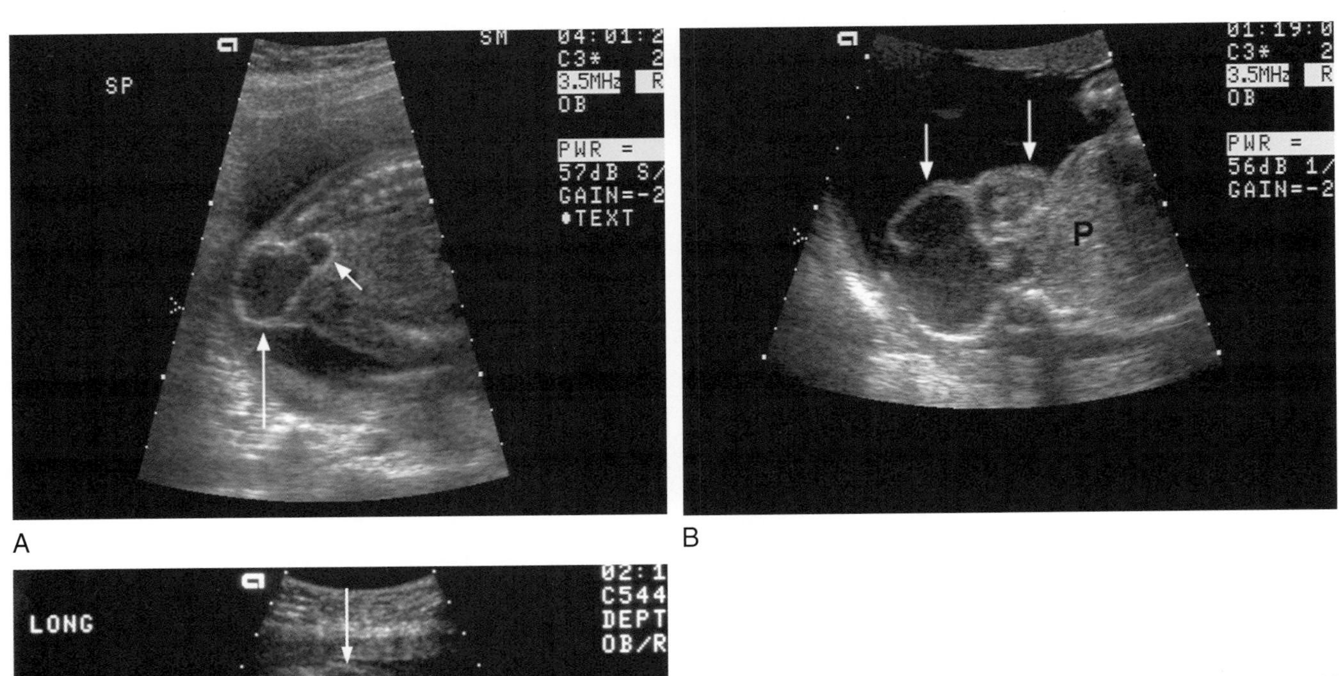

Figure 15-51 Sacrococcygeal teratoma: examples in two different fetuses. **A,** Sagittal image of pelvis of a 20-week fetus shows a sacrococcygeal teratoma with a small internal component *(short arrow)* and a larger external component *(long arrow).* **B,** Scan of same fetus performed 4 weeks after **A** shows the sacrococcygeal teratoma *(arrows)* has grown. It contains both cystic and solid components. P, pelvis. **C,** Sagittal image of distal spine *(short arrow)* of a different fetus, obtained during the third trimester shows a huge, predominantly external sacrococcygeal teratoma *(long arrows)* with cystic and solid (T) components.

isolated anomalies (unilateral or bilateral), they may also be part of a diffuse hydropic lymphatic obstruction, with additional signs of skin thickening and body cavity fluids (e.g., ascites) (Fig. 15-50). Cystic hygromas are highly deforming. When hydropic changes are also present, ultimate fetal or neonatal demise is highly likely. Over 60% are associated with chromosomal abnormalities: the best known is Turner's syndrome (XO karyotype), but other aneuploidies such as trisomy 21 and trisomy 18 are common. Lymphoceles do not always originate from the jugular lymph sac region. They can occur in any area of the body. While deforming, they are not then associated with chromosomal abnormalities or diffuse obstruction.

A teratoma with a variable proportion of solid areas (from combined cystic-solid to mostly solid) can be identified adjacent to the sacrum and coccyx and is termed a *sacrococcygeal teratoma* (Fig. 15-51). These teratomas may be divided into four types, from completely external (type 1) to completely internal (type 4). Type 4 is the most difficult to detect. In utero a sacrococcygeal teratoma can be markedly deforming but does not usually undergo malignant degeneration. After birth, if not removed, malignancy is possible and this likelihood increases the later the teratoma is detected and removed. The significance of these tumors is dictated by the extent of the involvement either directly or by compression of the surrounding tissues. Their size at time of delivery can necessitate a cesarean section. Vascular flow can be so extensive as to cause high-flow compromise to the fetus, and color Doppler examination is therefore suggested to determine the teratoma's extent. Teratomas may also occur in areas unrelated to the spine, such as the face, neck, and intracranially (see Figs. 15-26 and 15-38).

The differential diagnosis of a mass seen along the back of the fetal neck includes cephalocele, cystic hygroma, cervical teratoma, and, rarely, a cervical

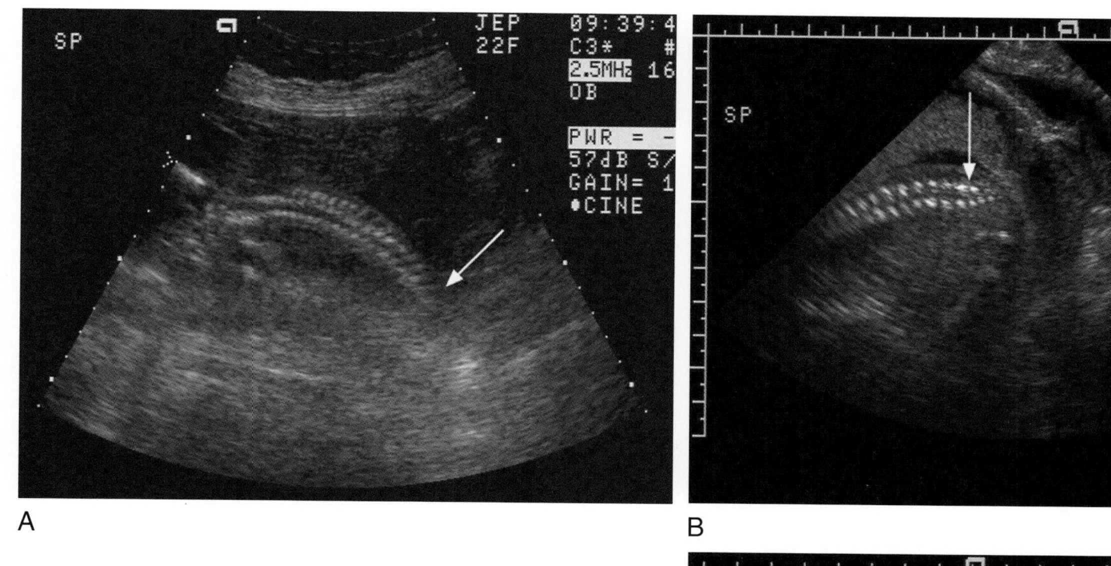

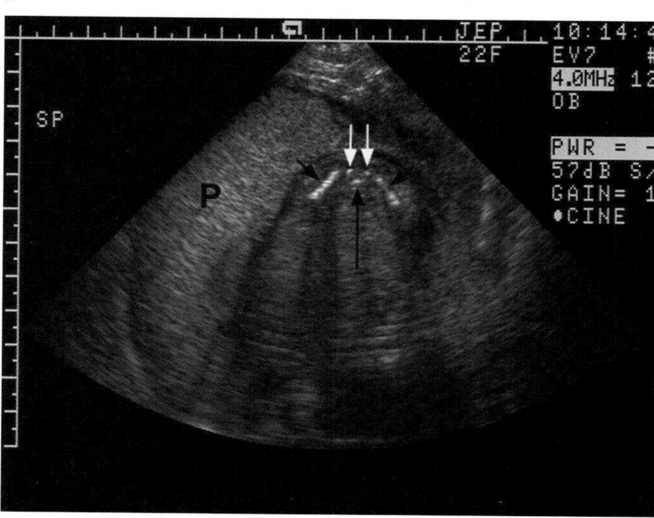

Figure 15-52 Value of transvaginal ultrasound for visualizing fetal anatomy. **A,** Sagittal transabdominal image of fetal spine at 19 weeks fails to adequately depict distal spine because of unfavorable orientation of spine in maternal pelvis. *Arrow,* region of poorly seen fetal spine. **B,** Sagittal transvaginal image of spine of same fetus as in **A** successfully demonstrates normal tapering of distal spine *(arrow).* **C,** Axial transvaginal image of lumbar spine successfully demonstrates normal convergence of posterior ossification centers *(short white arrows). Short black arrows,* iliac bones; *long black arrow,* vertebral body; P, placenta.

meningocele. Cephaloceles are distinguished from the other causes of masses in the neck region by identification of a calvarial defect and distortion of intracranial anatomy. A cystic hygroma contains septations but little if any solid tissue and is often associated with diffuse soft tissue thickening. A cervical teratoma typically contains large amounts of solid tissue intermixed with irregular fluid spaces and may have calcifications. Finally, a cervical meningocele is associated with a defect in the cervical spine.

There has been an attempt to evaluate the neurologic deficit caused by lumbosacral spinal defects (meningomyeloceles) and sacrococcygeal teratomas by observing the movement of the lower limbs and by the filling and emptying of the urinary bladder. At present these observations have not proven accurate in predicting function or outcome.

TRANSVAGINAL CENTRAL NERVOUS SYSTEM IMAGING

There are times when transabdominal scans cannot adequately evaluate the fetal structures occupying the lower uterine segment. In these circumstances, TV scanning should be considered. Its higher resolution capability and different scanning planes (frequently coronal and sagittal) can permit identification or more complete analysis of the fetus (Fig. 15-52).

Key Features

Anencephaly is easily diagnosed, even early in the second trimester, by absence of normal calvarium and brain above the orbits. Occasionally, residual dysmorphic brain called angiomatous stroma may remain above the orbits.

As a general rule, the more severe the polyhydramnios, the more likely there is a fetal problem. Mild polyhydramnios may be present in otherwise normal pregnancies. Moderate to marked polyhydramnios is often associated with fetal anomalies of the central nervous or gastrointestinal systems or with fetal hydrops.

Polyhydramnios accumulates slowly and may not be present, even when expected, until late in the pregnancy.

Fetal head measurements (BPD and HC) are accurate to ±1.2 weeks up to 24 weeks. Their accuracies decrease with advancing gestation and are ±3.8 weeks by the third trimester.

When a BPD is measured, the head shape should be considered. If the head is too oval or round, a correction factor should be included or an HC obtained.

The lateral ventricles are evaluated at their atria. The axial measurement should be less than or equal to 10 mm and the choroid plexus should occupy at least 60% of the ventricular atrium. A small or a "dangling" choroid plexus should alert the examiner to the possibility of ventriculomegaly.

An attempt to visualize both atria, in the near and far fields, should be made, especially when one ventricle appears enlarged.

Increased intracranial pressure (hydrocephalus) can be diagnosed by the presence of progressive ventriculomegaly and/or an enlarged head. However, in most cases the head size is normal. Other signs include a ruptured falx echo, third or fourth ventricular enlargement, and certain posterior fossa abnormalities.

Regardless of the severity of hydrocephalus, there is always a thin remaining cortical mantle. Hydranencephaly may mimic this appearance but instead is brain destruction. It is seen as a spectrum from irregular residual hyperechoic areas of tissue to complete absence of brain parenchyma in the frontal and parietotemporal regions.

Microcephaly (small brain and mental retardation) is clinically likely when the head measures more than 3 SD below the norm. It is caused by infections and developmental and genetic abnormalities. It is suggested when the BPD is smaller than the AD by 9 mm, the HC is smaller than the AC by 27 mm, or head size lags behind that of the body by 3 weeks.

Holoprosencephaly is a midline developmental anomaly that occurs in three forms: alobar, the most severe (frequently associated with many additional anomalies); semilobar; and lobar, the least severe. The lobar form frequently goes undiagnosed in utero because the absence of the frontal horns and cavum septi pellucidi is often not appreciated.

Facial anomalies can be isolated or associated with complex anomalies and karyotype abnormalities. Diagnoses of the interorbital diameter, lip and palate, and chin can be made and facial tumors detected.

Cephaloceles are protrusions of the intracranial structures through a calvarial defect and comprise a spectrum from small meningoceles to large encephaloceles. While frequently posterior with protrusion through the occipital bone, they can occur anywhere in the midline, including the ethmoidal sinus region. They are commonly associated with additional structural and chromosomal abnormalities.

Continued

Key Features—cont'd

In the normal posterior fossa, a normal bilobate cerebellum and a cisterna magna can be identified. A loss of the cisterna magna and/or a change in shape of the cerebellum to a "banana" configuration is proof of a neural tube defect with downward displacement of the cerebellum. An enlarged cisterna magna with splaying of the cerebellar hemispheres and a vermian defect is characteristic of Dandy-Walker abnormality.

A thin rim of nuchal skin, termed the nuchal fold, can be measured posterior to the occipital bone from 15 to 21 gestational weeks. A nuchal fold measurement of 6 mm or greater is a marker for trisomy 21.

Earlier in the second trimester, between 11 and 14 weeks, increased nuchal translucency has a high degree of associated aneuploidy and structural anomalies. The measurement varies with gestational age but is always abnormal when greater than 3 mm, even if the translucency resolves later in the pregnancy.

The choroid plexus may contain cysts. If any other abnormality is present or if the cysts are complex or large, the possibility of chromosomal abnormalities, in particular trisomy 18, is likely. On the other hand, an isolated cyst can be considered likely to be a normal variant, especially when an age-adjusted serum triple screen and an extended ultrasound examination show no abnormality.

Isolated CNS abnormalities can be detected by ultrasound. These include agenesis of the corpus callosum; cystic structures such as a vein of Galen aneurysm or arachnoid or porencephalic cyst; intracranial mass; and intracranial hemorrhage.

The fetal spine can be evaluated by a combination of α-fetoprotein measurements in the maternal serum or amniotic fluid and the ultrasound examination.

Ultrasound studies can evaluate the spine in three projections. Of these the most inclusive is the axial view at each vertebral level, which permits evaluation of their posterior elements and overlying posterior soft tissues. Most spinal defects occur in the lumbosacral region.

Secondary abnormalities of the head, the "lemon" and "banana" sign and hydrocephalus, often occur with spinal defects. Of these the "lemon" sign is the least specific and sensitive and often disappears after 24 gestational weeks.

Paraspinal abnormalities include teratomas in the lumbosacral area and cystic hygromas in the cervical region.

SUGGESTED READINGS

Achiron R, Yagel S, Rotstein Z, et al: Cerebral lateral ventricular asymmetry: Is this a normal ultrasonographic finding in the fetal brain? Obstet Gynecol 89:233, 1997.

Alagappan R, et al: Distal lateral ventricular atrium: Reevaluation of normal range. Radiology 193:405, 1994.

Allen LM, Silverman RK: Prenatal ultrasound evaluation of fetal diastematomyelia: Two cases of type 1 split cord malformation. Ultrasound Obstet Gynecol 15:78, 2000.

Anderson NG, Jordan S, McFarlane MR, et al: Diastematomyelia: Diagnosis by prenatal sonography. AJR Am J Roentgenol 163:911, 1994.

Babcock CJ, Chong BW, Salamat MS, et al: Sonographic anatomy of the developing cerebellum: Normal embryology can resemble pathology. AJR Am J Roentgenol 166:427, 1996.

Babcock CJ, McGahan JP, Chong BW, et al: Evaluation of fetal midface anatomy related to facial clefts: Use of US. Radiology 201:113, 1996.

Ball RH, et al: The lemon sign: Not a specific indicator of meningomyelocele. J Ultrasound Med 3:131, 1993.

Baumeister LA, et al: Fetal fourth ventricle: US appearance and frequency of depiction. Radiology 192:333, 1994.

Bennet GL, Bromley B, Benacerraf BR: Agenesis of the corpus callosum: Prenatal detection usually is not possible before 22 weeks of gestation. Radiology 199:447, 1996.

Benson CB, Doubilet PM: Sonographic prediction of gestational age: Accuracy of second- and third-trimester fetal measurements. AJR Am J Roentgenol 157:1275, 1991.

Bloom SL, Bloom DD, Dellanebbia C, et al: The developmental outcome of children with antenatal mild isolated ventriculomegaly. Obstet Gynecol 90:93, 1997.

Brace V, Grant SR, Brackley KJ, et al: Prenatal diagnosis and outcome in sacrococcygeal teratomas: A review of cases between 1992 and 1998. Prenat Diagn 20:51, 2000.

Bromley B, Benacerraf BR: Fetal micrognathia: Associated anomalies and outcome. J Ultrasound Med 13:529, 1994.

Bromley B, Benacerraf BR: Difficulties in the prenatal diagnosis of microcephaly. J Ultrasound Med 14:303, 1995.

Bromley B, Frigoletto FD Jr, Benacerraf BR: Mild fetal lateral cerebral ventriculomegaly: Clinical course and outcome. Am J Obstet Gynecol 164:863, 1991.

Bromley B, Nadel AS, Pauker S, et al: Closure of the cerebellar vermis: Evaluation with second trimester US. Radiology 193:761, 1994.

Browning BP, Laorr A, McGahan JP, et al: Proximal fetal cerebral ventricle: Description of US technique and initial results. Radiology 192:337, 1994.

Budorick NE, Pretorius DH, McGahan MC, et al: Cephalocele detection in utero: Sonographic and clinical features. Ultrasound Obstet Gynecol 5:77, 1995.

Budorick NE, Pretorius DH, Nelson TR: Sonography of the fetal spine: Technique, imaging, findings, and clinical implications. AJR Am J Roentgenol 16:421, 1995.

Cardoza JD, Goldstein BB, Filly RA: Exclusion of fetal ventriculomegaly with a single measurement: The width of the lateral ventricular atrium. Radiology 169:711, 1988.

Caughey AB, Kuppermann M, Norton ME, et al: Nuchal translucency and first trimester biochemical markers for Down syndrome screening: A cost effectiveness analysis. Am J Obstet Gynecol 187:1239, 2002.

Chervenak FA, et al: A prospective study of the accuracy of ultrasound in predicting fetal microcephaly. Obstet Gynecol 69:908, 1987.

Chinn DH, et al: Sonographically detected fetal choroid plexus cysts: Frequency and association with aneuploidy. J Ultrasound Med 10:255, 1991.

Crandall BF, Robinson L, Grau P: Risks associated with an elevated maternal serum alpha-fetoprotein level. Am J Obstet Gynecol 165:581, 1991.

Damato N, et al: Frequency of fetal anomalies in sonographically detected polyhydramnios. J Ultrasound Med 12:11, 1993.

Ecker JL, Shipp TD, Bromley B, et al: The sonographic diagnosis of Dandy-Walker and Dandy-Walker variant: Associated findings and outcomes. Prenat Diagn 20:328, 2000.

Eller KM, Kuller JA: Fetal porencephaly: A review of etiology, diagnosis, and prognosis. Obstet Gynecol Surv 50:684, 1995.

Estroff JA, Scott MR, Benacerraf BR: Dandy-Walker variant: Prenatal sonographic features and clinical outcome. Radiology 185:755, 1992.

Farrell TA, et al: Fetal lateral ventricles: Reassessment of normal values for atrial diameter at US. Radiology 193:409, 1994.

Goldstein I, et al: Sonographic evaluation of the normal developmental anatomy of fetal cerebral ventricles: I. The frontal horn. Obstet Gynecol 72:588, 1988.

Goldstein RB, Filly RA: Prenatal diagnosis of anencephaly: Spectrum of sonographic appearances and distinction from the amniotic band syndrome. AJR Am J Roentgenol 151:547, 1988.

Goldstein RB, LaPidus AS, Filly RA: Fetal cephaloceles: Diagnosis with US. Radiology 180:803, 1991.

Haimovici JA, Doubilet PM, Benson CB, et al: Clinical significance of isolated enlargement of the cisterna magna (>10 mm) on prenatal sonography. J Ultrasound Med 16:731, 1997.

Hata T, Yonehara T, Aoki S, et al: Three-dimensional sonographic visualization of the fetal face. AJR Am J Roentgenol 170:481, 1998.

Heling KS, Chaoui R, Bollmann R: Prenatal diagnosis of an aneurysm of the vein of Galen with three-dimensional color power angiography. Ultrasound Obstet Gynecol 15:333, 2000.

Heiserman J, Filly RA, Goldstein RB: Effect of measurement errors on sonographic evaluation of ventriculomegaly. J Ultrasound Med 10:121, 1991.

Hertzberg BS, et al: The three lines: Origin of sonographic landmarks in the fetal head. AJR Am J Roentgenol 149:1009, 1987.

Hertzberg BS, et al: Sonographic evaluation of fetal CNS: Technical and interpretive pitfalls. AJR Am J Roentgenol 172:523, 1999.

Hertzberg BS, et al: Fetal cerebral ventriculomegaly: Misidentification of the true medial boundary of the ventricle at US. Radiology 205:813, 1997.

Hilpert PL, Hall BE, Kurtz AB: The atria of the fetal lateral ventricles: A prospective study of normal size and choroid plexus filling. AJR Am J Roentgenol 164:731, 1995.

Hyett JA, Perdu M, Sharland GK, et al: Increased nuchal translucency at 10-14 weeks of gestation as a marker for major cardiac defects. Ultrasound Obstet Gynecol 10:242, 1997.

Jeanty P, et al: The binocular distance: A new way to estimate fetal age. J Ultrasound Med 3:241, 1984.

Johnson DD, Pretorius DH, Budorick NE, et al: Fetal lip and primary palate: Three-dimensional versus two-dimensional US. Radiology 217:236, 2000.

Kelly EN, Allen VM, Seaward G, et al: Mild ventriculomegaly in the fetus, natural history, associated findings and outcome of isolated mild ventriculomegaly: A literature review. Prenat Diagn 21:697, 2001.

Keogan MT, DeAtkine AB, Hertzberg BS: Cerebellar vermian defects: Antenatal sonographic appearance and clinical significance. J Ultrasound Med 13:607, 1994.

Kerner B, Flaum E, Mathews H, et al: Cervical teratoma: Prenatal diagnosis and long-term follow-up. Prenat Diagn 18:51, 1998.

Knutzon RK, et al: Fetal cisterna magna septa: A normal anatomic finding. Radiology 180:799, 1991.

Kolble N, Wisser J, Kurmanavicius J, et al: Dandy-Walker malformation: Prenatal diagnosis and outcome. Prenat Diagn 20:318, 2000.

Kurtz AB, et al: Ultrasound criteria for in utero diagnosis of microcephaly. J Clin Ultrasound 8:11, 1980.

Laing FC, et al: Sonography of the fetal posterior fossa: False appearance of mega-cisterna magna and Dandy-Walker variant. Radiology 192:247, 1994.

Lipitz A, Malinger G, Meizner I, et al: Outcome of fetuses with isolated cerebral borderline ventriculomegaly: Report of 31 cases and review of the literature. Ultrasound Obstet Gynecol 12:23, 1998.

Mahony BS, et al: The fetal cisterna magna. Radiology 153:773, 1984.

Mayden KL, et al: Orbital diameters: A new parameter for prenatal diagnosis and dating. Am J Obstet Gynecol 144:289, 1982.

Monteagudo A, Reuss ML, Timor-Tritsch IE: Imaging the fetal brain in the second and third trimesters using transvaginal sonography. Obstet Gynecol 77:27, 1991.

Noriega CA, Fleming AD, Bonebrake RG: A false-positive diagnosis of a prenatal encephalocele on transvaginal ultrasonography. J Ultrasound Med 20:925, 2001.

Nadel AS, et al: Isolated choroid plexus cysts in the second-trimester fetus: Is amniocentesis really indicated? Radiology 185:545, 1992.

Nelson NL, Callen PW, Filly RA: The choroid plexus pseudocyst: Sonographic identification and characterization. J Ultrasound Med 11:597, 1992.

Nyberg DA, et al: Holoprosencephaly: Prenatal sonographic diagnosis. AJNR Am J Neuroradiol 8:871, 1987.

Nyberg DA, Souter VL, El-Bastawissi A, et al: Isolated sonographic markers for detection of fetal Down syndrome in the second trimester of pregnancy. J Ultrasound Med 20:1053, 2001.

Pandya PP, et al: First-trimester fetal nuchal translucency thickness and risk for trisomies. Obstet Gynecol 84:420, 1994.

Pandya PP, Kondylios A, Hilbert L, et al: Chromosomal defects and outcome in 1015 fetuses with increased nuchal translucency. Ultrasound Obstet Gynecol 5:15, 1995.

Patel MD, et al: Isolated mild fetal cerebral ventriculomegaly: Clinical course and outcome. Radiology 192:759, 1994.

Patel MD, Goldstein RB, Tung S, et al: Fetal cerebral ventricular atrium: Difference in size according to sex. Radiology 194:713, 1995.

Pilu G, et al: Sonographic evaluation of the normal developmental anatomy of the fetal cerebral ventricles: II. The atria. Obstet Gynecol 73:250, 1989.

Pilu G, Falco P, Gabrielli S, et al: The clinical significance of fetal isolated cerebral borderline ventriculomegaly: Report of 31 cases and review of the literature. Ultrasound Obstet Gynecol 14:320, 1999.

Pilu G, Hobbins JC: Sonography of fetal cerebrospinal anomalies. Prenat Diagn 22:321, 2002.

Pilu G, Visentin A, Valeri B: The Dandy-Walker complex and fetal sonography. Ultrasound Obstet Gynecol 16:115, 2000.

Reiss I, Gortner L, Moller J, et al: Fetal intracerebral hemorrhage in the second trimester: Diagnosis by sonography and magnetic resonance imaging. Ultrasound Obstet Gynecol 7:49, 1996.

Schlembach D, Bornemann A, Rupprecht T, et al: Fetal intracranial tumors detected by ultrasound: A report of two cases and review of the literature. Ultrasou0nd Obstet Gynecol 14:407, 1999.

Sepulveda W, Kyle PM, Hassan J, et al: Prenatal diagnosis of diastematomyelia: Case reports and review of the literature. Prenat Diagn 17:161, 1997.

Shahabi S, Busine A: Prenatal diagnosis of an epidermal scalp cyst simulating an encephalocele. Prenat Diagn 18:373, 1998.

Sherer DM, Anyaegbunam A, Onyeije C: Antepartum fetal intracranial hemorrhage, predisposing factors and prenatal sonography: A review. Am J Perinatol 15:431, 1998.

Sherer DM, Fromberg RA, Rindfustz DW, et al: Color Doppler–aided prenatal diagnosis of a type 1 cystic sacrococcygeal teratoma simulating a meningomyelocele. Am J Perinatol 14:13, 1997.

Sherer DM, Onyeije CI: Prenatal ultrasonographic diagnosis of fetal intracranial tumors: A review. Am J Perinatol 15:319, 1998.

Sheth S, et al: Prenatal diagnosis of sacrococcygeal teratoma: Sonographic-pathologic correlation. Radiology 169:131, 1988.

Shipp TD, Bromley B, Benacerraf B: The ultrasonographic appearance and outcome for fetuses with masses distorting the fetal face. J Ultrasound Med 14:673, 1995.

Souka AP, Krampl E, Bakalis S, et al: Outcome of pregnancy in chromosomally normal fetuses with increased nuchal translucency in the first trimester. Ultrasound Obstet Gynecol 18:9, 2001.

Souka AP, Snidjers RJM, Novakov A, et al: Defects and syndromes in chromosomally normal fetuses with increased nuchal translucency thickness at 10-14 weeks of gestation. Ultrasound Obstet Gynecol 11:391, 1998.

Stoll C, Dott B, Alembik Y, et al: Evaluation of prenatal diagnosis of cleft lip/palate by fetal ultrasonographic examination. Ann Genet 43:11, 2000.

van den Hoff MC, et al: Evaluation of the lemon and banana signs in one hundred thirty fetuses with open spina bifida. Am J Obstet Gynecol 162:322, 1990.

Wald NJ, Watt HC, Hackshaw AK: Integrated screening for Down's syndrome based on tests performed during the first and second trimester. N Engl J Med 341:461, 1999.

Westerberg B, Feldstein VA, Sandberg PL, et al: Sonographic prognostic factors in fetuses with sacrococcygeal teratoma. J Pediatr Surg 35:322, 2000.

CHAPTER 16

Fetal Thorax

The antepartum obstetrical ultrasound standard recommends documentation of heart motion on every examination and a four-chamber view of the heart, including its position within the thorax, on every second- and third-trimester study. Further analysis of the heart and great vessels is, however, possible when the fetal position is appropriate. These additional views offer important information about cardiac anatomy.

In the normal fetus, the nonaerated lungs and the mediastinum blend together to assume a uniform hyperechoic echogenicity. Pulmonary and mediastinal abnormalities can be detected by a change in echogenicity or by a shift of the heart.

HEART

Rate and Rhythm

Heart motion defines a living conceptus. At 5 to 6 weeks, the heart rate averages 100 beats per minute, rising to 140 to 160 beats per minute by 8 weeks. Cardiac activity, often requiring the use of a transvaginal (TV) study, can be routinely detected in embryos with a crown-rump length of more than 5 mm (6.2 weeks) and not infrequently earlier.

This same heart rate is maintained throughout the second and third trimesters, not decreasing below 120 or increasing above 180 beats per minute, with slight normal slowing near term. A transient bradycardia can be normal, provided that it does not decrease below 60 beats per minutes or last longer than 15 to 20 seconds. Other rates and arrhythmias, while they may turn out to be of no consequence to the developing fetus, should however be documented and further evaluated.

The antepartum obstetrical ultrasound standard does not require routine hard-copy documentation of heart motion. Simply observation by real-time or color Doppler sonography will often suffice. However, an M-mode examination is desirable in any abnormal situation because, as a tracing, it can be more precisely analyzed. The ideal M-mode examination should be performed through an atrium and ventricle and include its atrioventricular valve. Pulsed Doppler analysis, because of its increased power levels, should be relegated to a role of confirming and detecting abnormal flow around cardiac valves, such as a right atrial tracing in suspected tricuspid insufficiency and determining flow through septal defects. A pulsed Doppler tracing can also be of value in analyzing the diastolic flow in the arterial waveforms of the ductus arteriosus and middle cerebral arteries.

All heart motion abnormalities should be examined for five properties: (1) rate, (2) rhythm—constant or variable, (3) normal atrial-to-ventricular association, (4) structural abnormalities—cardiac and noncardiac, and (5) evidence of fetal hydrops. The most common arrhythmia is produced by premature atrial contractions. These are usually benign but, if very frequent, can predispose to the development of a supraventricular tachycardia (Fig. 16-1). All other conduction abnormalities must be closely observed and occasionally treated.

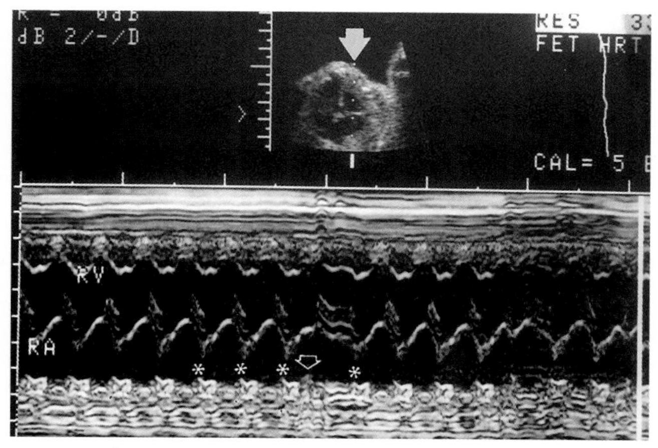

Figure 16-1 M-mode tracing of the fetal heart in a 22-week fetus with premature atrial contractions. The ultrasound image shows the position of the M-mode tracing through the right side of the heart, starting at the *arrow* and extending along the *dotted line.* The M-mode tracing shows the right ventricle (RV) and the right atrium (RA) separated by the tricuspid valve. At the bottom of the tracing *asterisks* denote normal contractions. Note the normal association between the atria and ventricles. The *open arrow* denotes a premature atrial contraction followed by a prolonged pause.

If a well-defined bradycardia or tachyarrhythmia is observed, a short M-mode tracing is sufficient for documentation. On occasion the heart rate may be normal and yet, because of unexplained hydrops, an intermittent conduction abnormality is suspected. A longer period of observation may then be necessary to document this suspected problem.

Normal Cardiac Structures

To identify cardiac position, a helpful starting point is the standard axial view of the upper abdomen. After identifying the liver and stomach, the transducer is moved up to the lower thorax, still in axial projection, to identify the four-chamber heart view. While after birth the apex of the heart points downward and the four-chamber view cannot be obtained in an axial projection, the in utero liver is proportionately so much larger that it elevates the cardiac apex.

Both the heart and stomach are normally on the left side of the fetus. The right and left sides of the fetus can be determined from the fetal presentation (cephalic or breech) and by the position of the fetal spine. With practice this assessment can be performed quickly and accurately.

Timing of the cardiac study is important. Transabdominally, the heart chambers are usually not identified clearly before 16 weeks; by 18 to 22 weeks it is possible to satisfactorily identify intracardiac anatomy in the majority of patients. In the four-chamber view, the cardiac apex points toward the left side of the fetus at an angle of approximately 45 degrees (Fig. 16-2). The right ventricle is the most anterior chamber. Occasionally, particularly when the fetus is positioned obliquely, it may be difficult to identify the right ventricle. A simple and usually successful approach to establishing chamber identity in the axial view is as follows: the descending thoracic aorta is immediately anterior and slightly to the left of the spine and directly anterior to it is the left atrium. From the left atrium, the right atrium and then their corresponding ventricles can be determined.

The four-chamber view (see Fig. 16-2) permits identification of the ventricles and their interventricular septa, the atria with their ostium secundum and foramen ovale, and the atrioventricular valves (mitral and tricuspid). The overall sizes of the atria and ventricles, both during systole or diastole, should exhibit a 1:1 relationship throughout the second and third trimesters. If needed, measurement tables are available, with the chamber sizes measured at their inner margins just above and below the atrioventricular valves. The examiner can encounter difficulty in full cardiac visualization if the fetal part closest to the transducer is the spine or in patients where the heart is more than 8 to 10 cm from the transducer (e.g., women of large girth or with polyhydramnios).

The transverse dimension or circumference of the heart, taken at the level of the atrioventricular valves, should not exceed 50% of a comparable measurement of

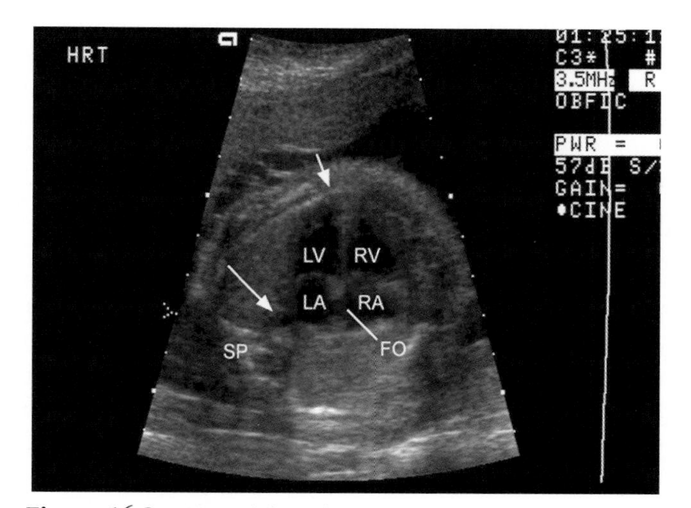

Figure 16-2 Normal four-chamber view in a second-trimester fetus. The cardiac apex *(short arrow)* points to the fetus' left side at an angle of approximately 45 degrees from the midline. The right ventricle (RV) is the most anterior chamber. The descending aorta *(long arrow)* is immediately anterior and slightly to the left of the spine (SP). The left atrium (LA) is anterior to the aorta. The interventricular septum is the echogenic line between the right (RV) and left ventricle (LV). The foramen ovale (FO) is seen between the left and right atria.

the fetal thorax. This is similar to the expected heart size relative to the thorax seen after birth on a posteroanterior chest radiograph.

Structural Abnormalities

With a family history of congenital heart disease, the risk of a cardiac anomaly, not necessarily of the same type, is increased in a subsequent child. The chance of recurrence increases by 10% if one parent (higher for an affected mother), by 3% if one sibling, and up to 10% if two siblings are affected. The risk of congenital heart disease is even higher if the mother had been affected with aortic stenosis: 13% to 18%.

Using only the four-chamber view, the overall detection rate for significant cardiac anomalies approaches 70%. However, the rate reported by some observers has been less, as low as 50%. Therefore, although the four-chamber view is valuable, it has limitations. It is only able to detect certain anomalies, and typically only the larger ones. These are listed by frequency (likelihood) of detection (Box 16-1). These anomalies can be classified into those affecting cardiac position (e.g., situs inversus and ectopia cordis), cardiac septa (e.g., ventricular septal defect), cardiac chambers (e.g., ventricular hypoplasia and Ebstein's anomaly), and masses (e.g., rhabdomyomas). Most are visualized directly, with the presence of others only inferred by the identification of a constellation of cardiac findings (e.g., that observed in the setting of pulmonary atresia). Because of its association with omphaloceles, ectopia cordis is discussed in Chapter 17.

The position of the heart is important. A right-sided heart may, on occasion, be an isolated finding but is much more likely associated with significant intracardiac and extracardiac anomalies. Similarly, a change in the angle of the heart from 45 degrees toward either 0 or 90 degrees (a rotational abnormality) has also been associated with increased cardiac anomalies.

A four-chamber view is good for identifying large septal defects, particularly ventricular or atrioventricular (AV) canal defects (Fig. 16-3). Smaller ventricular and most atrial defects, because of the normally patent foramen ovale, go undiagnosed in utero. On an apical four-chamber view, the region of the membranous septum, which is near the insertion of the mitral and tricuspid valves, may appear decreased in echogenicity or even absent (Fig. 16-4A). This is a technical artifact caused by the parallel orientation of this thin area to the ultrasound beam. Additional images can be obtained after adjusting the scan plane to prove the septum is intact (Fig. 16-4B).

Abnormal cardiac chambers are usually diagnosed on a four-chamber image. An "enlarged" right atrium that occurs in Ebstein's anomaly, a combination of the right atrium and the atrialized right ventricle, is readily detected (Fig. 16-5). Ventricular hypoplasia involving either the right or left ventricle is often diagnosed, provided proper technique is used (Fig. 16-6). In a true axial four-chamber view, the apices of both normal ventricles are seen to extend to the cardiac apex. Although an

Box 16-1 Abnormal Four-Chamber Heart View: The Frequency (Likelihood) of Cardiovascular Abnormality Detection

Frequently Detected

Hypoplastic right or left ventricle
Single ventricle
Atrioventricular (endocardial cushion) defect
Large ventricular septal defect
Double-outlet right ventricle
Ebstein's anomaly
Pulmonary atresia
Cardiac tumors
Ectopia cordis
Situs inversus

Less Frequently Detected

Large atrial septal defect
Tetralogy of Fallot
Cardiomyopathy
Aortic stenosis (severe)
Coarctation of aorta (severe)

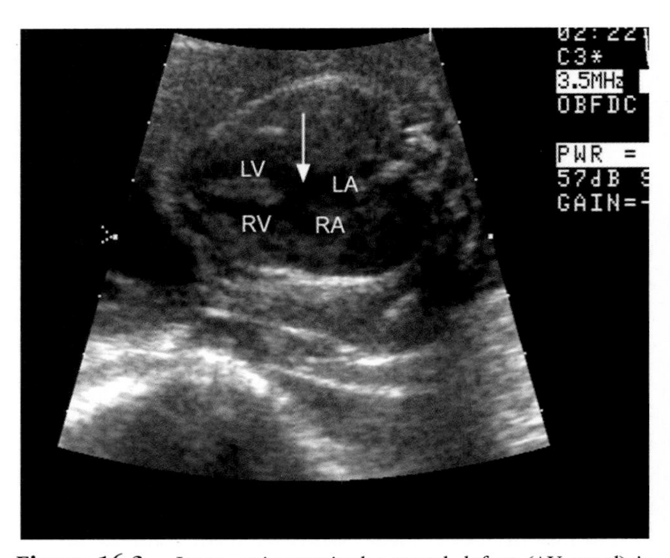

Figure 16-3 Large atrioventricular septal defect (AV canal) in a 17-week fetus with Down syndrome. Note the large defect *(arrow)* in both the upper part of the interventricular septum and the lower part of the interatrial septum. LV, left ventricle; LA, left atrium; RV, right ventricle; RA, right atrium.

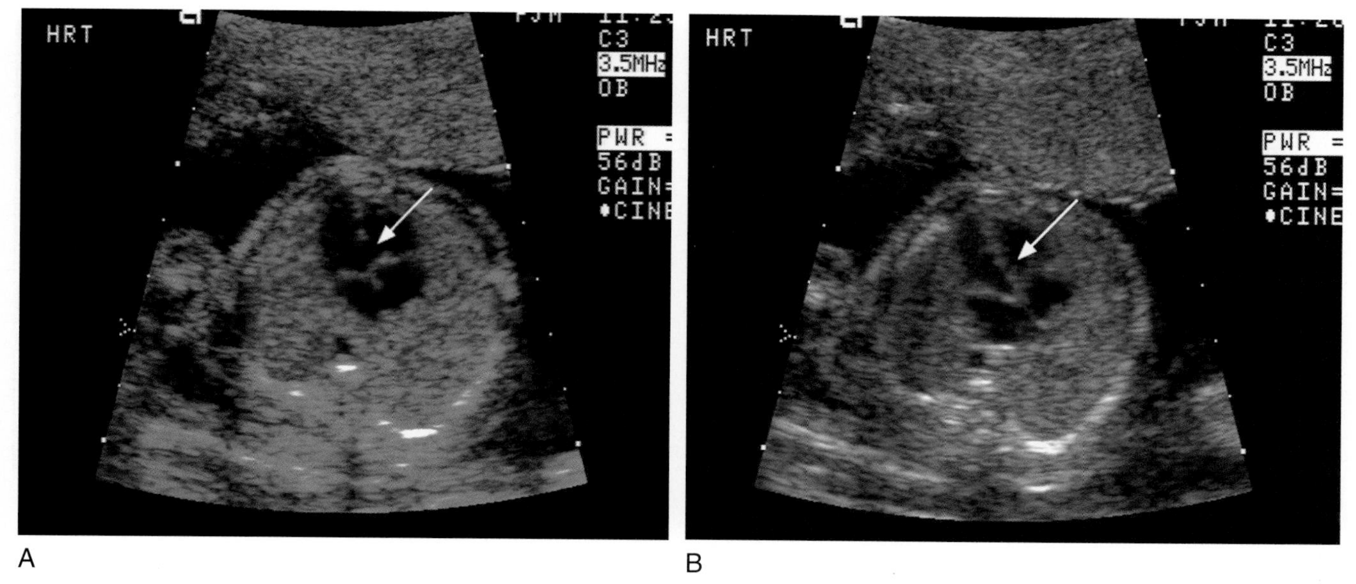

Figure 16-4 Four-chamber views in an 18-week fetus show apparent defect in a normal interventricular septum due to scan plane. **A,** Apparent defect *(arrow)* in the membranous part of the interventricular septum is caused by dropout due to the parallel orientation of the septum to the ultrasound beam. **B,** With a slight change in orientation, the septum *(arrow)* is shown to be normal.

offaxis (not axial) scan might incorrectly suggest ventricular asymmetry, the position of the ventricular apices would still be normal. In contradistinction, when true ventricular hypoplasia is present, the affected ventricular chamber is smaller and its apex shortened.

The four-chamber view can also identify cardiac masses. In particular, rhabdomyomas have been diagnosed (Fig. 16-7). These masses, typically associated with tuberous sclerosis, are hyperechoic and arise from the muscle of the walls or septa. If large, they can compress and narrow the cardiac chambers.

Small hyperechoic foci can be seen in either ventricle, the left more often than the right, or in both (Fig. 16-8). Although they do not cause shadowing, perhaps related to their small size and constant motion, they represent papillary muscle calcification, are of unknown cause, and are not associated with structural anomalies. However, there is now evidence to support an up to 2-fold increase in the overall incidence of trisomy 21 (Down syndrome) in the high-risk population. The ventricular echogenic focus is therefore considered a minor marker for Down syndrome. There are, however, currently insufficient data on the implications of this finding in low-risk populations to assess its significance in the low-risk patient. When no other findings of Down syndrome are present, this mildly increased risk is often not enough to require karyotype analysis.

The four-chamber view can overlook small or subtle intracardiac defects and cannot identify the aorta and pulmonary arteries. To overcome these shortcomings, additional images have been proposed that are not currently required as part of the routine antepartum obstetrical ultrasound standard. Nevertheless, the simplest two are a short-axis view of the great vessels at the base of the heart and a long-axis view of the left ventricular outflow tract (LVOT). The base view, obtained by moving the axial four-chamber view cephalad, identifies the normal perpendicular origins

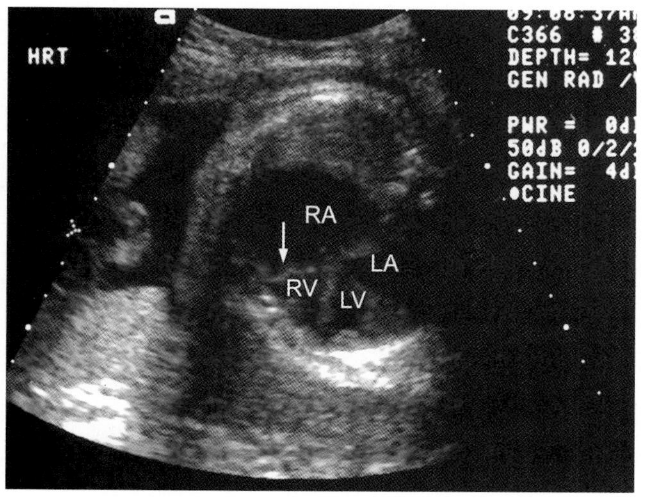

Figure 16-5 Ebstein's anomaly. Four-chamber view shows a markedly enlarged right atrium (RA) due to low insertion of tricuspid valve *(arrow)* and atrialization of much of the right ventricle (RV). LA, left atrium; LV, left ventricle.

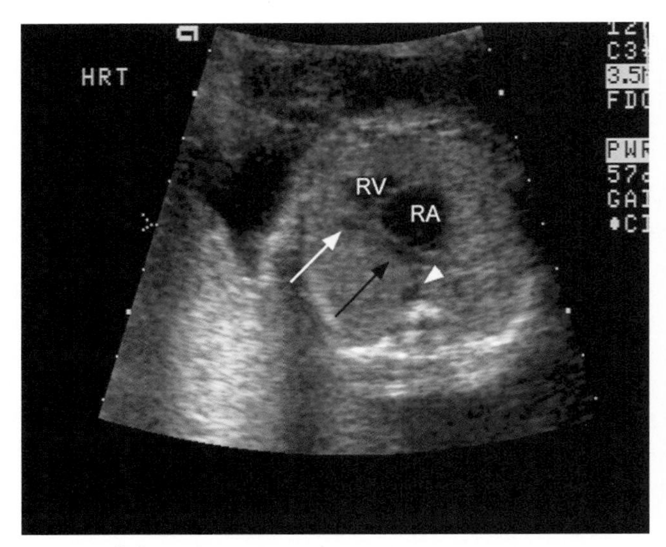

Figure 16-6 Hypoplastic left heart. Four-chamber view shows marked hypoplasia of the left heart. *White arrow,* left ventricle; *black arrow,* left atrium; RV, right ventricle; RA, right atrium; *arrowhead,* descending aorta.

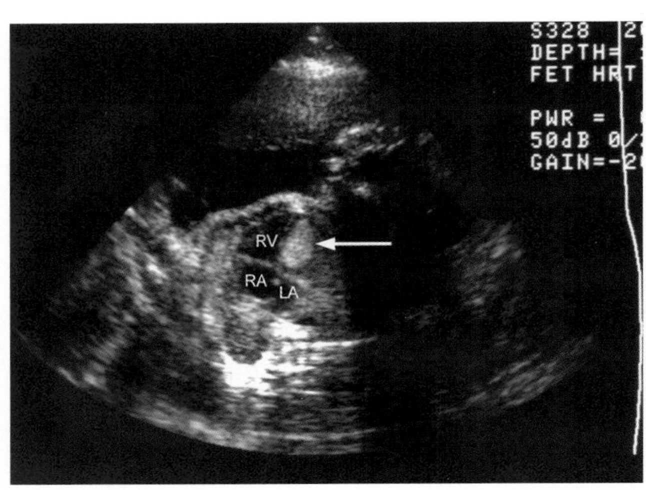

Figure 16-7 Cardiac mass in a 19-week fetus. A large hyperechoic mass *(arrow)* corresponding to a rhabdomyoma fills the majority of the left ventricle in this fetus with tuberous sclerosis. LA, left atrium; RA, right atrium; RV, right ventricle.

of the pulmonary artery and aorta (Fig. 16-9). It is important to identify proper great vessel orientation, because this rules out transposition of these vessels. The normal proportion of the overall sizes of the pulmonary artery and aorta is 1:1 throughout the second and third trimesters; size disproportionality can identify a number of abnormalities (Box 16-2). The pulmonary artery bifurcation into right and left pulmonary arteries can frequently be identified and the patent ductus arteriosus can be seen extending from the main pulmonary artery back to the descending thoracic aorta.

The long-axis view of the LVOT is obtained by scanning the left ventricle and then turning the transducer toward the fetal right shoulder (Fig. 16-10A and B). This

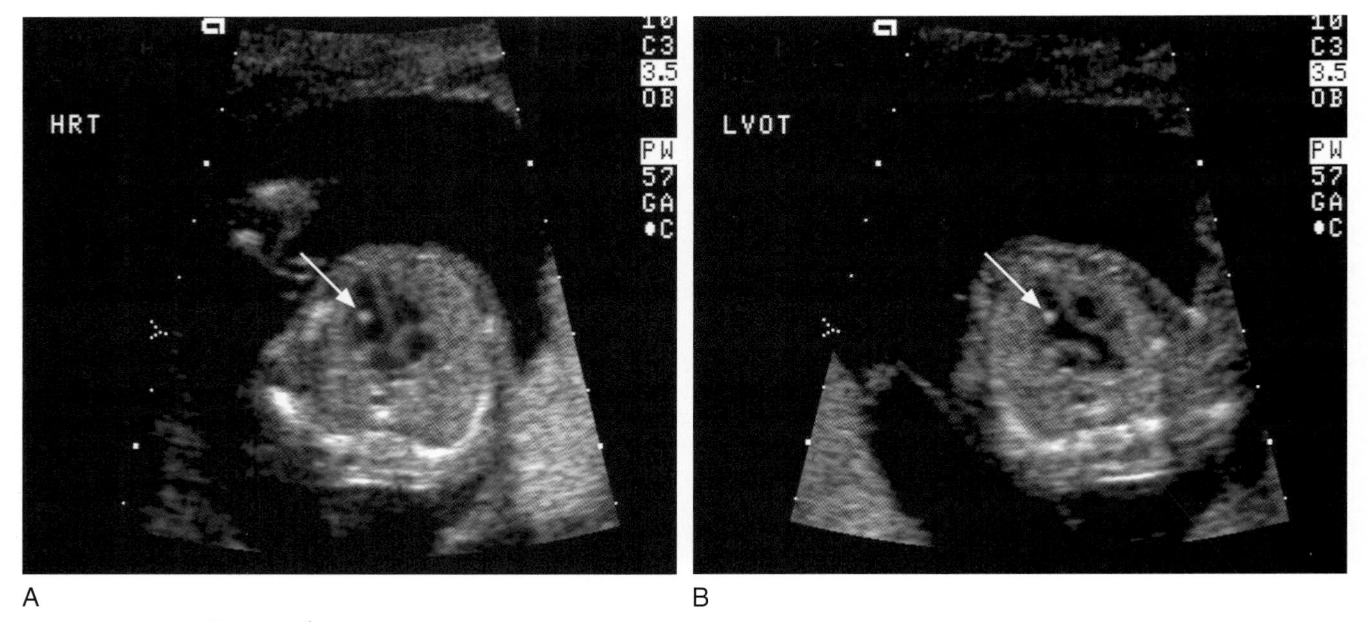

Figure 16-8 Left ventricular hyperechoic (echogenic) focus. A punctate highly echogenic focus *(arrow)* is seen in the left ventricle on the four-chamber (**A**) and left ventricular outflow tract (**B**) views.

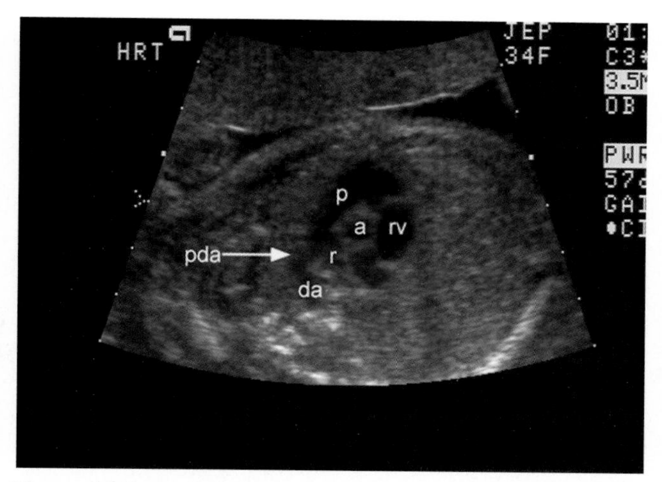

Figure 16-9 Normal axial short-axis view of the great vessels in a 26-week fetus. The pulmonary artery (p) is seen curving around the ascending aorta (a). This is the normal configuration for these vessels: the origins of the pulmonary artery and ascending aorta should not be oriented parallel to each other. Also note that the pulmonary artery and ascending aorta are similar in size. The pulmonary artery bifurcates into the right branch (r), and left branch (not shown). The patent ductus arteriosus (pda) extends posterior from the main pulmonary artery to join the descending aorta (da). rv, right ventricle.

view analyzes the continuity of the left ventricle with the ascending thoracic aorta and permits more complete evaluation of the ventricular septum. By turning the transducer in the other direction, a right ventricular outflow tract (RVOT) (see Fig. 16-10C) can also be imaged. With one or both of the outflow tract views, more ventricular septal defects and the overriding of the great vessels seen in tetralogy of Fallot can be identified (Fig. 16-11).

When these outflow tract and base views are added to the four-chamber view, the detection of cardiac anomalies, as cited in most series, increases to greater than 80%. However, the aortic arch and descending thoracic aorta, ductus arteriosus (in the long axis), the pulmonary veins, and the vena cava into the right atrium are still not imaged. These, too, can be imaged with additional practice in a number of cases.

A TV study of the heart can be performed earlier, at 12 to 16 weeks gestation. It, however, requires considerable skill. With smaller cardiac structures and poor fetal positioning problems, a combination of uterine fundal pressure with TV scanning permits more advantageous positioning of the fetus and, not infrequently, full imaging of the heart. Detection of many anomalies is possible, although many observers still prefer confirmation with an 18- to 22-week transabdominal evaluation.

If an examiner identifies a cardiac abnormality but does not feel certain of the diagnosis, videotape recording or recording of the heart on a cine loop on a digital system is recommended. This permits better documentation than freeze-frame imaging alone and allows for later review and consultation if needed. Recent attempts to perform 3-D imaging of the heart, using multiplanar reconstructions, have been found to be of promise in selected patients.

There are commonly extracardiac structural abnormalities and an increased incidence of chromosomal abnormalities (particularly trisomies) associated with congenital heart disease. Meticulous attention to the rest of the fetal structures and a karyotype analysis is often warranted when a fetus with a cardiac abnormality is detected. If the cardiac structural abnormality is severe enough to be incompatible with life and the pregnancy continues, the fetus should be observed serially for the assessment of fetal growth and for the detection of signs of heart failure (fetal hydrops). Medical treatments are available for certain cardiac arrhythmias (particularly digitalis and calcium channel blockers). These can be given to the mother, infrequently delivered into the amniotic fluid, or rarely even directly given into the fetus. Near term, decisions about the type of delivery and the type of hospital may be important.

Box 16-2 Disproportionate Size of the Great Vessels

Large Aorta

Tetralogy of Fallot
Truncus arteriosus

Small Aorta

Coarctation
Hypoplastic left heart

Small Pulmonary Artery

Hypoplastic right heart
Ebstein's anomaly with pulmonary hypoplasia

FETAL HYDROPS

Fetal hydrops (hydrops fetalis) is defined as excessive fetal body water. It is categorized as either immune or nonimmune hydrops. Immune-mediated hydrops is caused by maternal exposure to certain fetal antigens, resulting in a fetal hemolytic anemia. It is most commonly caused by rhesus (Rh) incompatibility.

Nonimmune hydrops consists of a heterogeneous group of abnormalities. It can be divided into five

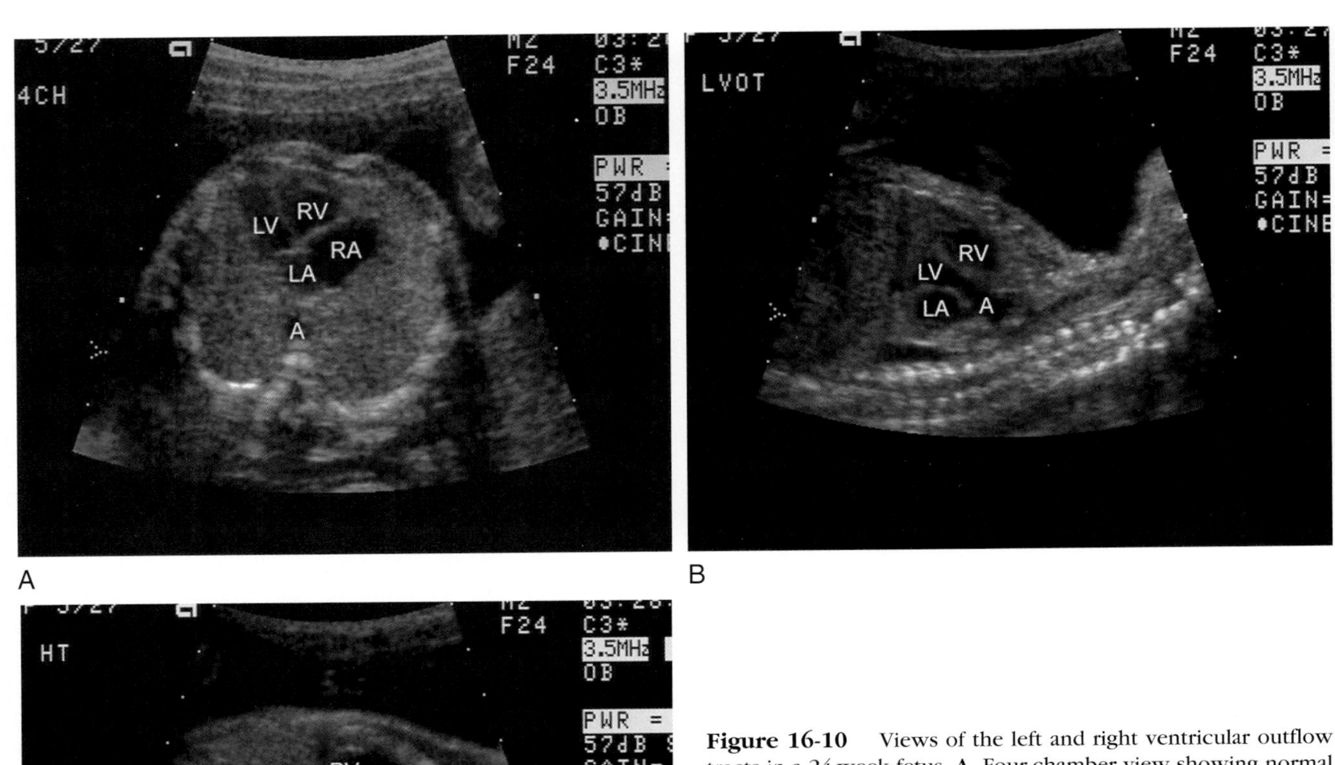

Figure 16-10 Views of the left and right ventricular outflow tracts in a 24-week fetus. **A,** Four-chamber view showing normal orientation and size of the cardiac chambers. **B,** Left ventricular outflow tract (LVOT) view is obtained by tilting and rotating the transducer toward the fetus' left shoulder from the four-chamber view. **C,** Right ventricular outflow tract (RVOT) view is obtained by rotating the transducer in the other direction. LV, left ventricle; LA, left atrium; RV, right ventricle; RA, right atrium; A, aorta; PA, pulmonary artery; PDA, patent ductus arteriosus.

categories: (1) cardiac (primary myocardial and high-output failure), (2) decreased plasma oncotic pressure, (3) increased capillary permeability, (4) obstruction of venous return, and (5) obstruction of lymphatic flow. The cardiac causes, constituting 22% to 40% of the nonimmune cases, comprise severe arrhythmias (either intermittent or constant), structural anomalies, severe anemias, myocarditis, arteriovenous shunts (usually resulting from fetal or placental tumors), and the twin-twin transfusion syndromes in multiple gestations. Decreased oncotic pressure resulting from decreased albumin formation or increased excretion (hepatitis or nephrotic syndrome, respectively), increased capillary permeability (anoxia), venous obstruction (congenital or space-occupying lesions), and generalized lymphatic obstruction (Turner's syndrome) may also lead to

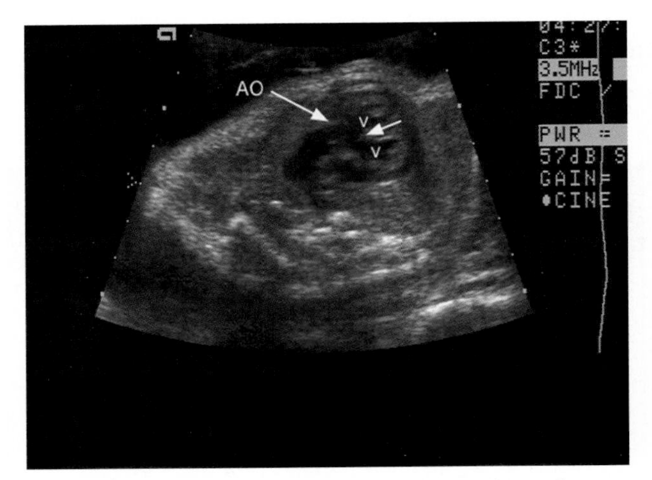

Figure 16-11 Tetralogy of Fallot. Left ventricular outflow tract view shows aorta (AO) overriding the left and right ventricles (V). A high ventricular septal defect *(short arrow)* is also seen. The four components of tetralogy of Fallot are a high ventricular septal defect, overriding aorta, pulmonic stenosis, and right ventricular hypertrophy.

nonimmune hydrops. In utero infections can present with fetal hydrops, usually caused by a combination of the causes just listed. Rarely, Down syndrome may present as a nonimmune hydropic fetus.

The classic sonographic findings of fetal hydrops are fluid in serous cavities (ascites, pleural and pericardial effusions), skin thickening (edema), placental enlargement, and polyhydramnios (Fig. 16-12). Hepatosplenomegaly may also be present, particularly in immune hydrops. In general, the more severe the hydrops, the more numerous and prominent the abnormalities. In any individual case, however, not all of these abnormalities are present and not all are equally prominent. It is uncommon to have fetal hydrops occur with only skin thickening (without serous fluid collections). Skin thickening alone is more often associated with gestational diabetes, sometimes in combination with placental enlargement and polyhydramnios.

Ascites, pleural effusions, and, rarely, pericardial effusions may be the first findings in fetal hydrops (Fig. 16-13). On occasion, however, these findings may be isolated and caused by more local problems. For example, ascites may be secondary to urinary tract

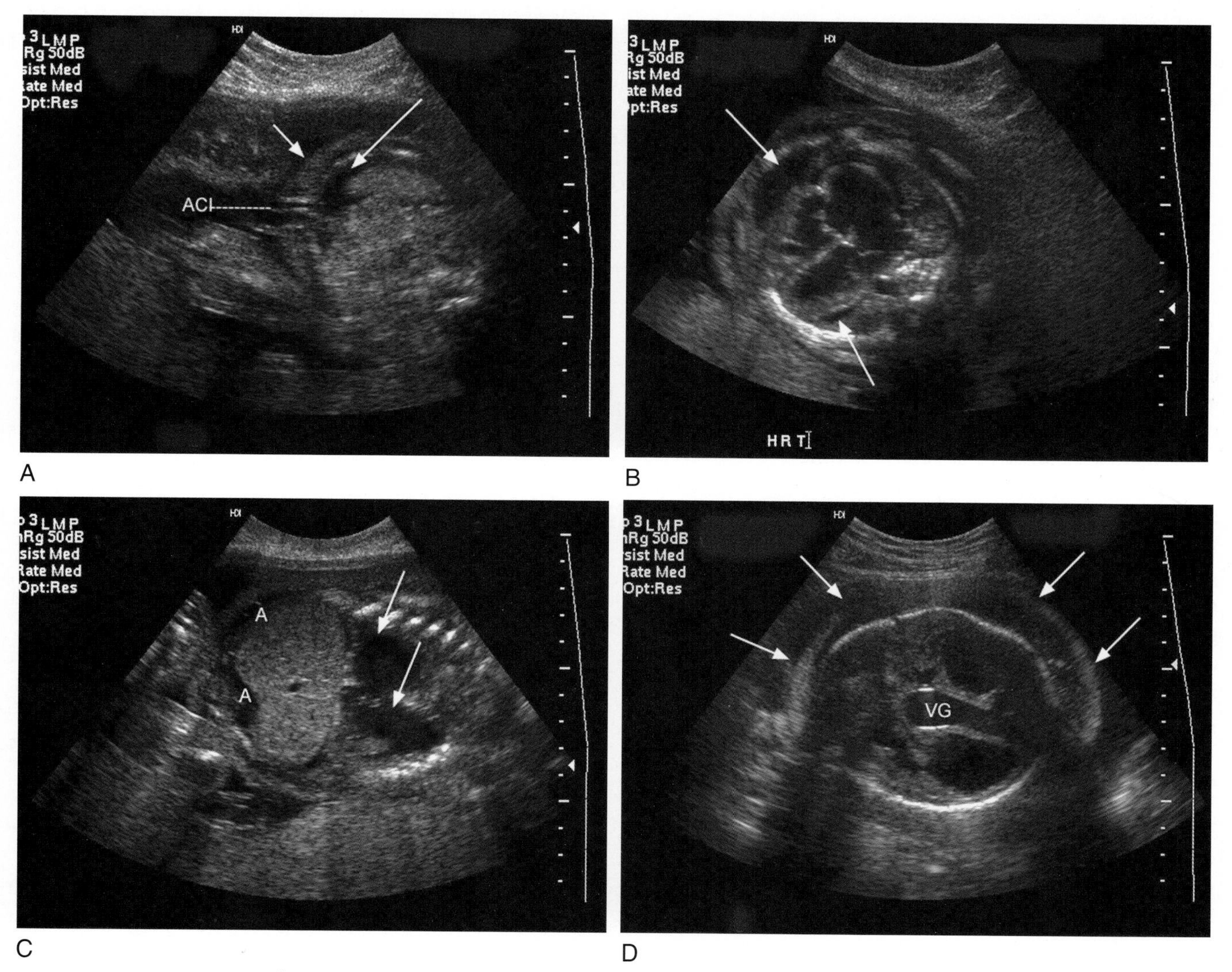

Figure 16-12 Fetal hydrops: typical findings. Typical ultrasound findings of hydrops are depicted in this third-trimester fetus with severe hydrops due to high output failure from a vein of Galen aneurysm. **A,** Axial image of abdomen shows ascites *(long arrow)* and skin thickening *(short arrow).* ACI, abdominal cord insertion. **B,** Axial image of thorax shows a pericardial effusion *(arrows)* and cardiomegaly. **C,** Coronal image of thorax and abdomen shows large bilateral pleural effusions *(arrows)* and ascites (A). **D,** Axial image of fetal head shows marked scalp edema *(arrows).* Also shown is the dilated vein of Galen (VG), which filled with color at color Doppler evaluation.

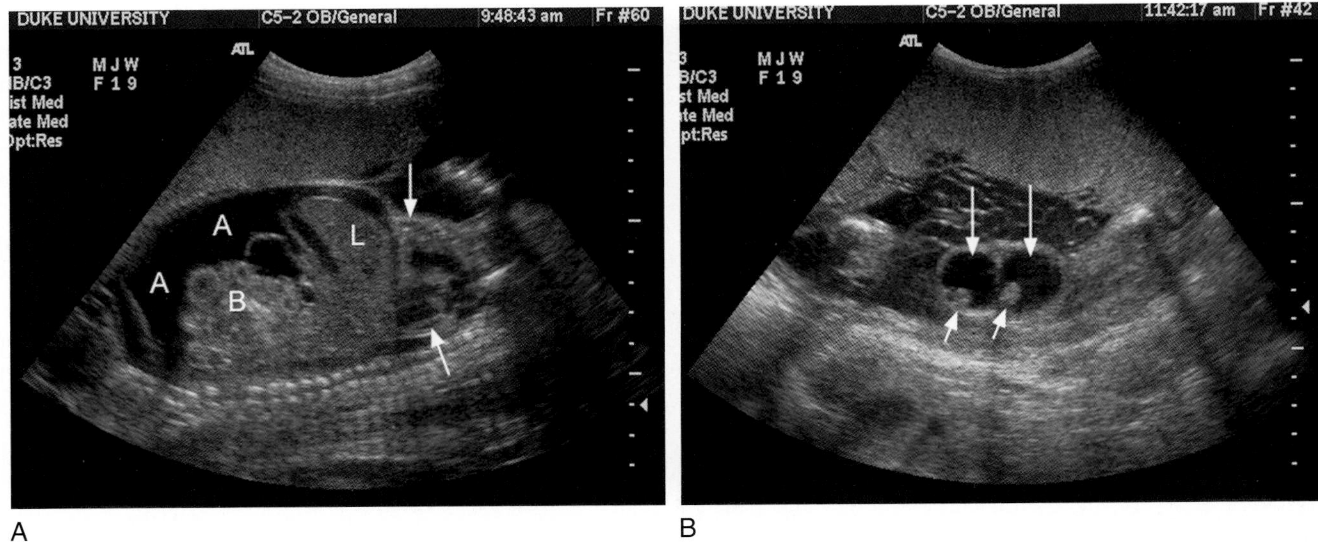

Figure 16-13 Fetal hydrops with predominant finding of ascites. **A,** Sagittal image of abdomen, pelvis, and chest shows a large amount of ascites (A). Ascites was the first sign of hydrops in this fetus with congenital syphilis. A very small pericardial effusion *(arrows)* is also seen. L, liver; B, bowel. **B,** Axial image through the scrotum shows large bilateral hydroceles *(long arrows).* Scrotal hydroceles are seen in some male fetuses with ascites because the processus vaginalis, which connects the abdominal and peritoneal cavities, is patent during part of pregnancy. *Short arrows,* testes.

rupture (urine ascites) or to meconium peritonitis. An isolated pericardial effusion is usually a normal finding if it is less than 2 mm in thickness. Even when more prominent (2 to 7 mm), if an isolated finding, it may not be associated with an adverse fetal outcome.

The overall prognosis for fetal hydrops is variable. In immune conditions, particularly those caused by Rh incompatibility, fetal survival rates are high if appropriate aggressive treatment, including fetal transfusions, is instituted. In nonimmune hydrops, the prognosis is poor unless the particular cause of the hydrops can be eliminated. This may only be possible in cases of severe arrhythmias controlled by medication or in anemias reversed by transfusions.

EXTRACARDIAC ABNORMALITIES

Major fetal thoracic extracardiac abnormalities can be detected by ultrasound. These are congenital diaphragmatic hernias (CDH), cystic adenomatoid malformations (CAM), bronchogenic cysts, duplication cysts, pleural effusions, sequestrations, and, rarely, laryngeal atresia. Congenital lobar emphysema and congenital bronchiectasis are typically detected after birth, not in utero.

To detect an extracardiac chest anomaly, either a shift in the cardiovascular structures (in particular the heart) or a change in echogenicity is needed. Commonly, both are present. Any deviation of the heart without a mass is a suspicious sign for an unusual situs (situs inversus or indeterminus) and is often associated with cardiac anomalies.

Congenital Diaphragmatic Hernia

CDH is the most common intrathoracic extracardiac fetal anomaly. It occurs sporadically, with an incidence of 1 in every 2000 to 3000 live births and is associated with abnormalities of all major organ systems and with an abnormal karyotype in 16% to 56% of cases. If growth restriction is present, the incidence of associated anomalies increases to 90%.

CDHs are usually posterolateral (90%) and are then called Bochdalek hernias. They are typically unilateral, are seven times more common on the left than on the right, and are rarely bilateral. The anteromedial or Morgagni hernia makes up the remaining 10%.

CDHs may be difficult to diagnose in utero. The typical presentation of a left-sided Bochdalek hernia is a cystic structure (the stomach) located on the left side of the chest, with no identifiable normal stomach bubble below the left hemidiaphragm (Fig. 16-14A). Often the heart is displaced upward or toward the right, or both (see Fig. 16-14B). Peristalsis or fluid-filled bowel loops within the chest are also diagnostic findings (see Fig. 16-14C). If the CDH contains only collapsed small bowel or mesentery, it is usually not detected.

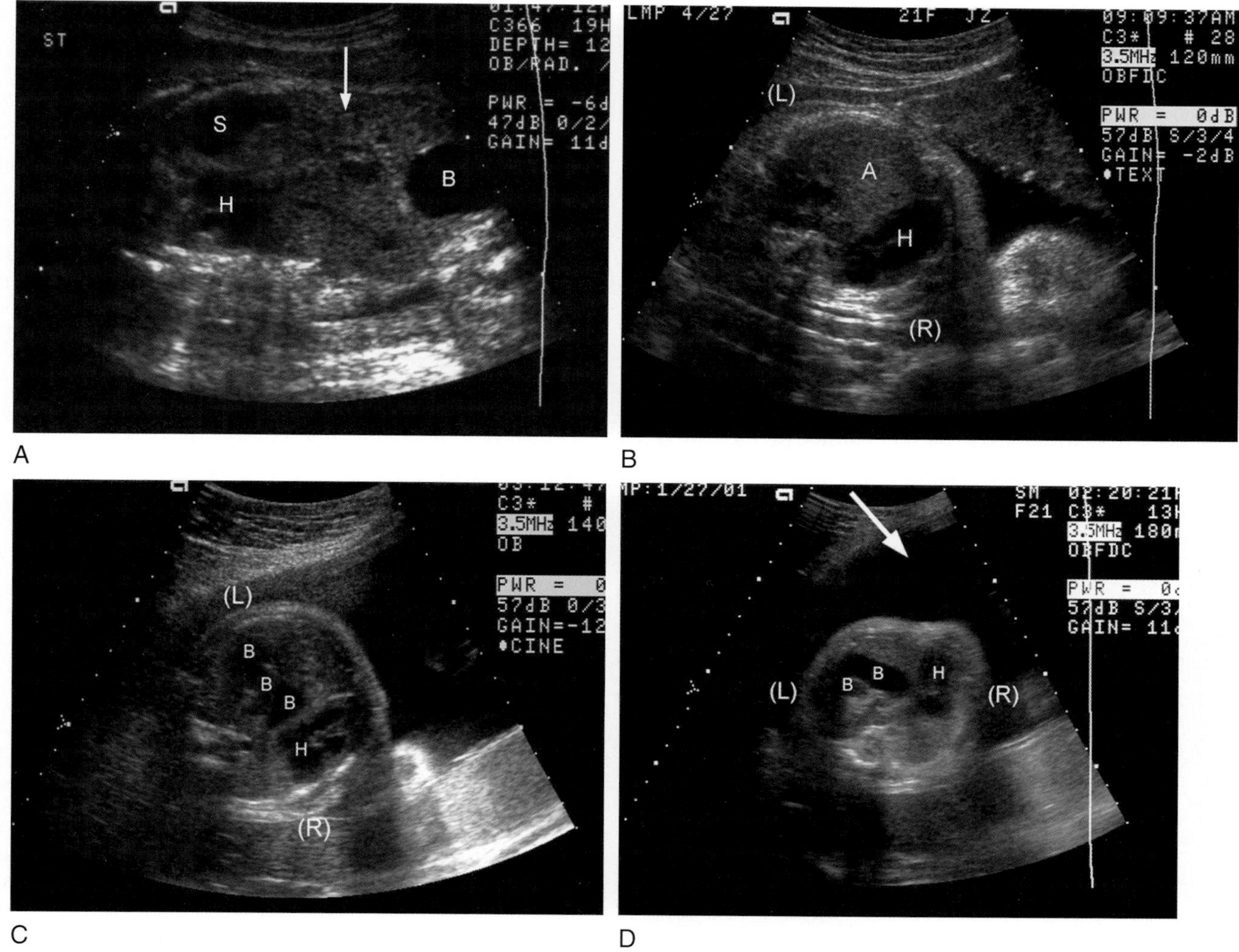

Figure 16-14 Ultrasound findings in four different fetuses with left-sided congenital diaphragmatic hernias. **A,** Longitudinal image shows absence of the stomach in expected location in left upper abdomen *(arrow)*. A cystic structure corresponding to the stomach (S) is seen in the thorax, at the same level as the heart (H). B, bladder. **B,** Axial image of thorax of a different fetus with a congenital diaphragmatic hernia reveals displacement of the heart (H) into the right hemithorax by herniated abdominal contents (A). The herniated abdominal contents appear solid because they consist of left lobe of liver and collapsed bowel loops. L, toward fetal left; R, toward fetal right. **C,** Axial image of thorax shows fluid-filled loops of bowel (B) in the chest, displacing the heart (H) to the right. At real-time evaluation, the bowel loops exhibited active peristalsis. L, toward fetal left; R, toward fetal right. **D,** Axial image of thorax reveals polyhydramnios *(arrow)* and congenital diaphragmatic hernia. The heart (H) is shifted into right hemithorax and dilated fluid-filled loops of bowel (B) are seen in left hemithorax. L, toward fetal left; R toward fetal right.

Left-sided hernias may also contain the spleen and left lobe of the liver.

The right-sided Bochdalek hernias are usually more difficult to detect. Typically, only the liver herniates into the chest, its echogenicity being similar to that of the mediastinum and nonaerated lungs. If anechoic structures such as the hepatic vascular structures (the hepatic and portal veins), the gallbladder, and fluid-filled bowel also enter the chest, detection is easier. Unless the hernia is large, the position of the heart is frequently undisturbed.

Morgagni hernias typically herniate into the pericardial sac. They are often very difficult to diagnose because only the liver herniates and the cardiac position remains undisturbed. As with right-sided Bochdalek hernias, the diagnosis is made easier if the same anechoic structures also enter the pericardium or if a pericardial effusion is present.

Any CDH obstruction of bowel loops may lead to polyhydramnios (Fig. 16-14D). Additionally, shift of the heart may cause obstruction of venous return from the inferior vena cava, leading to ascites.

The prognosis for a CDH is often poor, even when it is only an isolated anomaly. CDHs are usually larger than they appear and often continue to enlarge as the pregnancy progresses. Pulmonary hypoplasia may therefore be an important secondary problem and usually involves both lungs, especially when a significant cardiovascular shift is seen. Pulmonary hypoplasia is more completely discussed later in this chapter and in Chapter 18.

It would seem possible to diagnose a CDH by identifying a disruption in a hemidiaphragm. The hemidiaphragms, however, are curved, thin, hypoechoic bands that cannot be fully imaged and are normally often partially obscured by rib shadowing. As might therefore be expected, the diaphragmatic defect cannot be identified in utero. It has been suggested, however, that paradoxical diaphragmatic motion (the hemidiaphragm on the affected side moving in the opposite direction with respiration) might serve to reveal a CDH.

Diaphragmatic eventration is a developmental abnormality caused by muscular hypoplasia or aplasia. It is not a true hernia but represents an unusually elevated hemidiaphragm with the abdominal contents remaining intraperitoneally. The ipsilateral lung may be secondarily compressed. At least one lung will develop normally, however, unless the process is bilateral. An eventration is rarely associated with syndromes and triploidies.

Cystic Adenomatoid Malformation

CAM is a relatively uncommon dysplastic anomaly caused by hamartomatous involvement of the lung. In most cases the CAM involves only a sublobar area;

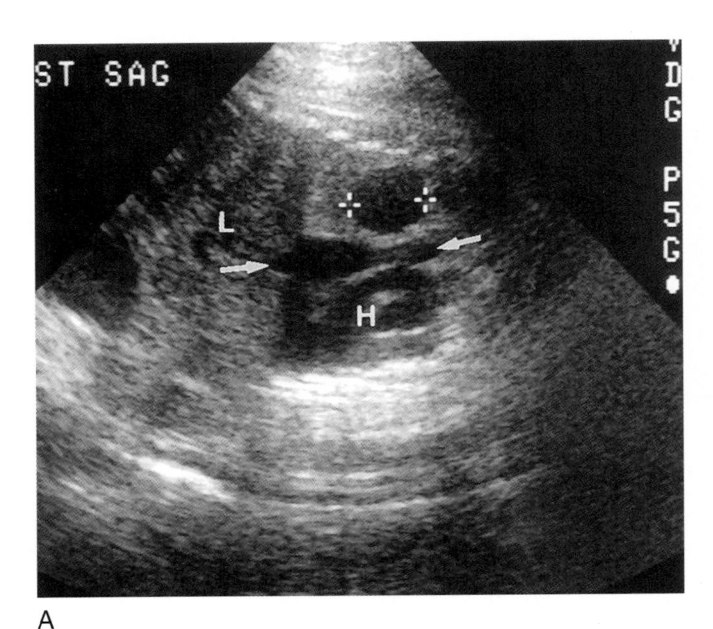

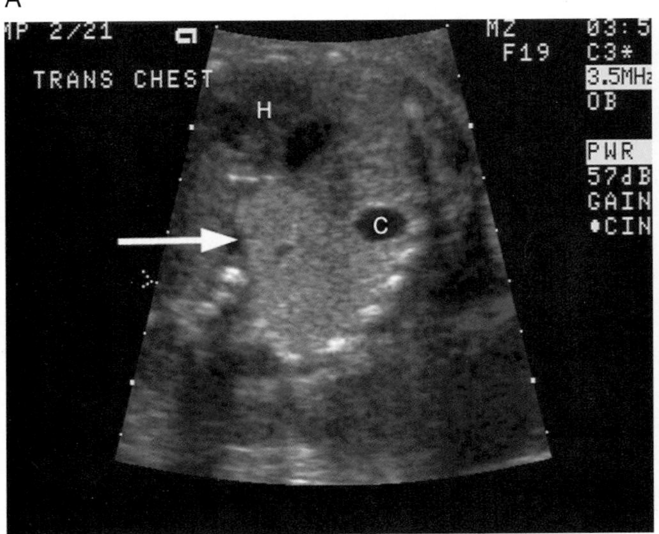

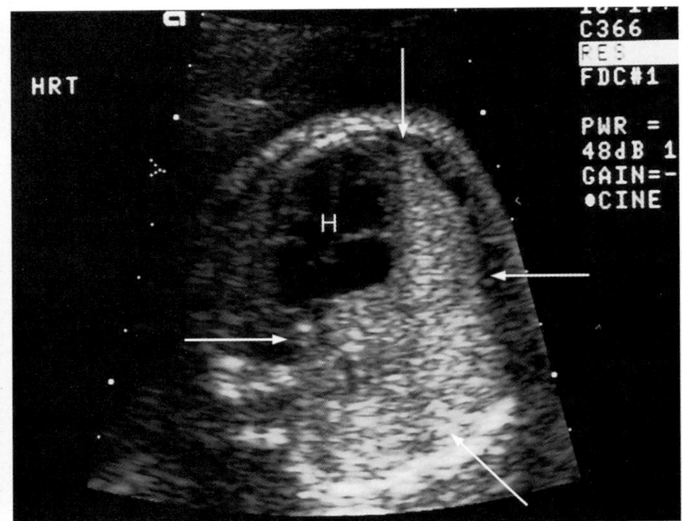

Figure 16-15 Three cases of cystic adenomatoid malformation (CAM). **A,** Type I CAM in an 18-week fetus. A sagittal-coronal view of the fetal body shows a well-defined cyst *(cursors)* surrounded by normal hyperechoic, nonaerated lung in the right hemithorax. There is slight displacement of the inferior and superior venae cavae *(arrows)*. The heart (H) is in a grossly normal position. The echoes within the cyst are artifacts. L, liver. **B,** Axial image of fetal chest with a type II CAM. Many of the cysts are too small to resolve so the dominant ultrasound pattern is that of a hyperechoic mass *(arrow)*, but a few small macroscopic cysts (C) were also seen. H, heart. **C,** Type III CAM. Axial image of chest shows a solid hyperechoic mass *(arrows)* in the left hemithorax displacing the heart (H) toward the right.

less frequently an entire lung and rarely both lungs are affected. CAMs can be divided into three types (I to III) on the basis of histologic, gross, and clinical characteristics.

Type I is the most common and consists of large cysts (2 to 10 cm in diameter) that are clearly identified by ultrasound (Fig. 16-15A). In type II, there are smaller macroscopic cysts usually less than 1.0 cm in diameter. Ultrasound detects most type II CAMs as multiple cysts, but when the cysts are too small they are instead identified as hyperechoic masses (see Fig. 16-15B). Type III consists of multiple small bronchiole-like structures (<0.5 cm in diameter) that are typically detected not as cysts but as a hyperechoic mass because of its multiple interfaces (see Fig. 16-15C). The echogenicity of all three types of CAM permits intrathoracic detection. Theoretically, a type III CAM could be isoechoic with the surrounding tissues.

Prognosis is related to the size of the CAM and the extent of involvement of the lung. While it was previously reported that type II CAMs were associated with renal, gastrointestinal, and other pulmonary abnormalities (<25% of the cases), it is now believed that there is no significant increase in anomalies. Karyotype abnormalities are not associated with CAMs. Often a CAM will become less prominent, or even appear to resolve, as pregnancy progresses. Despite the apparent improvement, if a postnatal CT scan is done, it will not uncommonly reveal a residual mass (Fig. 16-16). Alternately, an apparent hyperechoic mass in the lung that subsequently resolves may have been due to a temporarily obstructed bronchus from a mucus plug.

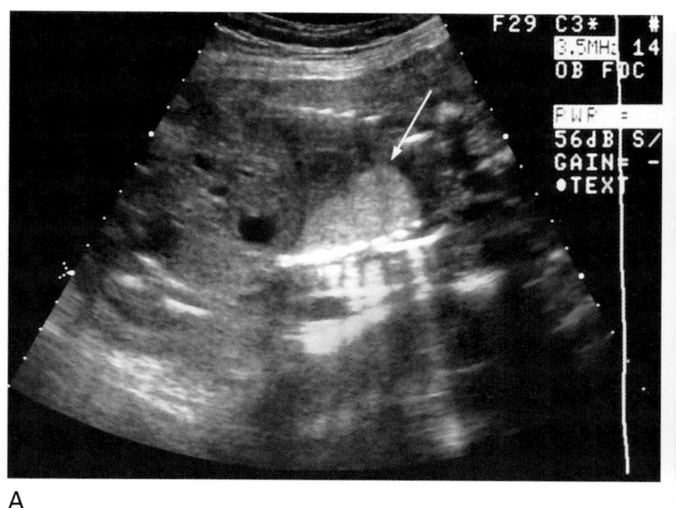

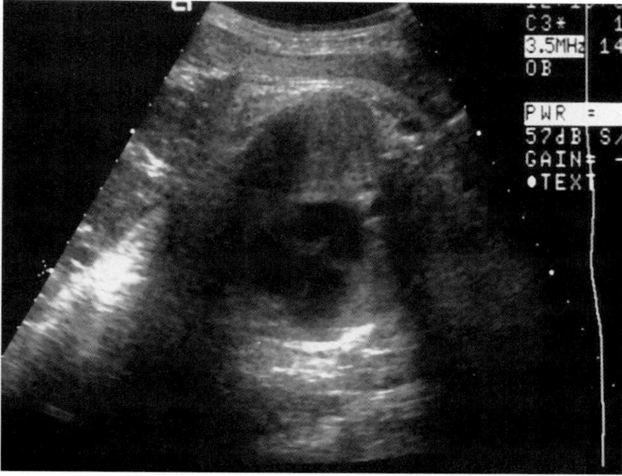

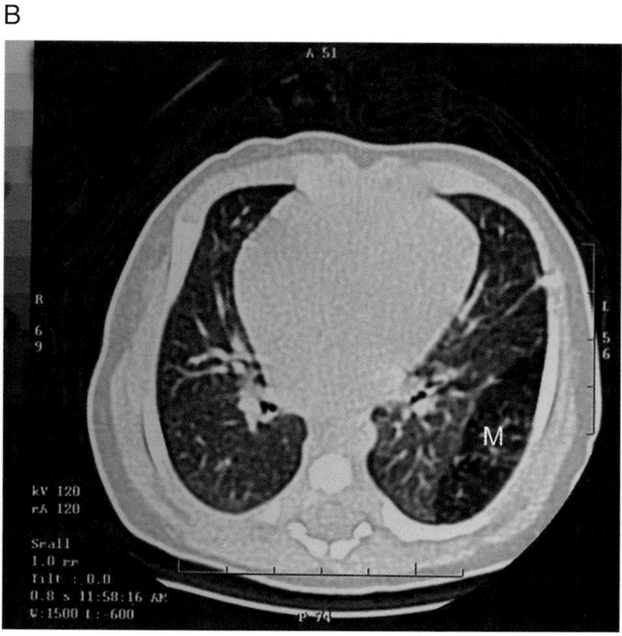

Figure 16-16 Apparent interval resolution of a cystic adenomatoid malformation (CAM), with postnatal documentation of a residual mass. **A,** Longitudinal image of left hemithorax at 22 weeks shows a large hyperechoic chest mass *(arrow)*. **B,** Axial image of chest at 31 weeks shows no evidence of the mass seen earlier in pregnancy. The mass could not be seen in multiple scan planes despite extensive attempts to document it. H, heart. **C,** Postnatal CT scan shows a residual mass *(M)* in left hemithorax. The mass was removed surgically, and the diagnosis of CAM was confirmed.

Bronchopulmonary Sequestration

Bronchopulmonary sequestrations are less common than CDHs and CAMs, constituting only 0.15% to 6.4% of all congenital pulmonary malformations. They form when a portion of the bronchopulmonary system develops separately. Sequestrations can be divided into two types on the basis of their pleural covering: the intralobar type without and the extralobar type with its own separate pleura. Sequestrations are often found in the lower lobes, in the posterior basal segments. They are more common on the left and are infrequently bilateral. Rarely, they are found below the diaphragm. While the intralobar type is more common in adults, it is rarely diagnosed in fetuses and neonates, raising the possibility that it is an acquired anomaly. Initially reported was an association with significant anomalies, in less than 60% of extralobar sequestrations; more recent studies have suggested no increase in abnormalities.

Ultrasound often detects a bronchopulmonary sequestration as a hyperechoic mass at the lung base (Fig. 16-17). Very infrequently, cystic components may also be present. Classically, the extralobar type is conical or triangular. It is common for the extralobar type to present as fetal hydrops or as a mass associated with a pleural effusion.

Color Doppler analysis may help make this diagnosis. The extralobar sequestration receives its arterial supply ectopically, usually from the descending thoracic or abdominal aorta. Identification of a feeding arterial vessel from the aorta favors an extralobar sequestration but is not a specific finding. A CAM may have a pulmonary arterial supply or be supplied by the aorta. Moreover, sequestration and CAM may coexist in the same lesion.

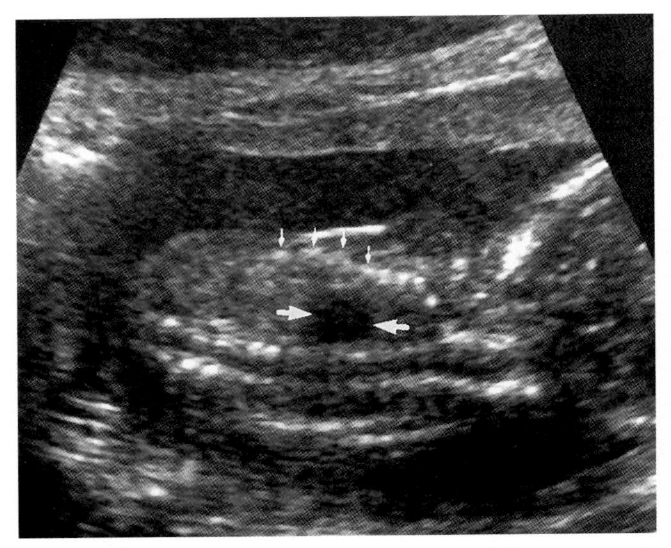

Figure 16-18 Bronchogenic cyst in a 20-week fetus. Long-axis view of the fetus with its head toward the right shows a cyst *(large arrows)* within the fetal thorax, in the area of the right lung. The heart is not significantly displaced. Although this appeared to be a type I cystic adenomatoid malformation, a simple bronchogenic cyst was found at birth. *Small arrows*, ribs.

Cysts

Primary bronchogenic (lung) cysts and duplication (gastrointestinal) cysts may also present as chest masses. They are commonly simple cysts and are usually solitary (Fig. 16-18). If large, they can cause cardiac displacement.

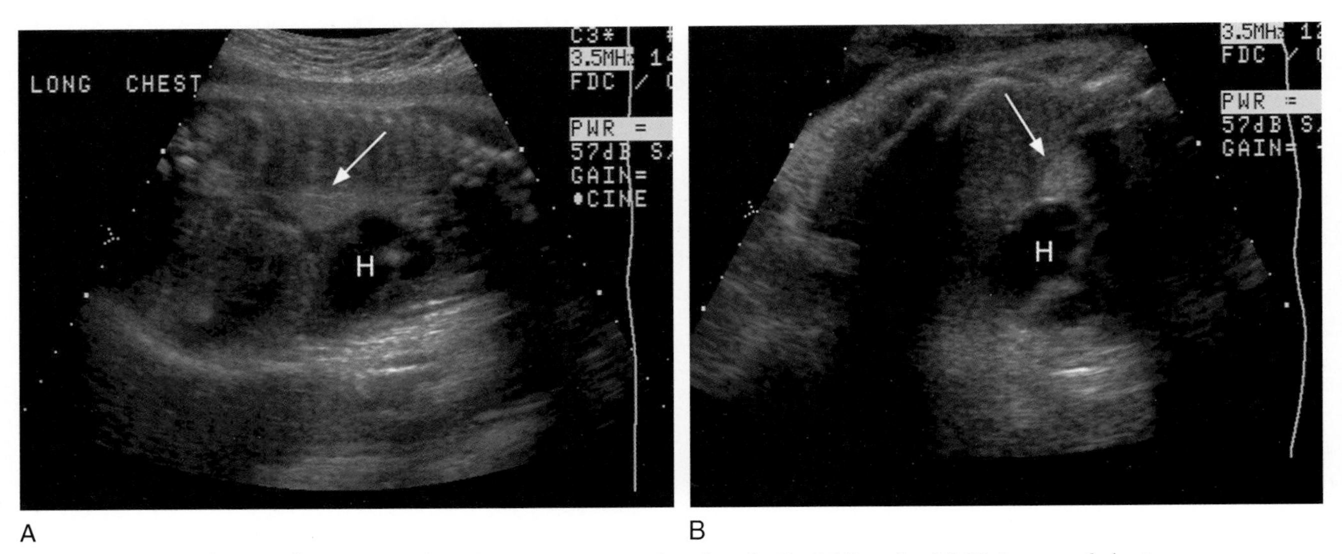

Figure 16-17 Bronchopulmonary sequestration. Longitudinal (**A**) and axial (**B**) images of chest of a 28-week fetus reveal an echogenic mass *(arrow)* in the posterior chest, which subsequently proved to be an extralobar sequestration. H, heart.

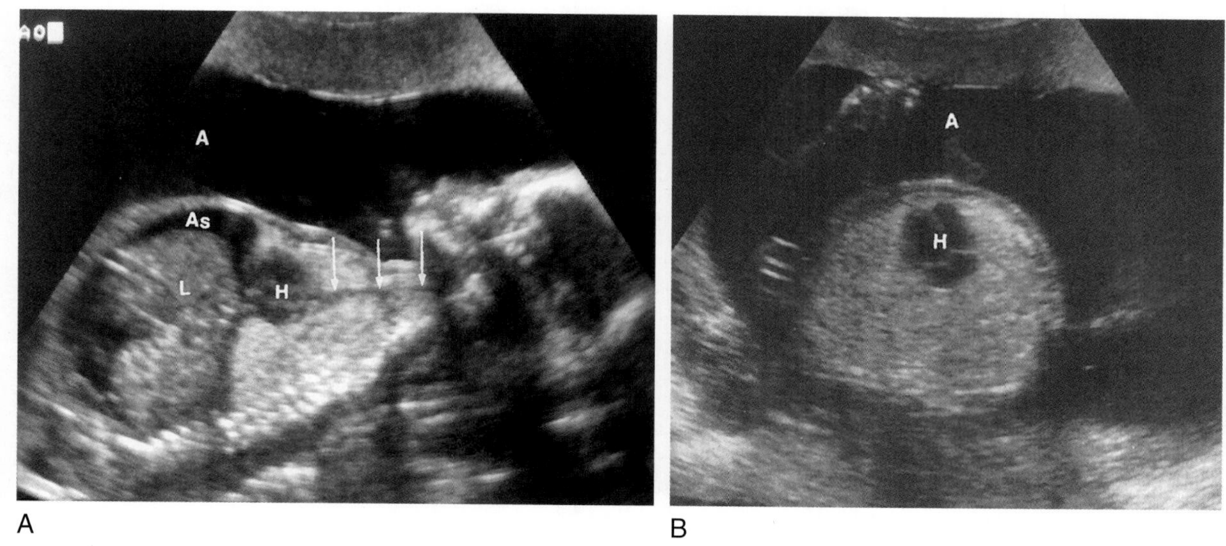

Figure 16-19 Laryngeal atresia in a 28-week fetus associated with polyhydramnios. **A,** Long-axis sagittal view shows markedly hyperechoic enlarged lungs. A fluid-filled hypopharynx and trachea is identified *(arrows)*. Ascites (As) surrounds the liver. **B,** Transaxial view through the fetal heart shows the heart (H) to be compressed by markedly hyperechoic enlarged lungs. A, amniotic fluid; H, heart; L, liver.

Laryngeal Atresia

Laryngeal atresia is a rare lethal entity. It is an obstruction of the tracheobronchial tree occurring anywhere from the larynx to the bronchi. Rarely, only one mainstem bronchus is involved. With obstruction, secretions from the lungs cannot be expelled. Both lungs (unless only one bronchus is involved) are found to increase in echogenicity and become enlarged, occasionally so large that they compress the heart and invert the hemidiaphragms (Fig. 16-19). The tracheobronchial tree can be identified as a tubular fluid-filled structure, filled with unexpelled secretions. Fetal hydrops and additional esophageal and tracheal abnormalities can also be present.

Pleural Effusions

Pleural fluid is readily detectable. It is typically anechoic, occasionally hypoechoic, and easily distinguished from the hyperechoic nonaerated lungs. When effusions are small, they are curvilinear collections (Fig. 16-20). When larger, the effusions are more rounded and compress the lungs toward the hila (Fig. 16-21). If they are large and left sided, the heart can be displaced and compressed.

Pleural effusions are often bilateral and associated with fetal hydrops. Less commonly, pleural effusions may be unilateral and are then often an indication of a more localized pathologic condition such as an extracardiac mass (e.g., extralobar sequestration) or a chylothorax. A chylothorax is a lymphatic obstruction that is more common on the left. It cannot pathologically be diagnosed as chylous antenatally, however, because no fat is present within the effusion in utero.

Bilateral pleural effusions can be severe enough to compromise the fetal lungs in one of two ways: (1) if

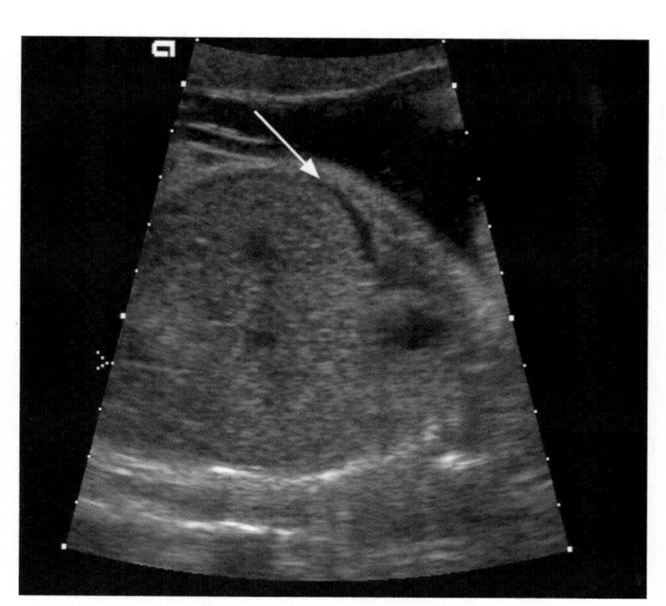

Figure 16-20 Small pleural effusion. Longitudinal image of chest and abdomen depicts a small pleural effusion as a curvilinear collection *(arrow)*.

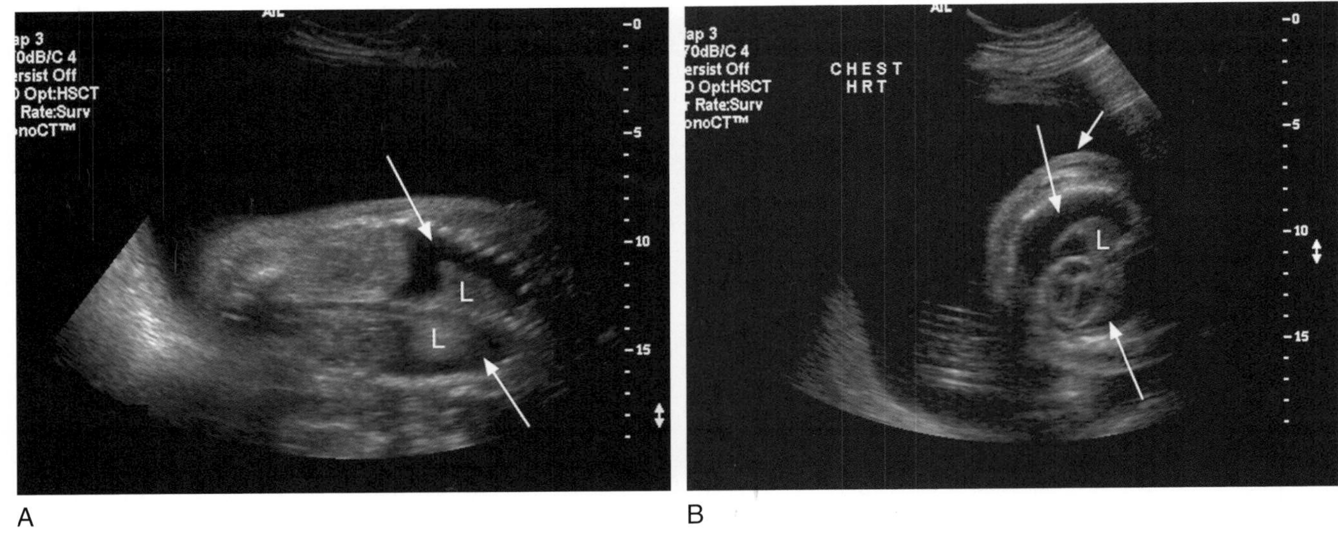

Figure 16-21 Large bilateral pleural effusions in fetus with hydrops and polyhydramnios. Longitudinal (**A**) and transverse (**B**) images show large bilateral pleural effusions *(long arrows)* that compress the lungs (L) toward the hila. Also note marked skin thickening *(short arrow)* due to hydrops.

prolonged, they can cause pulmonary hypoplasia; and (2) if present at birth, the lungs (even if normal) cannot expand. In the latter case, a thoracentesis performed just before delivery may be necessary to allow aeration of at least one lung when the newborn attempts to breathe.

Pulmonary Hypoplasia

The bronchial tree is fully developed by 16 weeks of fetal life. The distal airways continue to develop, with 20 million terminal air sacs forming by birth. The alveoli develop after birth and increase to 300 million by 8 years of age.

Anything that impedes the formation of the distal airways will cause the number of terminal air sacs, and ultimately the final number of alveoli, to be reduced. Any space-occupying process that compresses the lungs or any mass that involves part of the tracheobronchial tree will therefore inhibit lung development. Lung development also needs a large enough thoracic cage and a sufficient amount of amniotic fluid. A small chest or oligohydramnios, or both, will also spawn underdevelopment of the lungs.

It may be difficult to predict when pulmonary hypoplasia is severe enough to be life threatening. However, the more severe the visualized abnormality (by ultrasound) and the longer that it has been present, the greater the likelihood of serious pulmonary problems at birth. This issue has not been resolved by the use of measurements. The thoracic-to-abdominal circumference ratio, consisting of the circumference taken at the level of the four-chamber view of the heart and of the standard upper abdominal circumference, respectively, is normal if it is more than 0.75. The lung-to-hemithorax diameter is normal if it is more than 0.75. The chest area minus the heart area divided by the chest area normally exceeds 0.62. None of these ratios, however, has shown a high degree of accuracy in predicting significant lung compromise.

More recently, attempts to measure the lung length, its area, or its volume have been attempted to predict if the lung is sufficiently developed. At present, although this approach to direct lung measurement appears promising, there has not been adequate follow up to determine if it can successfully predict survival.

Key Features

The normal nonaerated lungs and mediastinum are hyperechoic and blend together. An abnormality can be detected by a change in echogenicity or by a mass effect on definable structures (usually the heart).

After 8 weeks the fetal heart rate is normally between 120 and 180 beats per minute. Transient bradycardia is a normal variant.

All other abnormal heart rates should be examined for rate, rhythm, concordance of the atria to the ventricles, structural abnormalities, and fetal hydrops.

An M-mode examination of the heart is not a necessary part of a normal study. It is suggested, however, to document and evaluate any abnormal rate or rhythm.

A routine four-chamber image of the heart, obtained as an axial view of the lower chest, evaluates the atria, ventricles, and their interposed septa.

Additional cardiac views of the base of the heart and ventricular outflow tracts identify and permit evaluation of the aorta and pulmonary arteries and improve detection of cardiac defects.

Fetal hydrops (immune and nonimmune) is caused by excessive fetal body water. Classically, its presenting signs consist of fluid in serous cavities, skin thickening, placental enlargement, and polyhydramnios. In any individual case, however, the number of abnormalities and their severity may vary.

Pericardial effusions less than 2 mm in thickness, if an isolated finding, are usually normal.

Cardiac causes of nonimmune hydrops are related to high-output failure (anemia and shunts), severe arrhythmias, structural anomalies, and myocarditis.

In utero infections and Down syndrome may present as fetal hydrops.

Extracardiac in utero masses can be divided into those that are primarily cystic and those that are primarily solid. The primarily cystic masses are Bochdalek congenital diaphragmatic hernias (CDHs), type I and perhaps type II cystic adenomatoid malformations (CAMs), bronchogenic cysts, duplication cysts, and pulmonary sequestration. The solid lesions are Morgagni and some Bochdalek CDHs, type III CAMs, and bronchopulmonary sequestration.

The heart is usually on the left side. Although there are occasions when a right-sided heart can be an isolated finding, a right-sided or indeterminate situs is more often associated with cardiac and/or extracardiac anomalies.

The most common intrathoracic extracardiac abnormality is the congenital diaphragmatic hernia (CDH). The most common CDH is a left-sided posterolateral hernia (Bochdalek hernia). In its classic form, the stomach is identified in the chest and the heart is displaced to the right.

A CDH may be difficult to diagnose in utero. When detected, it is generally more extensive than its sonographic appearance would suggest, and pulmonary hypoplasia is often a secondary complication. There is also an increased incidence of major organ abnormalities and abnormal karyotype.

Enlarged hyperechoic lungs are the presenting sign of laryngeal atresia, a rare lethal entity.

Pulmonary hypoplasia is caused by failure of normal bronchopulmonary development. A space-occupying process that either compresses or involves part of the bronchopulmonary tree, a very small chest, and/or prolonged significant oligohydramnios can adversely affect lung development.

It is not currently possible to accurately predict the severity of pulmonary hypoplasia.

SUGGESTED READINGS

Adzick NS, et al: Fetal cystic adenomatoid malformation: Prenatal diagnosis and natural history. J Pediatr Surg 20:483, 1985.

Adzick NS, et al: Diaphragmatic hernia in the fetus: Prenatal diagnosis and outcome in 94 cases. J Pediatr Surg 20:357, 1985.

Allen LD: A practical approach to fetal heart scanning. Semin Perinatol 24:324-330, 2000.

Axel L: Real-time sonography of fetal cardiac anatomy. AJR Am J Roentgenol 141:283, 1983.

Bahlmann F, et al: Congenital diaphragmatic hernia: Ultrasonic measurement of fetal lungs to predict pulmonary hypoplasia. Ultrasound Obstet Gynecol 14:162-168, 1999.

Barboza JM, et al: Prenatal diagnosis of congenital cardiac anomalies: A practical approach using two basic views. Radiographics 22:1125-1137, 2002.

Bromley B, et al: Fetal echocardiography: Accuracy and limitations in a population at high and low risk for heart defects. Am J Obstet Gynecol 166:1473, 1992.

Bromley B, et al: Fetal lung masses: Prenatal course and outcome. J Ultrasound Med 14:927, 1995.

Bronshtein M, et al: Early ultrasound diagnosis of fetal congenital heart defects in high-risk and low-risk pregnancies. Obstet Gynecol 82:225, 1993.

Bronshtein M, et al: Fetal cardiac abnormalities detected by transvaginal sonography at 12-16 weeks' gestation. Obstet Gynecol 78:374, 1991.

Brown DL, Roberts DJ, Miller WA: Left ventricular echogenic focus in the fetal heart: Pathologic correlation. J Ultrasound Med 13:613, 1994.

Brown DL, et al: Sonography of the fetal heart: Normal variants and pitfalls. AJR Am J Roentgenol 160:1251, 1993.

Budorick NE, et al: Spontaneous improvement of intrathoracic masses diagnosed in utero. J Ultrasound Med 11:653, 1992.

Bush A: Congenital lung disease: A plea for clear thinking and clear nomenclature. Pediatr Pulmonol 32:328-337, 2001.

Buskens E, et al: Efficacy of fetal echocardiography and yield by risk category. Obstet Gynecol 87:423, 1996.

Cass DL, et al: Cystic lung lesions with systemic arterial blood supply: A hybrid of congenital cystic adenomatoid malformation and bronchopulmonary sequestration. J Pediatr Surg 32:986, 1997.

Copel JA, Pilu G, Kleinman CS: Congenital heart disease and extracardiac anomalies: Associations and indications for fetal echocardiography. Am J Obstet Gynecol 154:1121, 1986.

Copel JA, et al: Fetal echocardiographic screening for congenital heart disease: The importance of the four chamber view. Am J Obstet Gynecol 157:648, 1987.

DiSalvo DN, et al: Clinical significance of isolated fetal pericardial effusion. J Ultrasound Med 13:291, 1994.

Dolkart LA, et al: Prenatal diagnosis of laryngeal atresia. J Ultrasound Med 11:496, 1992.

Frates MC: Sonography of the normal fetal heart: A practical approach. AJR Am J Roentgenol 173:1363-1370, 1999.

Friedman AH, et al: Diagnosis of cardiac defects: Where we've been, where we are and where we're going: Prenat Diagn 22:280-284, 2002.

Geipel A, et al: Perinatal diagnosis of cardiac tumors. Ultrasound Obstet Gynecol 17:17-21, 2001.

Guibaud L, et al: Fetal congenital diaphragmatic hernia: Accuracy of sonography in the diagnosis and prediction of the outcome after birth. AJR Am J Roentgenol 166:1196, 1996.

Hagay A, et al: Isolated fetal pleural effusion: A prenatal management dilemma. Obstet Gynecol 81:147, 1993.

Harrison MR, et al: A prospective study of the outcome for fetuses with diaphragmatic hernia. JAMA 71:382, 1994.

Hernanz-Schulman M, et al: Pulmonary sequestration: Diagnosis with color Doppler sonography and a new theory of associated hydrothorax. Radiology 180:817, 1991.

Holzgreve W, et al: Investigation of nonimmune hydrops fetalis. Am J Obstet Gynecol 150:805, 1984.

Hubbard AM, et al: Left-sided congenital diaphragmatic hernia: Value of prenatal MR imaging in preparation for fetal surgery. Radiology 203:636, 1997.

Johnson A, et al: Ultrasonic ratio of fetal thoracic to abdominal circumference: An association with fetal pulmonary hypoplasia. Am J Obstet Gynecol 157:764, 1987.

Kasales CJ, et al: Diagnosis and differentiation of congenital diaphragmatic hernia from other noncardiac thoracic fetal masses. Am J Perinatol 15:623-628, 1998.

Kirk JS, et al: Prenatal screening for cardiac anomalies: The value of routine addition of the aortic root to the four-chamber view. Obstet Gynecol 84:427, 1994.

Kirk JS, et al: Sonographic screening to detect fetal cardiac anomalies: A 5-year experience with 111 abnormal cases. Obstet Gynecol 89:227, 1997.

McGahan JP: Sonography of the fetal heart: Findings on the four-chamber view. AJR Am J Roentgenol 156:547, 1991.

Meagher SE, et al: Disappearing lung echogenicity in fetal bronchopulmonary malformations: A reassuring sign? Prenat Diagn 13:495-501, 1993.

Roggin KK, et al: The unpredictable character of congenital cystic lung lesions. J Pediatr Surg 35:801-805, 2000.

Saltzman DH, et al: Sonographic evaluation of hydrops fetalis. Obstet Gynecol 74:106, 1989.

Sbragia L, et al: Congenital diaphragmatic hernia without herniation of the liver: Does the lung-to-head ratio predict survival? J Ultrasound Med 19:845-848, 2000.

Shipp TD, et al: Levorotation of the fetal cardiac axis: A clue for the presence of congenital heart disease. Obstet Gynecol 85:97, 1995.

Sohaey R, et al: The fetal thorax: Noncardiac chest anomalies. Semin Ultrasound CT MR 17:34, 1996.

Thorpe-Beeston JG, et al: Cystic adenomatoid malformation of the lung: Prenatal diagnosis and outcome. Prenat Diagn 14:677, 1997.

van Leeuwen K, et al: Prenatal diagnosis of congenital cystic adenomatoid malformation and its postnatal presentation, surgical indications, and natural history. J Pediatr Surg 34: 794-798, 1999.

Vintzileos AM, et al: Comparison of six different ultrasonographic methods for predicting lethal fetal pulmonary hypoplasia. Am J Obstet Gynecol 161:606, 1989.

Walsh DS, et al: Fetal surgical intervention. Am J Perinatol 17:277-283, 2000.

Weston MJ, et al: Ultrasonographic prenatal diagnosis of upper respiratory tract atresia. J Ultrasound Med 11:673, 1992.

Wigton TR, et al: Sonographic diagnosis of congenital heart disease: Comparison between the four-chamber view and multiple cardiac views. Obstet Gynecol 82:219, 1993.

Winters WD, et al: Congenital masses of the lung: Prenatal and postnatal imaging evaluation. J Thorac Imag 16:196-206, 2001.

Winters WD, et al: Disappearing fetal lung masses: Importance of postnatal imaging studies. Pediatr Radiol 27:535-539, 1997.

Yagel S, et al: Examination of the fetal heart by five short-axis views: A proposed screening method for comprehensive cardiac evaluation. Ultrasound Obstet Gynecol 17:367-369, 2001.

CHAPTER 17

Fetal Gastrointestinal Tract

The antepartum obstetrical ultrasound standard recommends measurement of the upper abdomen in axial projection at the level of the liver and identification of the stomach. The standard also recommends identification of the anterior abdominal wall and its only identifiable landmark, the insertion of the umbilical cord.

Additional normal and abnormal gastrointestinal structures can be identified, but with varying success. It is not uncommon to diagnose abdominal masses, ascites, and upper gastrointestinal tract obstructions. Anomalies of the large bowel, however, are less frequently seen, and it is rare for the pancreas to be imaged.

THE UPPER ABDOMEN: LIVER AND STOMACH

In an axial view, the upper abdomen is round or oval. With the spine identified posteriorly, the right-sided liver (extending across the midline) and the left-sided stomach are constant landmarks. For the axial projection to be appropriate for an abdominal measurement, the umbilical portion of the left portal vein should be positioned within the liver equidistant from the sides of the abdomen. Ideally, the measurement should be obtained on an image in which the abdomen is round and the confluence of the left and right portal veins is seen as a curved structure (Fig. 17-1). Abdominal diameters or circumference can then be obtained from the perimeter of the soft tissues.

The fetal liver is normally prominent in utero. Because of its glycogen store and hematopoietic activity, it is proportionately larger than in postnatal life and is primarily responsible for the size of the upper abdomen and the position of the heart. The liver can enlarge in conditions causing fetal hydrops, particularly those with immune hydrops (isoimmunization), and is occasionally affected with congenital infections and, rarely, hepatic infiltrating disorders. The liver can decrease in size if asymmetric intrauterine growth restriction (IUGR) occurs. To evaluate changes in the liver size, liver length has been suggested as a sensitive method of assessment. The length of the right hepatic lobe is measured from its dome (immediately below the cardiac pulsation) to caudal tip (Fig. 17-2). The recommended technique is to first identify the abdominal aorta in long axis and then move the transducer toward the right side of the fetus. The caudal tip of the liver can usually be seen. The dome is more difficult to precisely identify, because it is often partially obscured by shadowing from the ribs or upper extremities. Despite this difficulty, this measurement of liver length should be considered whenever the upper abdominal measurements are not in proportion to the head and femur measurements and in cases of suspected fetal hydrops, particularly immune hydrops, and growth restriction (Table 17-1).

Liver echogenicity can also be assessed. As in postnatal life, the fetal liver has a normally uniform low-level echogenicity, interrupted only by blood vessels. In addition to the umbilical portion of the left portal vein, the main and right portal veins (see Fig. 17-1) and the gallbladder (Fig. 17-3) can often be identified.

Liver masses and calcifications are rarely seen in utero. They include cysts, which are typically anechoic, and hemangiomas, which are usually uniformly hyperechoic. Other benign (hemangioendothelioma and

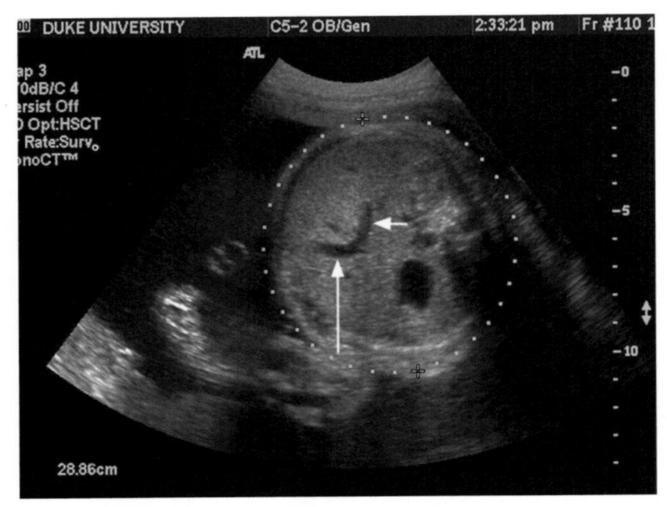

Figure 17-1 Measurement of abdominal circumference. Axial image of abdomen at 33 weeks shows scan plane for measuring abdominal circumference *(dotted line)*. The abdomen is round and the confluence of the left *(long arrow)* and right *(short arrow)* portal veins is seen as a curved structure.

Table 17-1 Fetal Liver Measurement*

Gestational Age	Long-Axis Measurement Mean	Range (2 SD)
20	27.3	20.9-33.7
21	28.0	26.5-29.5
22	30.6	23.9-37.3
23	30.9	26.4-35.4
24	32.9	26.2-39.6
25	33.6	28.3-38.9
26	35.7	29.4-42.0
27	36.6	33.3-39.9
28	38.4	34.4-42.4
29	39.1	34.1-44.1
30	38.7	33.7-43.7
31	39.6	33.9-45.3
32	42.7	35.0-50.2
33	42.8	37.2-50.4
34	44.8	37.7-51.9
35	47.8	38.7-56.9
36	49.0	40.6-57.4
37	52.0	45.2-58.8
38	52.9	48.7-57.1
39	55.4	48.7-62.1
40	59.0	—
41	49.3	46.9-51.7

*Measured in longitudinal plane from top of right hemidiaphragm to tip of right lobe of liver. Gestational age is in weeks, measurements in millimeters, and 2 SD = 5th percentile to 95% range.

From Vintzileos AM, et al: Fetal liver ultrasound measurements during normal pregnancy. Obstet Gynecol 66:477, 1985.

hamartoma) and malignant (hepatoblastoma and metastatic) masses are rare but have been reported. Discrete calcifications with or without shadowing have also been identified (Fig. 17-4). Although some have no known cause, liver parenchymal calcifications have been detected from TORCH infections (specifically toxoplasmosis, cytomegalovirus, and herpes simplex) and from varicella infections. Less commonly, benign and malignant liver tumors and peripheral liver emboli (caused by vascular accidents) can calcify. Rarely, calcified thrombi can be identified within vascular structures, particularly within the portal veins. These intraparenchymal calcifications need to be differentiated from perihepatic calcifications of meconium peritonitis (described later in this chapter).

Between the liver and the anterior abdominal wall, a hypoechoic curved line can often be identified just inside

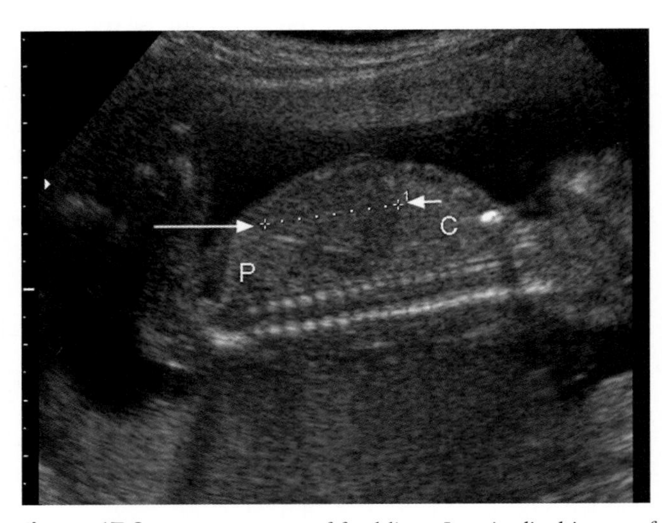

Figure 17-2 Measurement of fetal liver. Longitudinal image of fetal body at 16 weeks shows measurement of liver *(dotted line)*. The length of the right hepatic lobe is measured from the dome of the liver *(short arrow)* to its caudal tip *(long arrow)*. C, chest; P, pelvis.

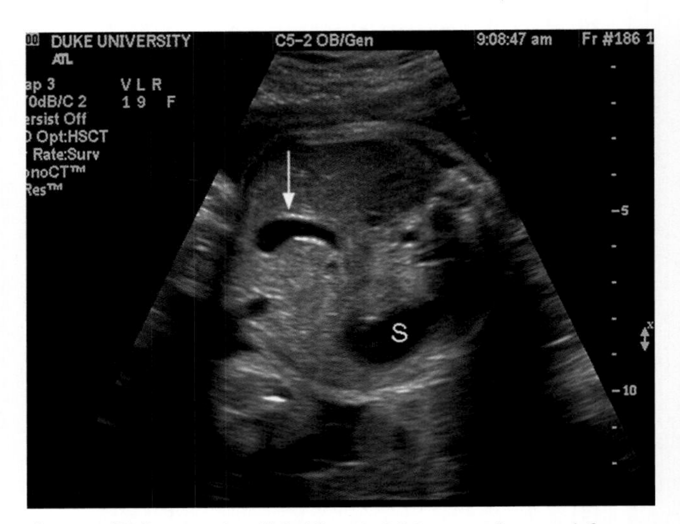

Figure 17-3 Fetal gallbladder. Axial image of normal fetus at 28 weeks depicts gallbladder *(arrow)* as a teardrop-shaped fluid-filled structure in the right upper quadrant. S, stomach.

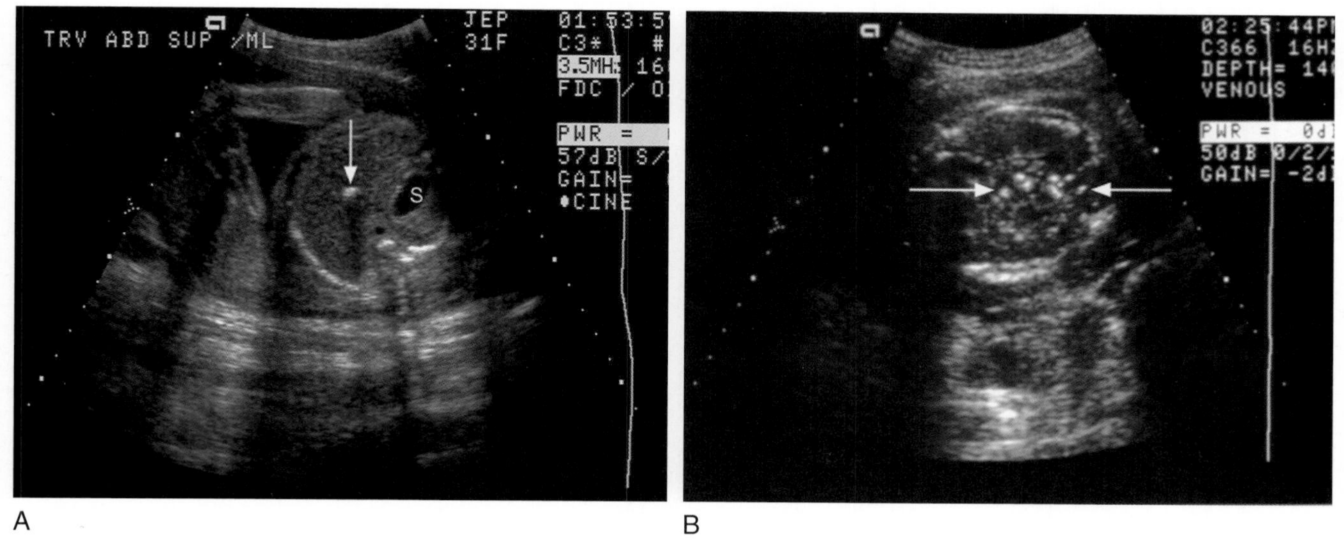

Figure 17-4 Liver calcifications. **A,** Idiopathic liver calcification. Axial image of fetal abdomen during second trimester shows a single calcification *(arrow)* with posterior shadowing in liver. The calcification was confirmed postnatally, the infant was asymptomatic, and the etiology of the calcification was never determined. S, stomach. **B,** Multiple liver calcifications due to cytomegalovirus. Axial image of fetal abdomen during second trimester shows multiple calcifications *(arrows)* in liver.

the hyperechoic soft tissues. This is a normal variant owing to hypoechoic abdominal wall musculature and is termed *pseudoascites.* Pseudoascites should be distinguished from true intraperitoneal fluid (ascites) (Fig. 17-5). Pseudoascites does not extend into the abdominal cavity deep to the ribs. Additionally, in the fetus with pseudoascites, only the lumen, not the outer echogenic walls of the intra-abdominal portion of the umbilical vein, is identified. With pseudoascites, fluid will not be seen surrounding abdominal organs. However, in the setting of ascites, the outer echogenic margins of the intra-abdominal portion of the umbilical vein and of the

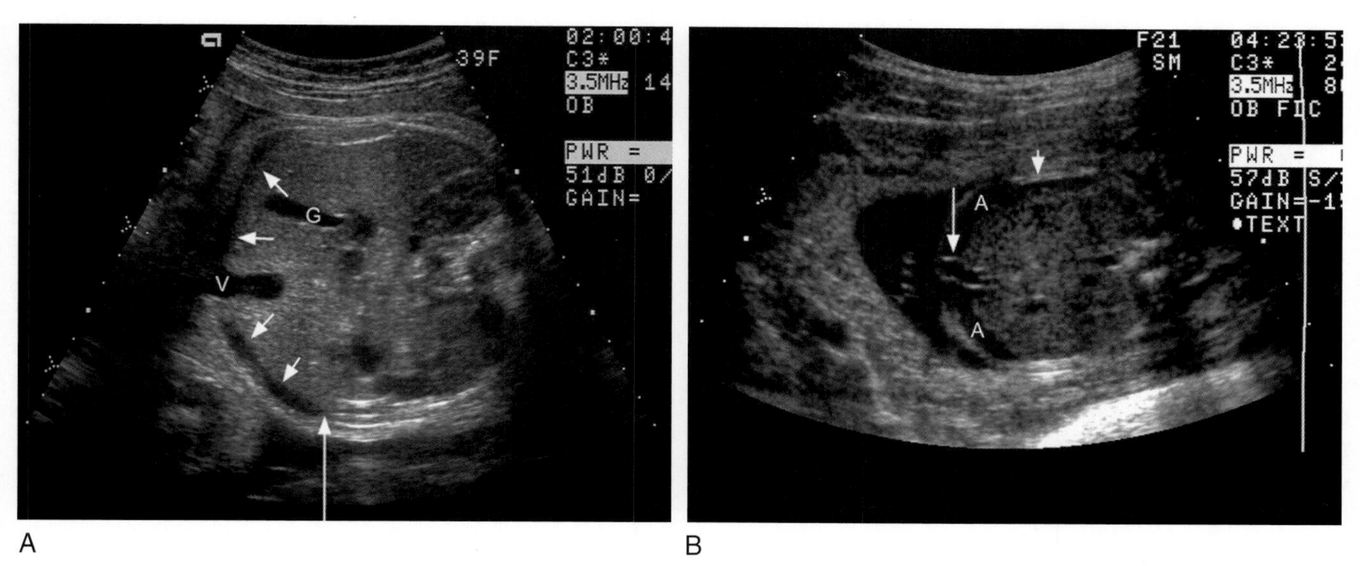

Figure 17-5 Pseudoascites versus ascites. **A,** Pseudoascites. Axial image of fetal abdomen shows a hypoechoic curved line *(short arrows)* just inside outer margin of abdominal wall. Note that the hypoechoic band does not extend beyond the ribs *(long arrow)* and does not surround intra-abdominal organs. Additionally, only the lumen of the abdominal portion of the umbilical vein (V) and not its echogenic outer wall is seen at the level of the pseudoascites. G, gallbladder. **B,** Ascites. Axial image of abdomen of fetus with true ascites shows ascites (A) extending beyond the level of the rib *(short arrow)* and outlining the echogenic walls *(long arrow)* of the intra-abdominal component of the umbilical vein.

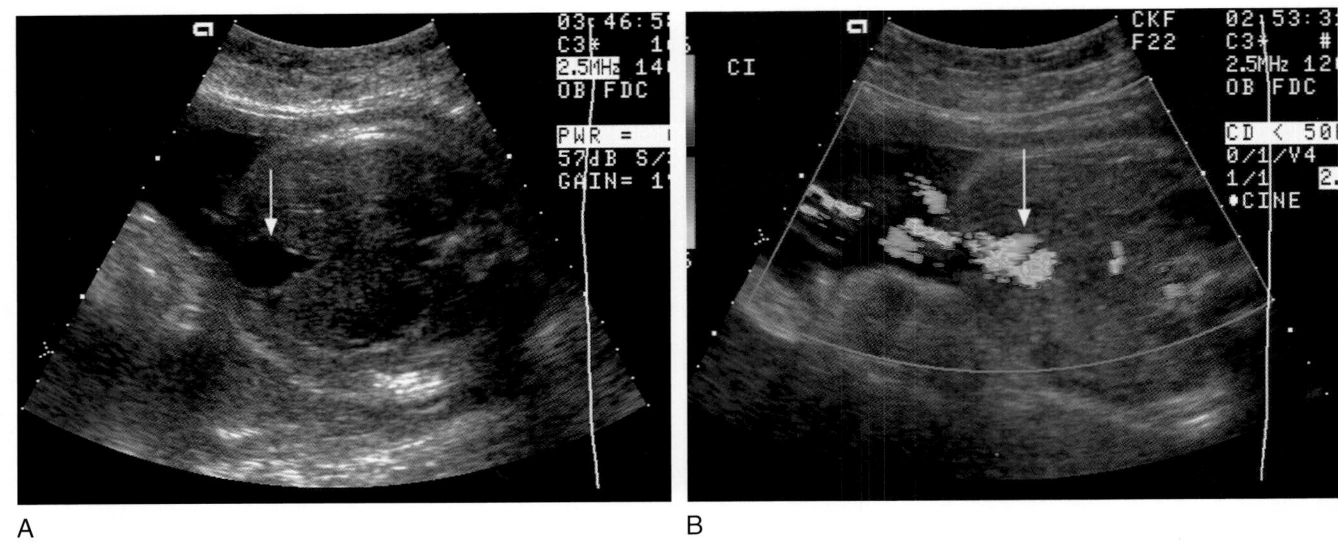

Figure 17-6 Umbilical vein varix. **A,** Gray-scale axial image of fetal abdomen during third trimester shows fluid collection in anterior portion of abdomen corresponding to focal dilatation *(arrow)* of intra-abdominal component of umbilical vein. **B,** Color Doppler image corresponding to **A** confirms the vascular nature of the umbilical vein varix *(arrow).*

falciform ligament can be seen and fluid may be identified surrounding portions of abdominal organs.

The intra-abdominal portion of the umbilical vein is normally small in caliber. It has parallel walls, and its diameter increases linearly from 3 mm at 15 weeks to 8 mm at term. A varix is an unusual enlargement of the extrahepatic portion of the vein (between the liver and anterior abdominal wall). It is typically observed to be large and round (Fig. 17-6). Although outcome is often normal in the fetus with an umbilical vein varix, in small series it has also been associated with fetal hydrops, structural anomalies, aneuploidy, and early third-trimester intrauterine demise.

The stomach is routinely identified as an anechoic (fluid-filled) structure in the left upper quadrant. Depending on the scan plane, it ranges from a round 4-mm-diameter structure to an ovoid or kidney-shaped 4-cm-long structure (Fig. 17-7A and B). Its size is somewhat dependent on gestational age, and it is typically larger in the third trimester. The position of the stomach is normally on the left side, immediately below the heart (situs solitus) (see Fig. 17-7C). If the stomach is on the right side or its position is indeterminate, this is commonly associated with complex structural abnormalities, particularly cardiac disorders. If the stomach is identified within the chest, this indicates the presence of a diaphragmatic hernia (usually the left-sided Bochdalek type). This is discussed in Chapter 16.

Occasionally, internal echoes are seen in the fetal stomach, caused by swallowed "debris" such as cells within the amniotic fluid. Echoes in the stomach can conglomerate into a rounded collection simulating a mass. This has been termed a *gastric pseudomass* (Fig. 17-8). A gastric pseudomass is usually a normal variant. However, the likelihood of visualizing a gastric pseudomass increases in fetuses with slowed transit through the gastrointestinal tract (as can occur with bowel obstructions) or with blood in the amniotic fluid (e.g., after placental abruption or amniocentesis).

The stomach fills every 10 to 45 minutes and empties in 5 to 30 minutes. The normal stomach is almost always identified, typically as early as when the abdomen is first imaged. If not seen or when persistently less than 1 cm in diameter (even though the latter finding may be normal), scanning should be repeated every 10 to 15 minutes up to 1 hour and/or within the next few days (Fig. 17-9). If the stomach is still not identified or remains small and amniotic fluid volume is normal or increased, there is a high probability of problems related to the inability of the fetus to swallow normally, as can be seen in association with severe central nervous system and high gastrointestinal (esophageal atresia, facial clefts, and swallowing) abnormalities. Another common cause of inability to depict the stomach or of a persistently small stomach is oligohydramnios (Fig. 17-10), owing to the decreased amount of amniotic fluid available for the fetus to swallow.

HIGH GASTROINTESTINAL TRACT OBSTRUCTION

The high gastrointestinal tract can be arbitrarily defined as the esophagus, stomach, and duodenum. The most proximal significant disorder is esophageal atresia, affecting 1 in 2500 to 4000 live births. There are five

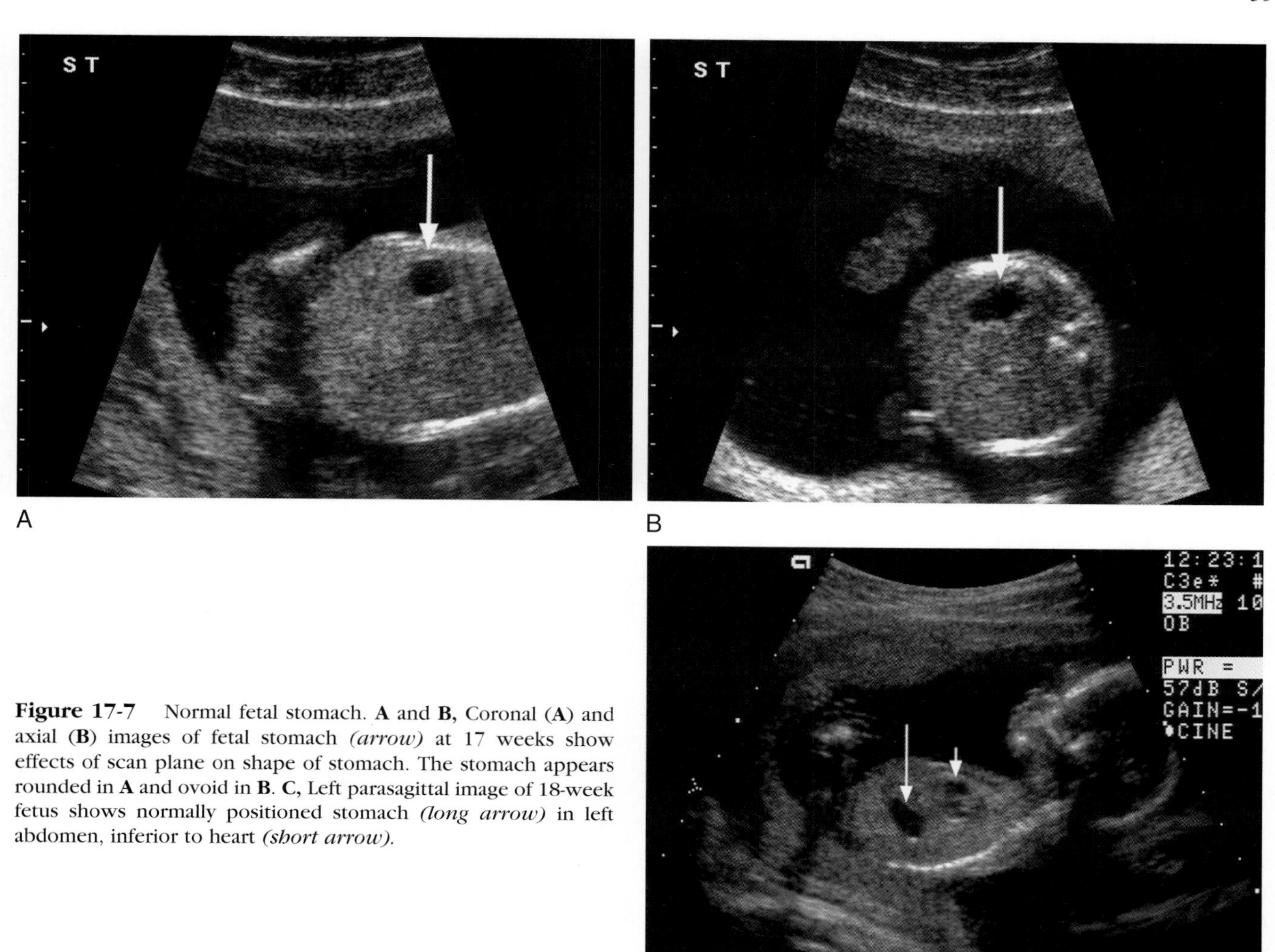

Figure 17-7 Normal fetal stomach. **A** and **B**, Coronal (**A**) and axial (**B**) images of fetal stomach *(arrow)* at 17 weeks show effects of scan plane on shape of stomach. The stomach appears rounded in **A** and ovoid in **B**. **C**, Left parasagittal image of 18-week fetus shows normally positioned stomach *(long arrow)* in left abdomen, inferior to heart *(short arrow)*.

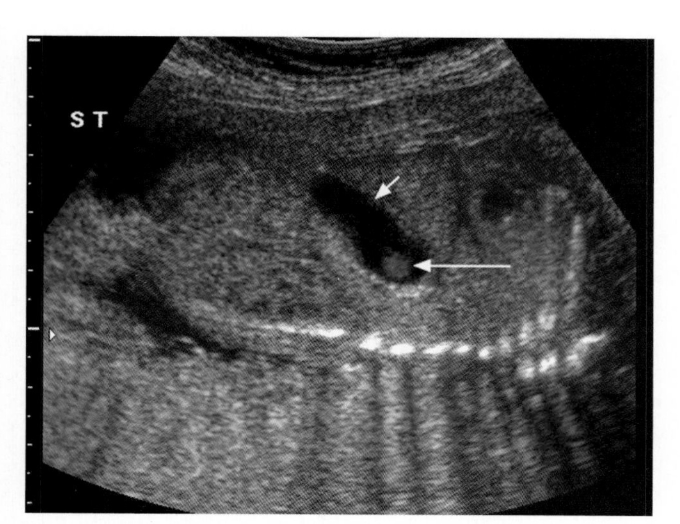

Figure 17-8 Gastric pseudomass. Longitudinal image of a normal 23-week fetus depicts a gastric pseudomass as a rounded collection of echoes *(long arrow)* in fetal stomach *(short arrow)*.

types, the most common associated with a tracheoesophageal fistula. The incidence of additional anomalies in the setting of esophageal atresia is high (50% to 70% of cases), and these comprise cardiac abnormalities, especially atrial and ventricular septal defects (24%), other gastrointestinal tract anomalies (28%), genitourinary tract disorders (13%), central nervous system disorders (7%), facial anomalies (6%), and chromosomal disorders including trisomy 21.

The two classic findings in esophageal atresia are polyhydramnios (60% to 90% of cases) and an absent stomach bubble (Fig. 17-11). In any individual case, however, one or both may not be appreciated, and the overall detection rate of esophageal atresia is surprisingly low at 50%. Moderate to marked polyhydramnios may not be noted until after 24 weeks. Infrequently, the stomach bubble is detected. This usually occurs when swallowed amniotic fluid enters the stomach through a tracheoesophageal fistula but rarely can occur in the

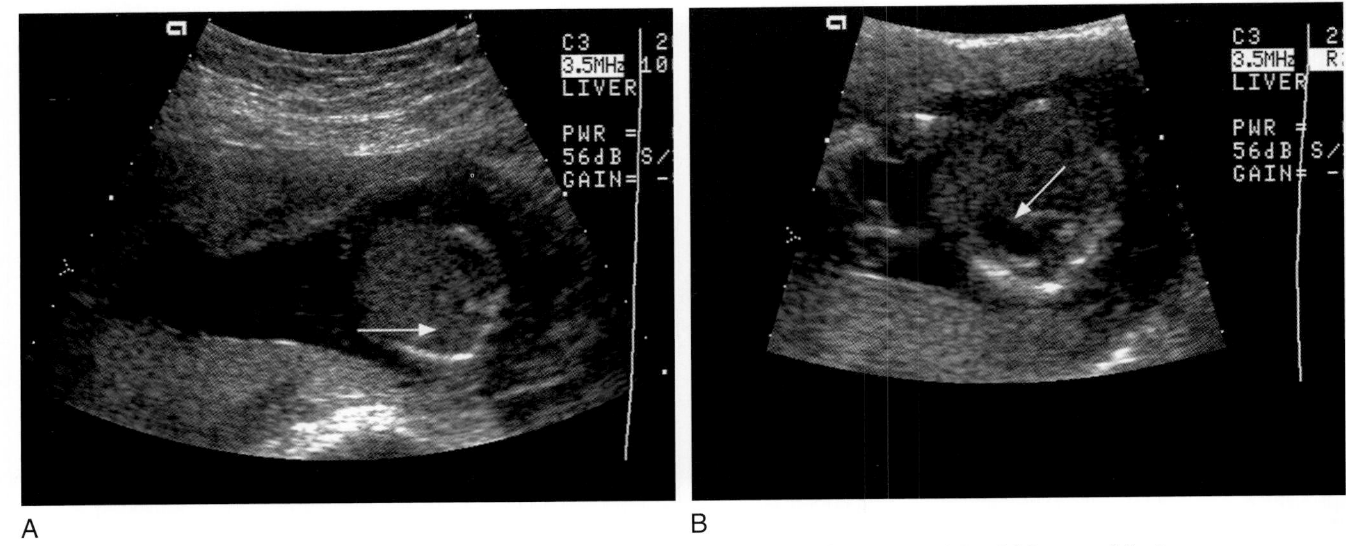

Figure 17-9 Transient gastric nonvisualization in a normal fetus. **A,** Initial axial image of fetal abdomen fails to depict stomach in expected location *(arrow)* in left upper quadrant. **B,** Axial view of same fetus, obtained approximately 30 minutes after **A**, shows normally distended stomach *(arrow)*.

absence of a tracheoesophageal fistula due to intrinsic gastric secretions.

Gastric obstruction is rare. Duodenal obstruction is more common and occurs in 1 in 5000 pregnancies. It is typically identified as two fluid-filled upper abdominal structures, the stomach and proximal duodenum, termed the *double-bubble sign* (Fig. 17-12). The fluid-filled stomach and duodenum should connect when the scan plane is adjusted. There is frequently also polyhydramnios. However, the overall detection rate for duodenal obstruction is low, approximately 50% of cases, because the typical findings are often not manifest until after 24 weeks. Duodenal obstructions are the result of intrinsic and extrinsic causes. The intrinsic abnormalities are atresia, diaphragmatic webs, and stenosis; the extrinsic causes are annular pancreas, malrotation, and bands. Duodenal atresia is the most common cause (42% of cases) and has a known link with trisomy 21 (33%). Other sonographic signs of Down syndrome (although only rarely associated) should therefore be sought, in particular increased nuchal skin thickness and cardiac abnormalities.

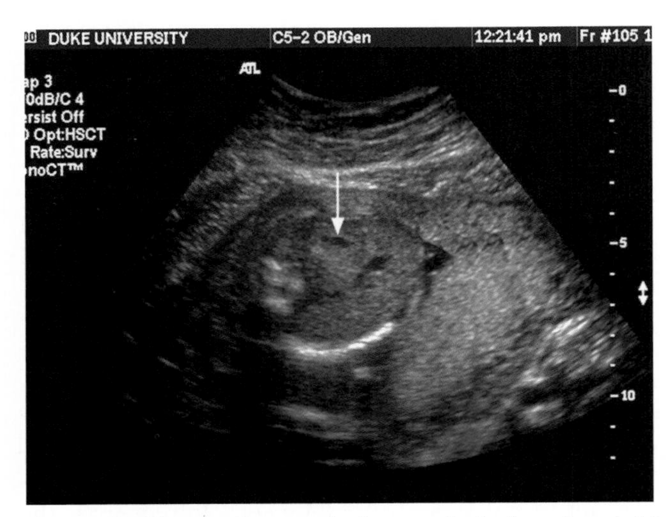

Figure 17-10 Small stomach due to oligohydramnios. Axial view of fetal abdomen in setting of oligohydramnios after premature rupture of membranes at 29 weeks shows small stomach *(arrow)*.

LOW GASTROINTESTINAL TRACT OBSTRUCTION

The low gastrointestinal tract can be defined arbitrarily as consisting of the jejunum, ileum, and colon. Jejunoileal obstructions are more common than those of the duodenum, occurring in 1 in 3000 to 5000 live births. They are usually caused by atresia, stenosis, volvulus, and meconium ileus.

Normal small bowel loops can be identified sonographically. They should not exceed 15 mm in length and 7 mm in diameter and occasionally exhibit peristalsis. Normal small bowel loops do not persist but instead appear and disappear and are more commonly seen in the third rather than the second trimester. Small bowel obstruction is not usually diagnosed in utero and, if detected, is typically not seen until after 24 weeks. A proximal jejunal obstruction can present as an anechoic upper abdominal structure, either a single long tube or three adjacent "cysts" (the stomach, duodenum, and upper jejunum) (Fig. 17-13); a more distal small

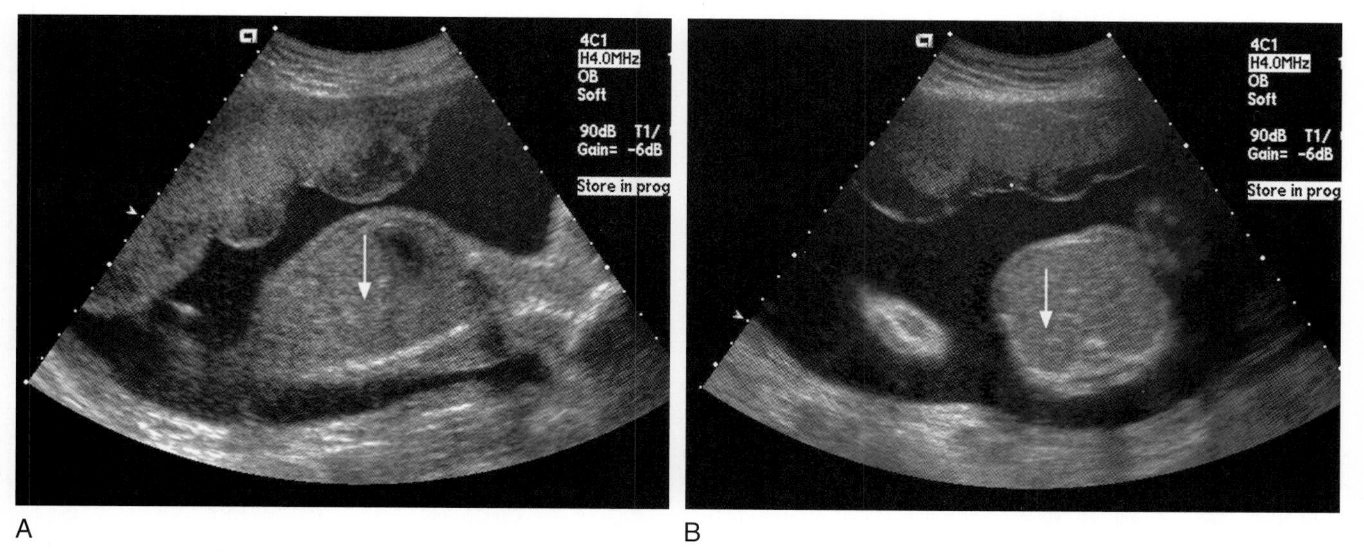

Figure 17-11 Esophageal atresia. **A** and **B,** Longitudinal (**A**) and axial (**B**) images of fetal abdomen in late second trimester show polyhydramnios and failure to depict stomach in its expected location in left upper quadrant *(arrow)* due to esophageal atresia.

bowel obstruction can present as either a solitary dilated segment of bowel immediately preceding the point of obstruction or as multiple persistent loops of small bowel (Fig. 17-14). Amniotic fluid may be normal or increased in volume. The reason for the paucity of bowel and amniotic fluid findings is not fully understood but is probably caused by the intestinal resorption of amniotic fluid and subsequent renal excretion. Resorption decreases the caliber of the small bowel, whereas both resorption and excretion maintain a normal amniotic fluid balance.

The large bowel is identified by its size, shape, position, and internal echogenicity (Fig. 17-15A and B). Its normal diameter increases linearly from approximately 5 mm at 20 weeks to approximately 15 mm at term, with a maximum diameter of no greater than 20 mm. The normal colon typically appears tubular, and it is often identified by its haustral markings (see Fig. 17-15B). The ascending and descending colons are seen in the flanks, adjacent to and below the kidneys; occasionally, the transverse colon can be detected in the mid abdomen. The normal colon can appear quite prominent during

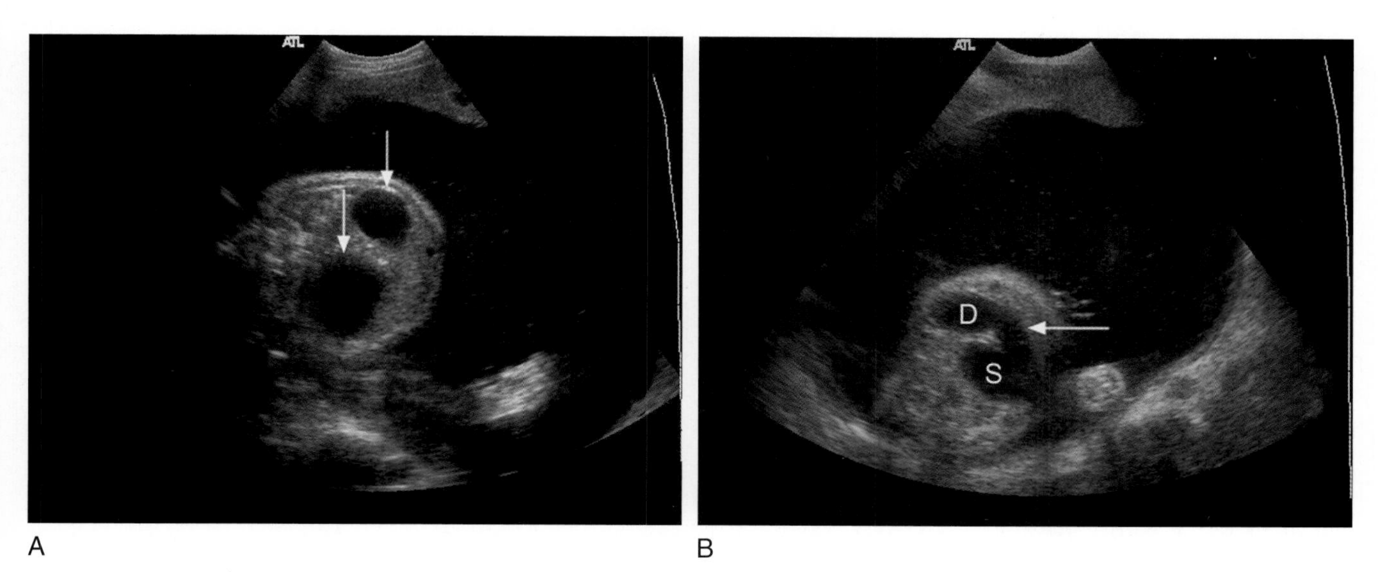

Figure 17-12 Duodenal atresia. **A,** Axial image of fetal abdomen during third trimester shows double-bubble sign *(arrows)* and marked polyhydramnios. **B,** Oblique image of abdomen shows the connection *(arrow)* between the dilated stomach (S) and duodenal bulb (D).

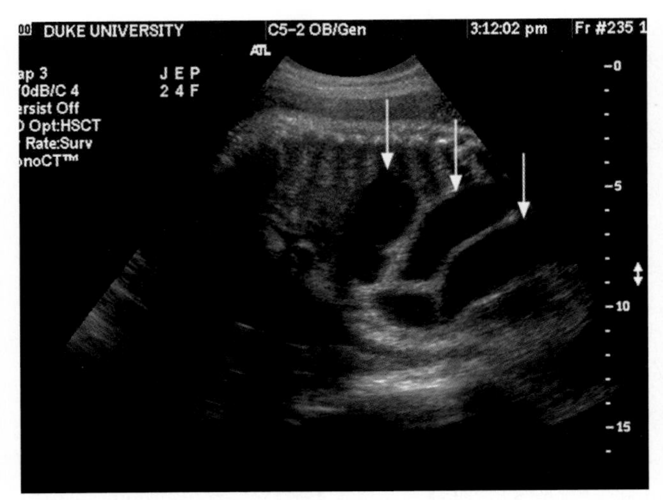

Figure 17-13 Jejunal atresia. Longitudinal image of abdomen of 35-week fetus with jejunal atresia shows several markedly dilated loops of bowel *(arrows)*. Although not shown here, there was also polyhydramnios.

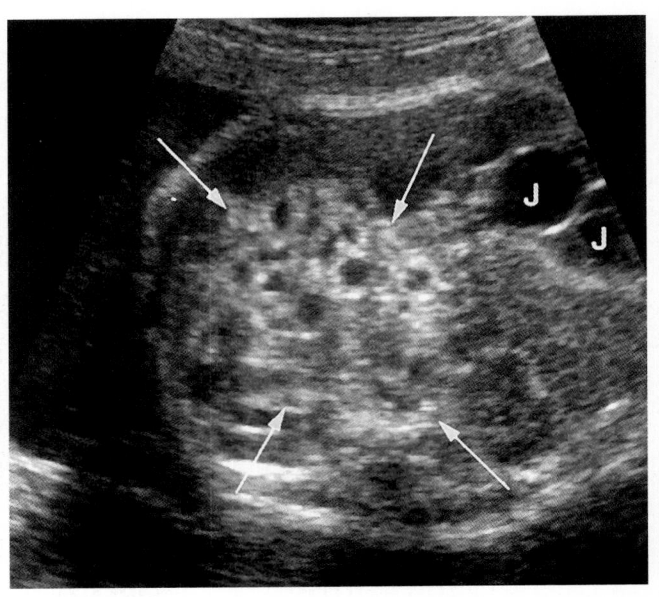

Figure 17-14 Ileal atresia. Note the mixed small bowel pattern on this transaxial view of the lower abdomen. Dilated cystic structures, toward the right, denote areas of jejunum (J), with multiple smaller anechoic spaces and hyperechoic mesentery consistent with additional matted loops of abnormal bowel *(arrows)* toward the left.

the third trimester. The echogenicity of the colonic contents (meconium) changes during the course of pregnancy: initially in the second trimester it is relatively echogenic, becoming progressively more hypoechoic by term. Although the change in echogenicity may be a sign of maturity, any meconium echogenicity is likely to be normal provided the colon size remains normal.

Large bowel abnormalities are rare, except in the anorectal region where malformations occur in 1 in 5000 live births. Most are due to developmental stenosis and atresia (e.g., imperforate anus). Rarely, the obstruction can be caused by a distal aganglionic segment (Hirschsprung's disease) or by a sigmoid mechanical obstruction (usually a volvulus).

Anorectal atresia is associated with additional abnormalities more than 75% of the time. Because of their common embryogenesis, the genitourinary tract is often involved. Two groups of disorders have been described: (1) the VACTERL syndrome of vertebral, anal, cardiovascular, tracheoesophageal, renal, and limb anomalies and (2) the caudal regression syndrome of renal agenesis or dysplasia, sacral agenesis, lower limb hypoplasia, and, rarely, sirenomelia.

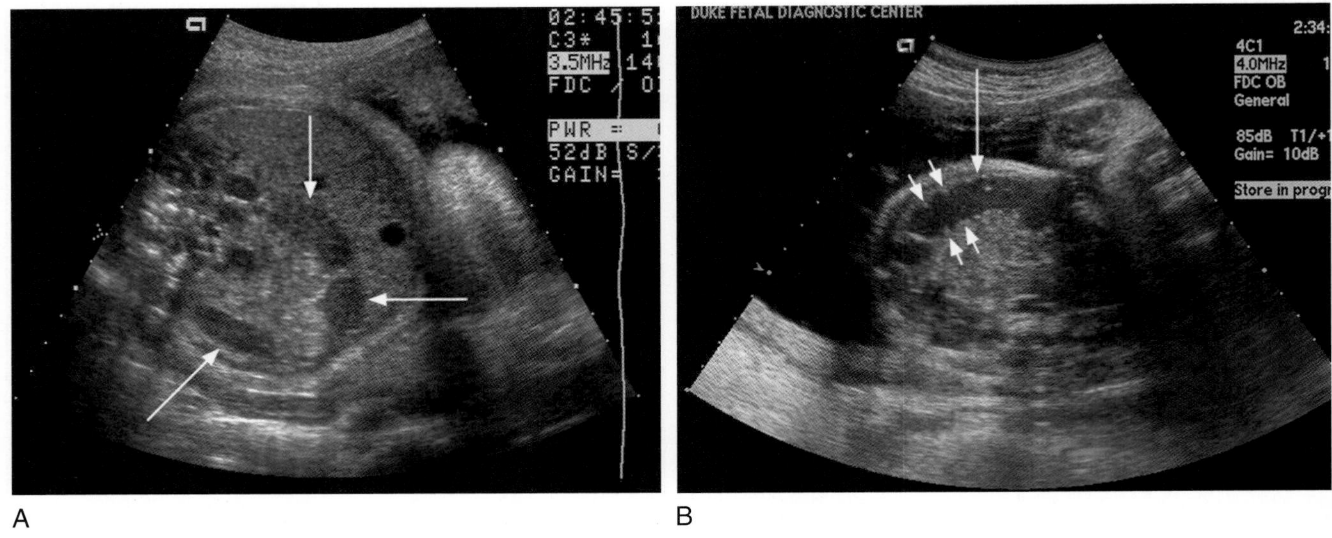

Figure 17-15 Normal colon in two third-trimester fetuses. **A** and **B,** The normal fetal colon is seen as a hypoechoic meconium-filled tubular structure *(long arrows)* in both of these late third-trimester fetuses. Haustral markings *(short arrows)* are seen in **B**.

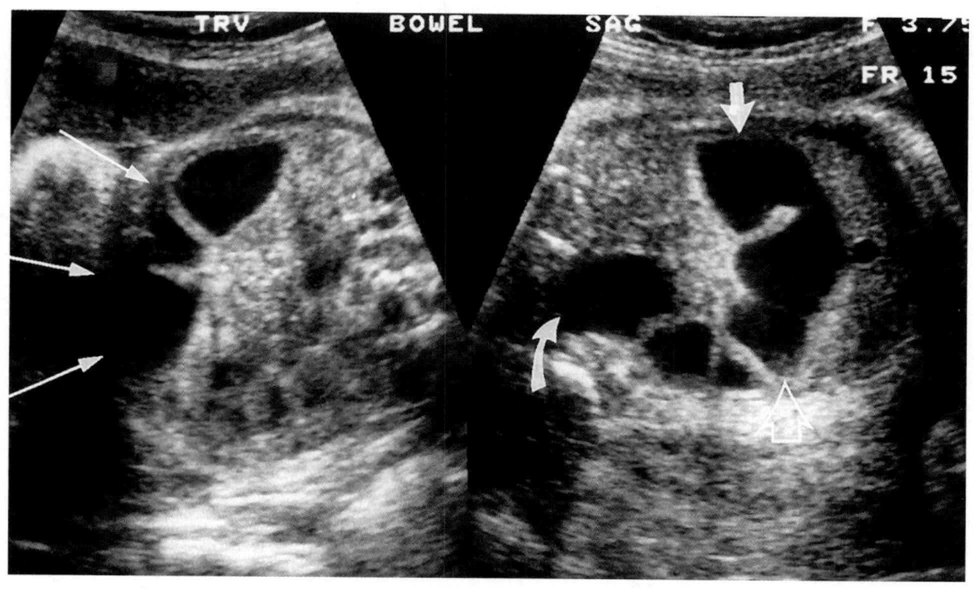

Figure 17-16 Anorectal atresia. Two views of the fetal abdomen. On the left is a transaxial view of the mid abdomen showing several dilated colonic loops extending along the edge of the flank *(long arrows)*. On the right is a sagittal-coronal view of the dilated colon extending from the rectum *(curved arrow)* up the left flank to the sigmoid flexure *(open arrow)*, with the transverse colon dilated to the hepatic flexure *(short closed arrow)*. Note that the hyperechoic septa do not extend completely across the bowel lumen but exhibit the typical haustral markings of the colon. No other abnormalities were detected, and the amniotic fluid was grossly normal in amount.

Sonographically, when a distal large bowel obstruction is present, the proximal colon may dilate down to the anorectal region (Fig. 17-16). The position of these dilated loops and the presence of haustral markings typically confirm the diagnosis. However, in many cases of distal large bowel obstruction, the colon does not dilate. In these cases, antenatal ultrasound may appear normal and the diagnosis may be missed. In some cases of anorectal atresia, the meconium may calcify. These calcifications may assume the appearance of punctate bright foci, and because they are small may not cause distal acoustic shadowing. Polyhydramnios is often present, although the reason for this is not well understood. Associated multiorgan abnormalities should be sought.

MECONIUM ILEUS AND PERITONITIS

Normal intraluminal bowel contents consist of swallowed amniotic fluid and a bowel mucopolysaccharide. This material is moved by peristalsis into the large bowel where the fluid is resorbed, leaving meconium. Meconium is most prominent by the third trimester.

Meconium ileus is an impaction of unusually thick and sticky meconium. It typically occurs in the distal ileum but on occasion may form within the colon. An impaction of abnormal meconium causes proximal bowel dilatation; more distally the bowel is typically collapsed. Almost all infants with meconium ileus prove to have cystic fibrosis, an autosomal recessive disorder affecting whites and occurring in 1 in 2000 births. Meconium ileus affects up to 15% of the infants with cystic fibrosis and, when present, is its earliest finding. Additional gastrointestinal tract complications develop in 50% of cases and consist of volvulus, atresia, bowel perforation, and meconium peritonitis.

Sonographically, the dilatation of the proximal bowel in meconium ileus is not typically identified until the third trimester. The intraluminal echogenicity varies. The bowel can be hyperechoic but is often heterogeneous (Fig. 17-17). Polyhydramnios is frequently present.

Meconium peritonitis is an intense sterile chemical inflammation caused by leakage of the intraluminal bowel contents into the peritoneal cavity. Approximately 50% of cases are caused by an underlying bowel disorder, usually small bowel abnormalities such as atresia, volvulus, and meconium ileus. Some cases have no obvious cause (idiopathic) and are most likely the result of vascular compromise and perforation of the bowel. The perforation can heal spontaneously. Intraperitoneal calcifications frequently develop in fetuses with meconium peritonitis.

Sonographically, the findings in meconium peritonitis are related to the extent of leakage and to the time interval before detection. Intraperitoneal calcifications have been reported in 85% of cases (Fig. 17-18A). They

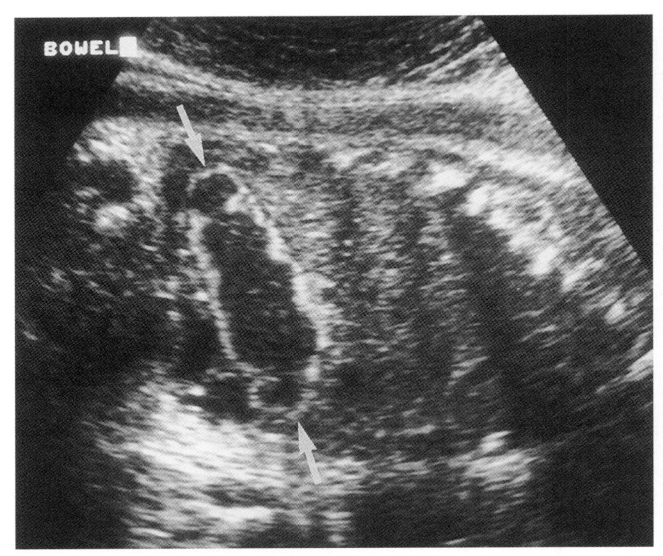

Figure 17-17 Meconium ileus in a 37-week fetus with cystic fibrosis. A solitary dilated loop of ileum *(arrows)* is seen with a low-level internal echogenicity. Multiple punctate intraluminal hyperechoic areas are seen, consistent with meconium calcifications; because of their small size, distal acoustical shadowing is not seen. The remainder of the abdomen appears unremarkable.

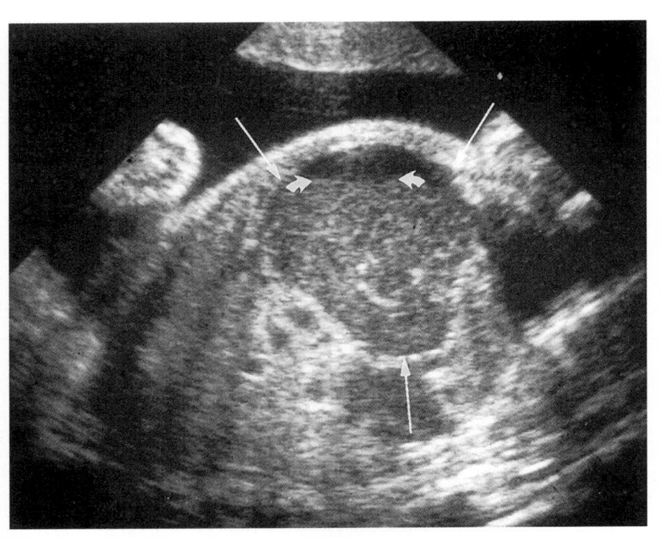

Figure 17-19 Meconium pseudocyst. Pseudocyst with well-defined walls *(arrows)* in the mid abdomen. Note the fluid-debris level *(curved arrows)*.

can be seen anywhere, particularly surrounding the liver and within the mesentery. In male fetuses, they can even extend through the patent processus vaginalis into the scrotum (see Fig. 17-18B). These calcifications are usually punctate, linear, or clumpy and sometimes exhibit acoustic shadowing. There is, therefore, a difference in appearance and position of intraparenchymal (organ) versus meconium ileus (bowel) calcifications.

Meconium peritonitis may also present as a meconium pseudocyst (Fig. 17-19) (14% of cases) and as bowel dilatation (27% of cases). The extent of the dilatation may suggest the position (and sometimes even the cause) of the underlying bowel abnormality. Ascites is common (see Fig. 17-18) (54% of cases) and usually contains internal echoes. If ascites is the only or the predominant finding, other causes of ascites should be considered (Box 17-1). One type of meconium peritonitis, the fibroadhesive form, may be extensive yet difficult to diagnose because no mass is present. Polyhydramnios is likely (65% of cases).

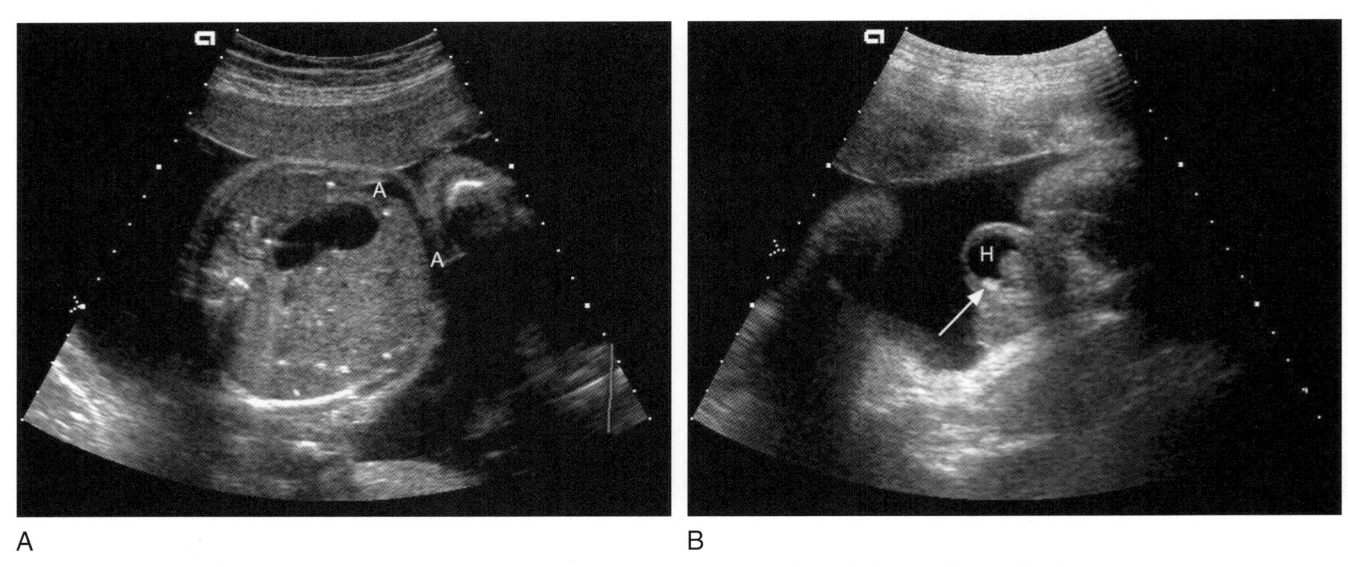

Figure 17-18 Meconium peritonitis. **A,** Axial image of fetal abdomen during third trimester shows a small amount of ascites (A) and multiple punctate highly echogenic foci due to calcification from meconium peritonitis. **B,** Axial image of scrotum shows hydrocele (H) and scrotal calcification *(arrow)*.

Box 17-1 Causes of Fetal Ascites

Generalized

Fetal hydrops*
Metabolic storage disease (e.g., Gaucher's disease, Wolman's disease)

Localized

Genitourinary (urine ascites)*
Obstruction—most common at urethrovesicular junction*
Nephrotic syndrome
Ovarian cyst with torsion
Intestinal*
Meconium peritonitis*
Volvulus and atresia
Hepatic
Hepatitis and fibrosis
Biliary atresia

*More common.

HYPERECHOIC BOWEL

Hyperechoic bowel probably represent a combination of small bowel and mesentery. It may be detected anywhere that small bowel is present. Most observers consider these hyperechoic areas normal if without mass effect, transient, and of an echogenicity less than the brightness of bone (the iliac crest or femur, for example). For the finding to be normal, no dilated loops of bowel can be seen, only prominent echogenicity. This echogenicity can be related to bowel wall interphases but can also be due to increased echogenicity of the contents of the bowel. Bowel echogenicity is a subjective finding and can spuriously appear increased when a relatively high scanning frequency is used (Fig. 17-20). Therefore, hyperechoic bowel should not be considered abnormal if it can only be seen at high transducer frequencies or with transvaginal ultrasound. It is more commonly seen on some ultrasound machines, probably related to different contrast enhancement from different image processors.

On the other hand, hyperechoic bowel is often significant (pathologic) if it produces a mass effect on adjacent structures, is consistently seen in different scan planes with different transducer frequencies, and has an echogenicity greater than or equal to that of adjacent bone. The region can be either uniformly hyperechoic or heterogeneous. When detected, there is a statistically increased incidence of cystic fibrosis, cytomegalovirus infection, a chromosomal abnormality (Fig. 17-21), growth retardation, and perinatal death. Although there are instances in which this increased echogenicity may resolve spontaneously, resolution cannot be construed as a sign of normalcy. Therefore, when this type of hyperechoic bowel is detected, a complete evaluation of all fetal structures to search for additional anomalies and at least one follow-up examination to look for growth restriction are indicated. Depending on the clinical situation, fetal karyotyping and other testing may be offered. Hyperechoic bowel

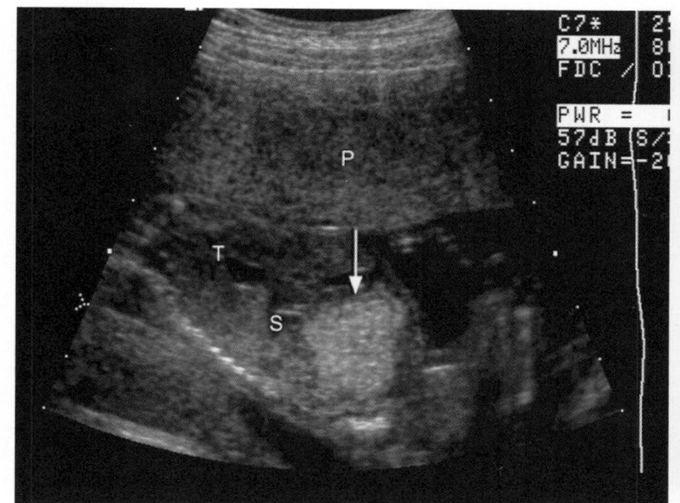

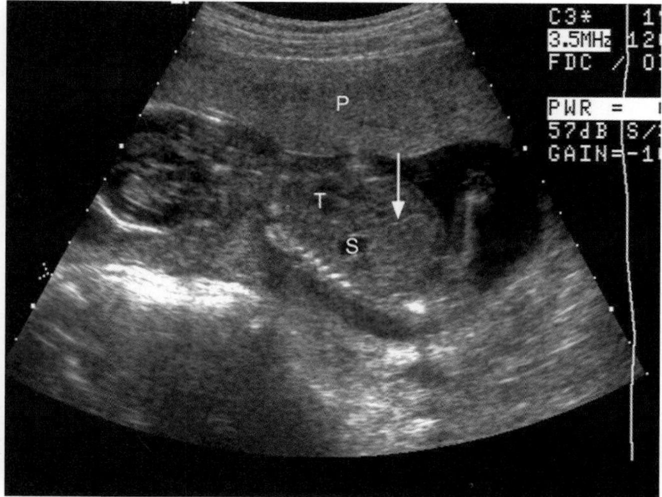

Figure 17-20 Increased bowel echogenicity due to use of a high-frequency transducer in a normal fetus. **A,** Longitudinal image of fetal body with 7.0-MHz transducer frequency shows echogenic bowel *(arrow)* in fetal pelvis and lower abdomen. S, stomach; T, thorax; P, placenta. **B,** Corresponding image of same fetus with 3.5-MHz transducer frequency shows normal bowel echogenicity *(arrow)*. S, stomach; T, thorax; P, placenta.

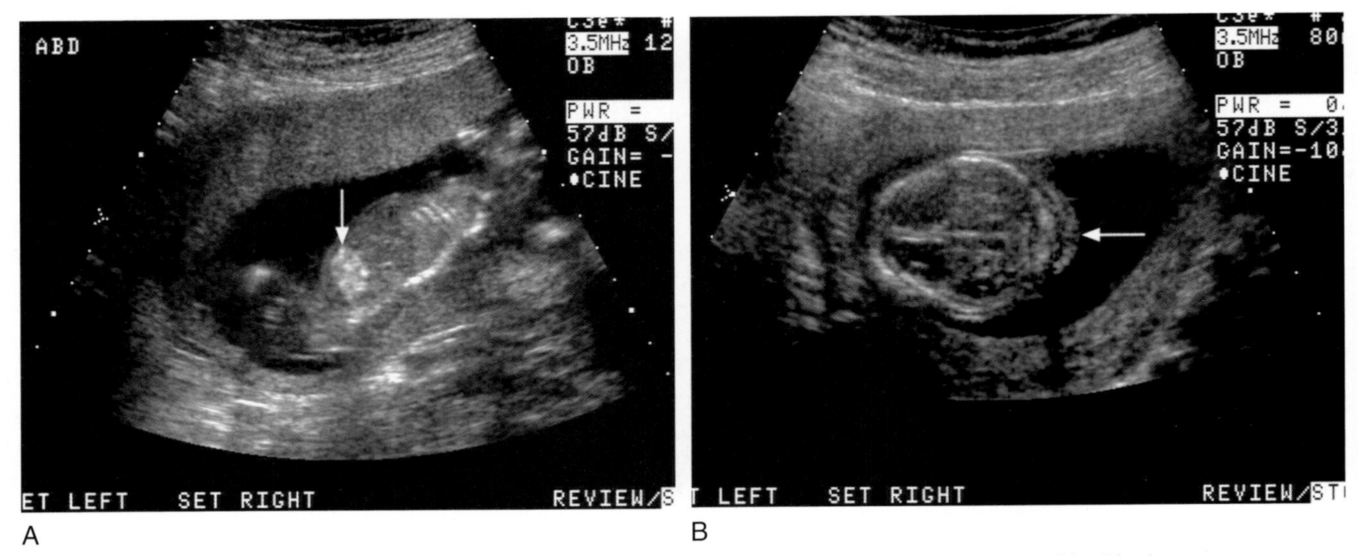

Figure 17-21 Hyperechoic bowel in fetus with trisomy 21. **A,** Longitudinal image of fetal body shows heterogeneous hyperechoic bowel *(arrow)* in lower abdomen. **B,** Axial image of fetal head demonstrates fetus also had nuchal thickening *(arrow).*

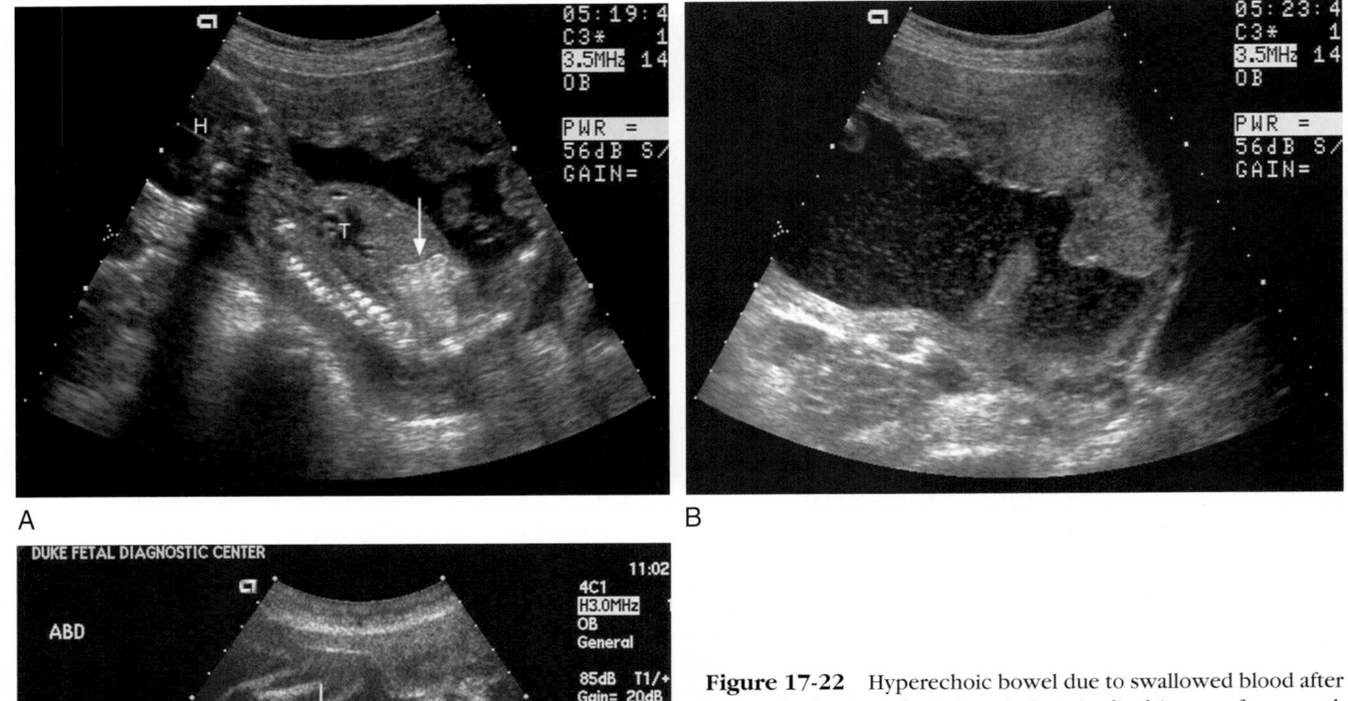

Figure 17-22 Hyperechoic bowel due to swallowed blood after marginal placental abruption. **A,** Longitudinal image of a second-trimester fetus shows heterogeneous hyperechoic bowel *(arrow)* in lower abdomen. T, thorax; H, head. **B,** Image of amniotic fluid obtained same day as **A** shows a large number of floating echoes corresponding to blood in amniotic fluid. **C,** Longitudinal image of fetal abdomen, taken approximately 1 month after **A** and **B** shows resolution *(arrow)* of the hyperechoic bowel previously seen in lower abdomen. T, thorax; B, bladder.

can also be seen as a transient phenomenon after the fetus swallows blood in the amniotic fluid (e.g., after a placental abruption or amniocentesis) (Fig. 17-22).

ANTERIOR ABDOMINAL WALL DEFECTS

There are four major anterior abdominal wall abnormalities: omphalocele, gastroschisis, pentalogy of Cantrell, and limb-body wall complex. All can be detected by careful evaluation of the anterior abdominal and lower thoracic wall. In all four the skin surface is disrupted, and all have elevated α-fetoprotein (AFP) levels in both the amniotic fluid and in maternal serum. After central nervous system anomalies, these anterior abdominal wall defects are the most common fetal structural cause of an elevated AFP level.

Omphalocele is the most common, occurring in 1 in 4000 live births. It is centrally positioned, caused by herniation of the intra-abdominal contents into the base of the umbilical cord, and covered by a thin amnioperitoneal membrane (Fig. 17-23). Ascites is frequently

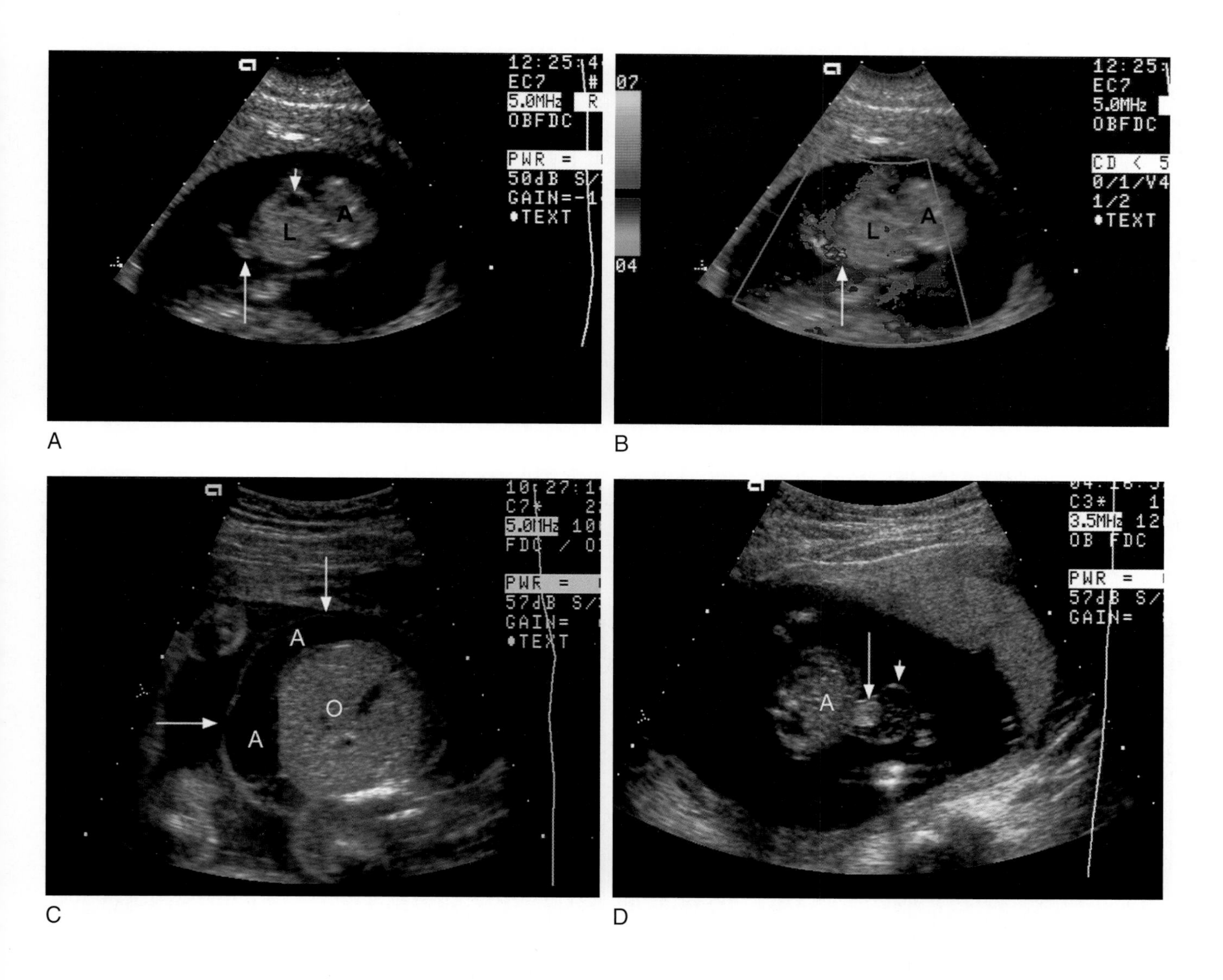

Figure 17-23 Omphaloceles. **A,** Large omphalocele at 15 weeks. Axial gray-scale image of fetal abdomen (A) shows central ventral abdominal wall defect with large omphalocele-containing liver (L) and stomach *(short arrow)*. The umbilical cord *(long arrow)* inserts into the anterior part of the defect. **B,** Color Doppler image corresponding to **A** confirms site of cord insertion *(arrow)* is on the omphalocele. A, fetal abdomen; L, liver. **C,** Large liver containing omphalocele (O) during the third trimester. Amnioperitoneal membrane *(arrows)* surrounds the omphalocele. Ascites (A) surrounds the eviscerated abdominal contents. The intact portion of the abdomen (not shown) was smaller than the omphalocele. **D,** Small omphalocele at 15 weeks. Axial image of fetal abdomen (A) shows herniation of a small amount of bowel *(long arrow)* into base of the umbilical cord *(short arrow)*.

present, confined within this membrane. Typically, the umbilical cord inserts into the anterior part of the defect; if the omphalocele is large, however, the cord insertion may be positioned at the side of the defect. The volume of amniotic fluid, often normal, is increased in one third of the cases.

There are two categories of omphalocele. The larger defects contain liver and usually bowel and stomach, and their presence suggests failure of primary abdominal wall closure. The umbilical cord insertion is often at the side of the defect. The smaller defects contain only bowel and probably represent a persistence of the primitive body stalk (failure of complete midgut rotation). The cord insertion is often midline. Unless causing bowel obstruction with dilatation, a small omphalocele might be missed unless a "cyst" of Wharton's jelly is identified at the site of the cord insertion. The first-trimester diagnosis of omphalocele is discussed in Chapter 14.

Theoretically, a small omphalocele might be difficult to differentiate from an umbilical hernia that is not of pathologic consequence. Both are defects that involve the base of the umbilical cord, but umbilical hernias rarely occur in utero. Very uncommonly a hemangioma at the base of the umbilical cord, of similar echogenicity to the bowel, could mimic a bowel-containing omphalocele.

Omphaloceles, on the other hand, are associated with a significantly increased incidence of chromosomal abnormalities, including trisomies. The mean incidence is 12% and is much greater in the setting of the smaller omphaloceles that contain only bowel. Structural defects are also present in approximately 75% of cases, more common in the larger defects: complex cardiac (30% to 50%), other gastrointestinal tract, and genitourinary tract anomalies. Associated central nervous system abnormalities and diaphragmatic hernia occur less frequently. The Beckwith-Wiedemann syndrome, an autosomal dominant disorder consisting of multiple anomalies including gigantism, renal tumors, hemihypertrophy, and macroglossia, accounts for 5% to 10% of all cases of omphalocele.

In the large defects, a careful evaluation of the anterior abdominal wall above and below the defect should include the position of the heart and urinary bladder. A heart detected outside the thorax or a bladder outside or open (extrophy) significantly worsens prognosis.

There is no normal "pot belly" appearance to the abdomen of a fetus. Any anterior abdominal wall "bulge" should therefore be further assessed. However, if during scanning the examiner inadvertently puts pressure on the fetal abdomen, or if a fetal limb or a fibroid pushes on the abdomen, an apparent bulge in the anterior abdominal wall (a pseudo-omphalocele) may appear (Fig. 17-24A). When this occurs, the anterior abdominal wall appears intact, and releasing the pressure allows the abdomen to return to a more rounded appearance without the anterior bulge (see Fig. 17-24B). This is more likely to occur in the third trimester when the fetus is large.

Gastroschisis is a less common disorder, occurring in 1 in 10,000 live births. It is typically a small defect, less

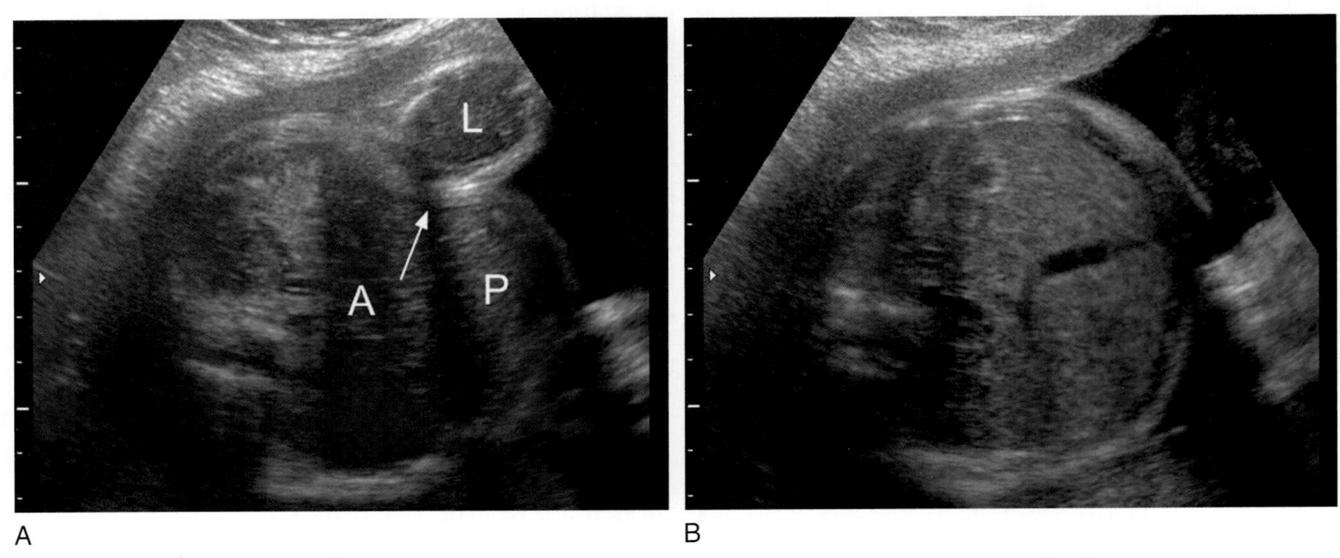

Figure 17-24 Pseudo-omphalocele. **A,** Axial image of fetal abdomen (A) at 29 weeks shows a pseudo-omphalocele (P) due to a bulge in contour of fetal abdomen secondary to pressure from an adjacent fetal limb (L), which transiently deformed the abdomen *(arrow)*. **B,** Axial image of abdomen obtained the same day as **A** after the limb had moved away from abdomen shows normal round abdominal contour.

than 4 cm in diameter, extending through all layers of the abdominal wall. It should not be confused with an omphalocele because it is paraumbilical, typically in the right lower quadrant, and the umbilical cord inserts normally on the abdomen (Fig. 17-25). Because it is not covered by a membrane, the protruding loops of bowel float freely in the amniotic fluid and ascites cannot occur. Associated anomalies and aneuploidy are rare.

Although the defect is small, the amount of eviscerated bowel varies. Small bowel always protrudes through the defect, and large bowel is often present. Protrusion of the stomach and parts of the genitourinary tract is uncommon, and the defect should not include herniated liver. The extruded bowel may appear thicker and more dilated than usual. The remaining intra-abdominally placed bowel may also dilate. At present there are no findings that can predict vascular bowel compromise, although small bowel dilatation is sometimes seen. The significance of bowel dilatation in the fetus with gastroschisis has not been fully worked out, however, and perhaps the thickness of the bowel wall and the use of Doppler (color and pulsed) imaging to evaluate mesenteric flow may prove to be of

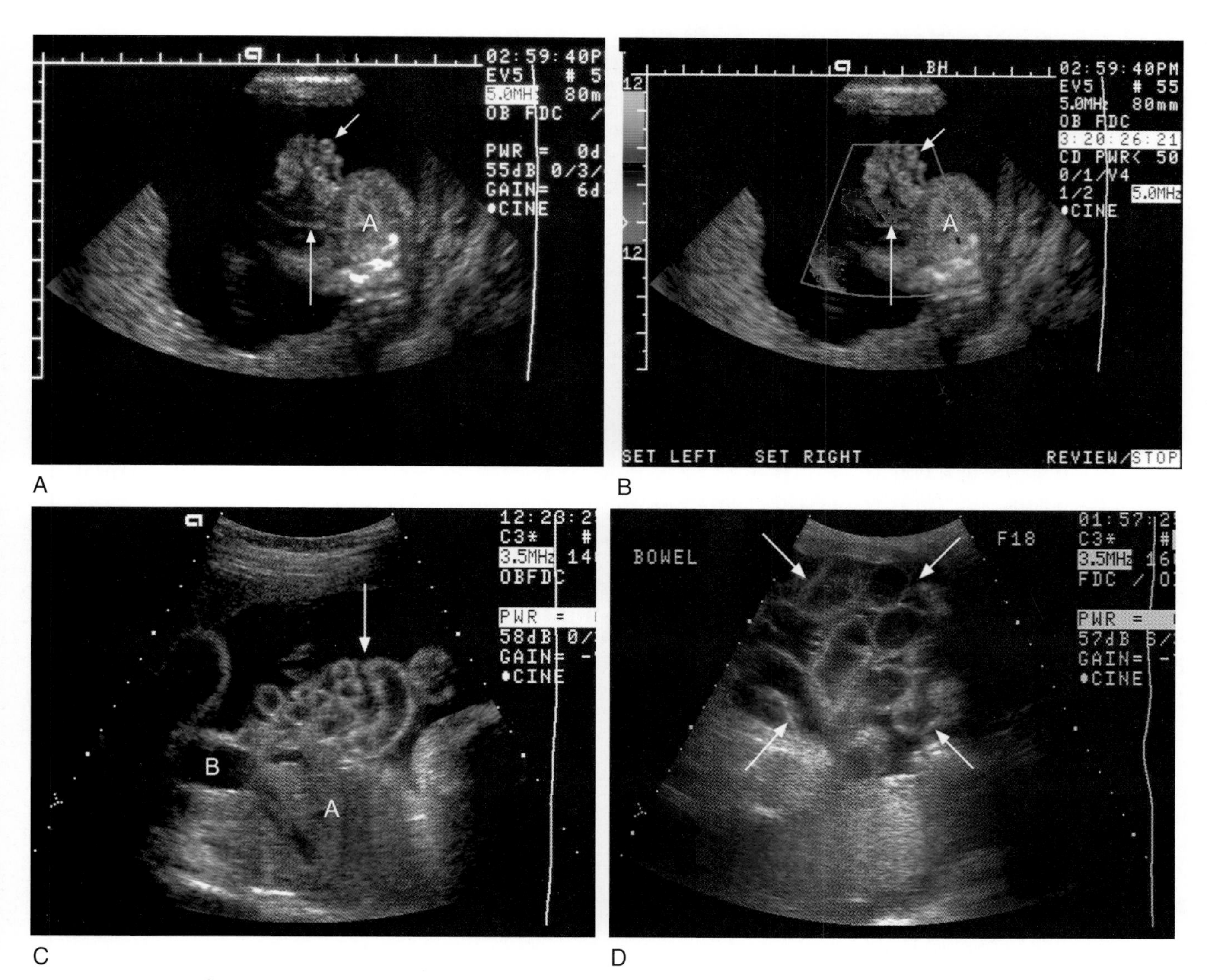

Figure 17-25 Gastroschisis. **A,** Axial gray-scale image of second-trimester fetal abdomen (A) shows umbilical cord *(long arrow)* inserting normally onto fetal abdomen. Eviscerated bowel loops *(short arrow)* are seen to the right of the cord insertion, floating in the amniotic fluid without a covering membrane. **B,** Color Doppler image corresponding to **A** confirms umbilical cord *(long arrow)* inserts directly onto fetal abdomen (A). *Short arrow,* eviscerated bowel loops. **C,** Moderate bowel dilation. Longitudinal image of abdomen (A) of a different fetus with gastroschisis shows moderately dilated bowel loops *(arrow)* floating in the amniotic fluid. B, bladder. **D,** Marked bowel dilatation. Multiple markedly dilated loops of bowel *(arrows)* are seen floating in amniotic fluid in this near-term fetus with gastroschisis.

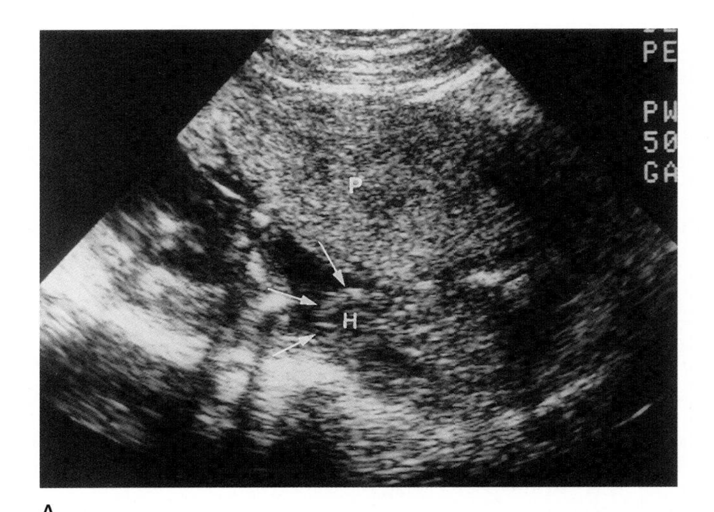

A

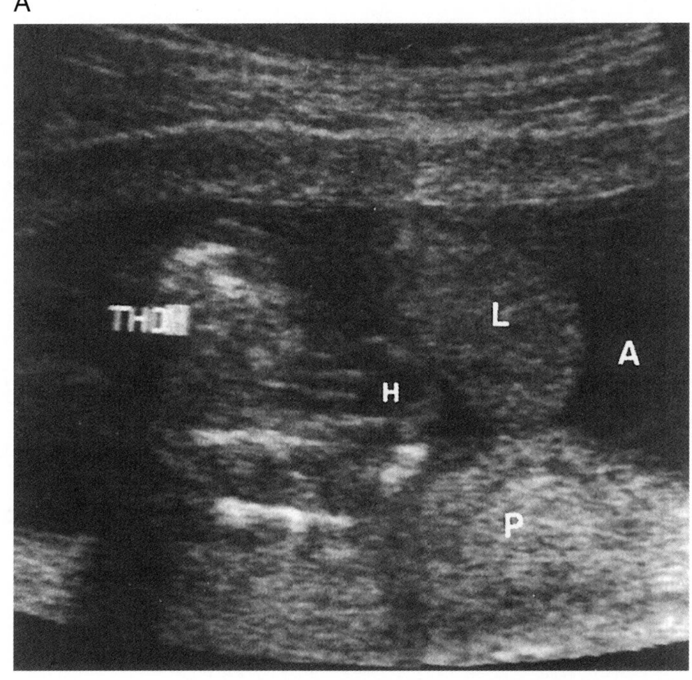

B

Figure 17-26 Two cases of ectopia cordis. **A,** Thoracic ectopia cordis in a 24-week fetus. This oblique image of the lower part of the fetal chest fails to show a normal anterior chest wall. Instead the heart (H) is pulsating against amniotic fluid (*arrows* indicate the anterior margin of the heart). P, placenta. **B,** Ectopia cordis caused by the amniotic band syndrome. This image of a severe asymmetric deformity of the anterior thoracic (THO) and abdominal walls shows the heart (H) and liver (L) without an omphalocele floating in the amniotic fluid (A). A severe scoliosis (not shown) was also present. P, placenta. (Courtesy of Kathryn Gumbach, Baltimore, MD.)

value. If the bowel perforates within the abdomen, meconium peritonitis may occur. Polyhydramnios is infrequent, except when bowel obstruction is present. Care must be taken not to mistake normal umbilical cord loops, adjacent to the abdomen, for a small gastroschisis.

The prognosis for both omphaloceles and gastroschisis is variable. If no additional structural or chromosomal abnormalities exist, the morbidity and mortality depend on the size of the defect and on the extent of the compromised bowel. The immediate problems in the neonatal period are related to heat loss and dehydration. A tertiary care center with facilities and experience to care for these newborns is therefore important for initial survival.

There is a uniformly poor prognosis for the other two anterior abdominal wall malformations: pentalogy of Cantrell and the limb-body wall complex. Ectopia cordis is a rare anomaly in which the heart is extrathoracic, causing it to pulsate against the amniotic fluid (Fig. 17-26A). Pentalogy of Cantrell represents a thoracoabdominal form of ectopia cordis because it is associated with an omphalocele, a diaphragmatic defect, a pericardial defect, and disruption of the sternum. Additional cardiac anomalies are frequently seen in association with pentalogy of Cantrell. The limb-body wall complex is a combination of abnormalities: a neural tube defect, an anterior abdominal wall defect, and limb anomalies. Although the spinal defect is not always present, severe scoliosis is common.

Amniotic bands can cause multiple and unusual fetal deformities. Although typically affecting the extremities, they can at times cause significant deformity of the abdomen and thorax (see Fig. 17-26B). This diagnosis may only be suspected on the basis of atypical asymmetric defects, because the bands are not always identified. The amniotic band syndrome is discussed in Chapter 19.

DISCRETE ABDOMINAL MASSES

Cystic masses are uncommon but can be identified within the fetal abdomen. In the mid and lower abdomen, a cystic mass can be an ovarian cyst or obstructed uterus and vagina (hydrometrocolpos) in a female fetus (Fig. 17-27A), a mesenteric or duplication cyst (see Fig. 17-27B), or a urachal cyst (originating from the dome of the bladder). If the mass is in the right upper quadrant, it may be associated with the liver or biliary system (choledochal cyst). If it is in the left upper quadrant, it may be associated with the spleen. Rare lymphangiomatous lesions have been reported.

Complex and solid gastrointestinal tract masses are rare except when associated with meconium peritonitis (meconium pseudocyst). They are more often associated with the genitourinary tract, usually the kidney and adrenal, and are discussed in Chapter 18.

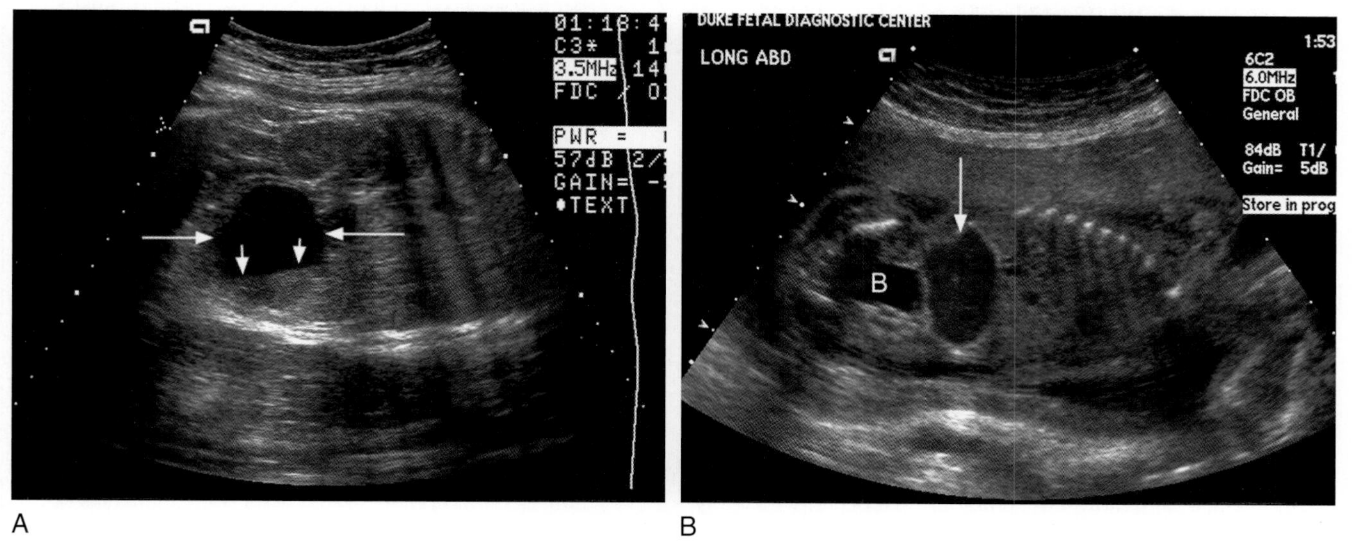

Figure 17-27 Cystic masses in fetal abdomen. **A**, Ovarian cyst with hemorrhage. Longitudinal image of abdomen of female fetus during third trimester shows a cystic mass *(long arrows)* with a fluid-fluid level *(short arrows)* due to hemorrhage into an ovarian cyst. **B**, Ileal duplication cyst. Longitudinal image of fetal abdomen late in second trimester shows a large predominantly cystic mass *(arrow)* filled with low-level echoes superior to the bladder (B). The mass corresponded to an ileal duplication cyst.

Key Features

The routine upper abdominal image is obtained through the liver in axial projection, just below the cardiac pulsation, at the confluence of the right and left portal veins. With this image, the stomach can be routinely identified and appropriate abdominal measurements obtained.

The most common causes of an enlarged liver are fetal hydrops and infections. The most common cause of a small liver is growth restriction. Although both can be suggested by an abnormal axial abdominal measurement, a direct measurement of liver length can also be used to evaluate liver size.

Pseudoascites, a hypoechoic band in the upper abdomen, should not be mistaken for ascites.

An umbilical vein varix may have a normal outcome but may be associated with fetal hydrops, structural anomalies, aneuploidy, and intrauterine demise.

If the stomach is not seen or remains persistently small, there is a high probability that the fetus is unable to swallow normally or has an upper gastrointestinal obstruction such as esophageal atresia. Nonvisualization of the stomach also occurs when there is oligohydramnios or when the abdomen is imaged during a period of physiologic gastric emptying in a normal fetus.

High gastrointestinal tract obstructions of the esophagus and duodenum are often associated with other anomalies. Polyhydramnios is commonly present but often not until after 24 weeks.

Low gastrointestinal tract obstructions may not be detected in utero. On occasion, a proximal dilated loop or polyhydramnios, or both, can be identified.

Anorectal obstructions are commonly associated with multiple additional abnormalities, sometimes presenting as proximal colon dilatation and polyhydramnios. However, many cases of anorectal obstructions are not detected at antenatal ultrasound.

Meconium ileus, an impaction of abnormally thick meconium, usually occurs in the terminal ileum. Proximal intestinal dilatation may not be identified until the third trimester. Causes include mechanical intestinal obstruction and cystic fibrosis.

Leakage of meconium into the peritoneal cavity leads to meconium peritonitis. This causes an intense reaction leading to intraperitoneal calcifications, meconium pseudocysts, bowel dilatation, ascites, and polyhydramnios.

Hyperechoic bowel can occur in either lower quadrant. If it is transient, less echogenic than adjacent bone, and without mass effect, it is probably a normal variant caused by normal bowel wall interfaces.

When hyperechoic bowel is of increased echogenicity (equal to or greater than the bone in brightness), often inhomogeneous, and often with mass effect, it should then be considered abnormal. It has been associated with cystic fibrosis, chromosomal abnormalities, growth restriction, swallowed blood and perinatal death.

The most common anterior abdominal wall defects are omphalocele and gastroschisis. Both are also associated with elevated α-fetoprotein levels.

Omphaloceles are defects that occur in the mid abdomen and are covered by a thin amnioperitoneal membrane. They can be divided into two types. The larger contains liver, usually stomach and bowel. The smaller contains only bowel and is at the base of the umbilical cord. An increased association with structural abnormalities and chromosomal abnormalities exists for both.

Gastroschisis, which is paraumbilical and usually in the right lower quadrant, does not have a covering membrane. The protruding bowel floats freely in the amniotic fluid. There are no associated anomalies or an abnormal karyotype.

Two other anterior abdominal wall malformations have uniformly poor prognosis: pentalogy of Cantrell and limb-body wall complex.

Discrete abdominal masses are usually cystic. In female fetuses they are often associated with the ovary. Both males and female may have mesenteric, duplication, or urachal cysts.

SUGGESTED READINGS

Al-Kouatly HB, et al: The clinical significance of fetal echogenic bowel. Am J Obstet Gynecol 185:1035, 2001.

Babcock CJ, et al: Gastroschisis: Can sonography of the fetal bowel accurately predict postnatal outcome? J Ultrasound Med 13:701, 1994.

Bair JH, et al: Fetal omphalocele and gastroschisis: A review of 24 cases. AJR Am J Roentgenol 147:1047, 1986.

Bejvan SM, et al: Prenatal evaluation of mesenchymal hamartoma of the liver: Gray scale and power Doppler sonographic imaging. J Ultrasound Med 16:22, 1997.

Bromley B, et al: Is fetal hyperechoic bowel on second-trimester sonogram an indication for amniocenteses? Obstet Gynecol 83:647, 1994.

Bronshtein M, Blazer S: Prenatal diagnosis of liver calcifications. Obstet Gynecol 86:73, 1995.

Bronshtein M, Zimmer EZ: Early sonographic detection of fetal intestinal obstruction and possible and possible diagnostic pitfalls. Prenat Diagn 16:20, 1996.

Brown DL, et al: Echogenic material in the fetal gallbladder: Sonographic and clinical observations. Radiology 182:7, 1992.

Brumfield CG, et al: Pregnancy outcomes following sonographic nonvisualization of the fetal stomach. Obstet Gynecol 91:905, 1998.

Corteville JE, et al: Bowel abnormalities in the fetus: Correlation of prenatal ultrasonographic findings with outcome. Am J Obstet Gynecol 175:72, 1996.

Daly-Jones E, et al: Fetal intraluminal gastric masses after second trimester amniocentesis. J Ultrasound Med 13:96, 1994.

Dicke JM, Crane JP: Sonographically detected hyperechoic fetal bowel: Significance and implications for pregnancy management. Obstet Gynecol 80:778, 1992.

Durfee SM, et al: Postnatal outcome of fetuses with the prenatal diagnosis of gastroschisis. J Ultrasound Med 21:269, 2002.

Fogata ML, et al: Prenatal diagnosis of complicated abdominal wall defects. Curr Probl Diagn Radiol 28:101, 1999.

Foster MA, et al: Meconium peritonitis: Prenatal sonographic findings and their clinical significance. Radiology 165:661, 1987.

Getachew MM, et al: Correlation between omphalocele contents and karyotypic abnormalities: Sonographic study in 37 cases. AJR Am J Roentgenol 158:133, 1991.

Harris RD, et al: Anorectal atresia: Prenatal sonographic diagnosis. AJR Am J Roentgenol 149:395, 1987.

Hashimoto BE, Filly RA, Callen PW: Fetal pseudoascites: Further anatomic observations. J Ultrasound Med 5:151, 1986.

Haynor DR, et al: Imaging of fetal ectopia cordis: Roles of sonography and computed tomography. J Ultrasound Med 3:25, 1984.

Hertzberg BS: Sonography of the fetal gastrointestinal tract: Anatomic variants, diagnostic pitfalls, and abnormalities. AJR Am J Roentgenol 162:1175, 1994.

Hertzberg BS: The fetal gastrointestinal tract. Semin Roentgenol 33:360, 1998.

Hertzberg BS, et al: Nonvisualization of the fetal gallbladder: Frequency and prognostic significance. Radiology 199:672, 1996.

Kalache DK, et al: The upper neck pouch sign: A prenatal sonographic marker for esophageal atresia. Ultrasound Obstet Gynecol 11:138, 1998.

Levine D, et al. Distention of the fetal duodenum: Abnormal findings? J Ultrasound Med 17:213, 1998.

Lindfors KK, McGahan JP, Walter JP: Fetal omphalocele and gastroschisis: Pitfalls in sonographic diagnosis. AJR Am J Roentgenol 147:797, 1986.

Mahony BS, et al: Varix of the fetal intraabdominal umbilical vein: Comparison with normal. J Ultrasound Med 11:73, 1992.

McKenna KM, Goldstein RB, Stringer MD: Small or absent fetal stomach: Prognostic significance. Radiology 197:729, 1995.

Millener PB, Anderson NG, Chisholm RJ: Prognostic significance of nonvisualization of the fetal stomach by sonography. AJR Am J Roentgenol 160:827, 1993.

Miro J, Bard H: Congenital atresia and stenosis of the duodenum: The impact of a prenatal diagnosis. Am J Obstet Gynecol 158:555, 1988.

Murao F, et al: Detection of intrauterine growth retardation based on measurements of size of the liver. Gynecol Obstet Invest 29:26, 1990.

Nyberg DA, et al: Echogenic fetal bowel during the second trimester: Clinical importance. Radiology 188:527, 1993.

Nyberg DA, et al: Fetal bowel: Normal sonographic findings. J Ultrasound Med 6:3, 1987.

Parulekar SG: Sonography of normal fetal bowel. J Ultrasound Med 10:211, 1991.

Patten RM, et al: Limb-body wall complex: In utero sonographic diagnosis of a complicated fetal malformation. AJR Am J Roentgenol 146:1019, 1986.

Paulson EK, Hertzberg BS: Hyperechoic meconium in the third trimester fetus: An uncommon normal variant. J Ultrasound Med 10:677, 1991.

Penna L, Bower S: Hyperechogenic bowel in the second trimester fetus: A review. 20:909, 2000.

Perez CG, Goldstein RB: Sonographic borderlands in the fetal abdomen. Semin Ultrasound CT MR 19:336, 1998.

Petrikovsky B, et al: Intra-amniotic bleeding and fetal echogenic bowel. Obstet Gynecol 93:684, 1999.

Pretorius DH, et al: Tracheoesophageal fistula in utero: Twenty-two cases. J Ultrasound Med 6:509, 1987.

Pretorius DH, et al: Sonographic evaluation of the fetal stomach: Significance of nonvisualization. AJR Am J Roentgenol 151:987, 1988.

Rahemtullah A, et al: Outcome of pregnancy after prenatal diagnosis of umbilical vein varix. J Ultrasound Med 20:135, 2001.

Richards DS, et al: The prenatal sonographic appearance of enteric duplication cysts. Ultrasound Obstet Gynecol 7:1, 1996.

Satoh S, et al: Antenatal sonographic detection of the proximal esophageal segment: Specific evidence for congenital esophageal atresia. J Clin Ultrasound 23:419, 1995.

Scioscia AL, et al: Second-trimester echogenic bowel and chromosomal abnormalities. Am J Obstet Gynecol 167:889, 1992.

Sepulveda W, et al: Fetal hyperechoic bowel following intra-amniotic bleeding. Obstet Gynecol 83:947, 1994.

Sepulveda W, et al: Fetal prognosis in varix of the intrafetal umbilical vein. J Ultrasound Med 17:17, 1998.

Stein B, et al: Fetal liver calcifications: Sonographic appearance and postnatal outcome. Radiology 197:48, 1995.

Strocker AM, et al: Fetal echogenic bowel: Parameters to be considered in differential diagnosis. Ultrasound Obstet Gynecol 16:519, 2000.

Vincoff NS, et al: Effect of ultrasound transducer frequency on the appearance of the fetal bowel. J Ultrasound Med 18:799, 1999.

Vintzileos AM, et al: Fetal liver ultrasound measurements during normal pregnancy. Obstet Gynecol 66:477, 1985.

Vintzileos AM, et al: Fetal liver ultrasound measurements in isoimmunized pregnancies. Obstet Gynecol 68:162, 1986.

White SP, et al: Prenatal diagnosis and management of umbilical vein varix of the intra-amniotic portion of the umbilical vein. J Ultrasound Med 13:99, 1994.

Zalel Y, et al: Varix of the fetal intra-abdominal umbilical vein: Prenatal sonographic diagnosis and suggested in utero management. Ultrasound Obstet Gynecol 16:476, 2000.

Zilianti M, Fernández S: Correlation of ultrasonic images of fetal intestine with gestational age and fetal maturity. Obstet Gynecol 62:569, 1983.

CHAPTER 18 Fetal Genitourinary Tract

The antepartum obstetrical standard recommends routine evaluation of the kidneys, urinary bladder, and amniotic fluid in the second and third trimesters. Together these parameters analyze the structure and, to some extent, the function of the fetal urinary tract. Evaluation of renal function depends on observing the urinary bladder and amniotic fluid. The cyclical changes in the size of the urinary bladder suggest that at least one kidney is producing an adequate volume of urine, although the type of urine cannot be determined. The amount of amniotic fluid, primarily produced through urine excretion after 16 weeks, should be appropriate for gestational age. Any significant abnormality of both kidneys or of the urinary bladder leads to oligohydramnios. The ureters cannot normally be identified, and their detection almost always means dilatation.

NORMAL FETAL KIDNEYS

The kidneys are normally situated on both sides of the spine just caudad to the liver. Typically, the kidneys have the same configuration as in postnatal life—round in axial and ovoid in long-axis views. Their appearance depends on the gestational age at which the study is performed (Fig. 18-1). In the early to middle second trimester, the renal cortex is poorly delineated from the renal sinus and the surrounding perinephric tissues, so the kidneys are depicted as ovoid hypoechoic structures in the flanks that can be difficult to identify. By the middle to late second trimester, the kidneys are better visualized because of increased hyperechoic interfaces (caused primarily by fat accumulation) in the perinephric and renal sinus regions. During the mid third trimester, further fat accumulation results in even more distinct hyperechoic renal borders and sinuses. Normal renal corticomedullary differentiation can often also be seen during the third trimester.

Fetal position affects the degree of renal visualization (Fig. 18-2). When the fetus is in a back-up position, both kidneys are easily detected in their paraspinal location. If the fetus is sideways to the transducer, the closer kidney is easily identified while the farther kidney is often partially obscured by shadowing from the spine. When the fetus is in a face-up position, it may be difficult to identify either kidney, particularly if the volume of amniotic fluid is decreased (degrading the ultrasound image) or if fetal limbs overlie and cast an acoustic shadow into the paraspinal regions.

Renal position and number may be atypical, and this can affect identification. Ptotic kidneys, either lower in the abdomen or in the pelvis (Fig. 18-3), crossed ectopia, agenesis of one kidney, and a horseshoe kidney can infrequently occur. When two renal outlines are not clearly identified in the paraspinal region, a careful search for the kidney or kidneys in unconventional places is therefore warranted. However, this search may not lead to clear identification, especially in the second trimester when the kidneys may not be well delineated from the surrounding tissues.

It is usually not necessary to measure the kidneys. A visual impression that they are less than one third the

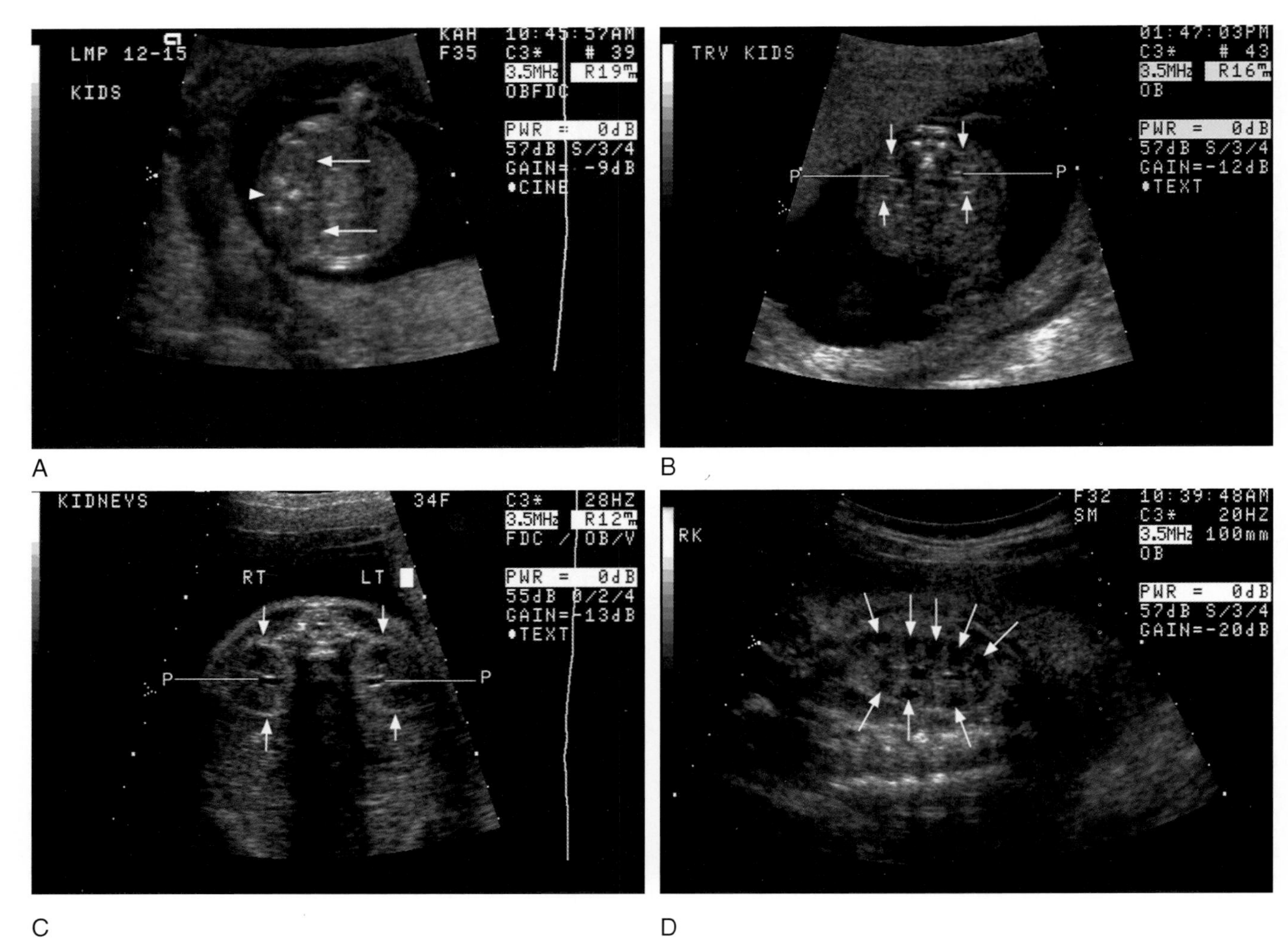

Figure 18-1 Normal kidneys at various stages of pregnancy. **A,** Early second trimester. Axial scan of kidneys *(arrows)* at 15 weeks shows they are hypoechoic and somewhat difficult to distinguish from the surrounding tissues. *Arrowhead,* spine. **B,** Mid second trimester. Axial scan at 22 weeks shows the kidneys are more readily identified due to visualization of a small amount of echogenic perinephric fat *(short arrows)* and depiction of the renal pelvis (P) bilaterally. **C,** Late second trimester. Axial scan at 27 weeks demonstrates even better delineation of the margins of the kidneys because of increased echogenic perinephric fat *(short arrows)*, which now surrounds the kidneys. P, small, normal amount of fluid in renal pelvis bilaterally. **D,** Third trimester. Longitudinal scan of right kidney at 32 weeks shows normal corticomedullary differentiation. The medullary pyramids are depicted as hypoechoic structures *(arrows)* at the corticomedullary junction and should not be mistaken for cysts or hydronephrosis.

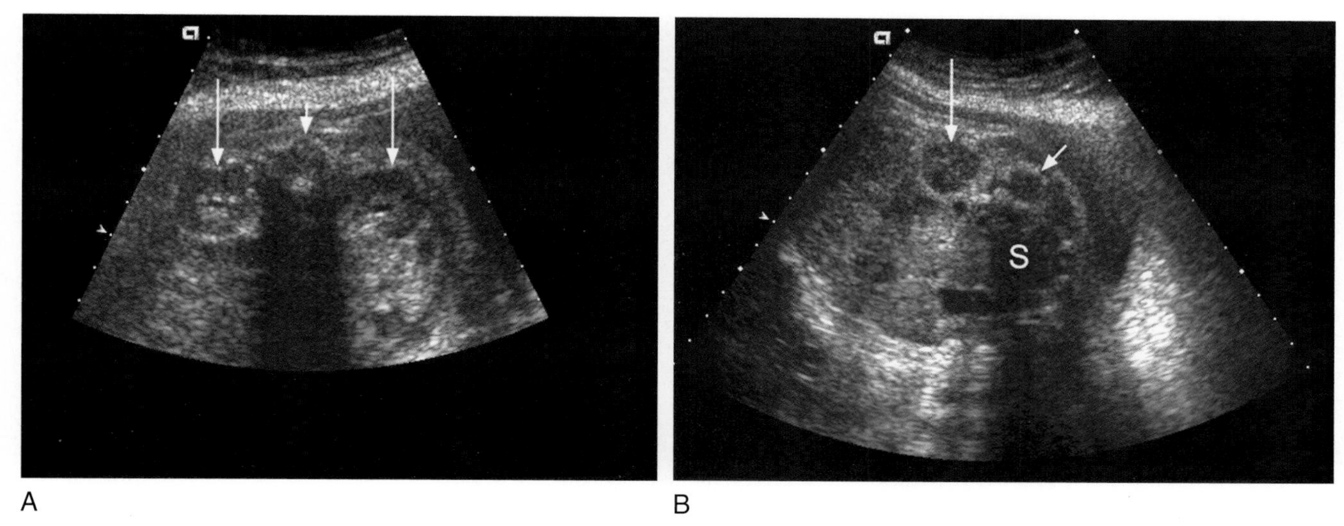

Figure 18-2 Effect of fetal position on visualization of kidneys. **A,** Axial image of kidneys during the third trimester with the fetus in a "back-up" position. Both kidneys *(long arrows)* are easily seen. *Short arrow*, spine. **B,** Same fetus as in **A**. With the fetal spine *(short arrow)* oriented sideways to the transducer, only the kidney located closest to the transducer *(long arrow)* is seen. The contralateral kidney is obscured by shadowing (S) from the spine *(short arrow)*.

abdominal size often suffices. If a measurement is needed, renal length can be obtained and compared with established standards for renal length during pregnancy (Table 18-1). The examiner must be careful not to inadvertently foreshorten the renal length because of acoustic shadowing from overlying bony structures. Alternately, a ratio of the kidney circumference to the abdominal circumference can be calculated. This ratio is relatively constant throughout the second and third trimesters, with average values between 0.27 and 0.30 (Fig. 18-4).

An anechoic space may develop within the renal sinus or collecting system. If only medial to the margin of the kidney, it is an extrarenal pelvis (a normal variant). If it spreads into the renal sinus, it is termed *pyelectasis* (Fig. 18-5). Pyelectasis can be unilateral or bilateral. Minimal pyelectasis in the absence of other urinary tract obstructive findings is typically not indicative of hydronephrosis, a mechanical obstruction. Instead, minimal pyelectasis is often physiologically normal in utero, provided the renal calices and ureters (structures that should not normally be seen) are not dilated. The anteroposterior dimension of the pyelectasis is therefore measured. There is controversy regarding the optimal threshold values above which abnormal dilatation should be suspected. Some practitioners use a cut-off of 4 mm up to 33 weeks and 7 mm after 33 weeks. Other observers consider these thresholds too restrictive and suggest higher cut-offs such as 5 mm up to 20 weeks, with progressively increasing thresholds with advancing gestation, and values as high as 10 mm considered normal at term. Although some ambiguity remains about the optimal upper limit measurements, clearly isolated pyelectasis measuring less than 4 mm can be considered normal at any stage of pregnancy. Of note is the observation that pyelectasis in the second trimester is also a minor marker for trisomy 21, which generally is not of concern as long as other ultrasound findings of Down syndrome such as nuchal skin thickening and humeral shortening (among others) are not also present. If in the third trimester the urinary bladder decreases in size (as the fetus spontaneously voids) and the renal central collecting systems show less prominence, the diagnosis of reflux should be considered.

If pyelectasis measures or appears too prominent, without other signs of obstruction, this should not be ignored. Instead, a follow-up study to identify progression is appropriate either later in the pregnancy or after delivery. Although no definite time interval has been established, generally a 4- to 6-week repeat study is suggested. If late enough in the third trimester that the follow-up examination should be delayed until after delivery, most studies are performed while the newborn is still in the hospital, generally within the first 3 days. Debates on the missed diagnosis of hydronephrosis in the newborn (because of dehydration) have raised the issue of a repeat examination within the first 3 months if the first postpartum study is normal. The issues of timing and number of these postnatal renal ultrasound examinations have not been completely worked out.

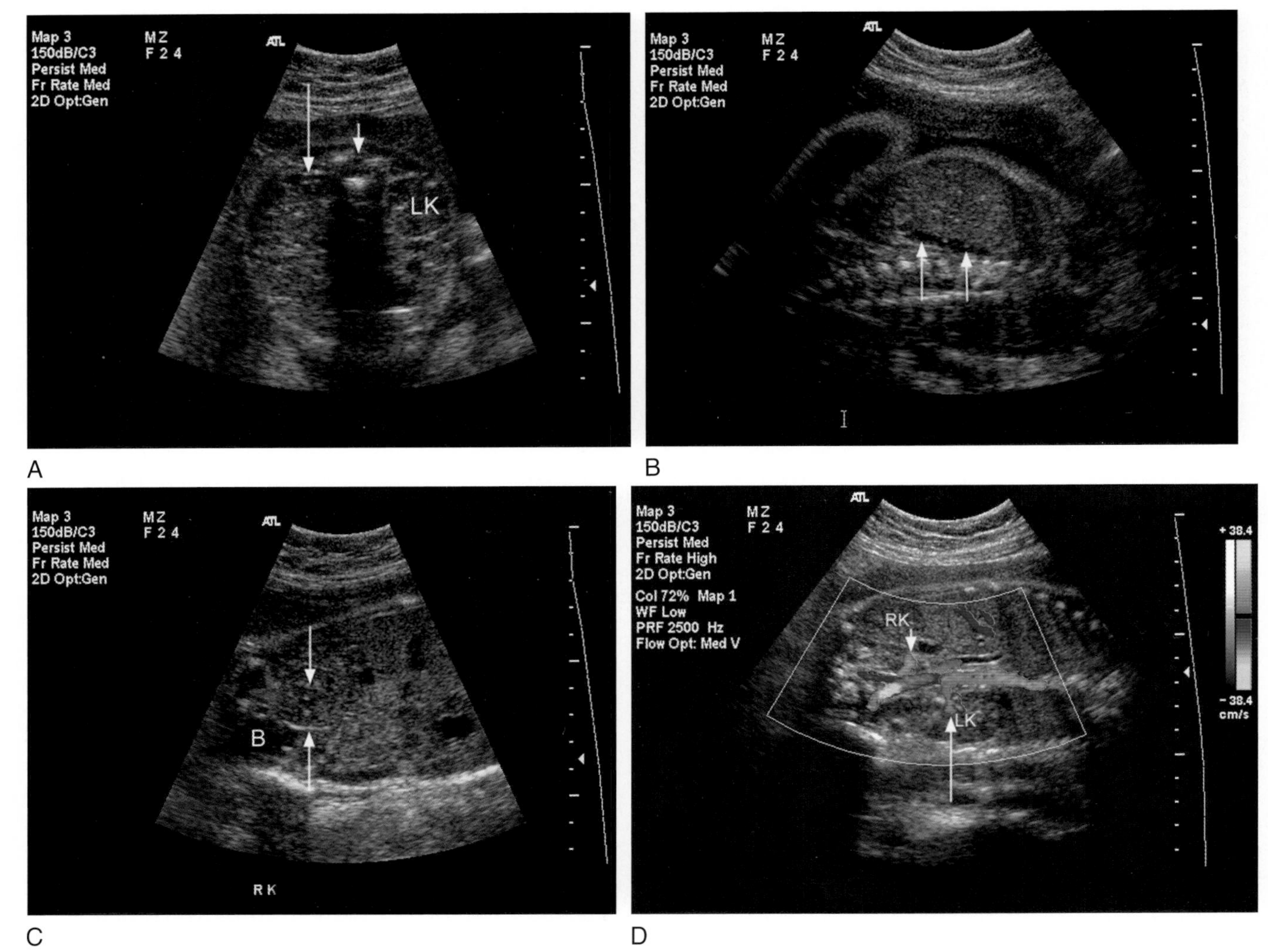

Figure 18-3 Pelvic kidney. **A,** Axial image of fetal abdomen at expected level of kidneys reveals left kidney (LK) in expected left paraspinal location but no evidence of a kidney in right flank *(long arrow). Short arrow,* spine. **B,** Longitudinal image of right flank confirms absence of right kidney in normal location. The adrenal gland *(arrows)* is seen in a paraspinal location. **C,** Longitudinal image of pelvis shows right kidney *(arrows)* in the pelvis, adjacent to the urinary bladder (B). Failure to identify a kidney in the expected location in the flank should prompt a careful search for an ectopic kidney. **D,** Coronal color Doppler image confirms normal location of renal artery and vein *(long arrow)* to left kidney (LK) and shows absence of renal blood vessels at corresponding level on the right. The renal artery *(short arrow)* feeding the pelvic right kidney (RK) is seen further caudad.

Table 18-1 Mean Renal Lengths for Various Gestational Ages*

Gestational Age (wk)	Mean Length (cm)	SD	95% CI	n
18	2.2	0.3	1.6-2.8	14
19	2.3	0.4	1.5-3.1	23
20	2.6	0.4	1.8-3.4	22
21	2.7	0.3	2.1-3.2	20
22	2.7	0.3	2.0-3.4	18
23	3.0	0.4	2.2-3.7	13
24	3.1	0.6	1.9-4.4	13
25	3.3	0.4	2.5-4.2	9
26	3.4	0.4	2.4-4.4	9
27	3.5	0.4	2.7-4.4	15
28	3.4	0.4	2.6-4.2	19
29	3.6	0.7	2.3-4.8	12
30	3.8	0.4	2.9-4.6	24
31	3.7	0.5	2.8-4.6	23
32	4.1	0.5	3.1-5.1	23
33	4.0	0.3	3.3-4.7	28
34	4.2	0.4	3.3-5.0	36
35	4.2	0.5	3.2-5.2	17
36	4.2	0.4	3.3-5.0	36
37	4.2	0.4	3.3-5.1	40
38	4.4	0.6	3.2-5.6	32
39	4.2	0.3	3.5-4.8	17
40	4.3	0.5	3.2-5.3	10
41	4.5	0.3	3.9-5.1	4

*Gestational age is an average of the gestational ages in weeks determined on the basis of biparietal diameter, femoral length, and abdominal circumference.

SD, standard deviation; 95% CI, 95% confidence interval; n, number of fetuses. A t distribution was used when $n < 30$.

Reprinted with permission from Cohen HL, et al: Normal length of fetal kidneys: Sonographic study in 397 obstetric patients. AJR Am J Roentgenol 157:545-548, 1991.

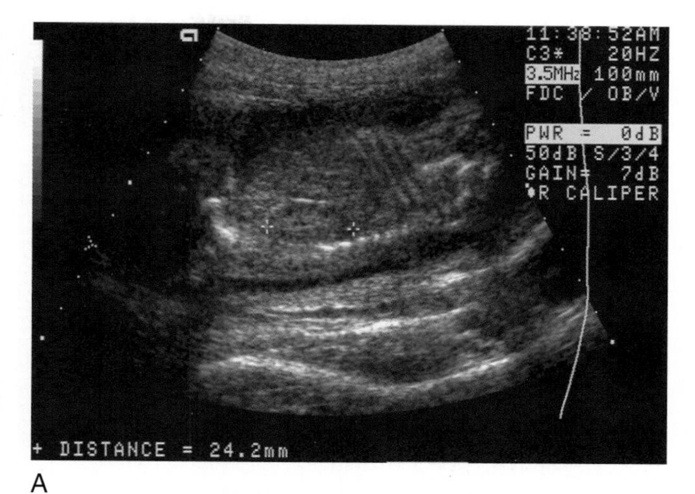

A

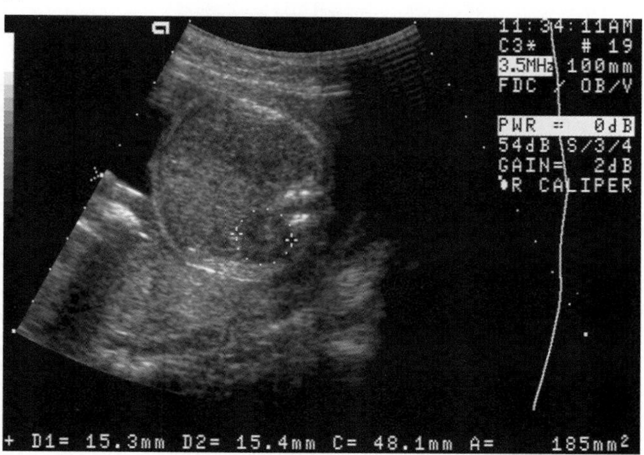

B

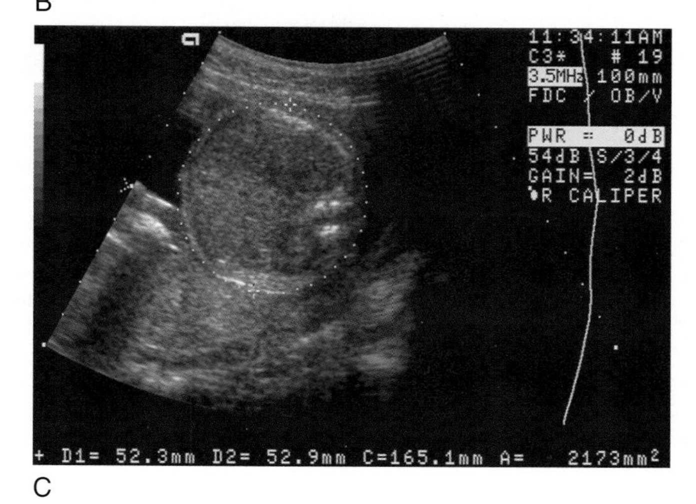

C

Figure 18-4 Measurement of fetal kidneys. Images of kidneys of a 20-week fetus depict technique for measuring renal length and obtaining ratio of kidney circumference to abdominal circumference. **A,** Longitudinal image of right kidney shows electronic calipers positioned on the upper and lower margins of the kidney *(cursors).* The length of 24.2 mm is normal for 20 weeks (see Table 18-1). **B** and **C,** Axial images of abdomen of same fetus as in **A** show measurement of renal (**B**) and abdominal (**C**) circumferences. The ratio of the renal circumference (48 mm) to the abdominal circumference (165 mm) is 0.29, which is within the normal range of 0.27 to 0.30.

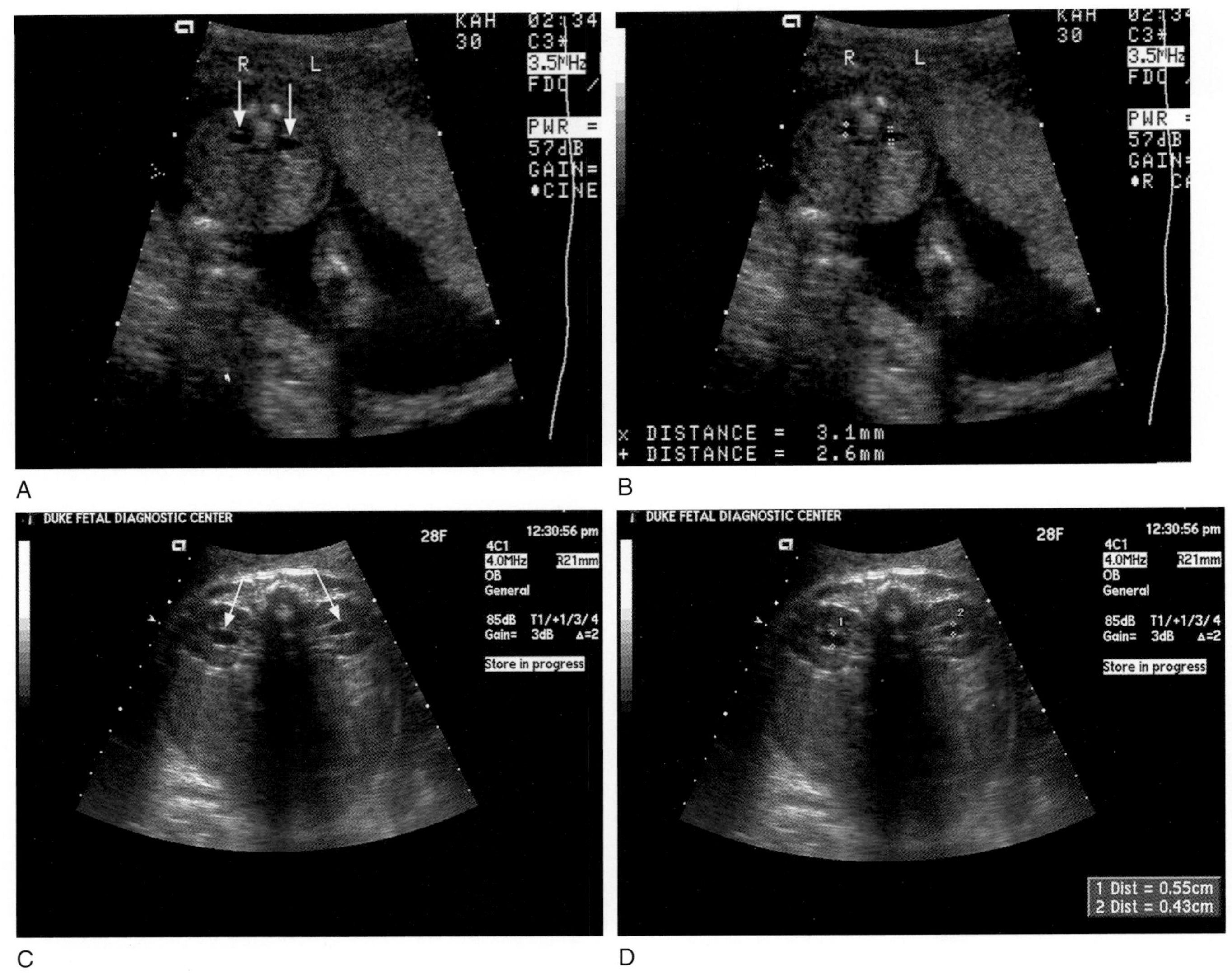

Figure 18-5 Examples of minimal pyelectasis, within normal limits for gestational age. **A,** Axial image of fetal kidneys at 19 weeks reveals minimal pyelectasis *(arrows)* bilaterally. **B,** Same fetus as in **A**. The anteroposterior diameter of the renal pelvis has been measured with electronic calipers *(cursors)*. Measurements of 2.6 mm on the right and 3.1 mm on the left are normal. **C,** Axial image of kidneys of a different fetus at 36 weeks reveals minimal pyelectasis *(arrows)* bilaterally. **D,** Same fetus as in **C**. The anteroposterior diameter of the bilateral renal pelves has been measured with electronic calipers *(cursors)*. The measurements of 5.5 mm and 4.3 mm are normal for a 36-week fetus.

THE URINARY BLADDER

The kidneys start to produce urine at approximately 10 weeks, and by 16 weeks fetal urination accounts for almost all of the amniotic fluid. The urinary bladder should be relatively easily identified not later than 16 weeks, and usually is seen earlier. The bladder is an oval or circular anechoic pelvic structure. When normally distended to 2 cm or more in diameter, it can be identified in any view (Fig. 18-6). When smaller, an axial pelvic view allows more consistent visualization. A fetal pelvic color Doppler image can also be helpful because in axial projection the iliac arteries can normally be seen surrounding the urinary bladder (Fig. 18-7A). This observation has a twofold value: it tells the observer that the identified cystic structure is definitely the bladder and that there is a normal three-vessel umbilical cord (two arteries and one vein). If only one iliac artery is identified (Fig. 18-7B), occasionally a technical problem, this suggests a two-vessel cord that has an increased incidence of associated anomalies.

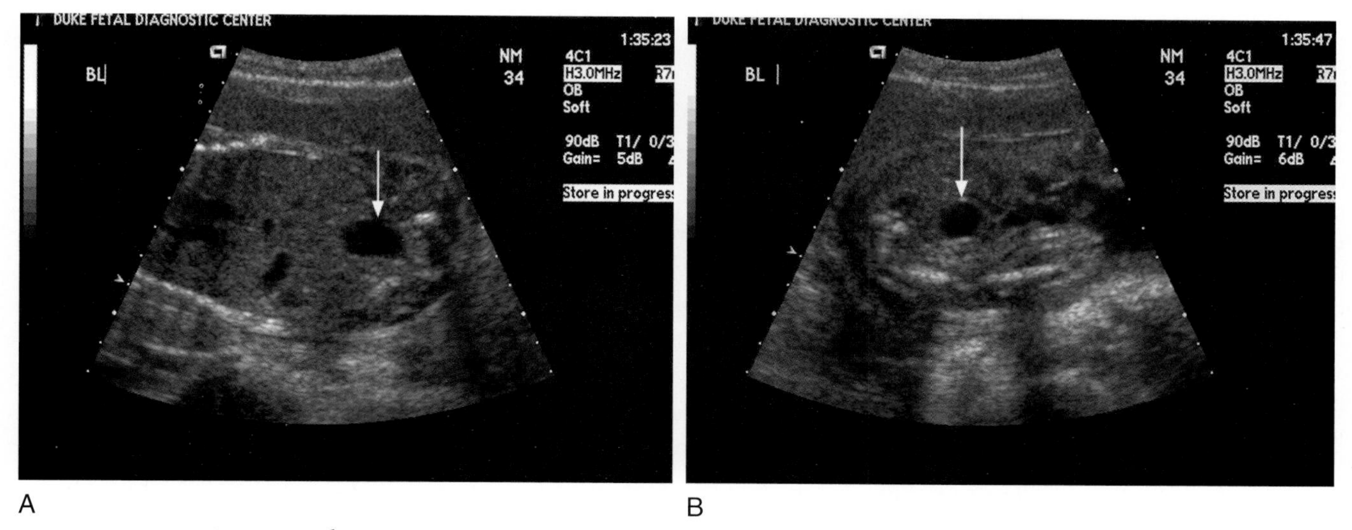

Figure 18-6 Normal urinary bladder. Longitudinal (**A**) and axial (**B**) images of pelvis in a 24-week fetus show the normal urinary bladder *(arrow)*. The bladder appears ovoid on the longitudinal view and rounded on the axial image.

A nonvisualized or very small bladder in an otherwise sonographically normal fetus is most likely normal. However, the urinary bladder has a normal cycle of 60 to 90 minutes. If the bladder is not initially seen or is less than 1 cm in diameter, sequential pelvic scans at 15 to 20 minutes for 1 hour are advised. If the bladder is still not identified or it remains persistently small, renal function is likely impaired. This suggests either a bilateral upper urinary tract abnormality or a more generalized fetal process such as growth restriction that impairs urine production. It is important for the examiner to keep in mind that a small pelvic cystic structure need not always be the urinary bladder. Rarely, a fluid-filled loop of bowel (rectosigmoid colon or small bowel) or pelvic pathology such as an ovarian or urachal cyst can instead be present.

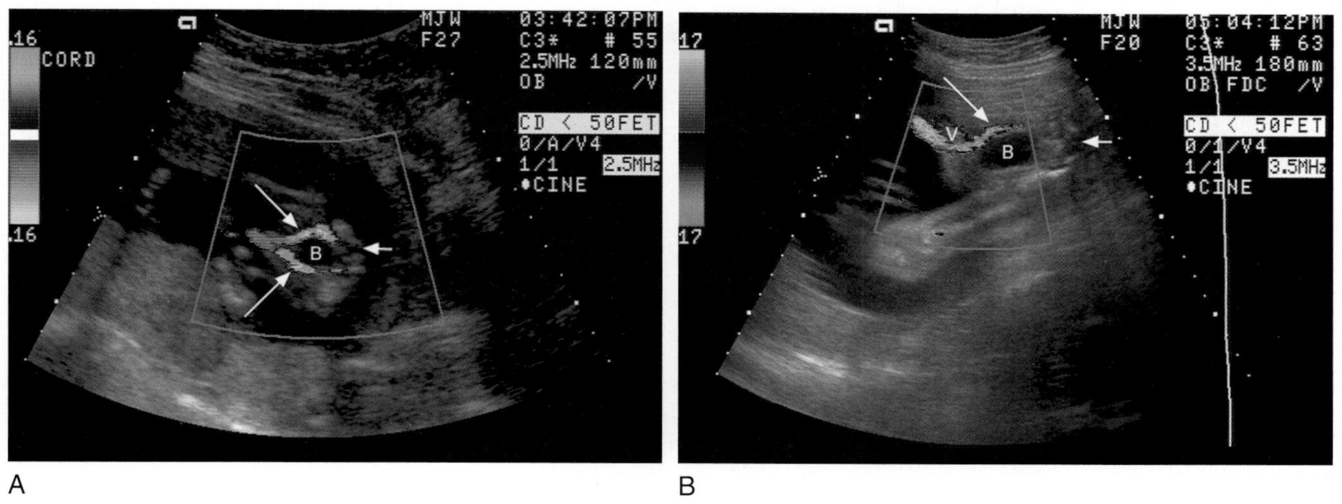

Figure 18-7 Color Doppler images of cord insertion and iliac arteries at level of urinary bladder. **A,** Fetus with normal three-vessel umbilical cord. Axial image of pelvis of a second-trimester fetus shows bilateral umbilical arteries emptying into the iliac arteries *(long arrows)* and coursing around the urinary bladder (B). Identification of the iliac arteries adjacent to a cystic structure in the pelvis confirms the structure is the urinary bladder. *Short arrow,* spine. **B,** Fetus with two-vessel umbilical cord. Axial image at level of bladder (B) shows an iliac artery *(long arrow)* on one side of the bladder, but no artery on the other side, consistent with a two-vessel umbilical cord. Short arrow, spine; V, umbilical vein.

OLIGOHYDRAMNIOS AND PULMONARY HYPOPLASIA

Oligohydramnios has a number of causes. These involve different pathologic processes, each of variable severity and time of onset (Table 18-2; Fig. 18-8). Complete urinary tract obstruction, either bilaterally at the renal or ureteric level or unilaterally at the bladder or urethral level, will cause severe oligohydramnios typically in the early to middle second trimester. Bilateral renal absence (agenesis) (Fig. 18-9), or significant bilateral renal malfunction or malformation (Fig. 18-10), will also cause early severe oligohydramnios.

The lungs need a number of factors to develop normally. One of the most important is amniotic fluid,

Table 18-2 Causes of Oligohydramnios

Causes	Usual Trimester	Typical Severity
Spontaneous rupture of membranes	Third	Mild to severe (sometimes normal)
Bilateral renal abnormality, dysfunction, or obstruction	Second	Severe
Obstruction at the urinary bladder level or below	Second	Severe
Significant growth retardation, commonly asymmetric	Third	Moderate
Fetal demise, ≥5 days	Either	Variable
Abdominal pregnancy (rare)	Either	Variable

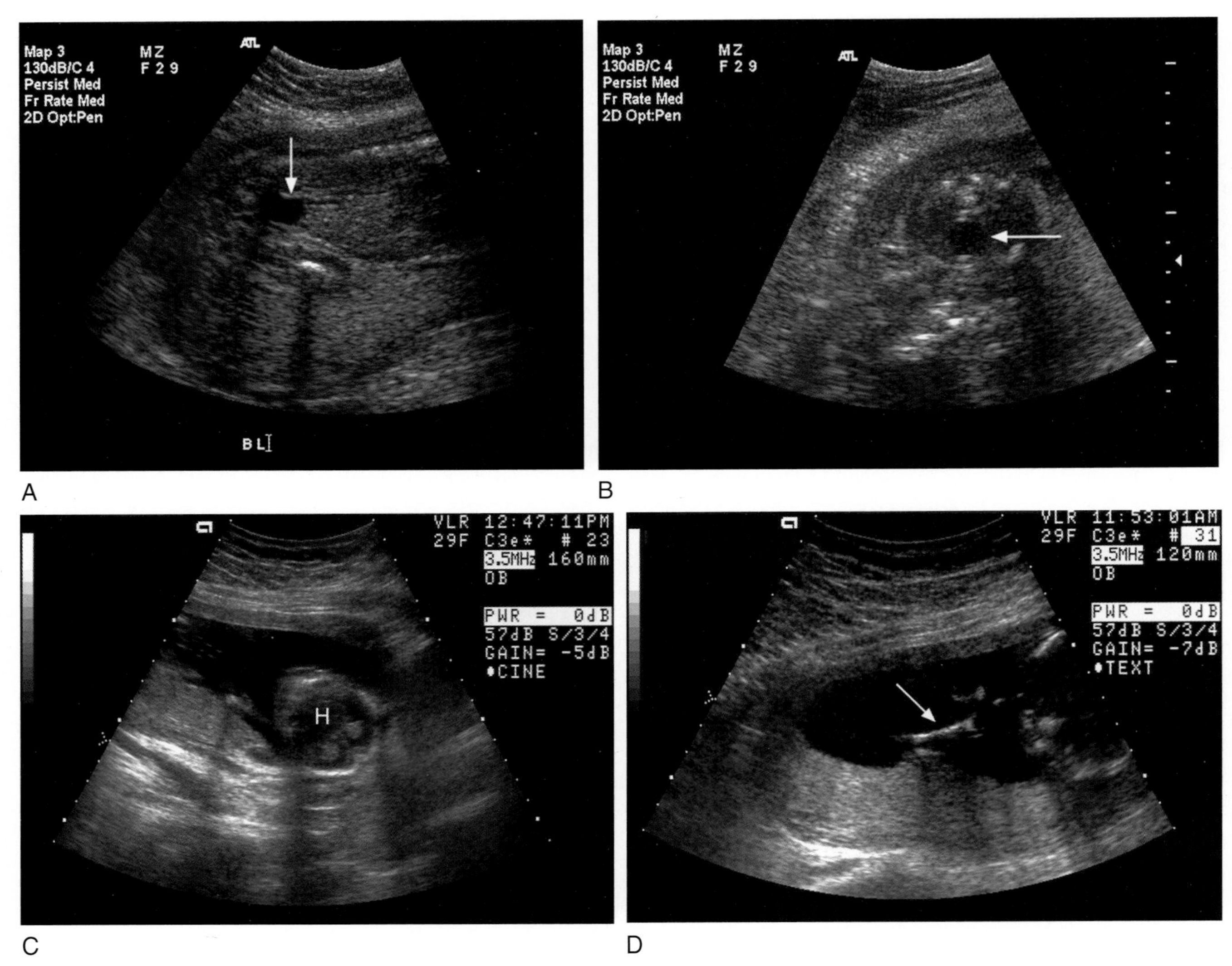

Figure 18-8 Oligohydramnios due to premature rupture of membranes. **A** and **B,** Longitudinal (**A**) and axial (**B**) images at level of urinary bladder *(arrow)* of 23-week fetus reveal severe oligohydramnios. **C** and **D,** Images of same fetus obtained at 17 weeks, before membrane rupture, show normal amniotic fluid volume. The bladder and kidneys are not shown but appeared normal. H, fetal head; *arrow,* humerus.

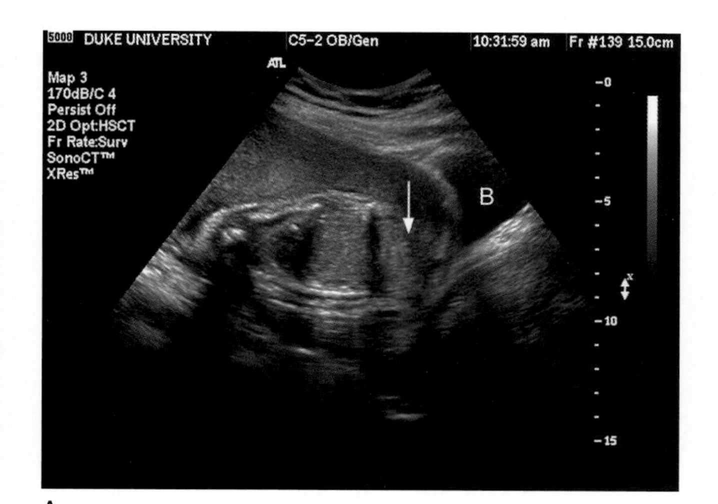

A

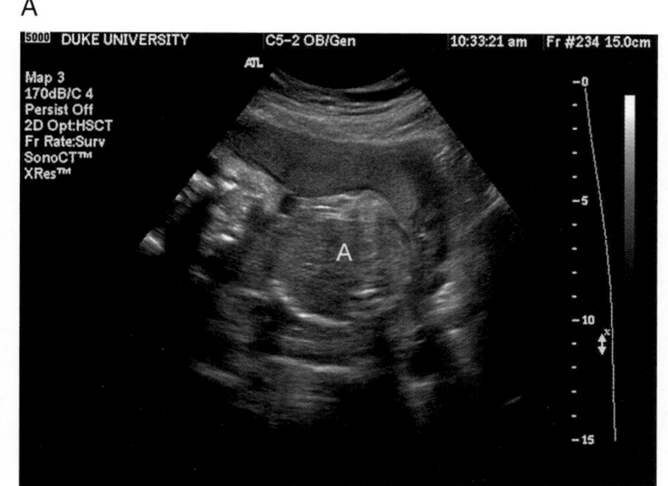

B

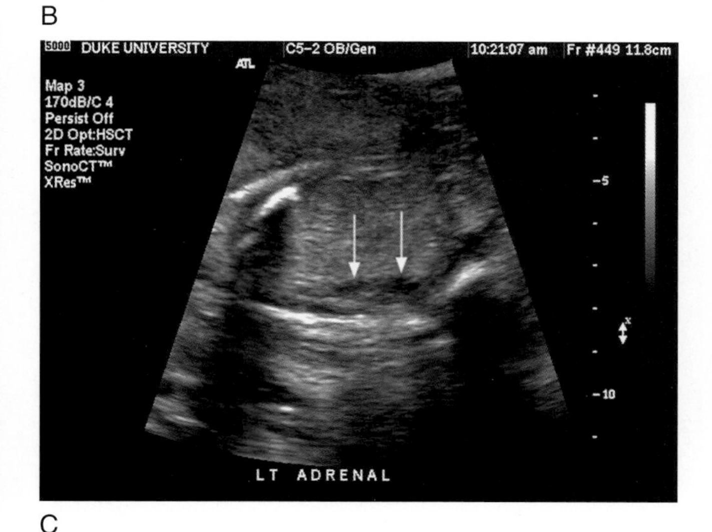

C

Figure 18-9 Oligohydramnios due to bilateral renal agenesis in a 24-week fetus. **A,** Longitudinal scan reveals absence of amniotic fluid and nonvisualization of urinary bladder in its expected location in pelvis *(arrow)*. B, maternal urinary bladder. **B,** Axial scan of fetal abdomen (A) confirms the absence of amniotic fluid and fails to show kidneys in the usual paraspinal location. **C,** Longitudinal image of left renal fossa shows left adrenal gland *(arrows)* as an elongated hypoechoic structure. The adrenal gland should not be mistaken for the kidney.

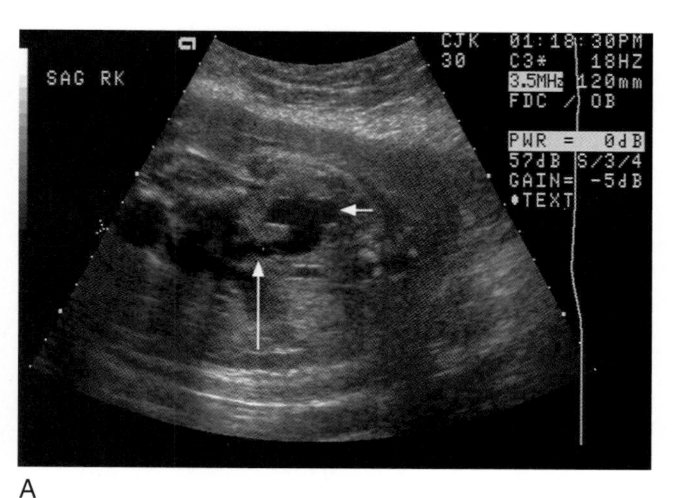

A

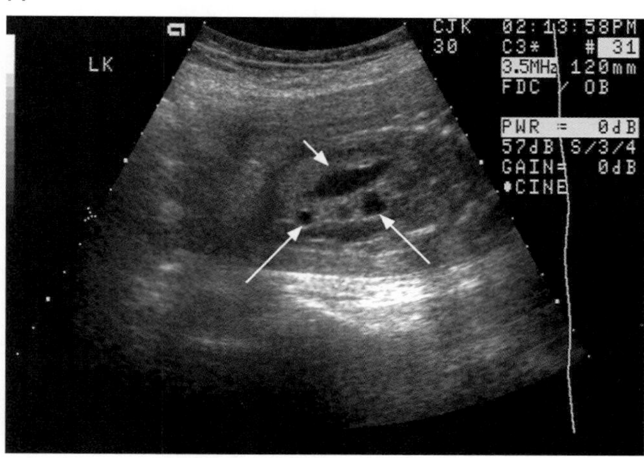

B

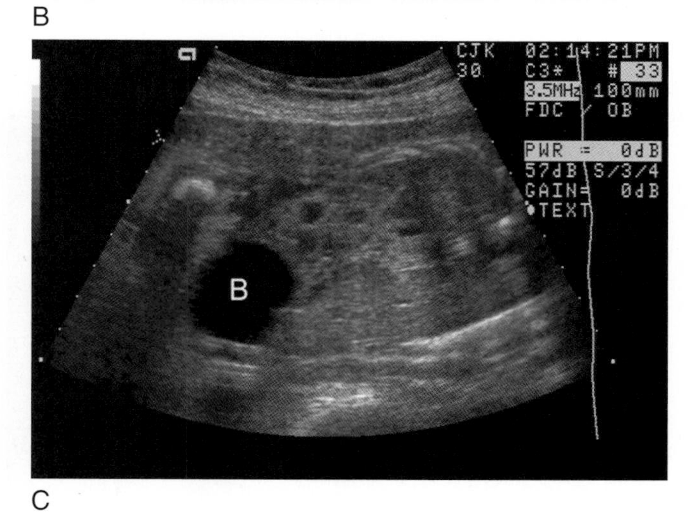

C

Figure 18-10 Oligohydramnios due to posterior urethral valves. **A,** Longitudinal image of right kidney reveals pelvocaliectasis *(short arrow)*, ureterectasis *(long arrow)*, and oligohydramnios. **B,** Longitudinal image of left kidney reveals pelviectasis *(short arrow)*, dysplastic renal cysts *(long arrows)*, and oligohydramnios. **C,** Coronal image of abdomen and pelvis shows enlarged urinary bladder (B) and further confirms the oligohydramnios seen in **A** and **B**.

which appears to have a directly positive effect on the development of the normal bronchial tree. Although the etiology is not clear, it has been suggested that the amniotic fluid, although primarily swallowed, is also aspirated and that this aspirate bathes the lungs and aids in lung differentiation.

Severe prolonged oligohydramnios has been shown to lead to pulmonary hypoplasia, especially when present from the beginning to mid second trimester. However, when less severe and/or of less duration, the effect on the lungs is not uniformly predictive. Although there have been attempts to measure the chest and lung volumes and to evaluate lung echogenicity, at present none of these has been consistently successful in the prediction of significant pulmonary hypoplasia.

BILATERAL RENAL ANOMALIES

Urinary tract obstruction can occur at any level from the kidneys to the urethra. Bilateral obstruction is usually caused by a blockage at the bladder outlet or urethra due to posterior urethral valves in a male fetus (see Fig. 18-10). Less commonly, a cloacal or urethral atresia causes bilateral obstruction in a female fetus. This obstruction typically occurs early. If it is prolonged and severe, it can lead to marked dilatation of the urinary tract. The renal parenchyma may be destroyed, in which case only large anechoic paraspinal sacs will remain (Fig. 18-11).

Dilated ureters may be identified as tubular structures in the lower abdomen. These can become very tortuous and may, on occasion, be mistaken for loops of bowel or for blood vessels. The differentiation from blood vessels can be easily shown with color Doppler analysis. The demonstration of a connection to the renal pelvis (see Fig. 18-10) differentiates dilated ureters from bowel. The obstructed urinary bladder is typically distended and may extend out of the pelvis even to the level of the kidneys (see Fig. 18-11). A dilated proximal urethra is often seen in a male fetus with posterior urethral valve obstruction as a keyhole-shaped structure to the caudal region of the bladder (Fig. 18-12). Because gender is therefore important, an evaluation of the genitalia (see Fig. 18-12) is indicated, although if there is oligohydramnios it may not be possible to image the genitalia.

Variants of bladder outlet obstruction exist. In some early cases of obstruction, instead of severe hydronephrosis, the fetus may initially present with marked dilatation of the urinary bladder and yet relatively mild renal bilateral pyelectasis or mild pelvocaliectasis. This is presumably caused by the somewhat "rigid" renal parenchyma in the early gestation. With time, the obstruction will cause the typical urinary tract dilatation. In long-standing obstruction, the urinary bladder may on occasion become hypertrophied and somewhat small (contracted) rather than dilated. The keyhole appearance of the proximal urethra is not always present and a subtle variant has been observed in a normal male fetus. If the obstruction is only partial, the urinary tract

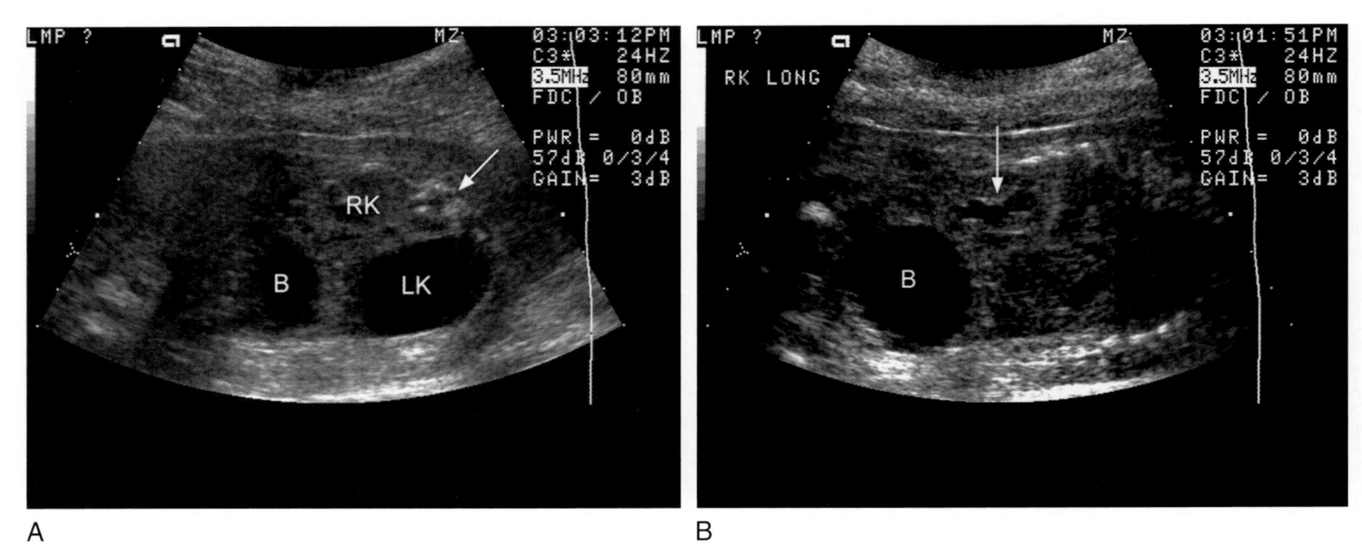

Figure 18-11 Posterior urethral valves resulting in asymmetric upper tract dilatation, with marked left hydronephrosis and mild right hydronephrosis. **A,** Axial image of fetal abdomen shows replacement of the left kidney by a large fluid-filled paraspinal anechoic sac (LK) without identifiable normal renal parenchyma due to destruction of the renal cortex secondary to severe obstruction. Also note the oligohydramnios. The urinary bladder (B) is so enlarged that it extends up to the level of the kidneys. RK, right kidney; *arrow,* spine. **B,** Longitudinal image of abdomen of same fetus as in **A** demonstrates mild right hydronephrosis *(arrow)* and enlarged urinary bladder (B). Oligohydramnios is again seen.

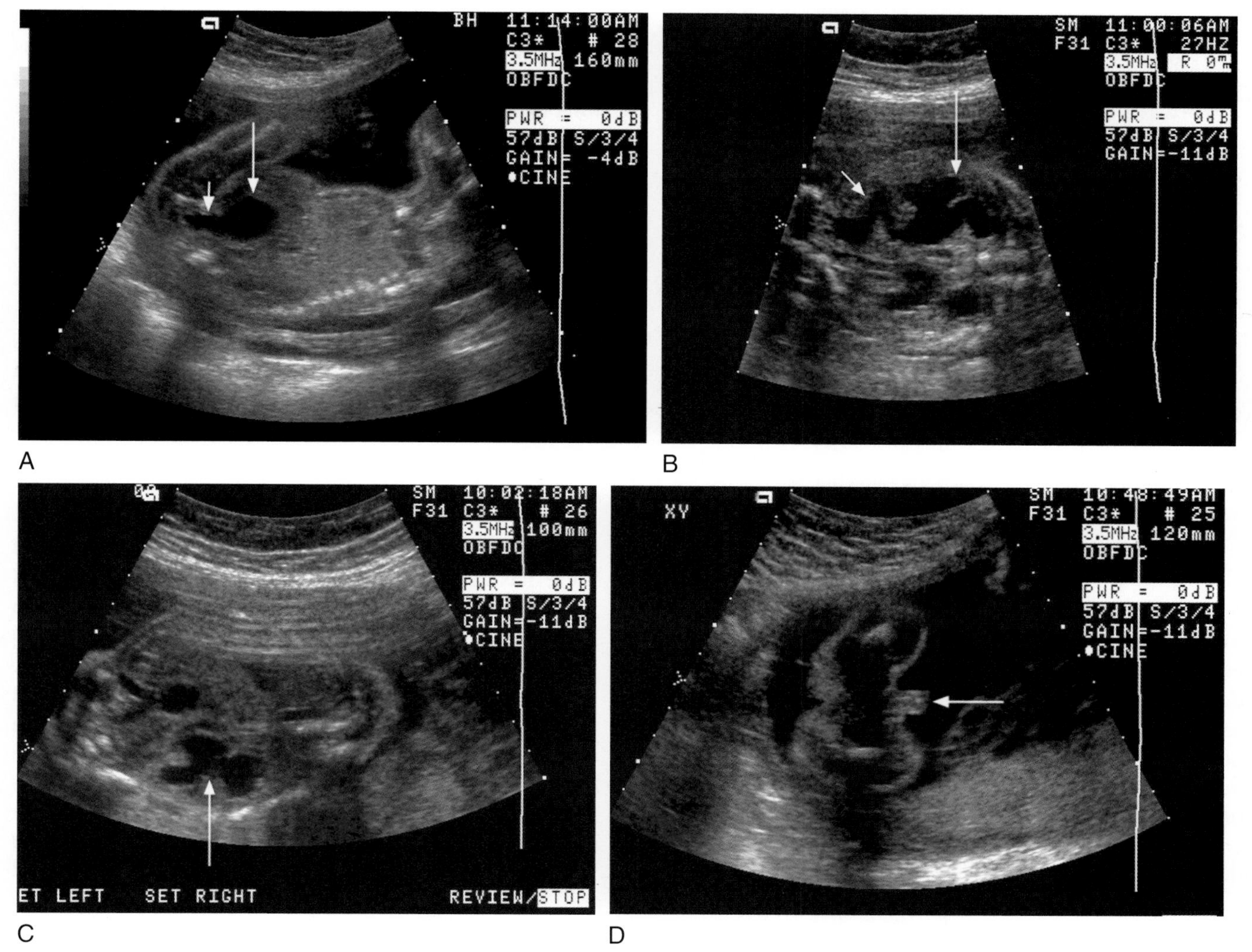

Figure 18-12 "Keyhole" configuration to bladder in a 25-week fetus with posterior urethral valves. **A,** Longitudinal image of bladder shows dilated proximal urethra *(short arrow)* connecting to bladder *(long arrow),* creating a "keyhole" configuration. **B,** Oblique image of right kidney shows severe hydronephrosis *(long arrow)* and a markedly dilated, tortuous ureter *(short arrow).* **C,** Oblique image of left kidney reveals left hydronephrosis *(arrow).* **D,** Image of the genitalia confirms this is a male fetus. *Arrow,* penis.

dilatation may not be severe and the amniotic fluid may not be appreciably decreased in volume. In these cases, pulmonary hypoplasia will often not evolve. Finally, urinomas can be seen as cystic structures next to the obstructed kidneys and may at times cause confusing appearances.

Bilateral severe renal dysfunction, most commonly caused by bilateral renal agenesis (see Fig. 18-9) and much less commonly by severe bilateral renal hypoplasia, presents as marked early second-trimester oligohydramnios. The urinary bladder is typically not seen but may on occasion be very small (<1 cm) and show no change on sequential scans. When the latter is present, the bladder contents are likely to be either mucosal secretions or residual urine in cases in which the kidneys had initially functioned and then became hypoplastic.

Bilateral renal agenesis is always lethal because of the pulmonary hypoplasia. Paraspinal reniform structures with a size and echogenicity similar to those of the kidneys can often be identified (particularly axially) in fetuses with renal agenesis (see Fig. 18-9). These are the normally prominent adrenal glands that descend into the empty renal fossae.

Infantile polycystic kidney (IPCK) disease is a bilateral renal disorder, an autosomal recessive abnormality, that typically manifests itself later in pregnancy (Fig. 18-13). *Polycystic* is an inadequate descriptive term because the renal abnormality in IPCK disease is not cystic as in adult

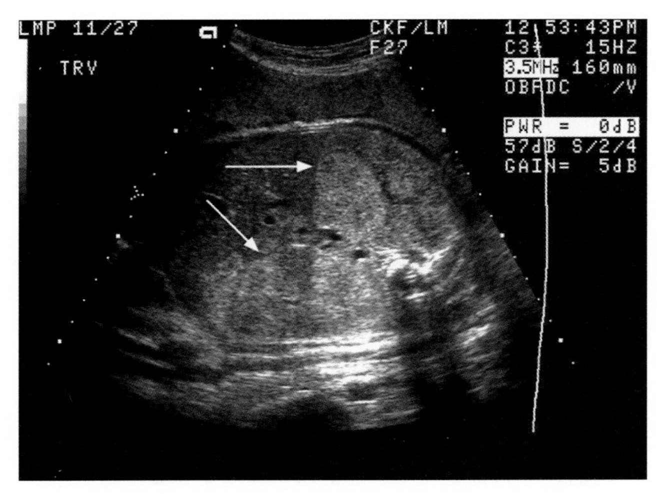

Figure 18-13 Infantile polycystic kidney disease. Axial image of abdomen of a third-trimester fetus with infantile (autosomal recessive) polycystic kidney disease shows markedly enlarged hyperechoic kidneys *(arrows)* and oligohydramnios.

polycystic renal disease but represents tubular ectasia. The kidneys in IPCK disease become progressively enlarged and uniformly hyperechoic, and their function decreases as the pregnancy progresses. However, the kidneys and volume of amniotic fluid are often relatively normal in the second trimester, with most of the findings occurring in the third trimester. The delay in onset of oligohydramnios can often minimize the deleterious effect of the decreased volume of amniotic fluid on the developing lungs.

The adult form of polycystic kidney disease is rarely detected in utero. It can present with hyperechoic kidneys (if the cysts are small) or with multiple identifiable cysts. In both infantile and adult polycystic disease, particularly when the kidneys are markedly enlarged and extend into the abdomen (sometimes filling the abdomen), proof of their renal origin is their extension to the paraspinal regions. Abdominal masses that are not retroperitoneal (renal or adrenal) in origin do not have a paraspinal component.

A careful analysis of the fetal head and hands should be performed when cystic or enlarged echogenic kidneys are identified. In the Meckel-Gruber syndrome, cystic kidneys are seen in conjunction with an abnormality of the head, frequently an encephalocele or microcephaly, and polydactyly (Fig. 18-14). Enlarged hyperechoic kidneys, polydactyly, and CNS anomalies can also be seen in fetuses with trisomy 13 (Fig. 18-15). Finally, mildly enlarged echogenic kidneys occasionally are a normal variant.

The prognosis for fetuses with IPCK disease is varied. Most die at or near birth from a combination of renal and pulmonary failure. Some survive into childhood and even adolescence, commonly then developing liver fibrosis. There are other cases, however, in which fetuses exhibit the appearance of IPCK disease in utero and yet have relatively normal renal function at birth. It is uncertain whether these infants will ultimately evolve to full-blown IPCK pattern or will have a milder form of the disorder.

PROGNOSTIC INDICATORS OF BILATERAL OBSTRUCTION

In utero obstructive uropathies can now be treated by surgical intervention. The placement of a percutaneous catheter from the obstruction into the amniotic cavity can partially or completely relieve the renal obstruction and increase the volume of amniotic fluid. This procedure can at least in theory prevent further renal and evolving pulmonary damage.

At the time of initial detection of a bilateral obstructive uropathy, it is important to accurately determine if there has been irreversible renal damage (dysplasia). If not, an invasive procedure to lessen the obstruction can be considered. While urine chemical analysis is highly specific, sonographic renal findings may also be of value. Two ultrasound renal characteristics have been found useful in predicting dysplasia when renal obstruction is present: renal cortical echogenicity greater than the liver and the identification of cortical or subcortical cysts in the remaining parenchyma. When one or both are detected, dysplasia has occurred (see Figs. 18-10B and 18-16). However, conversely, normal echogenicity and the absence of these cysts does not prove normalcy because dysplastic kidneys may have a normal appearance. Because of the importance of careful renal analysis and the difficulty in scanning when oligohydramnios is present, there may be selected cases in which the instillation of normal saline solution into the amniotic space could be considered to better visualize the fetus.

Direct analysis of the fetal urine can also be of value in assessing renal damage. By percutaneous puncture, usually into the dilated urinary bladder but occasionally into an obstructed renal collecting system, urine can be obtained and analyzed for multiple biochemical characteristics, in particular the sodium content, the urine osmolality, and the total protein content. If these values are low, normal renal function is present. If they are elevated, serial punctures should be performed to determine if these values decrease, because they may have been initially falsely elevated because of water resorption in the setting of a long-standing obstruction. If the urine values remain elevated, renal dysplasia exists. Additionally, during the puncture, amniotic fluid or urine can be obtained for karyotype analysis because there is a higher proportion of chromosomally abnormal fetuses in association with obstructive uropathies than in the general population.

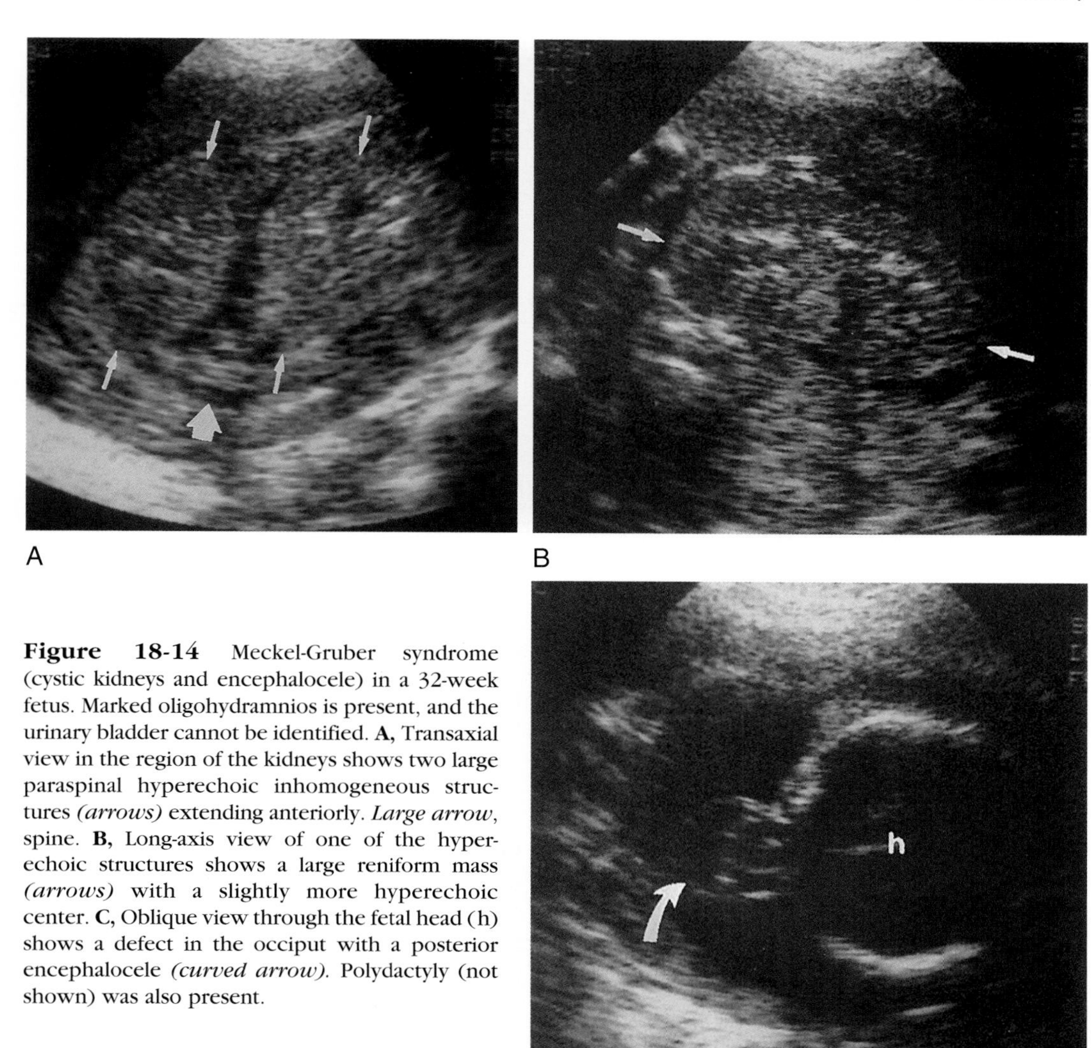

Figure 18-14 Meckel-Gruber syndrome (cystic kidneys and encephalocele) in a 32-week fetus. Marked oligohydramnios is present, and the urinary bladder cannot be identified. **A,** Transaxial view in the region of the kidneys shows two large paraspinal hyperechoic inhomogeneous structures *(arrows)* extending anteriorly. *Large arrow*, spine. **B,** Long-axis view of one of the hyperechoic structures shows a large reniform mass *(arrows)* with a slightly more hyperechoic center. **C,** Oblique view through the fetal head (h) shows a defect in the occiput with a posterior encephalocele *(curved arrow)*. Polydactyly (not shown) was also present.

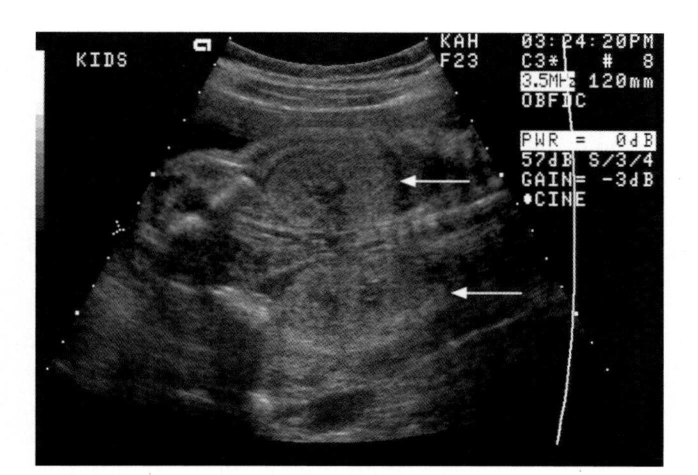

Figure 18-15 Enlarged echogenic kidneys in a fetus with trisomy 13. Coronal image of fetal abdomen reveals enlarged echogenic kidneys *(arrows)*. Multiple additional congenital anomalies were also seen, including holoprosencephaly, midline facial defects, polydactyly (see Fig. 19-11), and a complex cardiac anomaly.

Intervention in cases of obstructive uropathies is usually considered only when the following circumstances are present: progressive oligohydramnios, relatively normal renal function, no other anomalies, and a fetus too premature for delivery (usually <34 weeks). The treatment consists of the placement of a pigtail catheter that extends from the obstructed bladder (or less commonly from an obstructed kidney) into the amniotic space. It may first be necessary to instill saline solution into the amniotic cavity to provide a space for the catheter. These catheters do not always remain in place and have been found inside the fetus and in the amniotic space at birth. In other instances significant urine ascites has developed because of the puncture. Nevertheless, in some cases the procedure has been associated with no further deterioration in renal function. It is not possible, however, to determine with certainty if the procedure actually protected renal function in many cases.

The International Fetal Surgery Report has compiled a series of cases of treated obstructive uropathy.

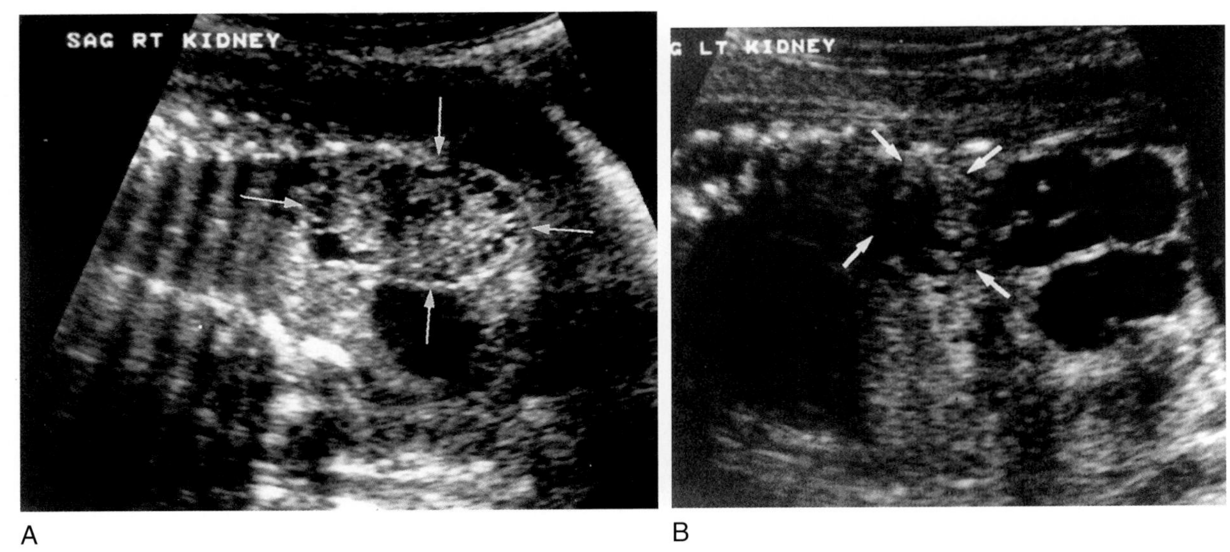

Figure 18-16 Dysplastic (irreversibly damaged) kidneys in two different fetuses. **A,** Long-axis view through the right kidney *(arrows)* shows an ill-defined hyperechoic kidney that is more echogenic than the liver. Multiple cysts are identified in a cortical-subcortical distribution. **B,** Long-axis scan through the region of the left kidney *(arrows)* shows a hyperechoic shrunken kidney. Dilated cystic structures seen more caudad (toward the right) represent a large tortuous ureter in a male fetus with posterior urethral valves. This might be confused with a multicystic dysplastic kidney. The urinary bladder was not identified; it was markedly hypertrophied and was very small.

From 1980 to 1985, 73 cases were reported: 21 posterior urethral valves, 3 urethral atresias, and 3 prune-belly syndromes (no other cause), with most of the remaining 46 of unknown cause. Chromosomal abnormalities occurred in 6 (8%). Only 30 (41%) of the fetuses survived, with the other 43 (59%) dying either as a stillborn or a neonate. Of the 29 neonatal deaths, 27 resulted from pulmonary hypoplasia. These poor results have made many examiners reluctant to perform invasive urinary procedures in most clinical settings.

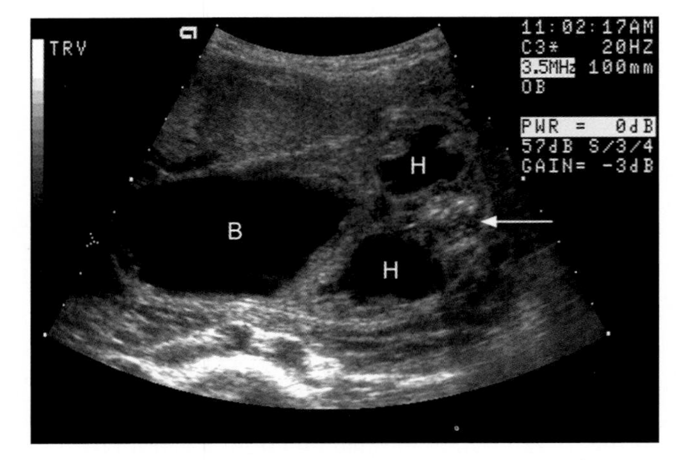

Figure 18-17 "Prune belly" configuration of abdomen due to posterior urethral valves with marked bladder distention. Axial image of the abdomen of a third-trimester fetus reveals severe bilateral hydronephrosis (H) and a markedly distended urinary bladder (B) associated with prominent anterior bulging of the abdominal wall due to flaccid abdominal musculature. *Arrow,* spine.

A further poor prognostic indicator may be suggested from the size and configuration of the abdomen. The abdominal wall is usually not affected by urinary tract problems, even when obstructive uropathies are present. However, if the obstruction is severe, particularly with a very distended urinary bladder, the abdomen may become much larger than normal. This results in flaccid abdominal musculature, called a "prune belly" appearance (Fig. 18-17). Whereas the flaccid and thinned abdominal musculature cannot be fully appreciated in utero, it can be suggested from the enlarged size and configuration of the abdomen. This secondary form of "prune belly," caused by overdistention of an intra-abdominal structure, is most commonly associated with a large bladder but can be seen secondary to long-standing and marked ascites or to any large mass such as an ovarian cyst. The flaccid musculature further complicates the course of the newborn.

A rare primary diffuse process of the abdominal musculature and internal smooth muscle is termed the *primary prune-belly syndrome* or *Eagle-Barrett syndrome.* This primary form overlaps with the secondary form, and the two can be difficult to distinguish. Eagle-Barrett syndrome is a heterogeneous group of disorders with different causes and presentations that has been postulated to be caused by abnormal mesenchymal development affecting the ureters, bladder, and abdominal wall. Affected infants present with abnormal abdominal laxity and marked wrinkling of the abdominal musculature in conjunction with an atypical-appearing obstructive uropathy and cryptorchism in a male fetus. As with the secondary form of "prune belly" appearance, only the abdominal enlargement without abdominal wall thinning may be appreciated in utero.

UNILATERAL RENAL ANOMALIES

Unilateral renal abnormalities are more common in fetal life than are bilateral anomalies. They are usually caused by either a multicystic dysplastic kidney (MCDK) or a ureteropelvic junction (UPJ) obstruction. Both are relatively easy to diagnose in utero.

The MCDK is an enlarged paraspinal structure composed of multiple noncommunicating cysts. The cysts may vary in size and usually look like a cluster of grapes (Fig. 18-18). No normal kidney is identified, but hyperechoic intervening tissue may be seen. A MCDK can enlarge or be stable in size during pregnancy. The ureter is atretic and is not identified. In contradistinction, the UPJ obstruction involves dilatation of the renal pelvis and calices (pelvocaliectasis). Both connect together to create the "glove" appearance of true hydronephrosis (Fig. 18-19). Because the obstruction is at the level of the renal pelvis, the ureter is normal in caliber below the UPJ and not identified. Careful scanning, particularly in the axial and coronal planes, can differentiate these two

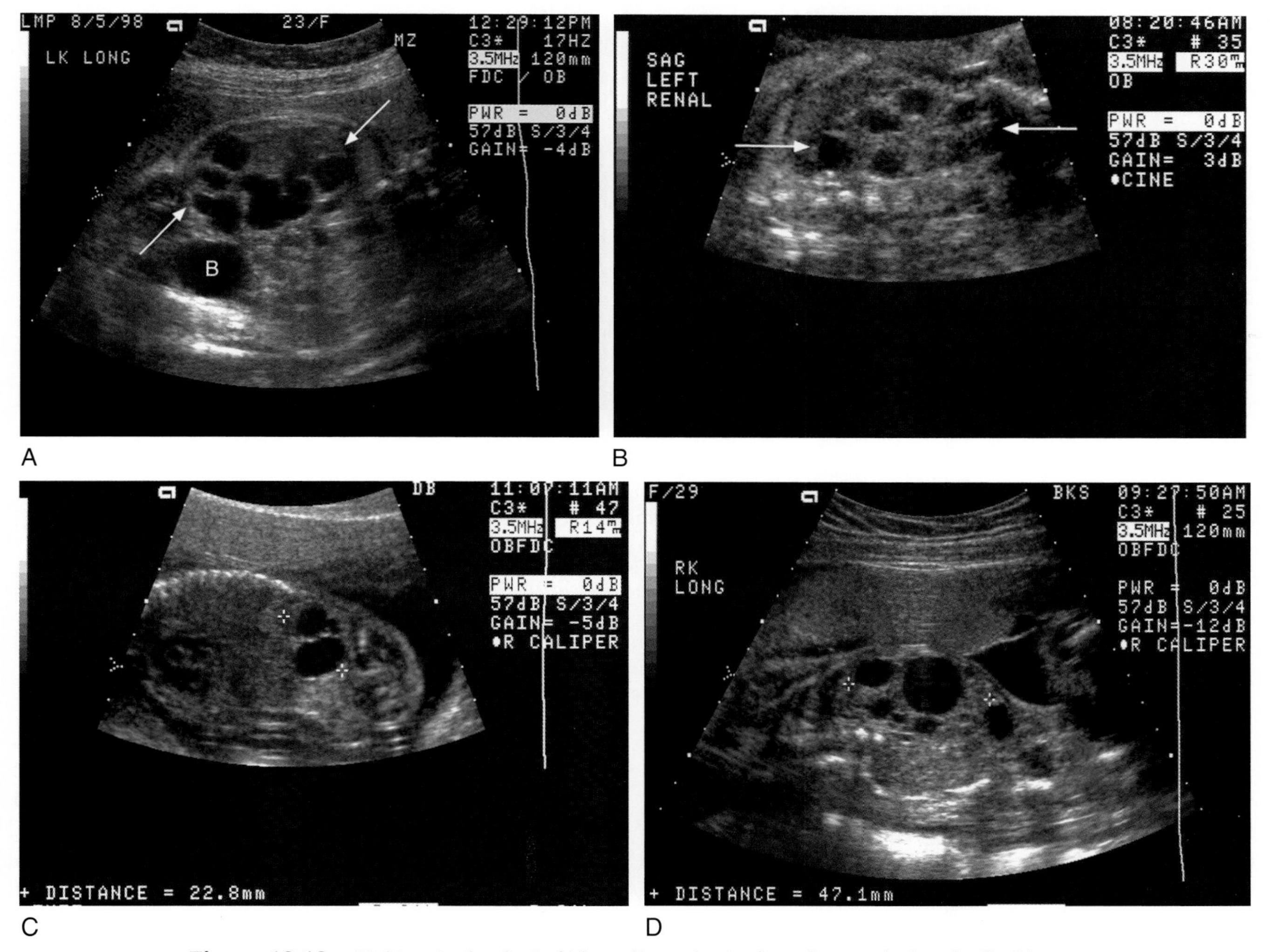

Figure 18-18 Multicystic dysplastic kidney: Examples in three fetuses. **A,** Longitudinal image of left multicystic dysplastic kidney *(arrows)* in a 30-week fetus shows enlarged kidney with multiple discrete cysts of varying sizes and shapes. B, bladder. **B,** Longitudinal image of left multicystic dysplastic kidney *(arrows)* in a 31-week fetus shows multiple small cysts that do not connect. Note the hyperechoic dysplastic soft tissue intervening between the cysts. **C** and **D,** Interval increase in size of a right multicystic dysplastic kidney during pregnancy. Longitudinal images of right kidney at 20 weeks (**C**) and 24 weeks (**D**) show multiple renal cysts. Note the interval increase in size of the kidney *(cursors)* and number of cysts between the two studies.

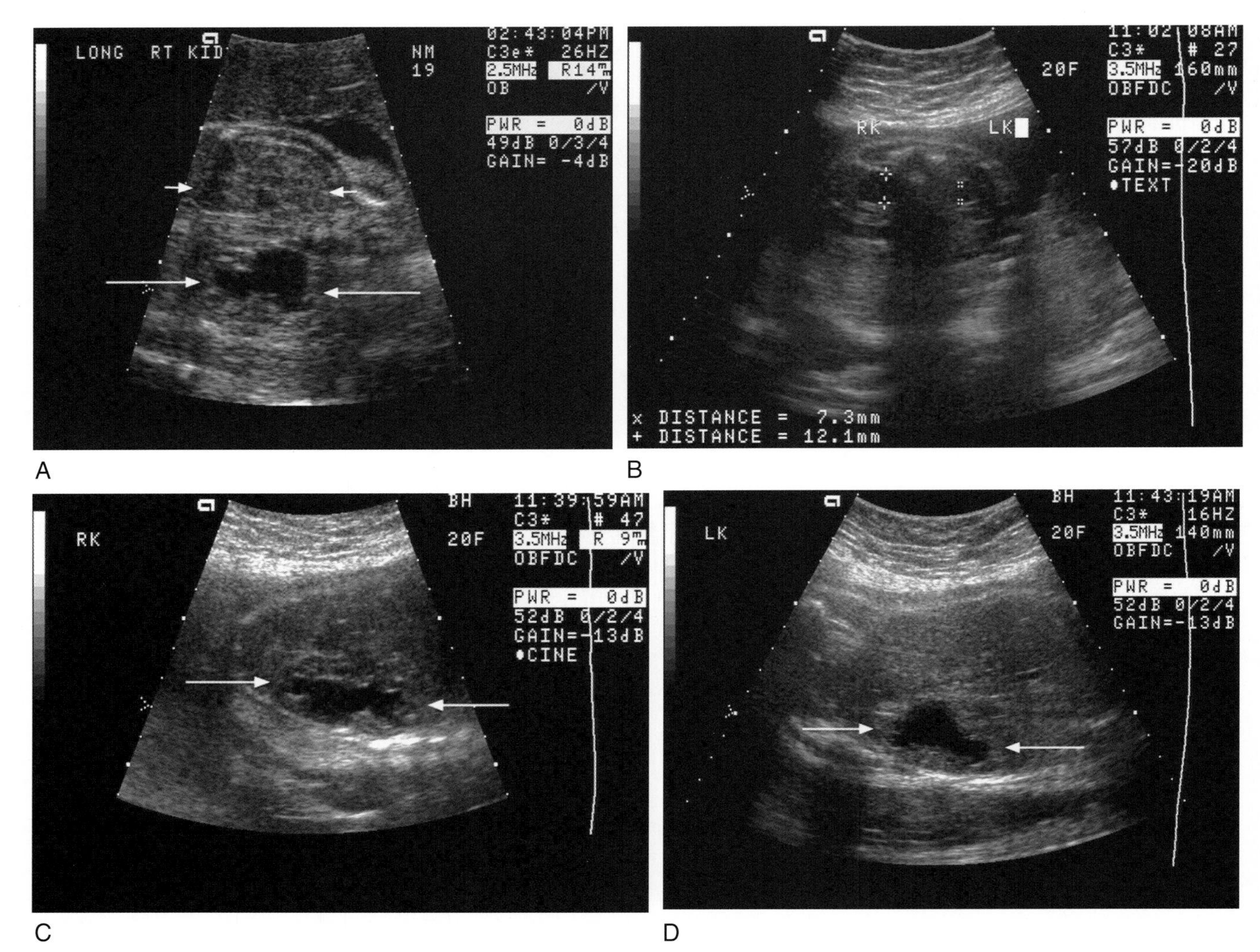

Figure 18-19 Examples of unilateral and bilateral ureteropelvic junction obstruction (UPJ). **A,** Unilateral UPJ obstruction in a 30-week fetus. Coronal image of kidneys shows a normal-appearing left kidney *(short arrows)* and a hydronephrotic right kidney *(long arrows).* Note the interconnections between the calyces and renal pelvis, which distinguish UPJ obstruction from a multicystic dysplastic kidney. A dilated ureter was not identified, favoring a UPJ obstruction over a more distal urinary tract obstruction. **B** to **D,** Bilateral UPJ obstruction in a 31-week fetus. **B,** Axial image of the kidneys reveals bilateral renal pelvic dilatation *(cursors).* Anteroposterior diameter of right renal pelvis is 12.1 mm and that of left renal pelvis is 7.3 mm. **C,** Longitudinal image of right kidney *(arrows)* shows dilated calyces connecting with a dilated renal pelvis. **D,** Longitudinal image of left kidney *(arrows)* demonstrates an appearance similar to the right kidney. Bilateral UPJ obstruction was confirmed postnatally.

entities by showing whether the cystic structures are separated (MCDK) or connected (UPJ). Rarely, a dilated tortuous ureter may present as a cystic mass, thus mimicking an MCDK (see Fig. 18-16B).

As long as the contralateral kidney is normal, the quantity of amniotic fluid will remain appropriate and the lungs will mature normally. However, there is a 20% incidence of a contralateral renal abnormality in fetuses with an MCDK, varying from subtle small (seemingly insignificant) cysts to another UPJ obstruction or a second MCDK. Occasionally, an MCDK can occur on one side and a UPJ obstruction on the other. Bilateral MCDK is lethal owing to oligohydramnios and pulmonary hypoplasia. Cysts are not normal in utero, and even solitary ones have been associated with renal dysplasia. However, these may not adversely affect renal function until after birth.

A unilateral obstruction may not always involve the entire kidney. A duplicated kidney may have an obstructed upper pole and a normal or a dilated lower pole (Fig. 18-20). Dilatation of the lower pole moiety is typically caused by reflux. The upper pole obstruction is caused by an ectopic ureter, which typically inserts lower and more medially toward the base of the bladder.

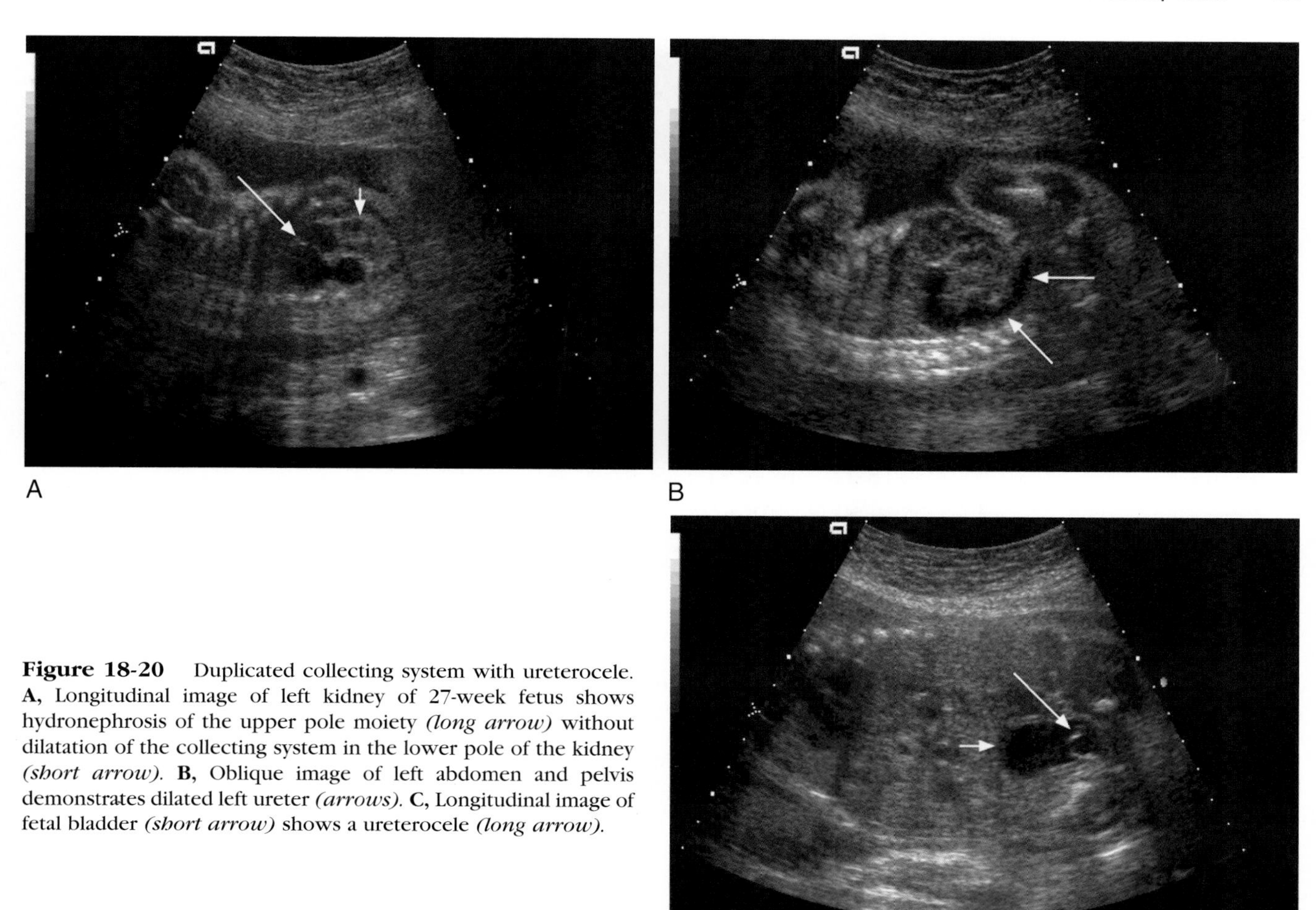

Figure 18-20 Duplicated collecting system with ureterocele. **A,** Longitudinal image of left kidney of 27-week fetus shows hydronephrosis of the upper pole moiety *(long arrow)* without dilatation of the collecting system in the lower pole of the kidney *(short arrow)*. **B,** Oblique image of left abdomen and pelvis demonstrates dilated left ureter *(arrows)*. **C,** Longitudinal image of fetal bladder *(short arrow)* shows a ureterocele *(long arrow)*.

On occasion, a ureterocele (the distal end of the ectopic ureter) can be identified as a cystic structure within the urinary bladder (see Fig. 18-20C). However, even when the ureterocele is not seen, the disparity between the obstructed upper pole and the normal or less dilated lower pole can suggest this diagnosis. This condition is rarely bilateral. Amniotic fluid remains normal in volume unless the ureterocele obstructs urine outflow at the bladder base. Surgical removal of the upper pole moiety, either unilateral or bilateral, can be performed successfully after birth without further sequelae.

MEGACALICES, MEGAURETERS, AND MEGACYSTIS

Primary abnormalities of the calices (megacalices), ureters (megaureters), or the urinary bladder (megacystis) are rare but can be identified at antenatal ultrasound. Dilated calices are identified as lateral cystic outpouchings from the renal pelvis and dilated ureters as tubular structures in the lower abdomen and pelvis (Fig. 18-21). Because the urinary bladder is normally prominent and there is not a well-established upper limit of normal, the diagnosis of megacystis is subjective.

When all three are dilated (calices, ureters, and urinary bladder), this is typically associated with an obstructive uropathy, most commonly a consequence of bladder outlet obstruction. Dilatation of the calices and pelvis alone is typically caused by a UPJ obstruction. For megacalices to be diagnosed, usually a unilateral developmental anomaly, the calices are disproportionately dilated, more than the remainder of the renal system.

When the ureters or urinary bladder, or both, are considerably more dilated than the pelvocaliceal system (megaureter and megacystis), this may still represent the early stage of a bladder outlet obstruction or the end stage of distal obstruction with dysplastic upper tracts (Figs. 18-21 and 18-22).

On occasion, an apparent obstructive uropathy is associated with a normal or increased volume of amniotic fluid (rather than with oligohydramnios). Normal amniotic fluid volume suggests either a less severe functional problem of the ureters and bladder

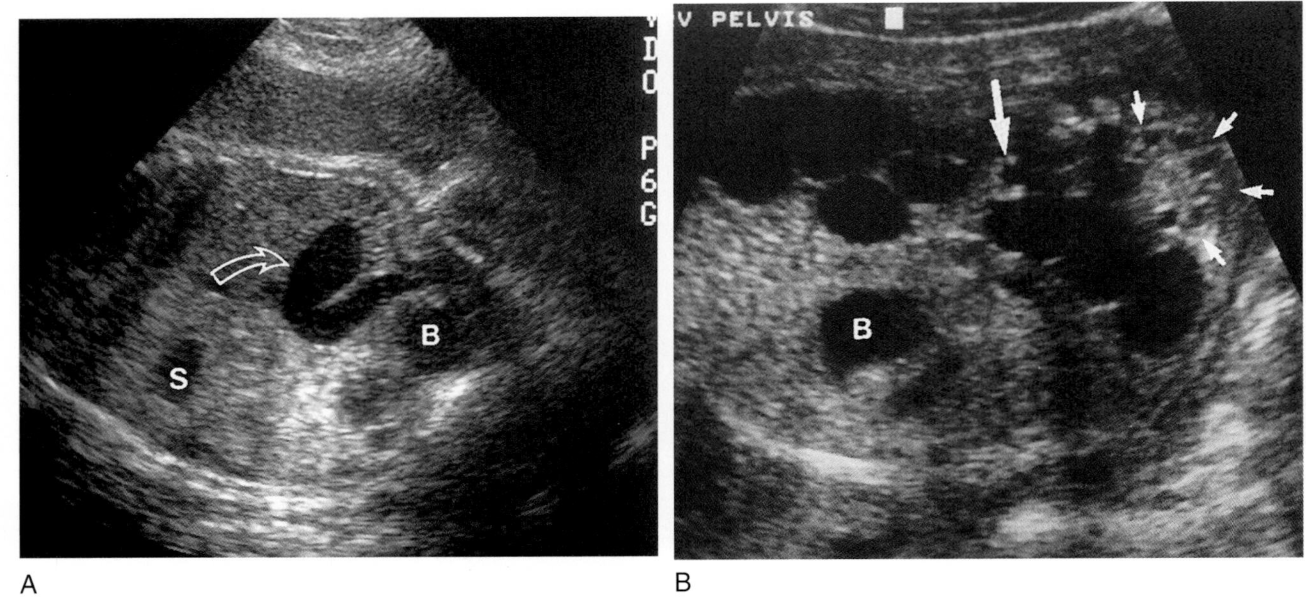

Figure 18-21 Dilated ureters resulting from different causes. **A,** Megaureter in a 32-week fetus. Long-axis image of the left side of the fetus shows a large "S"-shaped, anechoic, tubular structure *(curved open arrow)* above the small (but normal) urinary bladder (B). This persisted without change and with a normal-appearing kidney. S, stomach. **B,** Long-standing obstruction secondary to posterior urethral valves in a 38-week fetus. Transaxial-coronal view of the fetal abdomen shows a marked decrease in the volume of amniotic fluid. The upper part of the urinary bladder (B) and the fetal spine *(large arrow)* are seen. Multiple dilated cystic structures (the dilated ureters) are detected on both sides of the abdomen. The left kidney (on the right), denoted by *small arrows,* shows a small hyperechoic kidney with multiple cysts, a finding consistent with dysplasia.

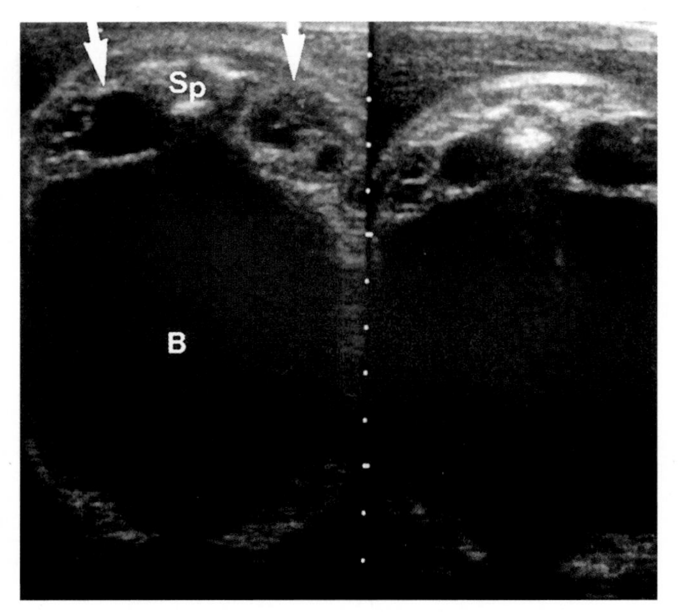

Figure 18-22 A case of markedly dilated bladder (B), or megacystis. Megacystis microcolon hypoperistalsis intestinalis in a 38-week fetus. Two images in a transaxial view show cystic structures *(arrows)* on both sides of the fetal spine (Sp), a finding consistent with obstructed hydronephrotic kidneys. The dilated bladder, however, is much more distended than the kidneys. On different images the amniotic fluid was noted to be markedly increased in volume.

(perhaps a prune-belly abnormality) or only a partial (incomplete) obstruction. Polyhydramnios would not be expected in the presence of the urinary tract abnormality unless a postobstructive diuresis or an additional anomaly, usually of the gastrointestinal tract or central nervous system, were also present. A rare entity called megacystis microcolon hypoperistalsis intestinalis, for example, includes polyhydramnios, an enlarged bladder, and often enlarged ureters (see Fig. 18-22). Although not always identified, intestinal obstruction is the presumed cause of the increased amniotic fluid volume.

THE ADRENAL GLANDS

The adrenal glands are normally quite prominent in utero and are approximately one half the size of the kidneys. They are often not detected until the third trimester, when they are identified axially as thin disc-like paraspinal structures above the upper poles of the kidneys (Fig. 18-23). The adrenal glands can sometimes also be seen in long-axis views as ovoid or triangular structures. Whereas their length and anteroposterior diameter have been evaluated, measurements are usually not important and are frequently underestimated

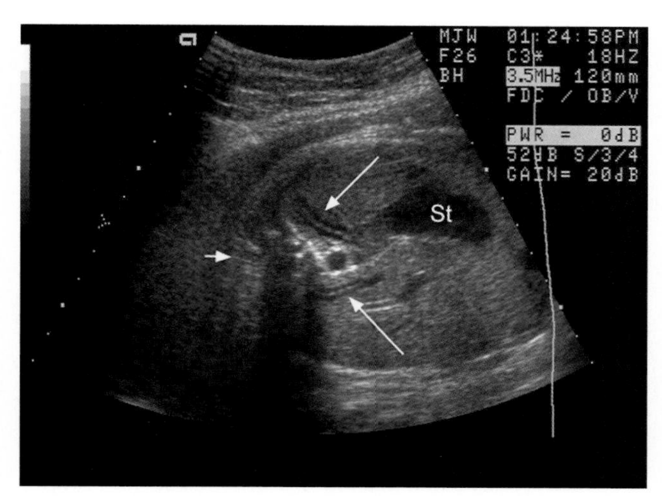

Figure 18-23 Normal adrenal glands in a third-trimester fetus. Axial image of fetal abdomen obtained at a level immediately superior to the kidneys shows the normal adrenal glands *(long arrows)* adjacent to the spine *(short arrow)*. Although the adrenal glands are different in shape and orientation than the kidneys, note their similar echo pattern, with a hyperechoic center and a hypoechoic periphery. St, stomach.

because rib shadowing often obscures at least part of the gland. The echogenicity of the adrenal glands is similar to that of the kidneys, with a hypoechoic cortex (periphery) and a hyperechoic medulla (center).

There are times when the adrenal glands can pose diagnostic problems. As previously discussed, when there is renal agenesis, the adrenals can assume an appearance in the renal bed mimicking that of the kidneys. The adrenal glands can also be abnormal. There have been documented cases of in utero adrenal hemorrhage (unilateral or bilateral) and rarely a solid neuroblastoma. Differentiation of hemorrhage from a solid mass is usually difficult unless a considerable change in their size or echogenicity, or both, is noted on a follow-up study; this suggests an evolving hemorrhage. Even then tumors may undergo necrotic or hemorrhagic changes. If an adrenal mass is large, it can displace the kidney so that the adrenal mass may be mistaken for a rare solid renal mass, the mesoblastic nephroma (hamartoma), and the rarer Wilms tumor. A definitive diagnosis must often await neonatal evaluation.

ADDITIONAL PELVIC ABNORMALITIES

Structures can be seen posterior to the urinary bladder. The rectosigmoid colon, either filled with meconium (normal) or obstructed, can be identified as a tubular structure.

In a female fetus a normally prominent uterus (under maternal hormonal influence) can infrequently be identified. No measurements are available. If the vagina is fluid-filled, vaginal atresia with an obstructed vagina is likely. In addition, if the uterus is also teardrop shaped or ovoid, the uterus is also obstructed. Often filled with blood, these are termed *hematocolpos* if only the vagina is involved and *hematometrocolpos* if the uterus is also involved (Fig. 18-24). Perineal images may show the

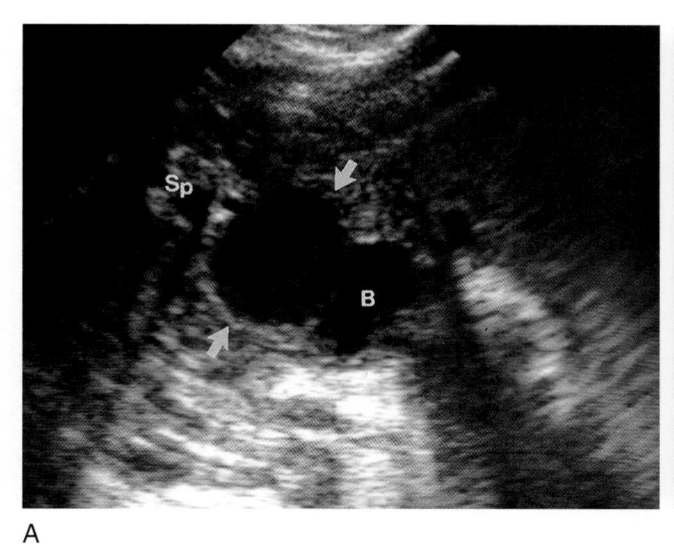

A

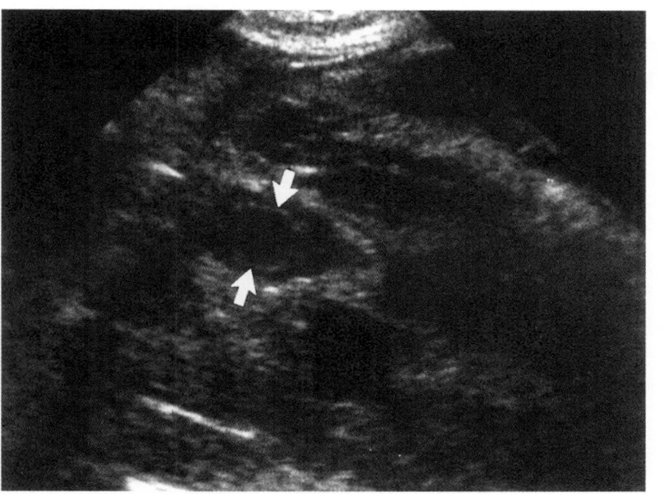

B

Figure 18-24 Hematometrocolpos, secondary to vaginal atresia, in a term female fetus. **A,** Transaxial view of the pelvis shows a cystic structure *(arrows)* immediately posterior to the urinary bladder (B). The bowel could be identified behind the cystic structure. The sagittal view (not shown) showed the cystic structure to be ovoid, a finding consistent with an obstructed uterus. Sp, fetal spine. **B,** Transaxial view through the perineum shows the cystic structure *(arrows)* extending down and spreading the labia, a finding consistent with an obstructed vagina.

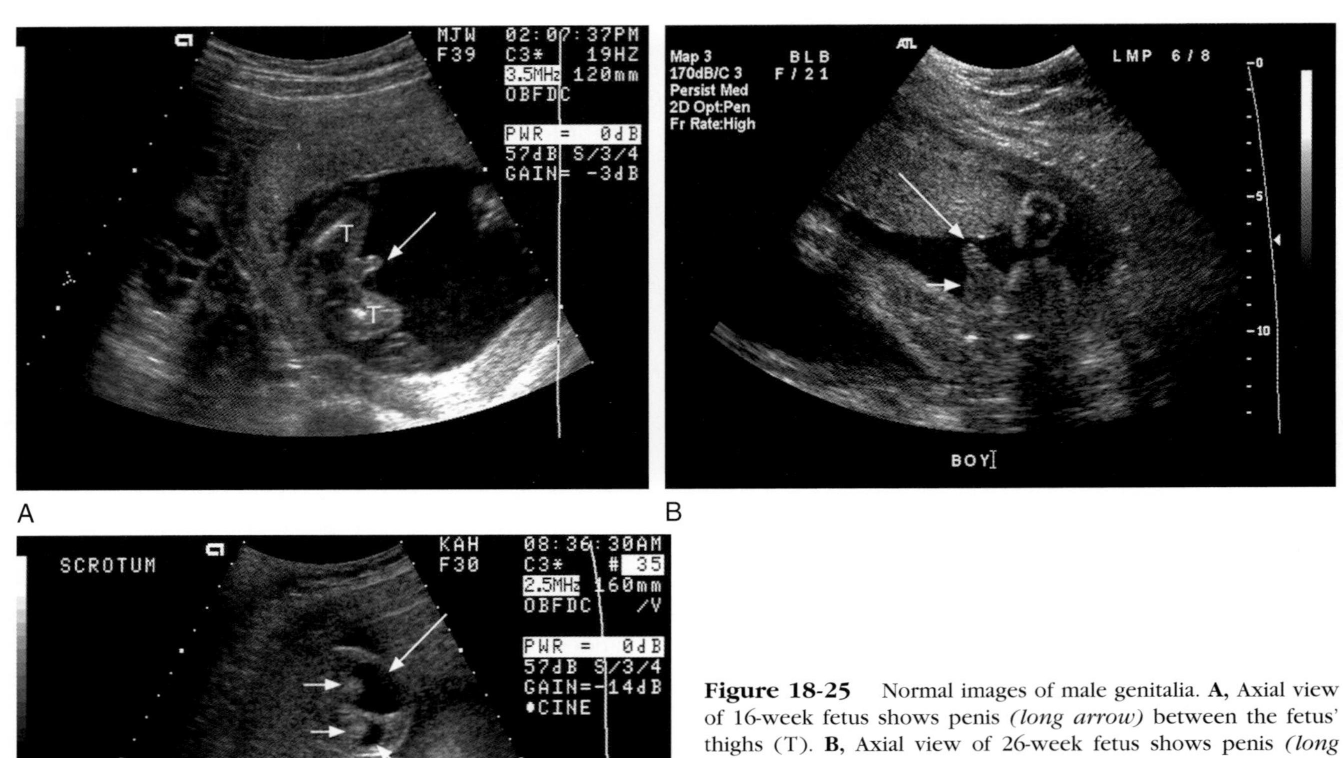

Figure 18-25 Normal images of male genitalia. **A,** Axial view of 16-week fetus shows penis *(long arrow)* between the fetus' thighs (T). **B,** Axial view of 26-week fetus shows penis *(long arrow)* and scrotum *(short arrow).* **C,** Image of scrotum of a 36-week fetus reveals small bilateral scrotal hydroceles *(long arrows),* a normal finding late in pregnancy. *Short arrows,* testes.

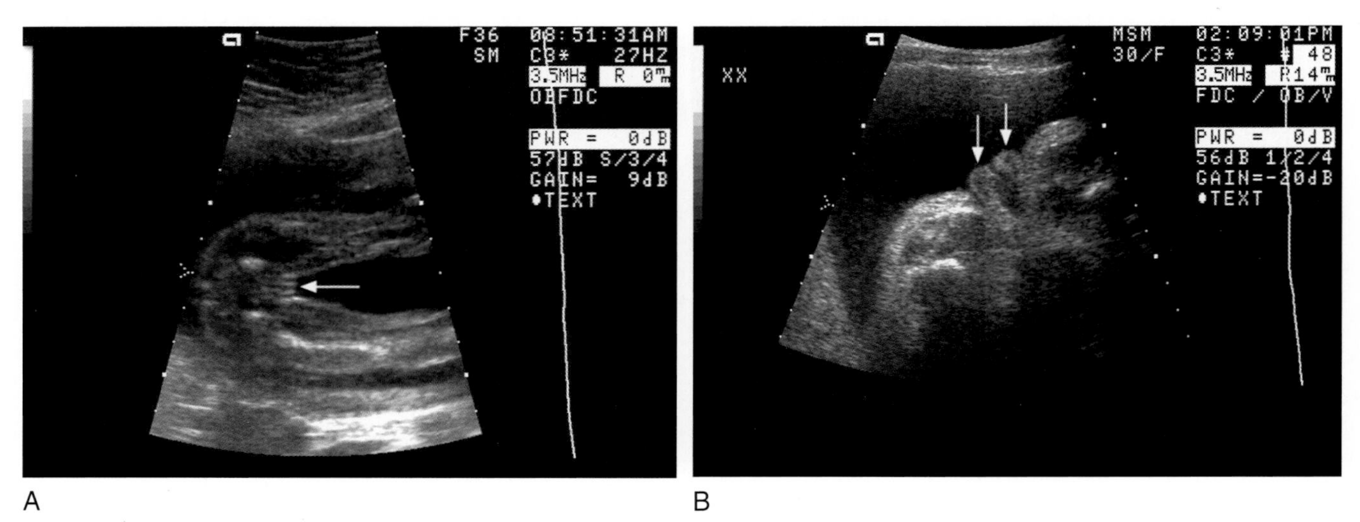

Figure 18-26 Normal images of female genitalia. **A,** Axial view of inferior portion of pelvis of 20-week fetus shows the labia as three parallel lines *(arrow).* **B,** Axial image of perineum in a late third-trimester fetus shows prominent labia *(arrows),* a normal finding. Prominence of the labia can resemble the appearance of the scrotum late in pregnancy, but the absence of the testes and penis distinguishes the labia from the scrotum.

hematocolpos bulging into the perineum. This can be corrected surgically at birth.

FETAL GENDER

The external genitalia can often be identified by scanning the perineum. By 16 weeks, and sometimes earlier, the identification of a scrotum or penis clearly indicates the fetus is male (Fig. 18-25A and B). Occasionally, anechoic fluid accumulates locally within the scrotal sac and outlines the testes (hydroceles) (see Fig. 18-25C). This typically resolves spontaneously after birth.

In the female fetus, the labia are more difficult to image (Fig. 18-26). On occasion they can be prominent and sometimes mimic the scrotum. Care must be taken not to confuse the umbilical cord between the legs as part of the genitalia.

In the late first and early second trimesters, a midline sagittal image can sometimes be used to identify the phallus in the male pointed cranially or vertically and the clitoris pointed caudally in females.

The overall accuracy of gender determination has not been fully established. There is obviously greater accuracy in the detection of males. This differentiation is not, however, of medical importance, unless a predisposition for a certain entity is of concern. For example, an obstructive uropathy caused by posterior urethral valves occurs only in a male fetus, and hemophilia (which cannot be detected in utero) occurs only in the male offspring of affected families.

Key Features

- In the second and third trimesters, it is recommended that the kidneys, urinary bladder, and amniotic fluid be routinely evaluated.
- The kidneys are paraspinal in location. Because of the accumulation of fat in the renal sinus and perinephric regions, the kidneys become progressively better seen as the pregnancy continues.
- Measurements of the kidneys are not usually needed. The simplest size evaluation is to measure renal length.
- Mild pyelectasis without caliectasis or other findings is often normal. There is controversy regarding the optimal threshold values above which abnormal dilatation should be suspected. Some practitioners use a cut-off of 4 mm up to 33 weeks and 7 mm after 33 weeks. Others use higher cut-offs such as 5 mm up to 20 weeks and values as high as 10 mm at term.
- The urinary bladder is routinely identified after 16 gestational weeks. If not seen, sequential scans over the course of 1 hour are indicated. Transient nonvisualization of the bladder in an otherwise normal obstetrical examination is likely normal.
- Oligohydramnios should not be considered a normal finding. It is likely associated with one of three conditions: spontaneous rupture of the membranes, bilateral renal or bladder abnormalities, or growth restriction.
- If the oligohydramnios is prolonged and severe, particularly if it continues from the second trimester, it is often associated with pulmonary hypoplasia.
- The most common bilateral renal anomalies are urethral obstruction (usually posterior urethral valves), renal agenesis, and infantile polycystic kidney disease. Bilateral ureteropelvic junction obstructions are also possible.
- Dilated ureters need to be differentiated from blood vessels by color Doppler analysis and from loops of bowel by real-time observation because bowel should change with time.
- An abdominal mass or masses that extend to the paraspinal areas are likely to be renal or adrenal in origin.
- The diagnosis of dysplasia (irreversible kidney damage) is made by chemical analysis of the urine. However, two ultrasound characteristics are associated with dysplasia: increased renal cortex echogenicity (greater than the liver) and subcortical cysts.
- Common unilateral renal problems include multicystic dysplastic kidney, reflux, and ureteropelvic junction obstruction. Some of these fetuses have an abnormality of the contralateral kidney.
- If obstruction is identified in the upper but not the lower pole of the kidney, a duplicated kidney with an ectopic ureterocele from the upper pole moiety should be considered.
- In marked distention of the urinary bladder (often related to obstruction) or to an abdominal process such as a cystic mass, the abdominal musculature may be distended more than normal, and this may lead to a thinning of the musculature, a prune belly appearance after birth.
- Megacalices, megaureters and megabladder are often associated with obstructive uropathies. If disproportionately dilated, they may be related to functional smooth muscle abnormalities of the fetus.
- Polyhydramnios is usually not associated with urinary tract abnormalities. If present, additional fetal structural abnormalities such as from the gastrointestinal tract should be sought.
- The normal adrenal glands can usually be identified in the third trimester. They become of diagnostic importance in the setting of renal agenesis, when they occupy the renal bed, and in the setting of adrenal masses, either neoplasms or hemorrhages.
- A prominent vagina (and uterus) may present as a pelvic mass, termed hematocolpos (or hematometrocolpos).

SUGGESTED READINGS

Anderson N, Clautice-Engle, Allen R, et al: Detection of obstructive uropathy in the fetus: Predictive value of sonographic measurements of renal pelvic diameter at various gestational ages. AJR Am J Roentgenol 164:719, 1995.

Arger PH, et al: Routine fetal genitourinary tract screening. Radiology 156:485, 1985.

Bowie JD, et al: The changing sonographic appearance of fetal kidneys during pregnancy. J Ultrasound Med 2:505, 1983.

Clautice-Engle T, Pretorius DH, Budorick NE: Significance of nonvisualization of the fetal urinary bladder. J Ultrasound Med 10:615, 1991.

Cohen HL, et al: Normal length of fetal kidneys: Sonographic study in 397 obstetric patients. AJR Am J Roentgenol 157:545, 1991.

Corteville JE, Gray DL, Crane JP: Congenital hydronephrosis: Correlation of fetal ultrasonographic findings with infant outcome. Am J Obstet Gynecol 165:384, 1991.

Du Bruyn R, Gordon I: Postnatal investigation of fetal renal disease. Prenat Diagn 21:984, 2001.

Gotoh H, Masuzaki H, Fukuda H, et al: Detection and assessment of pyelectasis in the fetus: Relationship to postnatal renal function. Obstet Gynecol 92:226, 1998.

Grannum P, et al: Assessment of fetal kidney size in normal gestation by comparison of ratio of kidney circumference to abdominal circumference. Am J Obstet Gynecol 136:249, 1980.

Hoffman CK, Filly RA, Callen PW: The "lying down" adrenal sign: A sonographic indicator of renal agenesis or ectopia in fetuses and neonates. J Ultrasound Med 11:533, 1992.

Johnson MP, et al: In utero surgical treatment of fetal obstructive uropathy: A new comprehensive approach to identify appropriate candidates for vesicoamniotic shunt therapy. Am J Obstet Gynecol 170:1770, 1994.

Kent A, Cox D, Downey P, et al: A study of mild fetal pyelectasia—outcome and proposed strategy of management. Prenat Diagn 20:206, 2000.

Kleiner B, et al: Multicystic dysplastic kidney: Observations of contralateral disease in the fetal population. Radiology 161:27, 1986.

Lazebnik N, Bellinger MF, Ferguson JE II: Insights into the pathogenesis and natural history of fetuses with multicystic dysplastic kidney disease. Prenat Diagn 19:418, 1999.

Lewis E, et al: Real-time ultrasonographic evaluation of normal fetal adrenal glands. J Ultrasound Med 1:265, 1982.

Mahony BS, Callen PW, Filly RA: Fetal urethral obstruction: US evaluation. Radiology 157:221, 1985.

Mahony BS, et al: Fetal renal dysplasia: Sonographic evaluation. Radiology 152:143, 1984.

Mandell J, et al: Structural genitourinary defects detected in utero. Radiology 178:193, 1991.

McHugo J, Whittle M: Enlarged fetal bladders: Aetiology, management and outcome. Prenat Diagn 21:958, 2001.

Mouriquand PD, Whitten M, Pracros JP: Pathophysiology, diagnosis and management of prenatal upper tract dilatation. Prenat Diagn 21:942, 2001.

Nimrod C, et al: The effect of very prolonged membrane rupture on fetal development. Am J Obstet Gynecol 148:540, 1984.

Persutte WH, Hussey M, Chyu J, et al: Striking findings concerning the variability in the measurement of the fetal renal collecting system. Ultrasound Obstet Gynecol 15:186, 2000.

Persutte WH, Klyle M, Lenke RR, et al: Mild pyelectasis ascertained with prenatal sonography is pediatrically significant. Ultrasound Obstet Gynecol 10:12, 1997.

Romero R, et al: The diagnosis of congenital renal anomalies with ultrasound: II. Infantile polycystic kidney disease. Am J Obstet Gynecol 150:259, 1984.

Romero R, et al: Antenatal diagnosis of renal anomalies with ultrasound: III. Bilateral renal agenesis. Am J Obstet Gynecol 151:38, 1985.

Seeds JW: Borderline genitourinary tract abnormalities. Semin Ultrasound CT MR 19:347, 1998.

Tsatsaris V, Gagnadous MF, Aubry MC: Prenatal diagnosis of bilateral isolated fetal hyperechogenic kidneys. Is it possible to predict long term outcome? Br J Obstet Gynecol 109:1388, 2002.

Van Eijk L, Cohen-Overbeek TE, den Hollander NS, et al: Unilateral multicystic dysplastic kidney: A combined pre- and postnatal assessment. Ultrasound Obstet Gynecol 19:180, 2002.

Vergani P, Ceruti P, Locatelli A, et al: Accuracy of prenatal ultrasonographic diagnosis of duplex renal system. J Ultrasound Med 18:463, 1999.

Wellesley D, How DT: Fetal renal anomalies and genetic syndromes. Prenat Diagn 21:992, 2001.

Wiener JS, O'Hara SM: Optimal timing of initial postnatal ultrasonography in newborns with prenatal hydronephrosis. J Urol 168:1826, 2002.

Wilcox DT, Chitty LS: Non-visualization of the fetal bladder: Aetiology and management. Prenat Diagn 21:977, 2001.

Willard DA, Gabriele OF: Megacystis-microcolon-intestinal hypoperistalsis syndrome in a male infant. J Clin Ultrasound 14:481, 1986.

Winyard P, Chitty L: Dysplastic and polycystic kidneys: Diagnosis, associations and management. Prenat Diagn 21:924, 2001.

Zeijl C, Roefs B, Boer K, et al: Clinical outcome and follow-up of sonographically suspected in utero urinary tract anomalies. J Clin Ultrasound 27:21, 1999.

CHAPTER 19

Fetal Musculoskeletal System

For Key Features summary see p. 484

The skeletal system is partially identified on every second- and third-trimester examination with the routine imaging of the fetal head, spine, and at least one femur. The antepartum obstetrical ultrasound standard recommends imaging the head to obtain head measurements (biparietal diameter [BPD] and head circumference [HC]) in axial projection and to identify the lateral ventricles with the choroid plexus and the posterior fossa, best imaged in slightly tilted axial projections. One femur is imaged in its long axis and its femoral length (FL) is measured. The spine is fully evaluated, which is usually accomplished in multiple projections: axial, sagittal, and occasionally coronal. These views of the skeleton allow gross evaluation of the bony calvarium, femur, and spine for size, shape, brightness, and, occasionally, anomalies. The overlying soft tissues, the muscles, and the subcutaneous tissues can be imaged but to date have only been incompletely studied.

Although not at present required as part of the routine ultrasound obstetrical examination, real-time high-resolution scanners can assess all the long bones: the other femur, the distal legs (tibiae and fibulae), the arms (humeri), and the forearms (radii and ulnae) (Fig. 19-1). An attempt should be made to identify all four extremities to rule out gross absence of an extremity. The normal relationship of lengths of the bones can be quickly assessed: an approximate 1:1 ratio between the bones of the forearm and the humerus and between the bones of the distal leg and the femur. Measurement tables are also available that show a normal but slight difference in length between the radius and the ulna and between the tibia and the fibula (with the radius and tibia longer). If measured, each of these bones should be individually evaluated.

Still smaller bones can be assessed. The hands and feet can be evaluated for shape and for the position and number of digits. The clavicles, ribs, and iliac crests can be identified, although this evaluation is not always complete.

The soft tissues have been measured in the mid upper arm or mid thigh in an attempt to determine when there is diffuse thickening. Whereas the exact sites of measurement have not been established, a diffuse thickening of more than 10 mm can occur in fetal hydrops and occasionally in the setting of maternal diabetes mellitus. Focal enlargement is usually secondary to a localized mass such as a hemangioma or lymphangioma (a lymphatic obstruction). If blood flow can be detected by Doppler analysis, then a vascular tumor is likely. The absence of detectable blood flow, however, is not diagnostic because avascular tumors and tumors with very slow flow (such as hemangiomas) typically have no detectable Doppler signal. Rarely, focal swelling may be a sign of constriction caused by an amniotic band.

Nuchal skin thickness that exceeds 6 mm in the mid second trimester is a marker for trisomy 21. This is discussed in Chapter 15.

There is no established lower limit for soft tissue thickness. Although decreased thickness is expected in the setting of asymmetric growth restriction (a state of fetal starvation), at present this diagnosis cannot be made by any modality.

FEMUR LENGTH MEASUREMENT AND ITS USES

Skeletal dysplasias are a varied and often confusing conglomerate of anomalies, with more than 200 types identified. Despite their number, they are relatively

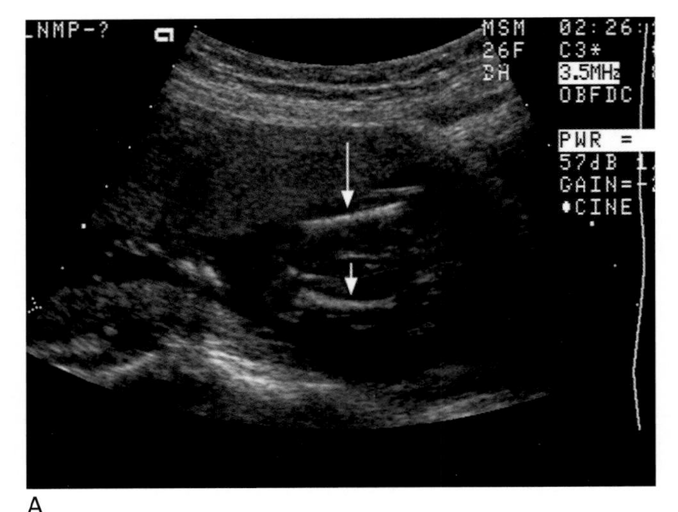

A

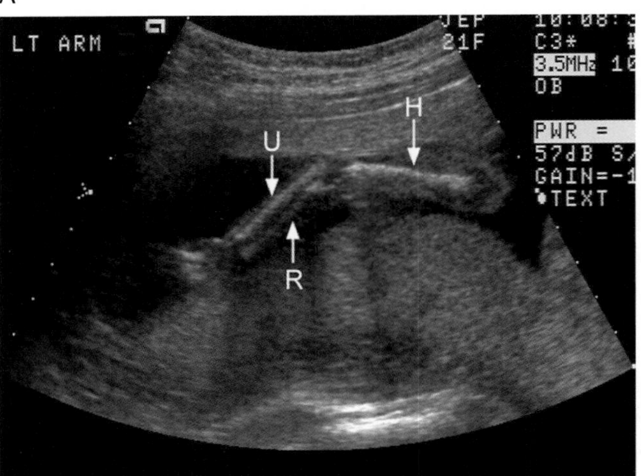

B

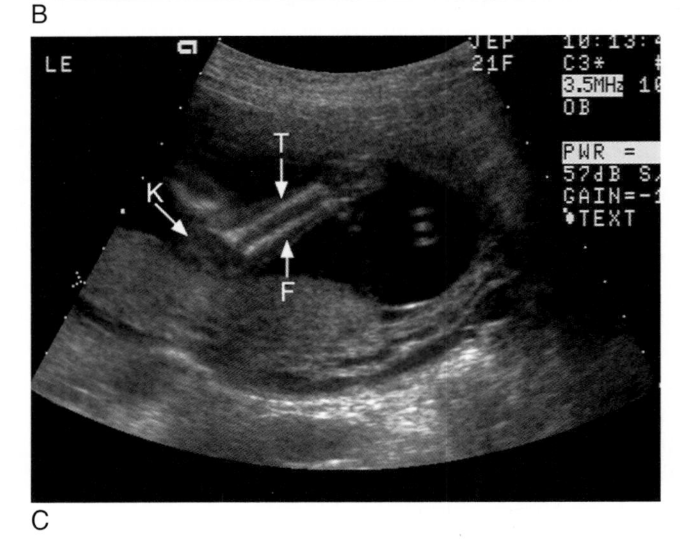

C

Figure 19-1 Normal images of long bones in the mid second trimester. **A,** Both femurs. Note that ultrasound preferentially images the lateral, straight margin of the femur closest to the transducer *(long arrow)* and the medial, curved margin of the femur farther from the transducer *(short arrow)*. **B,** Long bones of the arm, including humerus (H), radius (R), and ulna (U). The ulna can be distinguished from the radius because it is longer at the elbow. **C,** The tibia (T) can be distinguished from the fibula (F) because it is longer and wider at the knee (K).

uncommon and occur in less than 2.5 of every 10,000 births. While subtle deformities may be missed, most "significant" generalized dysplasias involve the long bones and present with short stature. The primary fetal parameter that relates to the length of the long bones is the FL, and the FL correlates directly with the length of the fetus. Therefore, the routine FL measurement detects most generalized skeletal dysplasias.

The femur is measured linearly from one end of the ossified shaft to the other (Fig. 19-2A). Although the femoral shaft also has a thickness (depth), this is usually not appreciated because the ultrasound beam is strongly attenuated after contacting the uppermost surface of the bone. Fibrous tissue surrounds the cartilaginous ends of the femoral shaft, at the nonossified head and at the condyles. If the ultrasound beam is perpendicular to the condylar fibrous tissue, an artifactual hyperechoic line can be imaged extending from the end of the femoral shaft (see Fig. 19-2B). It has been termed the *distal femur point* and is a potential source of error if included in the FL measurement. This error can be avoided, however, because this "point" is thinner than the shaft and will disappear with any change in the transducer orientation away from perpendicular. Another potential source of error near term is the normal distal femoral epiphyseal ossification. Although this will ultimately fuse with the femoral shaft to form the femoral condyles, it does not connect to the shaft in utero and should not be included in its measurement (see Fig. 19-2C).

An important value of the FL measurement is in its proportionality to the head (its value to obtain a gestational age is discussed in Chapter 12). Proportionality can be accomplished as either a direct comparison of the BPD and FL or as a ratio of the two. The direct comparison reveals that for every BPD there is an expected FL measurement at a mean and 2 SD range (see Table 12-7). Although only one femur needs to be routinely measured, if discrepancy is found (>2 SD difference), the other femur should be measured to determine if the process is unilateral or bilateral. When both femurs are elongated, it is typically a normal variant seen in the offspring of tall parents. If only one is elongated, however, this raises the possibility of unilateral hypertrophy seen in the Beckwith-Wiedemann syndrome, with its associated visceromegaly and renal anomalies (including Wilms' tumors).

If the femurs are short, either a constitutionally normally small fetus (frequently offspring of short parents), intrauterine growth restriction (IUGR) or a skeletal dysplasia is possible. Normal short fetuses exhibit only mild FL shortening, with appropriate interval growth and no additional structural abnormalities. Only when the femurs grow more slowly should heterozygous achondroplastic dwarfism be considered, often not diagnosed until after 24 weeks. Abnormal fetuses with

Figure 19-2 Measurement of the femur: landmarks and pitfalls. **A,** Femur length is measured by positioning calipers on the ossified ends of the femoral shaft *(cursors)*. The full thickness of the shaft is not seen due to shadowing *(arrows)* from the superficial surface of the bone. **B,** Distal femur point *(arrow)* is a hyperechoic line extending from the inferior edge of the femoral shaft along the outer edge of the superficial surface of the epiphysis. The distal femur point should not be included in the measurement of femur length. **C,** Distal femoral epiphysis (DFE) *(short arrow)* in a 37-week fetus. The DFE begins to ossify in the mid third trimester. This ossification center *(long arrow)* should not be included in the femur length measurement.

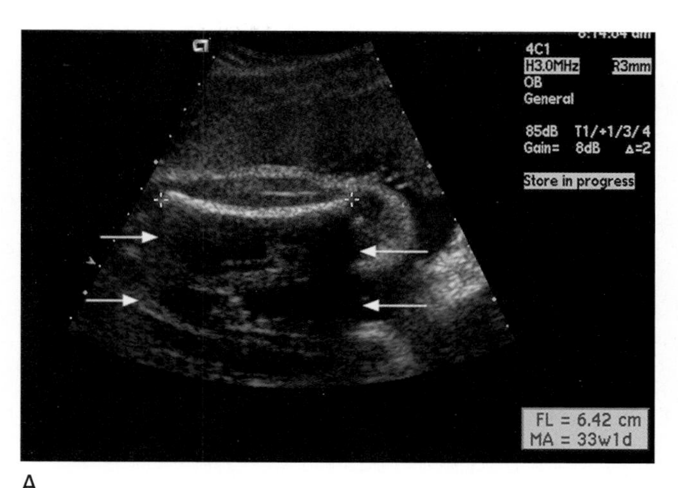

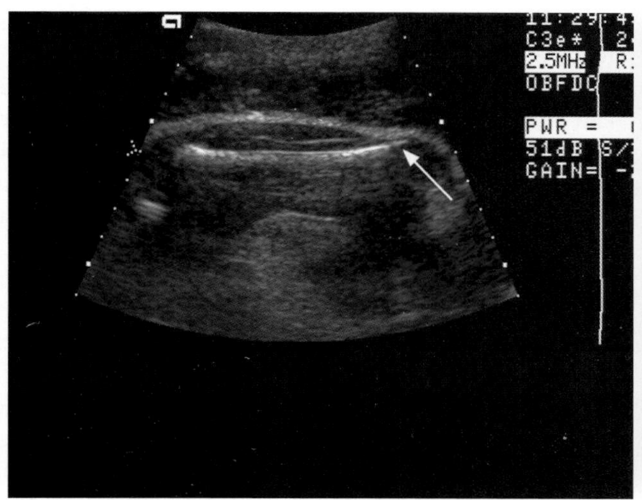

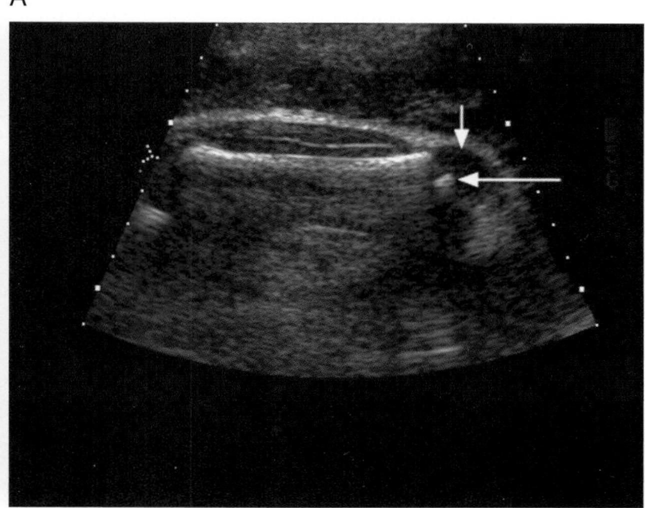

skeletal dysplasias have FLs greater than 5 mm below the 2 SD line (often considerably below 4 SD). They have additional major abnormalities, including a narrow thorax, fractures, and decreased bone brightness.

Shortened femurs or humeri, or both, have been described in association with chromosomally abnormal fetuses, in particular with trisomy 21. These have been detected by comparing the FL and humeral length (HL) to the gestational age or as a ratio of the BPD to either long bone, both at greater than 1.5 or 2 SD below the norm. Limitations with this analysis make it both insensitive and inaccurate. Normally, FLs and HLs are distributed in a bell-shaped curve, with a certain percentage of normal cases outside the arbitrary cut-off: for 2 SD, 5% of the normal cases lie outside—2.5% above (2.5 per 100 cases) and 2.5% below (2.5 per 100 cases)—whereas for 1.5 SD, 6.5 per 100 cases are above and below. Unless a significant separation of the normal from the abnormal cases can be shown, there will be too much overlap. In the majority of trisomy cases, their FLs and HLs "mix in" with normal cases, and their positive predictive values (i.e., true-positive values divided by true-positive plus false-positive values) are very low at only 3.5. Although the detection of abnormal cases is relatively good (true positives), far too many normal cases are incorrectly called abnormal (false positives). This is in contradistinction to a much higher positive predictive value of 44 for the finding of nuchal fold thickness of more than 6 mm in the detection of trisomy 21. Therefore, the FL and HL, separately or in combination with other characteristics, are not accurate enough to be used in the consistent prediction of chromosomal abnormality.

SKELETAL DYSPLASIAS

The in utero identification of skeletal dysplasias is important because of their association with significant physical deformity, mental retardation, or both. Some skeletal dysplasias are lethal conditions. All require genetic counseling before future pregnancies are attempted. Most skeletal dysplasias are anticipated

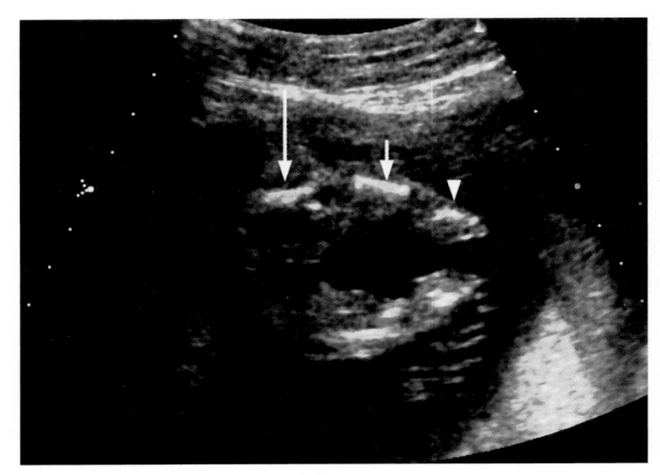

Figure 19-3 Severe micromelia in a second-trimester fetus with achondrogenesis. Note marked shortening of the entire lower extremity, both proximally and distally. *Long arrow,* femur; *short arrow,* tibia; *arrowhead,* deformed foot.

because of a family history of an affected parent or sibling. On occasion, though, a dysplasia may be discovered fortuitously as an incidental finding during ultrasound examination.

Significant generalized skeleton abnormalities typically exhibit at least one of three osseous findings: very shortened limbs, bony deformities (fractures and/or bowing), and decreased bone brightness (demineralization). If the entire limb is shortened both proximally and distally, the skeletal dysplasia has a micromelic pattern (Fig. 19-3); if only the proximal segment is shortened, a rhizomelic type of dysplasia is present. Both will be detected by the FL measurement. Only the less common isolated shortenings of the forearm and lower leg (mesomelia) and of the distal segment (acromelia) will be missed by FL analysis alone.

Fractures and bowing of the long bones are usually obvious. Only the medial (inner) aspect of the femoral shaft has a slight normal curve (see Fig. 12-10A and B). If this curve is accentuated or occurs along any other margin of the femur, it is abnormal (Fig. 19-4A). All other long bones are normally straight so that curves (bowing) or fractures should be considered abnormal (see Fig. 19-4B). Fractures or the bowing of other bones such as the ribs, however, may be difficult to appreciate.

Bone brightness (mineralization), another important feature, can be more difficult to assess. Quantification of bone brightness is not at present possible. The bones can only be considered abnormal if they are qualitatively decreased in brightness (Fig. 19-5A). Comparison with the scan of normal fetuses of the same gestational age and ideally on the same machine (with appropriate technique) can be helpful to determine if there is appropriate brightness of the osseous structures.

Four major types of skeletal dysplasias are most commonly encountered. They account for 66% of all dysplasias: thanatophoric dysplasia (28%), heterozygous achondroplasia (15%), osteogenesis imperfecta (OI; 14%), and achondrogenesis (9%). Heterozygous achondroplasia and approximately 50% of the cases of OI are nonlethal

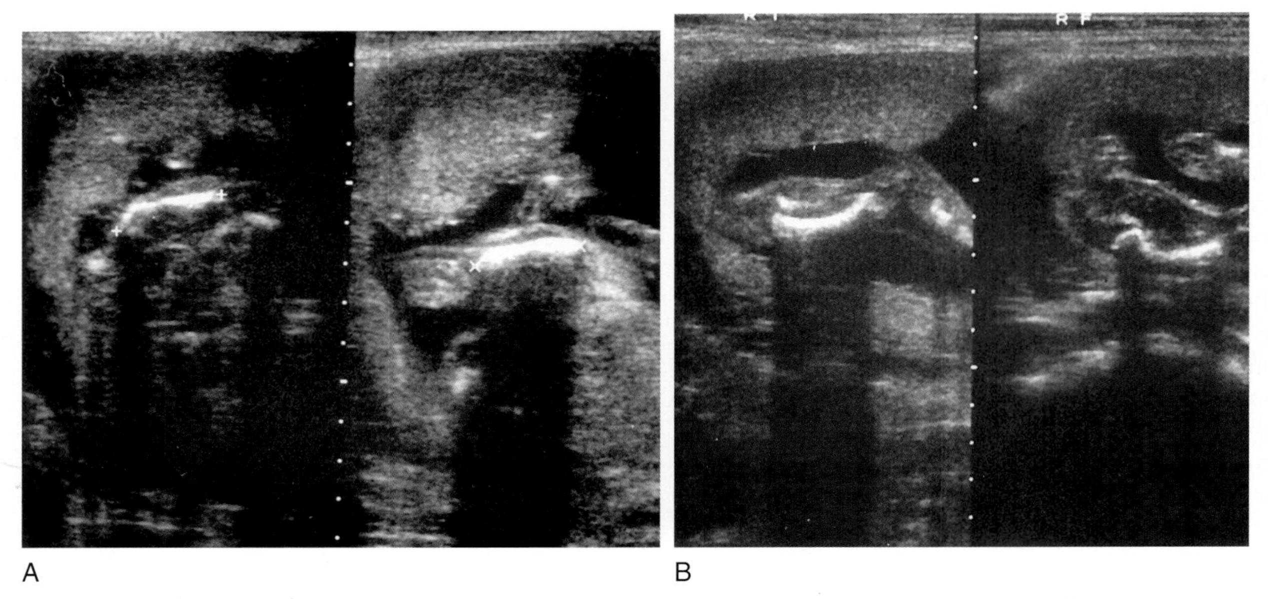

Figure 19-4 Abnormal curvature of long bones in fetuses with osteogenesis imperfecta. **A,** Thirty-one-week fetus with abnormal curvature and angulation of femur *(left)* and tibia *(right)* due to fractures. **B,** Eighteen-week fetus with abnormal bowing of tibia *(left)* and fibula *(right),* also due to fractures.

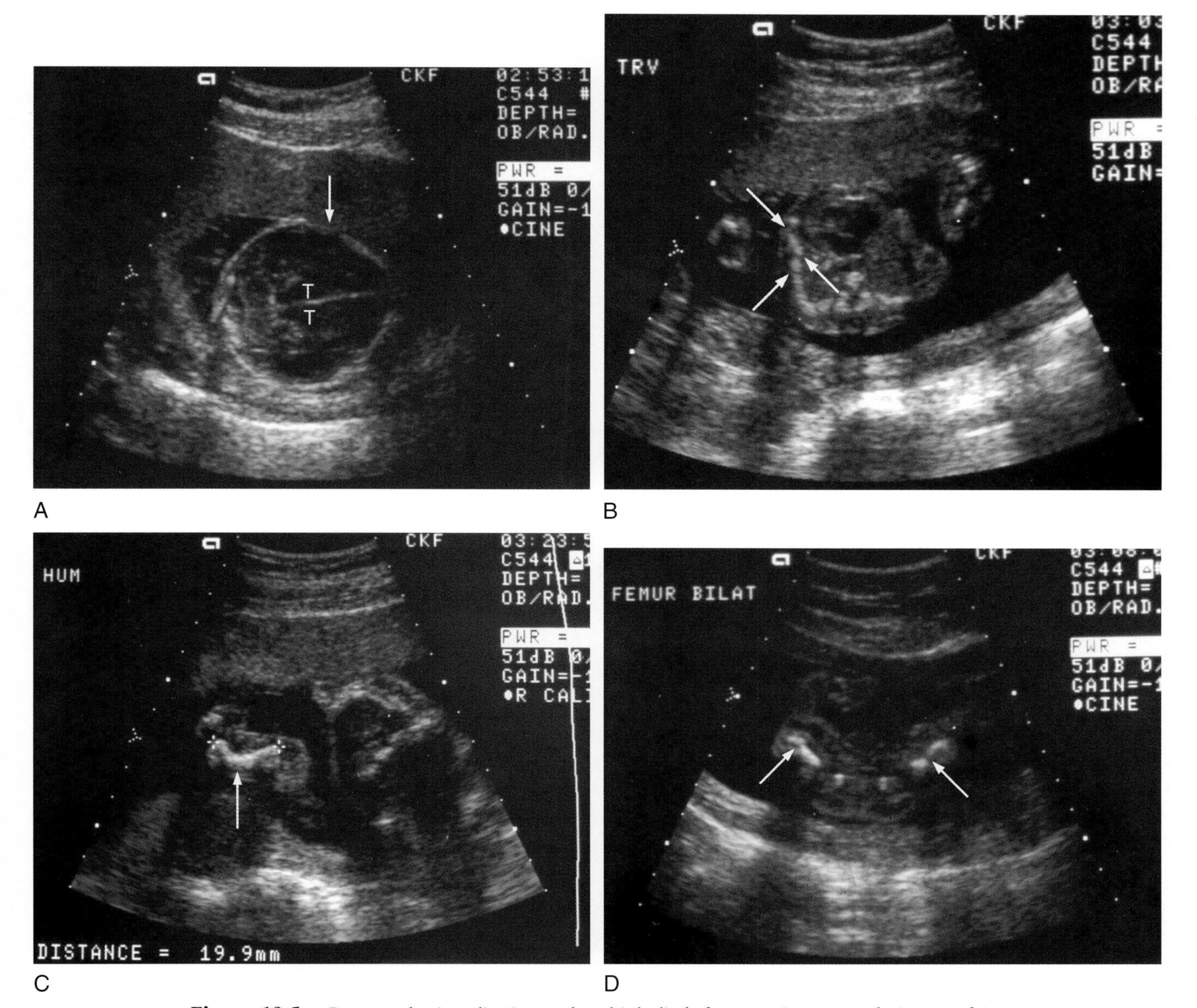

Figure 19-5 Decreased mineralization and multiple limb fractures in a second-trimester fetus with osteogenesis imperfecta. **A,** Axial image of fetal head at level of thalami (T) shows marked thinning and decreased brightness of the calvarium *(arrow).* **B,** Axial view of thorax shows rib fractures *(arrows).* **C,** Longitudinal image of humerus shows bowing *(arrow)* and shortening due to fractures. **D,** Longitudinal image of both femurs demonstrates marked shortening with fractures *(arrows).*

anomalies. Although all the other dysplasias listed earlier are lethal, their impact on the number of perinatal deaths is not great. They are responsible for only 1 in every 110 deaths: thanatophoric dysplasia, 44%; achondrogenesis, 18%; and osteogenesis imperfecta, 13%.

Heterozygous achondroplasia is the most common nonlethal skeletal dysplasia and is inherited as an autosomal dominant trait. One of the parents must be a heterozygous achondroplastic dwarf, and it would be expected that 50% of the offspring will be affected while the other 50% will be normal. If both parents are heterozygous achondroplastic dwarfs, there is still a 50% chance of an affected child with heterozygous dwarfism, with the other 50% divided equally between a normal child and a child with the more severe lethal homozygous achondroplastic dysplasia.

A person affected with heterozygous achondroplasia has a phenotypical appearance with proximal limb shortening (rhizomelic dwarfism) and additional skeletal deformities. In utero, however, the diagnosis can be made only by detecting a shortened femur. The initial FL shortening is often normal in the early to mid second trimester. It will grow slower and eventually fall below the 2 SD threshold, but this may not occur until the late second trimester. Therefore, in a fetus at risk for achondroplasia, when findings are initially normal, follow-up examinations should be continued up to 28 weeks before this type of dysplasia can be ruled out.

Osteogenesis imperfecta (OI) has four different types, most inherited as an autosomal dominant trait. Its fetal diagnosis can be made by the findings of skeletal deformities and demineralization. With an appropriate family history, assuming there has been no significant trauma to the fetus, any fracture or abnormal bowing will establish the diagnosis of OI (see Fig. 19-5B to D). Conversely, the diagnosis is not excluded if a normal fetus is identified because a fetus with OI may be unaffected in utero or may only exhibit subtle unappreciated deformities. Therefore, an abnormal finding is diagnostic; a normal study must be considered more cautiously particularly in a fetus at risk for this dysplasia.

Although osteoporosis is a hallmark of the severe forms of OI, the accurate ultrasound detection of bone brightness is variable. Obvious decreased brightness represents significant demineralization and strongly suggests the existence of the lethal types of OI (see Fig. 19-5A). Normal bone brightness, however, does not ensure that the bones will be found normal at birth. Without the appropriate history of OI, demineralization may instead suggest other rarer types of lethal dysplasias such as hypophosphatasia.

Achondrogenesis is an autosomal recessive dysplasia and is a lethal dysplasia. The fetus or newborn has the appearance of a cherub with very shortened extremities, short trunk, disproportionately large head, and a distended abdomen (Fig. 19-6A). The long bones are of

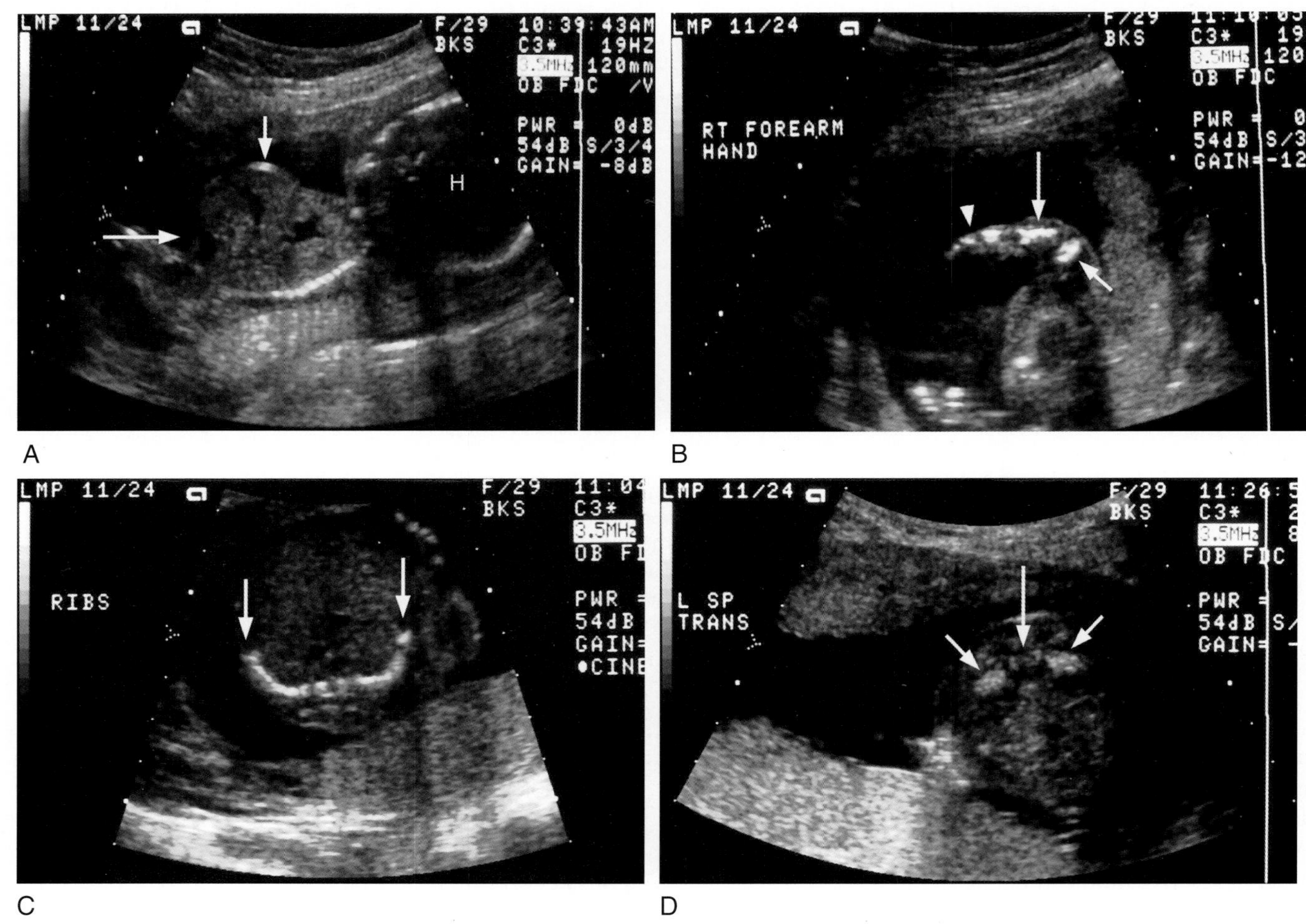

Figure 19-6 Achondrogenesis in a second-trimester fetus. **A,** Longitudinal image of fetus shows short trunk *(long arrow),* protuberant abdomen *(short arrow)*, and disproportionately large head (H). **B,** Image of right upper extremity shows markedly shortened long bones that are normal in brightness. *Short arrow,* humerus; *long arrow,* radius; *arrowhead,* hand. **C,** Axial image shows marked rib shortening *(arrows).* **D,** Axial view of lumbar spine *(long arrow)* shows markedly decreased spine ossification. *Short arrows,* iliac bones.

normal brightness, are severely shortened in a micromelic pattern, and are often deformed (see Fig. 19-6B). The shortening is so obvious that measurements are needed only for the sake of thoroughness.

The axial skeleton, however, can be either normal or markedly decreased in brightness with a chest narrowed in a bell-shaped appearance with short ribs (see Fig. 19-6C) and decreased spine ossification (see Fig. 19-6D). When the skeleton is of normal brightness, the differentiation of achondrogenesis from thanatophoric dysplasia may not be possible.

Thanatophoric dysplasia is a lethal condition, the word "thanatophoric" being derived from the Greek meaning "death." It is a sporadic noninherited disorder, and the bones of the fetus exhibit a normal brightness. The limbs show severe shortening (and often deformity) in a micromelic pattern (Fig. 19-7A). The entire ribs can be seen on one image, a sign that they are straight and markedly shortened. The skull has a cloverleaf shape (the kleeblattschädel deformity) due to craniosynostosis of the sutures (see Fig. 19-7B). Death is due to the markedly narrowed thorax, which gives the lungs little room to develop (see Fig. 19-7C); pulmonary hypoplasia results.

Ratios of the chest to abdomen (usually as circumferences) and intrathoracic ratios have been evaluated in an attempt to predict when pulmonary hypoplasia will result. Although no definite predictive number has been found, the lower the ratio (due to a narrowed chest), the greater the chance of serious pulmonary problems (see Chapter 16). Moderate to marked polyhydramnios is also typical, presumably caused by impaired swallowing secondary to the chest narrowing (see Fig. 19-7C).

Because of the lack of information about dysplastic fetal growth, in utero development of skeletal dysplasias is incompletely understood. Expected neonatal characteristics may not be present at the time of an ultrasound examination, and findings (even when present) may be

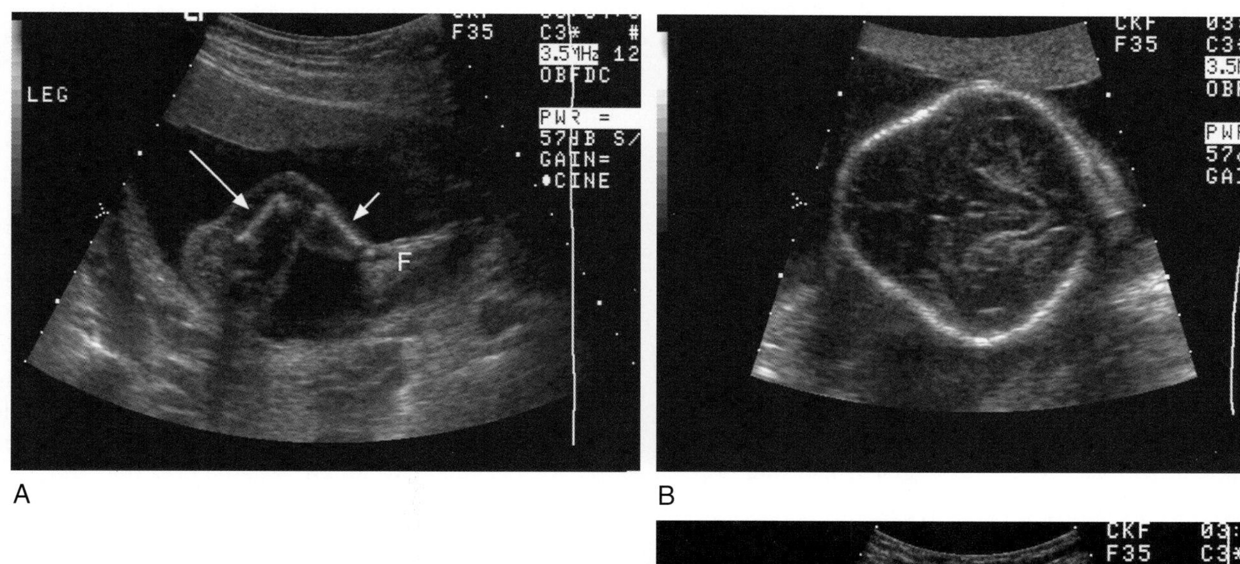

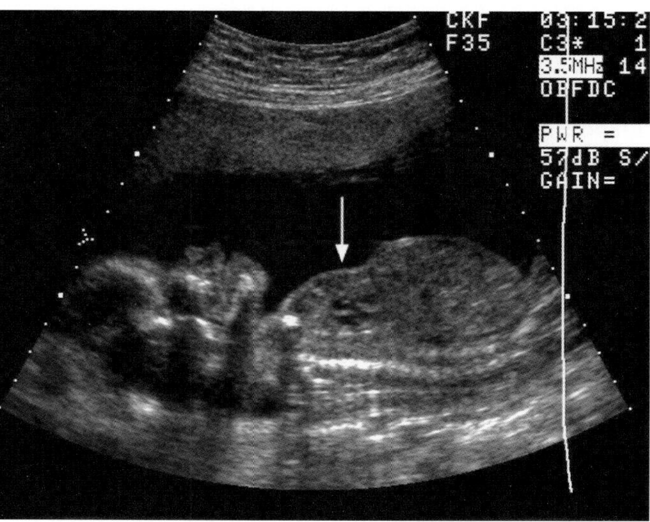

Figure 19-7 Thanatophoric dwarf during second trimester. **A,** Severe micromelic shortening of lower extremity. *Long arrow,* femur; *short arrow,* tibia; F, foot. **B,** Axial image of fetal head shows cloverleaf-shaped skull. **C,** Longitudinal image shows small thorax *(arrow)* and polyhydramnios.

too subtle to be appreciated. In addition, concomitant soft tissue abnormalities may not be detected. Despite these limitations, when an abnormal finding is discovered, particularly in the correct clinical setting, the diagnostic certainty is high.

The prediction of the lethality of any dysplasia is also clinically important. Although there are no absolute rules other than knowledge of the type of dysplasia involved, certain ultrasound findings strongly suggest incompatibility with life. These either individually or in combination include the following:

1. Shortening of both the proximal and distal parts of the extremities (micromelia)
2. Marked skeletal demineralization (decreased brightness)
3. Unusually small thorax

Because many skeletal dysplasias exhibit multiple characteristics, a thorough examination of the fetus should be performed, often going beyond the routine examination suggested in the antepartum obstetric ultrasound standard (see Chapter 12). The use of 3-D ultrasound in both multiplanar and surface rendering formats has helped to confirm some of the questionable and subtler abnormalities.

The head should be analyzed for the presence of calvarial and facial abnormalities. The calvarium can be demineralized. It can have a cloverleaf shape (the kleeblattschädel deformity), a deformity caused by the craniosynostosis of all the sutures and usually associated with mental retardation. It may be either an isolated anomaly (Fig. 19-8) or part of the thanatophoric dysplasia (see Fig. 19-7B). The transient lemon sign of frontal bone flattening often associated with spinal defects (see Chapter 15) and the strawberry-shaped skull described in cases of trisomy 18 can also be detected. In some skeletal dysplasias, the outer orbital diameter may be abnormally increased or decreased. Cleft lips and palates can also be found.

The vertebrae can be demineralized in certain dysplasias. The spine may be deformed, particularly with a sharply angled scoliosis or kyphosis. If there is no evidence of a meningocele or meningomyelocele, the deformity may instead be caused by vertebral body developmental anomalies, such as segmentation and fusion defects. Although often difficult to appreciate in utero, these problems can occur at any vertebral level, particularly in the thoracolumbar region (Fig. 19-9). Developmental anomalies are commonly isolated occurrences but can be associated with additional structural anomalies, which are frequently multiple, such as the VACTERL syndrome (vertebral, anal, cardiac, tracheal, esophageal, renal, radial, and limb anomalies).

The fetal pelvic bones have been studied. The iliac angle, iliac length, and anterior iliac separation have been analyzed. It has been found that the iliac angle and separation are increased in fetuses with trisomy 21 (Down syndrome).

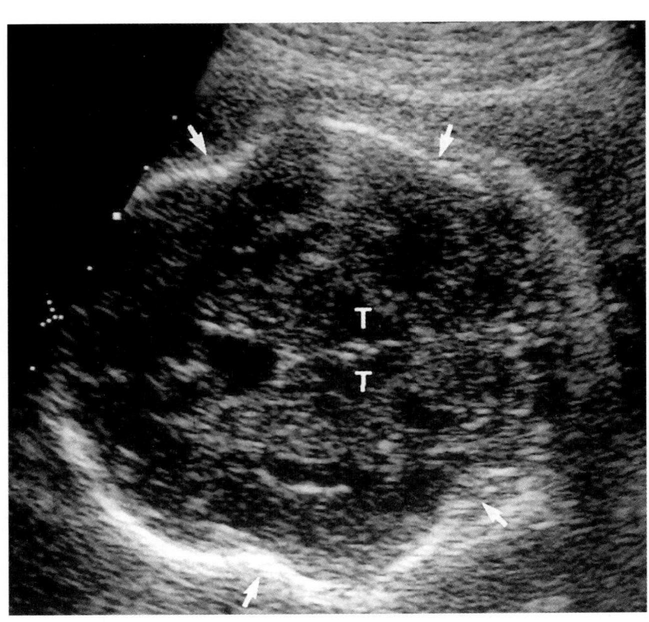

Figure 19-8 Cloverleaf skull (kleeblattschädel deformity) in a 20-week fetus, an isolated deformity not associated with thanatophoric dysplasia. Transaxial image of the fetal head through the area of the thalami (T) shows an unusual configuration of the calvarium. *Arrows* indicate unusual indentations in the frontal and parietal regions bilaterally, causing the head to be configured into three lobes.

Abnormalities of the hands and feet can be diagnosed with meticulous scanning technique. It is important to image not only the five metacarpals and metatarsals but also their phalanges (Fig. 19-10). In the hands, if more than five fingers are counted, polydactyly is present. The extra digits are usually on the ulnar side (adjacent to the little finger) but may be so rudimentary that they are difficult to appreciate (Fig. 19-11). Occasionally, the distal edge of the fifth metacarpal may be mistaken for an extra digit. Syndactyly is skin or bony fusion of adjacent digits such that a trident-type deformity of the hand may be seen, with the second and third fingers and the fourth and fifth fingers closely aligned. Clinodactyly is the sharp deviation of the fingers. Ectrodactyly, lobster-claw deformity, may also be identified (Fig. 19-12). A constantly clenched hand, especially with overlapping fingers, is seen in trisomy 18. Although some of these hand abnormalities can be isolated occurrences, they are not infrequently associated with generalized dysplasias.

Normally, the hands and feet are positioned neutrally and move freely (Fig. 19-13A). Clubhands and clubfeet are seen as sharply flexed distal extremities, remaining in fixed positions (see Fig. 19-13B and C). Although clubbing can be found in the setting of skeletal

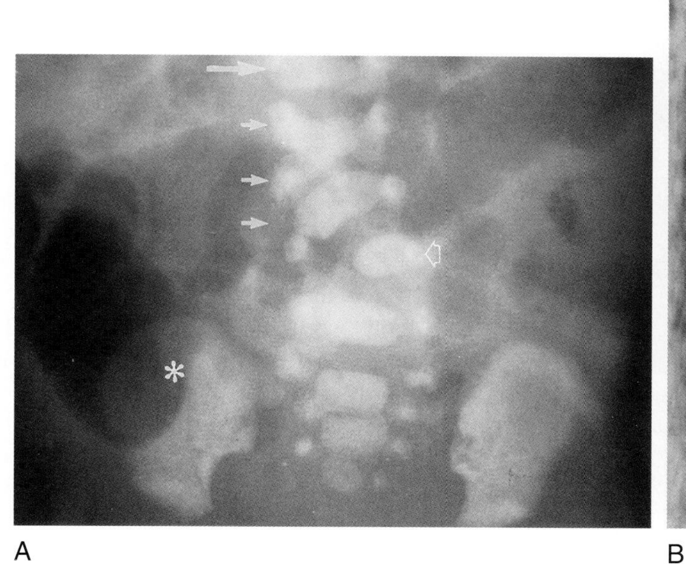

A

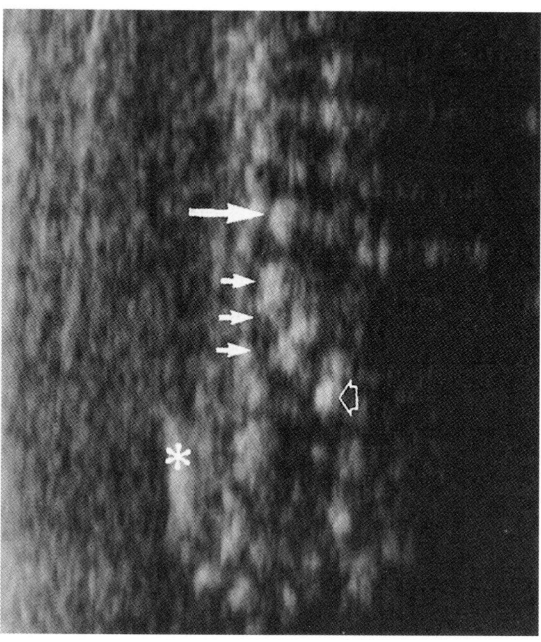

B

Figure 19-9 Complex segmental-fusion anomaly in a 22-week fetus. This was an isolated anomaly and not associated with additional fetal abnormalities. **A,** Anteroposterior abdominopelvic radiograph obtained at birth. **B,** Coronal image of the lumbosacral spine. Both images are oriented in the same plane. The *large arrow* indicates the last normal lumbar vertebral body, and the *asterisk* denotes the right iliac crest; *arrows* show a deformed vertebra and the *open arrow* shows a hemivertebra.

dysplasias, it can also be associated with musculoskeletal or neurologic conditions and is then called arthrogryposis. Prolonged severe oligohydramnios can also lead to secondary arthrogryposis, presumably caused by lack of fetal movement and the fixed position of the extremities. Arthrogryposis is not a true skeletal dysplasia but nevertheless causes significant deformity.

AMNIOTIC BANDS AND THE AMNIOTIC BAND SYNDROME

The fetus normally resides within the amniotic cavity, surrounded by a fused amnion and chorion. Rarely, because of conditions that are not well understood,

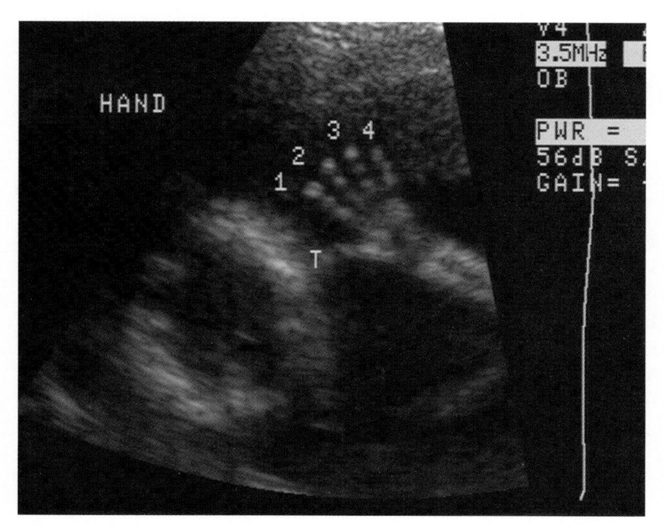

Figure 19-10 Normal hand at 17 weeks, 4 days. The phalanges in the five fingers are demonstrated. T, thumb; 1, 2, 3, 4, the other fingers.

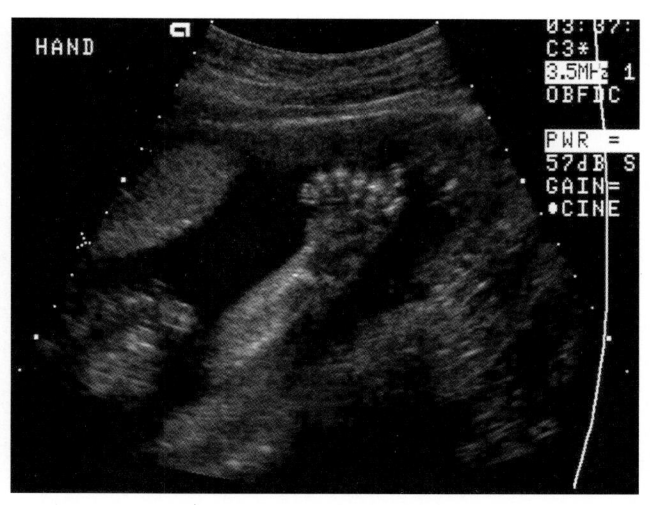

Figure 19-11 Polydactyly. Seven fingers are seen in this fetus with trisomy 13.

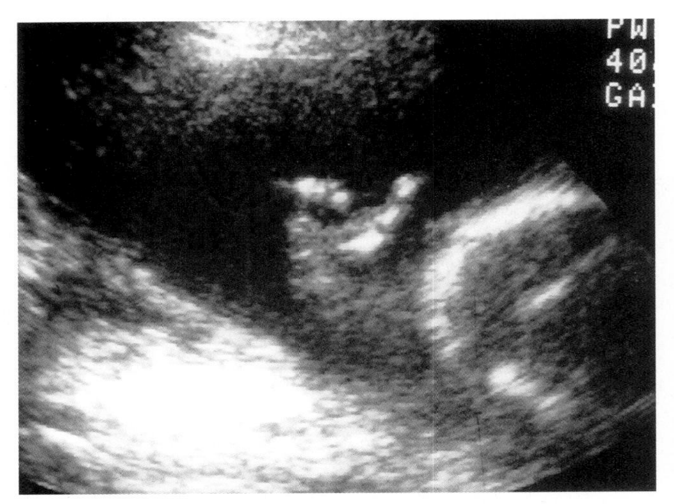

Figure 19-12 Fetus at approximately 20 weeks' gestation. "Lobster claw" deformity in the ectrodactyly-ectodermal dysplasia-clefting syndrome. As part of a complex series of anomalies, there are defects in the mid portion of both the hands and feet. On this image only three partially formed fixed digits are detected in a claw configuration.

there can be a rent or break in the amnion with the fetus then entering the space between the two membranes. Although this may not cause problems, there is a potential for the thin amniotic membrane to encircle fetal parts as bands. As these fetal parts grow, their motion can be restricted and the wrapped part deformed by these bands.

Amniotic bands are not always detected because they can be very thin. However, the gross deformities caused by these bands can be dramatic; and when seen in conjunction with amniotic bands, amniotic band syndrome can be diagnosed. The bands can involve any part of the fetus and typically cause asymmetric deformities; when involving the limbs, strangulation, deformity, and even amputation with pronounced soft tissue swelling are possible (Figs. 19-14 and 19-15).

The amniotic band syndrome is an isolated noninherited anomaly and is therefore not likely to recur in subsequent pregnancies. The deformities produced by

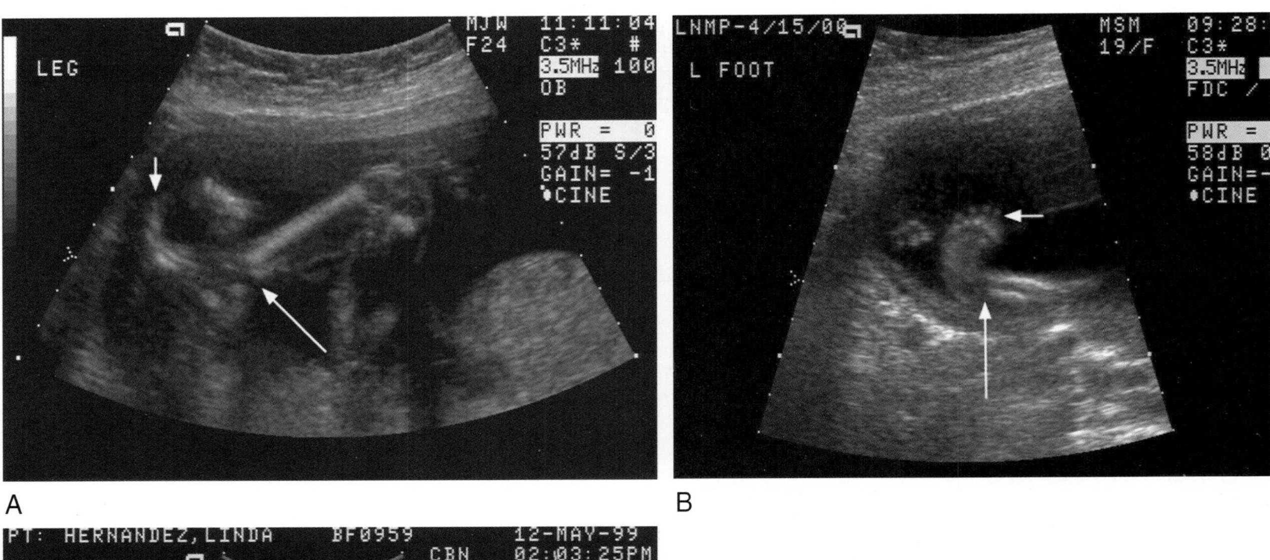

C

Figure 19-13 Normal and abnormally positioned feet. **A,** Long-axis image of a normal foot in a 22-week fetus. The foot moved normally at the ankle. *Long arrow,* ankle; *short arrow,* toes. **B** and **C,** Clubfoot in a fetus with a Chiari II malformation (**B**) and in a fetus with no other abnormalities (**C**). Note the unusual angulation of the foot at the ankle. The feet of both fetuses remained in a fixed position. *Long arrows,* ankles; *short arrows,* toes.

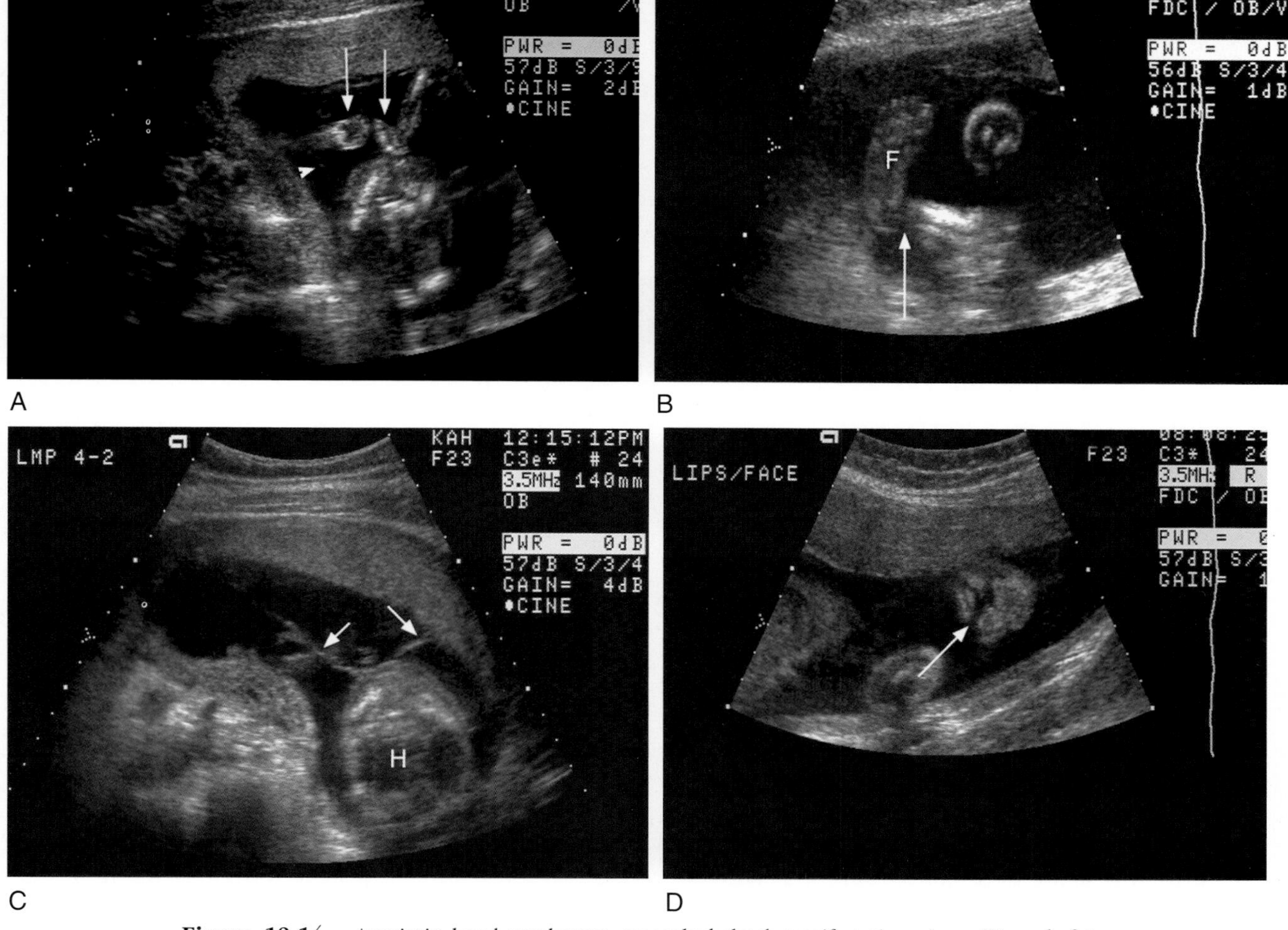

Figure 19-14 Amniotic band syndrome: musculoskeletal manifestations in a 17-week fetus. **A,** Both hands *(long arrows)* remained fixed together in clenched positions. Irregularly shaped amniotic bands *(arrowhead)* were seen in the amniotic cavity, extending to the hands, feet, and face. **B,** Foot (F) was clubbed and exhibited only limited mobility. *Arrow,* ankle. **C,** Amniotic band *(short arrows)* extending to fetal face. H, head. **D,** Large facial cleft *(arrow),* which was secondary to the amniotic band seen in **C**.

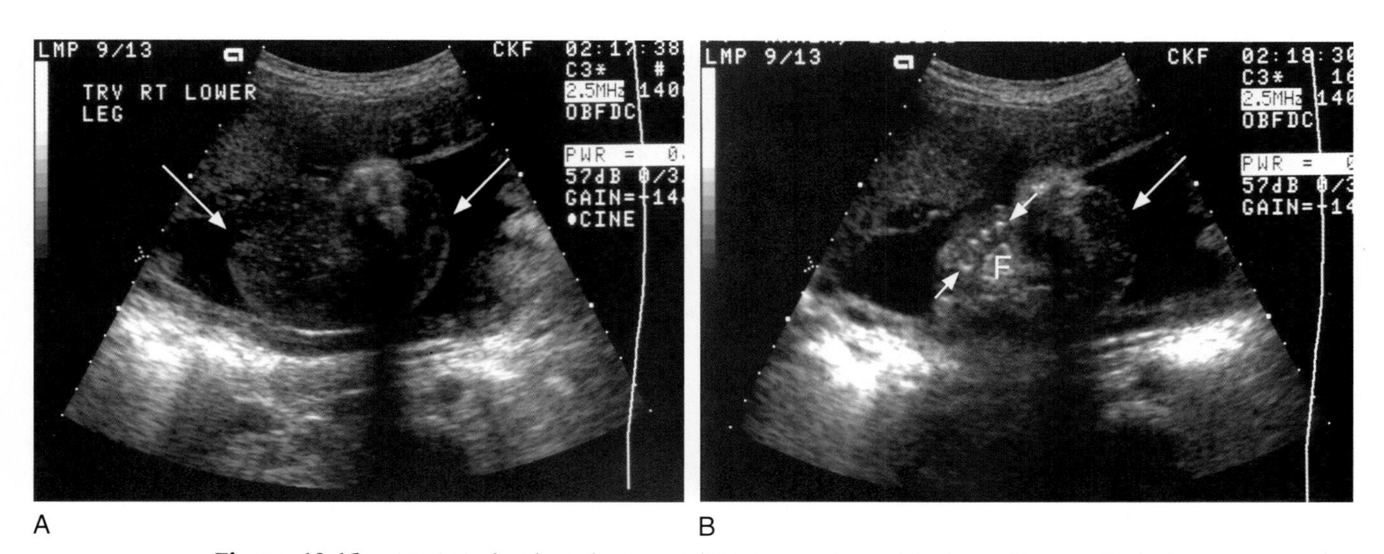

Figure 19-15 Amniotic band syndrome resulting in pronounced limb swelling. **A,** Marked swelling of soft tissues *(long arrows)* of right lower extremity resembles a mass. **B,** The foot (F) is deformed and fixated by the abnormal soft tissues *(long arrow).* Portions of several toes *(short arrows)* were amputated. Although amniotic bands were not seen at antenatal ultrasound, they were identified at the time of delivery.

the bands are not part of the spectrum of either skeletal dysplasias or any standard anomaly. Asymmetry and unusual nonembryologic patterns and combinations of defects can suggest the diagnosis even when the bands are not detected by ultrasound.

In the case of amniotic sheets, synechiae extend into the amniotic fluid. Because of their thickness (>2 mm) and multilayered appearance, these sheets should not be mistaken for amniotic bands. This is discussed more completely in Chapter 21.

Key Features

- Identification and measurement of at least one femur is a routine part of the obstetric ultrasound examination.
- Routine analysis of the skeletal system includes evaluation of the spine and the calvarium. An attempt should be made to identify all 4 extremities to rule out absence of an extremity.
- An important value of the femur length (FL) measurement is in its proportionality with other fetal structures, especially the head.
- Two appearances of the distal femur should not be included in its measurement: the distal femoral point and distal femoral epiphyseal ossification.
- If one femur measures abnormally short or long, the other femur should be measured to determine if the process is unilateral or bilateral.
- If both femurs are found to be short, a constitutionally normal fetus can usually be differentiated from one with dysplasia by FL interval growth assessment and evaluation of the remainder of the fetal structures.
- The femoral and humeral lengths do not have enough of a positive predictive value to be definitive in the consistent prediction of chromosomal abnormalities.
- The value of ultrasound in the investigation of skeletal dysplasias is primarily in three areas: limb shortening, bony deformity (fractures and/or bowing), and decreased bone brightness (demineralization). Ultrasound can also be used to determine if limb shortening is proximal, distal, or both. Experienced examiners can further assess more subtle changes in the hands, feet, face, spine, and other structures as indicated.
- There are four major skeletal anomalies, which account for two thirds of all dysplasias: heterozygous achondroplasia, osteogenesis imperfecta, achondrogenesis, and thanatophoric dysplasia.
- Heterozygous achondroplasia can be evaluated in utero by FL measurement and its interval growth. The FL can initially be normal but will exhibit slower than normal growth, which will typically fall below the 10th percentile at no later than 28 weeks' gestation.
- Osteogenesis imperfecta can only be detected if skeletal deformities (fractures and abnormal bowing) or demineralization is present.
- Achondrogenesis involves severe shortening of the limbs exhibiting a micromelic pattern. There are varying degrees of demineralization to the axial skeleton and chest narrowing.
- Thanatophoric dysplasia is a noninherited condition in which the bone brightness is normal. There is severe limb shortening and significant chest narrowing, usually in combination with pronounced polyhydramnios.
- As a general rule, any abnormal finding in a fetus examined for a skeletal dysplasia establishes the diagnosis of that dysplasia. A normal examination, however, must be considered cautiously because subtle or late developing abnormalities may not be appreciated.
- The amniotic band syndrome can often be differentiated from skeletal dysplasias and developmental abnormalities because the deformities that result are usually markedly asymmetric and atypical in appearance.

SUGGESTED READINGS

Avni EF, Rypens F, Zappa M, et al: Antenatal diagnosis of short-limb dwarfism: Sonographic approach. Pediatr Radiol 26:171, 1996.

Benacerraf BR, Frigoletto FD Jr: Sonographic observation of amniotic rupture without amniotic band syndrome. J Ultrasound Med 11:109, 1992.

Benacerraf BR, et al: Sonographic scoring index for prenatal detection of chromosomal abnormalities. J Ultrasound Med 11:449, 1992.

Benson CB, Doubilet PM: Sonographic prediction of gestational age: Accuracy of second- and third-trimester fetal measurements. AJR Am J Roentgenol 157:1275, 1991.

Bromley B, Benacerraf BR: Abnormalities of the hands and feet in the fetus: Sonographic findings. AJR Am J Roentgenol 165:1239, 1995.

Bulas DI, et al: Variable prenatal appearance of osteogenesis imperfecta. J Ultrasound Med 13:419, 1994.

Burton DJ, Filly RA: Sonographic diagnosis of the amniotic band syndrome. AJR Am J Roentgenol 156:555, 1991.

Camera G, Mastroiacovo P: Birth prevalence of skeletal dysplasias in the Italian multicentric monitoring system for birth defects. In Papadatos CJ, Bartsocas CS (eds): Skeletal Dysplasias. New York, Alan R. Liss, 1982.

Gaffney G, Manning N, Boyd PA, et al: Prenatal sonographic diagnosis of skeletal dysplasias: A report of the diagnostic and prognostic accuracy in 35 cases. Prenat Diagn 18:357, 1998.

Goldstein RB, Filly RA, Simpson G: Pitfalls in femur length measurements. J Ultrasound Med 6:203, 1987.

Kurtz AB, Wapner RJ: Ultrasonographic diagnosis of second-trimester skeletal dysplasias: A prospective analysis in a high-risk population. J Ultrasound Med 2:99, 1983.

Kurtz AB, et al: In utero analysis of heterozygous achondroplasia: Variable time of onset as detected by femur length measurements. J Ultrasound Med 5:137, 1986.

Kurtz AB, et al: Usefulness of a short femur in the in utero detection of skeletal dysplasias. Radiology 177:197, 1990.

Lemyre E, Azouz EM, Teebi AS, et al: Bone dysplasia series: Achondroplasia, hypochondroplasia and thanatophoric dysplasia: Review and update. Can Assoc Radiol J 50:185, 1999.

Mahony BS, et al: The amniotic band syndrome: Antenatal sonographic diagnosis and potential pitfalls. Am J Obstet Gynecol 152:63, 1985.

Malone FD, Marino T, Bianchi DW, et al: Isolated clubfoot diagnosed prenatally: Is karyotyping indicated? Obstet Gynecol 95:437, 2000.

Meizner I: Fetal skeletal malformations revisited: Steps in the diagnostic approach. Ultrasound Obstet Gynecol 10:303, 1997.

Patel MD, Filly RA: Homozygous achondroplasia: US distinction between homozygous, heterozygous, and unaffected fetuses in the second trimester. Radiology 196:541, 1995.

Pretorius DH, et al: Specific skeletal dysplasias in utero: Sonographic diagnosis. Radiology 159:237, 1986.

Rijhsinghani, Yankowitz J, Kanis AB, et al: Antenatal sonographic diagnosis of club foot with particular attention to the implications and outcomes of isolated club foot. Ultrasound Obstet Gynecol 11:103, 1998.

Schild RL, Hunt GH, Moore J, et al: Antenatal sonographic diagnosis of thanatophoric dysplasia: A report of three cases and a review of the literature with special emphasis on the differential diagnosis. Ultrasound Obstet Gynecol 8:62, 1996.

Shipp TD, Benacerraf BR: The significance of prenatally identified isolated clubfoot: Is amniocentesis indicated? Am J Obstet Gynecol 178:600, 1998.

Tretter AE, Saunders RC, Meyers CM, et al: Antenatal diagnosis of lethal skeletal dysplasias. Am J Med Genet 75:518, 1998.

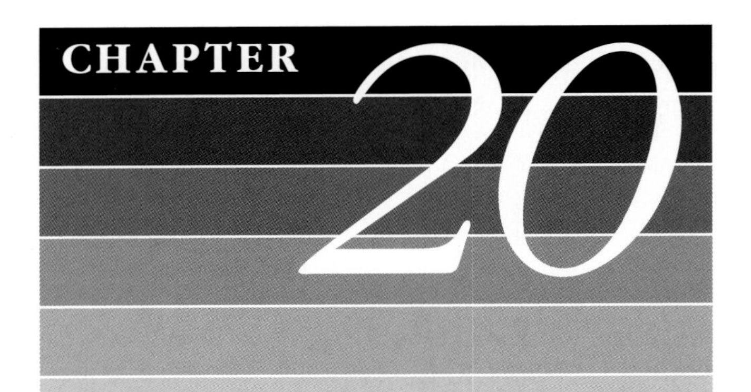

CHAPTER 20 Placenta, Umbilical Cord, and Cervix

The placenta should be evaluated as part of the second- and third-trimester examination. Its position, size, and echogenicity can be assessed, and any evidence of hemorrhage, infarction, or mass can be noted. Although not specifically mentioned in the antepartum obstetrical ultrasound standard, the cervix should be analyzed for possible incompetence. The number of vessels in the umbilical cord should be assessed. Doppler waveform analysis may be of diagnostic value in selected cases.

THE NORMAL PLACENTA

The early embryo (the blastocyst) embeds into the endometrium and sends out finger-like projections called chorionic villi. In response, the entire endometrial lining undergoes a decidual proliferation. Although most of these villi and decidua atrophy by the mid to late first trimester, the chorion frondosum and adjacent decidua basalis along a portion of the forming gestational sac margin proliferate, however, to form the placenta.

Sonographically, the placenta can be identified as early as 7 to 8 weeks and is routinely imaged by the end of the first trimester. The placenta is best appreciated when fundal, anterior, or lateral in position; when posterior, the fetus often overlies and frequently obscures full visualization. The placenta has a uniformly moderate echogenicity (Fig. 20-1). On its surface abutting the amniotic fluid, the chorionic plate (the chorioamnionic membrane) can be seen as a bright specular reflector when it is oriented perpendicular to the ultrasound beam. On its attachments with the uterine wall, the combined basilar-myometrial layer is sometimes identified as a hypoechoic band, best seen when the placenta is anterior or lateral. Serosal and juxtauterine veins can be identified at the margins of and immediately adjacent to the uterus, particularly laterally. These veins may be very prominent and will conform to the uterine wall without mass effect (Fig. 20-2).

Placental thickness is usually determined subjectively. If a measurement is needed, it is best obtained in mid position perpendicular to the placental surface from the chorionic plate to the beginning of the basilar-myometrial layer (Fig. 20-3A). When the umbilical cord inserts into the middle of the placenta, this measurement can be taken at its insertion site. Precise upper and lower values are not available, but the thickness is considered normal throughout the second and third trimesters if between 2 and 4 cm. Care must be taken not to measure either obliquely or near a uterine contraction, because the placental size can be altered, usually creating a false impression of enlargement (see Fig. 20-3B).

The placenta is a very vascular organ and consists of two blood supplies. From the fetus the umbilical arteries (typically two) carry blood from the fetal hypogastric arteries to the placenta and one umbilical vein carries blood back to the fetal left portal vein. From the mother, the branches of the uterine arteries (from the maternal hypogastric arteries) carry blood through the myometrium via the arcuate and radial arteries, through the basilar plate (the spiral arteries), and into the placenta; maternal blood leaves by comparable veins. Within the

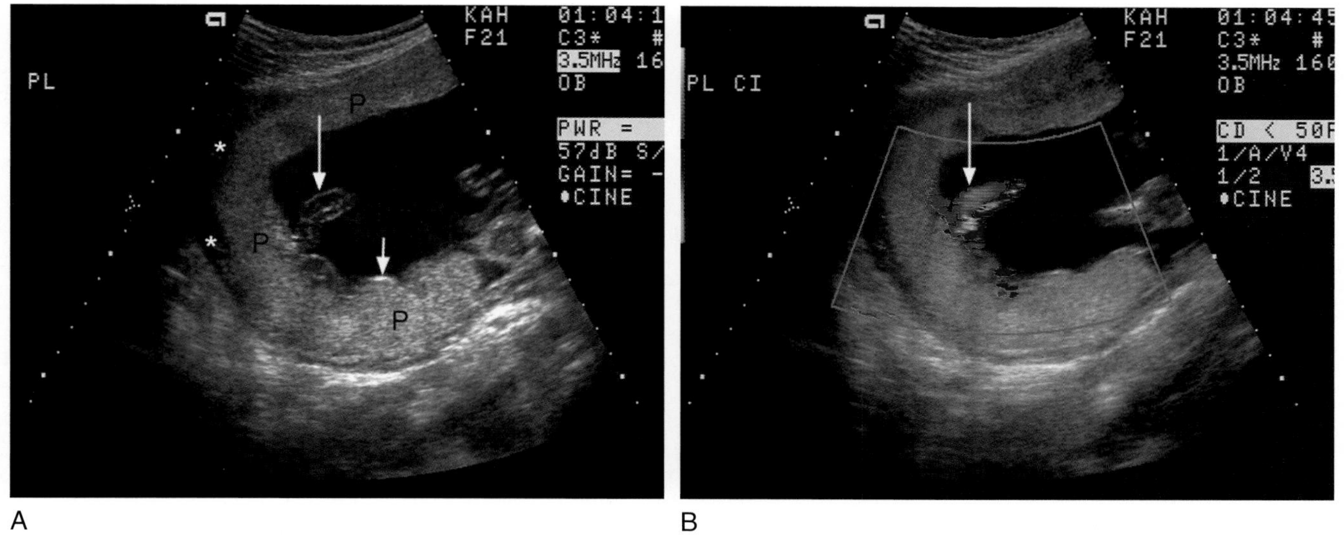

Figure 20-1 Normal placenta. **A,** Axial image of uterus at 19 weeks shows homogeneous echo pattern of a normal placenta (P). The chorionic plate *(short arrow)* is depicted as a bright specular reflector. The umbilical cord *(long arrow)* inserts centrally into the placenta. The hypoechoic myometrial-basilar layer (*) is seen behind the placenta. **B,** Color Doppler image of same patient as in **A** shows blood flow in the umbilical cord *(arrow)* at its insertion into the placenta.

placenta the two circulations intertwine but do not admix. With slow flow and large surface area, maximum exchange of nutrients for wastes and oxygenated blood for deoxygenated blood can take place.

Normal maternal venous channels (without fetal interconnections) are frequently seen as hypoechoic or anechoic spaces within the placenta. These are often focal and small but may infrequently be numerous and large, rarely even traversing the placenta from the basilar plate to the subchorionic region below the chorionic plate. Although given different monikers, including "venous lakes," these are best termed *intervillous connections* (Fig. 20-4). Blood flow can sometimes be observed by real-time observation and can be confirmed by its Doppler-detected venous flow.

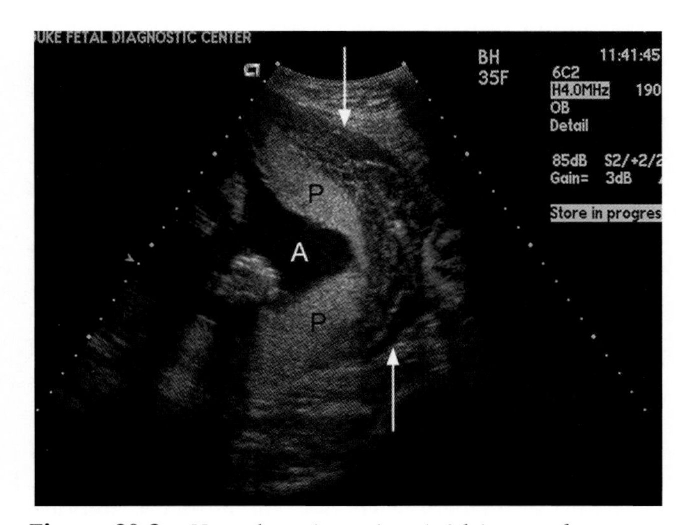

Figure 20-2 Normal uterine veins. Axial image of uterus at 26 weeks shows numerous normal, prominent blood vessels in the uterine wall *(arrows)*. Note that these blood vessels conform to the contour of the uterine wall and do not cause mass effect. P, placenta; A, amniotic fluid.

The placenta changes in appearance with advancing gestation. The normal uniform placental echogenicity is defined as grade 0 (Fig. 20-5A). In some women placental calcifications (hyperechoic foci) develop normally as the pregnancy matures (see Fig. 20-5B). Small diffuse speckled calcifications constitute grade 1 changes (≥30 weeks). Grade 2 changes are similar to grade 1 changes but include larger calcifications along the basilar plate (≥32 weeks) (see Fig. 20-5C). Grade 3 changes are similar to those of grade 2 but are more extensive and thicker, separating the placenta into areas called cotyledons (≥34 weeks) (see Fig. 20-5D). Grade 3 calcifications may cause significant shadowing, making the placental echogenicity appear falsely hypoechoic; increased gain will reveal its normal echogenicity. The placental grade is defined by its most advanced area.

Not all placentas undergo these maturation changes: up to 40% remain grades 0 to 1; 45%, grade 2; and 15%, grade 3. The lack of calcific changes has no clinical significance. Their presence, however, if too early, may signify placental dysmaturity and possible growth restriction. More work is needed to elucidate their significance (also discussed in Chapter 13), and, currently, most practices do not routinely use a placental grading system.

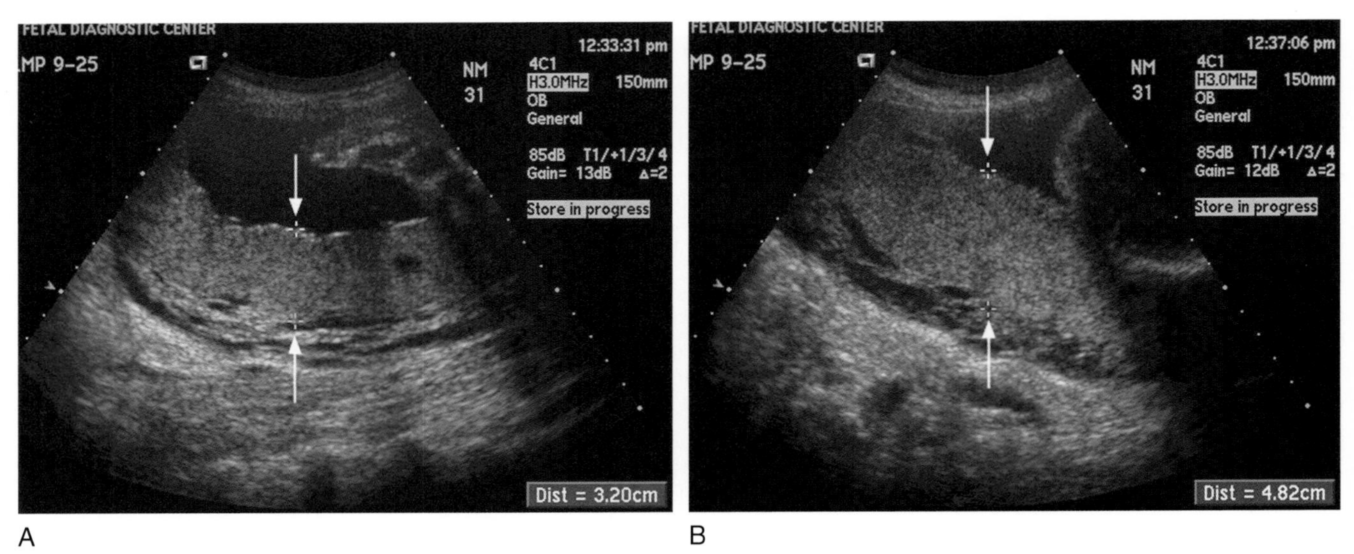

Figure 20-3 Measurement of placental thickness. **A,** Correct placement of calipers. Longitudinal image of placenta at 29 weeks shows measurement calipers *(arrows)* positioned on the mid portion of the placenta to measure placental thickness. The measurement should be made perpendicular to the placental surface, from the chorionic plate to the beginning of the basilar-myometrial surface. The measurement of 3.2 cm is normal. **B,** Incorrect scan plane and placement of calipers resulting in spuriously thickened placental measurement. Oblique image through the placenta causes it to appear thicker than in **A**. Measurement calipers *(arrows)* are oriented obliquely rather than perpendicular to the placenta. The combination of oblique scan plane and incorrect placement of measurement calipers results in a spuriously elevated placental thickness measurement of 4.8 cm.

TROPHOTROPISM

Trophotropism is a unifying concept that helps explain the occurrence of unusual placental shapes, eccentric umbilical cord insertions, and changes in placental position, particularly in relation to the internal cervical os. Initially, the placenta forms as a rounded disc with the umbilical cord at its center and with each portion of the placenta attaching to its underlying endometrium. If there is equal and good vascularity to all attachments, the placenta remains unchanged in position throughout pregnancy. If, however, the blood supply is unequal, preferential trophoblastic villi will proliferate into adjacent regions where the endometrial blood supply is better, with villous atrophy occurring in areas of poorer vascularity.

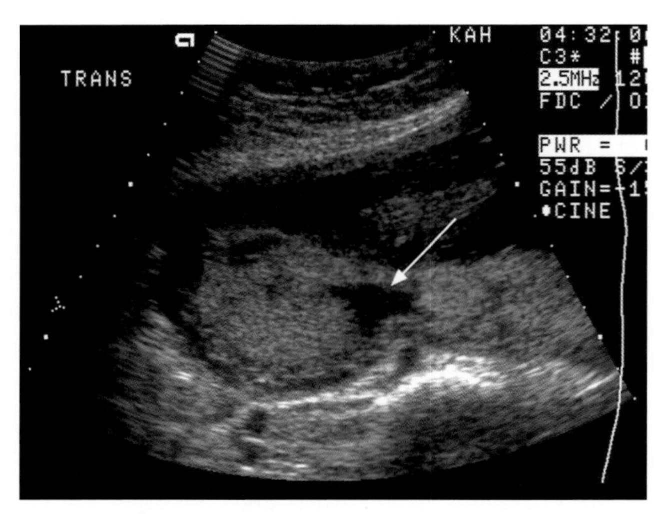

Figure 20-4 Normal intervillous connections (venous lake). Axial scan of placenta at 19 weeks shows a hypoechoic space *(arrow)* corresponding to a normal intervillous connection. Echoes were seen swirling within this space during real-time observation.

The poorest vascularity is typically (but not always) in the lower uterine segment, in areas of uterine scarring, and near large fibroids. In these conditions, placental remodeling or trophotropism results, and the following changes can then take place:

1. The placenta can shift relative to the umbilical cord insertion, leaving an eccentrically situated cord insertion. The insertion site may then be anywhere from the placental center to its edge (a marginal insertion). In the most extreme cases the placenta may be remodeled so that the cord insertion site is outside the placental margin (a velamentous cord insertion).
2. Unusual placental shapes including a bilobed placenta (Fig. 20-6) can occur. Rarely, a portion of the placenta (a succenturiate lobe) (Fig. 20-7) can separate from the main placental body.
3. A placenta previa can resolve.

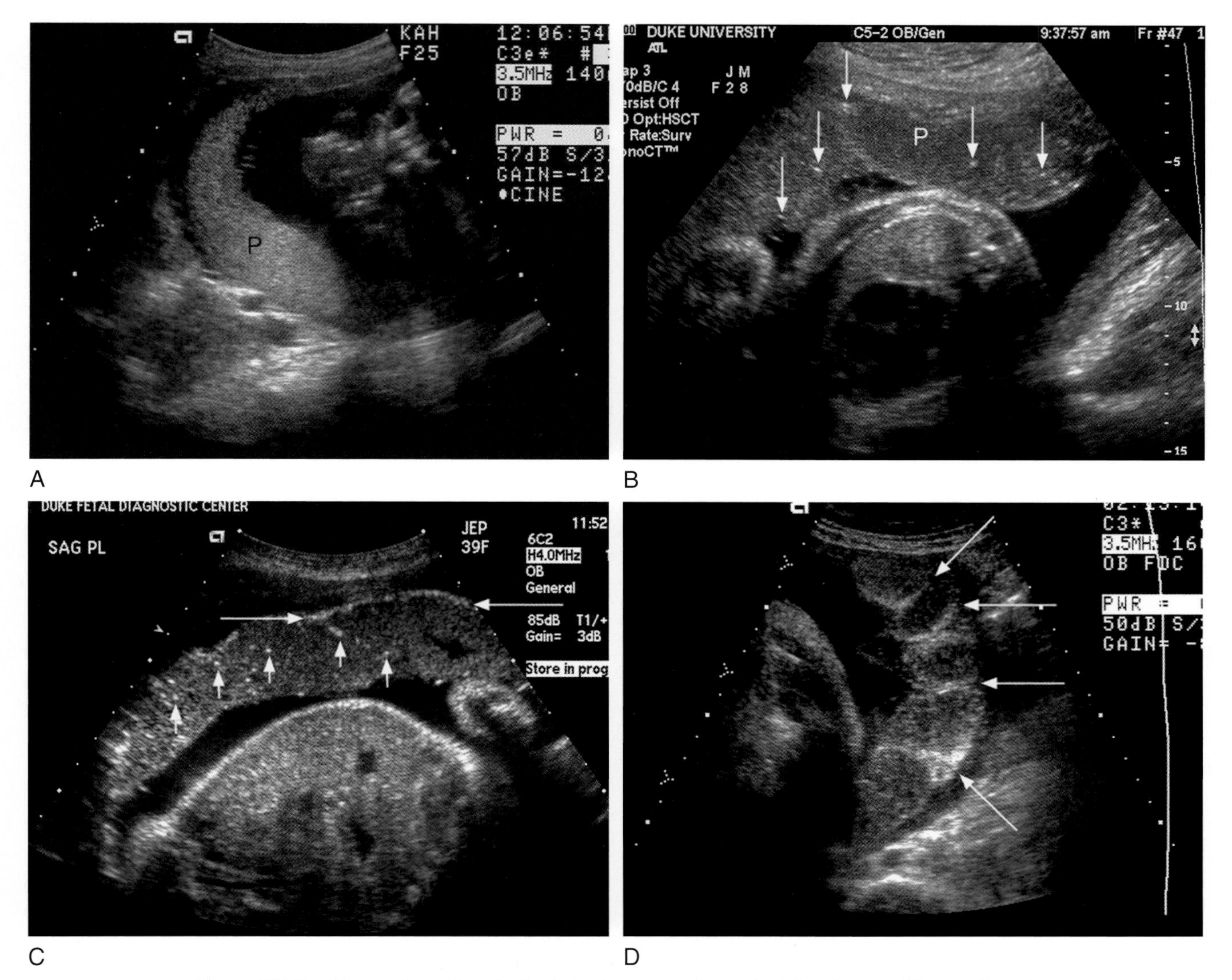

Figure 20-5 Placental grading. **A,** Grade 0 placenta at 17 weeks. The placenta (P) is uniform in echogenicity without calcifications. **B,** Grade 1 placenta at 34 weeks. Small punctate intraplacental hyperechoic foci *(arrows)* are scattered throughout the otherwise homogeneous placenta (P). **C,** Grade 2 placenta at 31 weeks. In addition to the scattered punctate intraplacental foci *(short arrows)* seen in a grade 1 placenta, note the larger areas of calcification along the basilar plate *(arrows).* **D,** Grade 3 placenta at 38 weeks. Calcifications are more extensive than in grades 0 to 2 and extend through the substance of the placenta *(arrows),* separating the placenta into areas called cotyledons.

THE UMBILICAL CORD

The umbilical cord is identified by the late first trimester and can be readily evaluated throughout the second and third trimesters (Fig. 20-8). Umbilical cord processes that can be assessed at ultrasound include placental insertion, cord length and twists, number of vessels, focal abnormalities, cord position, and fetal insertion.

The insertion of the umbilical cord into the placenta is considered normal if it remains within the placental substance (Figs. 20-1A and 20-9). In a velamentous cord insertion, with the insertion site located beyond the margin of the placenta, the umbilical cord's arteries and vein are not "anchored" into the placenta but instead are connected by a pedicle and covered only by the chorioamnionic membrane. Typically asymptomatic during the pregnancy, a fetal catastrophe can develop at delivery because these vessels are prone to rupture. In addition, a velamentous cord insertion if near the internal os can fix the umbilical cord and at delivery causes it to present in front of the fetus. Called an obligate cord presentation, this can lead to cord prolapse with potential loss of circulation to the fetus.

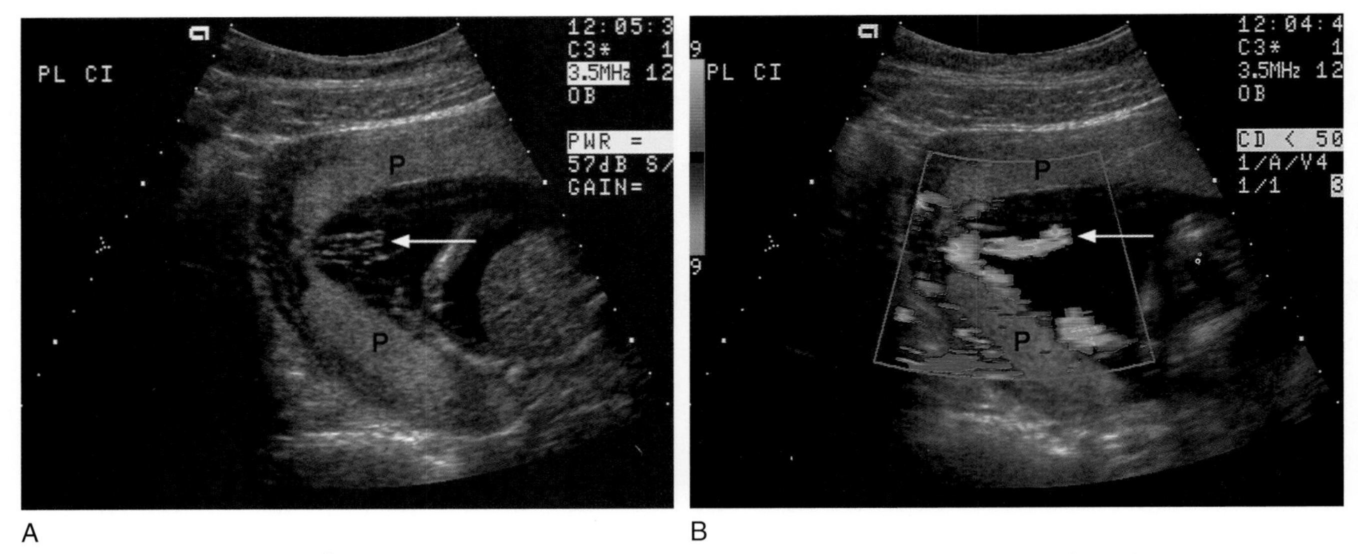

Figure 20-6 Bilobed placenta. **A,** Axial image of uterus shows a bilobed placenta (P). The umbilical cord *(arrow)* inserts on the thin rim of placental tissue bridging the placental lobes. **B,** Color Doppler image of the same region as in **A** confirms the umbilical cord *(arrow)* inserts between the two placental lobes (P).

Finally, if these fetal vessels cross the internal os, a vasa previa (fetal circulation over the internal os) will be present. While not a problem during pregnancy, severe fetal blood loss can occur at the time of rupture of membranes or delivery.

The umbilical cord length is also important. Cords that are too long or too short have been associated with problems of fetal circulation and fetal position. At present, cord length cannot be measured accurately; but if the entire cord can be imaged in one projection, it is too short. The umbilical cord is normally twisted like a braid, and the more uncommon untwisted cord has been associated with a higher incidence of perinatal morbidity and mortality (Fig. 20-10). Further work is needed to determine the full extent of the associated risk.

The number of umbilical blood vessels has prognostic importance. Easy to assess with an axial image of the cord, provided an adequate amount of amniotic fluid is present, more than 90% of singleton gestations have a

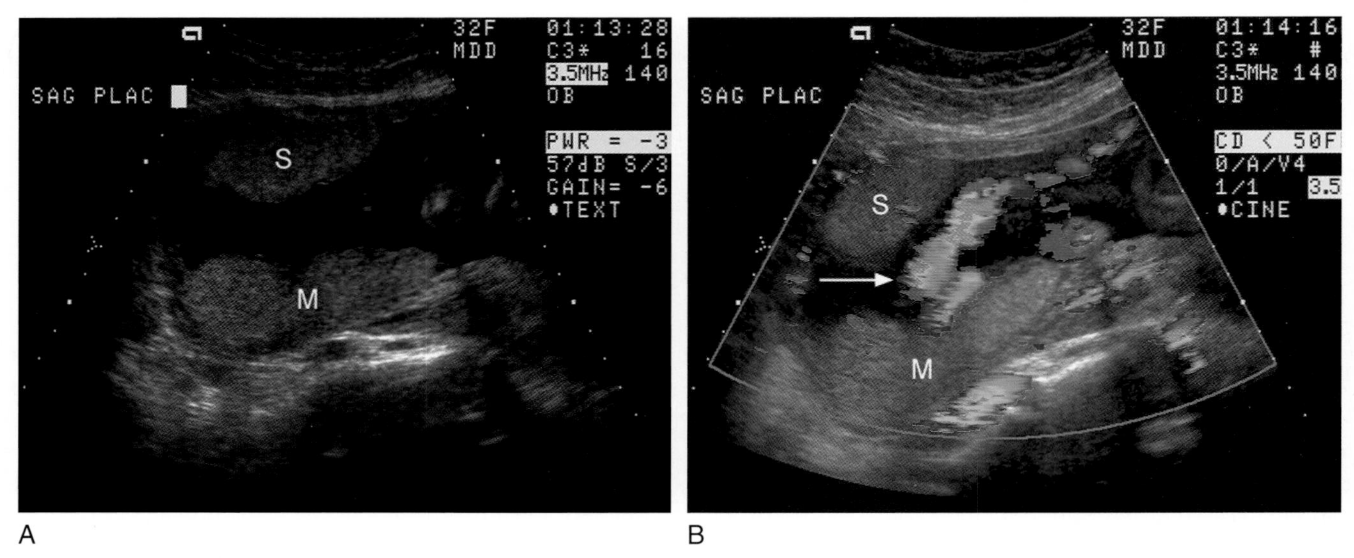

Figure 20-7 Succenturiate lobe. **A,** Sagittal image of uterus during second trimester shows two separate placental lobes. The main lobe (M) is located posteriorly and the succenturiate (accessory) lobe (S) is located anteriorly. There is no placental tissue bridging the two lobes. **B,** Color Doppler image shows the umbilical cord *(long arrow)* inserts on the main lobe (M) of the placenta. The succenturiate lobe (S) receives its blood supply from the main lobe of the placenta.

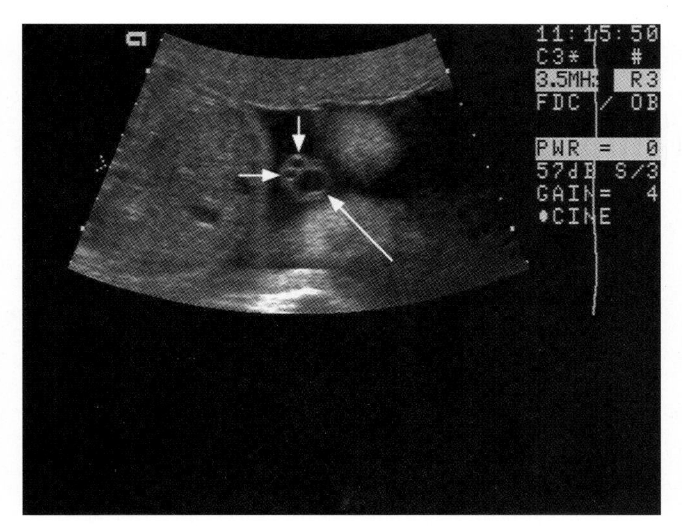

Figure 20-8 Normal umbilical cord. Cross-section of umbilical cord during third trimester shows normal configuration of two arteries *(short arrows)* and one vein *(long arrow).*

normal three-vessel cord: two arteries and one vein (see Fig. 20-8). In the remaining fetuses, only two vessels (one artery and one vein) are identified (Fig. 20-11). Because there is an increased incidence of structural abnormalities and growth restriction in fetuses with a two-vessel cord, a thorough fetal ultrasound evaluation including the face, extremities, and heart and a follow-up third-trimester study to assess fetal growth is indicated.

The accurate diagnosis of a two-vessel cord requires the identification of two vessels throughout the umbilical cord. If the umbilical cord has two vessels in one part (more commonly near the placenta), with reconstitution to three vessels in the rest (more commonly near the fetus), then the umbilical cord has the normal three vessels. An evaluation of the fetal pelvis to identify the two iliac arteries, one on each side of the bladder, is helpful; the absence of one perivesicular artery confirms the absence of one umbilical artery. In multiple gestations, a two-vessel cord is more common and is considered by some to be a normal variant. Nevertheless, others still advocate a more careful fetal evaluation.

Diffuse cord abnormalities can be present. The normal cord is less then 2 cm in overall diameter. An increased diameter is most often associated with excessive amounts of the normal Wharton's jelly but has also been reported in maternal diabetes mellitus, fetal hydrops (secondary to edema), and, rarely, fetal urachal (urine) extravasation.

Focal cord abnormalities can also be identified, usually seen closer to the fetal insertion. Typically cystic and avascular, they are more often a Wharton's jelly cyst (often associated with an omphalocele) or a developmental anomaly (e.g., allantoic duct cyst or urachal remnants) (Fig. 20-12). A hematoma and rarely a cystic remnant of a blighted twin from a dichorionic pregnancy may be seen adjacent to the placental insertion. The most common vascular cord mass is a hemangioma. It typically has a uniform low-level echogenicity similar to a bowel-containing omphalocele and if adjacent to the fetal body can lead to the erroneous diagnosis of an anterior abdominal wall defect. Doppler waveform analysis is

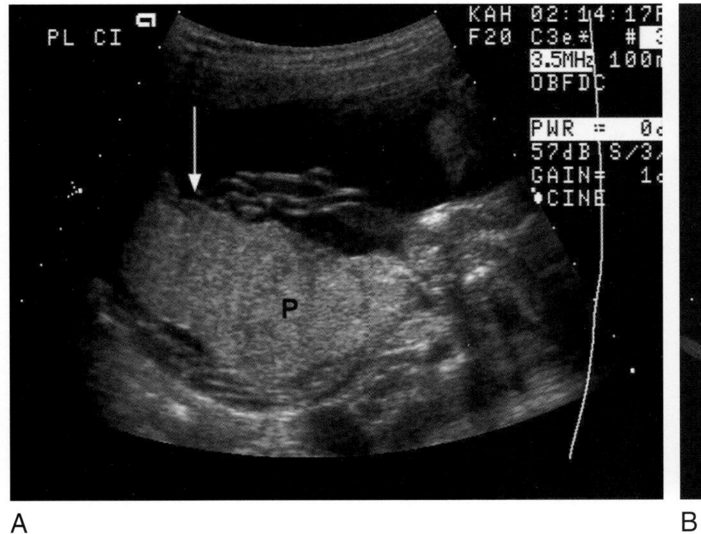

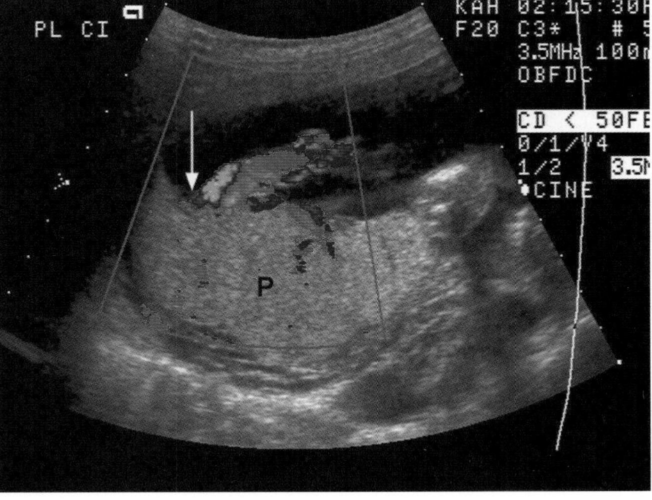

Figure 20-9 Normal, but eccentrically placed umbilical cord insertion. **A,** Longitudinal image of uterus during second trimester shows umbilical cord inserting eccentrically into the placental substance. **B,** Corresponding color Doppler image confirms the eccentric position of the cord insertion. P, placenta; *arrow,* cord insertion.

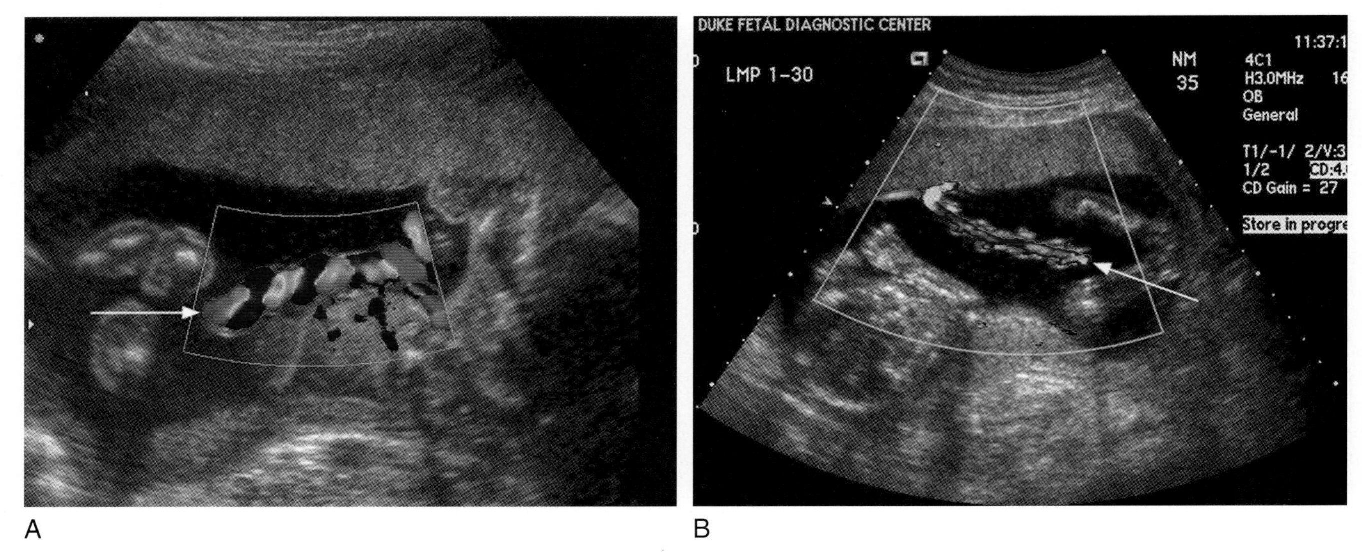

Figure 20-10 Umbilical cord: examples of a twisted and an "untwisted" cord. **A,** Longitudinal Color Doppler image of normal umbilical cord *(arrow* shows normal twisting of the blood vessels. **B,** Longitudinal Color Doppler image of untwisted umbilical cord shows a long segment of the umbilical vein *(arrow)* that does not exhibit the usual twisted appearance.

rarely of value because the blood flow in a hemangioma is typically too slow to be detected and prominent Doppler flow would suggest other pathologic processes.

The umbilical cord floats freely within the amniotic fluid. Often close to the fetus, it is not uncommon to identify the cord near the fetal neck. Termed a *nuchal cord,* defined as encircling the neck at least once, most observers neither look for nor report a nuchal cord since it has been seen in 20% of normal deliveries (Fig. 20-13). Nevertheless, if a nuchal cord is fortuitously found to significantly indent the soft tissues of the neck, this should be monitored as a sign of potential cord tightening.

BLEEDING OCCURRING IN OR AROUND THE PLACENTA

Because the placenta is a very vascular organ, spontaneous bleeding can occur within or around the placenta. Less commonly, bleeding can be caused by direct

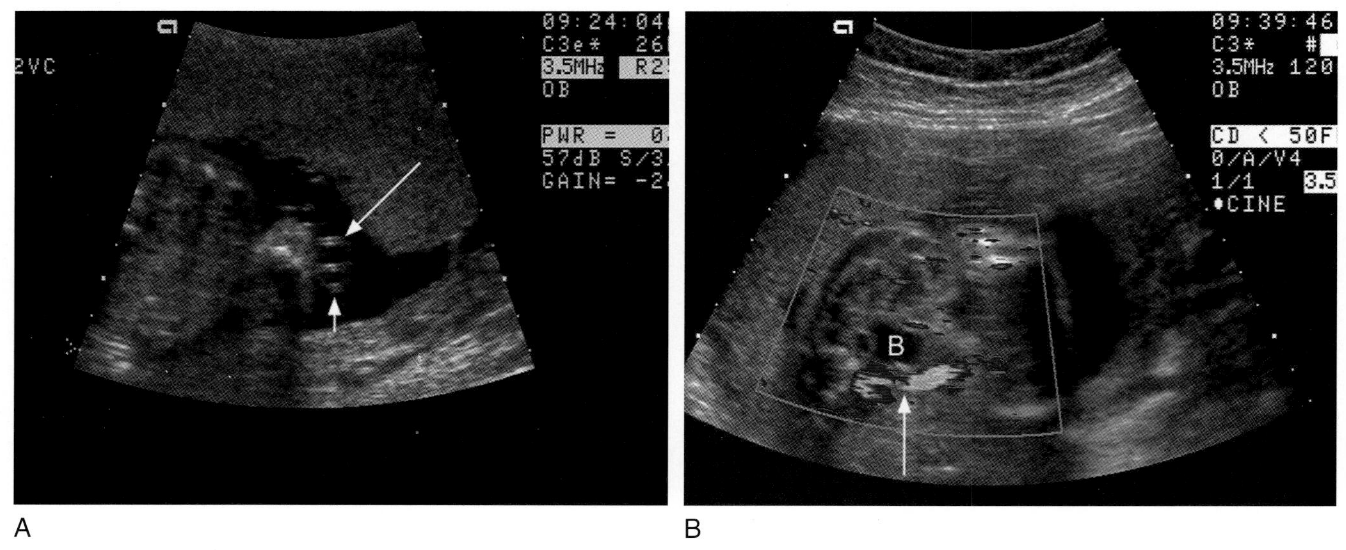

Figure 20-11 Two-vessel umbilical cord. **A,** Cross-section of a two-vessel umbilical cord in a second-trimester pregnancy shows one artery *(short arrow)* and one vein *(long arrow)*. **B,** Color Doppler axial image of pelvis shows an iliac artery *(arrow)* on one side of the urinary bladder (B) but no iliac artery on the other side.

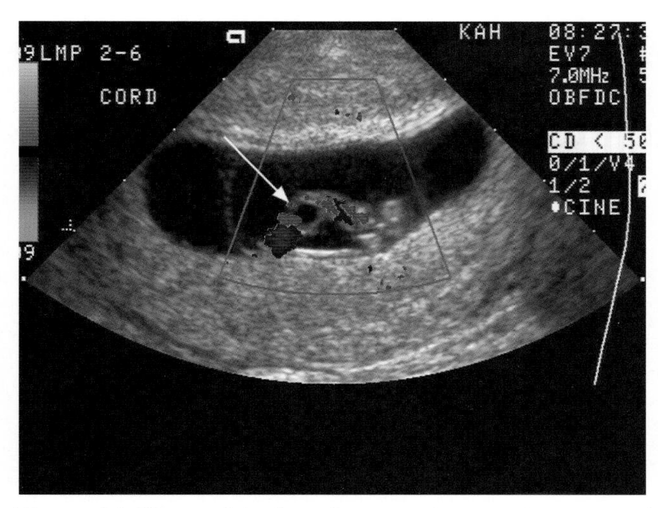

Figure 20-12 Umbilical cord cyst. Color Doppler image of umbilical cord of a 9-week embryo shows a small cyst *(arrow)* in the cord, owing to an allantoic cyst.

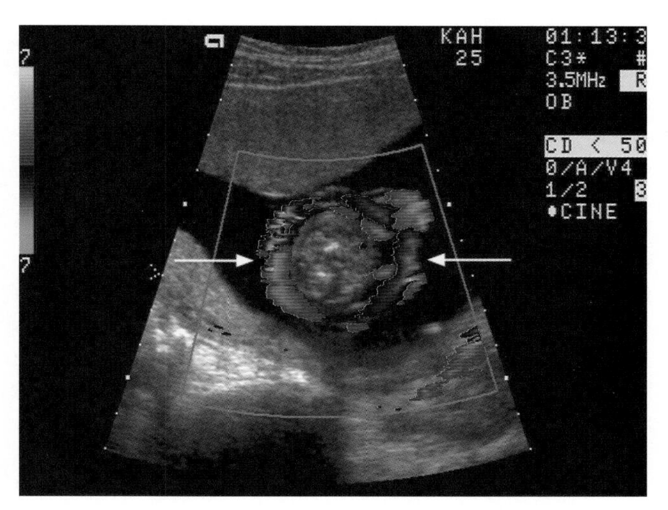

Figure 20-13 Nuchal cord. Axial color Doppler image of neck of a second-trimester fetus shows umbilical cord *(long arrows)* encircling the neck.

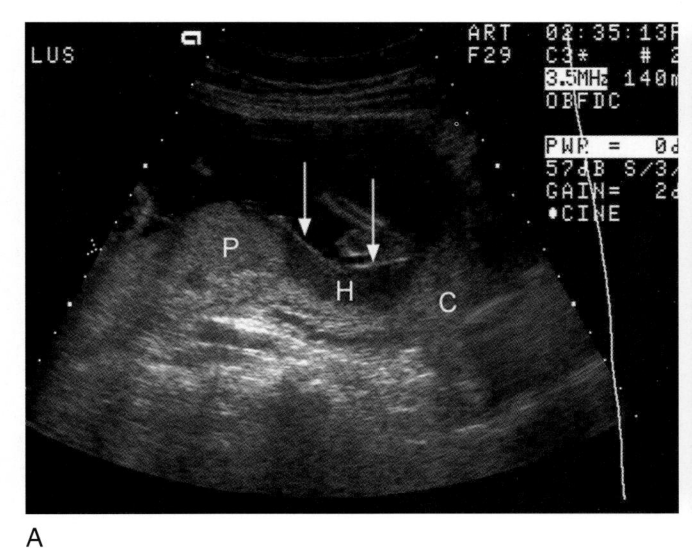

A

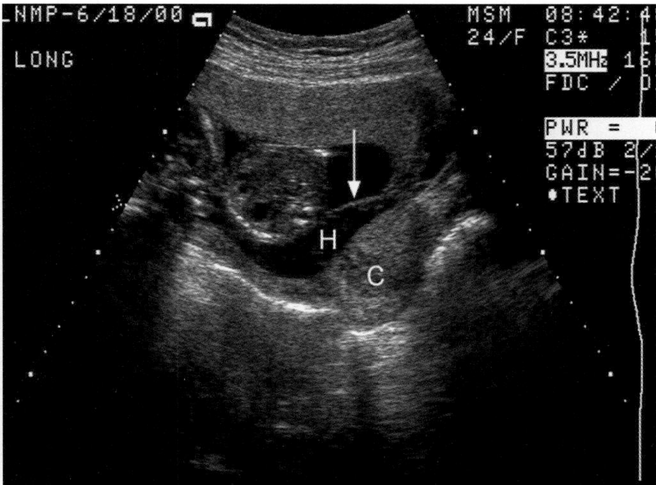

B

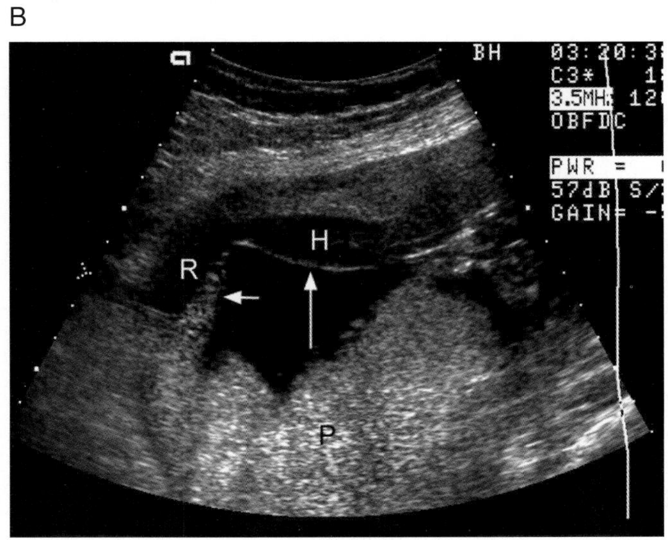

C

Figure 20-14 Examples of subchorionic hematomas during the second trimester. **A,** Longitudinal image of lower uterus shows a subchorionic hematoma (H) immediately adjacent to the placenta (P). The hematoma contains low-level echoes and is delineated by the amniochorionic membrane *(arrows).* It extends over a portion of the cervix (C). **B,** Longitudinal image of lower uterus of a patient who presented with several weeks of vaginal bleeding shows a subchorionic hematoma (H) delineated by a membrane *(arrow)* and extending over the cervix (C). Note that the hematoma is nearly completely anechoic, consistent with the chronic phase. **C,** Axial image of uterus shows a subchorionic hematoma (H) delineated by a membrane *(long arrow).* Note that although the hematoma is predominantly subchorionic, it has a smaller retroplacental component (R) that elevates the edge *(short arrow)* of the placenta (P) away from the uterine wall.

abdominal trauma or iatrogenically, either by placental puncture for the purpose of biopsy or transfusion or by an inadvertent or unavoidable placental puncture during amniocentesis. Regardless of the etiology, hemorrhages can occur in a number of sites. The most common sites are subchorionic and retroplacental. A subchorionic hematoma occurs at the margin of the placenta and extends between the chorioamnionic membrane and the uterus, elevating the chorioamnionic membrane from the uterine wall. A retroplacental hemorrhage occurs between the placenta and the uterine wall and is the site historically thought of as the location of a placental abruption (abruptio placentae). Occasionally, a hematoma will have both subchorionic and retroplacental components. The prognosis for any hemorrhage depends on its site and extent.

Blood classically evolves through three phases: hypoechoic to anechoic in the acute phase, hyperechoic and inhomogeneous as it organizes in the subacute phase, and again hypoechoic to anechoic as it lyses in the chronic phase. Because hemorrhages can clot within minutes, the first observable phase may be a subacute hemorrhage in which the blood appears hyperechoic. An occasionally helpful technique in an acute hemorrhage is to bounce the transducer directly over the suspected area. If it quivers or is compressible, then the blood has not yet organized. Rarely, blood can be seen to swirl as it enters an area of active bleeding.

Subchorionic hemorrhages are common. They usually present as vaginal bleeding but can be asymptomatic. They range from a small localized collection where the differential diagnosis is a cyst (perhaps the sequelae of prior hemorrhages) and a normal intervillous connection to a complete separation of the membranes from its attachments (Fig. 20-14). Hemorrhage can extend into the amniotic fluid (Fig. 20-15) and in the first trimester can enter and distend the endometrial canal (Fig. 20-16). Outcome after a subchorionic hematoma is often normal, although there is probably an increased chance of preterm labor and growth restriction and large first-trimester hematomas are associated with an increased risk of pregnancy loss.

Retroplacental hemorrhages can range from a small focal to a large extensive collection. An ultrasound examination can often detect the hematoma if it remains in its initial basilar position. However, if the blood dissects into other areas (Fig. 20-17), its appearance varies and if expelled may shrink so extensively that the placenta and surrounding area appears normal. In the subacute phase, the echogenicity of the hematoma may rarely be isoechoic and blend with the placenta (Fig. 20-18). Lastly, hemorrhage can recur and enlarge.

Women with retroplacental hemorrhages often present with vaginal bleeding, pelvic pain, and/or tenderness over the uterus. Although abruptions need to be considered, particularly in the predisposing clinical settings of maternal hypertension, collagen vascular disease, and abdominal trauma, these same symptomatologies can be caused by other conditions, some unrelated to the pregnancy. An incomplete list for pain includes degenerating fibroid and adnexal torsion and for bleeding includes cervical abnormalities such as polyps. Therefore, if ultrasound fails to detect a cause for the symptoms and an abruption is still a clinical possibility, a follow-up study within 2 to 4 weeks is recommended.

Doppler waveform analysis may prove of value. Umbilical artery Doppler imaging can be useful in

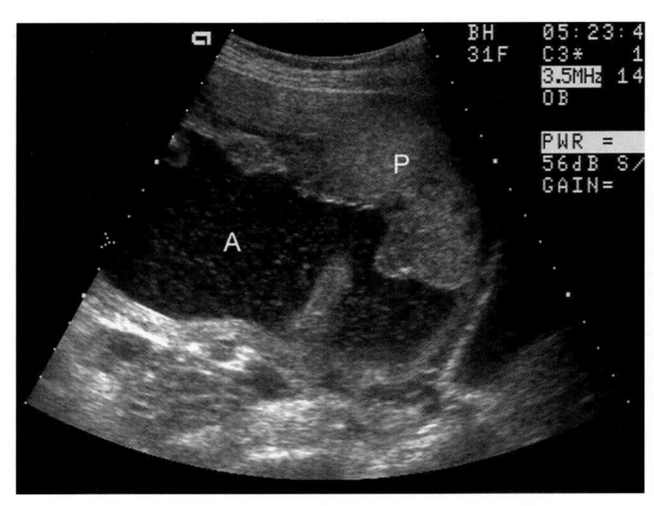

Figure 20-15 Intra-amniotic hemorrhage. Numerous echoes are seen floating in the amniotic fluid (A), corresponding to blood that extended into the amniotic cavity from a subchorionic hematoma. P, placenta.

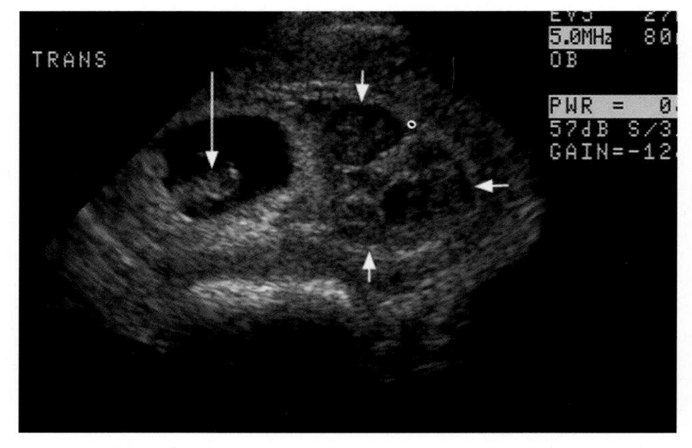

Figure 20-16 First-trimester hemorrhage distending the uterine cavity. Endovaginal ultrasound image shows a hematoma *(short arrows)* adjacent to the gestational sac, expanding the uterine cavity. A live embryo *(long arrow)* was also identified, and the pregnancy progressed normally to term.

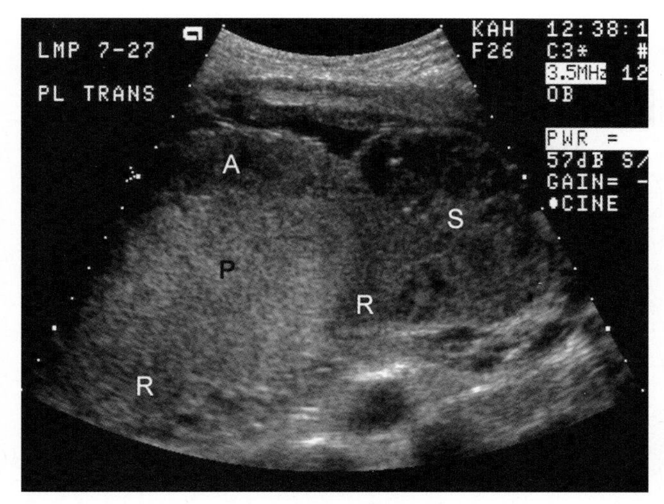

Figure 20-17 Retroplacental hemorrhage with extension beyond the retroplacental area. A large subacute hemorrhage is seen in the retroplacental region (R), elevating the edges of the placenta (P) and extending anterior to the placenta (A) and into the subchorionic space (S).

evaluating the fetus for vascular compromise (see Chapter 13). Because the maternal blood flow through the spiral arteries can be disrupted by retroplacental or intraplacental abruptions, in theory an analysis of the maternal arterial waveforms in the basilar plate would also be important. Intrafetal Doppler waveform analysis could be of use in evaluating fetal compromise. Further evaluation of the role of Doppler imaging in placental bleeding is therefore needed.

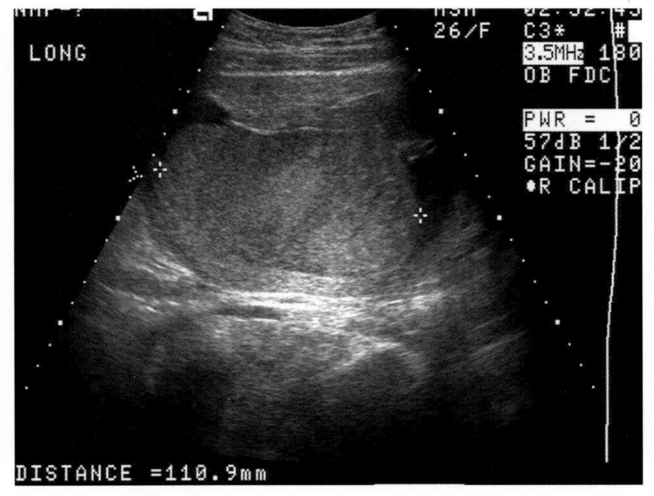

Figure 20-18 Hyperechoic hematoma indistinguishable from placenta. Longitudinal image of uterus of a 17-week gestation shows a large echogenic mass *(cursors)*. The mass is composed of a combination of placenta and hematoma from a placental abruption. The placental tissue cannot be definitely distinguished from the hematoma because they are similar in echogenicity.

Elevated maternal serum α-fetoprotein (MSAFP) levels are usually caused by inaccurate dates and less often by open structural fetal anomalies. When these have been ruled out, and particularly when the MSAFP levels are markedly elevated to greater than or equal to five multiples of the median, there remains an increased risk to the pregnancy of spontaneous loss and fetal growth restriction. The mechanism appears to be caused by increased placental permeability and in abruption has been postulated to be due to increased fetal-maternal blood connections.

PLACENTA ACCRETA, INCRETA, AND PERCRETA

The placenta normally attaches within the endometrium with the intact endometrium serving as a barrier to deeper placental (trophoblastic) extension. If the placenta attaches to a portion of the uterus where there is a deficient endometrial decidua, however, there is an increased risk for invasion to (accreta), into (increta), or through (percreta) the myometrium. This penetration anchors the placenta and at delivery prevents it from normally separating; if extensive and deep enough, this can lead to severe bleeding and even maternal demise. Although the obstetrician may attempt manual removal of the placenta, a hysterectomy is often necessary. With prior knowledge of this problem, delivery strategies can be planned to avoid an emergency operation.

Risk factors for placental invasion are prior uterine instrumentation or surgery that would have disrupted the endometrial layer. The most common risk profile is a woman with a previous cesarean section and the sonographic identification of a low-positioned anterior placenta with a placenta previa over the area of the uterine scar. Considerable attention should then be paid to the uterine hypoechoic basilar-myometrial layer, particularly in the region of the prior surgery. If this layer cannot be clearly identified or is present under one portion but not under another part of the placenta, suspicion for invasion should be heightened. The additional detection of a thinned or interrupted serosa, focal masses, and/or prominent irregular venous spaces at or near the point of invasion further suggests the presence of placental invasion (Fig. 20-19). Although the differentiation of an accreta from an increta and percreta is not currently possible, interruption of the serosal surface makes one of the latter two likely.

Transabdominal studies have shown that adequate urinary bladder distention is important to orient the anterior lower uterine segment perpendicular to the transducer so that the basilar-myometrial layer and

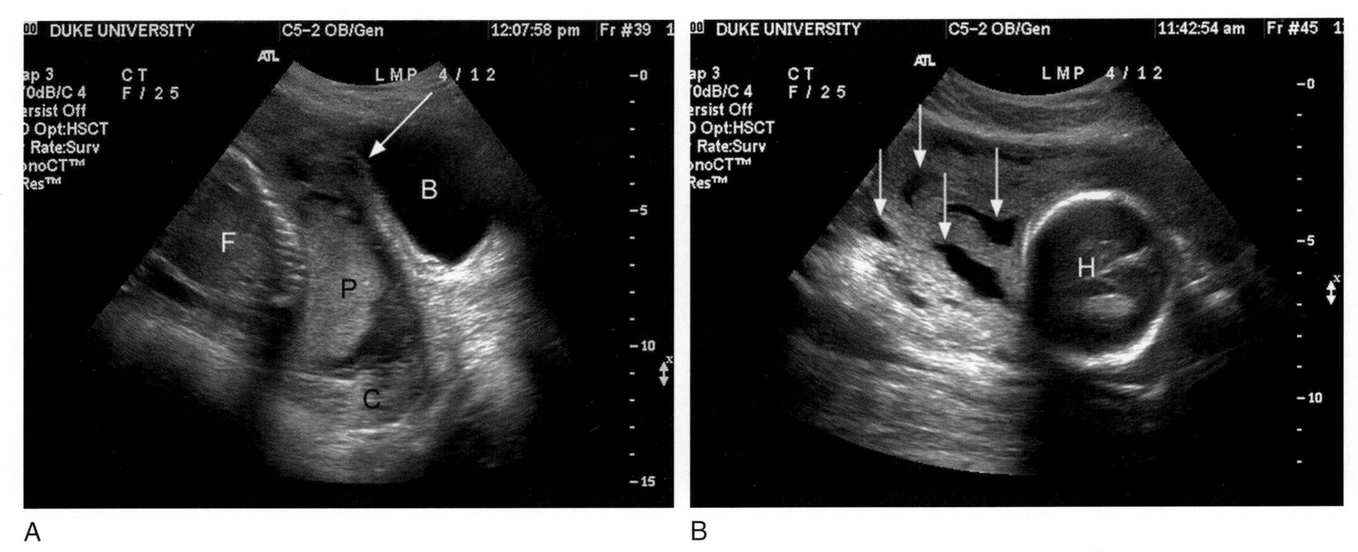

Figure 20-19 Placenta percreta. **A,** Longitudinal transabdominal image of lower uterus during the third trimester shows a complete placenta previa. The hypoechoic retroplacental basilar-myometrial layer is obliterated in the region of the prior cesarean section scar and the uterine serosa is interrupted by placental tissue *(arrow)*. The patient required an emergency cesarean hysterectomy at delivery. Histopathologic evaluation of the hysterectomy specimen confirmed placenta percreta. B, urinary bladder; P, placenta; C, cervix; F, fetus. **B,** Image of placenta of same fetus shows multiple irregular vascular spaces *(arrows)*. H, head.

serosal uterine surface can be studied. Both a transvaginal and Doppler study may be of value in equivocal cases, although they have not at present been shown to increase diagnostic accuracy.

PLACENTAL THICKNESS

Placental size, measured as thickness, normally decreases with increasing fetal age. The midportion of a normal placenta, however, should always remain thicker than 2 cm.

Abnormal placental thinning can be caused by maternal systemic vascular problems particularly associated with microinfarctions in cases of insulin-dependent diabetes and collagen vascular diseases and in severe hypertension. Because a thinned placenta could lead to insufficient fetal nutrition and oxygenation, the fetus in such circumstances should be considered at risk for growth restriction and hypoxia. False-positive diagnoses can occur in the setting of marked polyhydramnios, where the placenta is stretched and compressed along the inner surface of an enlarged uterus (Fig. 20-20).

Abnormally thickened placentas (>4 cm at its mid position) are most commonly associated with fetal hydrops, occurring in blood group incompatibilities (immune hydrops) particularly α-thalassemia, a congenital anemia, and in the congenital infections (nonimmune hydrops), particularly viral but also reported in syphilis (Fig. 20-21A and B). Gestational maternal diabetes mellitus for unknown reasons can also present as an enlarged placenta, associated with a macrosomic fetus with polyhydramnios but without signs of hydrops (see Fig. 20-21C and D). In all cases follow-up studies are indicated to assess potential fetal problems. Trophoblastic abnormalities (not to be confused with an enlarged placenta) are discussed later in the chapter.

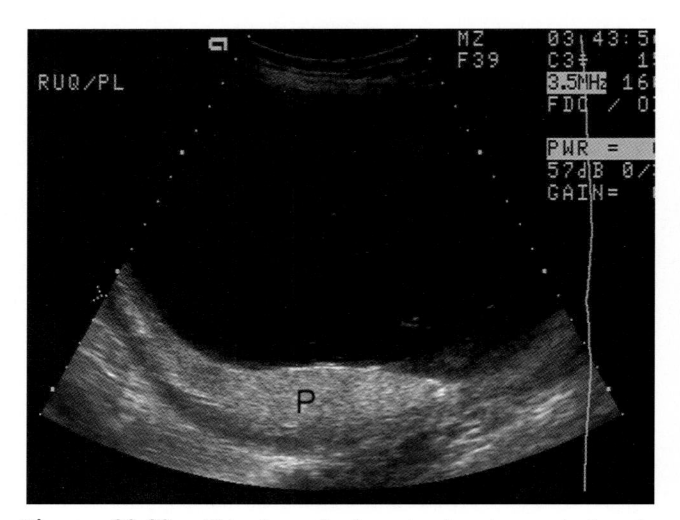

Figure 20-20 Thinning of placenta due to marked polyhydramnios. **A,** Longitudinal image of third-trimester uterus shows marked polyhydramnios. The placenta (P) appears thin because it is stretched and compressed along the inner surface of the enlarged uterus.

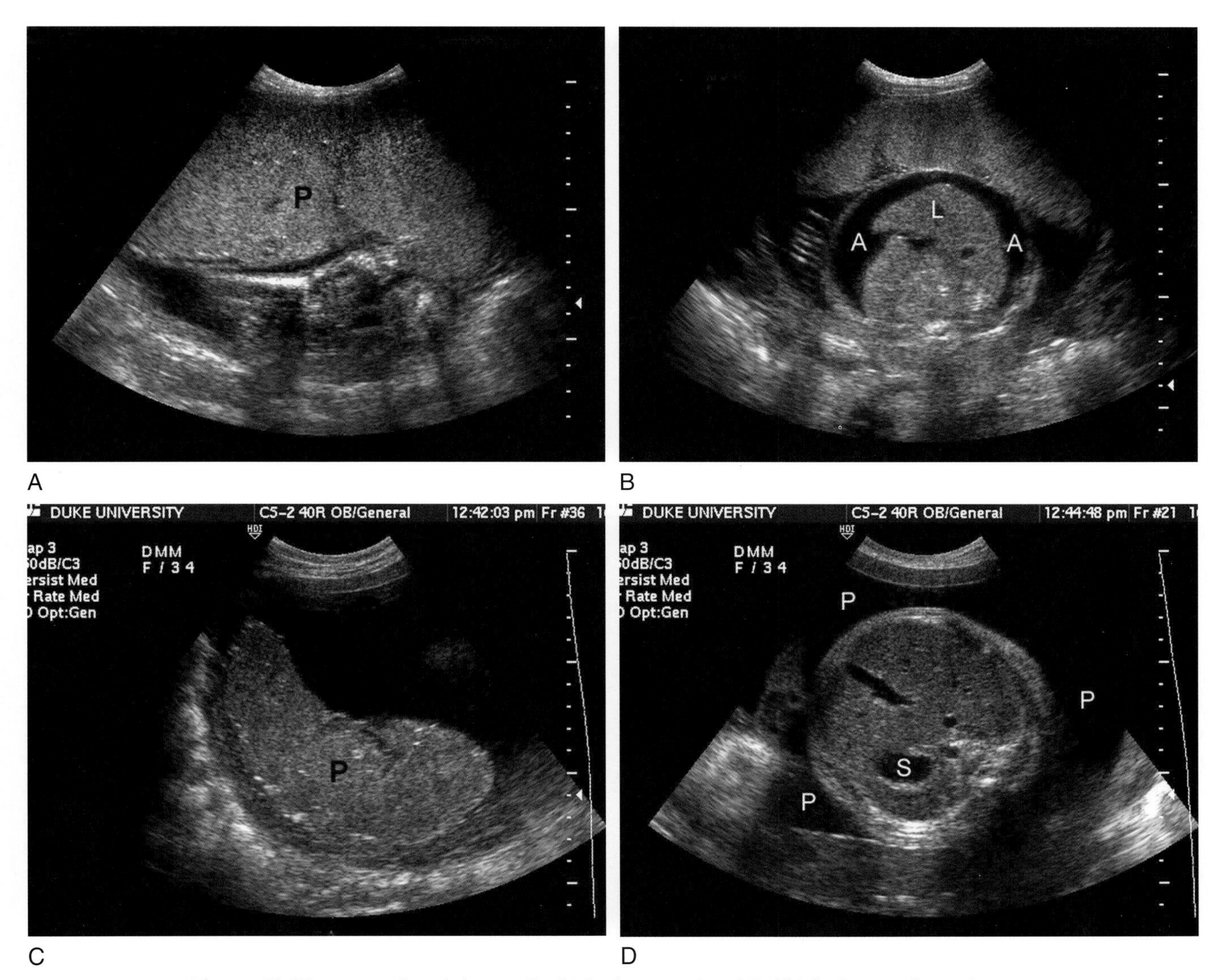

Figure 20-21 Examples of abnormally thick placentas. **A** and **B,** Thick placenta due to in utero infection. **A,** Axial image of uterus of second-trimester fetus with congenital syphilis shows marked placental thickening. P, placenta. **B,** Axial image of abdomen of same fetus as in **A** shows severe ascites (A) due to hydrops. The fetus also had a pericardial effusion. L, liver. **C** and **D,** Thick placenta due to gestational diabetes. **C,** Longitudinal image of placenta (P) during third trimester shows placental thickening. The mother had gestational diabetes. **D,** Axial image of abdomen of same fetus as in **C** shows polyhydramnios (P), also due to gestational diabetes. The fetus was large for gestational age. S, stomach.

UTERINE CONTRACTIONS

Myometrial contractions can occur at any time during pregnancy. They are more likely to be focal in the first and second trimesters, becoming more generalized (Braxton-Hicks contractions) as term approaches.

Contractions can occur any place within the uterine wall. They are typically seen as rounded "masses" that bulge into the amniotic space without changing the outer uterine contour (Fig. 20-22A). If located below the placenta, a contraction can cause the placenta to bow into the amniotic space (Fig. 20-23A). If a contraction occurs in the lower uterine segment or cervix and there is a low-positioned placenta, the placenta may appear to be falsely over the cervix with misdiagnosis of a placenta previa (Fig. 20-24).

Contractions are usually obvious. They are generally easy to differentiate from fibroids because fibroids are typically more inhomogeneous and frequently distort the outer uterine contour. However, because contractions can infrequently be inhomogeneous and rarely bulge the outer uterine contour, observing a change over time to prove that the area is a contraction

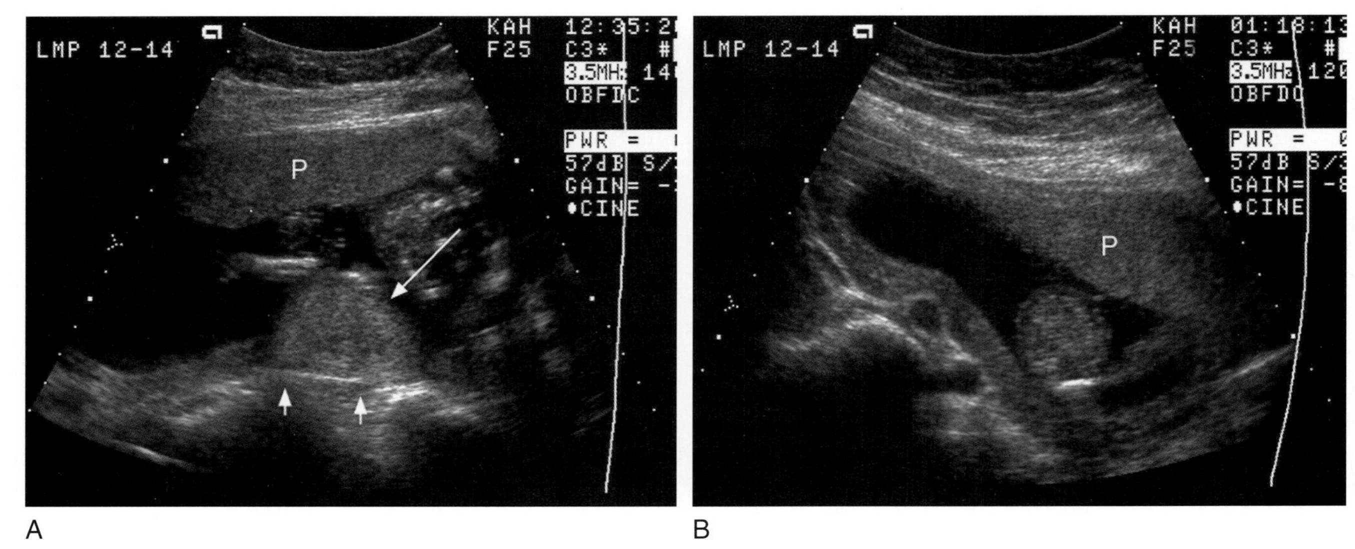

Figure 20-22 Uterine contraction. **A,** Longitudinal image of uterus at 18 weeks shows a rounded mass-like area *(long arrow)* bulging into the amniotic space, corresponding to a uterine contraction. Note that the outer uterine contour *(short arrows)* is not distorted by the contraction. P, placenta. **B,** Longitudinal image of uterus obtained 43 minutes after the image in **A** shows the contraction has resolved. Note the normal contour of the posterior uterine wall. P, placenta.

may be necessary (see Figs. 20-22B, 20-23B, and 20-24B). Contractions last variable amounts of time, rarely more than 1 hour, and a repeat study within 30 minutes often shows sufficient change to confirm the diagnosis. If a contraction persists, a longer interval of time, even a study on another day, may infrequently be needed.

PLACENTA PREVIA

Placenta previa occurs in 1 in 200 to 400 deliveries and is more common in multiparous women and women with pregnancies after a prior cesarean section. Placenta previa is a clinical diagnosis made at the time of delivery

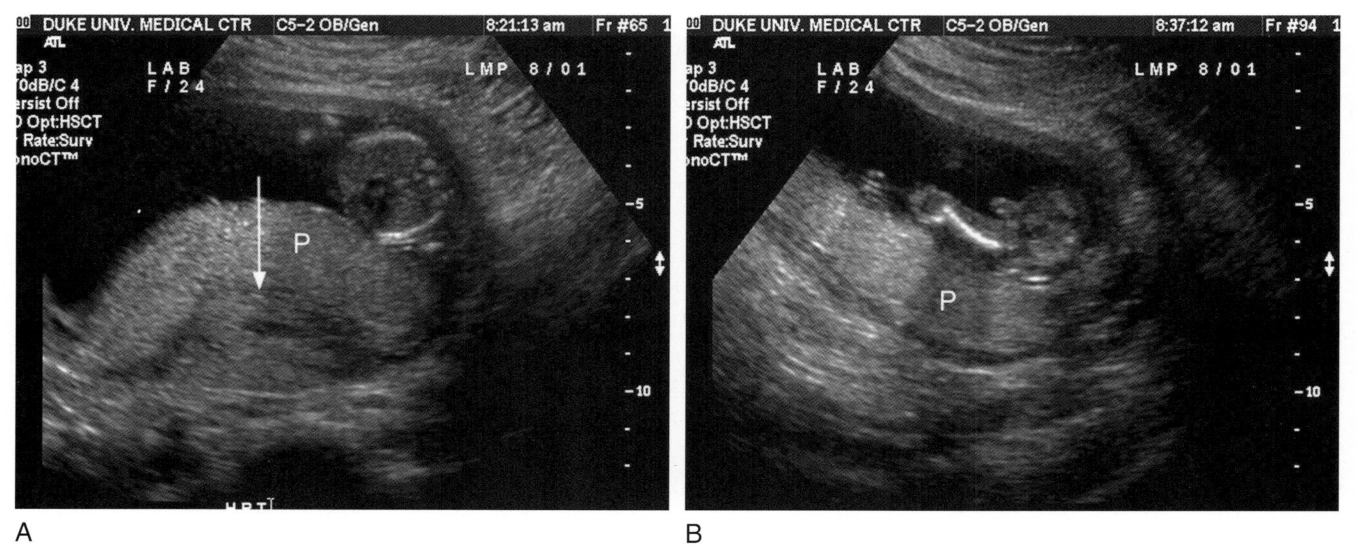

Figure 20-23 Retroplacental uterine contraction. **A,** Axial image of uterus of a 16-week gestation shows a retroplacental uterine contraction *(arrow)* that causes the placenta (P) to bulge into the amniotic cavity. **B,** Corresponding image obtained 14 minutes after the scan in **A** shows the contraction has resolved and the placenta (P) conforms to the normal contour of the amniotic cavity.

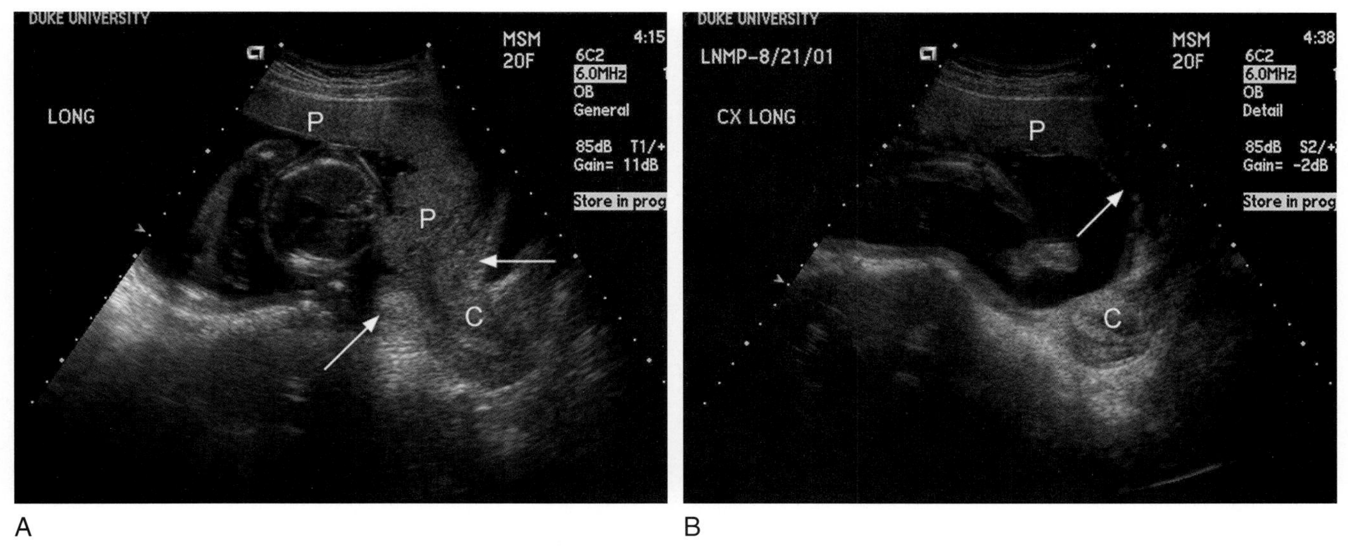

Figure 20-24 Spurious appearance of placenta previa due to lower uterine contraction. **A,** Longitudinal image of lower uterus shows placental tissue (P) extending over apparent region of cervix (C). Note, however, the presence of a circumferential contraction *(arrows)* in the lower uterus. **B,** Image of the lower uterus obtained 23 minutes later, after the contraction has resolved, shows lower edge *(arrow)* of placenta (P) is located far from the cervix (C).

and defined as the position of the placenta in relation to the dilated and effaced cervix. By palpation and visualization, the placenta is found to encroach on the dilated external os in one of three ways: in a marginal previa it extends to the edge of the os, in a partial previa it partially covers the os, and in a complete previa the os is totally covered.

These terms have been modified to make them applicable for ultrasound diagnosis in the second and third trimesters before the cervix dilates (Fig. 20-25). In a nondilated cervix, three ultrasound-based definitions are used in relation to the closed internal cervical os: a low-lying placenta where the placenta approaches but does not cover the os (Fig. 20-26A), a marginal (or partial) previa in which the placenta extends to the edge but does not cross the os (Fig. 20-26B), and a complete previa where the placenta crosses over and covers the internal os (Fig. 20-26C and D). Complete placenta previa can be further subdivided into two types. Asymmetric complete placenta previa occurs when the placenta is eccentrically situated over the internal cervical os, completely covering the os (Fig. 20-26C), whereas central complete placenta previa indicates the central portion of the placenta is implanted over the internal cervical os (Fig. 20-26D).

The definitions of all these terms are somewhat inexact. A low-lying placenta is often suggested when the lower margin of the placenta is within 2 cm of the internal os. The distinction between a marginal and a partial previa is too subtle, and these terms may be used interchangeably in utero. Lastly, the distinction between

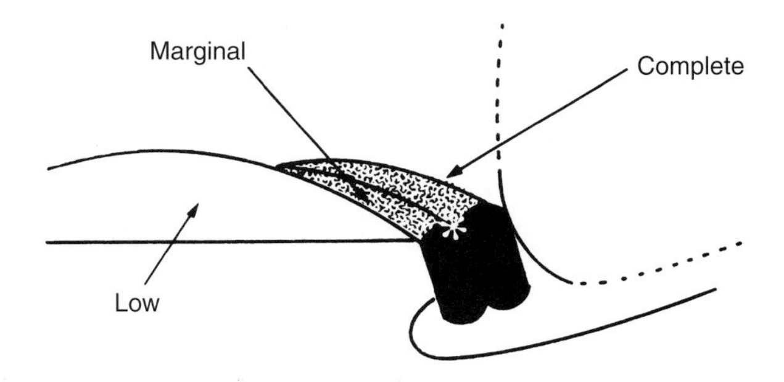

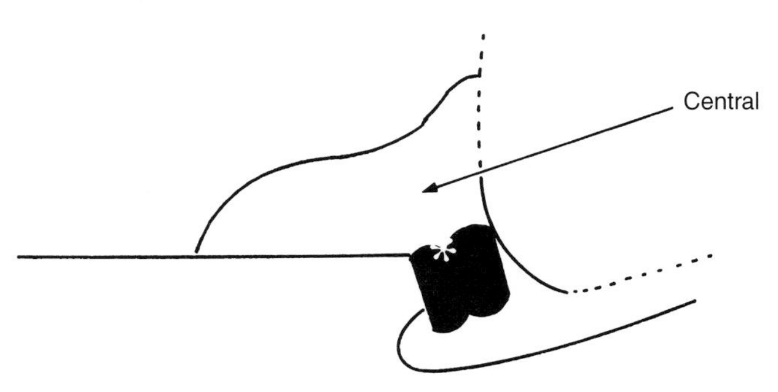

Figure 20-25 In utero representation of a low-lying placenta and of three types of placenta previa. The upper diagram shows a low-lying placenta and both a marginal and complete placenta previa in relation to the closed cervix (shown in black with an *asterisk* at the internal os). The lower diagram shows a central previa.

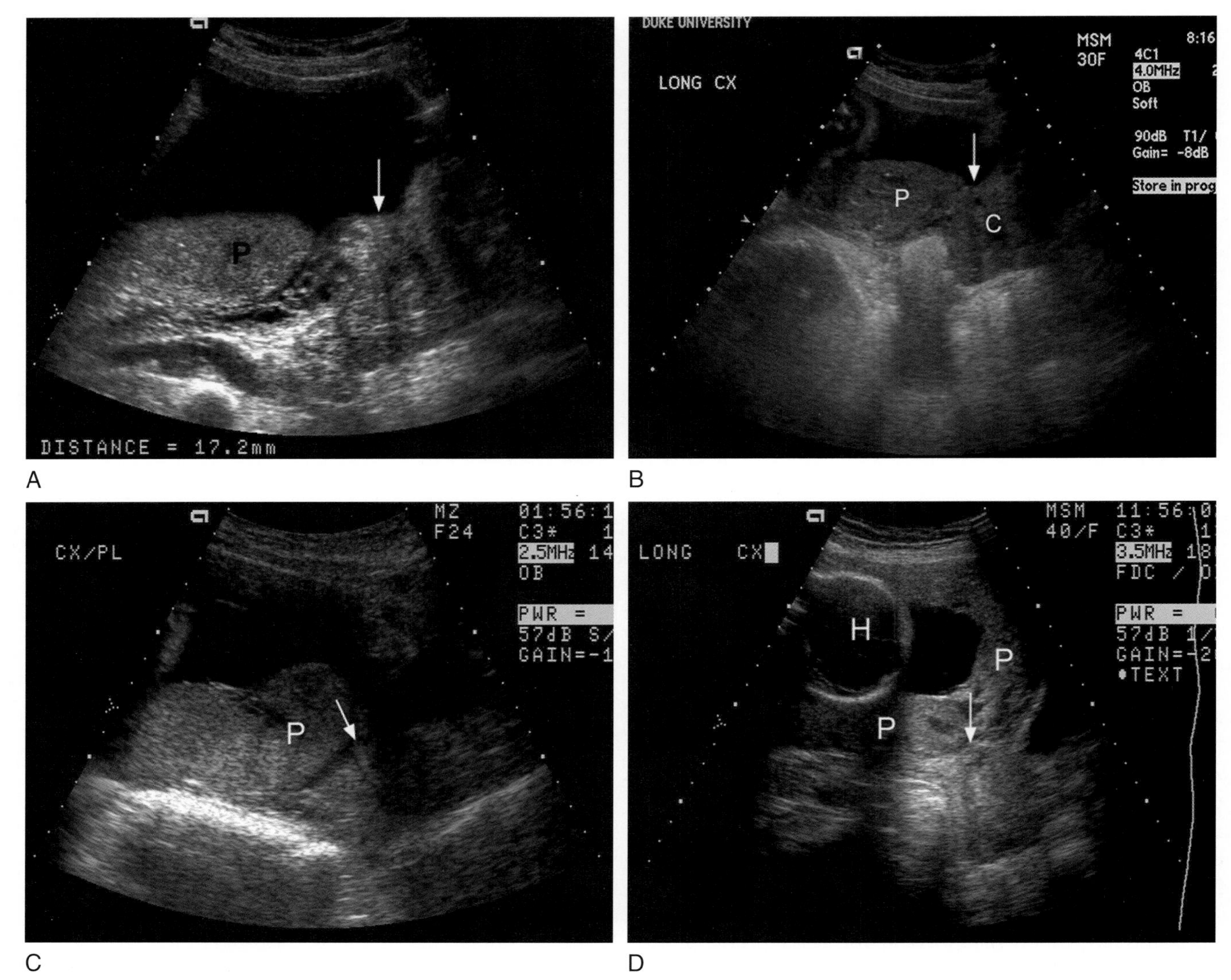

Figure 20-26 Placenta previa: examples of various grades of severity. **A,** Low-lying placenta without placenta previa. Transabdominal ultrasound image of lower uterus at 24 weeks shows a posterior placenta (P) implanted low in the uterus but not overlying the cervix. Distance between the lower edge of the placenta and the internal cervical os *(arrow)* was 1.7 cm. **B,** Marginal placental previa. Transabdominal image at 34 weeks shows a posterior placenta (P) that extends over a portion of the cervix (C) but does not cross the internal cervical os *(arrow)*. **C,** Complete placenta previa. Transabdominal scan at 29 weeks shows a posterior placenta (P) completely covering the internal cervical os *(arrow)*. Note that although the placenta covers the os, it is asymmetrically implanted in the lower uterus. **D,** Complete central placenta previa. Transabdominal image of lower uterus at 28 weeks shows the central portion of the placenta (P) implanted over and completely covering the internal cervical os *(arrow)*. H, fetal head.

a marginal and a complete previa is often not clear. These subtleties may not be important, however, because in these cases at least one follow-up study is indicated later in the pregnancy.

Two questions need answering. Because the cervix is closed (neither dilated nor effaced) during pregnancy, can ultrasound accurately detect a placenta previa? If a placenta previa is detected in utero, can ultrasound predict whether it will be present at birth? The answer to both questions is "yes," provided a proper scanning technique is used and trophotropism is taken into account.

The cervix must be visualized to properly evaluate for placenta previa. A full urinary bladder can serve as a sonic window that displaces the fetus cephalad, but a full bladder is not necessary to perform this assessment. Three empty-bladder techniques are also available and include transabdominal (TA), transvaginal (TV), and translabial (TL, also called transperineal) approaches. At any time in the pregnancy and using any of these four techniques, visualization of the cervix without placental tissue overlying it ensures that a previa will not be present during that pregnancy. The finding of a placenta positioned superior to the lower uterine segment without direct visualization of the cervix suggests there is no placenta previa but does not completely rule it out because it does not exclude the possibility of a succenturiate lobe of placenta overlying the cervix.

By the TA full urinary bladder technique, the following applies:

1. The internal os is better seen in the second trimester because the fetus is small relative to the amount of amniotic fluid. As the pregnancy progresses, the fetus becomes relatively larger and frequently obscures this region.
2. "Too much" placental tissue or "elevation" of the fetal parts in the lower uterine segment, or both, suggests a low-lying placenta and possible previa.
3. The distended bladder can compress and elongate both the cervix and the lower uterine segment, making them appear as an elongated cervix. A low-lying placenta can then falsely appear to cover the cervix (Fig. 20-27A).

If the initial evaluation is done with a full bladder and there is no placenta previa, previa is excluded. If, however, there appears to be a placenta previa but the bladder was full, the examination should be repeated after the bladder is empty (see Fig. 20-27B). This can be done by scanning through the amniotic fluid in a sagittal view angled downward from just below the umbilicus, or using TV or TL ultrasound. With the bladder empty the cervix often assumes a more vertical orientation at TA ultrasound analysis. Because the cervix can often be seen with an empty bladder, and a distended bladder can create a spurious appearance of placenta previa, many practices do not require a full bladder for obstetric ultrasound examinations.

If for either technical or anatomic reasons a placenta previa is still not ruled out, a TL or TV examination or a follow-up ultrasound study should be performed (Figs. 20-28 and 20-29). With an empty urinary bladder, a midline sagittal scan can almost always identify the internal cervical os and lower uterine segment and is therefore the only image needed to determine the presence of previa. Most observers favor the TV examination. Even in cases of active bleeding, a suspected previa, or a cervical abnormality, when care should be taken not to insert the probe too close to the external os, the TV study is not contraindicated. Although the TL examination is less invasive, visualization of the cervix during the TL examination may be suboptimal because the caudal portion of the cervix is often obscured by shadowing from bowel gas (see Fig. 20-28B), and a lower-frequency transducer than used during TV sonography must be employed. Despite these limitations, the TL examination is often diagnostic.

Because trophotropism can cause significant changes in placental position, a previa is usually not formally diagnosed before 20 weeks unless symptoms are present. When detected after 20 weeks in an asymptomatic

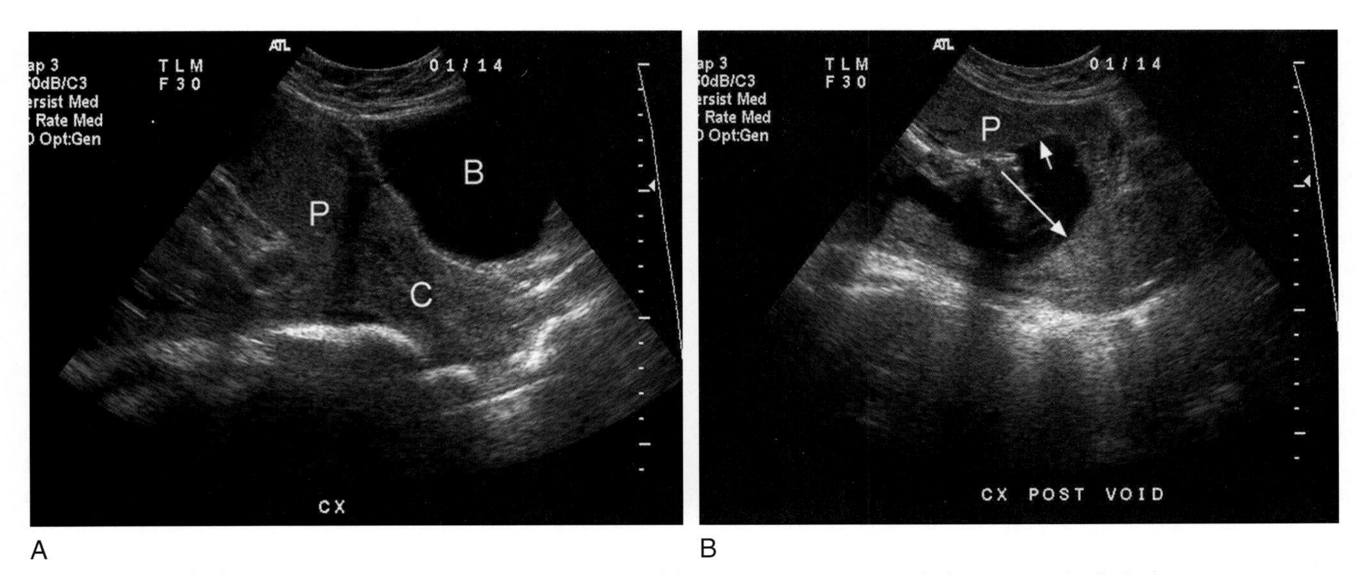

Figure 20-27 Full urinary bladder causing false-positive appearance of placenta previa. **A,** Longitudinal transabdominal ultrasound image of lower uterus obtained when the maternal urinary bladder (B) was full shows placental tissue (P) appears to cover the cervix (C). **B,** Corresponding image obtained after the patient emptied her bladder shows the lower edge *(short arrow)* of her anterior placenta (P) ends far from the internal cervical os *(long arrow)*.

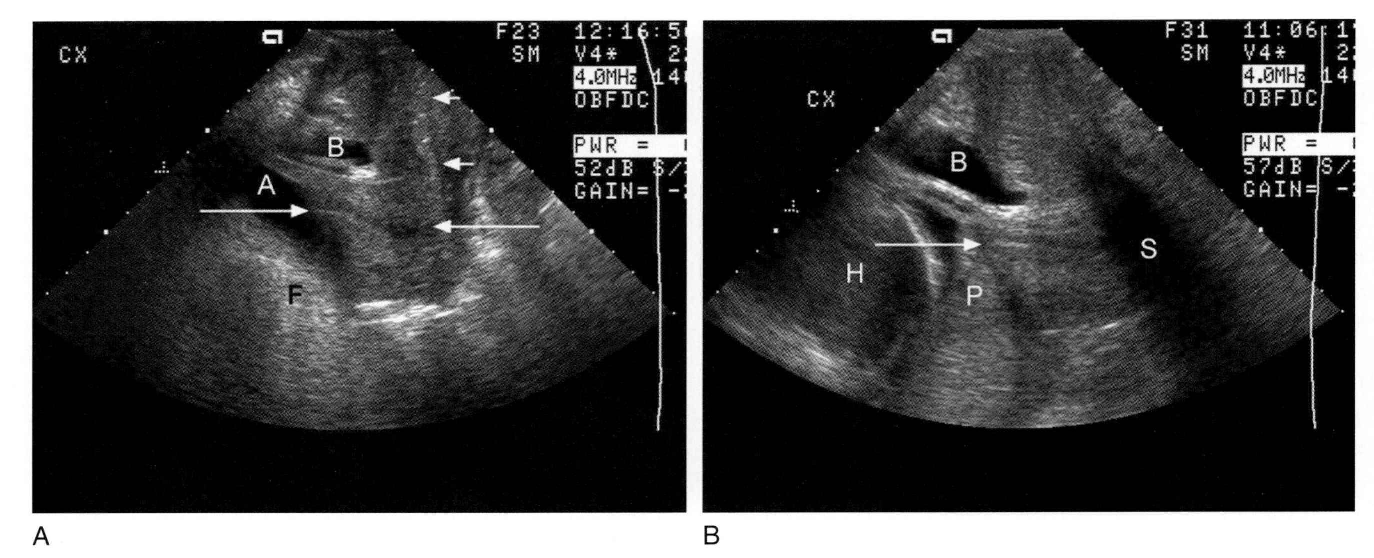

A B

Figure 20-28 Translabial ultrasound evaluation for placenta previa. **A,** No placenta previa. Sagittal translabial ultrasound image at 36 weeks shows amniotic fluid (A) overlying the internal surface of the cervix. The placenta was located in the uterine fundus, superior to the field of view. B, urinary bladder; F, fetal buttock; *long arrows,* endocervical canal; *short arrows,* vagina. **B,** Complete asymmetric placenta previa. Sagittal translabial ultrasound image at 27 weeks shows a posterior placenta (P) completely covering the internal cervical os *(arrow).* Note that only a thin segment of the inferior edge of the placenta overlies the cervix, consistent with an asymmetric complete placenta previa. The caudal portion of the cervix is obscured by shadowing (S) from gas in the rectum. Although this shadowing prevents accurate measurement of cervical length, the study is diagnostic for placenta previa because the internal surface of the cervix is well seen and is not obscured by shadowing. B, bladder; H, fetal head.

woman, a follow-up study should be performed at approximately 32 weeks (within 2 months of delivery) to determine if the previa is still present. If a woman is symptomatic, particularly vaginal bleeding, more frequent ultrasound studies are often necessary.

Blood vessels can be detected over the internal cervical os. Most are at the margins of a low-positioned placenta and are an admixture of fetal and maternal blood (Fig. 20-30). They are caused by juxtaplacental or marginal sinus blood vessels and should be treated clinically similar to a placenta previa. If, instead, blood vessels of a velamentous umbilical cord insertion or blood vessels extending between a succenturiate lobe and the main lobe of the placenta cross the internal os, this is called a vasa previa. These vessels are from the fetal circulation and can lead to significant fetal blood loss and fetal death at the time of rupture of membranes or delivery. They can be confirmed by Doppler examination (Fig. 20-31).

THE CERVIX AND EVALUATION FOR CERVICAL INCOMPETENCE

Ultrasound is able to identify the cervix and to evaluate it for incompetence or evidence of preterm labor. This analysis is important because cervical incompetence increases the risk of preterm loss or delivery. Incompetent cervix is defined as painless preterm dilatation of the cervix in the absence of uterine contractions. Both the appearance and measurement of the cervix are important. A midline sagittal view is the optimal image for evaluating the cervix and for identifying the internal os, the endocervical canal, and often the external os (Fig. 20-32).

Measured along its endocervical canal, the normal cervix averages 4.0 cm in length. From 20 weeks onward, the lowest acceptable normal length is 3.0 cm. There has been a debate about the length to be considered significantly (pathologically) shortened, with many institutions now using less than or equal to 2.5 cm (Table 20-1). The length of the nondistorted cervix, measured along the endocervical canal from the internal to external os, should typically be no longer than 5 cm.

Occasionally, only shortening of the cervical length is seen in cervical incompetence (Fig. 20-33A). More commonly, the incompetent cervix begins with dilatation of the internal os. The endocervical canal dilates next, causing "funneling" of the cervix and shortening the length of the remaining closed cervix (see Fig. 20-33B). The severity of funneling can be measured as % funneling, equal to the length of the open portion of the cervix measured from the internal os to the closed portion (O), divided by the length of the open portion (O) plus the length of the remaining closed

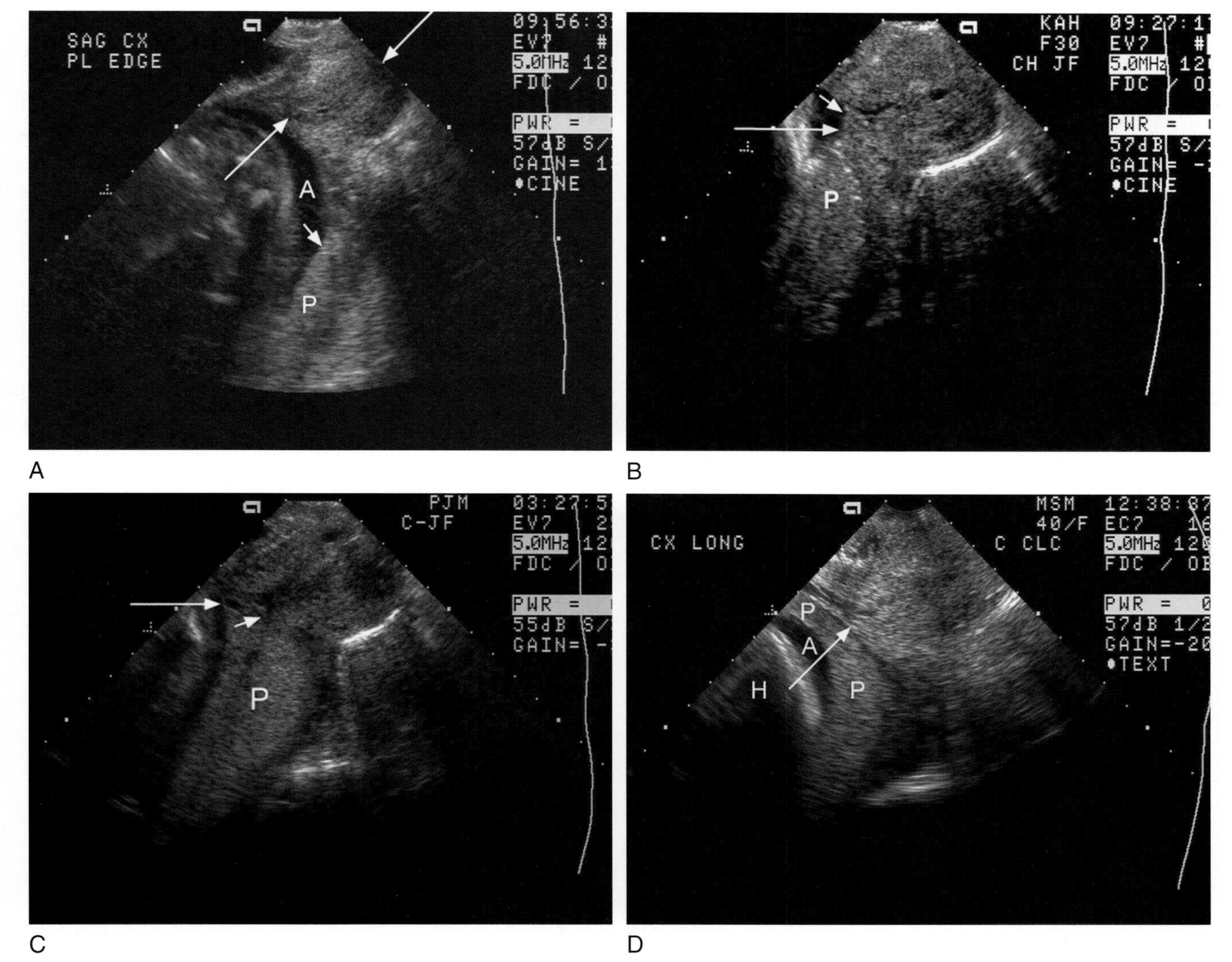

Figure 20-29 Transvaginal ultrasound evaluation for placenta previa. **A,** No placenta previa. Sagittal transvaginal ultrasound image at 23 weeks shows amniotic fluid (A) overlying the internal surface of the cervix. The lower edge *(short arrow)* of the placenta (P) ends above the level of the cervix. *Long arrows,* endocervical canal. **B,** Marginal placenta previa. Sagittal transvaginal ultrasound scan at 34 weeks shows the lower edge *(long arrow)* of the placenta (P) covering a portion of the cervix but not overlying the internal cervical os *(short arrow).* **C,** Complete asymmetric placenta previa. Sagittal transvaginal ultrasound image at 29 weeks shows a narrow segment of the lower edge *(long arrow)* of the placenta (P) completely covering the internal cervical os *(short arrow).* **D,** Complete central placenta previa. Axial ultrasound at 33 weeks shows placenta (P) centrally implanted over the cervix. *Arrow,* internal cervical os; A, amniotic fluid; H, fetal head.

endocervical canal (C) times 100. Hence, % funneling = $[O/(O + C) \times 100]$.

The timing of the examination may not be as important as initially thought. Originally in nulliparous women it was believed that the cervix should remain closed until the start of labor; conversely, in multiparous women the cervix might begin to dilate in the third trimester. If true, then the distinction between a normal cervix and true incompetence might not be possible in multiparous women. This concept, however, is controversial. Some observers now believe that the cervix should not dilate in any pregnancy until the start of normal labor and that the endocervical length should always be greater than or equal to 2.5 cm, regardless of both the time in the pregnancy and the past obstetrical history.

The cervical length is reported as the shortest endocervical length observed during the course of the full ultrasound examination. When there is funneling of the internal os, the length of the intact segment of cervix caudal to the funneled area should be measured

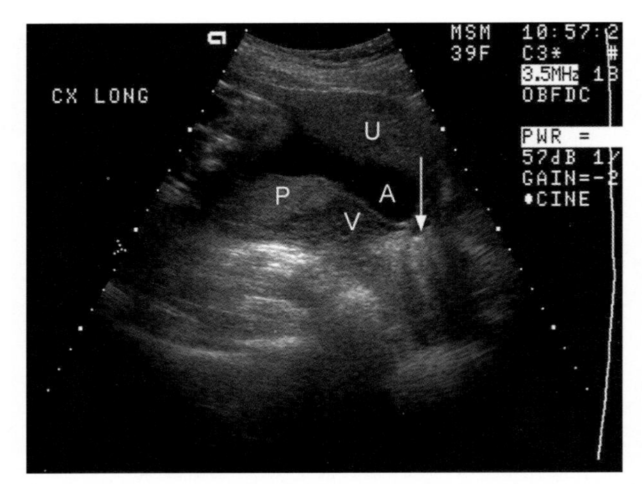

Figure 20-30 Juxtaplacental or marginal sinus blood vessels extending over cervix. Midline sagittal transabdominal scan of lower edge of placenta (P) and cervix shows blood vessels (V) crossing from the lower edge of the placenta over the internal cervical os *(arrow)*. Blood could be seen moving within these vessels during real-time evaluation. A, amniotic fluid; U, uterine contraction.

(see Fig. 20-33C). Gentle pressure can be applied to the uterine fundus during cervical scanning to determine if fundal pressure causes changes in the length or configuration of the cervix (Fig. 20-34). Although the full significance of cervical opening with fundal pressure is not certain, it is also considered abnormal. Likewise, the cervix is considered abnormal if it initially appears normal but spontaneously develops funneling and/or shortening during the period of observation (Fig. 20-35).

In the most severe cases of cervical incompetence, the endocervical canal dilates completely and is replaced by anechoic amniotic fluid. Fetal parts and the umbilical cord can then descend into the dilated cervix. If the cervix is maximally dilated, the entire endocervical canal opens to the external os and an "hourglass" deformity occurs in which the amniotic membranes are seen clinically to bulge into the vagina (Fig. 20-36). In these cases the appearance of the cervix, not its measurement, is most important because funneling is complete.

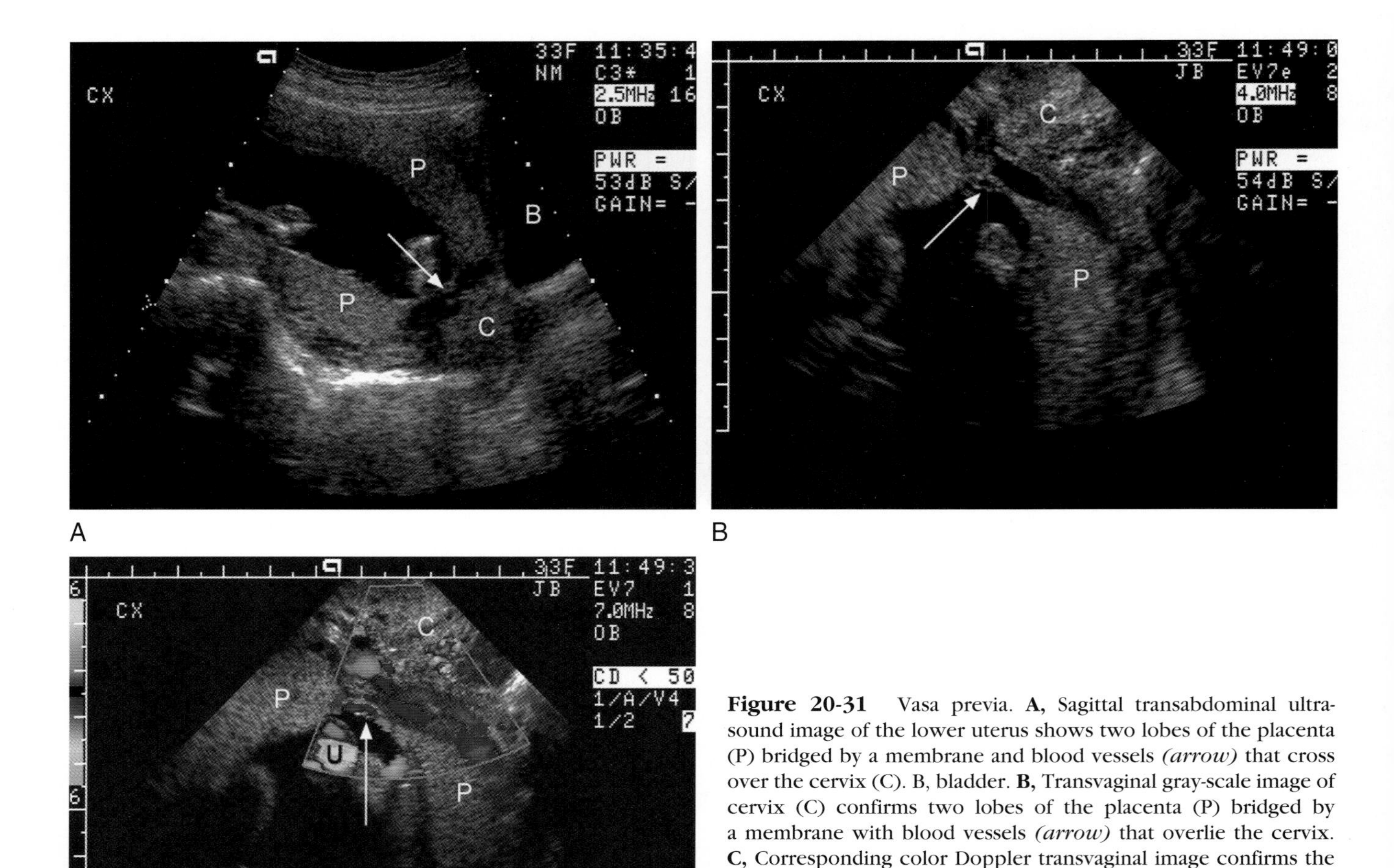

Figure 20-31 Vasa previa. **A,** Sagittal transabdominal ultrasound image of the lower uterus shows two lobes of the placenta (P) bridged by a membrane and blood vessels *(arrow)* that cross over the cervix (C). B, bladder. **B,** Transvaginal gray-scale image of cervix (C) confirms two lobes of the placenta (P) bridged by a membrane with blood vessels *(arrow)* that overlie the cervix. **C,** Corresponding color Doppler transvaginal image confirms the presence of blood vessels *(arrow)* overlying the cervix (C) and bridging the placental lobes (P). U, umbilical cord.

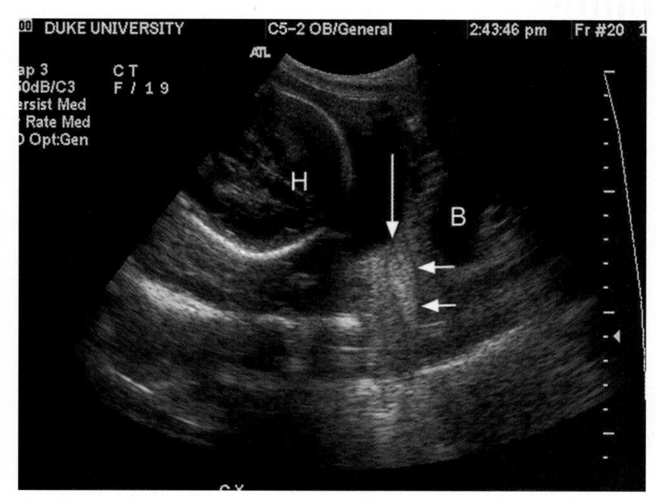

Figure 20-32 Normal cervix. Midline sagittal transabdominal image at 28 weeks shows normal appearance of cervix. *Long arrow,* internal cervical os; *short arrows,* endocervical canal; B, bladder; H, fetal head.

Table 20-1 Cervical (Endocervical) Length*	
Diagnosis	**Cervical Length (cm)**
Upper limit of normal	5.0
Average	4.0
Lower limit of normal	3.0
Pathologically decreased	2.5

*Measurement of the nondistorted cervix should be obtained using an empty maternal bladder technique, preferably transvaginal. The cervical (endocervical) length is measured along the endocervical canal, from the external to internal cervical os. If incompetence with funneling is noted, the remaining closed portion of the cervix along the endocervical canal to the external os should instead be measured.

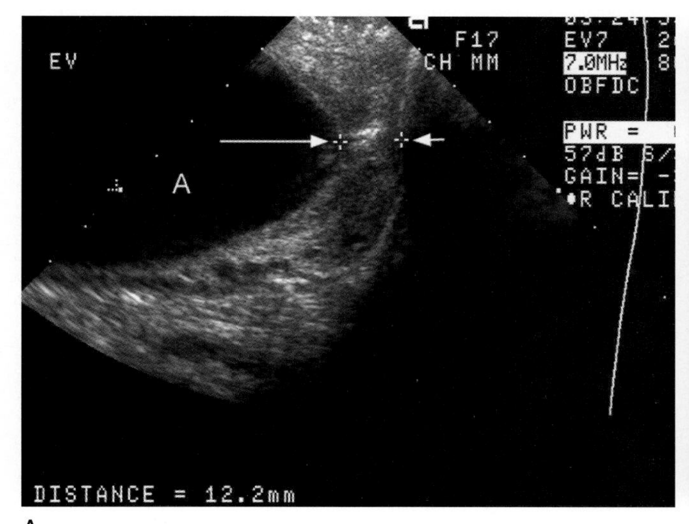

A

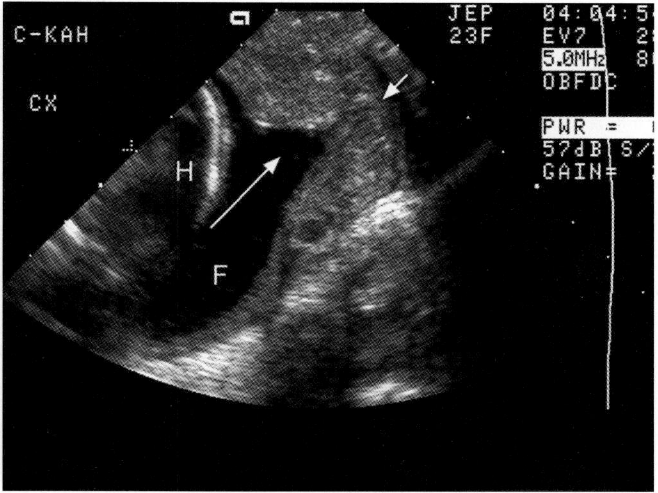

B

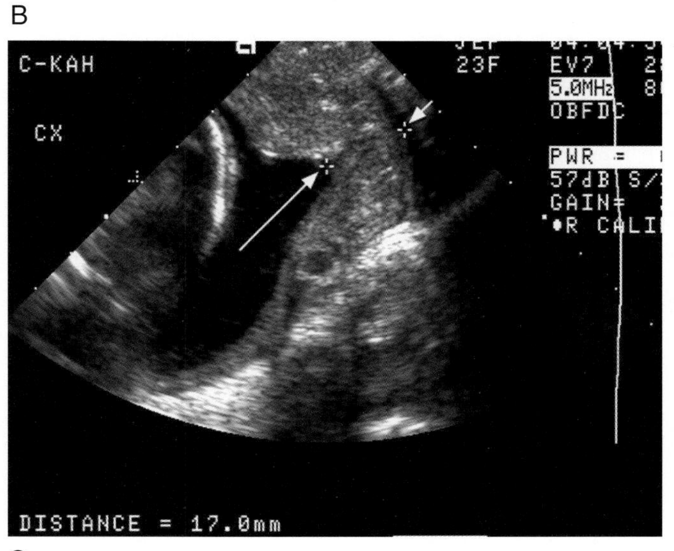

C

Figure 20-33 Examples of cervical incompetence. **A,** Midline sagittal transvaginal scan at 28 weeks shows a short cervix. Measurement calipers are positioned on the internal *(long arrow)* and external *(short arrow)* cervical os, and the corresponding measurement of 1.2 cm is abnormally short. A, amniotic fluid. **B,** Midline sagittal transvaginal ultrasound at 19 weeks shows "funneling" *(long arrow)* of the internal cervical os and endocervical canal. *Short arrow,* external os; F, amniotic fluid; H, fetal head. **C,** Technique to measure cervical length in same patient as in **B** with funneling of the internal cervical os. Note that electronic measurement calipers have been positioned at the inferior margin of the funneled area *(long arrow)* and on the external cervical os *(short arrow)* to measure the length of the intact segment of the cervix.

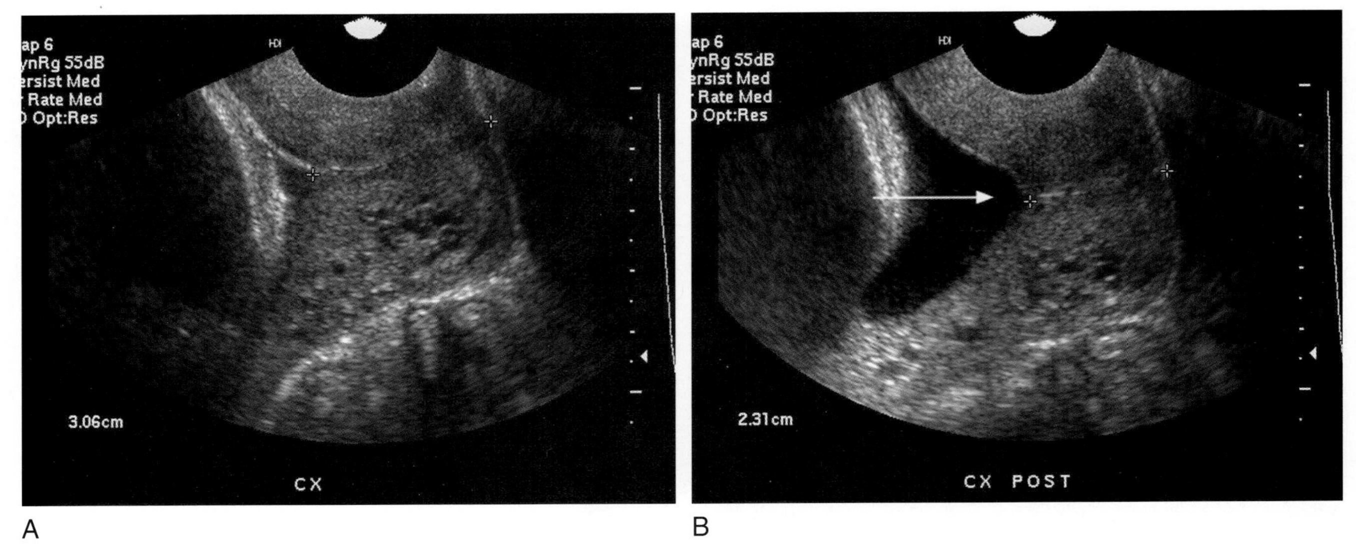

Figure 20-34 Fundal pressure causing cervical shortening. **A,** Midline sagittal transvaginal image of cervix at 26 weeks obtained before fundal pressure shows electronic calipers positioned on the cervix to measure cervical length. Cervical length of 3.1 cm is normal. **B,** Image of same cervix as in **A** obtained after fundal pressure shows decrease in cervical length to 2.3 cm and development of funneling of the internal cervical os *(arrow)* in response to fundal pressure.

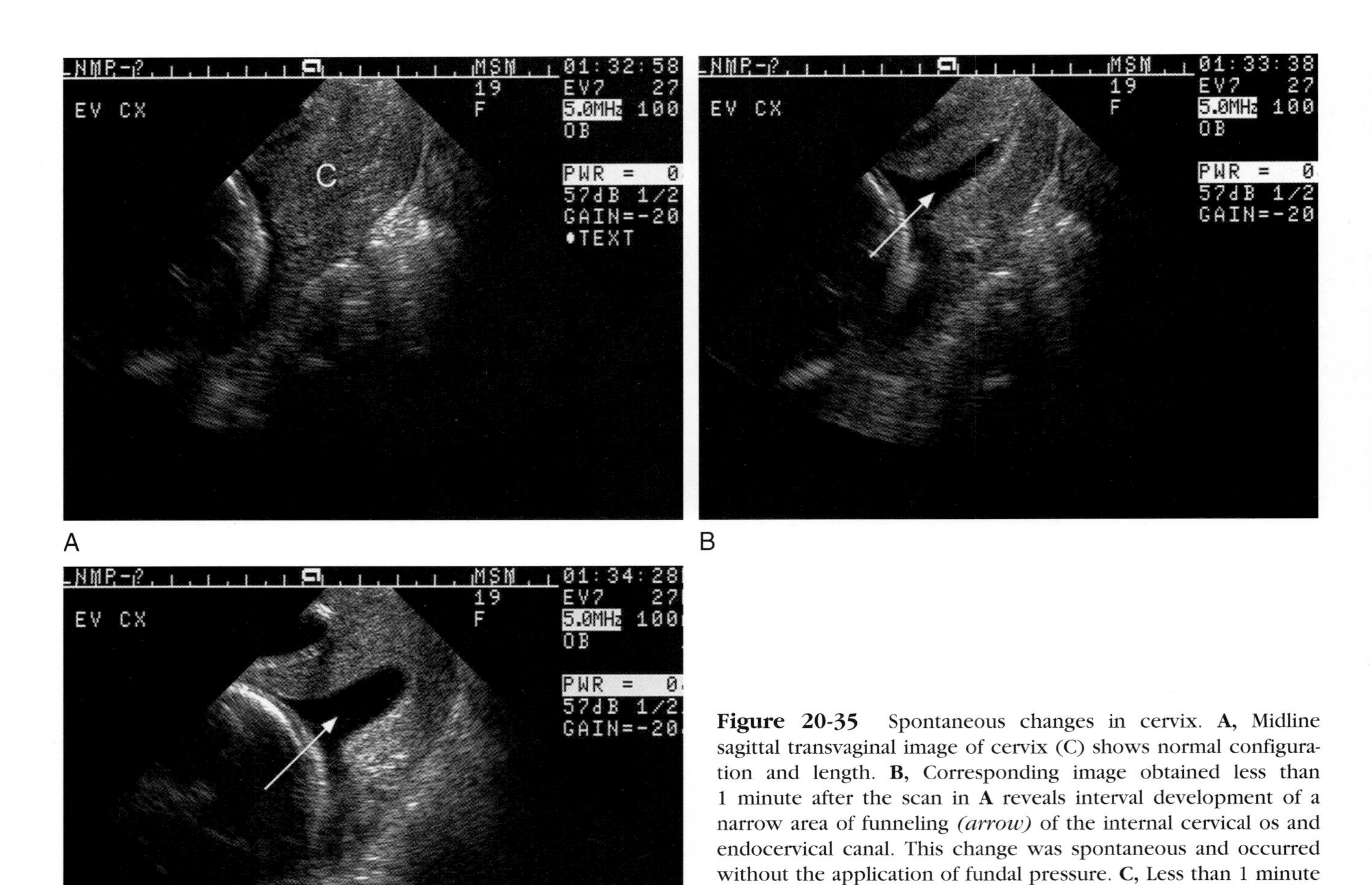

Figure 20-35 Spontaneous changes in cervix. **A,** Midline sagittal transvaginal image of cervix (C) shows normal configuration and length. **B,** Corresponding image obtained less than 1 minute after the scan in **A** reveals interval development of a narrow area of funneling *(arrow)* of the internal cervical os and endocervical canal. This change was spontaneous and occurred without the application of fundal pressure. **C,** Less than 1 minute after the image in **B**, the funneled segment *(arrow)* has become wider and more prominent.

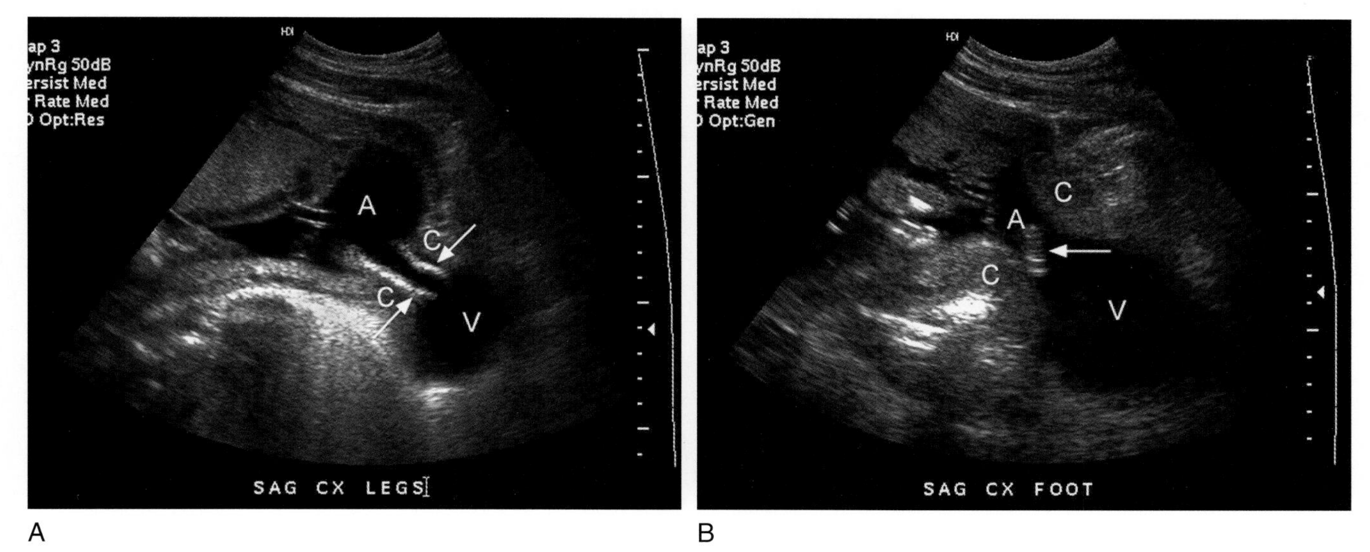

Figure 20-36 Hourglass configuration of amniotic cavity due to membranes bulging through dilated external cervical os. **A,** Midline sagittal transabdominal scan at 22 weeks shows completely dilated cervix (C) with amniotic fluid (A) bulging through the cervix into the vagina. V, component of amniotic cavity in vagina; *arrows,* fetal legs in endocervical canal. **B,** Corresponding image performed approximately 30 minutes after the image in **A** shows fetal foot *(arrow)* in the endocervical canal and increased amniotic fluid in the vagina (V). C, dilated cervix.

When advanced cervical incompetence is detected, with the cervix completely open and an "hourglass" configuration to the amniotic cavity in the lower uterus, cervix, and vagina, the obstetrician should be notified immediately. Ideally, the patient should be placed in reverse Trendelenburg position. In the event of an hourglass dilatation, however, spontaneous pregnancy loss is usually imminent.

Correlation between the clinical examination and the ultrasound findings is not always possible. This is understandable when one considers the different approaches of the two examinations. On physical examination the external os is identified and palpated, with the incompetent "soft" cervix diagnosed by the introduction of a finger through the external os. Sonographically, opening of the internal os or shortening of the cervical length are the first imaging findings of incompetence. When these two examinations are in agreement, treatment options are clear. When they are discrepant, treatment decisions are often based on past pregnancy history and the severity of all the findings.

The TA full-bladder technique is often sufficient to make the diagnosis of incompetence. However, on occasion an incompetent cervix may appear normal or its severity not fully appreciated because the distended bladder can compress the lower uterine segment (Fig. 20-37A). In the patient who has physical examination findings suggestive of incompetence or a history of incompetence in a past pregnancy, the lack of findings on the TA full-bladder examination may be misleading. The urinary bladder should then be emptied to complete the cervical evaluation (see Fig. 20-37B). Of the TV and TL techniques, the TV study performed with the probe inserted midposition into the vagina is particularly useful and is considered by most to be the procedure of choice in yielding additional information. However, aggressive maneuvering of the probe, particularly deeper penetration, should be avoided.

When incompetence is suggested, follow-up studies at close intervals are needed. These patients may require bed rest, tocolytic medication to decrease uterine contractions, and a cerclage (surgical sutures placed around the cervix). These sutures are placed through the vagina as high as possible around the proximal third of the cervix to the level of the pars vaginalis. A cerclage is not feasible if fetal parts or umbilical cord are already present within the dilated cervical canal. After cerclage placement, the clinical examination findings become less precise and ultrasound is needed to evaluate the extent and possible progression of endocervical canal dilatation. The hyperechoic cerclage sutures can often be identified (Fig. 20-38), and multiplanar 3-D reconstruction can be useful in evaluating the relationship of the sutures to the endocervical canal.

It is also important to evaluate the lower uterine segment and cervix for masses (i.e., fibroids) (Fig. 20-39). They may cause obstruction (dystocia) to a normal delivery at term. Cul-de-sac masses are usually ovarian in origin and, if large, even if benign, can cause similar problems at birth.

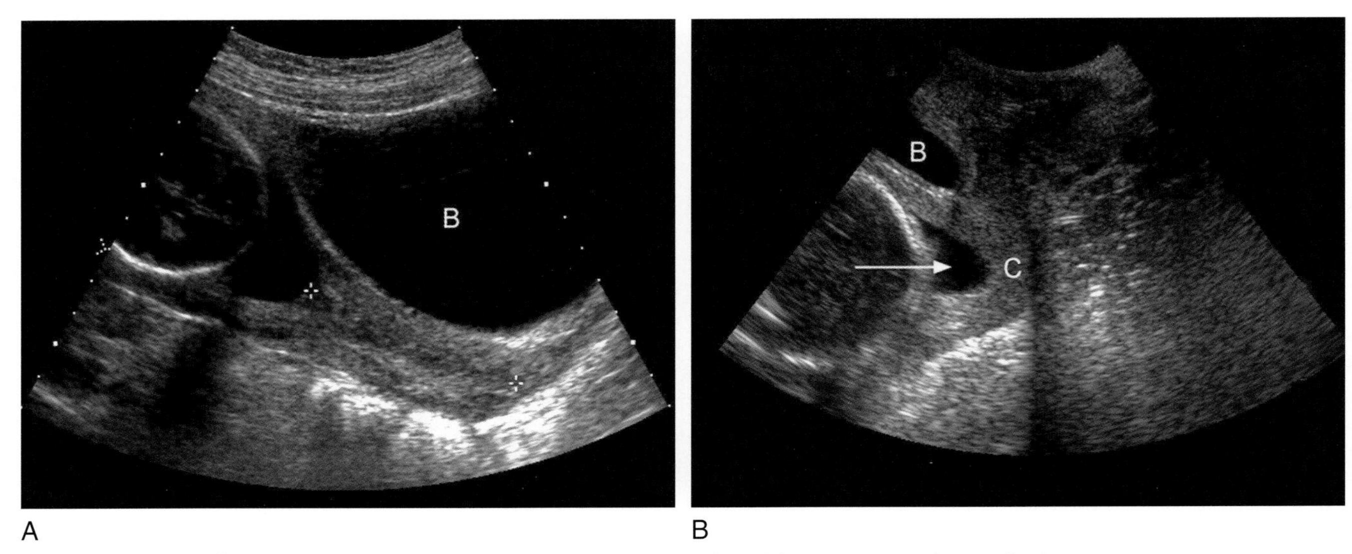

Figure 20-37 Overdistended urinary bladder: technical limitation in evaluation for incompetent cervix. **A,** Sagittal midline transabdominal scan in a patient with incompetent cervix at 28 weeks obtained when the urinary bladder (B) is markedly overdistended shows an apparently closed endocervical canal *(cursors).* This spurious appearance of a closed endocervical canal occurs because the overdistended bladder compresses and elongates the cervix and lower uterine segment. **B,** Post-void sagittal midline translabial scan on same patient as in **A** shows funneling *(arrow)* of the endocervical canal with only a short segment of intact cervix (C) caudad to the funneled area. B, bladder with a small amount of urine.

HYDATIDIFORM MOLES AND HYDROPIC CHANGES

The clinical manifestations of a classic or complete hydatidiform mole are abnormal vaginal bleeding, hyperemesis gravidarum, preeclampsia, and, occasionally, thyrotoxicosis. Physical examination reveals a large-for-date uterus and, rarely, passage of vesicular tissue. The human chorionic gonadotropin (hCG) levels are markedly elevated.

Molar pregnancies are usually detected in the second and third trimesters but have been discovered earlier (see Fig. 14-19). The ultrasound examination classically shows an enlarged uterus with uniformly hyperechoic tissue filling the endometrial canal. There is good through transmission because the multiple small cystic villi (hydropic changes) are often too small to be identified. If these cystic spaces are large (>2 cm), they give the mole a more inhomogeneous appearance. No fetus is seen. Pathologically, a mole has three properties: hydropic swelling of the chorionic villi, absent or inadequate development of villous vascularization, and variable degrees of hyperplasia and/or anaplasia of the chorionic epithelium.

Hydatidiform moles are noninvasive in 85% of the cases and remain confined to the endometrial canal. In the other 15%, 13% are locally invasive (termed *chorioadenoma destruens*) and extend into the myometrium. This extension cannot be determined by ultrasound. The remaining 2% metastasize and are termed *choriocarcinoma.* Because of the clinical symptoms and malignant potential, molar pregnancies are evacuated and observed closely for signs of recurrence by monitoring the hCG levels.

There are other causes for hydropic placental changes that can resemble the appearance of a complete mole: (1) twins with two separate sacs, one representing a normal pregnancy and the other containing a complete mole; (2) a partial (incomplete) mole associated with a triploid karyotype, a residual gestational sac, fetal tissue, and sometimes a coexisting living fetus (Fig. 20-40); and (3) hydropic degeneration of the placenta, either partial or complete, following a failed intrauterine pregnancy or with a coexisting living fetus (see Fig. 14-20B). Although all can manifest similar symptoms and laboratory results but without the passage of vesicular tissue, only the first possesses the same malignant potential as a complete hydatidiform mole. Differentiation of the other two, the partial mole and the hydropic changes, may not be possible in utero. Complete and partial moles both pose significant maternal problems during the pregnancy (preeclampsia or eclampsia) and at the time of delivery (vaginal bleeding). Partial moles are associated with significant potential fetal structural and chromosomal (particularly triploidy) abnormalities. Hydropic changes can be differentiated from a hydatidiform mole only by careful pathologic

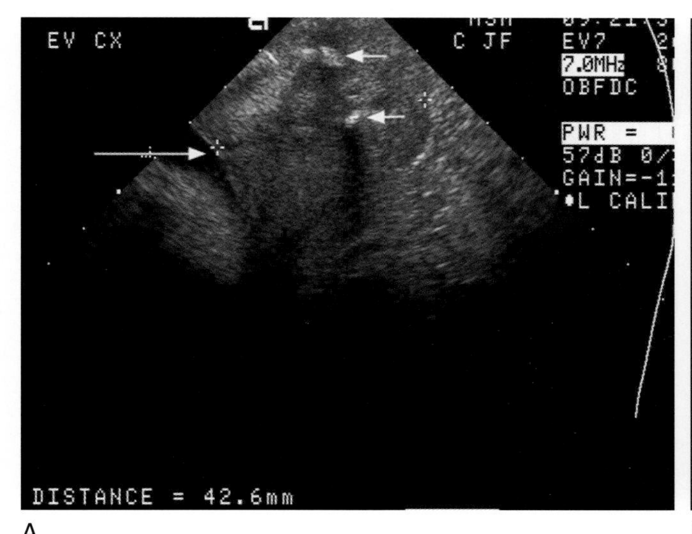

B

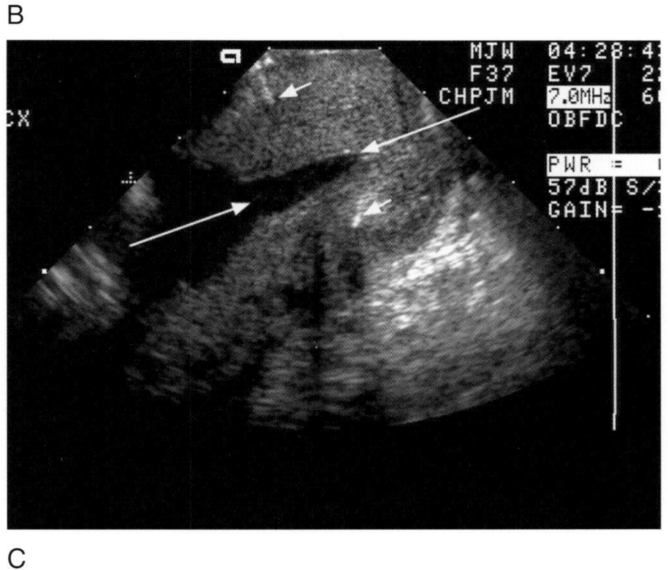

Figure 20-38 Cerclage suture: ultrasound evaluation of cervix after cerclage. **A,** Normal cervix. Transvaginal ultrasound image of cervix at 29 weeks shows normal length of 4.3 cm and no funneling of the internal os *(long arrow). Short arrows,* cerclage sutures. **B,** Mild funneling. Transvaginal ultrasound image of cervix of a different patient at 19 weeks shows mild funneling *(long arrow)* of the upper portion of the endocervical canal. The funneling ends above the level of the cerclage sutures *(short arrows).* **C,** Funneling extending caudal to sutures. Transvaginal ultrasound image of cervix at 23 weeks shows a long segment of funneling *(long arrows)* that extends caudad to the level of the cerclage sutures *(short arrows).*

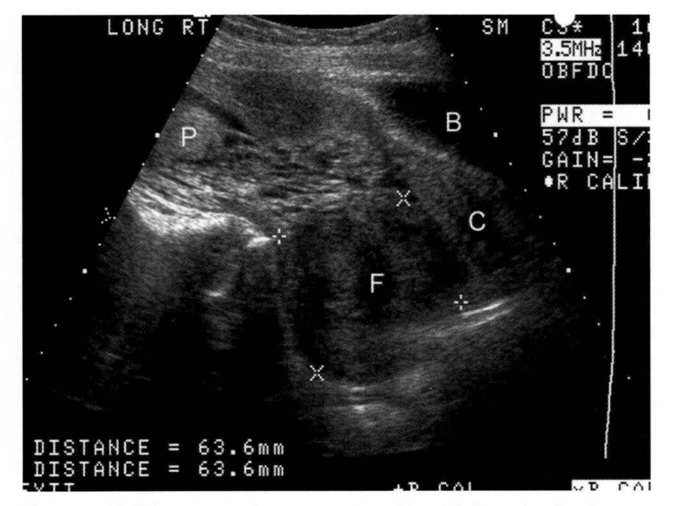

Figure 20-39 Large lower uterine fibroid. Longitudinal transabdominal image of lower uterus at 19 weeks shows a large lower uterine fibroid (F, *cursors*) extending caudad to the level of the cervix (C). The fibroid compresses and distorts the cervix. P, placenta; B, maternal bladder.

evaluation. Placental hydrops does not exhibit the chorionic epithelial hyperplasia and anaplasia.

Other abnormalities may infrequently mimic a partial hydatidiform mole or partial hydropic changes; these are an unresolved loculated abruptio placentae and an unusual-looking fibroid. Usually the clinical symptoms, physical examination findings, and hCG levels will establish the difference. When uncertainty persists, chromosomal analysis and careful fetal evaluation may be indicated.

Multicystic, multiseptated ovarian masses termed *theca-lutein cysts* (see Fig. 20-40C) are identified in association with some molar pregnancies. These theca lutein cysts are typically large and bilateral. They occur in fewer than half of patients with molar pregnancies. They can be so large as to be displaced out of the pelvis and can then be best identified by abdominal scanning. There may be hemorrhage into any of the cystic components, leading to changes in echogenicity. Ascites may also be present.

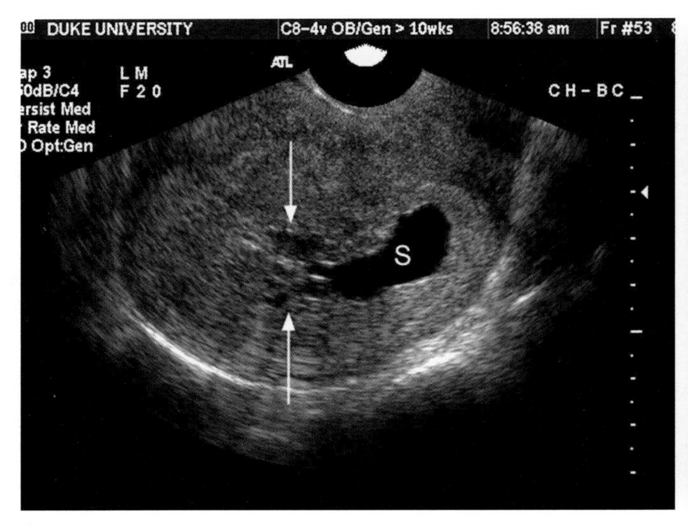

A

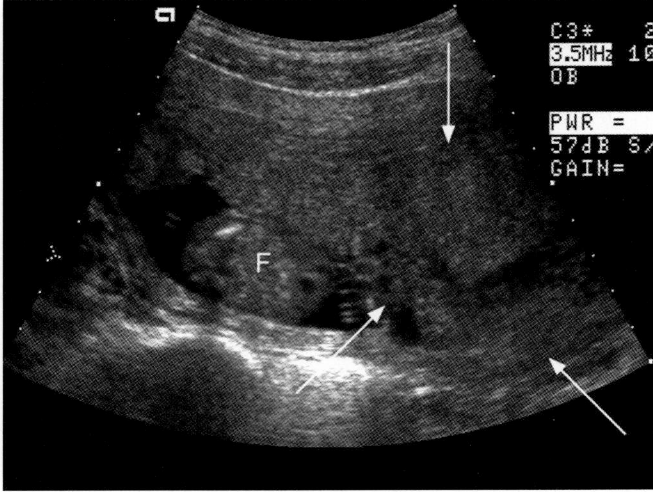

B

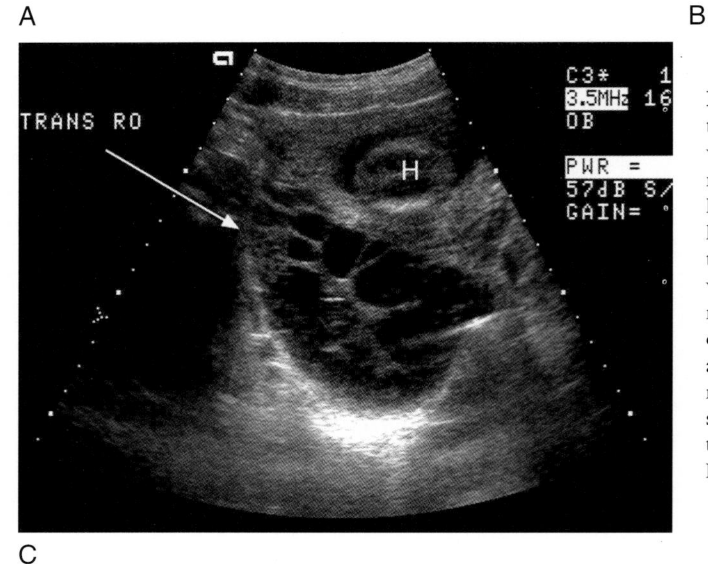

C

Figure 20-40 Examples of partial mole. **A,** During first trimester. Endovaginal ultrasound image of uterus of a 20-year-old woman with bleeding and a serum βhCG value of 42,005 mIU/mL reveals an irregularly shaped gestational sac (S) associated with hydropic changes *(arrows)* in a portion of the placenta. Pathologic evaluation revealed a partial mole. **B,** During second trimester. Longitudinal transabdominal image of uterus of a patient with a βhCG value of 1,120,714 mIU/mL at 16 weeks shows a markedly thickened and heterogeneous placenta *(arrows)* and a concomitant fetus (F). Dilatation and evacuation was performed and confirmed a partial mole. **C,** Theca lutein cysts and partial mole. Axial image of right side of pelvis of same patients as in **B** shows markedly enlarged multicystic right ovary *(arrow)* owing to theca lutein cysts. The left ovary was similar in appearance. H, fetal head.

PLACENTAL INFARCTS

Placental infarcts can be solitary or multiple. Most are too small to be detected by ultrasound. When seen, they are classically hypoechoic and 1 to 2 cm in diameter and can be indistinguishable from an intervillous connection (venous lake) or area of fibrin deposition. Some may be isoechoic or hyperechoic, and they frequently have a thick hyperechoic rim (Fig. 20-41).

The source of placental infarcts is not usually known, although they are more common in certain maternal vascular conditions such as collagen vascular diseases. If few in number, they should not impair fetal blood flow. If more than 50% of the placenta is affected, however, the pregnancy should be closely monitored for possible impaired fetal growth.

PLACENTAL TUMORS

Chorioangiomas are benign placental vascular neoplasms that are well circumscribed and usually solitary. When small, they are typically slightly hypoechoic relative to the normal placental tissue (Fig. 20-42A). When large, they are more commonly inhomogeneous. Chorioangiomas are either round or ovoid. Although they can be seen anywhere within the placental substance, they are more often at or near the chorionic plate and usually bulge into the amniotic fluid.

Chorioangiomas can have internal blood flow with arteriovenous shunting (see Fig. 20-42B). The fetus is at risk for hydrops (see Fig. 20-42C) caused by high-output congestive failure due to the arteriovenous shunting. The risk of hydrops is dependent on the size of the chorioangioma, the extent of atrioventricular shunting, and the amount of extra tissue the fetal heart must perfuse. This blood flow can be evaluated by a combination of color flow and pulsed Doppler analysis; the more the arterial flow, the closer the pregnancy should be observed for signs of fetal hydrops.

It is usually easy to differentiate chorioangiomas from fibroids. Although both may indent the placenta, they are situated in different areas (placenta versus myometrium). However, the Doppler findings may be similar. Although most fibroids have little appreciable vascularity, some exhibit considerable arterial flow.

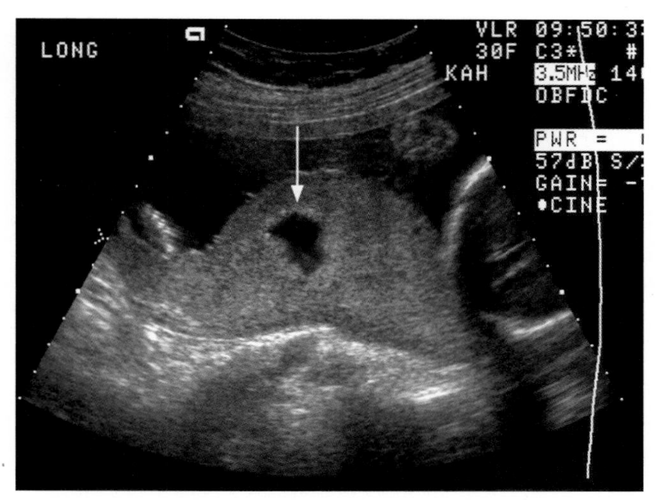

Figure 20-41 Placental infarct. Longitudinal transabdominal scan of the placenta of a 30-year-old patient with placental infarction due to abruption shows an irregular hypoechoic area surrounded by a rim of increased echogenicity *(arrow)* in the placenta corresponding to a placental infarct.

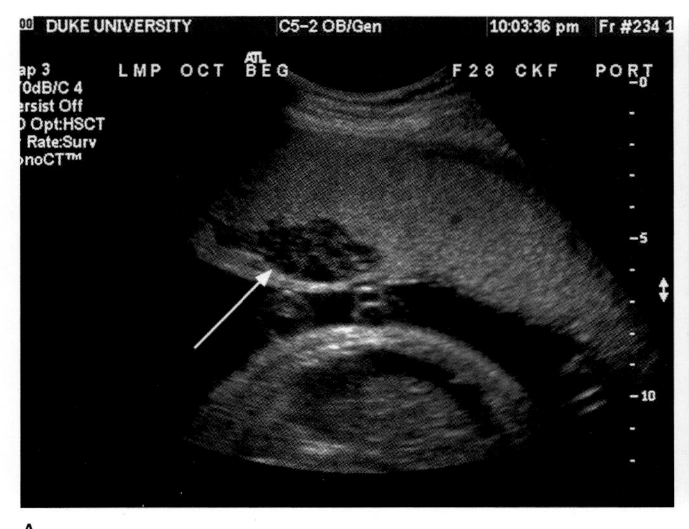

A

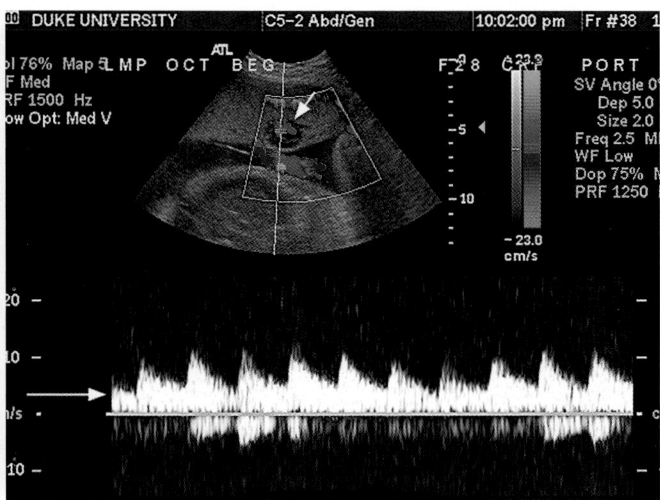

B

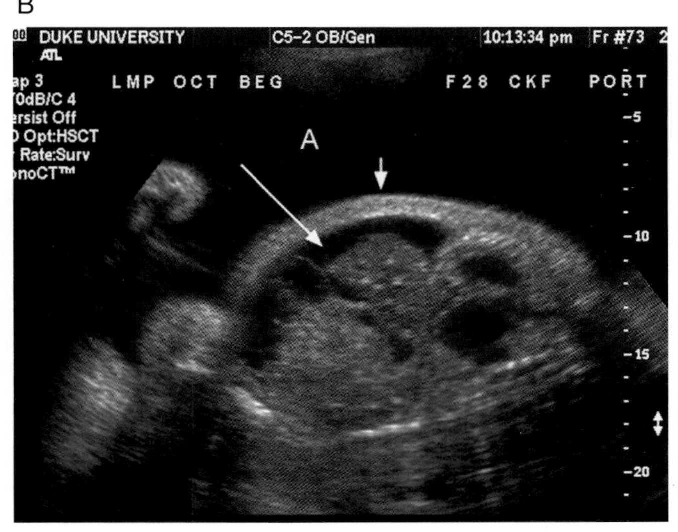

C

Figure 20-42 Chorioangioma associated with fetal hydrops. **A,** Transabdominal scan of placenta during third trimester shows a heterogeneous hypoechoic mass *(arrow)* due to a chorioangioma. **B,** Color Doppler evaluation reveals blood flow in the mass *(short arrow),* and spectral waveforms confirm the presence of low-resistance arterial flow *(long arrow)*. **C,** Longitudinal image of fetal abdomen shows hydrops, with ascites *(long arrow)* and skin thickening *(short arrow)*. There is also polyhydramnios. A, amniotic fluid.

Key Features

- The placenta normally has a low-level uniform echogenicity. On its outer surface is the thin hyperechoic chorionic plate (the chorioamnionic membrane) and on its inner border is the hypoechoic basilar-myometrial layer.
- The placenta is a very vascular organ made up of maternal and fetal blood supplies. Normal maternal venous channels can be seen as hypoechoic or anechoic spaces.
- Trophotropism, a concept of placental remodeling, can explain unusual placental shapes, eccentric umbilical cord insertions, and changes in placental position. Ideally, each part of the placenta attaches to an equally vascularized underlying endometrium. If the blood supply is uneven, however, modeling occurs, with villi proliferating into areas of good vascularity and villi atrophying in areas of poor vascularity.
- The umbilical cord is normally identified from the late first trimester onward. Its insertion is considered normal if within the placental substance. A marginal or velamentous cord insertion can cause serious fetal problems at delivery.
- The umbilical cord can also be evaluated for its length, a normally twisted state, and diffuse and localized processes.
- The umbilical cord normally contains three vessels: two arteries and one vein. A two-vessel cord—one artery and one vein—is associated with an increased incidence of fetal structural and karyotype abnormalities. Color Doppler imaging of the iliac arteries within the fetal pelvis, seen on both sides of the urinary bladder, confirms the number of umbilical arteries.
- Placental bleeding most commonly occurs in the subchorionic and retroplacental regions. Uncomplicated subchorionic hemorrhages are usually benign; retroplacental hemorrhages can cause considerable fetal and, infrequently, maternal problems.
- If placental bleeding is clinically suspected, even if not identified by ultrasound, a follow-up study may be helpful.
- Placental accreta, increta, and percreta are abnormal extensions of trophoblastic proliferation beyond the normal intact endometrium. These most commonly occur in areas of scarring, and the classic ultrasound finding is disruption or loss of the hypoechoic basilar-myometrial layer. Women at highest risk are those who have had previous cesarean sections and have a low-positioned anterior placenta with placenta previa.
- Placental thickness is usually evaluated subjectively, although a perpendicular measurement in its mid position can be attempted. The normal thickness is 2 to 4 cm. A thin placenta is most commonly seen in the maternal settings of hypertension, insulin-dependent diabetes, and collagen vascular disease. A thick placenta often occurs in the settings of fetal hydrops and gestational diabetes.
- Contractions can occur anywhere within the myometrial wall and at any time during pregnancy. Often obvious, they can at times cause uterine distortion and be confused with fibroids. Contractions usually change significantly within 30 to 60 minutes.
- Placenta previa is defined during an ongoing pregnancy as the position of the placenta in relation to a closed internal os. It is classified as low-lying, marginal (partial), or complete.
- The diagnosis of placenta previa may not be accurate before 20 weeks. Because of expected placental remodeling (except in a central previa, a subset of a complete previa), a repeat study should be performed.
- A full urinary bladder during transabdominal scanning may compress and elongate the cervix and lower uterine segment, making a low-lying placenta appear as a placenta previa. Having the patient empty the bladder, with scanning performed in any of three ways (transvaginally, transabdominally, and translabially) can confirm the existence of or rule out placenta previa.
- Vasa previa is the presence of *fetal* (not placental) blood vessels that cross the internal cervical os. This can occur in the settings of marginal or velamentous cord insertions and in succenturiate lobes and can cause serious fetal problems at delivery.
- Cervical incompetence is depicted as a shortened endocervical length to less than 2.5 cm, with or without cervical funneling. An incompetent cervix may look relatively normal during a distended urinary bladder study. When there is a clinical suspicion or a history of cervical incompetence, a nondistended bladder study with gentle fundal uterine pressure should be performed to evaluate the full extent of the incompetence.
- There can be discrepancies in the diagnosis of an incompetent cervix between the physical examination findings that rely on the detection of an abnormal *external* "soft" os and the ultrasound findings that rely on the detection of an abnormal *internal* os.

Continued

Key Features—cont'd

The classic or complete hydatidiform mole is noninvasive in approximately 85% of the cases, locally invasive in 13%, and metastatic (as choriocarcinoma) in 2%. It presents as an enlarged uterus that is typically filled with hyperechoic tissue (multiple small cysts) with good through transmission. Larger cysts give the mole an inhomogeneous appearance. No fetus is present.

Other types of trophoblastic disease can occur. One type consists of two separate sacs, with a normal pregnancy in one and a complete molar pregnancy (with malignant potential) in the other. A partial (incomplete) mole is associated with a low malignant potential but with very high risk of structural and chromosomal abnormalities, particularly triploidy.

Placental infarcts most commonly occur in certain maternal vascular conditions and may be too small to be identified by ultrasound. Infarcts can be seen when at least 1 to 2 cm in diameter and typically display a hypoechoic center with a hyperechoic rim. They may be of no clinical consequence unless multiple and occupying more than 50% of the placental substance.

Chorioangiomas are vascular placental tumors, which often have AV shunting. Commonly there is little, if any, adverse effect on the fetus. At their worst, high flow may lead to fetal high-output failure and hydrops.

SUGGESTED READINGS

Althuisius SM Dekker GA, van Geijn HP: Cervical incompetence: A reappraisal of an obstetric controversy. Obstet Gynecol 57:377, 2002.

Anderson HF, et al: Prediction of cervical cerclage outcome by endovaginal ultrasonography. Am J Obstet Gynecol 171:1102, 1994.

Avila C, Devine P, Lowre C, et al: Accuracy of prenatal ultrasonography in the diagnosis of placenta accreta, increta or percreta. Am J Obstet Gynecol 185:s256, 2001.

Ball RH, Buchmeier SE, Longnecker M: Clinical significance of sonographically detected uterine synechiae in pregnant patients. J Ultrasound Med 16:465, 1997.

Benson CB, Genest DR, Bernstein MR, et al: Sonographic appearance of first trimester complete hydatidiform moles. Ultrasound Obstet Gynecol 16:188, 2000.

Bergelin I, Valentin L: Normal cervical changes in parous women during the second half of pregnancy—a prospective, longitudinal ultrasound study. Acta Obstet Gynecol Scand 81:31, 2002.

Bowie JD, Andreotti RF, Rosenberg ER: Sonographic appearance of the uterine cervix in pregnancy: The vertical cervix. AJR Am J Roentgenol 140:737, 1983.

Budorick NE, Kelly TF, Dunn JA, et al: The single umbilical artery in a high-risk patient population: What should be offered? J Ultrasound Med 20:619, 2001.

Catanzarite V, Maida C, Thomas W, et al: Prenatal sonographic diagnosis of vasa previa: Ultrasound findings and obstetric outcome in ten cases. Ultrasound Obstet Gynecol 18:109, 2001.

Chou MM, Tseng JJ, Hwang JI, et al: Sonographic appearance of tornado blood flow in placenta previa accreta/increta. Ultrasound Obstet Gynecol 17:362, 2001.

Chow JS, Benson CB, Doubilet PM: Frequency and nature of structural anomalies in fetuses with single umbilical arteries. J Ultrasound Med 17:765, 1998.

Crandall BF, Robinson L, Grau P: Risks associated with an elevated maternal serum α-fetoprotein level. Am J Obstet Gynecol 165:581, 1991.

Dashe JS, McIntire DD, Ramus RM, et al: Persistence of placenta previa according to gestational age at ultrasound detection. Obstet Gynecol 99:692, 2002.

Devsa R, Muñoz A, Torrents M, et al. Prenatal diagnosis of vasa previa with transvaginal color Doppler ultrasound. Ultrasound Obstet Gynecol 8:139, 1996.

Di Salvo DN, Benson CB, Laing FC, et al: Sonographic evaluation of the placental cord insertion site. AJR Am J Roentgenol 170:1295, 1998.

Dudiak CM, Salomon CG, Posniak HV, et al: Sonography of the umbilical cord. Radiographics 15:1035, 1995.

Elchalal U, Ezra Y, Levi Y, et al: Sonographically thick placenta: A marker for increased perinatal risk—a prospective cross-sectional study. Placenta 21:268, 2000.

Finberg HJ, Williams JW: Placenta accreta: Prospective sonographic diagnosis in patients with placenta previa and prior cesarean section. J Ultrasound Med 11:333, 1992.

Gielchinsky Y, Rojansky N, Fasouliotis SJ, et al: Placenta accreta—summary of 10 years: A survey of 310 cases. Placenta 23:210, 2002.

Gossett DR, Lantz ME, Chisholm CA: Antenatal diagnosis of single umbilical artery: Is fetal echocardiography warranted? Obstet Gynecol 100:903, 2002.

Guzman ER, et al: A new method using vaginal ultrasound and transfundal pressure to evaluate the asymptomatic incompetent cervix. Obstet Gynecol 83:248, 1994.

Guzman ER, Vintzileos AM, McLean DA, et al: The natural history of a positive response to transfundal pressure in women at risk for cervical incompetence. Am J Obstet Gynecol 176:634, 1997.

Harris RD, Barth RA: Sonography of the gravid uterus and placenta: Current concepts. AJR Am J Roentgenol 160:455, 1993.

Heath VCF, Southal TR, Souka AP, et al: Cervical length at 23 weeks' gestation: Prediction of spontaneous preterm delivery. Ultrasound Obstet Gynecol 12:312, 1998.

Heifetz SA: Single umbilical artery: A statistical analysis of 237 autopsy cases and review of the literature. Perspect Pediatr Pathol 8:345, 1984.

Hertzberg BS, et al: Diagnosis of placenta previa during the third trimester: Role of transperineal sonography. AJR Am J Roentgenol 159:83, 1992.

Hertzberg BS, Kliewer MA: Vasa previa: Prenatal diagnosis by transperineal sonography with Doppler evaluation. J Clin Ultrasound 26:405, 1998.

Hertzberg BS, Kliewer MA, Farrell TA, et al: Spontaneously changing gravid cervix: Clinical implications and prognostic features. Radiology 196:721, 1995.

Hertzberg BS, Livingston E, DeLong DM, et al: Ultrasound evaluation of the cervix: Transperineal versus endovaginal imaging. J Ultrasound Med 20:1071, 2001.

Hoddick WK, et al: Placental thickness. J Ultrasound Med 4:479, 1985.

Hoffman-Tretin JC, et al: Placenta accreta. Additional sonographic observations. J Ultrasound Med 11:29, 1992.

Iams JD, Goldenberg RL, Meis PJ, et al: The length of the cervix and the risk of spontaneous premature delivery. N Engl J Med 334:567, 1996.

Jauniaux E: Ultrasound diagnosis and follow-up of gestational trophoblastic disease. Ultrasound Obstet Gynecol 11:367, 1998.

Jauniaux E, Campbell S, Vyas S: The use of color Doppler imaging for prenatal diagnosis of umbilical cord anomalies: Report of three cases. Am J Obstet Gynecol 161:1195, 1989.

Karis JP, Hertzberg BS, Bowie JD: Sonographic diagnosis of premature cervical dilation: Potential pitfall due to lower uterine mature cervical dilatation. J Ultrasound Med 10:83, 1991.

Katz VL, et al: The clinical implications of subchorionic placental lucencies. Am J Obstet Gynecol 164:99, 1991.

Korbin CD, Benson CB, Doubilet PM: Placental implantation on the amniotic sheet: Effect on pregnancy outcome. Radiology 206: 773, 1998.

Lazarus E, Hulka C, Siewert B, et al: Sonographic appearance of early complete molar pregnancies. J Ultrasound Med 18:589, 1999.

Liu CC, Pretorius DH, Scioscia AL, et al: Sonographic prenatal diagnosis of marginal placental cord insertion: Clinical importance. J Ultrasound Med 21:627, 2002.

Macdonald R, Smith P, Vyas S: Cervical incompetence: The use of transvaginal sonography to provide an objective diagnosis. Ultrasound Obstet Gynecol 18:211, 2001.

McGahan JP, et al: Sonographic spectrum of retroplacental hemorrhage. Radiology 142:481, 1982.

Mahony BS: Ultrasound of the cervix during pregnancy. Abdom Imaging 22:569, 1997.

Murakawa H, et al: Evaluation of threatened preterm delivery by transvaginal ultrasonographic measurement of cervical length. Obstet Gynecol 82:829, 1993.

Mustafa SA, Brizot ML, Carvalho MH, et al: Transvaginal ultrasonography in predicting placenta previa at delivery: A longitudinal study. Ultrasound Obstet Gynecol 20:356, 2002.

Nomiyama M, Toyota Y, Kawano H: Antenatal diagnosis of velamentous umbilical cord insertion and vasa previa with color Doppler imaging. Ultrasound Obstet Gynecol 12:426, 1998.

Prapas N, Liang RJ, Hunter D, et al: Color Doppler imaging of placental masses: Differential diagnosis and fetal outcome. Ultrasound Obstet Gynecol 16:559, 2000.

Pretorius DH, Chau C, Poeltier DM, et al: Placental cord insertion visualization with prenatal ultrasonography. J Ultrasound Med 15:585, 1996.

Rinehart BK, Terrone DA, Taylor CW, et al: Single umbilical artery is associated with an increased incidence of structural and chromosomal anomalies and growth restriction. Am J Perinatol 17:229, 2000.

Rozenberg P, Gillet A, Ville Y: Transvaginal sonographic examination of the cervix in asymptomatic pregnant women: Review of the literature. Ultrasound Obstet Gynecol 19:302, 2002.

Sepulveda W, Avioles G, Carstens E, et al: Prenatal diagnosis of solid placental masses: The value of color flow imaging. Ultrasound Obstet Gynecol 16:554-558, 2000.

Sepulveda W, Leible S, Ulloa A, et al: Clinical significance of first trimester umbilical cord cysts. J Ultrasound Med 18:95, 1999.

Sherer DM, Anyaegbunam A: Prenatal ultrasonographic morphologic assessment of the umbilical cord: A review: I. Obstet Gynecol 52:506, 1997.

Sherer DM, Anyaegbunam A: Prenatal ultrasonographic morphologic assessment of the umbilical cord: A review: II. Obstet Gynecol 52:515, 1997.

Shukunami K, Tsunezawa W, Hosokawa K, et al: Placenta previa of a succenturiate lobe: A report of two cases. Eur J Obstet Gynecol Reprod Biol 99:276, 2001.

Strong TH Jr, Finberg HJ, Mattox JH: Antepartum diagnosis of noncoiled umbilical cords. Am J Obstet Gynecol 170:1729, 1994.

Verdel MJC, Exalto N: Tight nuchal coiling of the umbilical cord causing fetal death. J Clin Ultrasound 22:64, 1994.

Weissman A, Drugan A: Sonographic findings of the umbilical cord: Implications for the risk of fetal chromosomal anomalies. Ultrasound Obstet Gynecol 17:536, 2001.

Zalel Y, Weisz B, Gamzu R, et al: Chorioangiomas of the placenta: Sonographic and Doppler flow characteristics. J Ultrasound Med 21:909, 2002.

Zorzoli A, et al: Cervical changes throughout pregnancy as addressed by transvaginal sonography. Obstet Gynecol 84:960, 1994.

CHAPTER 21

Twin (Multiple) Gestations

For Key Features summary see p. 528

On average, the worldwide incidence of twinning is 1 in every 85 births. Triplets, quadruplets, and quintuplets are much less common. Triplets occur naturally in 1 of every 7,629 births; and quadruplets and quintuplets occur in 1 in every 670,734 and 41.6 million births, respectively. These numbers have somewhat increased due to fertility treatments.

This incidence of multiple births varies by nation and by race. The highest and lowest birth rates for twin gestations, for example, are in South America: the maximum in Chile at 1:51 and the minimum in Venezuela at 1:294. Twin gestations also vary by race, with incidences in the United States for blacks, whites, and Asian populations of 1:76, 1:86, and 1:92 births, respectively.

The lay terminology of fraternal and identical twins is well known. Fraternal twinning caused by the production of two ova (dizygotic) and their separate fertilization yields twins of the same or different gender and are in most instances phenotypically dissimilar after birth. Identical twinning is caused by the fertilization of one ovum (monozygotic) and then its separation. These twins are usually similar in appearance and are always of the same gender. The incidence of identical or monozygotic twins is the same, one for every five twin gestations (20%). The variation in numbers of twins is therefore related to the incidence of fraternal or dizygotic twinning. Fertility drug-induced pregnancies have been responsible for increasing the incidence of dizygotic gestations, by increasing the number of ova available for fertilization.

Twin pregnancies will be the focus of the remainder of this chapter because twins have been studied the most completely and serve as a model for all multiple gestations. Larger numbers of gestations (e.g., triplets) exhibit similar growth and in utero complications as twin gestations but with a greater tendency for earlier delivery and the inherent problems related to prematurity.

CHORIONICITY AND AMNIONICITY

The terms *dizygotic* and *monozygotic* (fraternal and identical) do not fully describe a twin pregnancy. Instead it is more relevant to determine the chorionicity and amnionicity of the twinning because this permits a more accurate anticipation of potential risk factors.

When two ova are fertilized separately (dizygotic twinning), each embryo develops within its own sac surrounded by its own amnion and chorion. As the two layers of the one sac abut on the two layers of the other, four layers appose and usually fuse. These four interposed layers define this type of twinning as *dichorionic-diamniotic* (Di-Di twinning). The embryos are the same or different genders. Di-Di twinning can also occur less frequently after fertilization and separation of a single ovum (monozygotic twinning) when the blastomere separates early within the first day after fertilization. In these 20% to 30% of monozygotic twinning conceptions the embryos develop within their own chorionic-amniotic sacs and are also Di-Di pregnancies but always of the same gender. All Di-Di twins are affected by the least risk factors of any type of twinning because each embryo develops within its own environment with its own placenta.

The remaining 70% to 80% of the monozygotic twins separate later, causing a shared environment and placental circulation, either partial or complete. Almost all of these (70% to 75%) separate within 1 to 7 days after fertilization. The two embryos then share a common chorion but have their own amniotic sacs. The two interposed amniotic layers define this type of twinning as *monochorionic-diamniotic* (Mono-Di twinning).

When the monozygotic separation occurs still later, between 7 to 13 days (1% to 3% of the cases), the two embryos are then surrounded by a common amnion and chorion. They have no interposed membrane, and this type of twinning is termed *monochorionic-monoamniotic* (Mono-Mono twinning).

The rarest group of monozygotic twins, fortunately far less than 1%, separates after 13 days. Not only is this a Mono-Mono twinning but also the embryos fail to completely separate. The twins are therefore conjoined.

TWIN GESTATIONS

The two primary questions to ask about twin gestations are (1) why is it important to diagnose twins in utero and (2) why is it important to classify the twins by their amnionicity and chorionicity? In the United States the perinatal death rate for singleton gestations is 33 in 1000 whereas in twins this risk is increased fourfold to 138 per 1000. The anticipation of twin births is therefore important because of the following complications: prematurity, each twin smaller than a singleton infant, and a prolapsed cord and ensuing anoxia in the second-born twin. There is also a suggestion of increased incidence of growth restriction, in one or both fetuses, and perhaps of increased incidence of structural anomalies, although the incidence and types have not been established. The importance of further classification by their amnionicity and chorionicity is that in a comparison of perinatal death rates for Di-Di twins and Mono-Mono twins there is a further increase from 75 to 191 per 1000 twin deaths, a 2.5-fold further increase if monochorionic twinning is present. Monochorionic twins (whether monoamniotic or diamniotic) share the same placental circulation and are at risk for twin-twin transfusions and acardiac twinning. In addition, the Mono-Mono twins, because they do not have an intervening membrane, are at risk for two more complications: entanglement of the umbilical cords and conjoining.

Therefore, not only should twins be detected, but also (if possible) they should be described in terms of their chorionic and amniotic membranes. When more than two gestations are detected, particularly after fertilization treatment, all are likely to be Di-Di gestations. However, careful analysis of each sac is needed because of the possibility of a spontaneous monochorionic gestation.

SECOND- AND THIRD-TRIMESTER EVALUATION

In the second and third trimesters, five characteristics can be used to determine the type of twinning: placental number, fetal genders, type of interposed membranes, presence or absence of the lambda (twin peaks) sign, and volume of amniotic fluid. The amniotic fluid is discussed later under the complications of monochorionic pregnancies.

If two completely separate placentas are identified, this ensures the existence of a Di-Di pregnancy (Fig. 21-1A). However, because of the physical constraints of the uterine cavity, it is common to identify only one placental site. This single-appearing placenta can be either the two separate but apposed placentas of a dichorionic pregnancy or the fused placenta of a monochorionic pregnancy (Fig. 21-1B). At present these two cannot be definitively differentiated; perhaps in the future, Doppler sonography may help differentiate placental circulations.

The "lambda" sign is also helpful in diagnosing the Di-Di twin pregnancy. The lambda sign is so named because of the triangular area of normal placental tissue that extends between the two dichorionic sacs and resembles the shape of the Greek letter lambda (Fig. 21-1C). Also called the "twin peaks" or "triangle" sign, it is only seen in Di-Di twinning. The lambda sign is particularly useful when a single placental site is detected. It should not be present in a monochorionic pregnancy because its single chorionic membrane surrounds both sacs and prevents the placenta from extending between the sacs. In the second and third trimesters the lambda sign, when present, has been shown to accurately predict a Di-Di pregnancy.

The evaluation of the external genitalia is often not possible until the mid second trimester. However, the detection of different genders, discussed in Chapter 18, confirms Di-Di twinning.

The identification and types of the interposed membrane have been well studied. A Di-Di membrane, two layers of chorion and two layers of amnion, is characteristically well defined and at least 2 mm in thickness (Fig. 21-1D). Although not often seen, when the two layers of one twin's membrane (its amnion and chorion) do not completely fuse to the two layers of the other, this finding is also characteristic of a Di-Di twinning (Fig. 21-1E). A Mono-Di membrane, composed of only two thin layers of amnion, appears thin and wispy

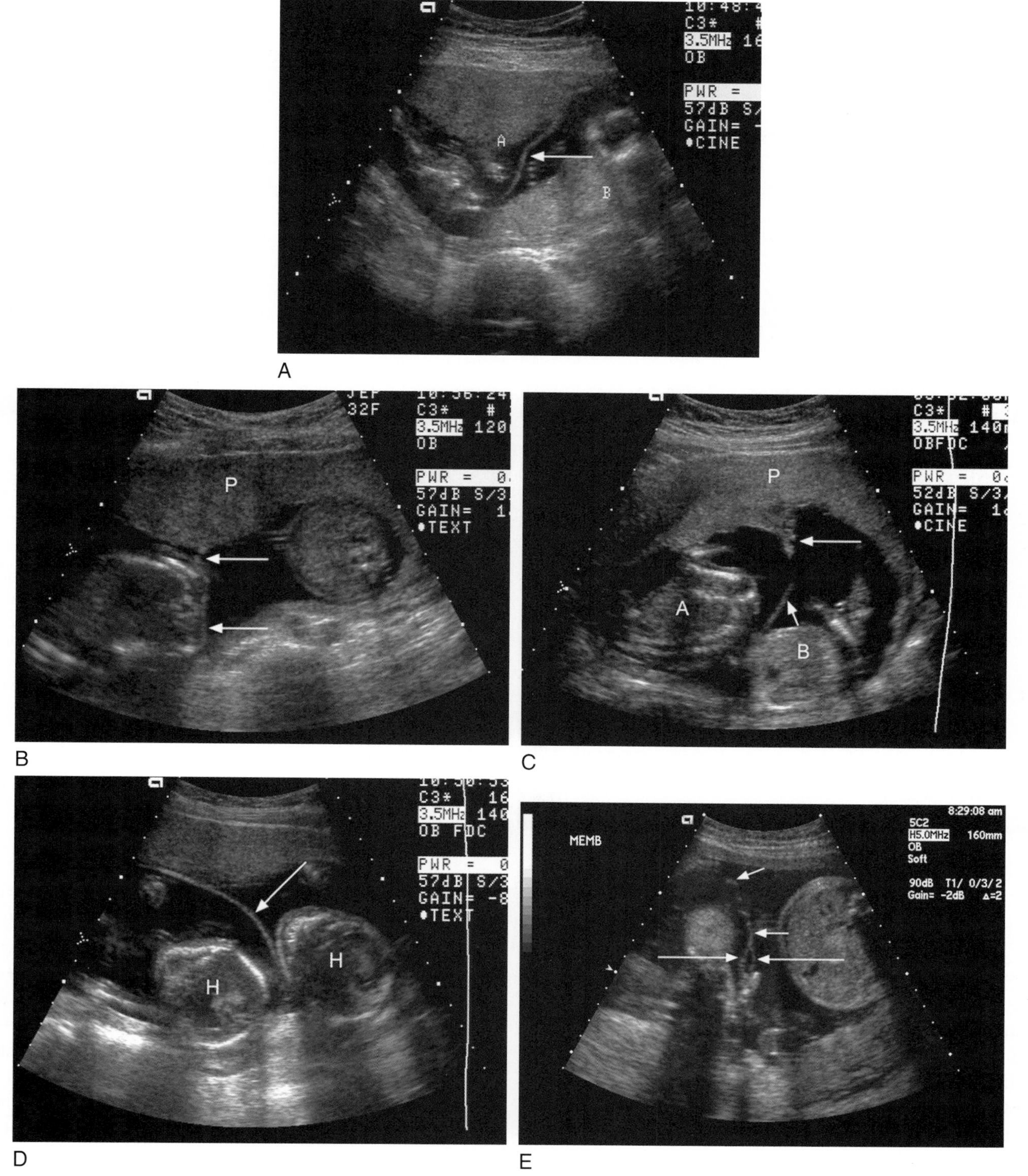

Figure 21-1 Dichorionic-diamniotic twinning: ultrasound findings. **A,** Identification of two separate placental sites is diagnostic of dichorionic-diamniotic twinning. In this example, one placenta (A) is anterior and the other (B) is posterior. A thick membrane *(arrow)* is seen between the twins. **B,** Only a single placental site (P) is seen even though these are dichorionic-diamniotic twins, because the two separate placentas are directly apposed. A thick membrane *(arrows)* is also seen. **C,** Lambda (twin peaks) sign. A triangular area of normal placental tissue *(long arrow)* extends between the two dichorionic sacs. The bodies of both twins (A, B) are seen on either side of the thick dividing membrane *(short arrow)*. Only a single anterior placental site (P) is seen, but the lambda sign and thick membrane are consistent with dichorionic-diamniotic twinning. **D,** Thick dividing membrane *(arrow)* due to imaging two layers of chorion and two layers of amnion. Fetal heads (H) are seen on either side of the membrane. **E,** Incomplete fusion of dichorionic-diamniotic membrane. A thick membrane *(short arrows)* is seen, but in a small focal area the amnion and chorion of one sac are not fused with the membranes of the other sac *(large arrows)*.

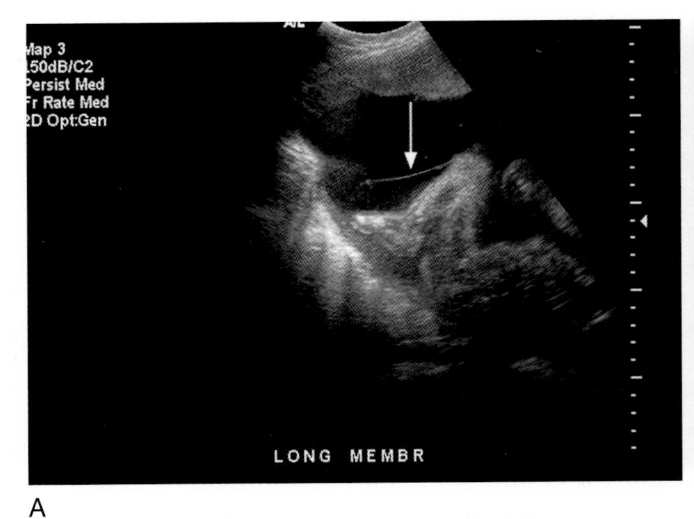

A

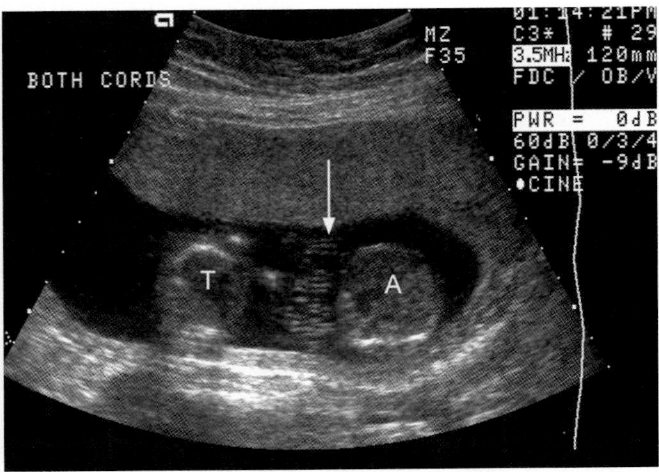

B

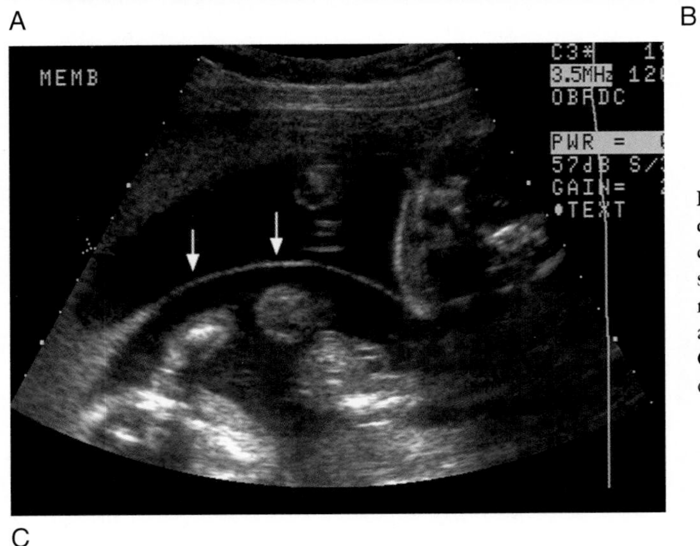

C

Figure 21-2 Membrane: value in establishing amnionicity and chorionicity. **A,** Thin and wispy membrane *(arrow)* in a monochorionic-diamniotic pregnancy. **B,** No interposed membrane is seen in this monochorionic-monoamniotic twin pregnancy. Only multiple loops of umbilical cord *(arrow)* are seen between the abdomen (A) of one twin and the thorax (T) of the other twin. **C,** Thick, well-defined membrane *(arrow),* consistent with dichorionic-diamniotic twin pregnancy.

(like a spider web) and is approximately 1 mm thick (Fig. 21-2A). In a Mono-Mono pregnancy, no interposed membrane can be detected (Fig. 21-2B).

In all trimesters (see Fig. 21-2C), a well-defined thick membrane is a diagnostic sign of a Di-Di pregnancy. However, false-positive and false-negative diagnoses do occur. If a thin membrane is perpendicular to the ultrasound beam and the gain is set unusually high, it may appear falsely thick and mimic a Di-Di membrane (Fig. 21-3A and B). Conversely, a thick Di-Di membrane can sometimes appear thinner, particularly in the third trimester, perhaps "thinned" or stretched by the increased volume of amniotic fluid (Fig. 21-3C); these membranes still appear intermediate in thickness and are almost always still Di-Di membranes. Last, although the absence of a membrane strongly suggests a Mono-Mono pregnancy, it is not always possible to appreciate a very thin diamniotic membrane, particularly late in pregnancy (Fig. 21-3D).

FIRST-TRIMESTER EVALUATION

Separate gestational sacs can sometimes be seen early in the pregnancy. This is a diagnostic sign of a dichorionic (Di-Di) pregnancy (Fig. 21-4A). In addition, the membrane thickness, the number of placental sites, and the lambda sign can also be used to analyze chorionicity and amnionicity in the first trimester (Fig. 21-4B). By transabdominal ultrasound, two placental sites or a thick membrane, or both, can correctly diagnose Di-Di pregnancies in over 95% of cases (Fig. 21-4C). This high accuracy suggests that the first trimester is the best time in pregnancy to establish chorionicity. The lambda sign, while not fully studied in the first trimester, would be anticipated to be an accurate sign of a Di-Di twinning. Nevertheless, an intermediate or thin membrane can infrequently be seen, indicating an overlap with monochorionic pregnancies. A thin membrane

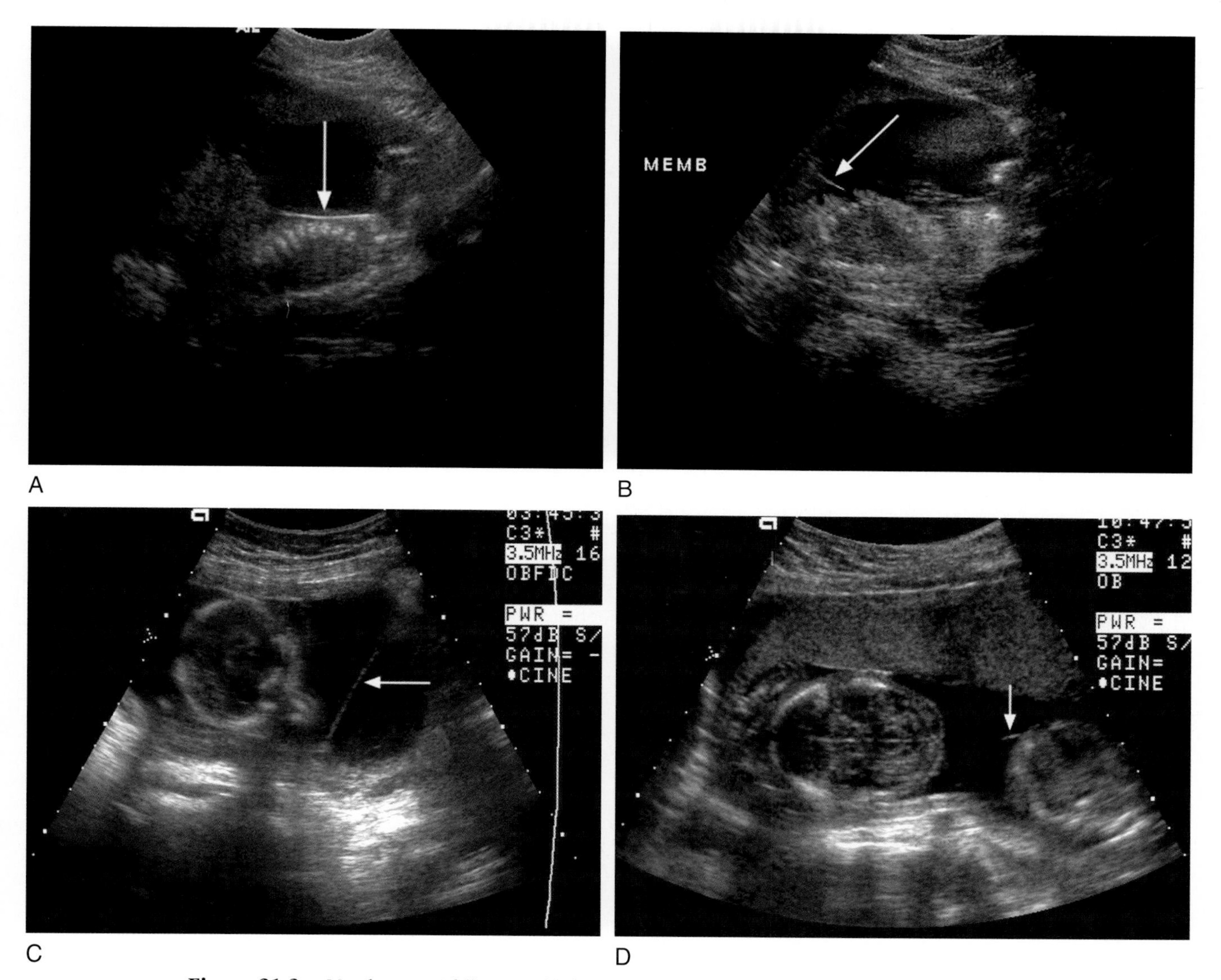

Figure 21-3 Membrane: pitfalls in establishing amnionicity and chorionicity. **A,** Thin membrane of a monochorionic-diamniotic pregnancy appears falsely thick *(arrow)* because it is oriented directly perpendicular to the ultrasound beam. **B,** Same patient as in **A**. After changing the orientation of the ultrasound beam, the membrane *(arrow)* appears thin, consistent with a monochorionic-diamniotic pregnancy. **C,** Membrane *(arrow)* in a late second-trimester dichorionic-diamniotic pregnancy appears relatively thin. This pitfall in assigning chorionicity based on membrane thickness is most common late in pregnancy and typically occurs when the membrane is "stretched" by a large amount of amniotic fluid. **D,** Monochorionic-diamniotic pregnancy with very thin membrane that was extremely difficult to visualize. Only a very short segment of the membrane *(arrow)* is seen here.

(and one placental site) is seen in over 85% of Mono-Di pregnancies (Fig. 21-5). However, very infrequently, no membrane is seen (overlapping a Mono-Mono pregnancy) or there is a membrane of intermediate thickness (overlapping a Di-Di pregnancy).

Higher-frequency transducers and different imaging planes of section are used in the transvaginal examination. This technique should be utilized to reevaluate any apparently thin or absent membrane before the final diagnosis of a monochorionic twinning (with its increased risk) is made (Fig. 21-6). On the other hand, because detection of two placental sites or a thick membrane or both by transabdominal examination confirms the presence of a dichorionic pregnancy, there is often no need for further evaluation.

PITFALLS IN DIAGNOSIS

There are potential intrauterine spaces in the first trimester. These can mimic an abnormal second sac and are due to fluid within the endometrial canal, the normal

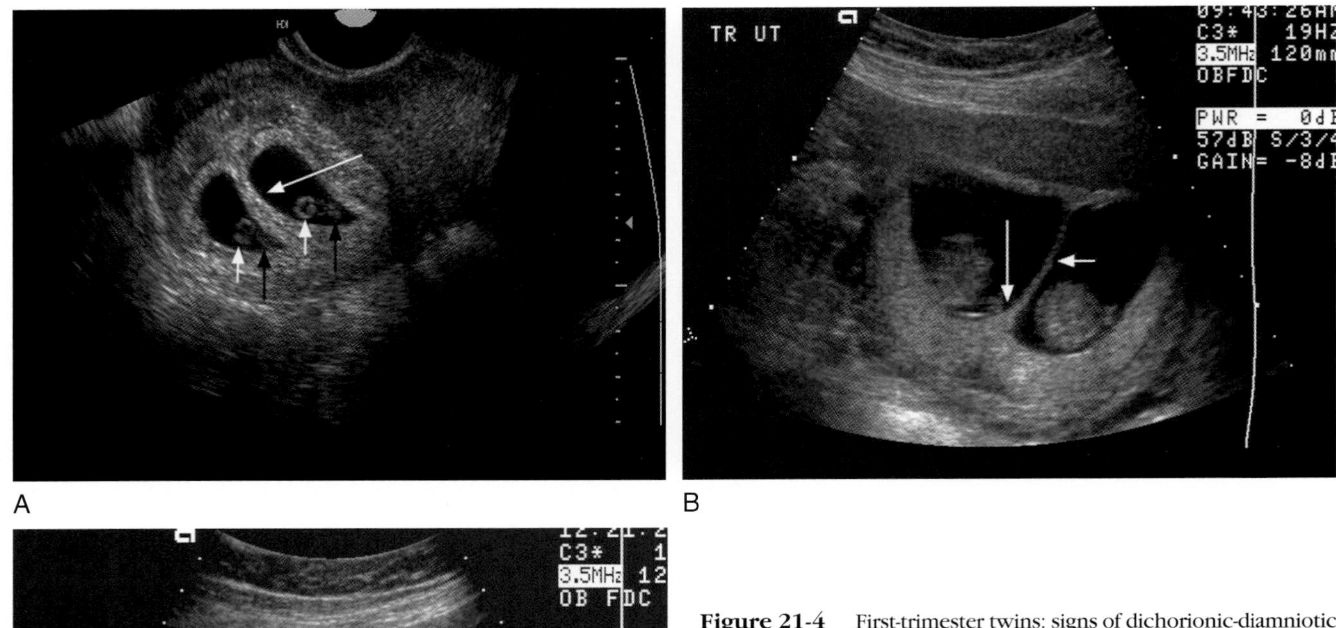

Figure 21-4 First-trimester twins: signs of dichorionic-diamniotic twinning. **A,** Transvaginal ultrasound image of early first trimester twins shows two discrete, separate gestational sacs with thick intervening tissue *(long white arrow),* diagnostic of dichorionic-diamniotic twinning. A yolk sac *(short white arrows)* and 6-week embryo *(black arrows)* was seen in each gestational sac. **B,** Thick dividing membrane *(short arrow)* and lambda sign *(long arrow)* are depicted on this axial transabdominal ultrasound study of twins at 11 weeks, consistent with dichorionic-diamniotic twinning. **C,** Two placental sites (P) and very thick dividing septum *(arrow)* are seen on this axial transabdominal ultrasound of twins at 12 weeks, diagnostic of dichorionic-diamniotic twinning.

chorioamnionic separation, an implantation bleed, and a necrotic fibroid. These are discussed in Chapter 14. Additionally, the "vanishing twin" sign is the first-trimester detection of a twin pregnancy where there is a normal developing embryo in one sac and a second abnormal sac is identified. This second sac, usually in a Di-Di and much less commonly in a Mono-Di pregnancy, contains either an abnormal embryo or more commonly is a distorted empty sac (Fig. 21-7). It is called a vanishing twin sign because with time, usually by the second trimester, this second sac will have disappeared, leaving a singleton gestation.

In the second and third trimesters an unusually thick membrane called an amniotic sheet or shelf can sometimes be identified within the amniotic cavity, usually in a singleton gestation (Fig. 21-8A). This is a synechia, a fibrous band caused prior to the pregnancy by endometrial instrumentation or infection, or by both, or the margin of a circumvallate placenta. It extends into the amniotic space and is covered by a single layer of normal amnion and chorion. Because of its thickness, this shelf should not be confused with any other membrane, even a Di-Di membrane, and frequently exhibits two additional characteristics: a bulbous-free end within the amniotic fluid (Fig. 21-8B) and a "Y"-shaped split at its endometrial margin (Fig. 21-8C). The singleton fetus typically moves freely and is unaffected by the shelf. The shelf can also extend across the amniotic cavity, appearing to divide it into two sacs, with the fetus then either unusually positioned or remaining only on one side of the shelf, or both. The fetus should still be normal at birth.

COMPLICATIONS OF MONOCHORIONIC PREGNANCIES

In all monochorionic pregnancies there is a single fused placenta with arterial and venous interconnections. Some of these interconnections are small and inconsequential to the twins; others are large and can become very important as the pregnancy progresses. Although

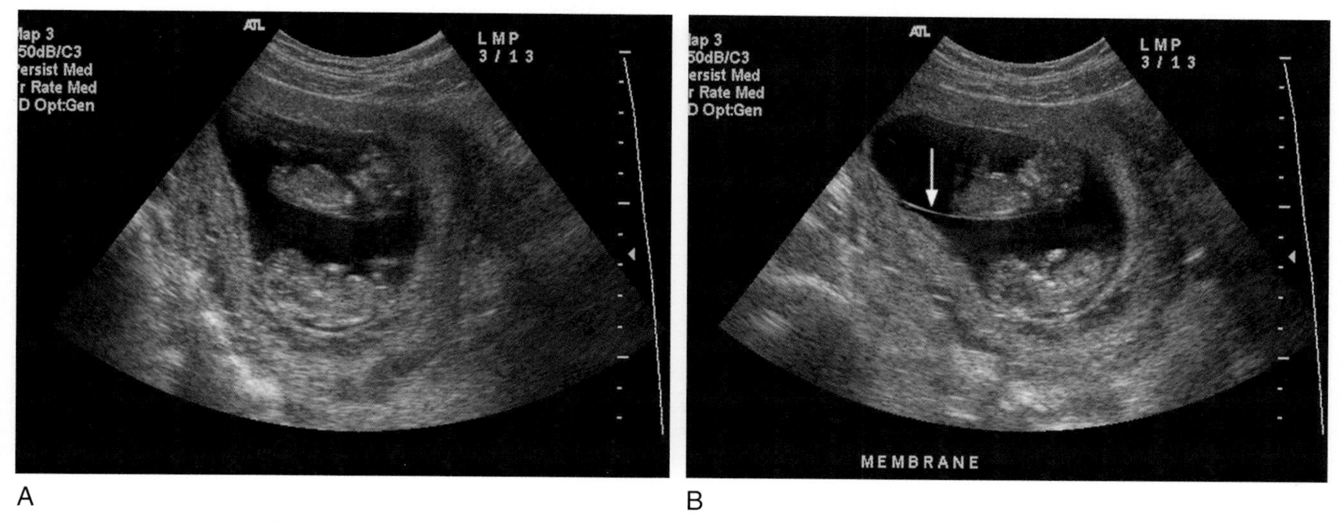

Figure 21-5 Monochorionic-diamniotic twins during the first trimester. **A,** Initial transabdominal images of twins at 11 weeks failed to show a membrane, suggesting the possibility of monochorionic-monoamniotic twinning. **B,** Additional images obtained in a slightly different scan plane demonstrated a thin membrane *(arrow)*, consistent with monochorionic-diamniotic twinning.

their extent should be predictive of major vascular monochorionic twin risk factors, at present these interconnections cannot be fully assessed even with color or power Doppler imaging. Their significance must instead await detection of abnormal intrauterine findings, typically the late manifestations of the twin-twin transfusion syndrome.

The twin-twin transfusion syndrome occurs in 15% to 30% of the monochorionic twin gestations. In its full-blown (most severe) form, one fetus receives or "steals" blood, becoming larger and plethoric, frequently with hydropic changes; the other fetus gets less blood and becomes smaller and anemic (Fig. 21-9). Although a twin-twin transfusion can occur at any time after the first trimester, it is commonly not appreciated until the late second or early third trimester. The direction of Doppler flow in the umbilical arteries and veins is in the correct directions: arterial flow away from and venous flow toward the fetus.

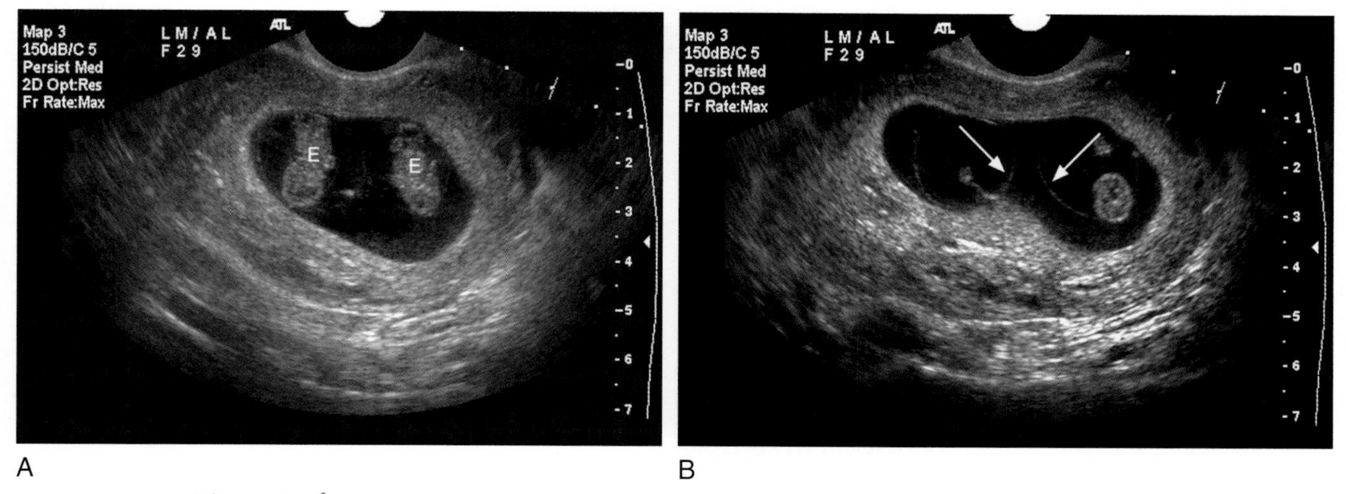

Figure 21-6 Transvaginal evaluation of amnionicity and chorionicity of first-trimester twins. **A,** Initial transvaginal images demonstrate two 9-week embryos (E) but fail to depict a membrane. **B,** Additional transvaginal images in a different orientation demonstrate the amnion *(arrows)* surrounding each gestational sac, consistent with monochorionic-diamniotic twinning. This case underscores the importance of searching for the membrane in multiple scan planes when initial images fail to depict a membrane.

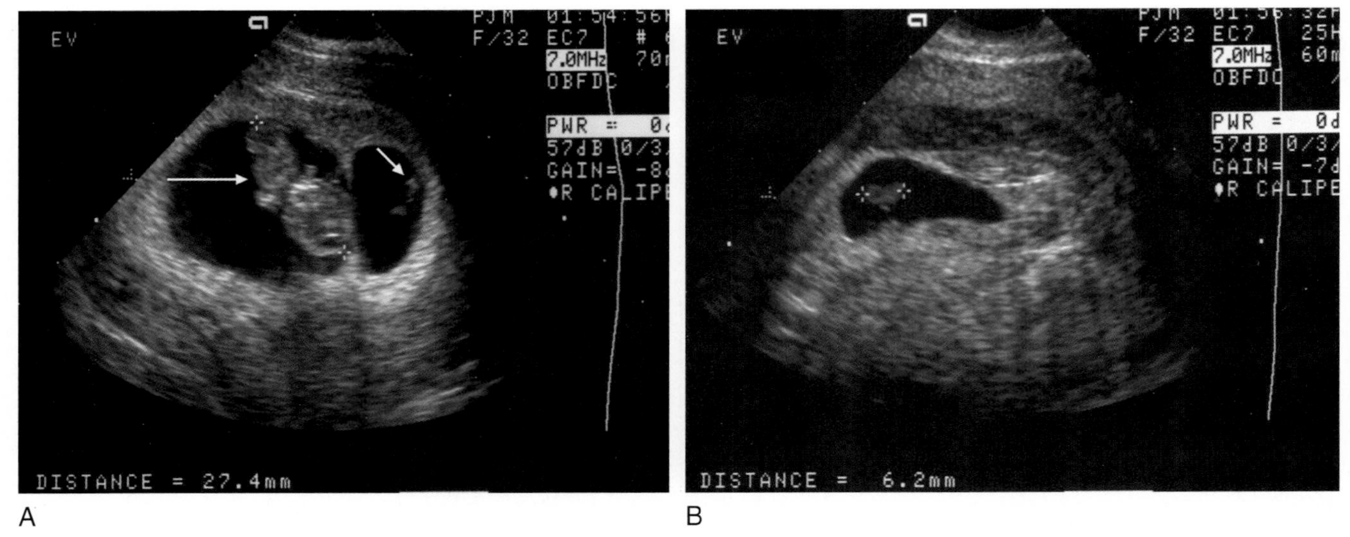

Figure 21-7 "Vanishing" twin. **A,** Transvaginal ultrasound of first-trimester twins shows two gestational sacs. The larger sac contains a normal twin *(long arrow)* with a crown-rump length (CRL) of 27.4 mm, which corresponds with 9.6 weeks. The smaller sac contains a much smaller embryo *(short arrow),* which did not have cardiac activity and eventually was resorbed, hence the term "vanishing" twin. **B,** CRL of the smaller, "vanishing" twin *(cursors)* was only 6.2 mm, corresponding to 6.4 weeks.

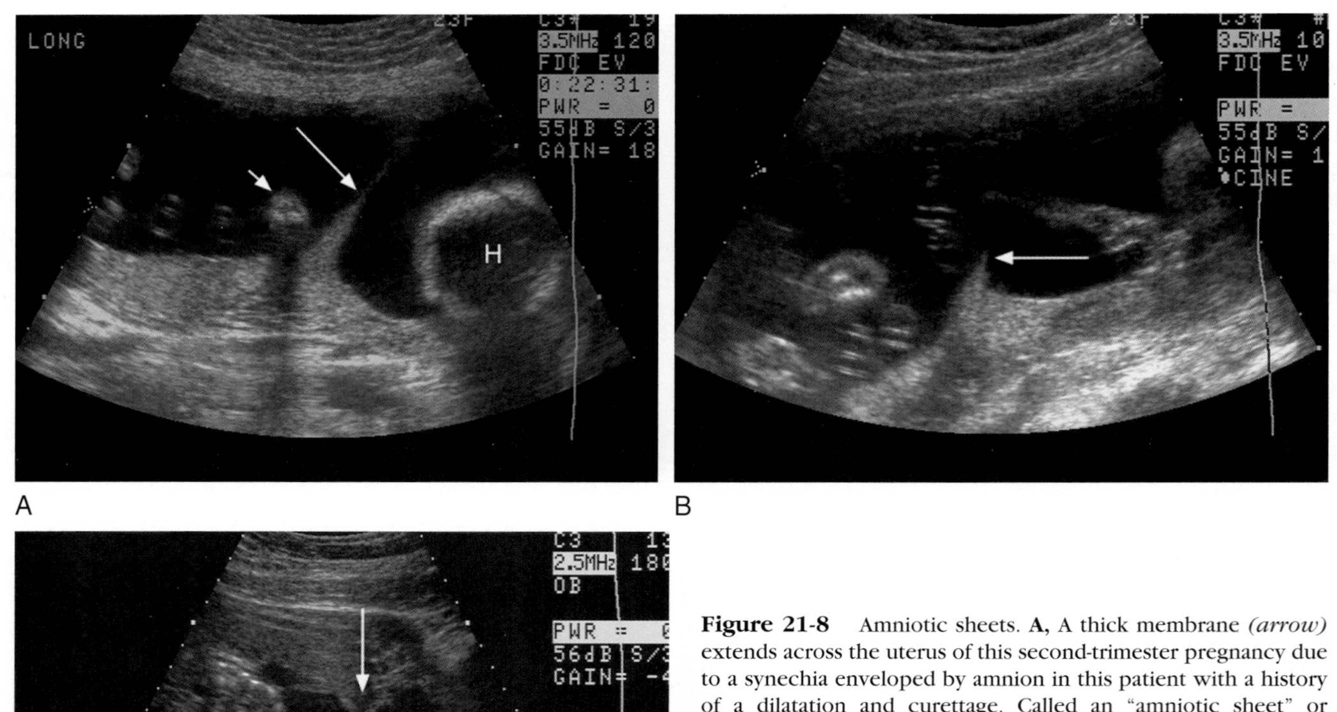

Figure 21-8 Amniotic sheets. **A,** A thick membrane *(arrow)* extends across the uterus of this second-trimester pregnancy due to a synechia enveloped by amnion in this patient with a history of a dilatation and curettage. Called an "amniotic sheet" or "amniotic shelf," it should not be mistaken for the membrane seen in a twin pregnancy. A fetal extremity *(short arrow)* is seen to the left of the membrane and moved freely on either side of it. H, fetal head. **B,** In a different scan plane, the amniotic sheet seen in **A** has a bulbous free edge *(arrow).* **C,** Longitudinal image of uterus of a different patient during second trimester shows an amniotic sheet *(short arrow)* in lower uterus with characteristic "Y"-shaped split at endometrial margin *(long arrow).*

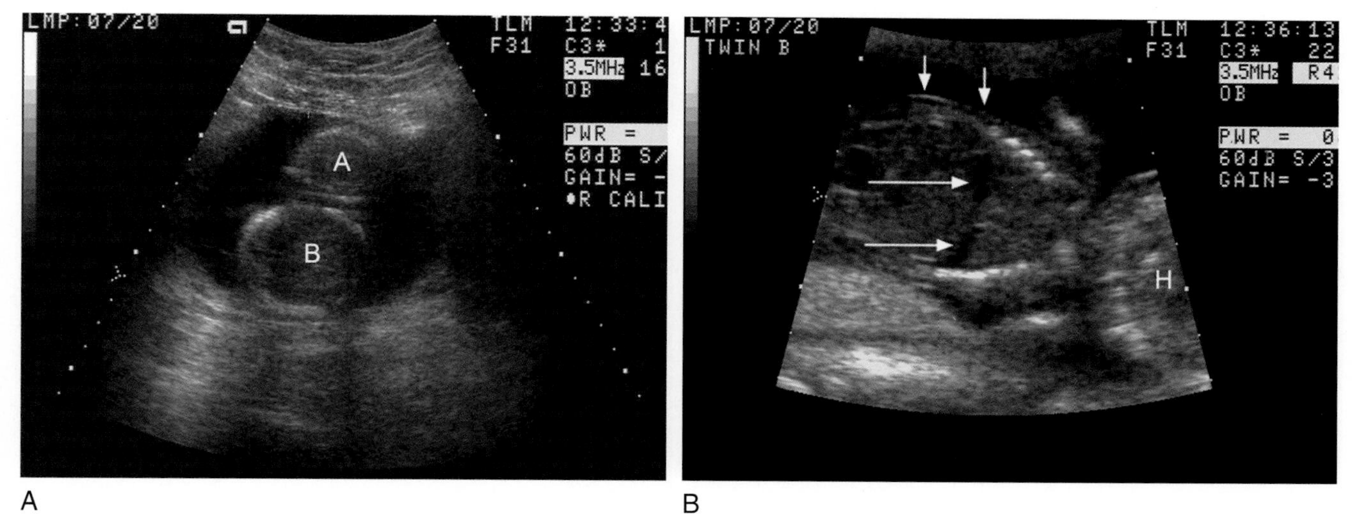

Figure 21-9 Twin-twin transfusion syndrome. **A,** Image at level of fetal heads shows marked discrepancy in size. Twin A is smaller and anemic; twin B is larger and was hydropic. **B,** Coronal view of body of twin B confirms hydrops, with bilateral pleural effusions *(long arrows)* and skin thickening *(short arrows)*. H, fetal head.

If the twins have their own amniotic sacs (i.e., a Mono-Di pregnancy), then differences in the amount of surrounding amniotic fluid can be appreciated. In its most typical and severe form, polyhydramnios is associated with the larger fetus and oligohydramnios with the smaller fetus. If the oligohydramnios surrounding the smaller twin is severe, it may appear to be "stuck" or fixed to a margin of the uterine cavity by the thin diamniotic membrane (Fig. 21-10). A number of variations can also occur. One fetus may look completely normal and the other smaller, both with a normal volume of amniotic fluid, or one fetus may look normal while the other smaller fetus is affected by significant oligohydramnios. It may be difficult to differentiate either of these patterns of findings from growth restriction of the smaller fetus. In another permutation one fetus may be normal and the other fetus larger and/or exhibit signs of hydrops. Preliminary studies of the fetal heart and blood vessels, in particular the right ventricular ejection fraction and the inferior vena cava Doppler waveform, have shown promise in determining potential fetal cardiovascular compromise. More work is needed, however, before these can be used as prognostic indicators.

Once the ultrasound findings of a twin-twin transfusion syndrome are detected, the prognosis is not good for either fetus, with the reported mortality rates frequently exceeding 50%; usually the prognosis is worse for the smaller fetus. Frequent follow-up examinations should be performed, because these fetuses are in a hostile environment and should be delivered as soon as clinically possible to prevent further deterioration. Therapeutic amniocentesis of the sac containing polyhydramnios will not infrequently benefit both fetuses, permitting re-accumulation of fluid in the oligohydramnionic sac. Another newer treatment that is under investigation consists of laser ablation of the placental vascular interconnections between the twins.

A rarer complication of a monochorionic pregnancy is a very unfortunate condition called acardiac twinning. In it, one fetus is normal and the other, the acardiac twin, exhibits an unusual lack of development of the upper parts of the fetus, including head, upper extremities, and part of the thorax down to and sometimes including the heart (Fig. 21-11). Marked skin thickening is usually present. The mid trunk through the lower extremities is typically less affected but can still be markedly abnormal. The shared blood supply is artery-to-artery and vein-to-vein with arterial blood flow toward and venous blood flow away from the acardiac twin. This aberrant flow pattern can be detected with Doppler waveform analysis. The normal fetus must perfuse both itself and the acardiac twin, both continuing to grow. This burden to the normal fetus can become an increasing problem, which can lead to cardiac decompensation by the third trimester.

The overall volume of amniotic fluid in all twin pregnancies is more than that for a singleton gestation. However, in most twin pregnancies, the volume of amniotic fluid for each fetus is normal. The fluid is estimated in each sac if a membrane separating the fetuses can be seen. Then an overall subjective estimate of the fluid surrounding each fetus and a comparison of the two can be made. Quantitatively, the largest pocket can be measured. It is not considered standard practice or accurate to attempt an amniotic fluid index on each sac.

In the setting of a twin-twin transfusion syndrome, polyhydramnios may be present and significantly

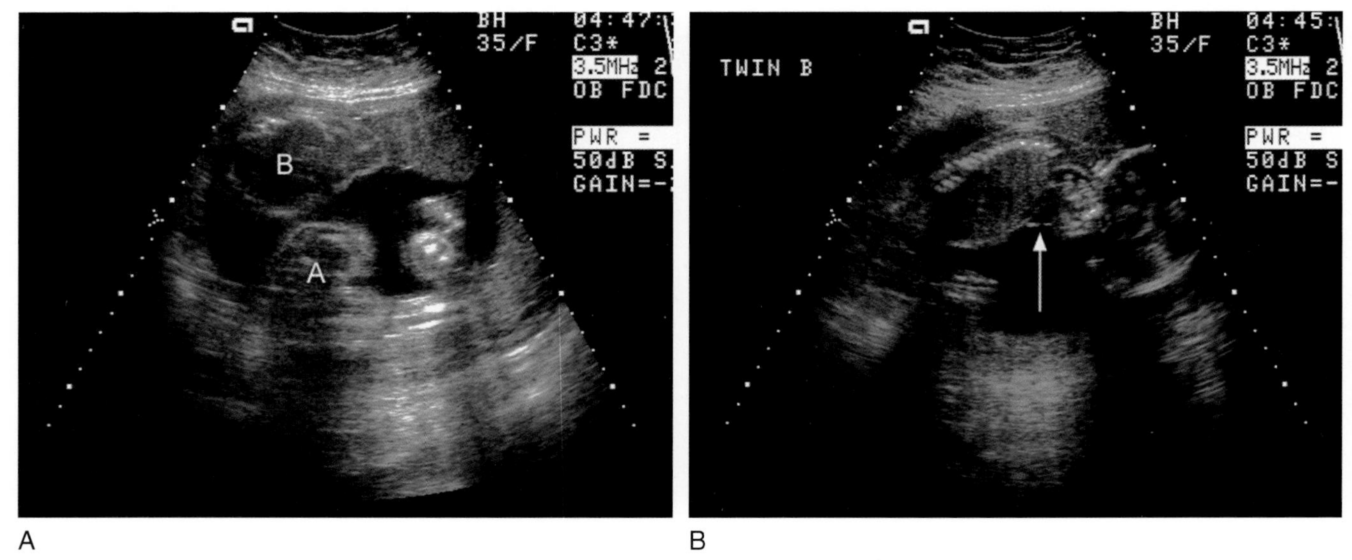

A B

Figure 21-10 "Stuck" twin. **A,** Axial image of monochorionic-diamniotic twin pregnancy shows mild polyhydramnios surrounding twin A, with such severe oligohydramnios surrounding twin B that it appears to be "stuck" to the anterior uterine wall. **B,** A short segment of the thin monochorionic-diamniotic membrane *(arrow)* is seen immediately apposed to the body and upper extremities of twin B. Because the membrane is often closely apposed to the oligohydramnionic twin in the setting of "stuck" twin, it can be difficult to identify, creating the spurious impression of absent membrane and monochorionic-monoamniotic twinning. If however, one twin is moving freely in ample amniotic fluid, and the other exhibits relatively little movement and appears confined to a localized portion of the amniotic cavity, "stuck" twin should be considered. A concerted effort should then be made to demonstrate the membrane in the vicinity of the "stuck" twin.

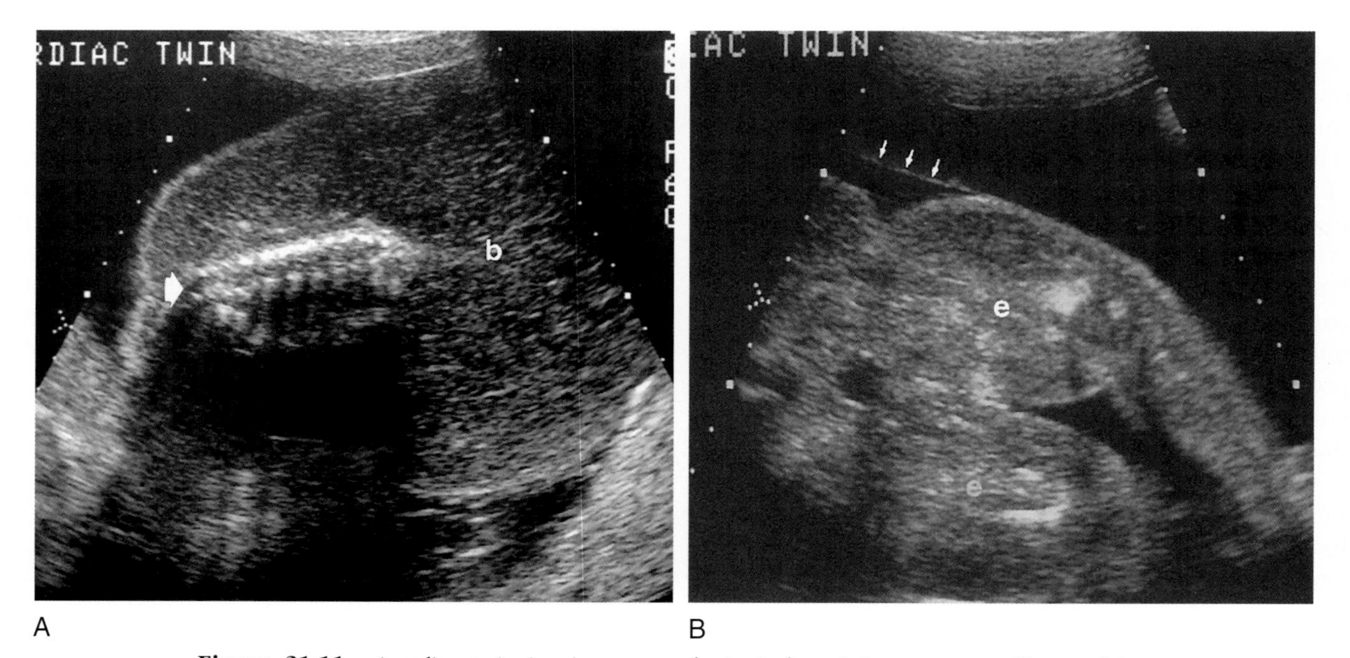

A B

Figure 21-11 Acardiac twinning in a monochorionic-diamniotic pregnancy. Two real-time images show the abnormal acardiac twin. **A,** The acardiac body (b) is seen as an edematous amorphous mass. Only the partially developed lower spine (*arrow* denotes its distal end) can be identified. **B,** The lower extremities (e) are identified with normal bony structures and edematous soft tissues. *Small arrows* denote thin diamniotic membrane.

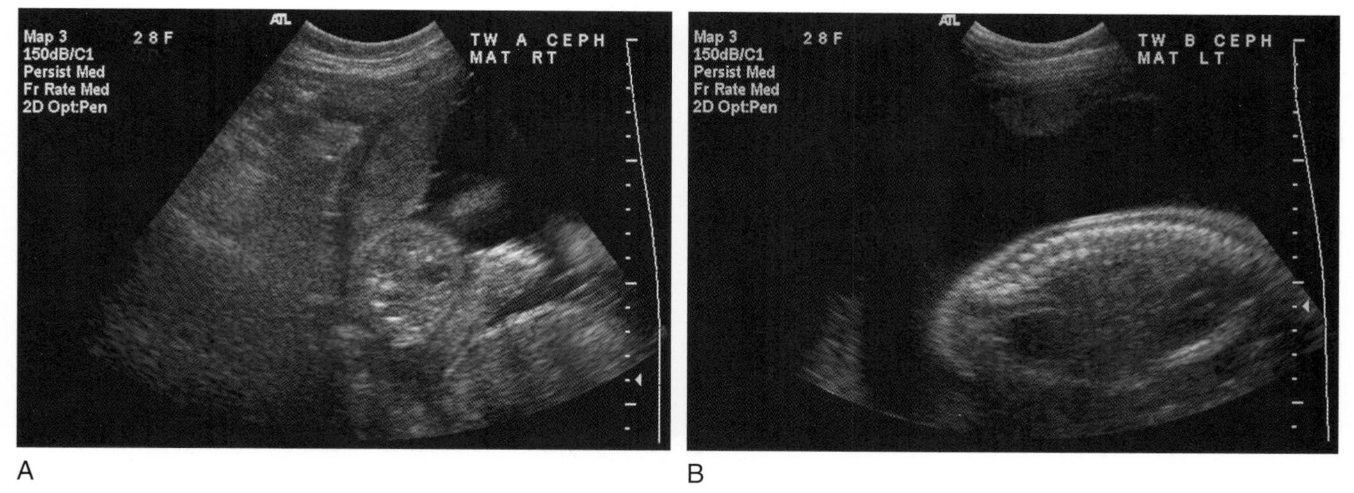

Figure 21-12 Polyhydramnios in twin-to-twin transfusion syndrome. **A,** Image of twin A shows it is directly apposed to the uterine wall. Twin A was also much smaller than twin B. **B,** Twin B is surrounded by severe polyhydramnios.

increased in the sac of the larger twin (Fig. 21-12). In addition, severe polyhydramnios can occur in uncomplicated Mono-Mono pregnancies, of unknown etiology.

Of the two additional monoamniotic complications, entangled umbilical cords can occasionally be diagnosed antenatally (Fig. 21-13). The other complication, conjoined twins, can however be detected throughout most of pregnancy (Fig. 21-14). Although the most common type is thoracopagus in which the fetuses are joined at the chest, conjoining can occur anywhere from the head to the hips. The type of conjoining should not affect the survival of the twins in utero, but it is important in terms of the type of delivery, the twins' chances for separation and their quality of life after birth. At one extreme, if the connection is only at the pelvis, it is likely that the twins can be separated successfully. At the other extreme, interconnection of the vital organs such as the brain or heart may preclude separation. If the abdomens are conjoined, a combined umbilical cord containing two sets of blood vessels can sometimes be identified. There will always be two umbilical veins, but the number of umbilical cord arteries can vary from two to four.

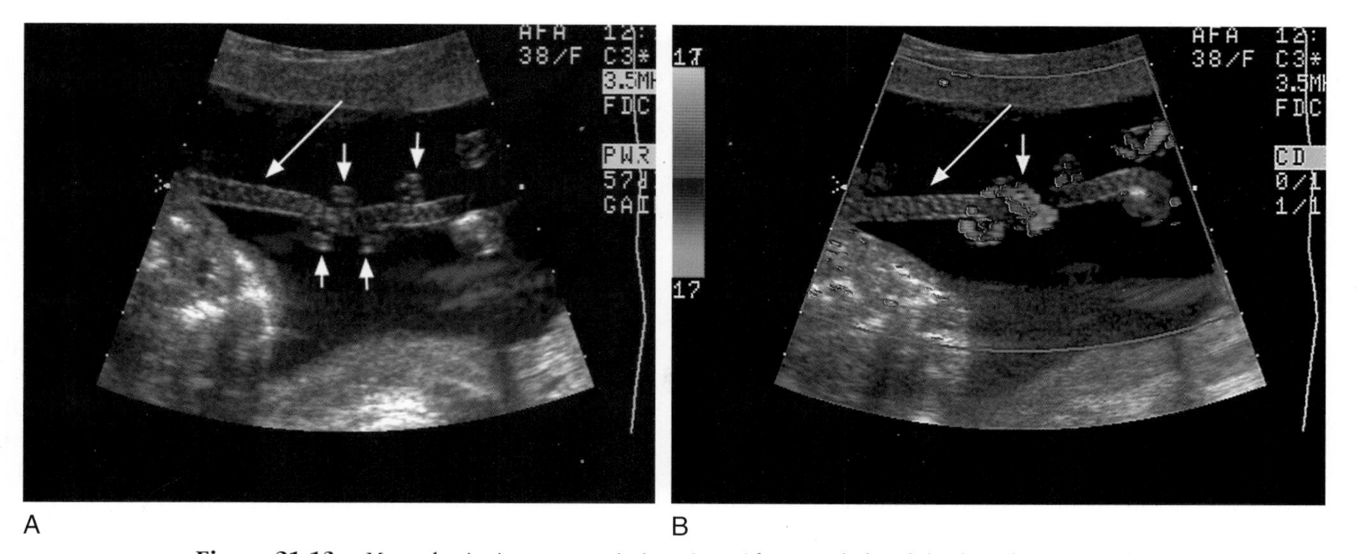

Figure 21-13 Monochorionic-monoamniotic twins with entangled umbilical cords at 18 weeks. **A,** Gray-scale ultrasound image shows umbilical cord of one twin *(short arrows)* wrapped around umbilical cord *(long arrow)* of other twin. Both twins died several days later. **B,** Color Doppler image confirms umbilical cord of one twin *(short arrow)* is wrapped around umbilical cord of other twin *(long arrow)*. There is decreased blood flow in the encircled umbilical cord.

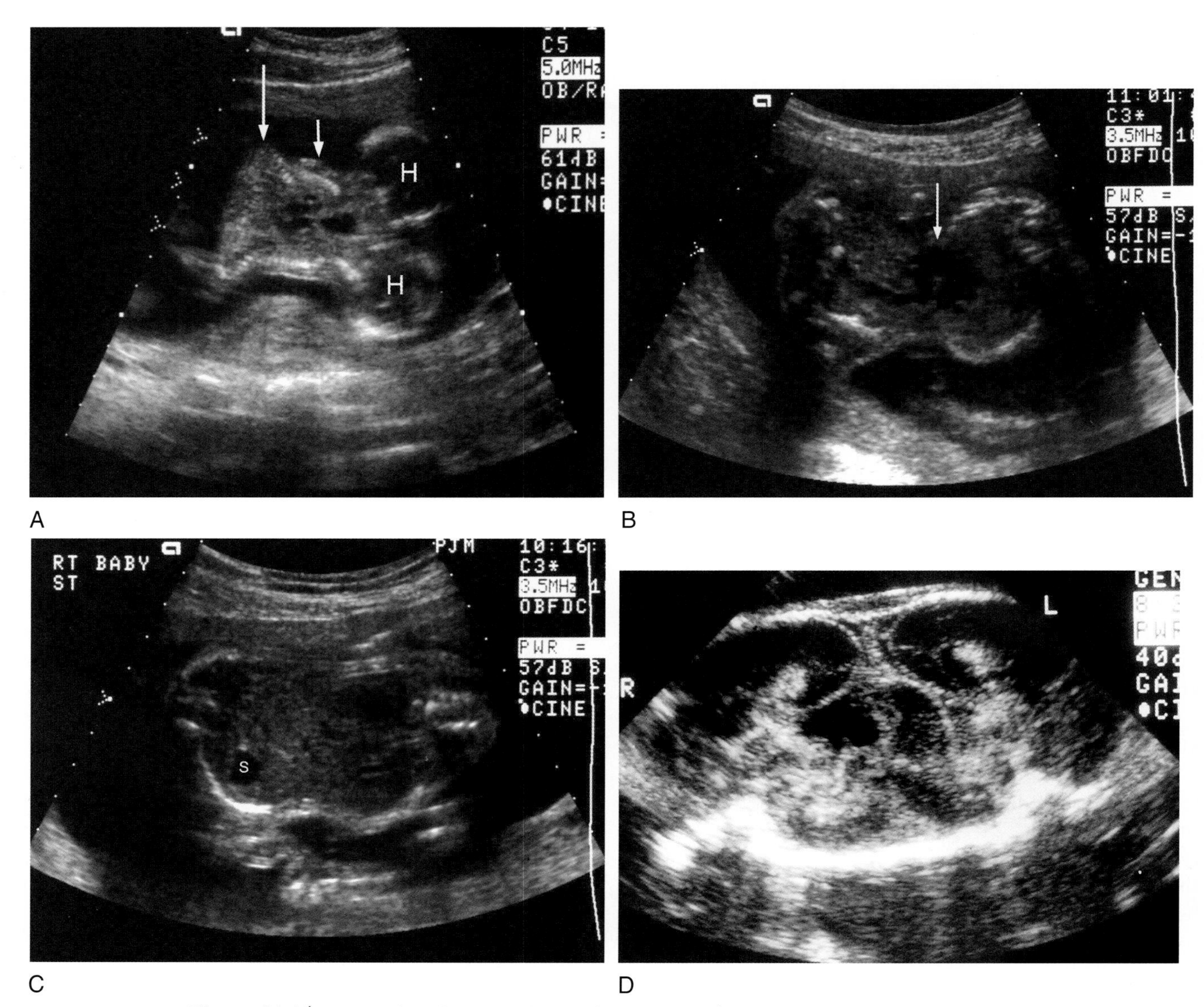

Figure 21-14 Examples of conjoined twins. **A,** Twins at 14 weeks with conjoined chests *(short arrow)* and abdomens *(long arrow).* The heads (H) are separated. **B** and **C,** Axial images of a different set of conjoined twins during the mid second trimester show the twins connected anteriorly at the chests (**B**) and abdomens (**C**). *Arrow,* shared heart; S, stomach of fetus on maternal right. **D,** Craniopagus detected in the mid third trimester. Transabdominal scan through the joined fetal heads imaged coronally shows significant interconnection of the ventricles and brain parenchyma. Although not shown, the chests, abdomens, and pelves are all separate.

INTRAUTERINE DEMISE IN TWIN PREGNANCIES

Embryonic loss is most common in the first trimester, affecting either one or rarely both pregnancies. As with singleton gestations, the loss of either of the twins occurs (on average) in 20% to 25% of the cases. Many of these demises go undetected, are typically not evident at birth, and have been described as the "vanishing twin" phenomenon (see Fig. 21-7).

When, more uncommonly, an intrauterine demise of one of the twins occurs in the second or third trimester, the fetal material is less likely to disappear. In the second trimester a small thin remnant of the dead twin can often be identified as residual bone and soft tissue, frequently along a margin of the uterine cavity. This is called a fetus papyraceus, with *papyracia* meaning "like paper." If the demise occurs in the late second or third trimester, the fetus undergoes autolysis and maceration and is clearly identified at the time of delivery. Death of one twin during the second and third trimester is associated with increased mortality and morbidity in the surviving fetus. A third-trimester demise may also occasionally induce labor.

The risk to the surviving twin depends on the extent of the shared circulation. In a Di-Di pregnancy the risk to the surviving fetus (in its separate environment) is negligible, provided there are no other uterine problems such as subchorionic collections or fibroids. However, when a later demise occurs, there is a risk of premature labor and of the macerated fetus obstructing delivery. In monochorionic gestations, because of their vascular interconnections, the surviving fetus is at considerably greater immediate potential risk of suffering twin embolization syndrome and disseminated intravascular coagulation or demise. The risk of a second demise should decrease with time. However, signs of embolization or disseminated intravascular coagulation may not be apparent in the surviving twin until after birth.

GESTATIONAL MEASUREMENTS OF TWINS

It is important to determine the fetal age of the twins. As with singleton pregnancies, this should be established by the first ultrasound examination, preferably before 24 weeks. Assignment of a single fetal age for both twins can at times be difficult, however.

If the twins have the same measurements, the same crown-rump lengths in the first trimester or the same head measurements in the second trimester, establishing a single mean and range for both twins is straightforward. If there are discrepancies in the measurements, however, a single fetal age can be established by one of three methods: (1) by averaging the means and taking the outer limits of the ranges, (2) by picking the mean and range closer to the menstrual dates if the menstrual dates are accurate, or (3) by assigning the gestational age of the larger fetus to both twins. On all subsequent examinations the age of the twins is determined by adding the first established age to the number of intervening weeks since that study.

It is also important to establish the position of each twin and to keep this constant throughout pregnancy, perhaps by labeling the fetuses "A" and "B." If problems develop for either fetus, such as discrepancies in measurements, structural abnormalities, or abnormalities in position, these can then be monitored without confusion as to which twin is affected.

Measurements and growth in twin pregnancies have not been as well studied as they have been for singleton pregnancies. The number of articles and the numbers of cases per study are much smaller. As might be expected, evaluation of the more uncommon triplet and quadruplet pregnancies is further limited by even smaller numbers of cases per series.

However, the literature on twin gestations is still quite extensive, and a number of issues about twins have been resolved. First, the growth of dichorionic and monochorionic twins is similar, provided there are no complications such as a twin-twin transfusion syndrome. Second, normal twins closely parallel each other in their size and growth. Third, the growth of the twins closely parallels that of singleton gestations until at least 30 weeks. Fourth, if normal slowing of growth occurs after 30 weeks, it should not decrease below the lower 10th percentile for singleton growth. The findings from much larger studies on singleton gestations are therefore applicable to the analysis of twins, and these singleton measurement tables are also recommended for twin assessments.

Because twins parallel each other in their growth, can we define a limit beyond which twins can be considered discrepant in size? Arbitrary but useful rules are as follows: embryos should be within 5 mm of each other. The biparietal diameters should normally be within 5 mm of each other and the interval growths within 3 mm per week of each other. If head circumferences are used, they should be within 15 mm ($3 \text{ mm} \times \pi$).

Abdominal circumferences and weights have been evaluated in an attempt to predict twin growth discordance. Both are limited in their ability to identify discrepancy, even when wide discordances are found. At present, when the abdominal circumferences differ by more than 20 mm, the positive predictive value (true-positive value divided by the true-positive plus false-positive values) is only 80%. The positive predictive values for weight discrepancies of more than 20% (the smaller from the larger) are even more disappointing, only approaching 75%. Therefore, even when large measurement differences are used, 20% to 25% of the cases are still not correctly diagnosed!

If discrepancies in the twin biparietal diameters are detected (or in the abdominal circumferences), femur lengths should be analyzed more carefully. The femur length correlates directly with fetal length, and the lengthwise growth of twins does not slow, even in the late third trimester. As twins crowd each other, particularly in the third trimester, the head and body measurements may become less accurate. Although discrepancies in the biparietal diameter can be partially corrected by either an area-corrected biparietal diameter or a head circumference, and an unusually shaped body partially corrected by an average abdominal diameter or circumference, these corrections only rectify inaccuracies in two dimensions. The third dimension of the head, from the vertex to the base, and of the body, from the diaphragm to the pelvis, cannot be corrected without the use of volume measurements; at present, volume calculations have only been provided in small series and their validity is unsubstantiated. The femur length, on the other hand, is unaffected by crowding. In addition, in the third trimester, the femur length is more accurate than a head measurement in establishing fetal ages. Therefore, when the other measurements show discrepancies, femur lengths within 5 mm of each other which continue to grow normally favor that the twins are developing normally.

SUGGESTED READINGS

Barss VA, Benacerraf BR, Frigoletto FD Jr: Ultrasonographic determination of chorion type in twin gestation. Obstet Gynecol 66:779, 1985.

Barth RA, et al: Conjoined twins: Prenatal diagnosis and assessment of associated malformations. Radiology 177:201, 1990.

Benson CB, Doubilet PM, Vivek D: Prognosis of first-trimester pregnancies: Polychotomous logistic regression analysis. Radiology 192:765, 1994.

Blickstein I: The twin-twin transfusion syndrome. Obstet Gynecol 76:714, 1990.

Brown DL, et al: Twin-twin transfusion syndrome: Sonographic findings. Radiology 170:61, 1989.

Bruner JP, et al: Twin-to-twin transfusion syndrome: A subset of the twin oligohydramnios-polyhydramnios sequence. Am J Obstet Gynecol 169:4, 1993.

Doubilet PM, et al: "Appearing twin": Undercounting of multiple gestations on early first trimester sonograms. J Ultrasound Med 17:199, 1998.

Finberg HJ: The "twin-peak" sign: Reliable evidence of dichorionic twinning. J Ultrasound Med 11:571, 1992.

Finberg HJ: Uterine synechiae in pregnancy: Expanded criteria for recognition and clinical significance in 28 cases. J Ultrasound Med 10:547, 1991.

Grumbach K, et al: Twin and singleton growth patterns compared using US. Radiology 158:237, 1986.

Hertzberg BS, et al: Significance of membrane thickness in the sonographic evaluation of twin gestations. AJR Am J Roentgenol 148:151, 1987.

Key Features

Twin (multiple) gestations are defined by their chorionicity and amnionicity. This helps predict potential risk factors both in utero and at time of birth.

Twins in completely separate environments are surrounded by their own chorionic and amniotic membranes and are called dichorionic-diamnionic (Di-Di) twins.

When twins are surrounded by one chorion (monochorionic), they partially or completely share the same environment. If still within their own amniotic membrane, they are monochorionic-diamniotic (Mono-Di) twins. When there is no separating membrane, they are monochorionic-monoamniotic (Mono-Mono) twins.

In the first trimester a Di-Di pregnancy is diagnosed by the type of interposed membrane or by separate placentas. Transvaginal scanning may be of value in determining membrane thickness.

In the second and third trimesters, five characteristics can be used to differentiate the types of twinning: the number of placentas, the fetal genders, the type of interposed membranes, the presence or absence of the "lambda (twin peaks)" sign, and, occasionally, by the amount of amniotic fluid. Separate placentas, different fetal genders, a thick Di-Di membrane, or a combination of these findings, confirms a Di-Di pregnancy.

All twin pregnancies have an increased incidence of the following: twins smaller than singleton infant (even at term), prematurity, growth restriction, and a possible increased incidence of structural anomalies.

The most common complication of monochorionic pregnancies is twin-twin transfusion through a single fused placenta. This has variable presentations. If one twin is small or is within an oligohydramnionic sac, without other findings, it will be difficult to differentiate this from growth restriction. In its most severe form, the smaller twin will be in an oligohydramnionic sac (a "stuck" twin) and the larger twin will be hydropic and in a polyhydramnionic sac. When this is detected, the prognosis for both twins is poor, with mortality rates approaching 50%.

Monochorionic-monoamniotic twins have a further increased incidence of entangled cords.

In Mono-Mono twinning, the twins should be carefully studied to be certain that they are not conjoined.

The identification of an in utero twin death and its complications is related to the trimester in which the death occurs and the type of twinning. The earlier the demise, the more likely that there will be complete resorption of the demised fetus.

The following is known about twin gestational growth: the twins grow similarly regardless of their chorionicity and amnionicity, twins closely parallel each other in their growth, and twins closely parallel singleton gestations in growth until at least 30 weeks when they tend to slow down toward (but not below) the normal lower 10th percentile.

Hill LM, et al: The sonographic assessment of twin growth discordance. Obstet Gynecol 84:501, 1994.

Kurtz AB, et al: Twin pregnancies: Accuracy of first-trimester abdominal US in predicting chorionicity and amnionicity. Radiology 185:759, 1992.

Langlotz H, Sauerbrei E, Murray S: Transvaginal Doppler sonographic diagnosis of an acardiac twin at 12 weeks' gestation. J Ultrasound Med 10:175, 1991.

Mahony BS, Filly RA, Callen PW: Amnionicity and chorionicity in twin pregnancies: Prediction using ultrasound. Radiology 155:205, 1985.

Mahony BS, et al: The "stuck twin" phenomenon: Ultrasonographic findings, pregnancy outcome, and management with serial amniocenteses. Am J Obstet Gynecol 163:1513, 1990.

Monteagudo A, et al: Early and simple determination of chorionic and amniotic type in multifetal gestations in the first fourteen weeks by high-frequency transvaginal ultrasonography. Am J Obstet Gynecol 170:824, 1994.

Randel SB, et al: Amniotic sheets. Radiology 166:633, 1988.

Scardo JA, et al: Prospective determination of chorionicity, amnionicity, and zygosity in twin gestations. Am J Obstet Gynecol 173:1376, 1995.

Su LL: Monoamniotic twins: Diagnosis and management. Acta Obstet Gynecol Scand 81:995-1000, 2002.

Trop I: The twin peak sign. Radiology 220:68-69, 2001.

van den Brand SF, et al: Prenatal ultrasound diagnosis of conjoined twins. Obstet Gynecol Surv 49:656, 1994.

Weissman A, et al: Sonographic growth measurements in triplet pregnancies. Obstet Gynecol 75:324, 1990.

Wood SL, et al: Evaluation of the twin peak or lambda sign in determining chorionicity in multiple pregnancy. Obstet Gynecol 88:6 1996.

CHAPTER 22

Pelvis and Uterus

The female pelvis can be evaluated by two ultrasound techniques: transabdominal (TA) and transvaginal (TV). The TA examination is performed from the anterior abdominal wall, using transducers with frequencies of up to 5 MHz. Scans typically use the distended urinary bladder as a "sonic" window to identify the uterus and adnexa and as an overview of the other pelvic structures.

The TV examination is performed with the patient's bladder empty using higher transducer frequencies of 7.5 MHz or more. These higher frequencies have better near-field focusing and resolution, which often permits greater detail of the uterus and adnexa. However, the intracavitary position of the TV probe limits movement of the transducer and the ultrasound beam penetrates only 8 to 10 cm from the transducer face. Findings farther away from the transducer may be either not fully appreciated or may go undetected.

For an initial study of the female pelvis, especially if the patient has not been previously studied, it is recommended that a TA study be initially performed. Even when the urinary bladder is only partially distended or is empty, a TA scan may still help as an overview to the pelvic structures. The TV examination provides more detailed evaluation, especially of areas not fully identified by the TA study. For subsequent studies, however, because of prior knowledge of a patient's particular pelvic anatomy or pathologic condition, often only one of the two diagnostic techniques is needed and this determination can often be made by the history, physical examination, and the expected findings from the first ultrasound study.

The TA pelvic examination is best initiated by first identifying the urinary bladder and allows an evaluation of its walls and lumen (Fig. 22-1A). Even when a patient claims to have completely voided, often identifiable residual fluid still remains with the bladder lumen (Fig. 22-1B). It is important to definitely identify the urinary bladder to rule out the possibility of a midline cystic or complex mass, usually of ovarian origin, that can infrequently occupy the lower pelvis. Such a mass can inadvertently be mistaken for the bladder (Fig. 22-2). The bladder shape may be helpful because a well-distended urinary bladder typically has a triangular or elongated shape on midline sagittal scans with a posterior impression from the uterus, whereas a cystic ovarian mass typically has a rounded or ovoid contour. If there is any question as to whether a cystic structure in the pelvis represents the bladder, the identity of the bladder should be confirmed by emptying or filling it.

The uterus should then be identified in its long axis. This may not be in a true anatomic sagittal plane because the uterus can normally deviate toward either the right or the left. Once the uterine long axis is established, parallel sagittal scans are then obtained to its right and left to evaluate the uterine margins and the adnexa. The transducer should then be turned 90 degrees so that axial or axial-coronal images can be obtained. If the orientation is lost, which is a particular problem during the TV study, the examiner should restart the evaluation with a long-axis uterine image.

The TA probes are end-firing transducers. The beam is emitted directly from the end of the probe like a flashlight beam, and as the examiner moves the ultrasound probe the imaged body part is directly below the probe. This makes the examination easy to conceptualize. With TV scanning, however, the ultrasound beam is often set

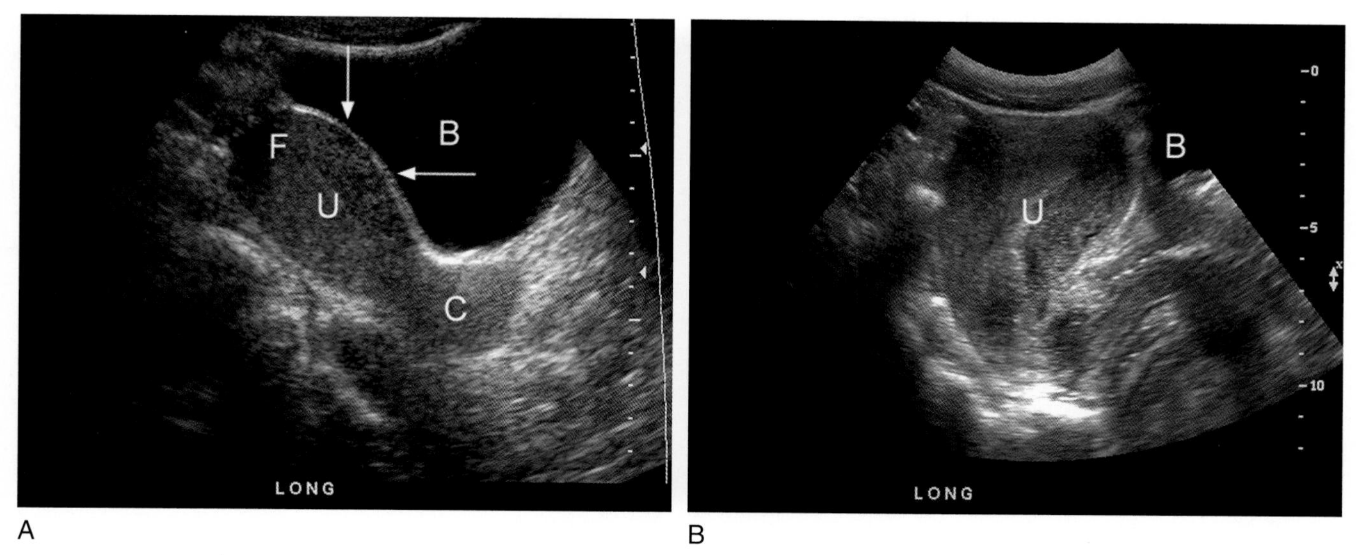

Figure 22-1 Urinary bladder. **A,** Midline sagittal transabdominal image shows a distended urinary bladder (B) anterior to the uterus (U). Note the elongated configuration of the bladder and the relative narrowing of the superior portion of the bladder due to a posterior impression on it *(arrows)* from the uterus. F, uterine fundus; C, cervix. **B,** Post-void midline sagittal image shows a small amount of residual urine in the bladder (B). U, uterus.

at an angle of between 30 to 60 degrees from the end of the probe. This angle was created because of the usual anteverted position of the uterus relative to the vaginal canal. Therefore, in the sagittal plane the anteriorly angled beam helps to fully image the uterus and anteriorly positioned ovaries. However, when the uterus is tilted posteriorly or the ovaries are in the cul-de-sac, full visualization may not be possible unless the probe is turned a full 180 degrees. If the examiner has difficulty visualizing an upside-down image, the image can be flipped 180 degrees by pushing the invert button on the machine. Similar problems occur in axial or axial-coronal views. When the transducer is turned to the right, the angle of the beam can prevent full visualization of the left side unless the same 180-degree maneuver is used. Before the use of an intracavitary probe the examiner should inquire about the angle of the beam.

There are no universally established gynecologic contraindications to the use of the TV probe, although it is recommended that transvaginal evaluation not be performed in patients who have never been sexually active. After the probe is appropriately soaked in an antibacterial and often antiviral solution and after a sheath (usually a condom) is placed over the transducer, the probe is typically inserted about halfway into the vagina. With carefully insertion, the probe will not touch the cervix. The TV study is therefore considered relatively noninvasive and, when clinically or sonographically considered appropriate, can be performed in the evaluation of any gynecologic abnormality.

Doppler waveform analysis (color or pulsed) may be of value. It can help differentiate vascular from nonvascular tubular structures and can help define normal anatomic characteristics. Its use in the evaluation of adnexal masses is discussed in Chapter 23.

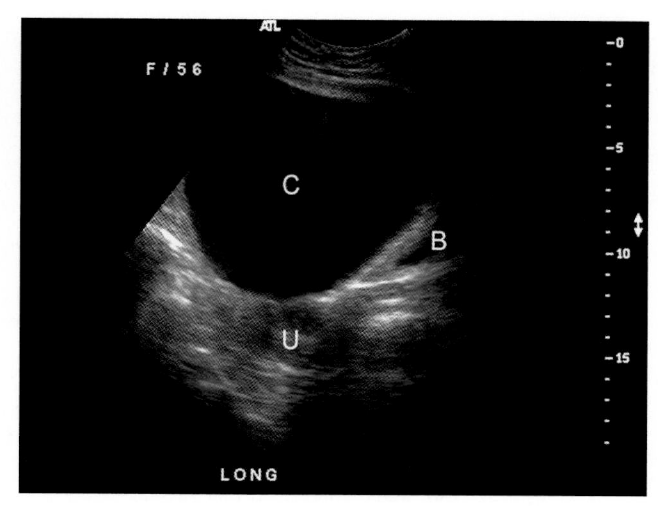

Figure 22-2 Cystic ovarian mass resembling urinary bladder. Midline sagittal transabdominal image of pelvis of a postmenopausal female shows a large cystic mass (C) between the uterus (U) and anterior abdominal wall. Although this mass superficially resembles a distended urinary bladder, it is rounder than a typical bladder. Additionally, a small amount of urine is seen in the true bladder (B). Histopathologic evaluation revealed the cystic mass was a serous cystadenoma.

NORMAL FERTILE YEARS FINDINGS

Most women examined during their fertile years, typically between 14 and 50 years of age, are undergoing monthly menstrual cycles. These cycles cause continuing and often predictable changes in the endometrium and the ovaries (discussed in Chapter 23).

During midline sagittal scanning, the vagina is usually identified as a thin hyperechoic line (Fig. 22-3A). If a tampon, fluid, or blood causes the canal to spread, it becomes thicker and may have a hypoechoic center (Fig. 22-3B to D).

The endometrial stripe (also called the endometrial complex) is composed of the endometrial canal surrounded by two layers of endometrium. The brightness

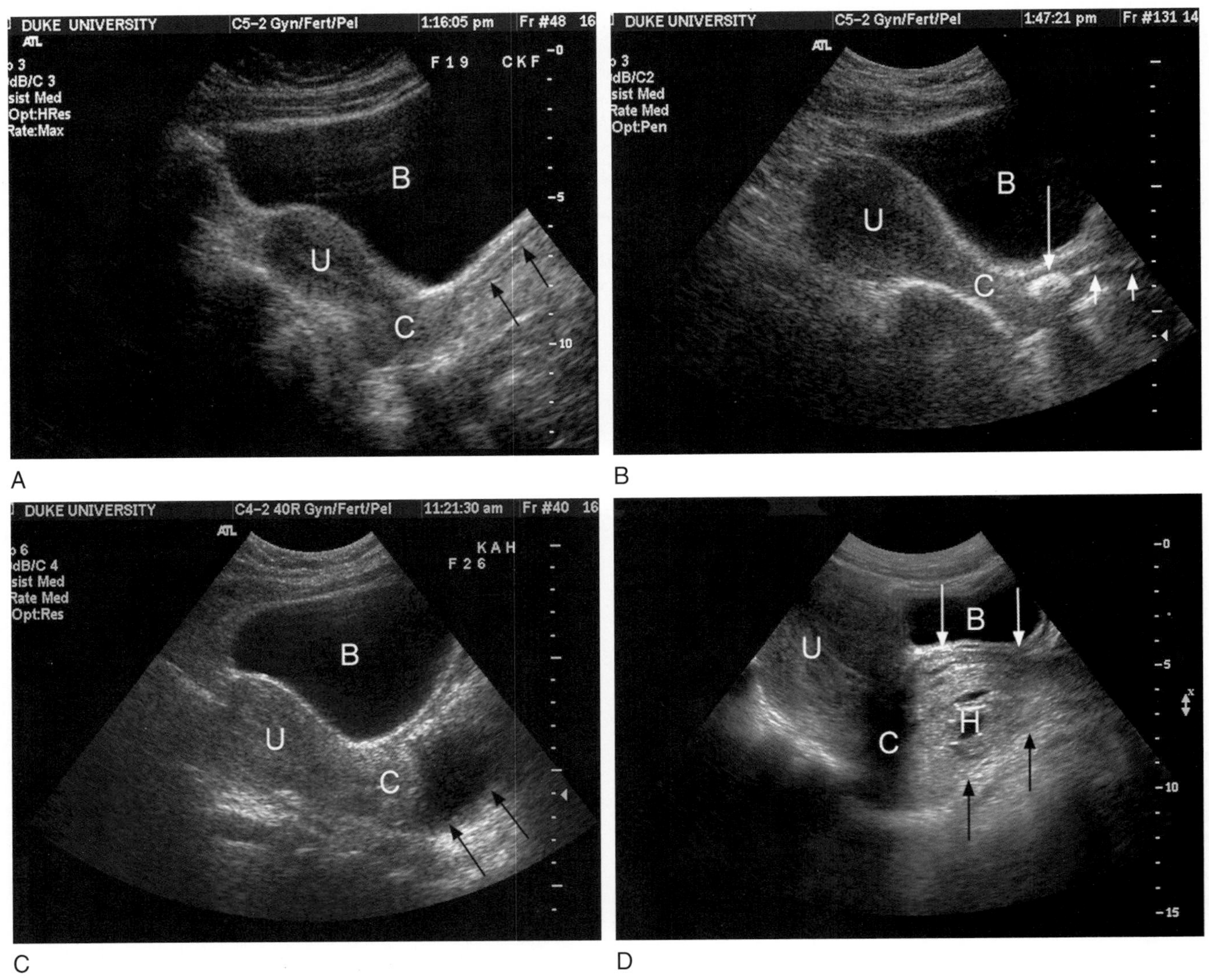

Figure 22-3 Vagina: ultrasound appearances. **A,** Normal appearance. Midline sagittal transabdominal scan depicts the normal vagina as a hyperechoic stripe *(arrows)* posterior to the bladder (B) and caudal to the cervix (C). U, uterus. **B,** Tampon in vagina. Midline sagittal transabdominal scan depicts tampon in the upper vagina as a thick echogenic structure *(long arrow)* with posterior shadowing. A normal vaginal stripe *(short arrows)* is seen caudal to the tampon. B, bladder; U, uterus; C cervix. **C,** Fluid distending vagina. Midline sagittal transabdominal image of pelvis shows fluid distending the vagina *(arrows)* due to inadvertent introduction of sterile saline into the vagina through a Foley catheter that was initially inserted into the vagina instead of the bladder. U, uterus; B, bladder; C, cervix. **D,** Blood and products of conception distending vagina. Midline sagittal transabdominal scan of pelvis shows marked distention of vagina by heterogeneous material (H) corresponding to blood clots and products of conception. Patient was in the midst of spontaneous miscarriage at the time of the ultrasound. *Black arrows,* posterior surface of vagina; *white arrows,* anterior surface of vagina; U, uterus; C, cervix; B, bladder.

and thickness of this stripe depends primarily on the time in the patient's menstrual cycle. At the end of menses the endometrial stripe is a discrete thin hyperechoic line that is usually only 2 to 3 mm thick (Fig. 22-4A). Between then and the onset of ovulation, termed the *proliferative (estrogen) phase*, the stripe becomes thicker, as much as 8 mm, and remains uniformly hyperechoic and distinct (Fig. 22-4B). Occasionally, a striated appearance (also called the *triple layer* or trilaminated appearance) may be detected; this consists of three hyperechoic lines surrounding two hypoechoic layers and is typically seen at mid cycle (Fig. 22-4C). Although the overall thickness of both patterns is similar, the striated appearance seems to signify a time when the endometrium is particularly receptive to implantation. Fertility medications control the number

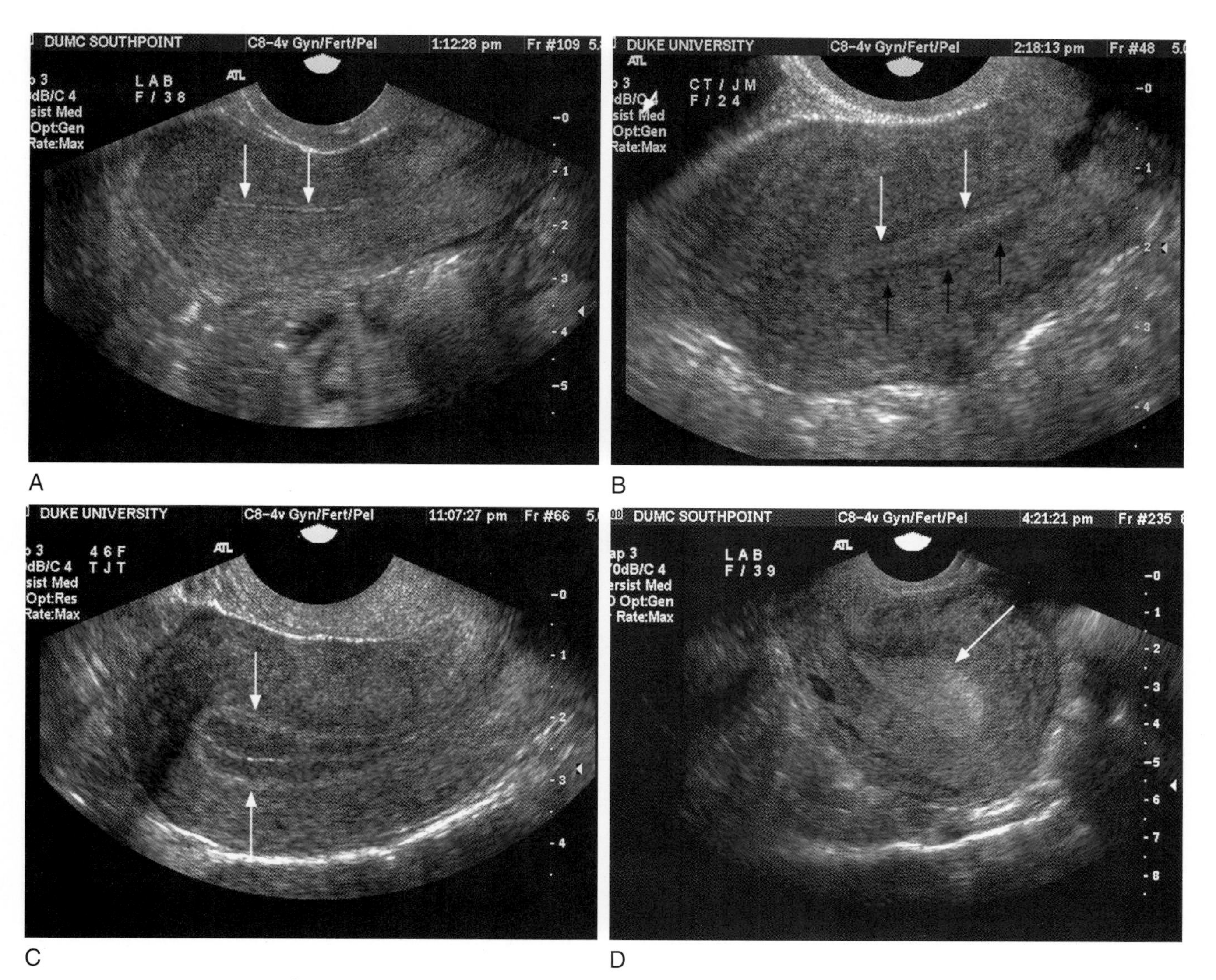

Figure 22-4 Endometrium: examples of normal endometrium at different stages of menstrual cycle. **A,** After menses. Longitudinal transvaginal scan of the uterus obtained 2 days after cessation of menses depicts endometrium as a discrete thin hyperechoic line *(arrows)*. **B,** Proliferative phase. Longitudinal transvaginal scan of uterus obtained during proliferative phase shows uniformly hyperechoic endometrium *(white arrows)*. A hypoechoic layer *(black arrows)* is seen deep to the endometrium, corresponding to the junctional zone. Note the endometrium is thicker than in the patient scanned 2 days after menses in **A**. **C,** Triple layer, striated appearance. Longitudinal transvaginal scan of uterus at mid cycle, late in proliferative phase and immediately before ovulation shows a triple-layer appearance of the endometrium *(arrows)* with three hyperechoic lines surrounding two hypoechoic layers. **D,** Secretory phase. Longitudinal transvaginal scan of retroflexed uterus during secretory phase of menstrual cycle shows normal hyperechoic thick endometrium *(arrow)*.

of days of the proliferative phase and the timing of ovulation. If the proliferative phase is lengthened, the endometrial complex may be thicker.

From ovulation until the start of the menses, termed the *secretory (progesterone) phase*, the endometrium further thickens to as much as 15 mm and sometimes more (Fig. 22-4D). Although uniformly hyperechoic, its boundaries may be less well defined. As menses begins, the endometrium sloughs, the stripe thins out, and the cycle starts again.

If there is fluid within the endometrial canal, and a small amount of fluid is normal, it should not be included in the endometrial stripe measurement. Both endometrial walls are then measured separately and added together.

A distended urinary bladder during TA scanning may complicate these appearances because it can cause occasional compression and distortion of the uterus. If this is observed, a follow-up TA or TV examination after bladder emptying should be performed.

A thin hypoechoic layer, commonly called the *junctional zone*, is identified deep to the endometrium (see Fig. 22-4B). It is anatomically either the boundary between the endometrium and myometrium or the innermost margin of the myometrium. Although not always detected by ultrasound, it is an important landmark because the junctional zone is distorted in the settings of adenomyosis (the uterine form of endometriosis), diffuse fibroids, and invasive endometrial carcinoma. The junctional zone is more consistently identified by MRI, which can perhaps better differentiate among these processes.

The myometrium (the uterine muscle) is identified beyond the junctional zone. It is the largest component of the uterus and gives the uterus its shape. During the fertile years the uterine body and fundus are more prominent than the cervix, but before puberty the cervix is similar in size or more prominent than the uterine body and fundus (Fig. 22-5). The normal myometrium has a uniform low-level echogenicity that is less than that of the endometrium.

The serosal surface is usually not appreciated. Occasionally, subserosal veins may appear as prominent anechoic spaces (Fig. 22-6). This is a normal variant, usually identified in multiparous women.

There is a wide range of normal uterine sizes, and these are due to a variety of factors, particularly previous pregnancies. The nulliparous uterus typically measures approximately 7 by 5 by 3 cm, respectively, in its length, width, and anteroposterior dimensions, with the anteroposterior measurement obtained perpendicular to the uterine length (Table 22-1). In parous women the uterus is typically larger in all three dimensions, increasing with each pregnancy up to six. It may then be more than 10 cm long. As long as the echogenicity is normal and all uterine layers are maintained, uterine size alone is not an indicator of uterine abnormalities.

The normal uterus may have different positions. It is most commonly anteverted with the entire uterus (from the cervix to the fundus) tilted forward toward the anterior abdominal wall (Fig. 22-7A). When the urinary bladder is distended during TA scanning, the anteverted uterus is often pushed backward (Fig. 22-7B). A markedly distended bladder can push the uterus into a

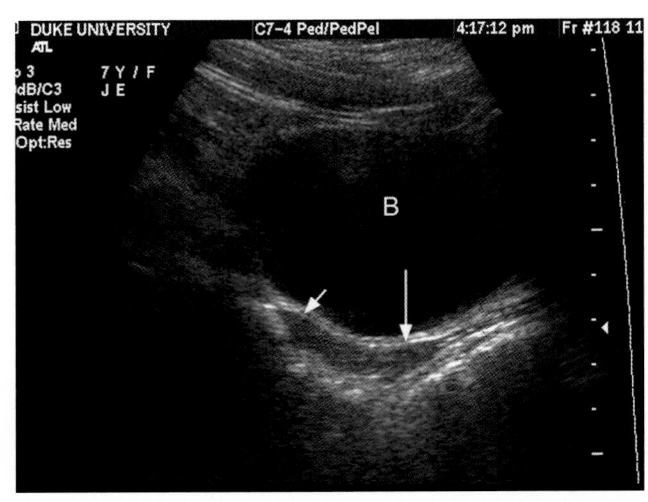

Figure 22-5 Normal uterus in a child. Midline transabdominal scan of uterus of a 7-year-old girl shows normal prepubertal uterine configuration. Uterine fundus *(short arrow)* is less prominent than cervix *(long arrow)*. Compare with Figure 22-1A, which shows normal uterine configuration during childbearing years in which uterine fundus and body are more prominent than cervix. B, bladder.

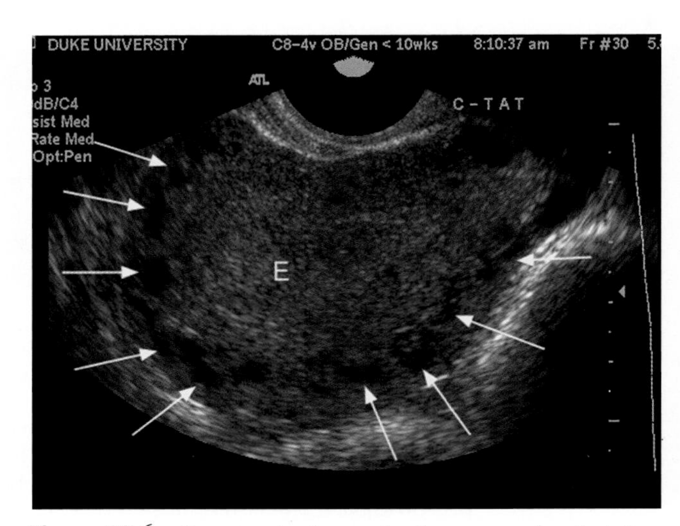

Figure 22-6 Prominent subserosal veins, a normal variant. Longitudinal transvaginal image of uterus shows serpiginous hypoechoic structures *(arrows)* around the periphery of the uterus between the myometrium and serosal surface, corresponding to subserosal veins. E, endometrium.

Table 22-1 Normal Anatomic Uterine Dimensions in Adult Women During Their Fertile Years According to Parity

	Mean (±SD)		
Parity	Length (cm)	Anteroposterior (cm)	Width (cm)
0	7.7 (1.1)	2.9 (1.1)	4.7 (0.6)
1	8.6 (1.5)	3.5 (1.0)	5.0 (1.0)
2-3	9.2 (1.3)	3.9 (1.3)	5.6 (1.3)
4-5	9.4 (1.1)	4.2 (1.1)	5.8 (1.1)
6	9.7 (1.1)	4.2 (1.1)	5.9 (1.1)

Adapted from Langlois PL: The size of the normal uterus. J Reprod Med 4:221, 1970.

horizontal position. Although the uterus is then perpendicular to the ultrasound beam and would seem to be ideally positioned to be imaged through the bladder, because the distended bladder can also compress and distort the uterus, empty-bladder scans may be needed to evaluate the true size and shape of the uterus.

In some women the uterus is retroverted, tilted posteriorly from the vaginal vault. Another common normal variant position of the uterus is termed *flexion*. Rather than tilted entirely forward or backward, the uterine body is folded in on itself, anteflexed if folded anteriorly and retroflexed if folded posteriorly (Fig. 22-8). The overall ultrasound appearance is similar to that of an anteverted and retroverted uterus except that there is a sharp angle to both the uterine body and the endometrial complex at the point of flexion. Because the endometrial stripe of a retroverted or retroflexed uterus is oriented approximately parallel to the ultrasound beam at TA ultrasound, it can be difficult to image, creating the spurious impression of a large posterior hypoechoic fibroid (see Fig. 22-8A). By adjusting the orientation of the transducer, the normal endometrial stripe can be better appreciated (see Fig. 22-8B). TV ultrasound can then be used to confirm the absence of a fibroid (see Fig. 22-8C).

The gynecologist is often not able to differentiate version from flexion on the basis of clinical findings. If evacuation of the endometrial cavity is planned, knowledge of flexion is important because the angle may interfere with effective treatment of the upper half of the canal. With correct probe angulation, perhaps performed under ultrasound guidance, more complete insertion is usually possible with less chance of uterine perforation.

An interesting observation about uterine position relative to the TA and TV techniques has recently been described. It had always been assumed that a horizontal-positioned uterus identified on a TA study with a

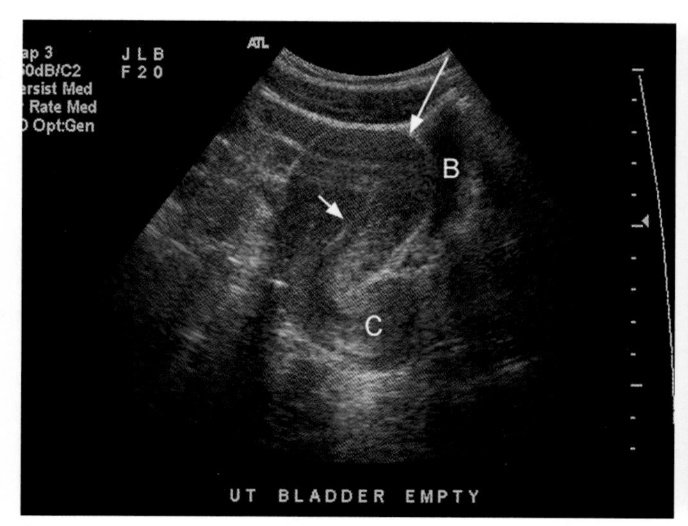

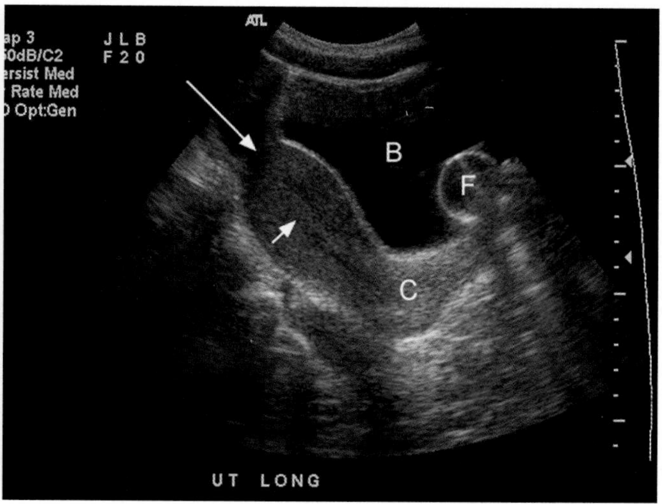

Figure 22-7 Effect of urinary bladder distention on uterine configuration. **A,** Midline sagittal transabdominal scan performed post void with only a minimal amount of fluid in the bladder (B) shows the anteverted configuration of uterus typically seen when the bladder is empty. The uterine fundus *(long arrow)* is tilted forward toward the anterior abdominal wall. C, cervix; *short arrow,* endometrial stripe. **B,** Corresponding image obtained with the bladder (B) distended shows the uterine fundus *(long arrow)* has been displaced posteriorly, away from the anterior abdominal wall. This is the typical configuration seen when the bladder is full. When the bladder is markedly overdistended, the uterus can be pushed into a more horizontal configuration. C, cervix; *short arrow,* endometrial stripe; F, balloon on Foley catheter.

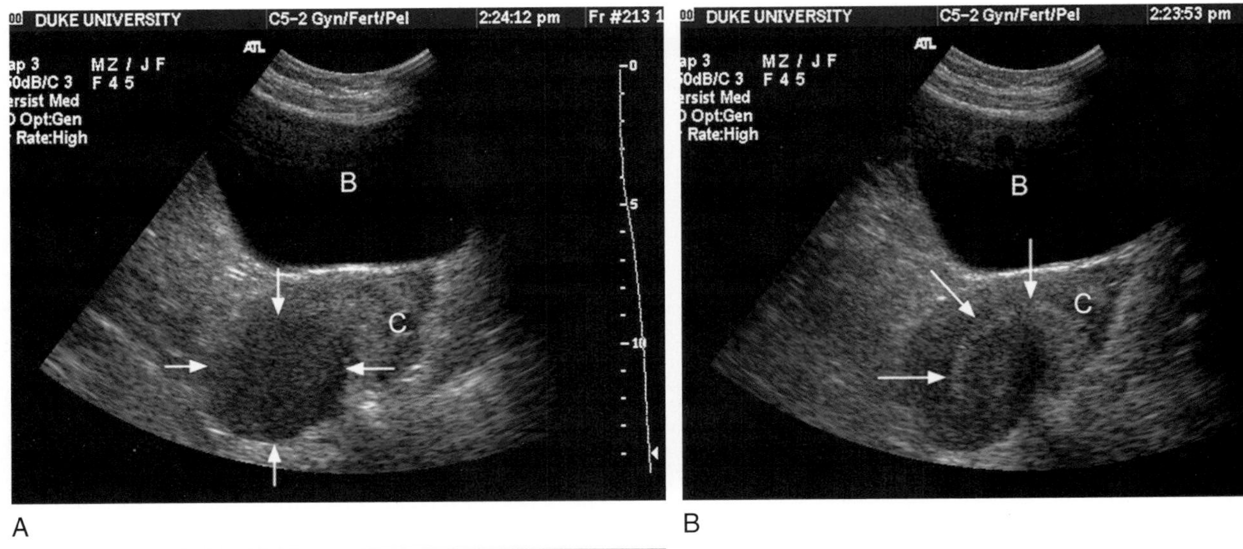

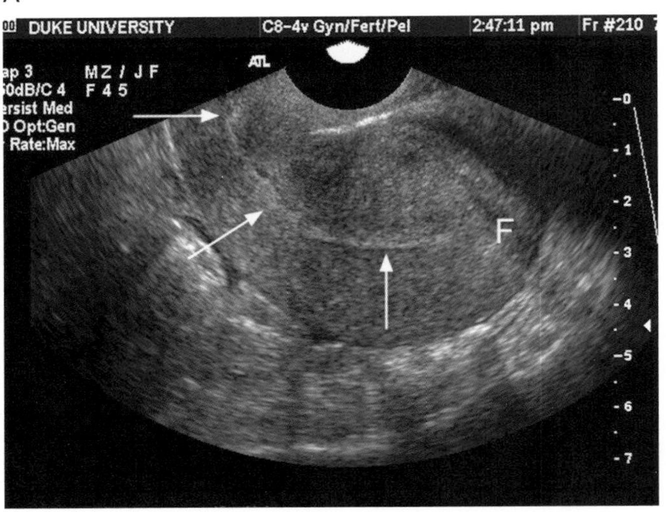

Figure 22-8 Retroflexed uterus causing spurious impression of fibroid. **A,** Midline longitudinal transabdominal scan of uterus shows a large hypoechoic structure *(arrows)* with an appearance resembling a fibroid. B, bladder; C, cervix. **B,** Corresponding transabdominal image obtained after minor adjustment to orientation of transducer shows the endometrial stripe *(arrows)* coursing posteriorly within the area that resembled a fibroid in **A**. There is no evidence of a fibroid. The uterine body is folded on itself, consistent with a retroflexed uterus. B, bladder; C, cervix. **C,** Sagittal transvaginal ultrasound image performed on same patient as shown in **A** and **B** confirms the absence of a fundal fibroid and the retroflexed configuration of the uterus. Note that the uterine fundus (F) points to the right side of the image, which is the orientation expected with a retroflexed uterus. An anteflexed uterus would point to the left side of the image on a sagittal transvaginal scan. *Arrows,* endometrial stripe.

distended urinary bladder would become anteverted (move anteriorly) when the bladder was emptied. In a comparative study of the full-bladder TA to the empty-bladder TV examination, however, this was not always found. On occasion, the TV study showed an apparently retroverted or retroflexed uterus. Because the true neutral position of the uterus must be considered as present when the urinary bladder is empty, it is best to predict the uterine position with an empty bladder, either on a TA or TV study.

There are a number of congenital uterine anomalies, ranging from a simple uterine septation to a bicornuate and didelphys uterus. Occasionally, only one horn of the uterus (a unicornuate uterus) develops. These abnormalities are all related to müllerian duct anomalies and are not infrequently reported to be associated with ipsilateral renal anomalies. Although most uterine and cervical anomalies are detected by a combination of physical examination and radiographic hysterogram findings, an ultrasound examination may reveal an abnormality by showing two endometrial canals, two uterine horns, an unusually broad and "squared-off" uterus in an axial view, and/or ptosis or absence of a kidney (Fig. 22-9). TV ultrasound, 3-D ultrasound, and saline-infusion sonohysterography can offer a great deal of additional information; and, on occasion, MRI may help confirm the malformation.

TV imaging is not always needed when scanning the uterus. It should be used when expected TA findings are not detected or are equivocal or when abnormal findings require further evaluation (Fig. 22-10). TV scanning permits different orientations, its resolution is better, and a more "neutral"-appearing uterus is possible because the urinary bladder is not distended. The endometrial stripe is often more completely identified by TV scanning, especially when the uterus is retroverted or

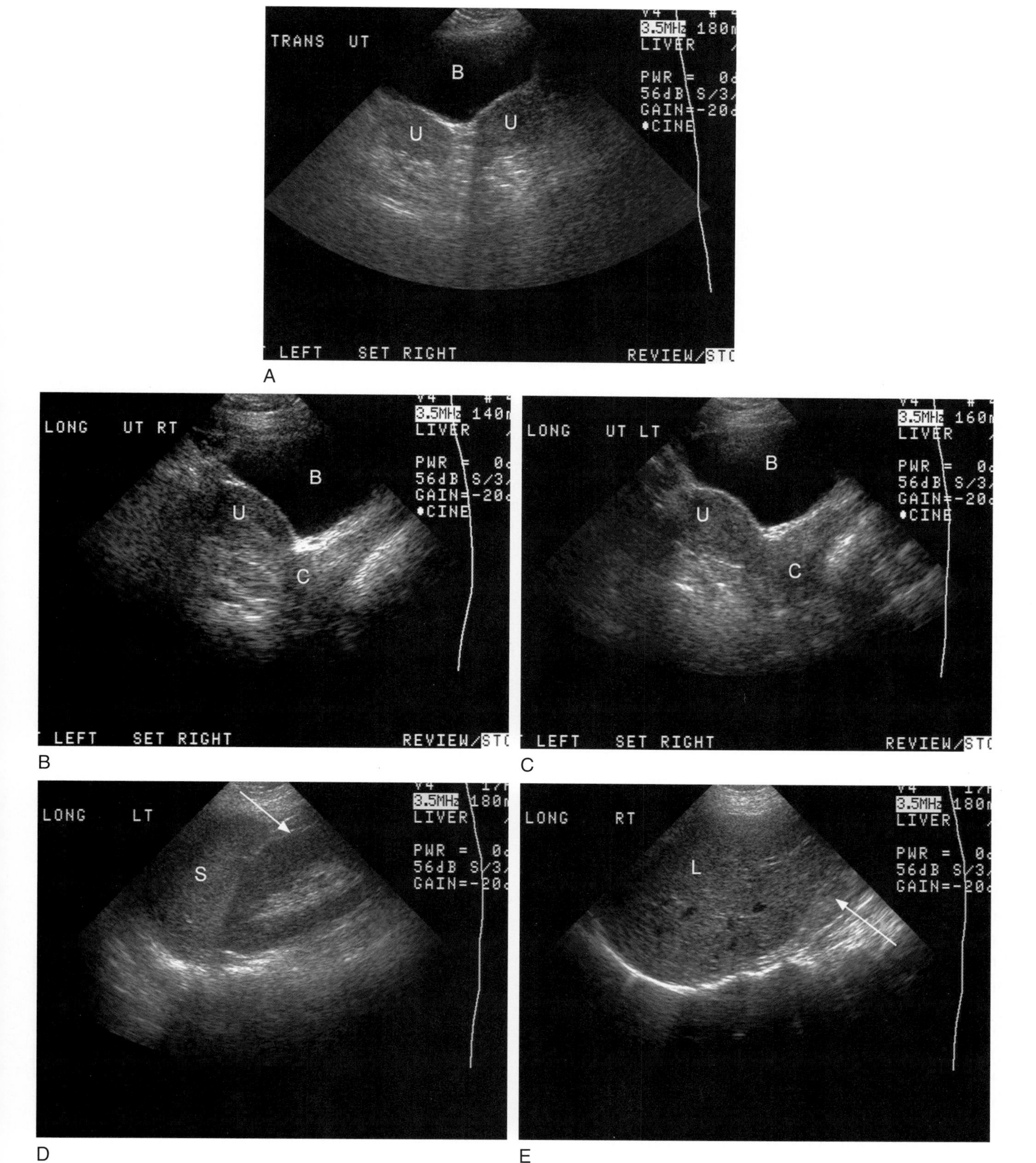

Figure 22-9 Uterus didelphys associated with right renal agenesis. **A,** Axial transabdominal scan of pelvis shows two discrete uterine bodies (U). B, bladder. **B** and **C,** Longitudinal transabdominal images of the right (**B**) and left (**C**) pelvis confirm the presence of two complete duplicated uteri (U) and two cervices (C). B, bladder. **D,** Longitudinal image of left upper quadrant shows left kidney *(arrow)* in normal position, immediately inferior to spleen (S). **E,** Longitudinal image of right upper quadrant shows absence of the right kidney in its expected location in the right flank *(arrow)*. Additional images of the abdomen and pelvis also failed to identify an ectopic kidney. L, liver.

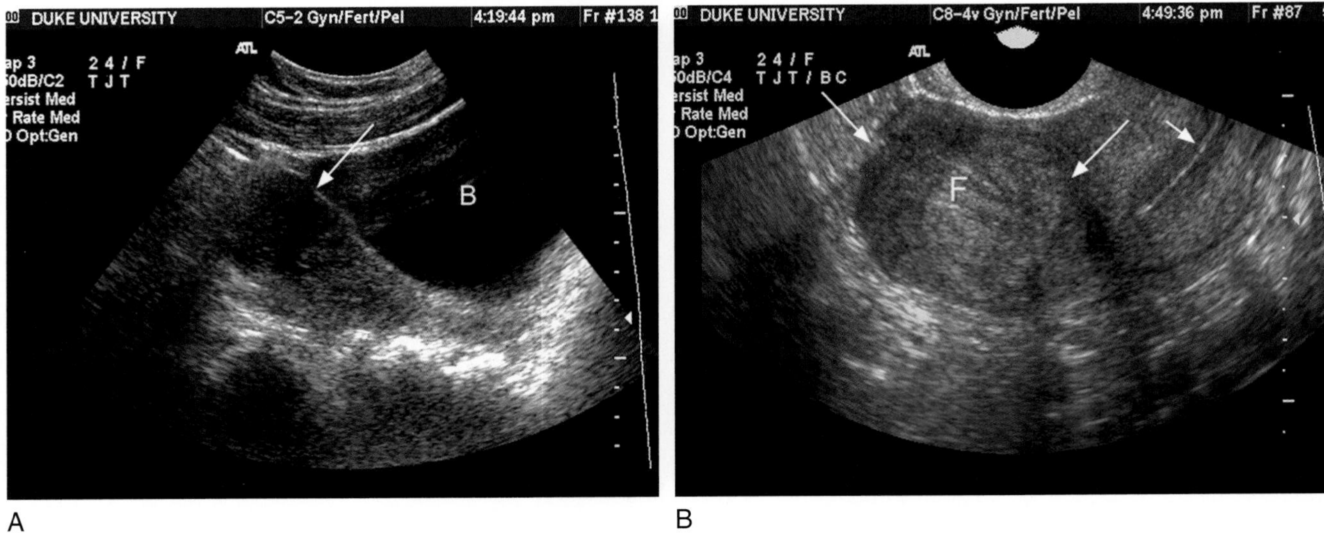

A B

Figure 22-10 Value of transvaginal ultrasound in imaging pelvic abnormalities. **A,** Longitudinal transabdominal scan shows a poorly defined hypoechoic area *(arrow)* along superior aspect of uterus. The area is not seen adequately at transabdominal ultrasound to determine if it is cystic or solid. **B,** Longitudinal midline transvaginal image of same patient shows the abnormality seen in **A** *(long arrows)* is solid and originates from the uterine fundus, consistent with a fibroid (F). Also note the improved visualization of the endometrial stripe *(short arrow)* on the transvaginal image.

retroflexed. The stripe may occasionally appear thicker, however, perhaps because the bladder is not compressed by the uterus.

POSTPARTUM FINDINGS

The greatly enlarged postpartum uterus normally begins to involute immediately after delivery and continues for 6 to 7 weeks. Changes in uterine size can be evaluated transabdominally by measuring the uterine length. At mean times of 1.4 days, 2.7 weeks, and 6.7 weeks after delivery, the uterus decreases in length from a mean and 1 SD of 19.9 ± 2.1 cm, to 11.2 ± 2.0 cm, and then to 8.7 ± 1.2 cm, respectively. Most of the involution is completed by 3 to 4 weeks; by the seventh postpartum week, the uterus has returned to its baseline size.

The technique of scanning is important, particularly in the early postpartum period when the uterus is large, "spongy," and very easily compressible. Even slight transducer pressure can change the uterine size or distort its configuration. Additionally, the uterus is so large that it extends out of the pelvis into the abdomen, forming an angle over the sacral promontory. To measure uterine length in the first 2 postpartum weeks, two long-axis measurements taken along the endometrial canal, one from the fundus to the sacral angle and the other from this angle to the cervix, can be added together. The width and anteroposterior dimensions are not consistent in the early postpartum period because of spontaneous uterine contractions. By 3 to 4 weeks, the uterus has decreased enough in size that it has returned to the pelvis and its length can be evaluated by a single linear measurement.

The length of the postpartum uterus is strongly influenced by the number of previous pregnancies (the woman's parity) during the early and middle (up to 3 to 4 weeks) postpartum periods (Table 22-2). No other factors, not even infant birth weight and breast-feeding have been convincingly shown to affect uterine size or the timing of its involution.

The postpartum uterus need not be routinely studied. However, a pelvic ultrasound may be performed in the event of unexplained fever or pelvic pain. The primary

Table 22-2 Postpartum Uterine Size: Increase in Uterine Length in the Early (Mean, 1.4 Days) and Middle (Mean, 2.7 Weeks) Postpartum Periods Caused by Increasing Parity

	Sagittal Dimensions (cm) (±SD)	
Parity	Early	Middle
1	19.1 (1.7)	10.4 (0.4)
2	19.7 (2.1)	10.9 (0.3)
3	20.7 (2.0)	11.4 (0.4)
4	21.6 (1.8)	11.9 (0.6)

From Wachsberg RH, et al: Real-time ultrasonographic analysis of the normal postpartum uterus: Technique, variability, and measurements. J Ultrasound Med 13:215, 1994.

concern is for retained placenta or endometritis. Endometritis is an important clinical concern when significant uterine tenderness is present. Sonographically, the normal postpartum endometrium appears thin, typically less than 15 mm and often less than 10 mm. Thickening above these numbers is not normal, and retained products, hemorrhage, or infection, should be considered (Fig. 22-11). A fluid collection or gas in the endometrial canal is an important and supportive finding of endometritis. However, bright endometrial reflectors (gas) with either a "dirty" or "clean" shadow can be seen in 15% of clinically normal (without symptoms) postpartum women in the first 3 to 4 postpartum weeks (Fig. 22-12). If the focus of gas is small, a discrete shadow may not be detected. It is still likely to be gas if its brightness is equal to that of gas in adjacent loops of bowel.

In the postpartum period, periuterine abnormalities may also be clinically confused with endometritis. An ovarian vein thrombus almost always occurs on the right side and can cause pain and fever. It can be detected by an imaging study, more often by CT and MRI but also with ultrasound. Hematomas can accumulate after either a vaginal or cesarean delivery and can also cause pain and sometimes fever. They are typically identified as hypoechoic masses in the anterior abdominal wall or in a bladder flap after a cesarean section (Fig. 22-13). A bladder flap hematoma arises between the urinary bladder (initially dissected away from the uterus) and the uterus. If secondarily infected, their appearance may not change unless gas is present.

PREMENSTRUAL AND POSTMENOPAUSAL NORMAL FINDINGS

The premenstrual period commences at birth and continues until the time of menses. Although not quantified, the neonatal uterus, which is affected by maternal hormones, remains prominent for several weeks after birth and has the shape of a fertile uterus, with the body and fundus larger than the cervix. After the hormone effects dissipate, the fundus involutes, leaving a prominent cervix (see Fig. 22-5). The uterus is then small but enlarges as the fertile years approach (Table 22-3). The endometrial stripe is not routinely identified but can infrequently be seen as a very thin hyperechoic stripe.

The menopausal period is defined as beginning 1 year after cessation of menses. The postmenopausal uterus progressively atrophies and decreases to its prepubertal size by 15 to 20 postmenopausal years with the body and fundus remaining more prominent than the cervix. The endometrial stripe is normally thin and hyperechoic or difficult to identify. It is considered normal in thickness when it measures 5 mm or less. Any focal thickening or an overall thickness greater than 5 mm is considered by most examiners to warrant an endometrial biopsy. Causes of a thickened endometrium in a postmenopausal woman include endometrial carcinoma, endometrial polyp, and endometrial hyperplasia. With hormone replacement therapy (primarily estrogens), the uterus and endometrium may not involute and may have an

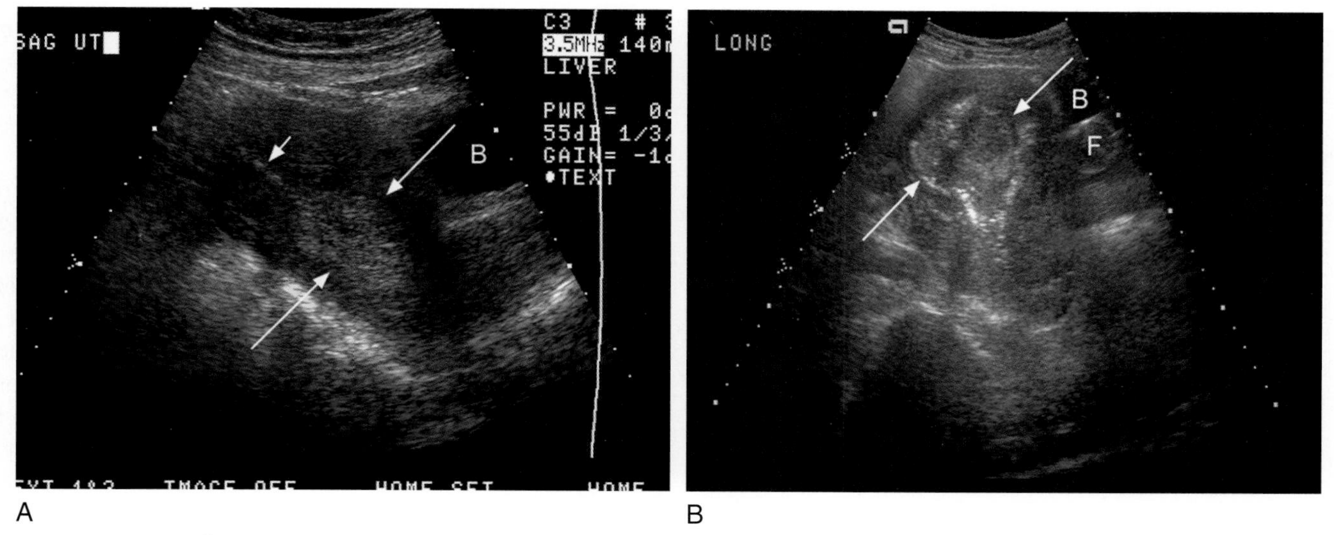

Figure 22-11 Retained placenta. **A,** Sagittal transabdominal image of postpartum uterus shows echogenic tissue distending the mid and inferior portions of the endometrial cavity *(long arrows)*. This tissue corresponded to retained placenta at surgery. The upper portion of the endometrial cavity *(short arrow)* is not affected. B, bladder. **B,** Sagittal transabdominal ultrasound image of a different postpartum patient shows a heterogeneous mass *(arrows)* distending uterine cavity. Histopathologic evaluation confirmed the mass corresponded to retained placenta. B, bladder; F, balloon on Foley catheter in bladder.

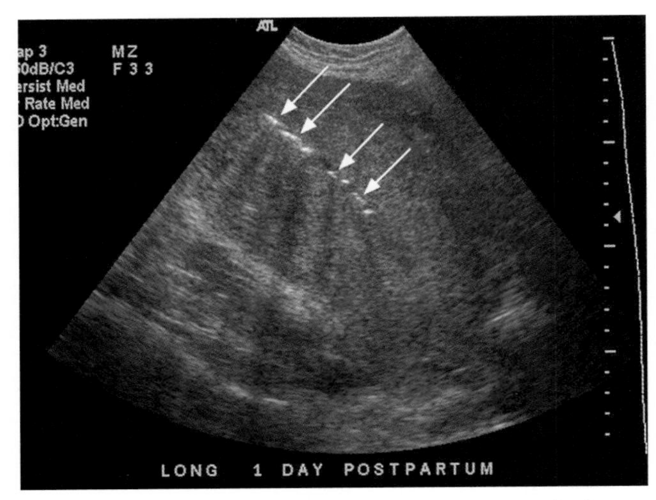

Figure 22-12 Normal postpartum uterus. Longitudinal transabdominal image of pelvis obtained 1 day post partum shows enlarged uterus, consistent with postpartum state. The endometrial cavity contains echogenic foci *(arrows)* with posterior shadowing, corresponding to normal postpartum air in the cavity.

Table 22-3 Normal Uterine and Cervical Dimensions in Pediatric (Premenstrual) Age Groups

Age (yr)	Length (cm), Mean (±SD)	Anteroposterior Dimension of Corpus (cm), Mean (±SD)	Anteroposterior Dimension of Cervix (cm), Mean (±SD)
2-7	3.3 (0.4)	0.7 (0.2)	0.8 (0.2)
8	3.6 (0.7)	0.9 (0.3)	0.8 (0.2)
9	3.7 (0.4)	1.0 (0.3)	0.9 (0.2)
10	4.0 (0.6)	1.3 (0.5)	1.1 (0.3)
11	4.2 (0.5)	1.3 (0.3)	1.1 (0.3)
12	5.4 (0.8)	1.7 (0.5)	1.4 (0.5)
13	5.4 (1.1)	1.6 (0.5)	1.5 (0.2)

From Orsini LF, et al: Pelvic organs in premenarchal girls: Real-time ultrasonography. Radiology 153:113-116, 1984.

appearance more typical of a fertile woman. The type of hormonal therapy, and if applicable the stage of the cycle, should be considered when interpreting the sonogram.

There are transitional periods between the premenstrual and fertile years and between the fertile and postmenopausal years. These transitions last an unpredictable number of years but usually occur between 9 to 13 years of age and last for 5 to 10 years after the cessation of menstrual periods, respectively. During these times the uterine size, shape, and endometrial shape are intermediate in appearance.

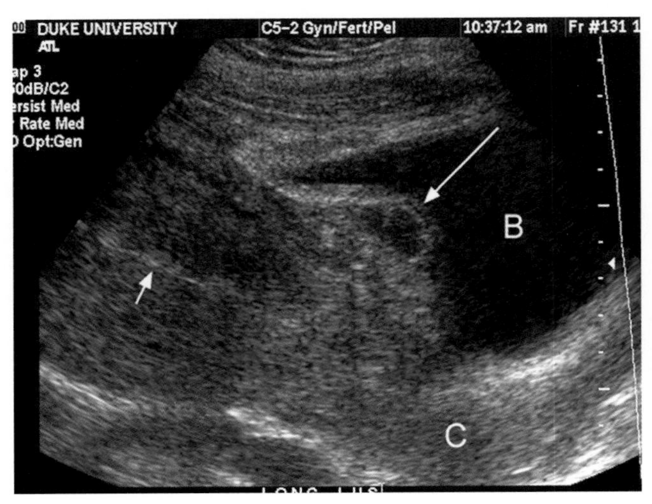

Figure 22-13 Bladder flap hematoma. Sagittal transabdominal image of uterus obtained 6 days after cesarean section shows a heterogeneous collection *(long arrow)* between the lower uterine segment and urinary bladder, consistent with a bladder flap hematoma. *Short arrow,* endometrial stripe; B, bladder; C, cervix.

ENDOMETRIAL ABNORMALITIES

Two questions should be considered when evaluating an endometrial abnormality: (1) Is the patient premenstrual, fertile, or postmenopausal? (2) Is the abnormality an unusually thick endometrium, or is it a collection that is spreading the endometrial canal?

An abnormality is very uncommon during the premenstrual years. If present, it is almost always a collection within the vaginal canal, caused by vaginal (colpos) and occasionally additional proximal uterus (metrocolpos) obstruction. In the neonate, mucosal secretions and fluid collect behind a vaginal atresia, vaginal septum, or an imperforate hymen. Later in premenstrual life, near the time of menses, blood can accumulate behind an imperforate hymen or vaginal septum (Fig. 22-14). Surgical repair commonly allows the uterus and vagina to return to normal.

In the fertile years a small amount of fluid can occasionally be seen in the endometrial canal during menstruation. Occasionally, blood (hematometros) or pus (pyometros) distends the cavity due to cervical stenosis (Fig. 22-15) and/or pelvic inflammatory disease. Most other endometrial fluid collections in the fertile years are related to pregnancy, either intrauterine or extrauterine, and almost all are detected in the first trimester. These are discussed in Chapter 14. Briefly, they include normal and abnormal intrauterine gestational sacs, pseudogestational sacs associated with ectopic pregnancy, fluid collections after miscarriages (spontaneous abortions), and retained products of conception (POCs).

Retained POCs assume varied appearances. It is important to detect retained POCs because they can lead to uterine infection and to the formation of synechiae and metaplasia. The ultrasound appearances

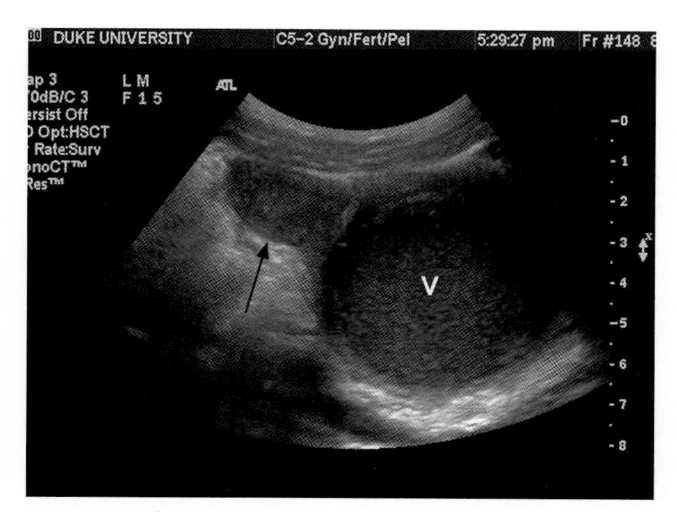

Figure 22-14 Hematocolpos. Sagittal transabdominal image of 15-year-old patient at menarche shows markedly distended vagina (V) filled with blood due to obstruction by a vaginal septum. The blood does not extend into the uterus *(arrow)*.

of first-trimester POCs are a gestational sac (with or without a nonliving embryo), a round to ovoid fluid collection, and a thickened hyperechoic endometrial stripe of more than 5 mm. A thinner endometrial stripe of less than 5 mm, particularly when it is less than 2 mm, favors only retained blood.

In the postmenopausal years a thickened endometrium is a well-established sign of endometrial malignancy (Fig. 22-16). This is often related to a patient's symptomatology, particularly vaginal bleeding. If ultrasound shows a thin endometrium in a postmenopausal patient with vaginal bleeding, the etiology of the bleeding is likely endometrial atrophy. The differential diagnosis for a hyperechoic endometrial thickening of more than 5 mm is carcinoma, hyperplasia (Fig. 22-17) and polyps (Fig. 22-18). A uniformly thickened endometrium more likely signifies glandular hyperplasia whereas focal thickening is more typically in cancer and polyps. However, this distinction is not absolute. Color Doppler sonography sometimes reveals a prominent blood vessel supplying the polyp (see Fig. 22-18). Disruption of the junctional zone (more consistently seen with MRI) may be an important sign. Of these three hyperechoic processes, it would be expected in the setting of invasive cancer. Disruption of the junctional zone occurs more typically in the presence of fibroids and adenomyosis. Both are more typically isoechoic or hypoechoic. If a fibroid is focal and near the endometrial complex, it may be submucosal (Fig. 22-19) or may prolapse into the endometrial canal, both causing focal endometrial thickening or disruption of the endometrial stripe.

TV ultrasound with the instillation of sterile saline into the endometrial canal is called a saline-infusion sonohysterogram (Fig. 22-20). This technique can have significant impact on the diagnosis of endometrial and submucosal abnormalities, especially when focal, in both the fertile and postmenopausal years. Because of the normal proliferation of the endometrial lining during each menstrual cycle, however, it is preferable that menstruating women should have this procedure performed only within the first week of their cycle to ensure that the normal endometrial lining is as thin as possible.

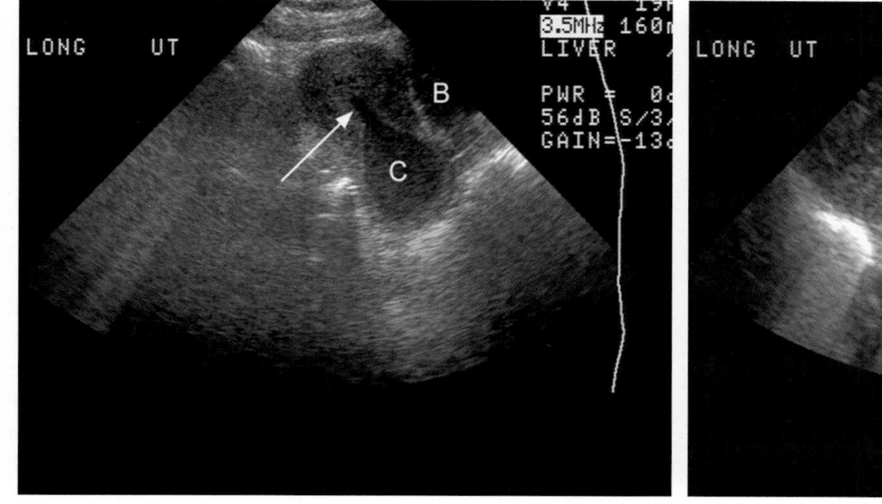

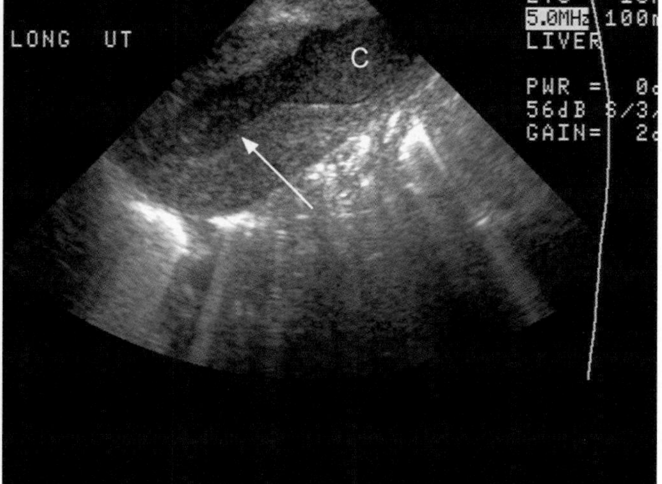

Figure 22-15 Hematometros due to cervical stenosis. **A,** Midline transabdominal image of uterus of a 47-year-old woman reveals fluid with low-level echoes distending the endocervical (C) and endometrial *(arrow)* canals. Cervical stenosis was found at surgery. There was no evidence of tumor or infection. B, bladder. **B,** Sagittal transvaginal image on same patient demonstrates transvaginal appearance of hematometros distending the endocervical (C) and endometrial *(arrow)* canals.

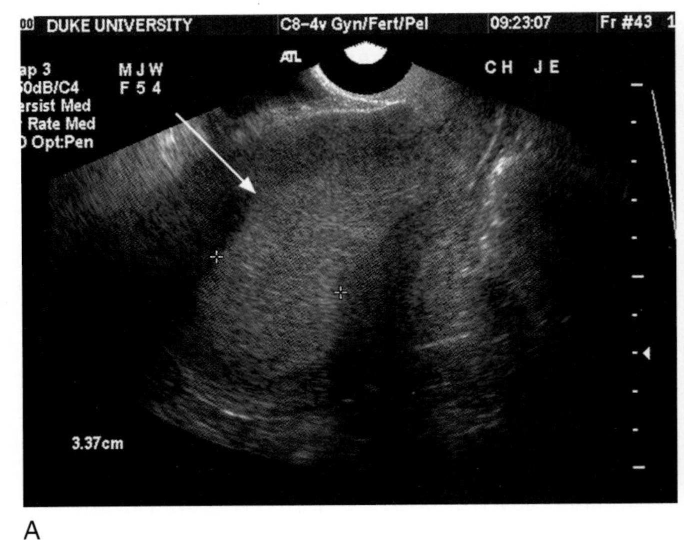

A

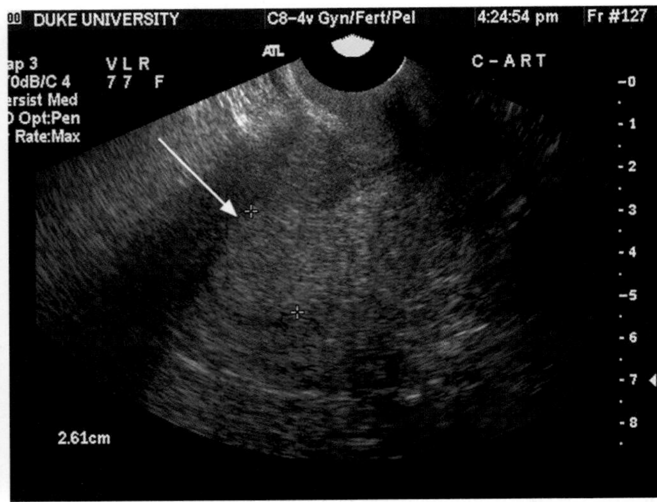

B

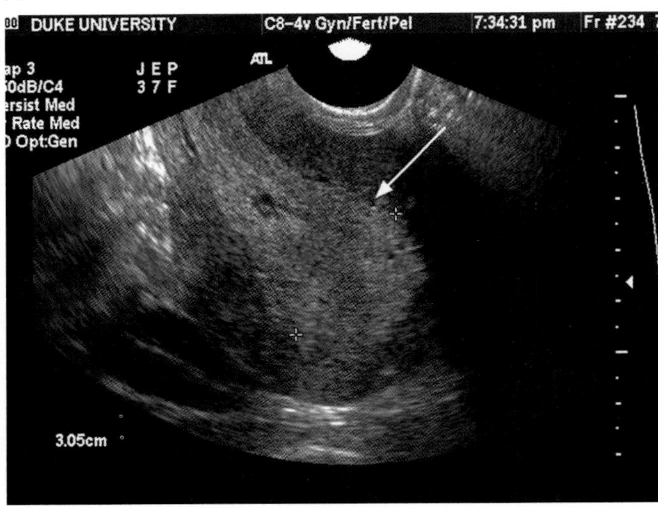

C

Figure 22-16 Endometrial carcinoma: examples. **A,** Sagittal transvaginal scan of uterus of a 54-year-old postmenopausal patient with vaginal bleeding shows markedly thickened endometrium *(arrow)* measuring 33.7 mm due to endometrial carcinoma. **B,** Sagittal transvaginal image of uterus of 77-year-old woman with vaginal bleeding shows marked thickening of the endometrium *(arrow)* to 26.1 mm, also due to endometrial carcinoma. **C,** Sagittal transvaginal image of retroverted uterus of a 37-year-old woman with abnormal vaginal bleeding shows heterogeneity and marked thickening of the endometrium *(arrow)* that measures 30.5 mm. Histopathologic evaluation revealed well-differentiated adenocarcinoma. Endometrial carcinoma can occur during the fertile years, although it is relatively uncommon in this age group.

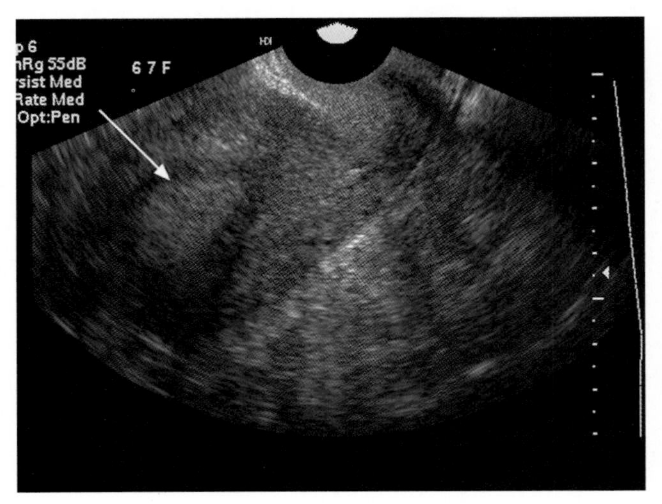

Figure 22-17 Endometrial hyperplasia. Transvaginal sagittal ultrasound image of uterus of a 67-year-old woman shows marked endometrial thickening *(arrow),* raising concern for endometrial carcinoma. Dilatation and curettage was performed and revealed endometrial hyperplasia with no evidence of malignancy.

A more experimental technique called endoluminal sonography employs a transducer at the end of a catheter. This could be of value in selected cases where the extent of an endometrial or subendometrial process needs more complete sonographic evaluation.

A postmenopausal endometrial canal collection (Fig. 22-21) is never a normal finding. It can be due to cervical stenosis or an obstructing malignant tumor (not always identified) such as endometrial or cervical cancer. The endometrial collections range in echogenicity from hypoechoic to hyperechoic and can have a number of causes (serous, mucin, or blood). Any collection can be secondarily infected and would then be called a *pyometra*. If a pyometra goes untreated, serious consequences, including sepsis and uterine rupture, can result.

Many patients with breast cancer are treated with tamoxifen. Although tamoxifen is beneficial in suppressing recurrence of breast cancer, its estrogenic

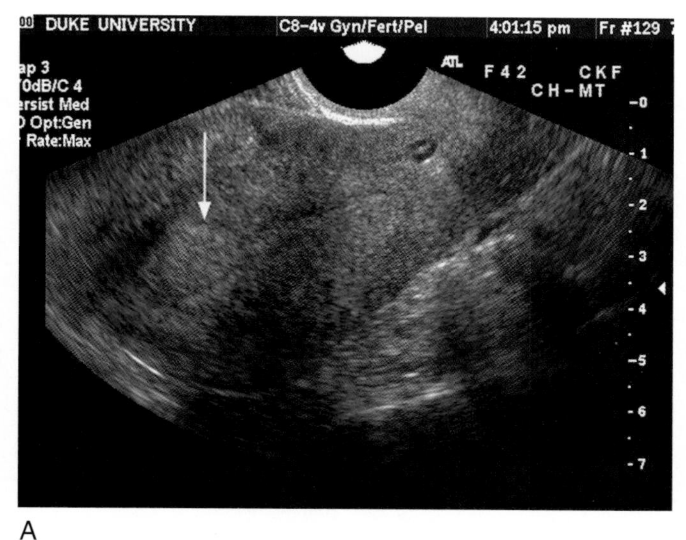

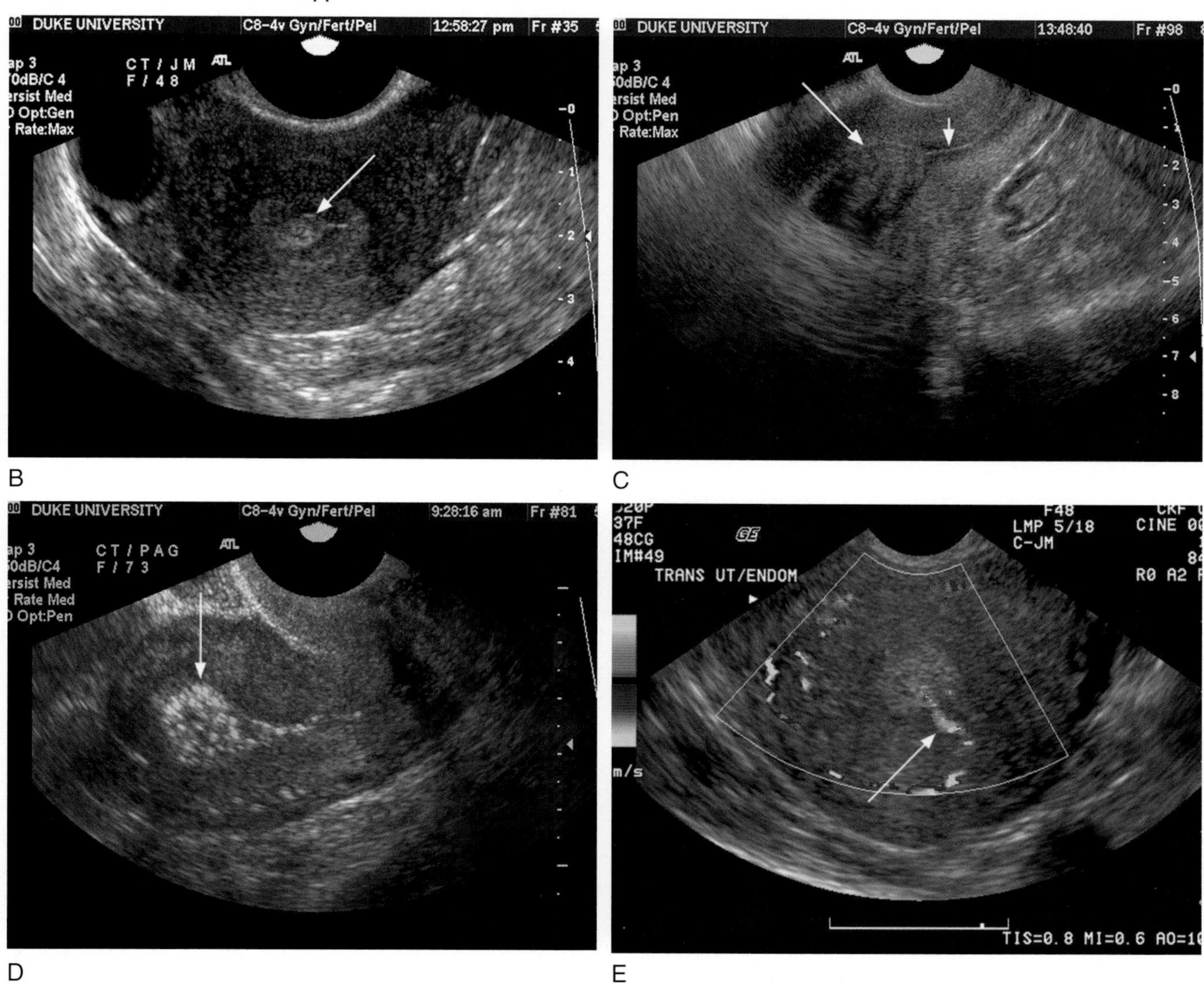

Figure 22-18 Endometrial polyps: examples of pathologically proven benign polyps. **A,** Transvaginal longitudinal image of uterus of a 42-year-old woman shows a focal homogeneously hyperechoic mass *(arrow)* in the endometrium. **B,** Transvaginal axial image of uterus of a 48-year-old woman shows a small echogenic mass *(arrow)* in endometrium. **C,** Transvaginal longitudinal image of uterus shows a large mass *(long arrow)* causing focal enlargement of the endometrial canal. Note the normal appearance of the endometrium *(short arrow)* caudad to the polyp. **D,** Transvaginal longitudinal image of uterus of a 73-year-old woman shows thickening of endometrium *(arrow)* by a heterogeneous mass containing numerous highly echogenic foci. **E,** Color Doppler transvaginal axial image of uterus of a 48-year-old woman shows a prominent blood vessel *(arrow)* supplying a focal endometrial polyp.

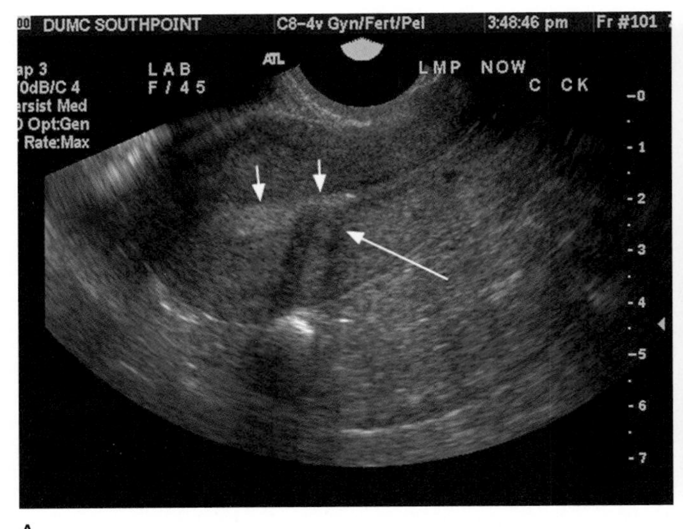

A

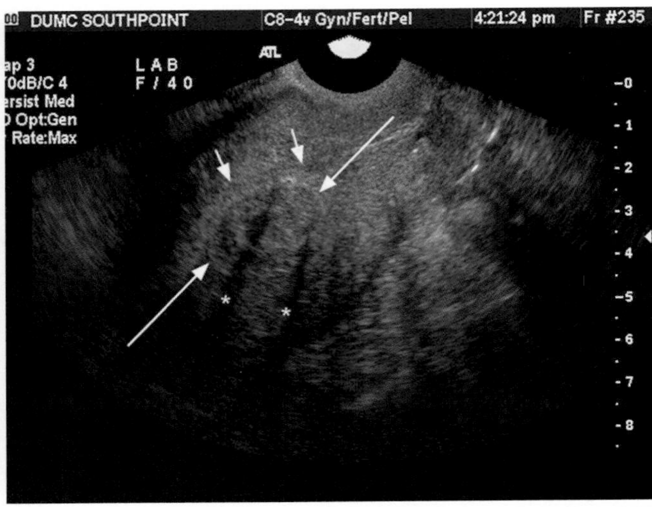

B

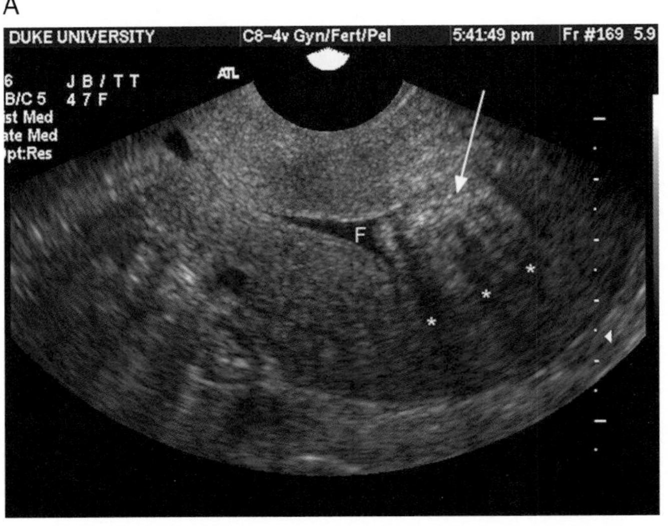

C

Figure 22-19 Submucosal fibroids. **A,** Longitudinal transvaginal scan of uterus of a 45-year-old woman with abnormal vaginal bleeding shows a small hypoechoic fibroid *(long arrow)* pushing on the endometrial stripe *(short arrows)*. **B,** Longitudinal transvaginal image of uterus of a 40-year-old woman with prolonged vaginal bleeding shows a large hypoechoic mass *(long arrows)* disrupting and thickening the endometrial stripe *(short arrows)*. Note that the mass causes recurrent well-defined posterior shadows (*), a shadowing pattern typical of a fibroid. **C,** Longitudinal transvaginal scan of a 47-year-old woman with a retroverted uterus demonstrates a focal submucosal fibroid *(arrow)* projecting into the endometrial canal. The endometrial canal and the fibroid are outlined by a small amount of endometrial fluid (F). The fibroid creates a typical shadowing pattern (*).

effect on the endometrium can cause hyperplasia and increased risk for endometrial carcinoma. Tamoxifen-induced ultrasound changes include endometrial thickening and cystic changes (Fig. 22-22). Cysts can also extend into the subendometrial region. Unfortunately, ultrasound frequently depicts these changes but does not distinguish between cystic endometrial hyperplasia and endometrial carcinoma in this patient population.

There may be a role for Doppler imaging in the evaluation of suspected endometrial abnormalities. Some observers have found that endometrial cancers exhibit abnormal arterial waveforms with elevated peak systole and unusually high diastolic flow. These Doppler abnormalities are thought to be signs of tumor invasion and neovascularity. However, the findings are not always present, and their sensitivity and positive predictive values have not yet been established. Polyps may have a characteristic stalk identified by color Doppler analysis, and occasionally fibroids may have markedly increased flow, their findings then similar to those of endometrial cancer.

INTRAUTERINE CONTRACEPTIVE DEVICES (IUCD)

The use of intrauterine contraceptive devices (IUCDs) has declined significantly in certain parts of the world, including North America, for two reasons: they are only moderately effective as a contraceptive and they do not protect against gynecologic infections. Sometimes IUCDs are even responsible for causing infections. Nevertheless, their ultrasound appearances are important because IUCDs are still prescribed in selected instances.

In a woman who is known to have an IUCD, the most common clinical problem is to determine whether the IUCD is in its correct position (in situ) or if it has been spontaneously expelled. This is particularly pertinent

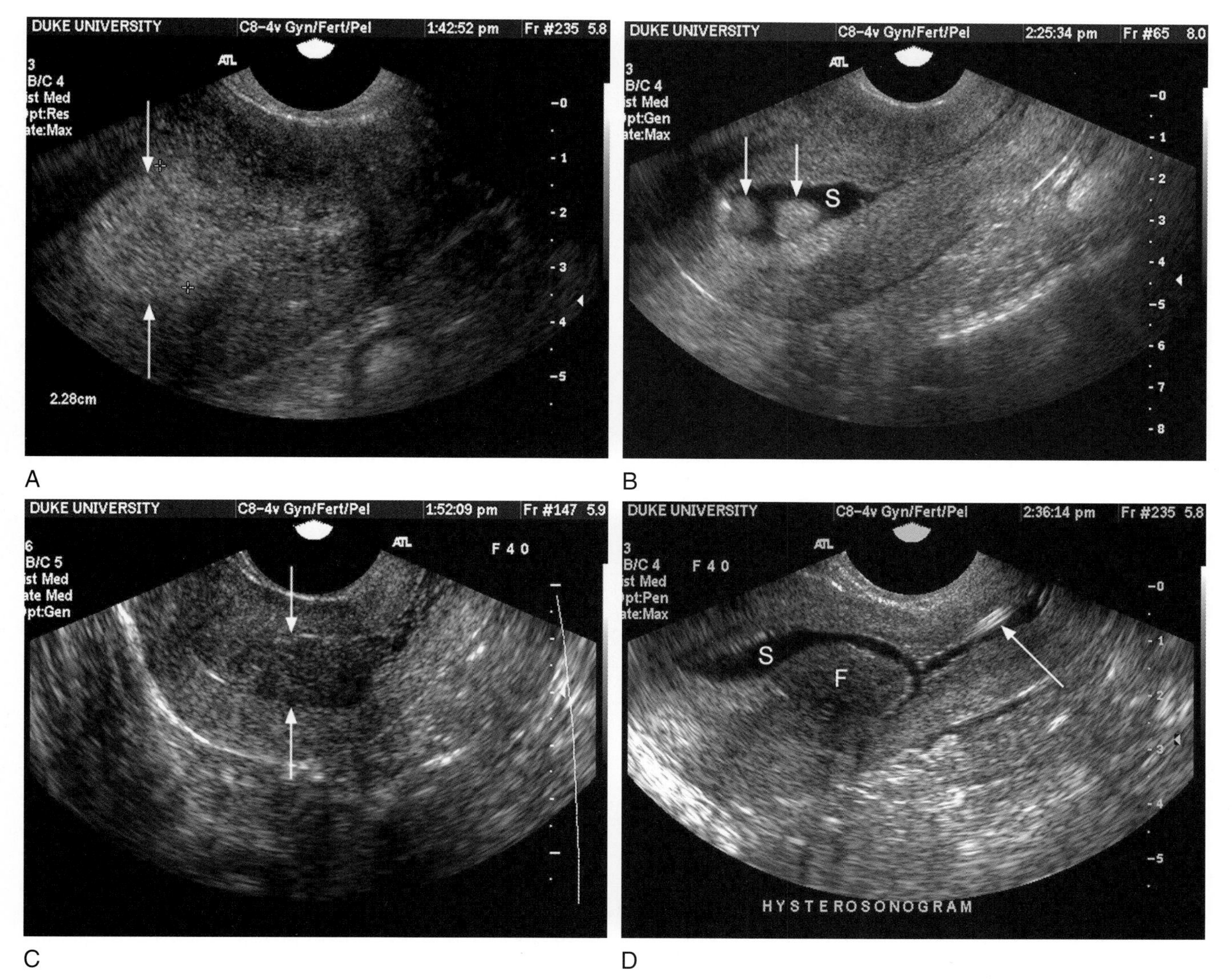

Figure 22-20 Value of saline infusion sonohysterogram. **A** and **B,** Endometrial polyps. **A,** Sagittal transvaginal image of uterus obtained before saline sonohysterography shows a thickened hyperechoic endometrial stripe *(arrows).* **B,** Transvaginal image obtained after instillation of sterile saline (S) into the endometrial canal reveals the endometrial thickening in **A** is caused by two endometrial polyps *(arrows).* **C** and **D,** Submucosal fibroid. **C,** Sagittal transvaginal image of uterus of a 40-year-old woman obtained before saline sonohysterography shows a hypoechoic thickened endometrial stripe *(arrows).* **D,** Transvaginal image obtained after instillation of sterile saline (S) into the endometrial canal reveals the endometrial thickening in **C** is due to a submucosal fibroid (F) bulging into the endometrial cavity. *Arrow,* sonohysterogram catheter in cervix.

when the string from the IUCD is no longer identified in the vagina. A woman with an IUCD may also be studied because of unexplained pelvic pain for IUCD perforation or pelvic inflammatory disease and when a pregnancy is suspected.

Ultrasound can determine whether an IUCD is present within the uterus and is normally in the midline position within the endometrial canal, equidistant from the uterine margins (Fig. 22-23). Only when fibroids are present does an off-center position still favor the IUCD is within the canal.

The sonographic appearance of an IUCD is related to its shape and the material from which it is composed, plastic or metal (copper) or both. Most IUCDs are now shaped like a "7" or a "T." Previous shapes included a serpiginous "S"-like configuration termed a Lippe loop. The IUCD materials are easily differentiated. Plastic is seen as two parallel lines of equal intensity (called an *entrance-and-exit echo*). Metal, usually wound around the plastic, is seen as a single bright line with a posterior reverberation artifact consisting of multiple repeating lines of lessening intensity that fade into the posterior

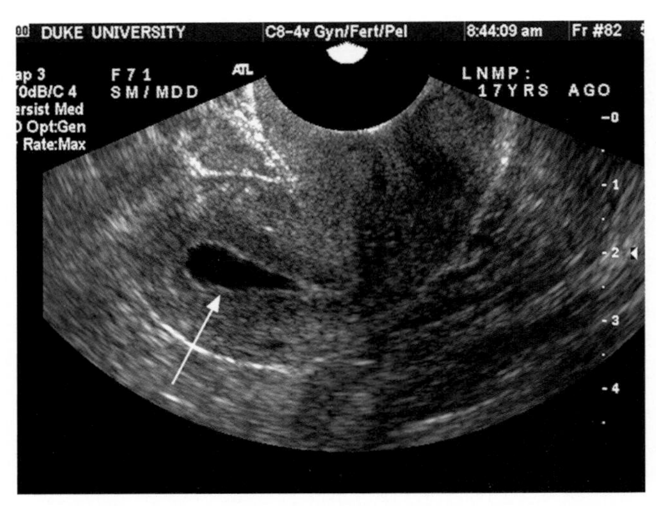

Figure 22-21 Postmenopausal endometrial fluid collection. Longitudinal transvaginal scan of the uterus of a 71-year-old woman shows fluid *(arrow)* distending the endometrial cavity due to cervical stenosis. Other causes of fluid in the endometrial cavity of a postmenopausal patient include endometrial and cervical carcinoma. Endometrial carcinoma would be unlikely in this patient because the endometrium surrounding the fluid is thin.

soft tissues. These are best seen when the ultrasound beam is perpendicular to the IUCD. An additional sharp shadow is created by both materials but only in the short axis of the IUCD, relating to disrupting the Z axis of the ultrasound beam.

Ultrasound can detect some, but not all, malpositioned IUCDs (Fig. 22-24). When ultrasound does not detect an IUCD, this is usually a sign of unrecognized expulsion. But on occasion it can indicate that the IUCD has perforated into or through the myometrium. It is difficult to diagnose perforation, and the ultrasound signs of perforation can vary from an unexplained obliquely positioned IUCD to indefinite visualization. If distorted by fibroids, an abnormal IUCD position can mimic the appearance of partial perforation. Bright adjacent bowel gas can mimic (or mask) the appearance of complete perforation. If the ultrasound findings are normal but there is still clinical concern that the IUCD has perforated, an anteroposterior pelvic radiograph or CT would determine whether the radiopaque IUCD is still present within the pelvis.

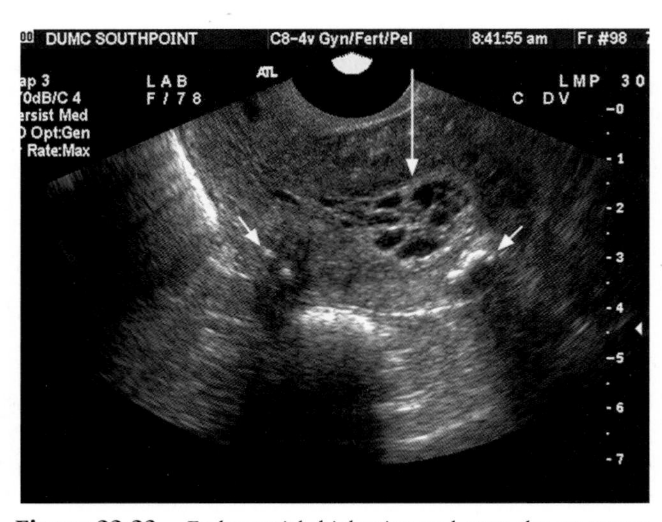

Figure 22-22 Endometrial thickening and cysts due to tamoxifen therapy. Longitudinal transvaginal image of retroverted uterus of a 78-year-old woman undergoing tamoxifen therapy for breast cancer shows marked thickening and cystic change in endometrium *(long arrow)*. This is a frequent appearance in patients on tamoxifen therapy. A few small calcified fibroids *(short arrows)* are also seen.

If a woman with an IUCD has pelvic pain, the area around the uterus needs to be assessed to determine whether pelvic inflammatory disease is present. Dilated fallopian tubes (usually hydrosalpinx) and related abscesses are discussed in Chapter 23.

On occasion, a pregnancy occurs despite the "protection" of the IUD. If it is an intrauterine pregnancy, an ultrasound examination is needed to identify the gestational sac and determine whether the IUCD is still present (Fig. 22-25). The IUCD can provide a nidus for infection during the pregnancy, so when possible it is usually removed. Removal is best accomplished transcervically under ultrasound guidance and is most successful (without causing pregnancy loss) when the IUCD is adjacent to or below the sac. When above the sac, the sac can be considerably distorted during IUCD removal and miscarriage is more likely. Because the incidence of an extrauterine pregnancy is increased in women with IUCDs, though the reason for this is not fully understood, the possibility of an ectopic pregnancy must be considered whenever the pregnancy test results are positive but no intrauterine gestation is seen.

FIBROIDS (LEIOMYOMAS) AND ADENOMYOSIS

Fibroids are the most common myometrial abnormality. They are benign soft tissue tumors that more frequently affect women in certain racial groups, particularly African-Americans, and women of advancing age. However, fibroids can develop in all women and at all ages. Fibroids can be solitary or multiple, small or large, and located anywhere from completely within the myometrium, to exophytic, to prolapsing into the endometrial canal (Fig. 22-26). Fibroids usually continue to grow until menopause; after which they often involute. Rarely, sarcomas may develop within the myometrium, either de novo or secondary to fibroid degeneration.

The most common sonographic appearance of a fibroid is a hypoechoic solid mass (Fig. 22-26). However,

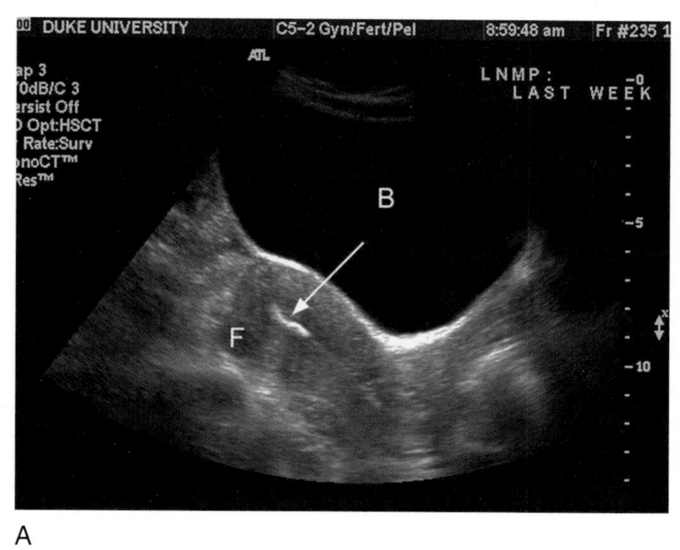

A

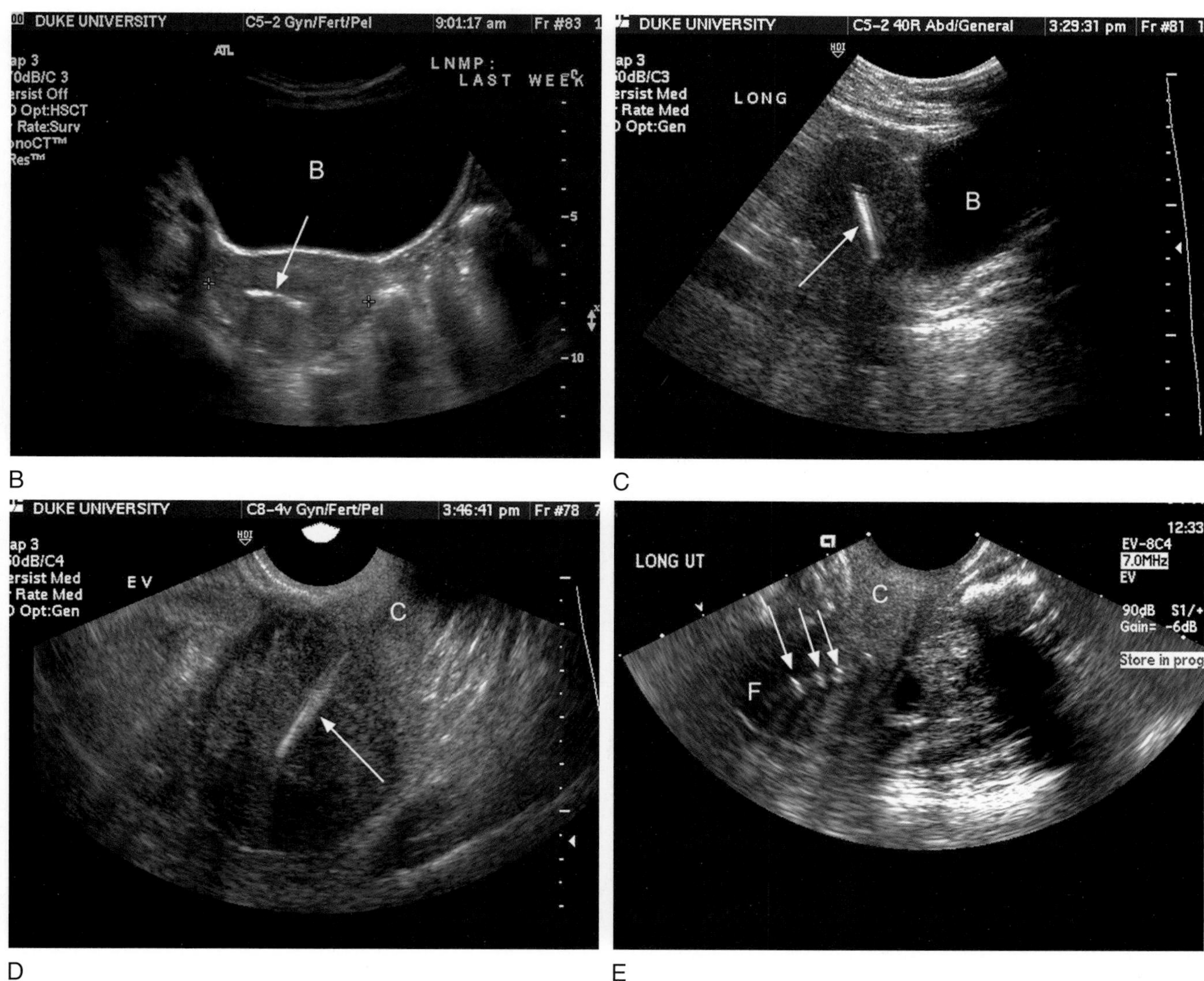

B

C

D

E

Figure 22-23 Intrauterine contraceptive device (IUCD). Examples of correct positioning. **A** and **B,** Longitudinal (**A**) and axial (**B**) images of uterus show a T-shaped IUCD *(arrows)* correctly positioned in the endometrial cavity. A small fibroid (F) is also seen along the posterior surface of the uterus. B, bladder. **C** and **D,** Longitudinal transabdominal (**C**) and transvaginal (**D**) images of uterus show a Cu7 IUCD *(arrows)* correctly positioned in the endometrial cavity. B, bladder; C, cervix. **E,** Longitudinal transvaginal image of uterus shows a Lippe loop IUCD *(arrows)* correctly positioned in the endometrial cavity. C, cervix; F, uterine fundus.

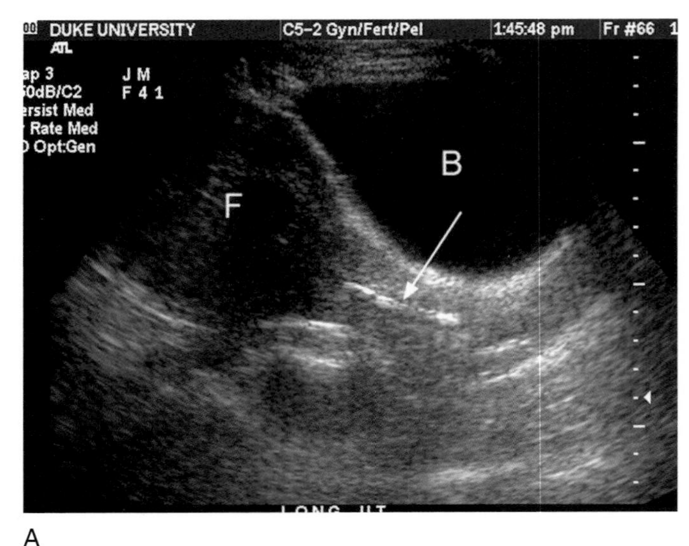

A

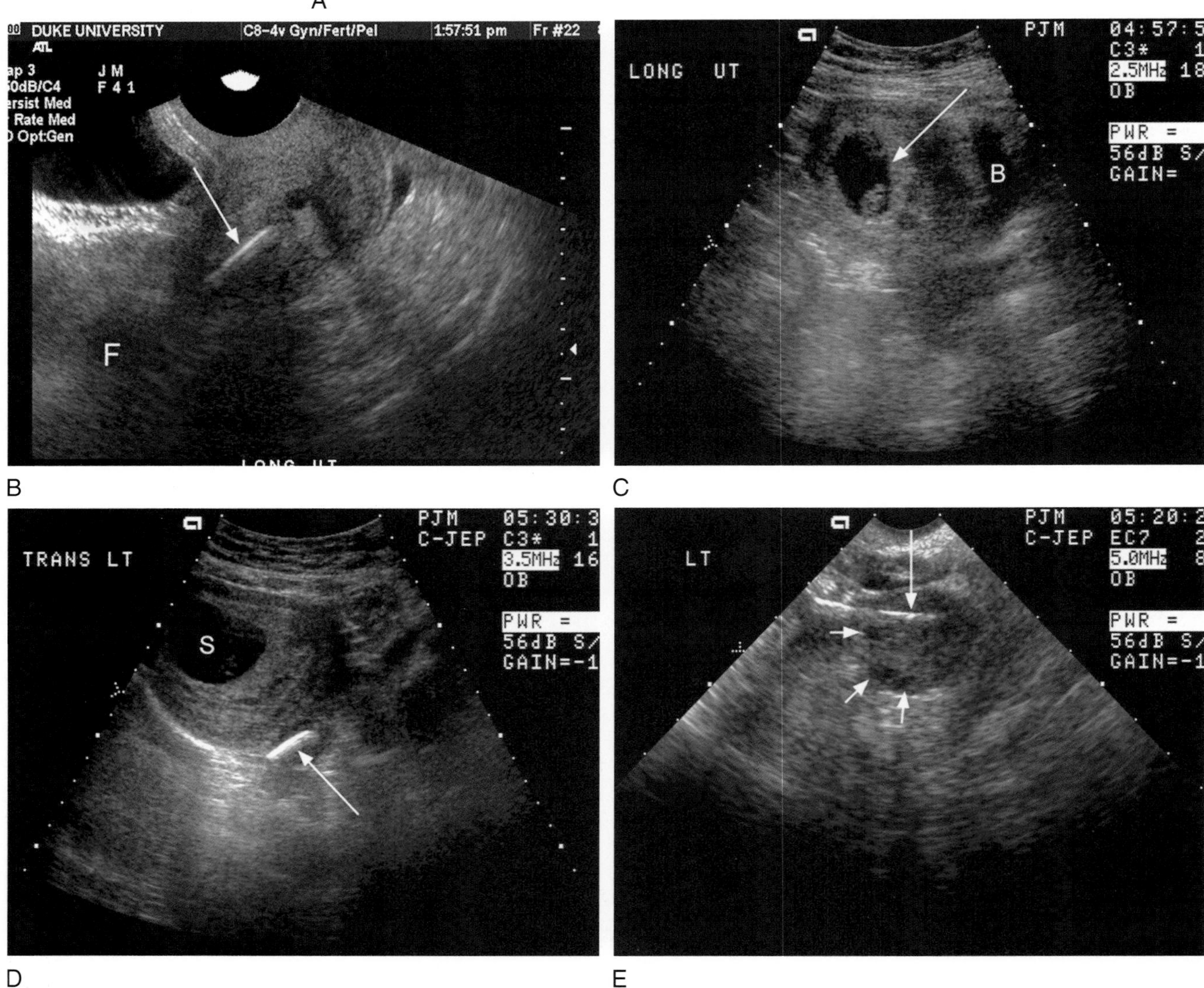

B C D E

Figure 22-24 Incorrectly positioned IUCDs. **A** and **B,** IUCD in cervix. Longitudinal transabdominal (**A**) and transvaginal (**B**) images of uterus of 41-year-old woman with a large fundal fibroid (F) show IUCD *(arrow)* positioned too low, in the cervix and lower uterus. B, bladder. **C** to **E,** Perforation of IUCD into adnexa. **C,** Longitudinal midline transabdominal scan of uterus in patient with an IUCD during first trimester of pregnancy does not show the IUCD. *Arrow,* gestational sac; B, bladder. **D,** Axial transabdominal scan of pelvis angled toward the left shows the IUCD *(arrow)* outside the uterus, in region of left adnexa. S, gestational sac. **E,** Axial transvaginal scan confirms location of IUCD *(long arrow)* in left adnexa, extending into left ovary. *Short arrows,* follicles on left ovary.

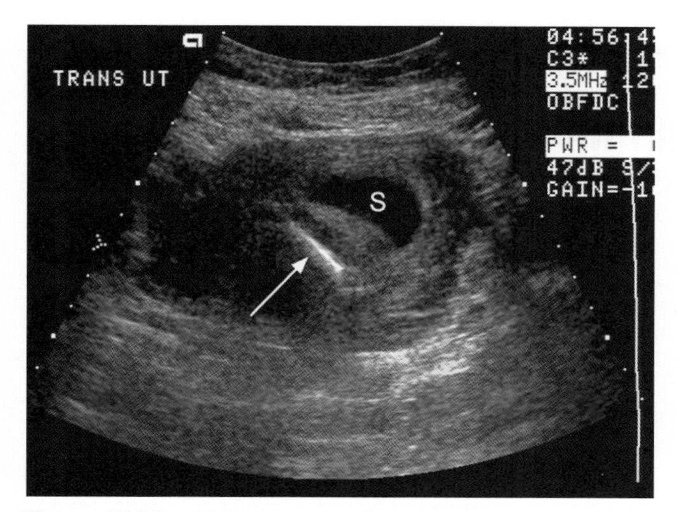

Figure 22-25 IUCD in uterus during pregnancy. Axial transabdominal scan of uterus during first trimester shows an IUCD *(arrow)* adjacent to the gestational sac (S). The IUCD was subsequently removed, and the pregnancy progressed normally to term.

the echogenicity can vary from heterogeneous to hyperechoic, not infrequently within the same mass. Fibroids can also calcify and necrose, thus further complicating their sonographic appearances. Because fibroids are solid masses (unless necrotic), they absorb sound and cause some degree of acoustic shadowing.

It is not always possible to differentiate a single large fibroid from a close grouping of multiple smaller fibroids (Fig. 22-27). Usually this distinction is not important unless a uterine-sparing myomectomy is being contemplated. Then MRI is of value to better define the extent of the fibroid (or fibroids) and to determine how much normal myometrium remains.

The clinical symptoms and the appearance of fibroids depend on their position, size, and number. The symptoms are usually most pronounced when the fibroids are submucosal or prolapse into the endometrial canal (see Fig. 22-19). Pain and vaginal bleeding are then common, often occurring irregularly and unrelated to the menstrual cycles. If a fibroid is exophytic, it is useful if possible, to differentiate between a pedunculated fibroid on a thin stalk (Fig. 22-28A) and a subserosal fibroid with a broad-based attachment to the uterus (Fig. 22-28B). Of these two, the pedunculated fibroid, particularly if it is large and mobile, can torse and necrose and cause pain. This distinction may not be possible at ultrasound evaluation, but if the examiner can identify and palpate the exophytic fibroid and on physical examination can move the fibroid, it is likely a pedunculated fibroid.

Most fibroids develop in the middle of the myometrium. Depending on their size, they may bulge the uterine contour and distort the junctional zone. Distortion of the uterine contour, even when the uterine echogenicity is normal, makes fibroids (usually small) likely.

As previously described, a retroverted or retroflexed uterus is normally more globular in shape and attenuates more of the ultrasound beam than an anteverted uterus. It may initially give the impression of a single large hypoechoic fibroid. Increasing the ultrasound gain, adjusting the orientation of the transducer, and TV scanning can usually show the uterus to be normal (see Fig. 22-8).

Fibroids may calcify, sometimes heavily (Fig. 22-29). These calcifications are usually dense and clumped and, when numerous, confluent. They have a typical sonographic appearance consisting of well-defined hyperechoic areas with sharp acoustic shadowing. The calcifications can often be identified within the confines of the fibroid but are occasionally the only presenting sign of a fibroid. If the calcifications become extensive, they may completely obscure the uterus and a pelvic radiograph is then needed to establish the diagnosis of a myomatous uterus.

Fibroids may necrose, giving an ultrasound appearance of hypoechoic or anechoic irregular spaces within an otherwise solid mass (Fig. 22-30). If the appearance is very atypical and/or if the mass is unusually large, especially when associated with ascites, a sarcoma should be considered. This distinction is otherwise not possible. The differentiation of a fibroid from an endometrial carcinoma is usually straightforward unless the endometrial carcinoma has extensively invaded the myometrium.

Adenomyosis is the uterine correlate of endometriosis. Adenomyosis is the pathologic extension of endometrial rests (usually microscopic) into the myometrium. Adenomyosis typically causes pain, particularly around the time of menstruation, and can be identified by MRI and occasionally by ultrasound primarily by the finding of a distorted junctional zone and often a distorted myometrium. Ultrasound studies have shown that the junctional zone in adenomyosis is lost and replaced by multiple small hypoechoic solid masses (<10 to 15 mm in diameter) that give a "moth-eaten" heterogeneous appearance to the myometrium (Fig. 22-31). This, however, can also occur with multiple small fibroids, although less commonly. An enlarged uterus that exhibits abnormal echogenicity but shows no discrete mass could be a sign of diffuse leiomyomatosis involvement but could also be due to adenomyosis. MRI can be helpful in distinguishing fibroids from adenomyosis. Another, perhaps more definitive, pattern of adenomyosis is the identification of small subcentimeter cysts within the myometrium (Fig. 22-31B and C).

When fibroids cause the uterus to enlarge, the ovaries are displaced from their normal position, usually into the

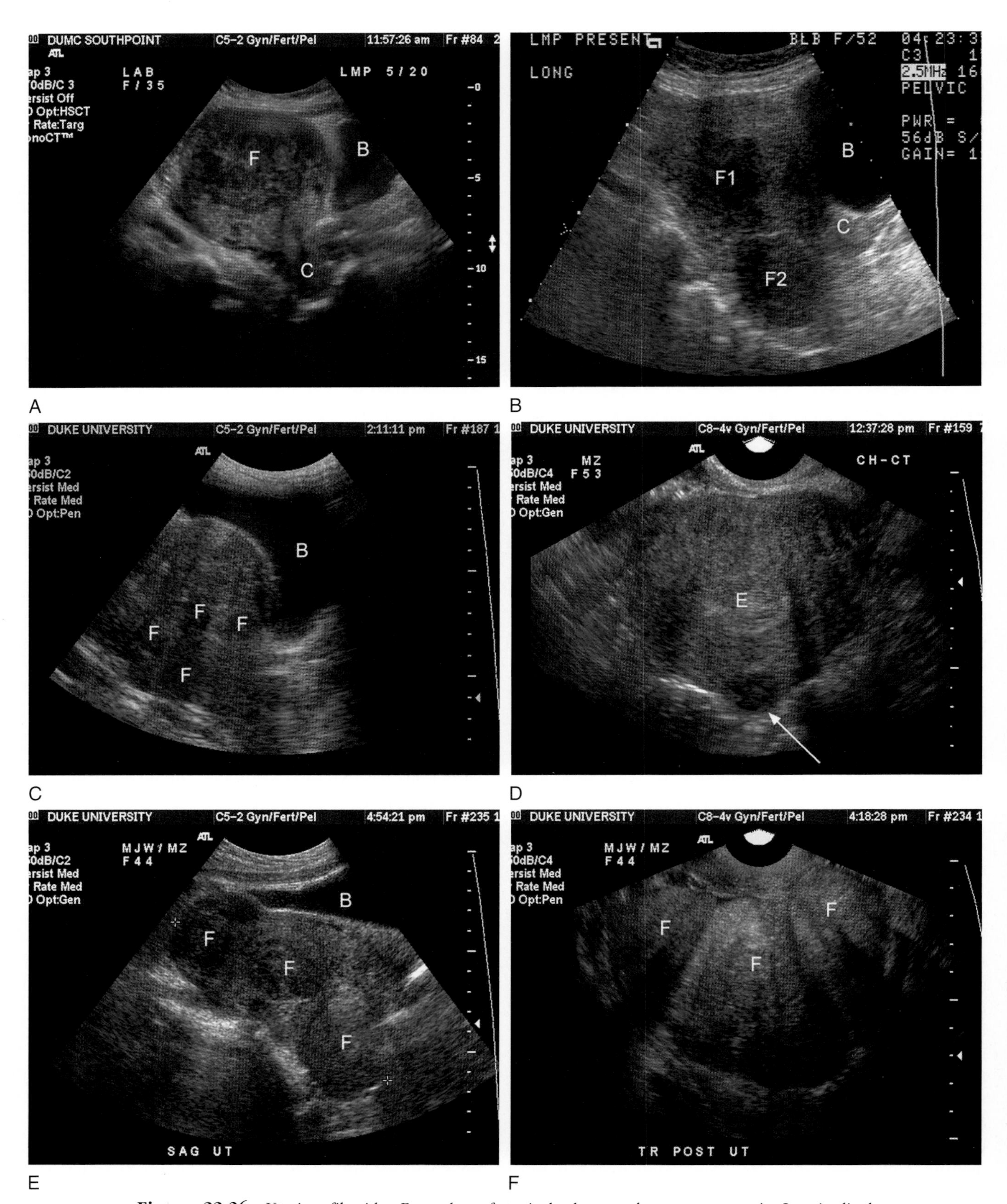

Figure 22-26 Uterine fibroids. Examples of typical ultrasound appearances. **A,** Longitudinal transabdominal scan shows a focal heterogeneous, predominantly hypoechoic fibroid (F). B, bladder; C, cervix. **B,** Longitudinal transabdominal scan shows two focal hypoechoic fibroids (F1, F2) that cause uterine enlargement. One fibroid (F2) extends posterior to the cervix (C) into the cul-de-sac. B, bladder. **C,** Longitudinal transabdominal image shows multiple poorly defined fibroids (F) that result in an enlarged, lobulated appearance to the uterus. B, bladder. **D,** Small hypoechoic subserosal fibroid *(arrow)* is shown on this transverse transvaginal image. E, endometrium. **E** and **F,** Longitudinal transabdominal (**E**) and axial transvaginal (**F**) scans of uterus show marked enlargement of uterus and lobulation of uterine contour due to multiple large fibroids (F). The large fibroids distort and obscure the endometrium, preventing its evaluation by ultrasound. B, bladder.

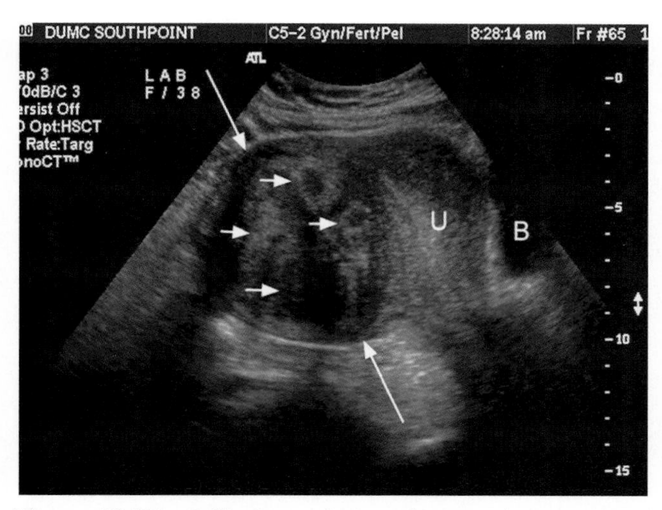

Figure 22-27 Difficulty in distinguishing single large fibroid from close grouping of multiple small fibroids. Longitudinal transabdominal scan of pelvis shows large mass *(long arrows)* causing focal bulging of posterior aspect of uterus (U). It is not clear if this represents a single large fibroid or a close grouping of multiple smaller fibroids *(short arrows)*. B, bladder.

upper pelvis/abdomen, but infrequently they become fixed in the cul-de-sac. Although the ovaries continue to lie adjacent to the enlarged uterus, distortion of the uterine contour often makes identification of the ovaries difficult. Unless typical follicles are present, the area of the presumed ovary might be a small fibroid. However, even if the ovaries are not definitively identified, it is at least possible to survey the area around the uterus to rule out the existence of an extrauterine mass, which if ovarian would typically be cystic or complex.

Fibroids can present clinically, sonographically, or both for the first time during pregnancy (Fig. 22-32). Although their development is not caused by the pregnancy, their growth is often accelerated. If the fibroid is in the lower uterine segment or at the site of placental attachment, it should be carefully monitored throughout the remainder of that pregnancy for potential problems at delivery (dystocia) or effects on fetal growth.

FIBROIDS—THE PELVIC MIMICKER

Although the sonographic appearance of fibroids is usually straightforward, it may mimic other pelvic conditions both normal and abnormal in less than 5% of the cases. Fibroids can assume the appearance of uterine variants, uterine abnormalities, pregnancy-related conditions, IUCD perforation, and adnexal masses.

Fibroids can mimic the appearance of uterine duplication and obstruction (Fig. 22-33). If a fibroid extends directly lateral to the body of the uterus, usually into the broad ligament, it may have the approximate shape and size of a second uterine horn. If necrotic, a large fibroid may look like a fluid collection in an obstructed uterus. If multiple and small, fibroids may mimic the appearance of adenomyosis.

Atypical fibroid appearances may mimic pregnancy-related conditions or distort their appearance, primarily

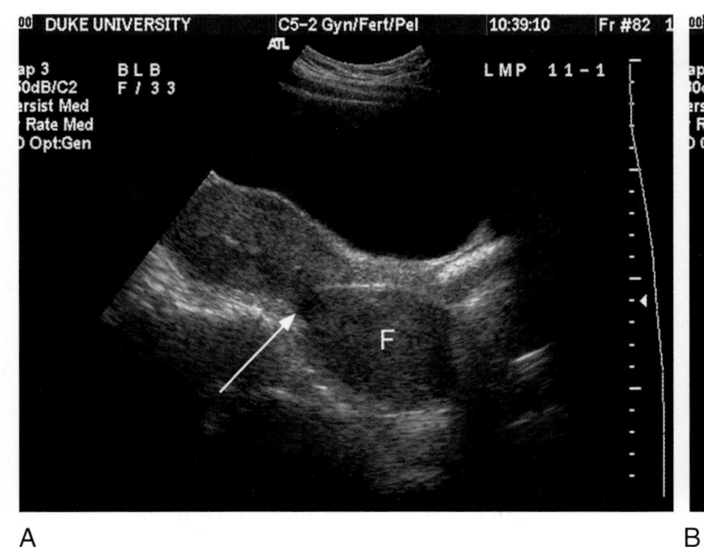

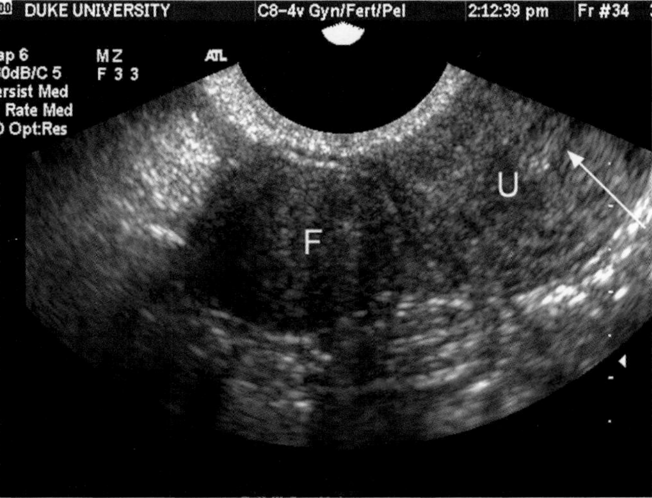

Figure 22-28 Exophytic fibroids. **A,** Pedunculated. Longitudinal transabdominal scan of pelvis shows large fibroid (F) extending into cul-de-sac from posterior aspect of uterus. Note the hypoechoic stalk *(arrow)* that connects the fibroid to the uterus. **B,** Subserosal. Axial transvaginal image of uterus (U) shows a large exophytic subserosal fibroid (F) originating from the right side of the uterus. *Arrow,* endometrial stripe. Note that an exophytic fibroid such as the one shown here can mimic the appearance of an adnexal mass.

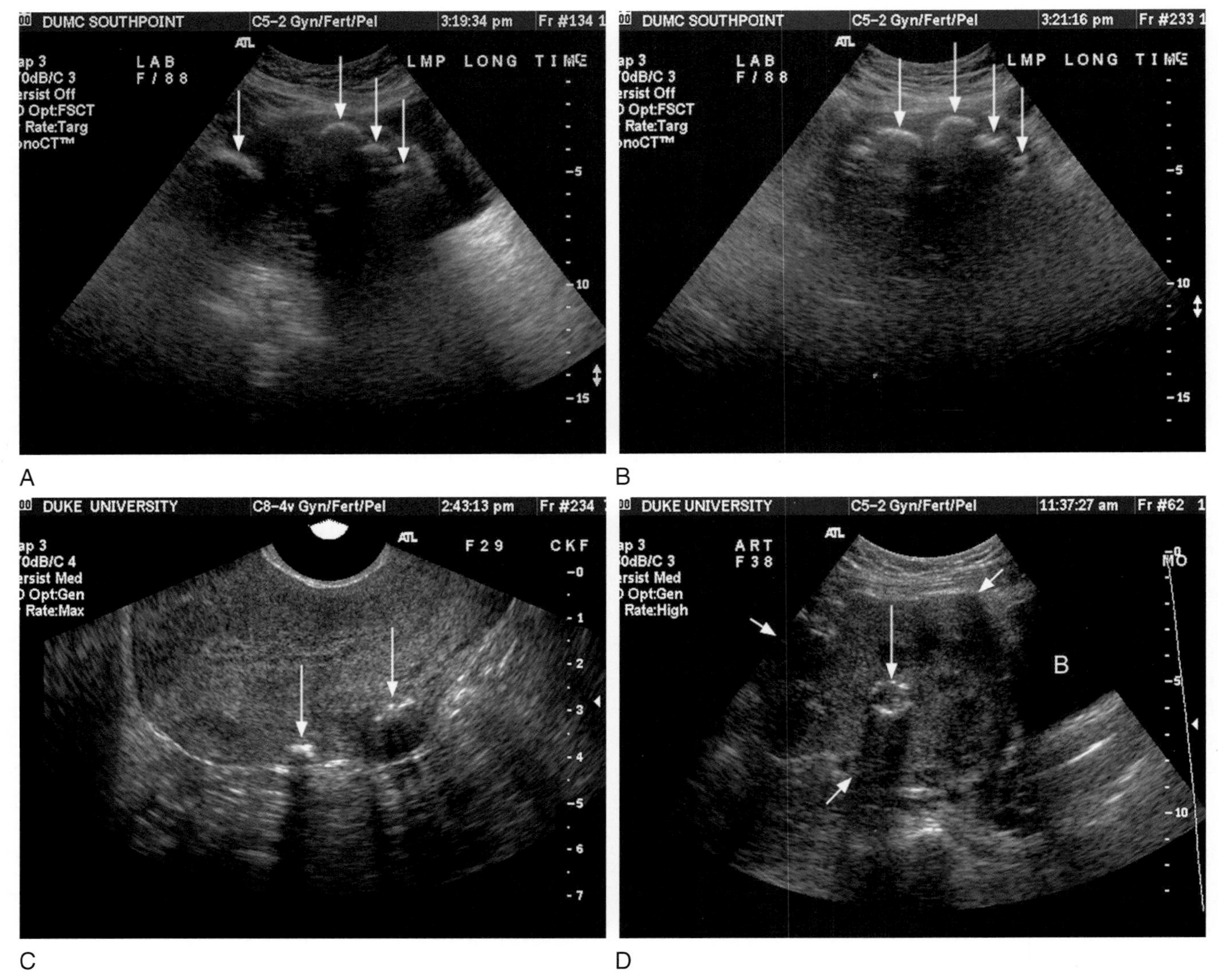

Figure 22-29 Calcified fibroids. **A** and **B,** Longitudinal (**A**) and axial transabdominal (**B**) images of myomatous uterus of an 88-year-old woman show enlarged uterus due to multiple densely calcified fibroids *(arrows)* with posterior acoustic shadowing. **C,** Midline longitudinal transvaginal scan of uterus of 29-year-old woman shows two small calcified fibroids *(arrows)* with posterior shadowing. **D,** Longitudinal transabdominal image of pelvis of a 38-year-old woman shows a markedly enlarged lobulated uterus *(short arrows)* with a centrally located fibroid outlined by a rim of peripheral calcification *(long arrow)*. B, bladder.

in the first trimester. Multiple fibroids can surround a small gestational sac. A fibroid can have a necrotic center that looks like a gestational sac (Fig. 22-34). If the fibroids are large and very hyperechoic, they can occasionally mimic the appearance of a hydatidiform mole. A fibroid that calcifies along its rim may be mistaken for the calvarium of a fetal head (Fig. 22-35). Fibroids may so distort the position of a single normal gestational sac that the sac appears to be at the edge of or outside the uterus, then falsely appearing in an ectopic position.

An IUCD is expected to be in the middle of the uterus, within the endometrial canal. As already stated, fibroids can distort the canal, making an IUCD appear partially perforated into the uterine wall.

When fibroids are primarily exophytic, they can mimic the appearance of adnexal masses (see Fig. 22-28B). Their appearances may be so atypical that the diagnosis of fibroids is not considered unless other more typical appearing fibroids are also present. Fibroids can mimic the cystic and complex appearances of dermoids, endometriomas, cystadenomas, hemorrhagic cysts, and

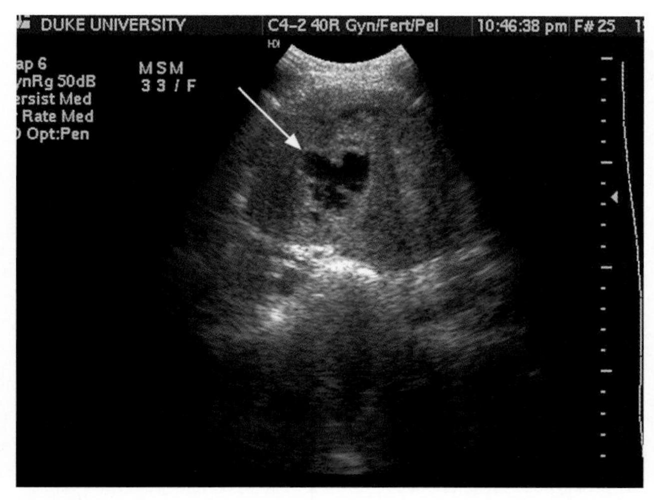

Figure 22-30 Necrotic fibroid. Axial transabdominal image of uterus shows an irregularly shaped fluid collection *(arrow)* in the uterus, due to necrosis in a fibroid.

even ovarian malignant tumors. Solid ovarian masses are less common, however; and when a solid mass is detected in the adnexa, a fibroid is more likely.

Even pelvic Doppler findings may be misleading. Some fibroids, similar to some ovarian cancers, have a low-resistance arterial waveform showing elevated peak systole and high diastolic flow (Fig. 22-36). This is discussed further in Chapter 23.

When the diagnosis of a fibroid is uncertain, TV scanning may be helpful. Although not always able to image the entire uterus (especially when the uterus is enlarged), TV imaging may show that there are additional more typical appearing fibroids and even identify the connection of an exophytic fibroid to the uterus. Additionally, fibroids often exhibit a typical shadowing pattern in which multiple well-defined recurring shadows originate from the mass (Figs. 22-19B and C and 22-37). These shadows arise from transition zones

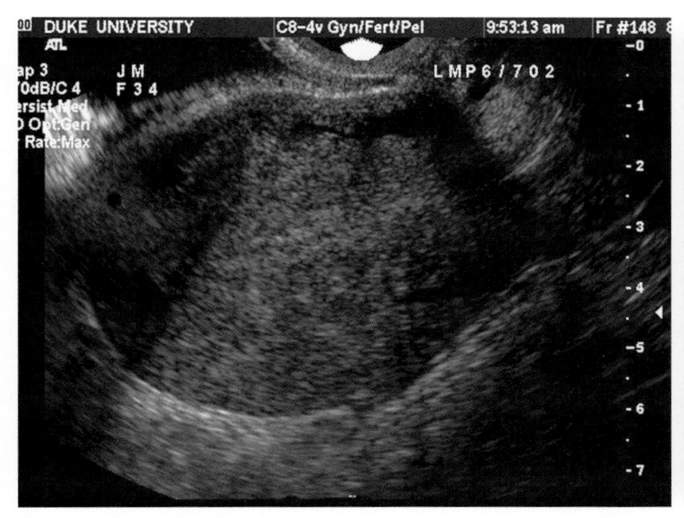

A

B

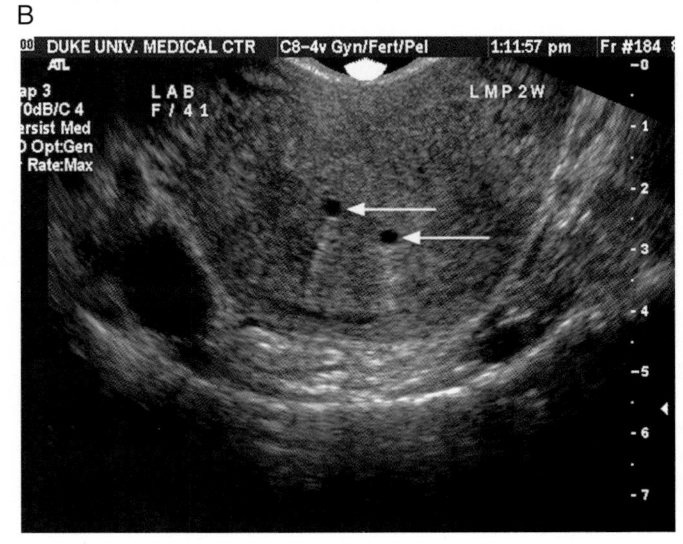

C

Figure 22-31 Adenomyosis. **A,** Longitudinal transvaginal image of uterus of a 39-year-old patient with dysfunctional bleeding due to adenomyosis shows enlarged heterogeneous appearance of the myometrium. No focal fibroids are seen. **B,** Longitudinal transvaginal image of the uterus of a 42-year-old patient with heavy menses secondary to adenomyosis shows heterogeneous myometrial echo pattern, with a small myometrial cyst *(arrow)*. **C,** Axial transvaginal scan of uterus of a 41-year-old patient with painful heavy menses and adenomyosis shows myometrial cysts *(arrows)*.

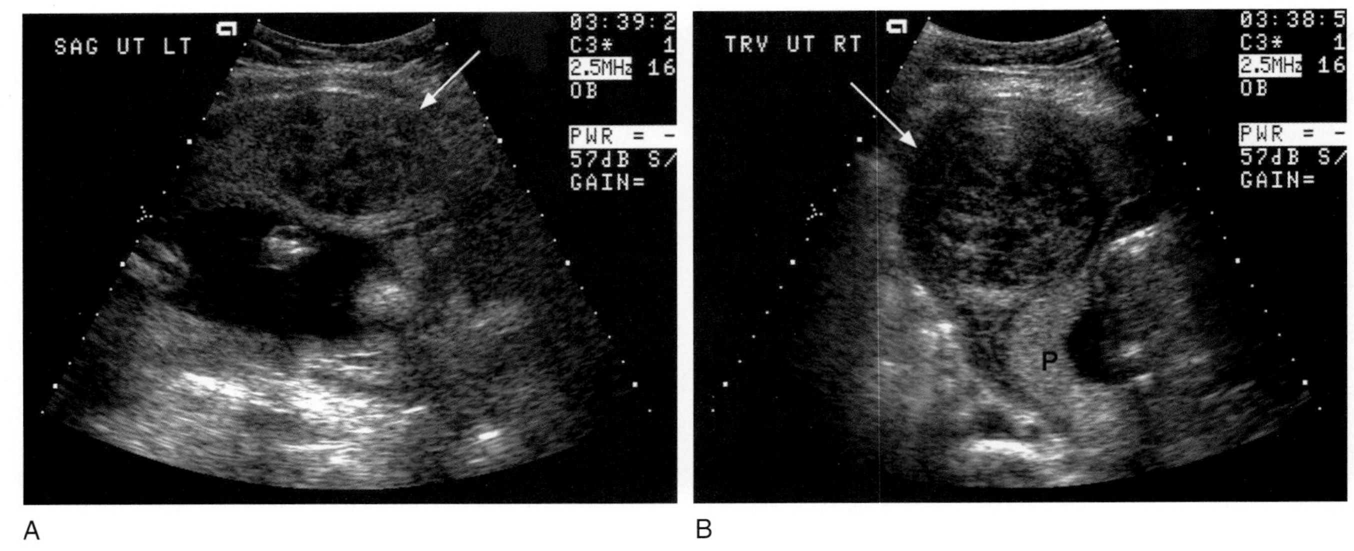

Figure 22-32 **A** and **B**, Fibroids during pregnancy. Longitudinal transabdominal image of left side of uterus (**A**) and axial image of right side of uterus (**B**) of a 19-week gestation show two fibroids *(arrows)* that were first recognized during pregnancy. P, placenta.

between different tissue types within the mass. They are sometimes seen by TA ultrasound but are more commonly identified at TV ultrasound. Identification of this shadowing pattern increases the likelihood that a mass is a fibroid. Finally, although not as yet fully evaluated, 3-D ultrasound may be able to be reconstructed in planes of section that show the attachment of an atypical exophytic fibroid to the uterus.

On occasion, a woman is found to have a large solid pelvoabdominal mass. If the uterus is not detected and the mass has no other site of origin, a fibroid should be considered.

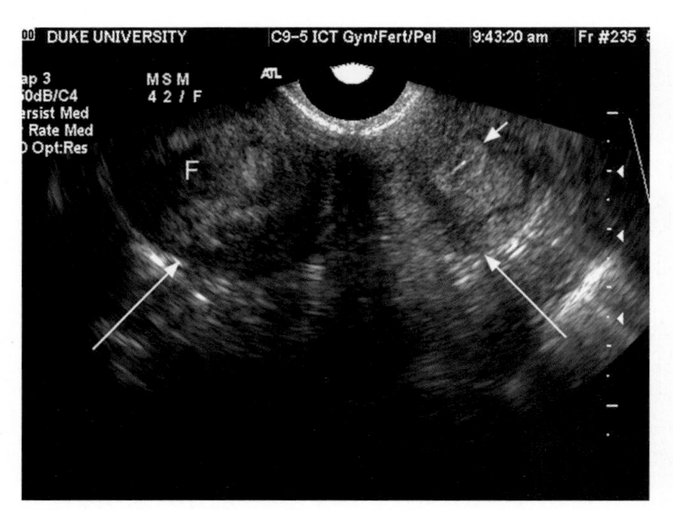

Figure 22-33 Pedunculated fibroid mimicking duplicated uterus. Axial transvaginal scan of pelvis shows two rounded solid structures *(long arrows)*, each with configuration similar to that of a uterus, resembling the appearance of a bicornuate or didelphys uterus. Note, however, the well-defined normal-appearing endometrial stripe *(short arrow)* in the true uterus (on the right of the image). A similar-appearing endometrial stripe is not seen in the fibroid (F).

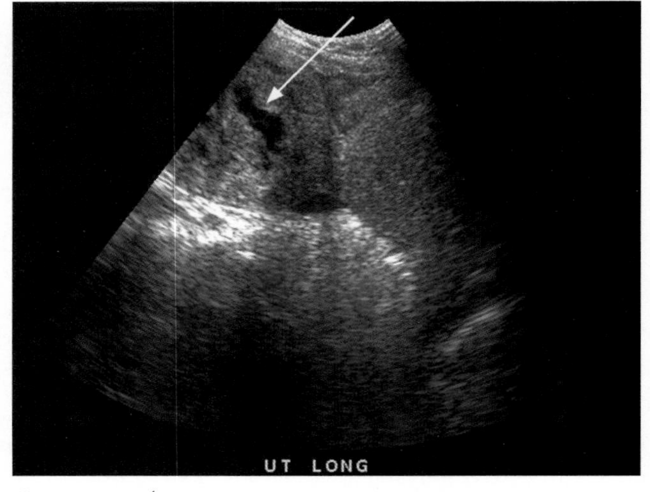

Figure 22-34 Necrotic fibroid resembling gestational sac. Midline longitudinal transabdominal scan of pelvis shows an irregular fluid collection *(arrow)* in the uterus with appearance suggestive of abnormal gestational sac. This fluid collection corresponded to the necrotic center of an infarcted fundal fibroid.

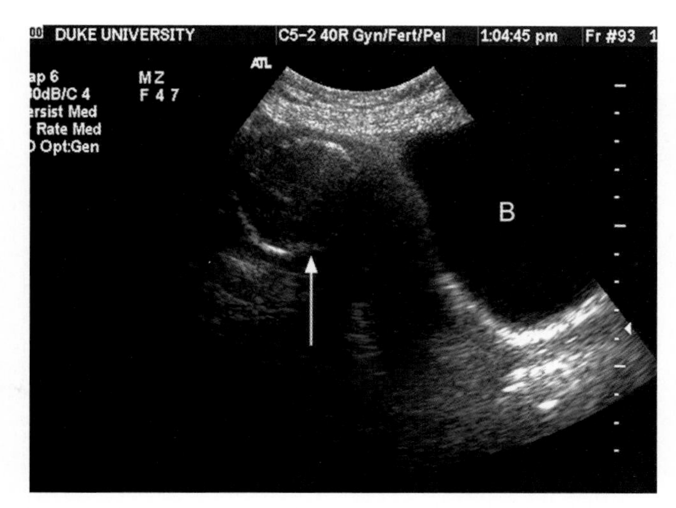

Figure 22-35 Fibroid with peripheral rim of calcification resembling fetal head. Midline longitudinal transabdominal scan was performed to rule out retained products following a therapeutic abortion. Rim of calcification *(arrow)* has sonographic appearance similar to that of a fetal calvarium but actually corresponds to calcification along the outer margin of a fibroid. B, bladder.

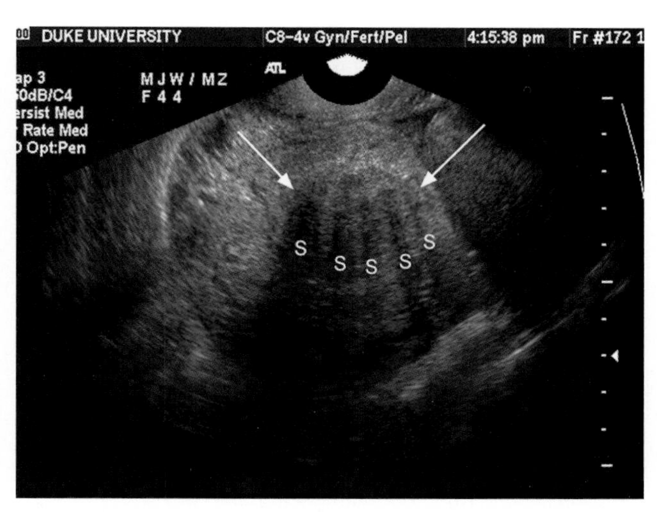

Figure 22-37 Fibroid with characteristic pattern of recurrent shadows. Axial transvaginal scan of uterus shows a central fibroid *(arrows)* causing typical pattern of multiple recurrent shadows (S).

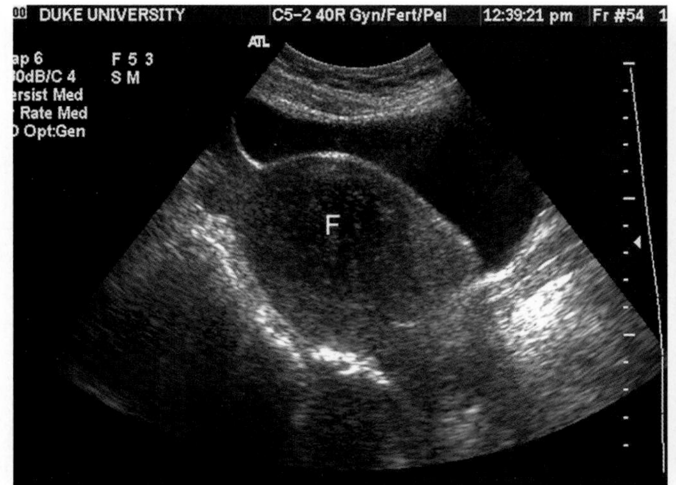

A

B

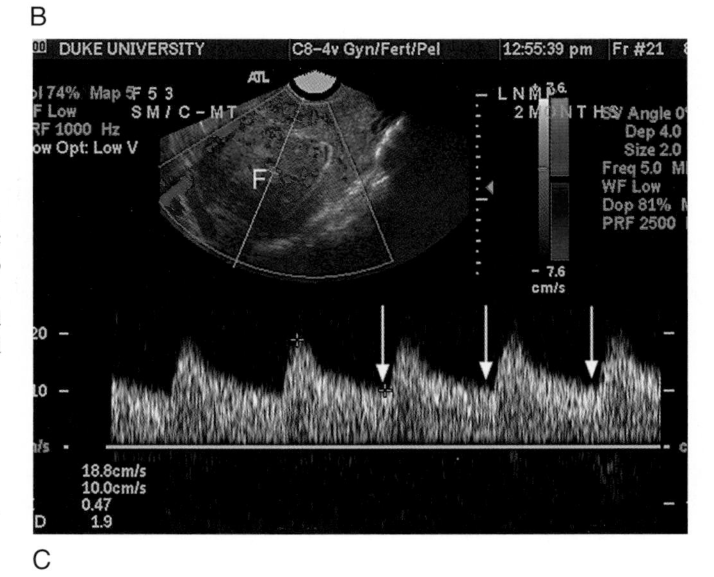

C

Figure 22-36 Fibroid with low-resistance arterial blood flow. **A,** Longitudinal transabdominal scan of uterus shows a large hypoechoic fibroid (F). **B,** Color Doppler image corresponding to the scan in **A** shows the fibroid (F) is highly vascular. B, bladder. **C,** Longitudinal transvaginal color Doppler image of the fibroid (F) with spectral waveform reveals a low-resistance arterial waveform with high diastolic fluid *(arrows)*.

Key Features

Two pelvic ultrasound techniques can be used: the transabdominal (TA) study and the transvaginal (TV) examination. The TA study obtains an overview of pelvic structures. The TV scan shows structures in greater detail but has limited movement of the transducer and depth of field.

On any initial examination, especially without a prior study, it is preferable to perform the TA scan with the TV study used for a more detailed evaluation. It may only be necessary to use the more diagnostic technique on a follow-up examination.

There is often an angle to the ultrasound beam as it exits from the TV probe. This must be taken into account when imaging the pelvis, especially if there is difficulty in identifying an anticipated structure.

There is no universally established gynecologic contraindication to the use of the TV probe.

In the fertile years, typically between ages 14 and 50, the uterus should be evaluated for the following: its overall position and size, the endometrial complex for its echogenicity and thickness, the junctional zone, and the myometrial echogenicity.

In the estrogen or proliferative phase, the endometrium has either a uniformly hyperechoic or a striated appearance and is typically 8 mm or less thick. In the progesterone or secretory phase, the endometrium continues to thicken (up to 15 mm and sometimes more) and is typically uniformly hyperechoic.

There is a wide range of normal uterine sizes and uterine positions.

It may be important to differentiate uterine version where the uterus is tilted but the endometrial canal is straight from flexion where the uterine body folds (is flexed) on itself if the woman is to undergo evacuation of the endometrial canal.

Congenital uterine anomalies range from a simple uterine septation to a unicornuate, bicornuate, or didelphys uterus. These may be associated with renal anomalies including absence or ptosis. Ultrasound may reveal a number of these uterine abnormalities, especially if TV ultrasound is combined with 3-D or saline-infusion sonohysterography.

The postpartum uterus involutes rapidly, with most of the size decrease occurring during the first 3 to 4 weeks. The uterus returns to normal by the seventh week. The postpartum uterus can be reliably measured in its long axis.

The postpartum endometrium is typically less than 15 mm in thickness. Retained products of conception, hemorrhage, or infection should be considered when the endometrium remains thicker. If gas is detected in the first 4 weeks, it may be a normal finding unless associated with the physical findings suggestive of endometritis (usually marked uterine pain).

After the early neonatal period during which the uterus is affected by the maternal hormones, the premenstrual uterus is small. The cervix is larger than the body and fundus, whereas the endometrial canal is thin and may not be identified.

The postmenopausal uterus (in the absence of hormone replacement therapy) progressively involutes. By 15 to 20 years after cessation of menses, the uterus has involuted to a size similar to that of a premenstrual uterus except the fundus and body remain larger than the cervix.

The postmenopausal endometrial stripe is either not identified or is hyperechoic and thin. Any focal thickening or enlargement over 5 mm should be considered for endometrial biopsy, particularly in a patient with vaginal bleeding.

When an abnormality of the endometrium is encountered, two questions need to be answered: (1) Is the patient premenstrual, fertile, or postmenopausal? (2) Is the abnormality an unusually thick endometrium, or is it a collection within the endometrial canal?

Abnormalities of the endometrium in the premenstrual period are frequently related to a vaginal obstruction. In the fertile years they are often related to pregnancies or retained products and present as either a thickened endometrium or a collection. In the postmenopausal years a thickened endometrium and obstruction are frequently associated with endometrial or cervical cancer.

A saline-infusion sonohysterogram has been shown to be of value in evaluating endometrial and submucosal abnormalties, especially when focal.

Tamoxifen, a treatment for breast cancer with an estrogenic effect on the endometrium, can cause hyperplasia and increase the risk of endometrial cancer. Cystic changes of the endometrium and subendometrium are also seen.

In a woman who is known to have an intrauterine contraceptive device (IUCD), scans are performed primarily to determine whether the device is in place and well positioned. Its absence suggests spontaneous expulsion, although perforation is often difficult to identify. Additionally, evidence of associated pelvic inflammatory disease (fallopian tube abnormalities or an abscess) and pregnancy (intrauterine or extrauterine) should be sought.

A typical fibroid is a hypoechoic solid mass that is positioned within the myometrium. There is tremendous variability in echogenicity, size, number, and position of fibroids.

Adenomyosis can initially appear as multiple small hypoechoic areas that distort the junctional zone (the outer layer of the endometrium/inner layer of the myometrium) and sometimes the myometrium

Continued

Key Features—cont'd

itself. Sonographically, they can mimic the appearance of small fibroids.

Often when an enlarged myomatous uterus is identified, the ovaries cannot be clearly defined unless typical follicles are seen.

During pregnancy, fibroids may become evident and often enlarge. If critically placed, such as in the lower uterine segment, they should be closely watched for potential problems related to fetal growth and delivery.

Fibroids are the great pelvic mimicker. They may assume the appearance of a number of pelvic conditions: uterine variants, uterine abnormalities, pregnancy-related conditions, IUCD perforation, and adnexal masses. An early intrauterine pregnancy may be so displaced by the fibroid as to appear in an ectopic position. Even Doppler evaluation can be misleading.

When a solid abdominopelvic mass is identified without an obvious site of origin, a fibroid uterus should be considered a possible source.

SUGGESTED READINGS

Baker ME, Bowie JD, Killam AP: Sonography of post-cesarean-section bladder-flap hematoma. AJR Am J Roentgenol 144:757, 1985.

Baltarowich OH: Female pelvic organ measurements. In Goldberg BB, Kurtz AB (eds): Atlas of Ultrasound Measurements. Chicago, Year Book Medical Publishers, 1990.

Baltarowich OH, et al: Pitfalls in the sonographic diagnosis of uterine fibroids. AJR Am J Roentgenol 151:725, 1988.

Breckenridge JW, et al: Postmenopausal uterine fluid collection: Indicator of carcinoma. AJR Am J Roentgenol 139:529, 1982.

Carter JR, et al: Gray scale and color flow Doppler characterization of uterine tumors. J Ultrasound Med 13:835, 1994.

Cicinelli E, et al: Transabdominal sonohysterography, transvaginal sonography, and hysteroscopy in the evaluation of submucous myomas. Obstet Gynecol 85:42, 1995.

Dubinsky TJ, et al: Transvaginal hysterosonography in the evaluation of small endoluminal masses. J Ultrasound Med 14:1, 1995.

DuBose TJ, et al: Sonography of arcuate uterine blood vessels. J Ultrasound Med 4:229, 1985.

Goldberg BB, et al: Endoluminal gynecologic ultrasound: Preliminary results. J Ultrasound Med 10:583, 1991.

Haynor DR, et al: Changing appearance of the normal uterus during the menstrual cycle: MR studies. Radiology 161:459, 1986.

Kupfer MC, et al: Transvaginal sonographic evaluation of endometrial polyps. J Ultrasound Med 13:535, 1994.

Kurtz AB, et al: Detection of retained products of conception following spontaneous abortion in the first trimester. J Ultrasound Med 10:387, 1991.

Langlois PL: The size of the normal uterus. J Reprod Med 4:221, 1970.

Mitchell DG, et al: Zones of the uterus: Discrepancy between US and MR images. Radiology 174:827, 1990.

Najarian KE, Kurtz AB: New observations in the sonographic evaluation of intrauterine contraceptive devices. J Ultrasound Med 5:205, 1986.

Orsini LF, et al: Pelvic organs in premenarchal girls: Real-time ultrasonography. Radiology 153:113, 1984.

Pellerito JS, et al: Diagnosis of uterine anomalies: Relative accuracy of MR imaging, endovaginal sonography, and hysterosalpingography. Radiology 183:795, 1992.

Shalev J, et al: Continuous sonographic monitoring of IUD extraction during pregnancy: Preliminary report. AJR Am J Roentgenol 139:521, 1982.

Siedler D, et al: Uterine adenomyosis: A difficult sonographic diagnosis. J Ultrasound Med 6:345, 1987.

Strobelt N, et al: Natural history of uterine leiomyomas in pregnancy. J Ultrasound Med 13:399, 1994.

Thickman D, et al: Sonographic assessment of the endometrium in patients undergoing in vitro fertilization. J Ultrasound Med 5:197, 1986.

Togashi K, et al: Adenomyosis: Diagnosis with MR imaging. Radiology 166:111, 1988.

Tongson T, Pongnarisorn C, Mahanuphap P: Use of vaginosonographic measurements of endometrial thickness in the identification of abnormal endometrium in peri- and postmenopausal bleeding. J Clin Ultrasound 22:479, 1994.

Varner RE, et al: Transvaginal sonography of the endometrium in postmenopausal women. Obstet Gynecol 78:195, 1991.

Wachsberg RH, Kurtz AB: Gas within the endometrial cavity at postpartum US: A normal finding after spontaneous vaginal delivery. Radiology 183:431, 1992.

Wachsberg RH, et al: Real-time ultrasonographic analysis of the normal postpartum uterus: Technique, variability, and measurements. J Ultrasound Med 13:215, 1994.

CHAPTER 23

Adnexa

For Key Features summary see p. 584

The adnexa contain the ovaries, with their mesosalpinges, fallopian tubes, and broad ligaments. There are also bilateral uterine and ovarian blood vessels.

Sonographically, the normal ovaries are almost always detected, especially during the fertile years. The normal nondilated fallopian tubes are not identified, although thin hypoechoic soft tissue bands containing the tubes can often be imaged adjacent to the lateral margins of the uterine fundus. The normal mesosalpinges and broad ligaments are not seen sonographically. Although normal-caliber uterine and ovarian arteries and veins are not distinctly identified at gray-scale ultrasound, their Doppler flow can be detected particularly along the lateral uterine margins and adjacent to the ovaries.

OVARIAN POSITION

The position of the ovaries, the only truly intraperitoneal adnexal structures, is not constant (Fig. 23-1). They are usually identified directly lateral to the body of the uterus in shallow depressions called the ovarian fossae. These fossae are bordered laterally and anteriorly by the external iliac blood vessels and posteriorly by the ureter and internal iliac (hypogastric) blood vessels. However, when the uterus is deviated toward the right or left (a normal variant), the ovary on that side is usually displaced superiorly, taking a position lateral or superior to the uterine fundus. Occasionally, it may instead be identified within the cul-de-sac. When the uterus is tilted posteriorly, the ovaries sometimes follow and appear as "rabbit ears" at the top of the uterine fundus.

With uterine enlargement (including pregnancy), the ovaries are displaced, typically into a more superior and lateral position. After a myomectomy or after delivery, the ovaries often remain in their new position, rather than returning to the ovarian fossae. On occasion an ovary (either normal or abnormal) becomes fixed in the cul-de-sac. After hysterectomy the ovaries usually assume a more caudad position, medial and directly superior to the vaginal cuff.

NORMAL OVARIES IN THE FERTILE PERIOD

The fertile (ovulating) woman is usually between 14 and 50 years of age. With each menstrual cycle, the ovaries vary in size because of the changing number and size of their follicles (functional cysts). The ovary is classically ovoid (not round). It has a low-level uniform echogenicity with multiple small follicles in women of childbearing age (Fig. 23-2).

Many observers express the ovarian size as a volume. Using three perpendicular (orthogonal) measurements, the volume is calculated from the formula for a prolated ellipse: length (L) times width (W) times anteroposterior (AP) dimension times 0.5 ($L \times W \times AP \times 0.5$). This formula yields reported maximum volumes of 9.0 and 15.0 mL for nulliparous and parous women, respectively (Table 23-1). Because multiple follicles are incorporated

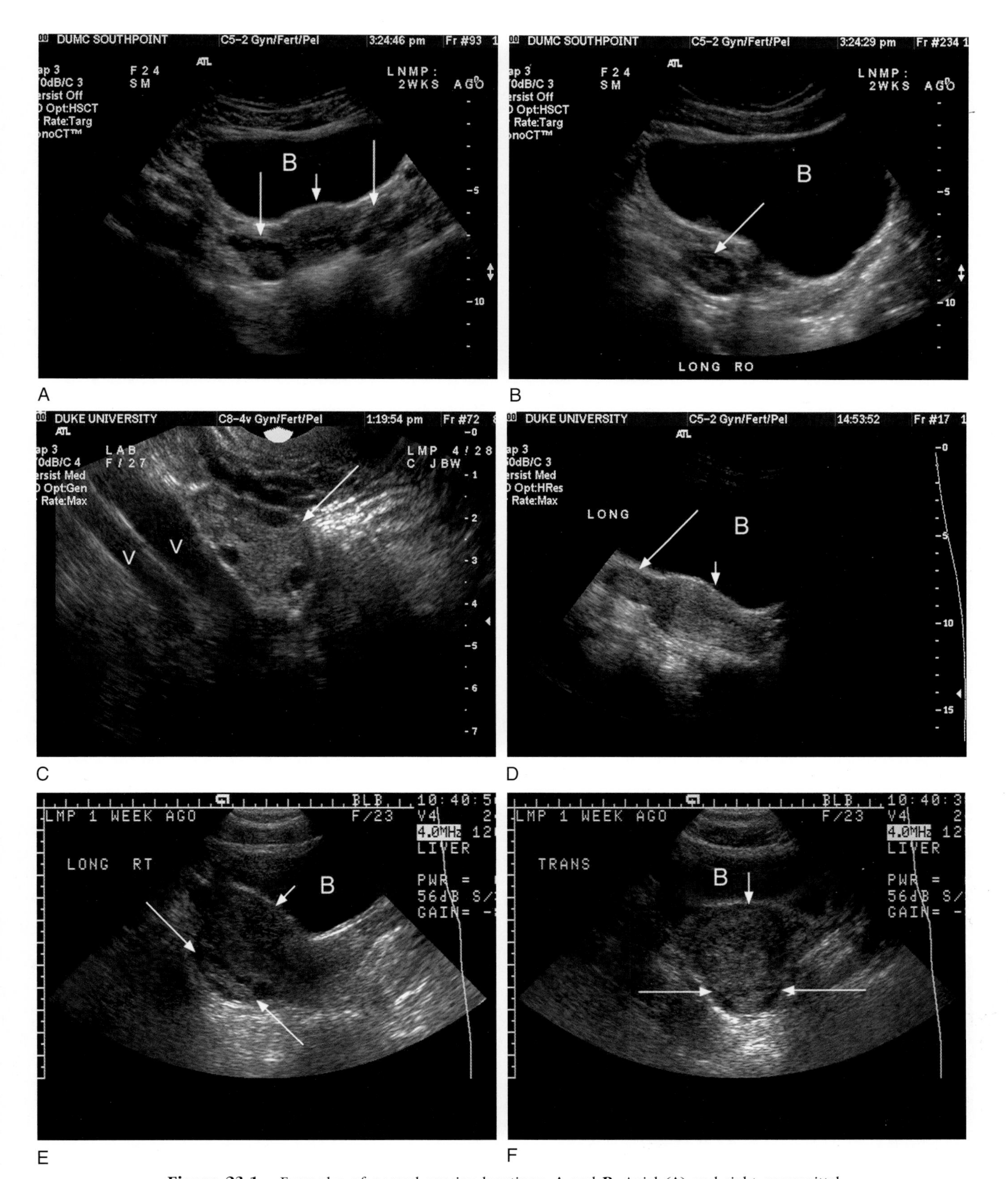

Figure 23-1 Examples of normal ovarian locations. **A** and **B,** Axial (**A**) and right parasagittal (**B**) transabdominal images show typical location of ovaries *(long arrows)* lateral to uterus *(short arrow).* B, bladder. **C,** Axial transvaginal ultrasound angled to the right shows right ovary *(arrow)* immediately anterior to the iliac blood vessels (V). **D,** Midline longitudinal transabdominal scan shows right ovary *(long arrow)* located immediately superior to uterus *(short arrow).* B, bladder. **E** and **F,** Midline longitudinal (**E**) and axial (**F**) transabdominal scans show right ovary *(long arrows)* in cul-de-sac, posterior to uterus *(short arrow).* B, bladder.

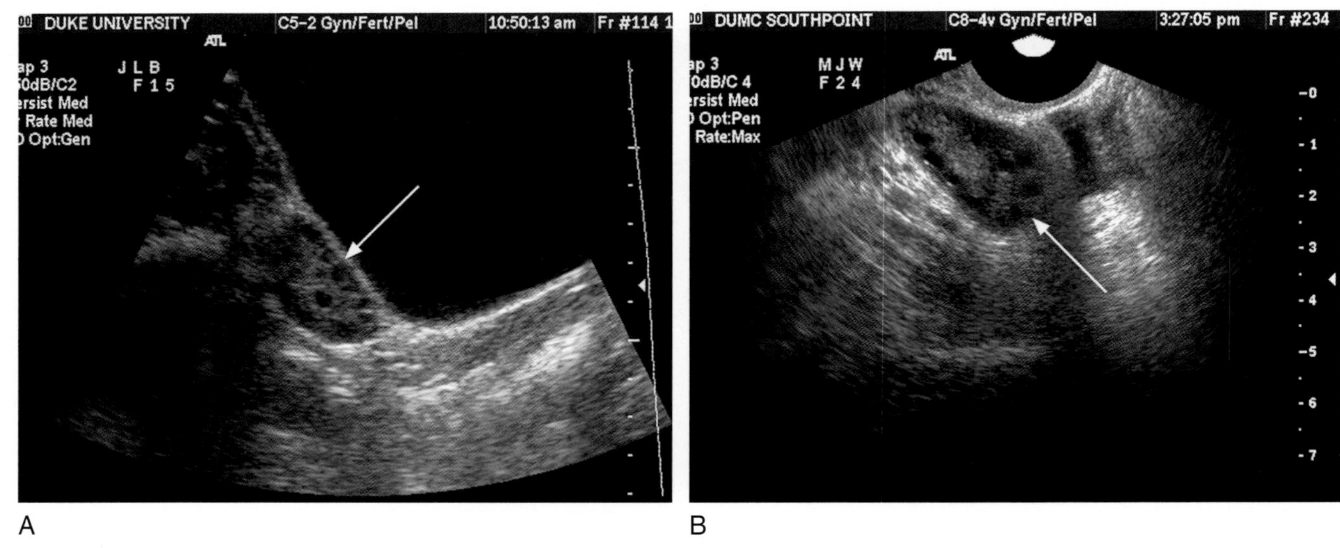

Figure 23-2 Normal ovaries. Transabdominal (**A**) and transvaginal (**B**) images of normal ovaries *(arrows)* in women of childbearing age. Note the ovoid shape of the ovaries and the presence of multiple tiny cysts corresponding to follicles.

in the ovarian measurements for *both* the young nulliparous and older parous women, the ovarian dimensions and calculated volumes can be larger and still normal. Therefore, if the remaining ovarian tissue appears normal, ovarian volumes can be considered normal up to 15 mL and even up to 20 mL for both groups.

There is no statistically significant difference in the size of the right and left ovaries. Their volumes, however, may be discrepant by as much as 14 mL.

The ovaries in the normally fertile woman go through cycles lasting approximately 28 days. These menstrual cycles can be divided into two phases: *the estrogen phase* before ovulation and *the progesterone phase* after ovulation. In the estrogen phase, at the time of menstruation, the ovaries are at their smallest and contain follicles that are typically less than 5 mm in diameter and occasionally are too small to be detected. By day 10 of the cycle, one follicle begins to dominate and increases in size. Most of the other bilateral follicles remain small or regress. By mid cycle the dominant follicle attains a diameter approaching 20 to 25 mm or greater. It then contains a mature ovum or egg. This can be detected as a small hyperechoic soft tissue or cyst-like area along the inner margin of the follicle and is termed the *cumulus oophorus* (Fig. 23-3).

The luteinizing hormone surge at mid cycle causes the mature follicle to rupture and release its egg. All the other follicles begin to shrink in the progesterone phase. The ruptured follicle loses its fluid, rapidly shrinks, and becomes a corpus luteum. A small amount of fluid can often then be detected in the cul-de-sac. On occasion, the ruptured follicle bleeds internally and re-expands, even becoming large enough to present as a mass (Fig. 23-4). This "mass" is termed a *hemorrhagic cyst* and usually resolves within one to two menstrual cycles (discussed further in the section on complicated cysts). By the end of the progesterone phase, as menstruation begins, all the follicles have involuted and the cycle starts again.

Table 23-1 Approximate Top Normal Ovarian Linear Dimensions and Volumes During the Fertile (Ovulatory) Years

Patient Category	Dimensions (L × W × AP)*	Volume†
Young adult, nulliparous	3 × 3 × 2‡	9‡
Adult, parous	5 × 3 × 2	15

*The three perpendicular orthogonal diameters in centimeters: L, length; W, width; AP, anteroposterior.

†Volume calculated by the prolated ellipse equation in cubic centimeters: L × W × AP × 0.5.

‡From Harris L. Cohen, MD: Personal communications.

From Baltarowich OH: Female pelvic organ measurements. In Goldberg BB, Kurtz AB (eds): Atlas of Ultrasound Measurements. Chicago, Year Book Medical Publishers, 1990.

FERTILITY MEDICATIONS

Fertility medicines such as clomiphene citrate (Clomid) overdrive the ovaries and force the maturation of many follicles, often bilateral. With successful treatment it is not uncommon for the ovaries to show multiple follicles of 20 mm or more in diameter by mid cycle.

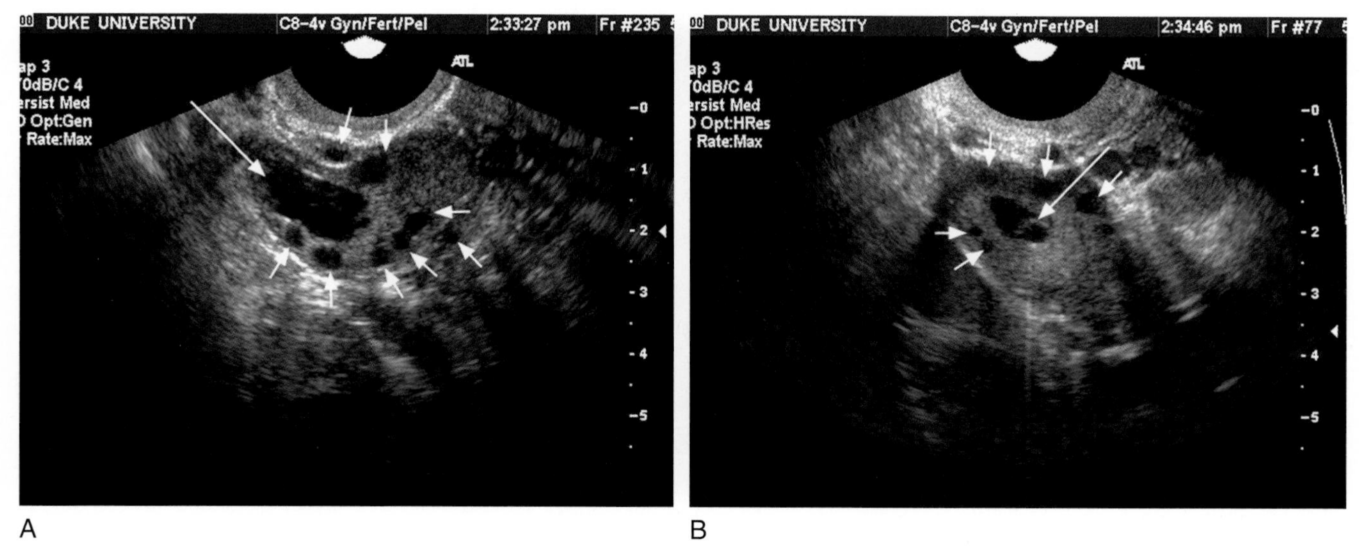

Figure 23-3 Dominant follicle. **A,** Development of the dominant follicle. Axial transvaginal scan of right ovary on day 12 of menstrual cycle shows a developing dominant follicle *(long arrow)* as well as multiple small nondominant follicles *(small arrows).* **B,** Cumulus oophorus. Longitudinal transvaginal scan of right ovary of a different patient at mid cycle depicts the cumulus oophorus as a cyst-like structure *(long arrow)* protruding into the dominant follicle. *Short arrows,* nondominant follicles.

The role of ultrasound is to identify and measure these follicles. If the follicles are of appropriate size, even if multiple, the woman can then be stimulated with luteinizing hormone or the follicles can be harvested by cyst aspiration.

Infrequently the ovaries can be overstimulated so that an ovarian hyperstimulation syndrome (OHS) develops. OHS is often caused by increased dosage of medication. It can, however, be idiopathic, occurring even after the same dose of medication in one cycle but not in the preceding or subsequent cycle. OHS is a clinical syndrome in which both ovaries become so enlarged with multiple follicles that they are easily palpable (Fig. 23-5). The ovaries may be so large that each measures greater than 20 cm in maximum length alone. The follicles leak fluid across their walls, causing transudative ascites and even

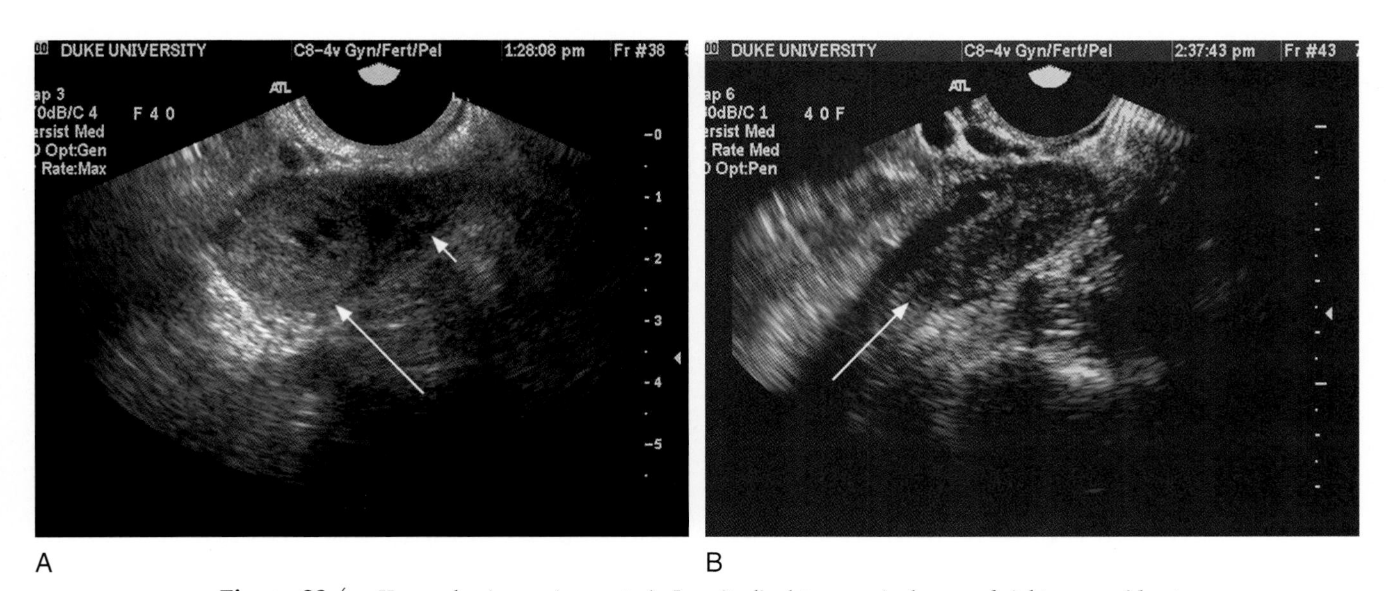

Figure 23-4 Hemorrhagic ovarian cyst. **A,** Longitudinal transvaginal scan of right ovary *(short arrow)* shows a heterogeneous intraovarian mass *(long arrow)* due to hemorrhage into a corpus luteal cyst. **B,** Longitudinal transvaginal scan performed 6 weeks after the scan in **A** shows interval resolution of the hemorrhagic ovarian cyst. The right ovary *(arrow)* is normal in appearance with no evidence of a residual mass.

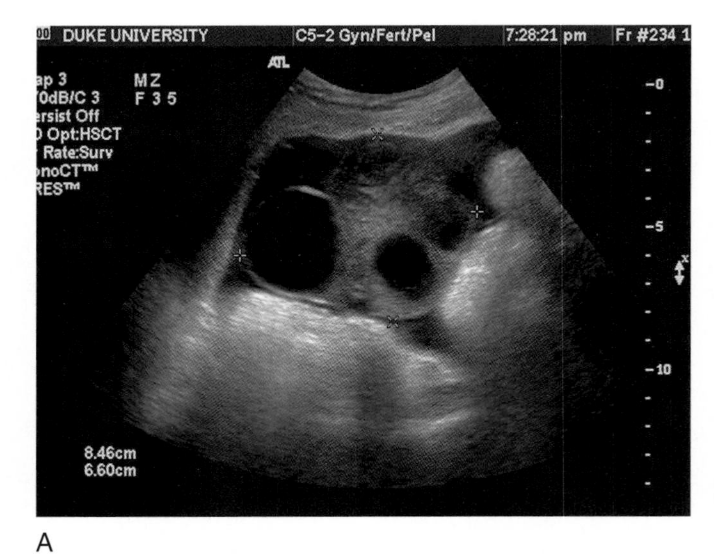

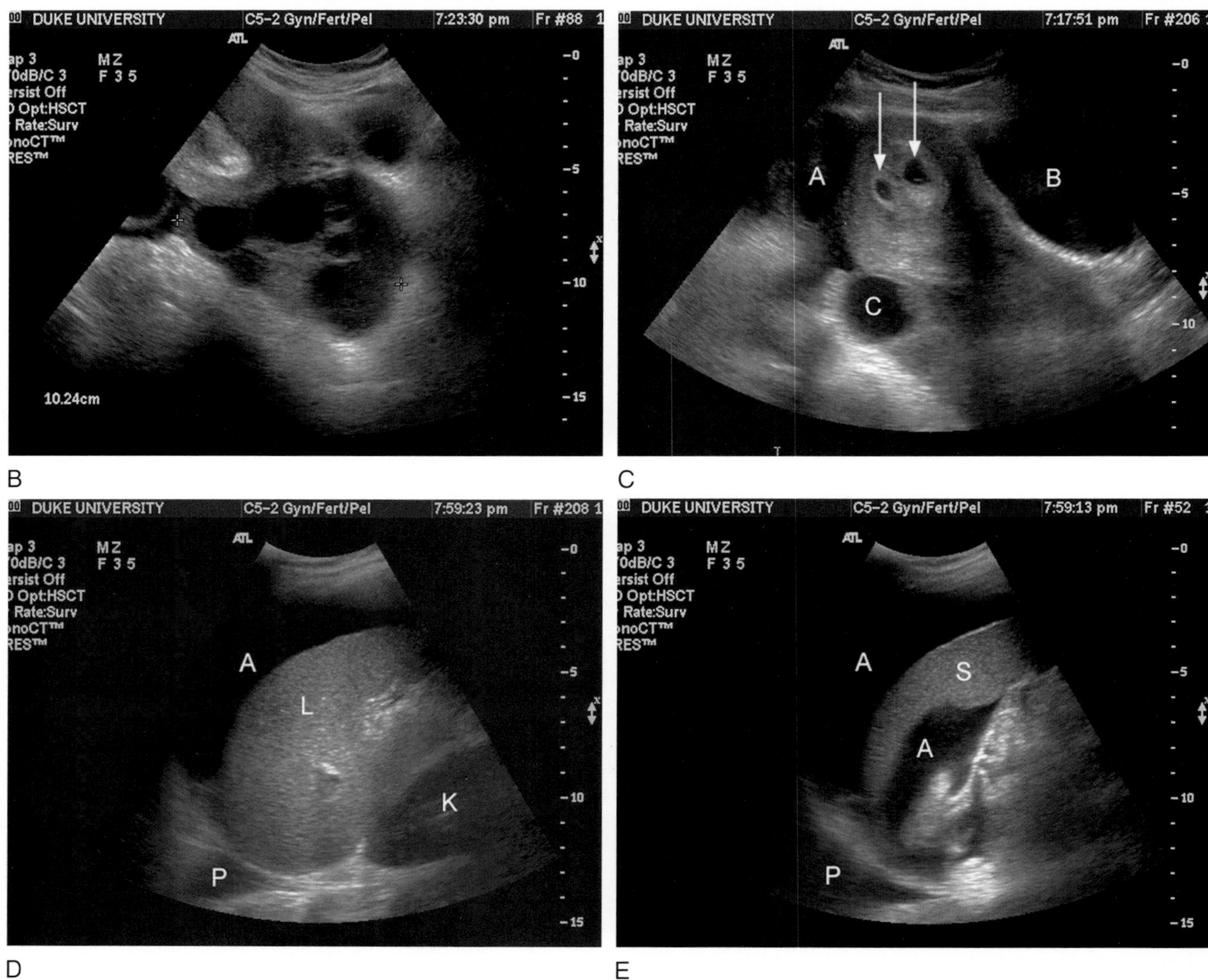

Figure 23-5 Ovarian hyperstimulation syndrome. **A** and **B,** Transabdominal images of right (**A**) and left (**B**) adnexa show bilaterally enlarged ovaries with numerous cysts secondary to ovarian hyperstimulation from infertility medication. **C,** Longitudinal transabdominal image of pelvis shows pelvic ascites (A). Two intrauterine gestational sacs *(arrows)* are seen, corresponding to a twin pregnancy. B, bladder; C, ovarian cyst. **D** and **E,** Longitudinal transabdominal images of the right (**D**) and left (**E**) upper quadrants reveal a large amount of ascites (A) and bilateral pleural effusions (P). L, liver; S, spleen; K, kidney.

Table 23-2 Normal Ovarian Volumes in Pediatric (Premenstrual) Age Groups

Pediatric Groups	Age	Volume (mL) Mean (±SD)
Neonatal	1 day to 3 mo	1.06 (0.03-3.56)*
Infancy	4 to 12 mo	1.05 (0.18-2.71)*
	6 wk-2 yr	0.67 (0.15-1.68)*
Early childhood	2-8 yr	0.9 (0.3)†
Late childhood	9 yr	2.0 (0.8)†
	10 yr	2.2 (0.7)†
	11 yr	2.5 (1.3)†
	12 yr	3.8 (1.4)†
	13 yr	4.2 (2.3)†
Puberty	13-14 yr	4.1 (3.0)†

*From Cohen HL, Shapiro M, Mandel F, Shapiro M: Normal ovaries in neonates and infants: A sonographiic study of 77 patients 1 day to 24 months old. AJR Am J Roentgenol 160:583-856, 1993, at mean and 2 standard deviations.
†From Baltarowich OH: Female pelvic organ measurements. In Goldberg BB, Kurtz AB (eds): Atlas of Ultrasound Measurements. Chicago, Year Book Medical Publishers, 1990, at mean and 1 standard deviation.

pleural effusions. If a woman with OHS becomes pregnant, the hyperstimulation may persist and even worsen. The pregnant woman may suffer considerable hemodilution and electrolyte disturbances and require prolonged care or hospitalization during her pregnancy. The condition can even be life threatening.

Ultrasound can easily detect these hyperstimulated ovaries, even before they become clinically obvious. Before gross enlargement, the ovaries have already increased in size and are completely replaced by follicles. When no identifiable ovarian tissue remains, luteinizing hormone stimulation and pregnancy induction should be avoided until the ovaries revert to normal.

NORMAL OVARIES IN THE PREMENSTRUAL (PEDIATRIC) PERIOD

In the premenstrual period (before puberty), the ovaries are relatively quiescent. Nevertheless, size changes (calculated as volumes) can be divided into four groups: neonatal (up to 3 months), infancy (6 months to 2 years), early childhood (2 to 8 years), and late childhood (9 to 13 years) (Table 23-2). Because ovaries less than 1 mL are rarely identified, a transabdominal examination may not detect them in early childhood unless they exceed this threshold. More rapid growth begins by 8 years of age, with doubling of the ovarian volume between 8 and 9 years of age and then again between 9 and 13 years of age as puberty approaches. From age 9 onward, the ovaries should therefore be routinely imaged.

The ovaries in the premenstrual period may contain follicles, and many ovaries have a normal polycystic appearance (Fig. 23-6). True follicles occur in all pediatric age groups, most measuring between 4 and 8 mm (range, 1 to 17 mm). Most of these when larger than 5 mm should be identified.

NORMAL OVARIES IN THE POSTMENOPAUSAL PERIOD

Menopause is most commonly defined as commencing 1 year after the complete cessation of menses. After menopause the ovaries steadily atrophy (Table 23-3). The size of a postmenopausal ovary is considered abnormal (even without a mass) if it exceeds the upper limits of normal or if it is twice the size of the other ovary, even if both are still within normal limits. Atrophy is slowed in women receiving hormone replacement therapy. It may be difficult to detect postmenopausal ovaries. Although the literature states that one or both postmenopausal ovaries can be identified in 80% to 90% of women (whether studied transabdominally or transvaginally), this still means that numerous ovaries may not be seen (Fig. 23-7). There are additional cases in which the structure identified as the ovary was not confirmed at surgery or laparoscopy. This is particularly a problem in the very elderly woman who is more likely to have atrophic ovaries without follicles. Therefore, the true incidence of detection is not known but should be considerably lower than 80%.

Small simple cysts (less than 3 cm) are seen in up to 15% to 20% of postmenopausal women. On follow-up studies these cysts can exhibit a range of changes: some cysts remain stable, others regress or disappear, and some ovaries develop new cysts. Although a small simple postmenopausal cyst is usually a normal benign finding, it should be followed closely to exclude the possibility of a developing ovarian cancer.

Some examiners have stated that when postmenopausal ovaries are not visualized by either the transabdominal (TA) or transvaginal (TV) technique, a normal physical examination rules out an abnormality. This argument is fraught with potential error because ultrasound can detect subtle size or echogenicity changes, both possible early signs of a malignancy, which physical examination may not identify.

TRANSABDOMINAL VERSUS TRANSVAGINAL SCANNING

Sonographically, the technique for evaluating the adnexa is the same for both the TA study performed through the distended urinary bladder and the TV

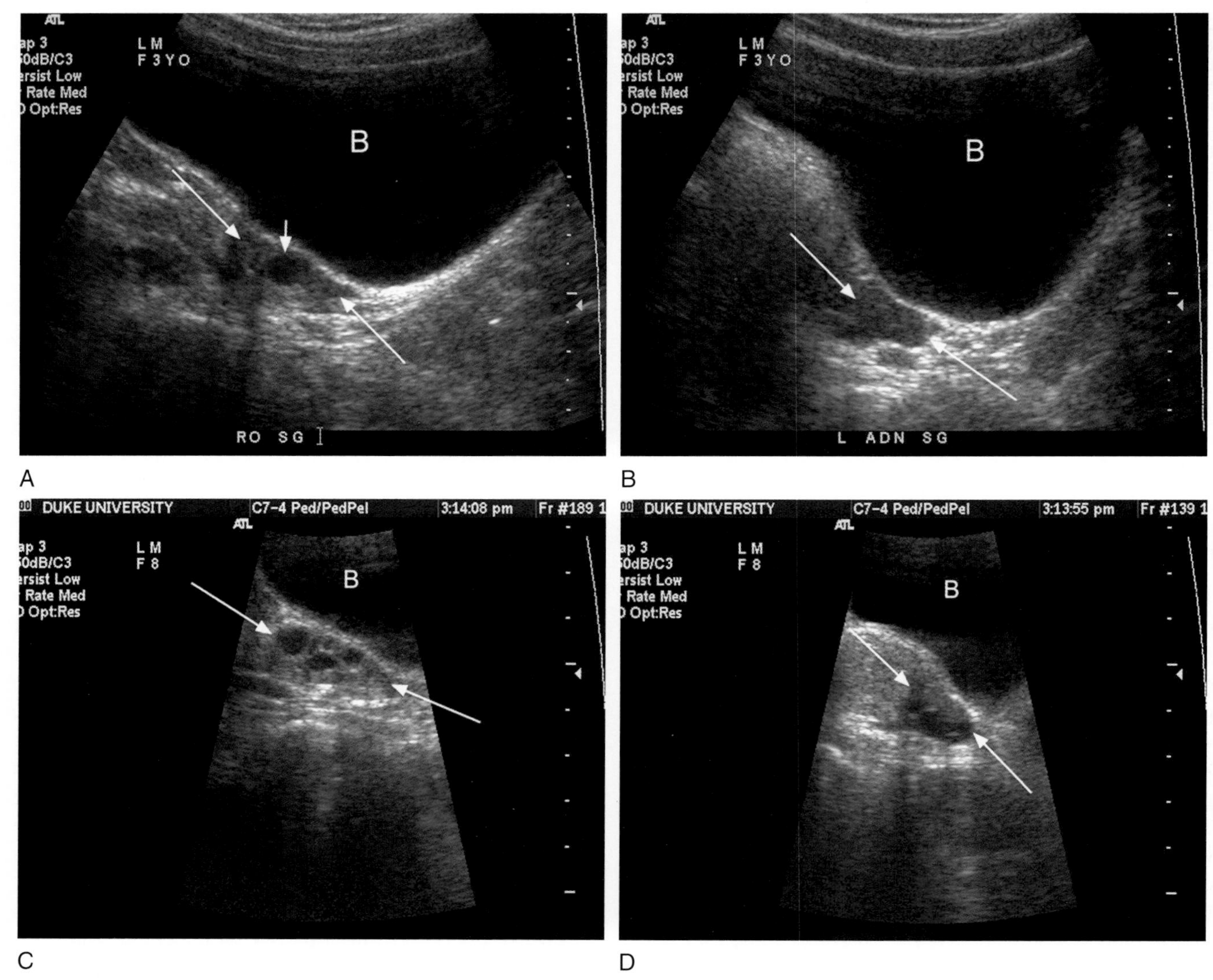

Figure 23-6 Normal ovary in a child. **A** and **B**, Longitudinal transabdominal scans of the right (**A**) and left (**B**) ovaries of a 3-year-old girl show a follicle *(short arrow)* on the right ovary but no demonstrable follicle on the left. *Long arrows,* ovaries; B, bladder. **C** and **D**, Longitudinal transabdominal scans of the right (**C**) and left (**D**) ovaries *(arrows)* of an 8-year-old girl show numerous follicles bilaterally. B, bladder.

examination performed with the bladder empty. After the long axis of the uterus is identified, parallel sagittal scans are obtained laterally to image the long axis of the adnexa and identify the ovaries. Axial-coronal views of the adnexa are then obtained.

Two issues with regard to TV scanning discussed in Chapter 22 need reemphasis. First, the TV transducer beam usually exits from the probe at an angle. Although this is excellent for evaluating anteverted structures in their long axis, it can cause difficulties in imaging ovaries when they are positioned posteriorly. The left adnexa can be similarly difficult to image when the probe is turned toward the right in the axial-coronal plane. In both cases it may be necessary to turn the probe a full 180 degrees. Second, although there are no universally established contraindications to TV scanning, it is recommended that TV sonography not be done in patients who have never been sexually active. The transducer is typically placed only part of the way into the vagina, and there is no undue pressure on the adnexal regions.

The TA and TV techniques have been compared in their abilities to image the adnexa to determine which is better for the following: to identify an abnormality, to analyze its ultrasound characteristics, and to determine its site of origin. In general, TV ultrasound has been found to be superior for identifying and characterizing most lesions (Figs. 23-8 and 23-9). There are, however, exceptions in which TA ultrasound detects an

Table 23-3 Postmenopausal Ovarian Volumes

Years Since Menopause	No.	Chronologic Age (Mean) (yr)	Ovarian Volume (mL) Mean ± SD
Perimenopausal	33	50.67	8.6 ± 2.3
1-2	56	54.1	6.2 ± 2.7
3-4	30	55.5	5.2 ± 1.6
5-6	36	57	4.0 ± 1.8
7-8	36	58.25	3.1 ± 1.3
9-10	31	60.25	2.8 ± 2.1
11-12	28	62.6	2.4 ± 1.3
13-14	27	66.37	2.2 ± 1.3
≥ 15	34	70.55	2.2 ± 1.4

Portions of table from Tepper R, Zalel Y, Markov S, et al: Ovarian volume in postmenopausal women—suggestions to an ovarian size nomogram for menopausal age. Acta Obstet Gynecol Scand 74:208, 1995. Reprinted with permission.

abnormality not seen at TV ultrasound (Fig. 23-10). These exceptions generally are attributable to the limited field of view afforded by TV ultrasound. A mass that is high in the pelvis, beyond the field of view of the TV probe, will be missed.

It is therefore recommended that TA scanning be performed first in a patient who has not undergone a previous pelvic ultrasound study. This allows visualization of the entire pelvic area. If the TA study findings are deemed completely normal or a well-defined anomaly and its site of origin are detected, it is often possible to stop the examination. However, the TV study should always be considered when the TA findings are uncertain or when a patient has normal findings but is at high risk for abnormalities. For example, a woman with normal ovaries but with a strong family history of ovarian cancer should have a TV study.

It has not been shown that the TV examination should be performed instead of the TA study for an initial pelvic study. In fact, in patients with large abnormalities, very distorted anatomic features and abnormalities more than 8 cm from the TV probe, the TV study may miss the findings or the TV findings may be misinterpreted in the absence of a TA study. On a subsequent study, however, it is often appropriate to use only TV scanning because the pelvic anatomic characteristics and the ultrasound appearance can now be anticipated.

FUNCTIONING AND NONFUNCTIONING OVARIAN CYSTS

Functioning cysts (follicles) are affected by the cyclic hormonal changes that occur during the menstrual cycle. These cysts are benign and usually 25 mm or less in diameter. They may rarely, however, attain a diameter of up to 40 or even 50 mm. Because they are under hormonal influence, follicles should regress by the beginning of the next menstrual cycle.

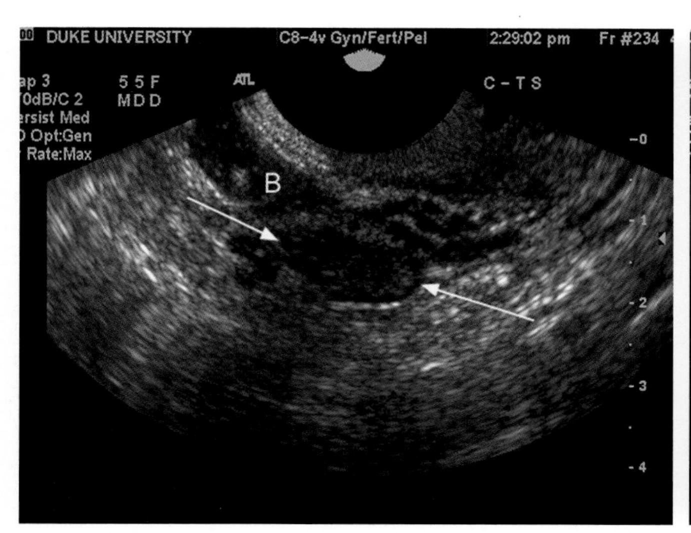

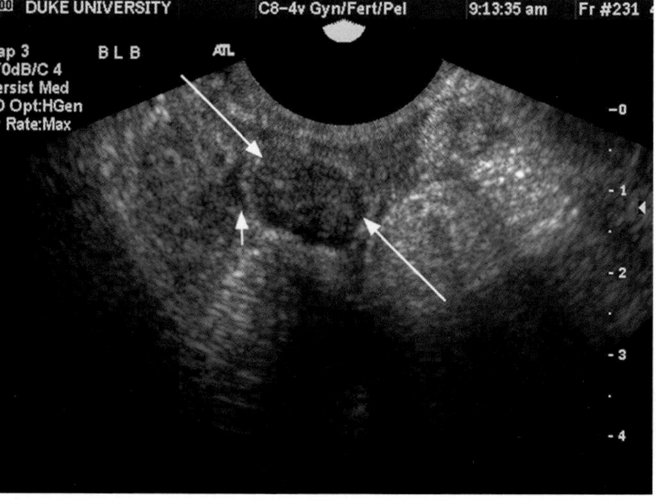

Figure 23-7 Normal ovaries in postmenopausal women. **A,** Sagittal transvaginal image of left ovary *(arrows)* in a 55-year-old woman. Because the follicles are small and atrophic, the ovary is difficult to distinguish from adjacent loops of bowel (B). The contralateral ovary could not be seen. **B,** Axial transvaginal image of right ovary *(long arrows)* in a 71-year-old woman with a previous hysterectomy and left oophorectomy. The right ovary was distinguishable from surrounding bowel because of a subtle difference in echo texture and the observation of bowel peristalsis at real-time evaluation. A small amount of fluid *(short arrow)* is seen in a loop of bowel adjacent to the ovary.

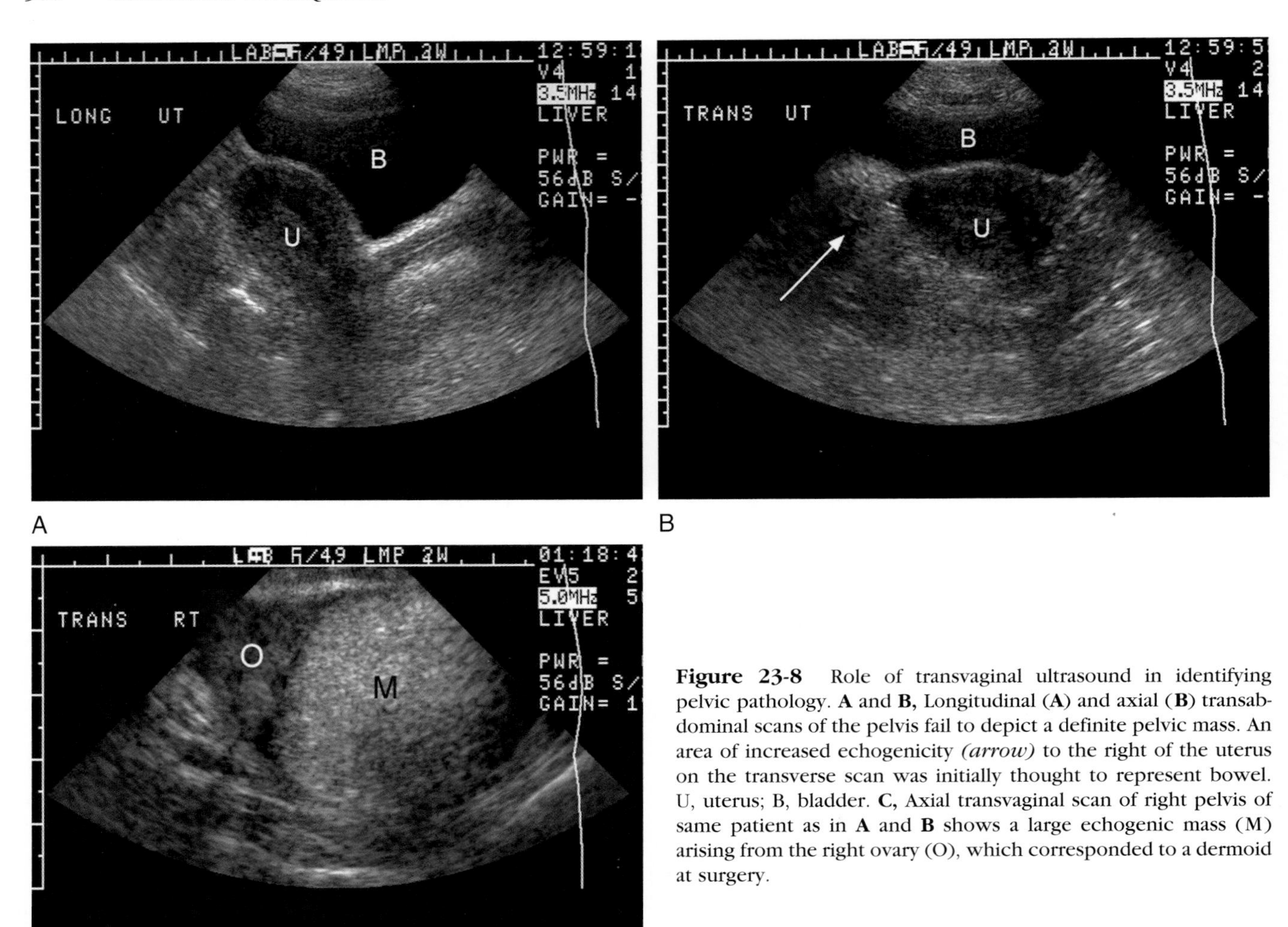

Figure 23-8 Role of transvaginal ultrasound in identifying pelvic pathology. **A** and **B,** Longitudinal (**A**) and axial (**B**) transabdominal scans of the pelvis fail to depict a definite pelvic mass. An area of increased echogenicity *(arrow)* to the right of the uterus on the transverse scan was initially thought to represent bowel. U, uterus; B, bladder. **C,** Axial transvaginal scan of right pelvis of same patient as in **A** and **B** shows a large echogenic mass (M) arising from the right ovary (O), which corresponded to a dermoid at surgery.

Most follicles do not need to be reexamined. However, if their appearance (e.g., with internal echoes) or size is unusual, it is recommended that a follow-up study wait until the start of the next one or two menstrual cycles. There is no well-defined interval in premenopausal (fertile) women who have had either a hysterectomy or who have very irregular menstrual periods and in all postmenopausal women. A 6-week follow-up study is often then taken as an arbitrary waiting period between examinations.

If a simple cyst persists and either does not change or increases in size, it is then considered nonfunctioning (not under hormonal influence). It is usually of ovarian or paraovarian or paratubal in origin (Fig. 23-11). A cyst is considered simple if it is anechoic without wall thickening or internal echoes and has good distal acoustic enhancement. A persistent simple nonfunctioning cyst less than 5 cm is almost always benign but should be followed to confirm stability. If the cyst is more than 5 cm and persists, the likelihood of malignancy increases. Therefore, even if simple, it may be considered for surgical removal. In the differential diagnosis are a cystic neoplasm (usually a cystadenoma) and an endometrioma. Either can be simple or complex in appearance. Dermoid and nongynecologic masses are less likely considerations because they are usually heterogeneous complex masses.

Polycystic ovaries present as multiple small nonfunctioning cysts. This appearance is often (but not always) identified in infertile women and may be part of the Stein-Leventhal syndrome (SLS), which includes obesity and hirsutism. SLS is based on clinical and laboratory findings, and not infrequently the women have additional systemic problems. SLS does not usually require ultrasound confirmation, although ultrasound is sometimes performed. At ultrasound, polycystic ovaries present a

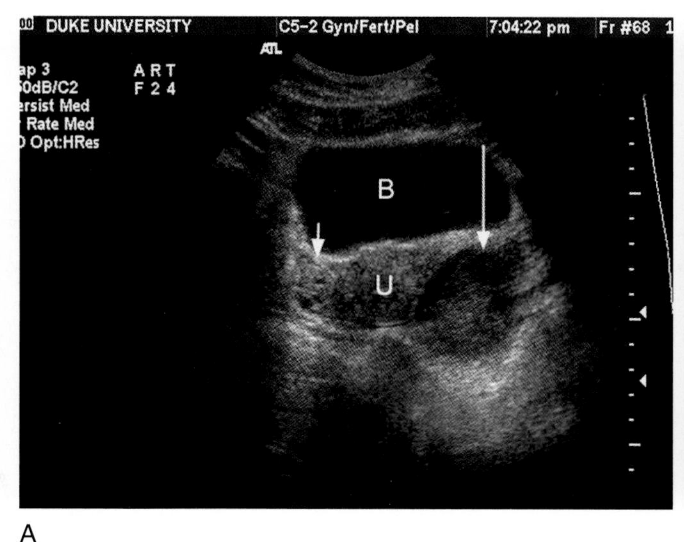

A

B

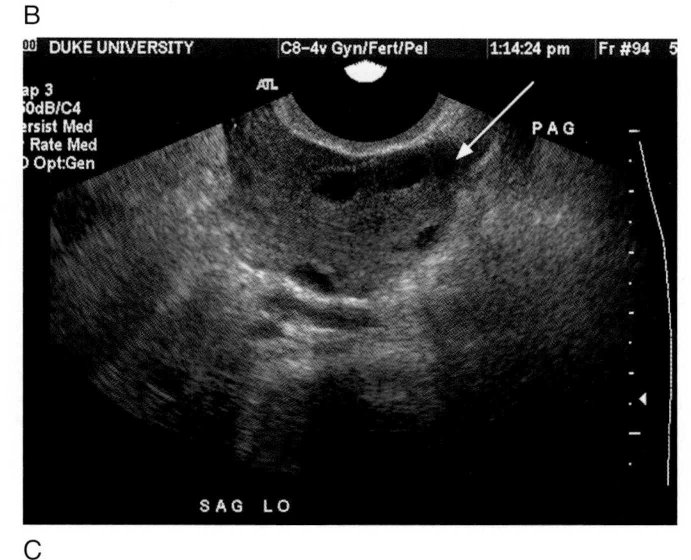

C

Figure 23-9 Role of transvaginal ultrasound in characterizing pelvic pathology. **A,** Axial transabdominal scan of pelvis shows a hypoechoic mass *(long arrow)* in the left adnexa. The internal characteristics of the mass are poorly demonstrated, and it is not clear if the mass arises from the ovary. B, bladder; U, uterus; *short arrow,* right ovary. **B,** Axial transvaginal scan of uterus (U) and left adnexa shows ovarian tissue with follicles *(short arrows)* compressed around the periphery of the mass, indicating it is ovarian in origin. Internal septations and a fluid-fluid level *(long arrows)* are visualized only on the transvaginal scan. **C,** Follow-up transvaginal scan of left ovary *(arrow)* performed 7 weeks after the scans in **A** and **B** shows the mass has resolved, consistent with resolution of a hemorrhagic ovarian cyst.

range of appearances. These ovaries are typically rounder than normal ovaries and may have a bright thick hyperechoic capsule. The classic appearance is enlarged ovaries with numerous small cysts that are typically less than 5 mm in diameter and line up in the periphery, just inside the capsule, in a "string-of-pearls" configuration (Fig. 23-12). However, other patterns such as normal ovaries, large solid-appearing ovaries, and so on, can also be seen (see Fig. 23-12). In the past, women with SLS were treated for their infertility with wedge resection of the fibrous capsule, thus allowing the release of developing follicles. Now, only fertility medication is needed.

COMPLEX CYSTS

A complex cyst retains some of the properties of a simple cyst. It can be irregular or have thickened walls and internal echoes or septations, as long as good through transmission is maintained. If the mass absorbs sound, it is most likely to be solid.

The differential diagnosis includes a wide spectrum of adnexal abnormalities: hemorrhagic cyst (either functioning or nonfunctioning), endometrioma, dermoid, ovarian torsion, abscess, pyosalpinx or hydrosalpinx, and cystic neoplasm (benign and malignant). Less commonly, a nongynecologic complex cyst such as a duplication or mesenteric cyst may be seen in the pelvis. Although very uncommon, necrotic fibroids may present as a complex adnexal mass.

The possibility of malignancy needs to be considered whenever a complex cystic mass is detected. Analysis of its wall thickness, the structure of its inner wall, the presence and thickness of septa, and its echogenicity has been studied and quantitated (Table 23-4). As might be expected, the more abnormal and numerous the ultrasound properties, the greater the likelihood of malignancy. The complementary use of Doppler imaging is

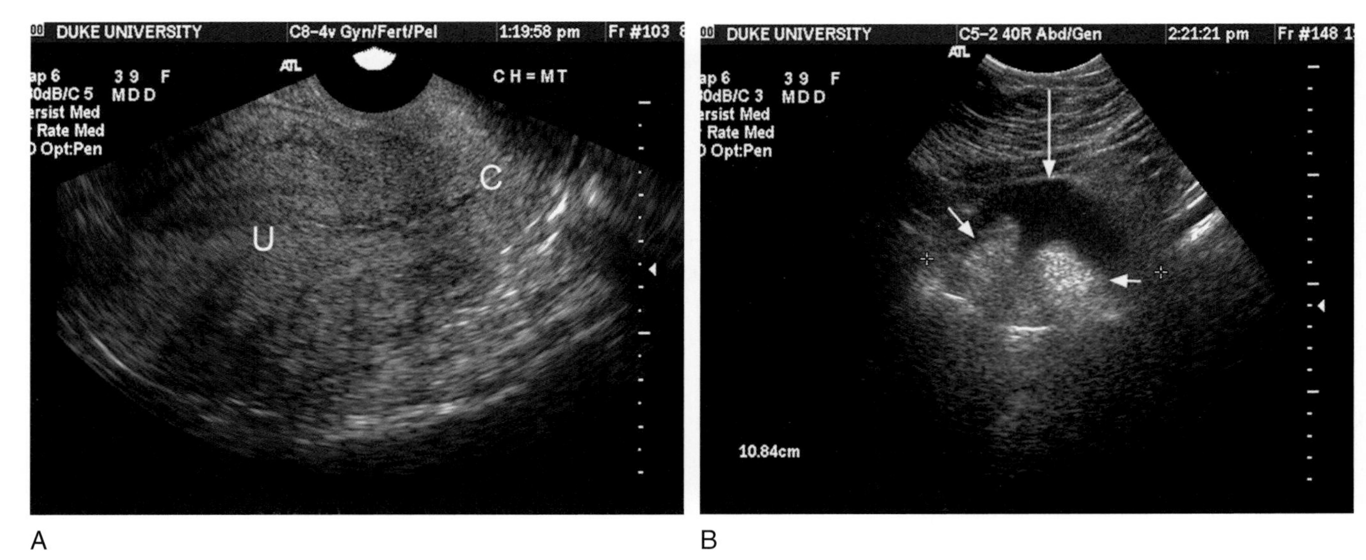

Figure 23-10 Adnexal mass identified at transabdominal but not transvaginal ultrasound. **A,** Longitudinal transvaginal scan of pelvis of a woman with a palpable right adnexal mass shows heterogeneity of the uterine echotexture due to adenomyosis but no evidence of a pelvic mass. Additional extensive transvaginal imaging of the adnexal regions also failed to detect a mass. U, uterus; C, cervix. **B,** Longitudinal transabdominal scan obtained high in the pelvis, above the level of the uterus and urinary bladder shows a large heterogeneous mass *(long arrow)* containing highly echogenic components *(short arrows)*. The mass was not seen at transvaginal ultrasound due to its high position in the pelvis, beyond the field of view of the transvaginal probe. It was surgically removed and corresponded to a dermoid.

discussed later in the section on ovarian malignancy. At present, however, although Doppler findings may be suggestive and additive they are not specific enough to be used by themselves.

Hemorrhagic ovarian cysts exhibit widely variable patterns (Fig. 23-13; see also Figs. 23-4 and 23-9). They may mimic the appearance (size and echogenicity) of a number of other adnexal masses. Because they are predominantly cystic, hemorrhagic ovarian cysts exhibit good through transmission. Additionally, they frequently contain internal echoes, strands and septations, or blood clots, depicted as more solid-appearing focal components along the inner wall or as sheets of echogenicity traversing the middle of the lesion. Because the echogenic internal components correspond to blood products in the lesion, they do not contain flow at Doppler evaluation. Another typical pattern is a uniformly hyperechoic mass that can look like the dermoid plug in a cystic teratoma except that there is surprisingly good through transmission rather than absorption of sound. Hemorrhagic cysts, however, can be of any size (up to 15 cm) and can be of any echogenicity. Unless malignancy is strongly indicated by clinical or ultrasound criteria, or both, it is often prudent to wait one to two menstrual cycles before rendering a diagnosis because almost all hemorrhagic cysts will resolve within 1 to 2 months.

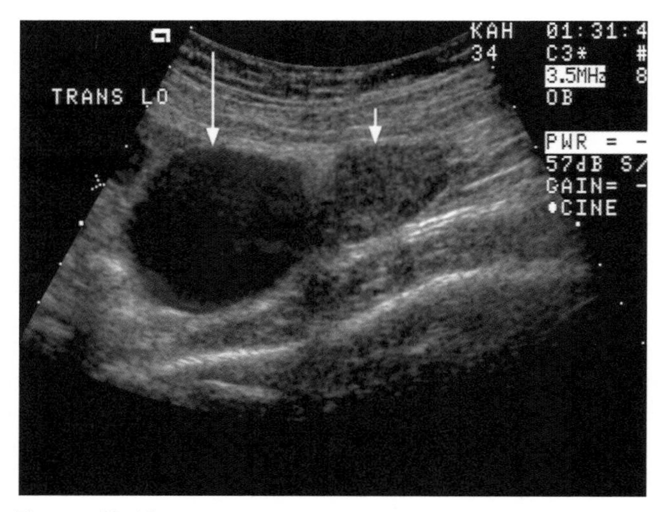

Figure 22-11 Paraovarian cyst. Axial transabdominal scan of left pelvis shows a simple paraovarian cyst *(long arrow)* adjacent to the left ovary *(short arrow)*.

CYSTIC TERATOMA (DERMOID)

Cystic teratomas or dermoids account for 10% to 15% of all ovarian neoplasms. They are benign ovarian tumors and are bilateral in 10% of cases. Dermoids are composed of mature epithelial elements: a combination of skin, hair, desquamated epithelium, and teeth. Their

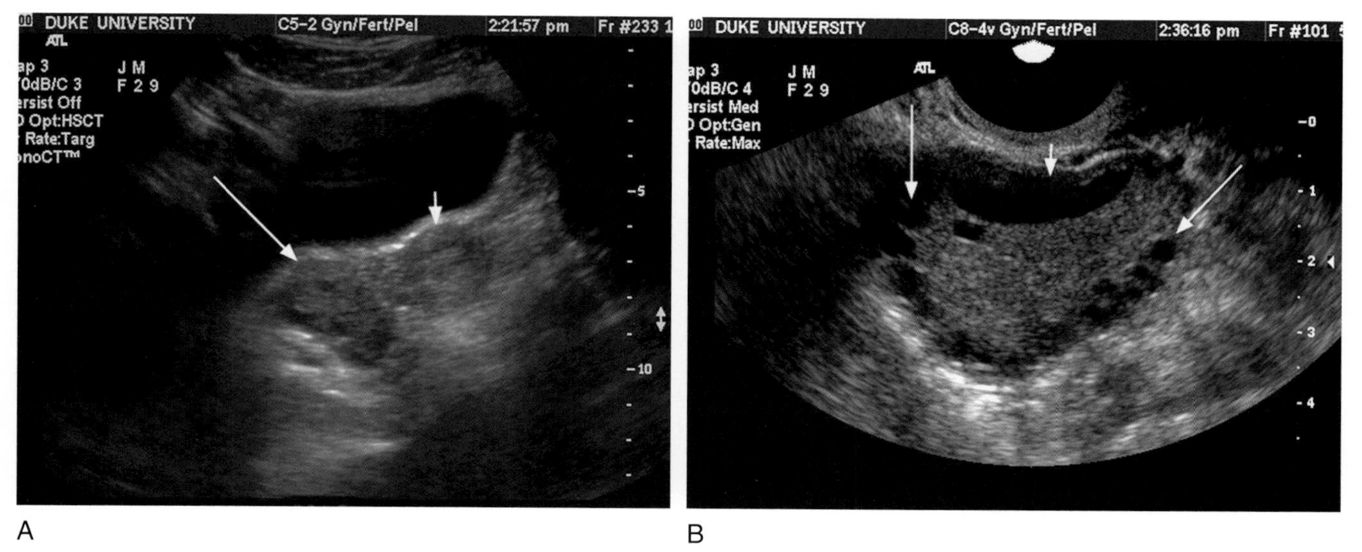

Figure 23-12 Polycystic ovary disease. **A**, Axial transabdominal scan of pelvis in a woman with polycystic ovary disease shows an enlarged right ovary *(long arrow)*. Note the disproportionate size of the ovary compared to the uterus *(short arrow)*. The left ovary *(not shown)* was also enlarged. **B**, Axial scan of right ovary of same patient as in **A** shows "string of pearls" configuration *(long arrows)* due to numerous small cysts just inside the capsule. A larger elongated cyst *(short arrow)* is also seen.

Table 23-4 Scoring System for the Evaluation of Adnexal Masses, Either Ovarian or Extrauterine Masses (If of Uncertain Origin)*

Variables	Mass Evaluation
Wall Thickness	
Thin (≤3mm)	1
Thick (>3mm)	2
Not applicable, mostly solid	3
Inner Wall Structure	
Smooth	1
Irregularities	2
Papillary projections >3 mm	3
Not applicable, mostly solid	4
Septa	
No septa	1
Thin (≤3 mm)	2
Thick (>3 mm)	3
Echogenicity	
Anechoic	1
Low echogenicity	2
Low echogenicity with hyperechoic core	3
Mixed echogenicity	4
Hyperechoic	5

*To calculate the total score, add up the individual scores for all four variables (minimum score = 4; maximum score = 15). Benign = 4. The higher the number > 5, the more likely malignant.

Adapted from Sassone AM, et al: Transvaginal sonographic characterization of ovarian disease: Evaluation of a new scoring system to predict ovarian malignancy. Obstet Gynecol 78:70, 1991.

lucency may be detected on radiographs and is due to the presence of pure sebum (a fluid of lipid density).

Dermoids are present from birth. Because of their slow growth, they are typically not detected until the second and third decades of life. Dermoids are relatively soft masses and on physical examination may be difficult to palpate and are frequently either missed or underestimated in size. If large, a dermoid may torse, and then present as acute abdominal pain. They are rarely malignant.

Dermoids range in size and echogenicity (Fig. 23-14). Depending on the extent and admixture of their epithelial elements, the ultrasound patterns can vary markedly, even within a single mass. There are, however, some typical patterns. The two "classic" dermoid appearances are the "tip of the iceberg" sign (Fig. 23-14A and B), caused by absorption of most of the ultrasound beam at the top of the mass (because of multiple internal interfaces) and the "dermoid plug" sign (Figs. 23-14C to F), which has the appearance of one or more hyperechoic rounded areas within a hypoechoic mass. The "tip of the iceberg" sign helps differentiate a typical dermoid from a typical hemorrhagic cyst .

Another less commonly seen, but more specific, dermoid appearance is identification of interlacing linear and punctate echoes corresponding to crossing strands of hair within the mass (Fig. 23-14G). Occasionally, a dense calcification corresponding to a completely

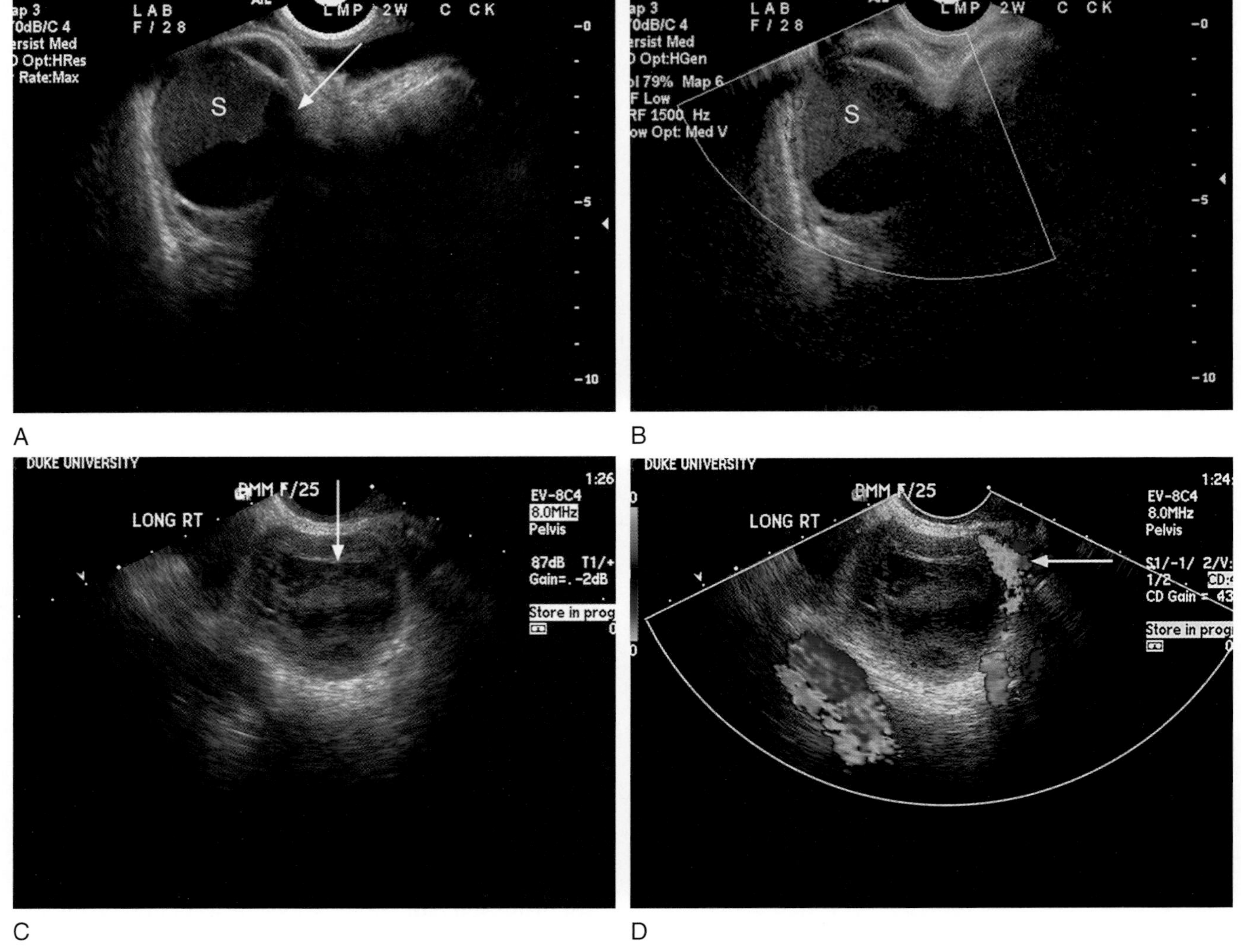

Figure 23-13 Examples of hemorrhagic ovarian cysts. Axial ultrasound images of hemorrhagic ovarian cysts that subsequently resolved demonstrate a wide range of appearances. (For additional examples see Figures 23-4 and 23-9.) **A,** Ovarian cyst *(arrow)* containing a more solid-appearing component (S) due to blood clot along inner wall. **B,** Color Doppler scan of the same cyst as in **A** shows no evidence of blood flow within the solid-appearing component (S) in the cyst. The absence of blood flow in the solid-appearing component favors blood clot in a hemorrhagic cyst; blood flow in the solid-appearing component would favor other causes such as a neoplasm. **C,** Ovarian cyst *(arrow)* containing irregular bands of internal echoes due to hemorrhage in the cyst. **D,** Color Doppler scan of the same cyst as in **C** shows no blood flow in cyst. Blood flow *(arrow)* is seen in the ovarian tissue at the periphery of the cyst.

Continued

formed or rudimentary tooth is seen (see Fig. 23-14H) and can be confirmed to be a tooth by a pelvic radiograph or a CT scan (see Fig. 23-14H). Rarely, a lipid-fluid level can be identified within the mass (see Fig. 23-14I) and the fluid level may shift position when the patient moves. Very rarely, dermoids can be almost completely anechoic; this is encountered most commonly in adolescent girls.

A dermoid is often removed in an attempt to save what remains of that ovary. Surgical removal should, however, be delayed 1 or 2 months if a hemorrhagic cyst is a reasonable diagnostic alternative.

ENDOMETRIOSIS

Endometriosis is the presence of endometrial glands or stroma, or both, in abnormal locations. It has two forms. The more common is the external or indirect form, also called endometriosis, which occurs outside

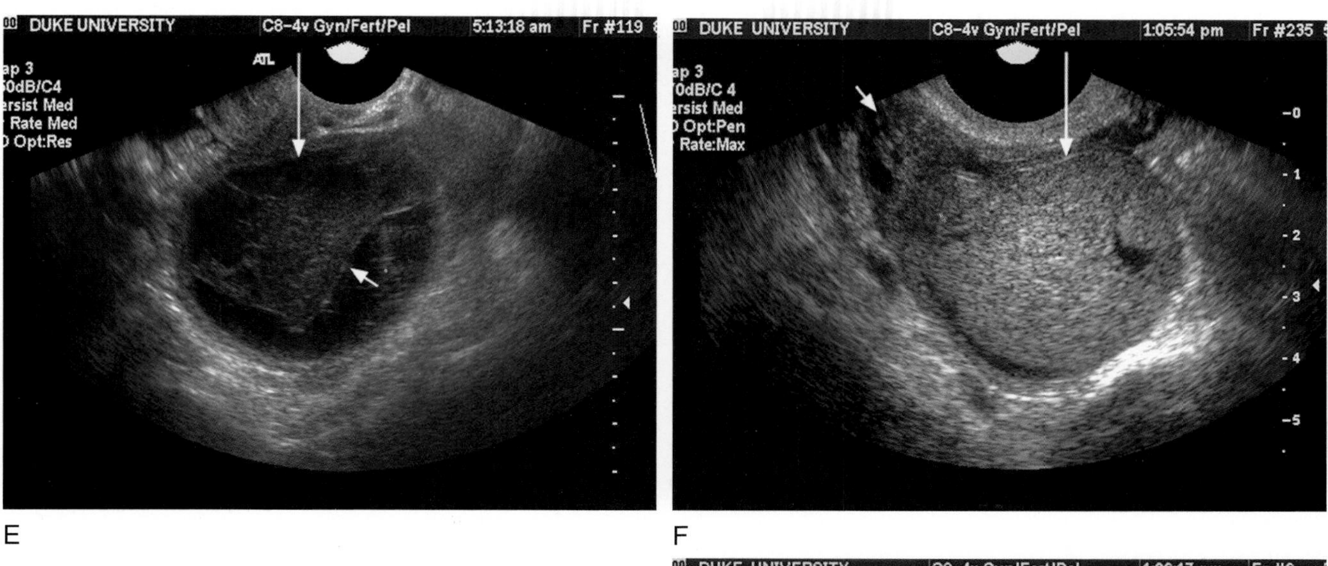

E

F

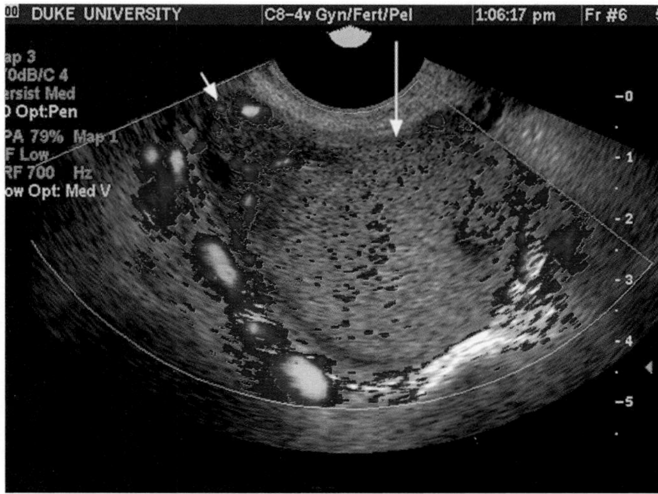

G

Figure 23-13, cont'd **E,** Ovarian cyst *(long arrow)* containing irregular region of solid-appearing tissue *(short arrow)* due to hemorrhage. **F,** Hyperechoic mass *(long arrow)* originating from ovary *(short arrow)* has appearance similar to an echogenic dermoid. The increased through transmission, however, favors a hemorrhagic cyst. **G,** Power Doppler image of the mass seen in **F** shows blood flow in the unaffected portion of the ovary *(short arrow)* but no blood flow in the hemorrhagic cyst *(long arrow)*. (See also Plate 107B, D, and G.)

the uterus. This external form is usually confined to adnexal structures but may be widely distributed and vary in extent from small foci to widespread sheets of tissue to focal masses (endometriomas). The second form, called the internal or direct form, is also called adenomyosis and is less common. It remains confined within the uterus, invading the junctional zone and the myometrium. Adenomyosis is discussed in Chapter 22.

Both forms of endometriosis may occur in any menstruating female. Classically, the presenting symptoms of endometriosis are the triad of infertility, dysmenorrhea, and dyspareunia. However, this triad is only present in 10% of patients. Symptoms depend on the location and extent. Patients can be asymptomatic if the condition is confined to the ovaries or they can suffer severe pain if it is widespread. Usually the most severe symptoms are associated with adenomyosis. Although typically associated with infertility, endometriosis may even be identified in a pregnant patient.

The ability of ultrasound to identify and confirm the clinical diagnosis of endometriosis is variable. If the process is extrauterine, endometriosis is rarely detected sonographically unless a focal mass called an endometrioma is present. The echogenicity of endometriomas varies from cystic to solid and their size varies widely from less than 1 cm to more than 10 cm in diameter. The masses are the result of multiple episodes of bleeding. As a result, a common appearance is that of a rounded mass with homogeneous internal echoes and increased through transmission (Fig. 23-15A). Fluid-fluid levels (Fig. 23-15B) and internal septations (Fig. 23-15C) are frequently seen. Some endometriomas are multiloculated, often with varied internal echo patterns (Fig. 23-15C) and/or interconnecting loculations (Fig. 23-15D). Endometriomas may be multiple and present in both adnexa (Fig 23-15E). As a general rule, the more unusual or varied the echogenicity and the more ovoid or irregular the shape, the more likely the

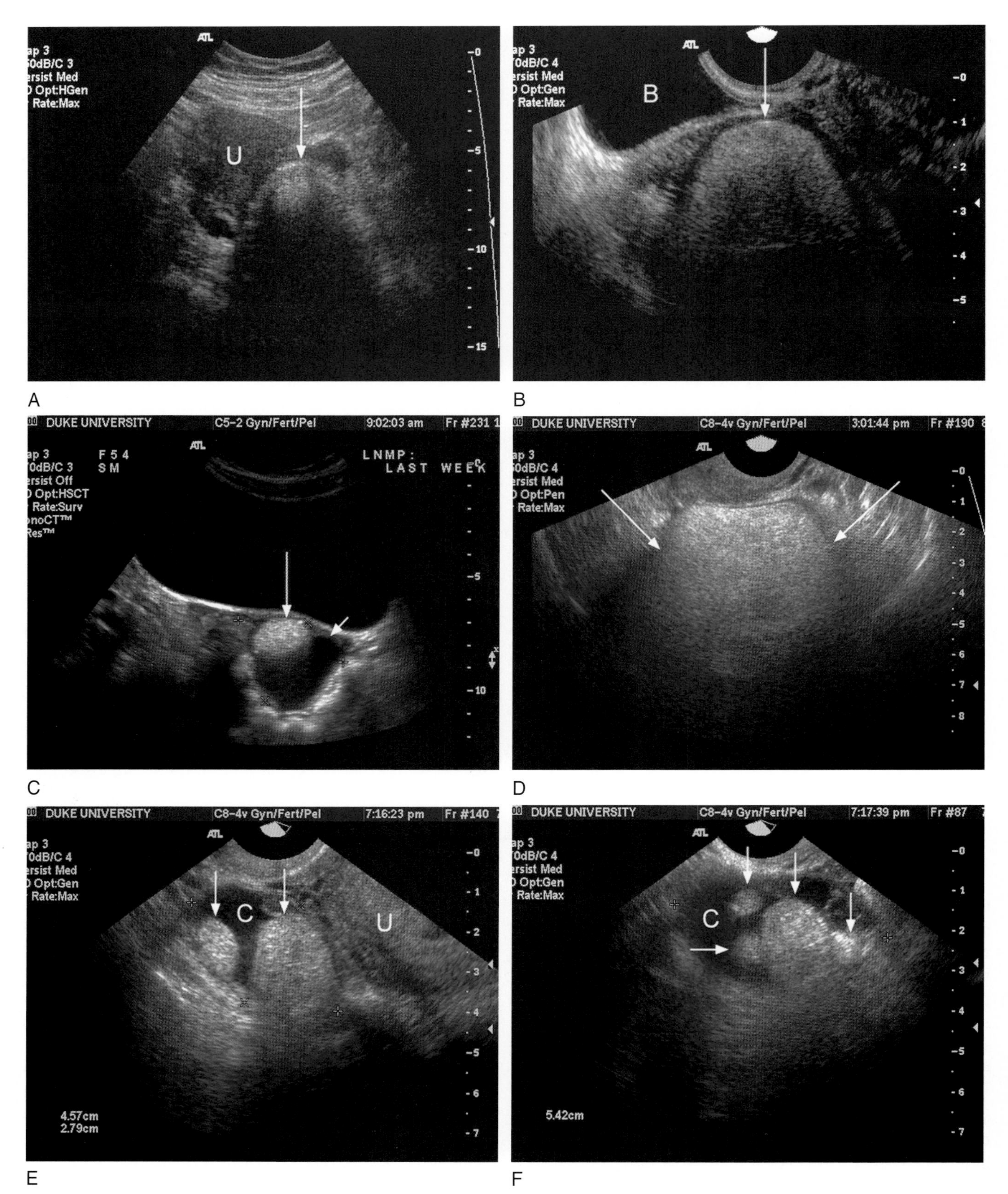

Figure 23-14 Examples of dermoids. **A** and **B,** Tip of iceberg sign. Axial transabdominal (**A**) and transvaginal (**B**) scans of a left ovarian dermoid clearly depict the echogenic superficial portion of the mass ("tip of the iceberg") *(arrow).* The remainder of the mass is not seen due to rapid attenuation of the ultrasound beam. U, uterus; B, bladder. **C,** Small dermoid plug. Longitudinal transabdominal scan of dermoid shows a small hyperechoic area *(long arrow)* corresponding to a dermoid plug in a larger cystic mass *(short arrow).* **D,** Large dermoid plug. Axial transvaginal scan of left ovarian dermoid shows a large rounded echogenic dermoid plug *(arrows)* comprising the majority of the mass. **E** and **F,** Multiple dermoid plugs. Axial (**E**) and longitudinal (**F**) transvaginal scans of a right ovarian dermoid show a complex mass composed of cystic components (C) and multiple rounded echogenic structures *(arrows)* corresponding to dermoid plugs. U, uterus.

Continued

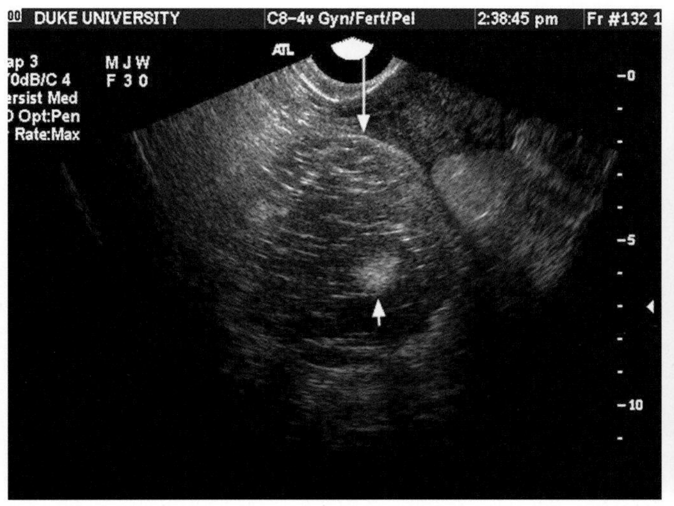

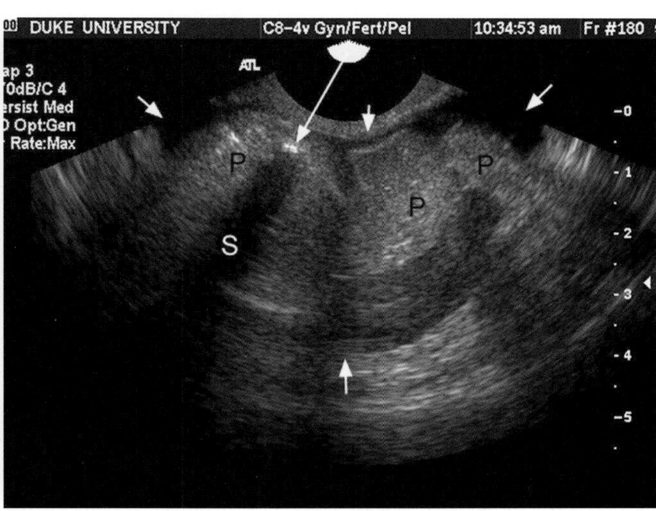

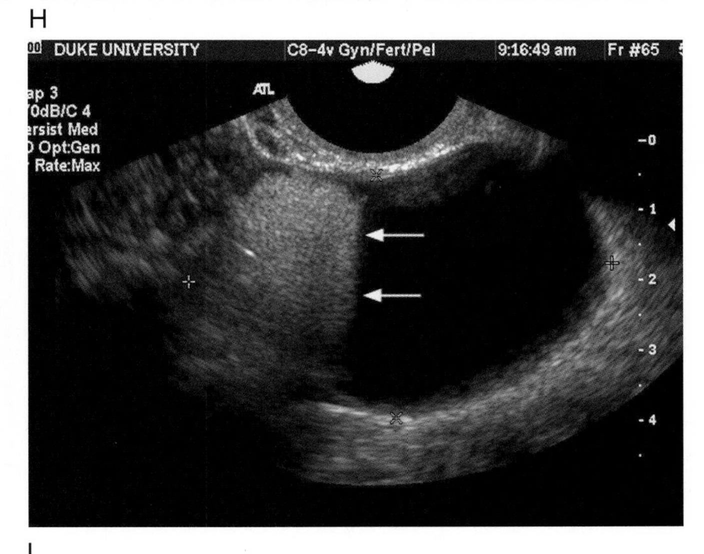

Figure 23-14, cont'd **G,** Hairball. Longitudinal transvaginal scan of right ovarian dermoid *(long arrow)* shows multiple linear and punctate echoes in the mass due to interlacing strands of hair. A small dermoid plug *(short arrow)* is also seen. **H,** Tooth. Axial transvaginal scan of large dermoid *(short arrows)* shows a complex mass with multiple dermoid plugs (P) and a highly echogenic focus *(long arrow)* with posterior shadowing (S) corresponding to a tooth. **I,** Fat-fluid level. Longitudinal transvaginal scan of left ovarian mass shows an abrupt linear change in echogenicity *(arrows)* due to fat-fluid level in dermoid.

mass is an endometrioma. However, on occasion, inflammation (abscess), trophoblastic tissue (ectopic pregnancy), and dermoids can exhibit similar appearances.

PELVIC INFLAMMATORY DISEASE

In the acute phases of pelvic inflammatory disease (PID), salpingitis and, less commonly, endometritis are often clinically apparent, and treatment options have been standardized. An ultrasound examination may not be needed in the acute phase. However, when PID is subacute or chronic, particularly in patients who have not responded appropriately to antibiotics, an ultrasound study may be requested to evaluate for persistent disease and abscess formation. Because PID always involves the fallopian tubes, a search for dilated (damaged) tubes and for pelvic fluid in the cul-de-sac and abscesses should be performed. In addition, if there are abdominal symptoms, an abdominal ultrasound to look for similar infective processes should be performed.

Sonographically, normal fallopian tubes are not identified. Sometimes a normal thin (5-mm) hypoechoic soft tissue band originating from the uterine fundus can be imaged in an axial-coronal view. If distinct tubular structures are instead seen, hydrosalpinges (dilated tubes) are diagnosed (Fig. 23-16A). Although both tubes are almost always damaged, this damage may be asymmetric and only the more dilated tube appreciated sonographically. Although contrast-enhanced salpingography is the definitive test, ultrasound appears accurate in identifying this pathologic process, particularly when performed transvaginally. Occasionally, prominent blood vessels may be present in the adnexa. Although these may initially be misinterpreted as a hydrosalpinx, color or pulsed Doppler imaging will show blood flow in an

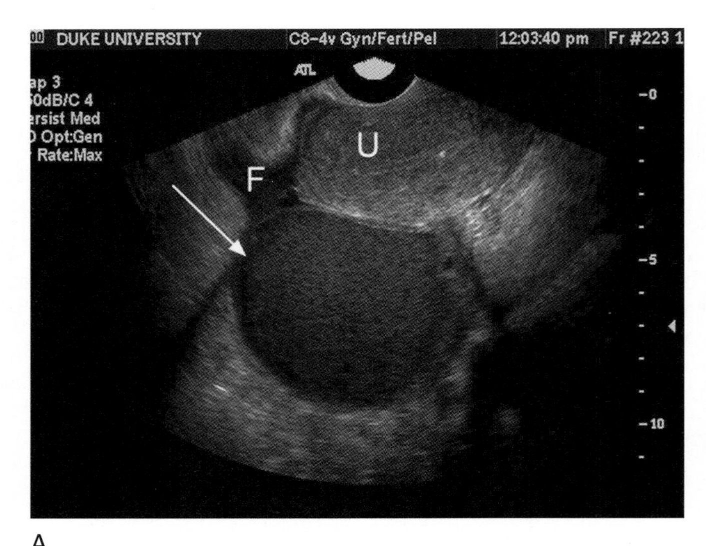

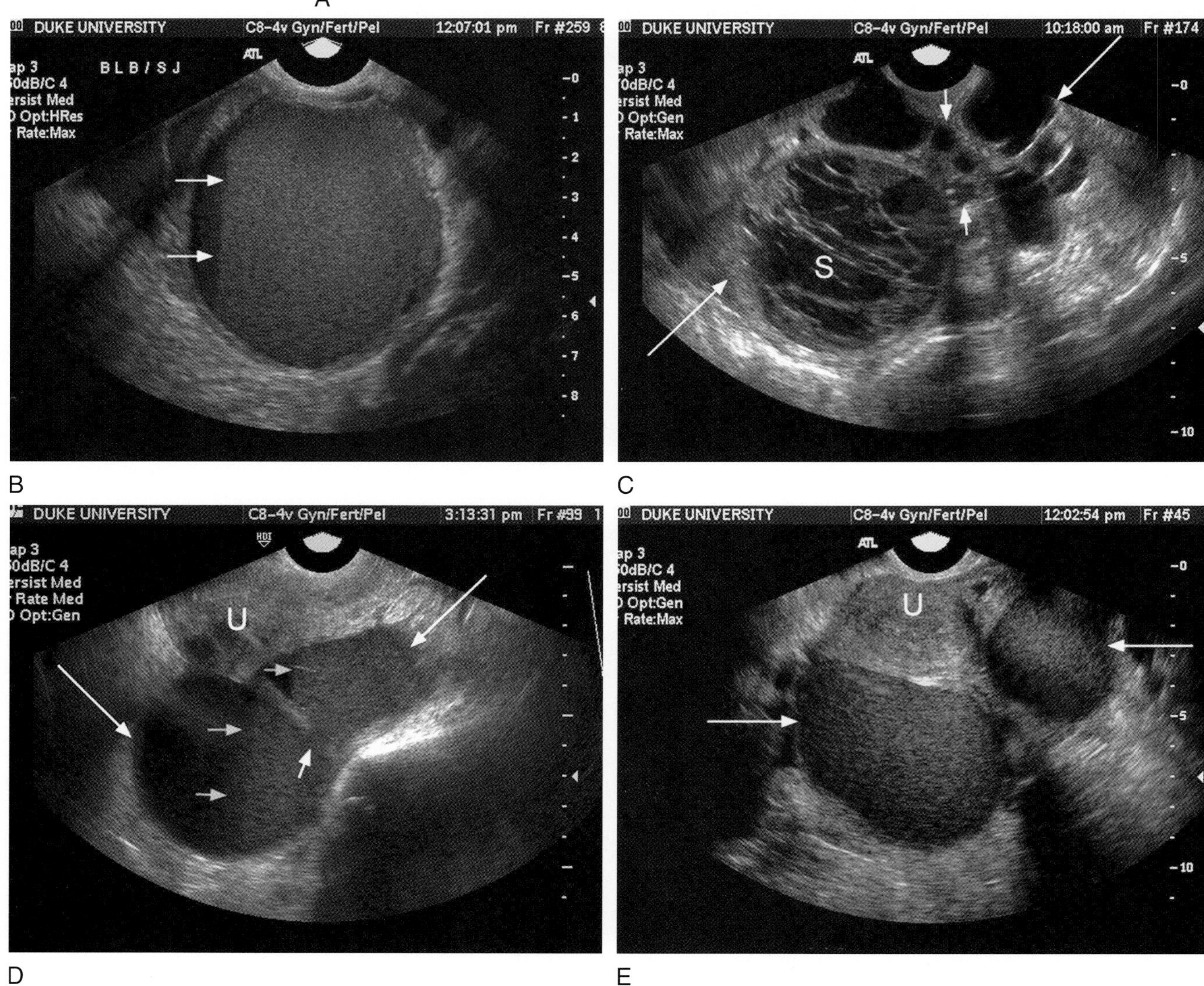

Figure 23-15 Examples of endometriomas. **A,** Longitudinal transvaginal scan shows a rounded mass *(arrow)* with homogeneous internal echoes and increased through transmission. U, uterus; F, small amount of free pelvic fluid. **B,** Longitudinal transvaginal scan depicts a fluid-fluid level *(arrows)* corresponding to settling of blood products in an endometrioma. **C,** Axial transvaginal image shows a large multiloculated endometrioma *(long arrows)* surrounding the left ovary *(short arrows)*. The endometrioma contains components of varying echogenicity, one of which contains numerous internal septations (S). **D,** Longitudinal transvaginal scan shows a biloculated endometrioma *(long white arrows)* with fluid-fluid level *(short gray arrows)* and an interconnection *(short white arrow)* between the loculations. **E,** Axial transvaginal scan shows bilateral ovarian endometriomas *(arrows)*. U, uterus.

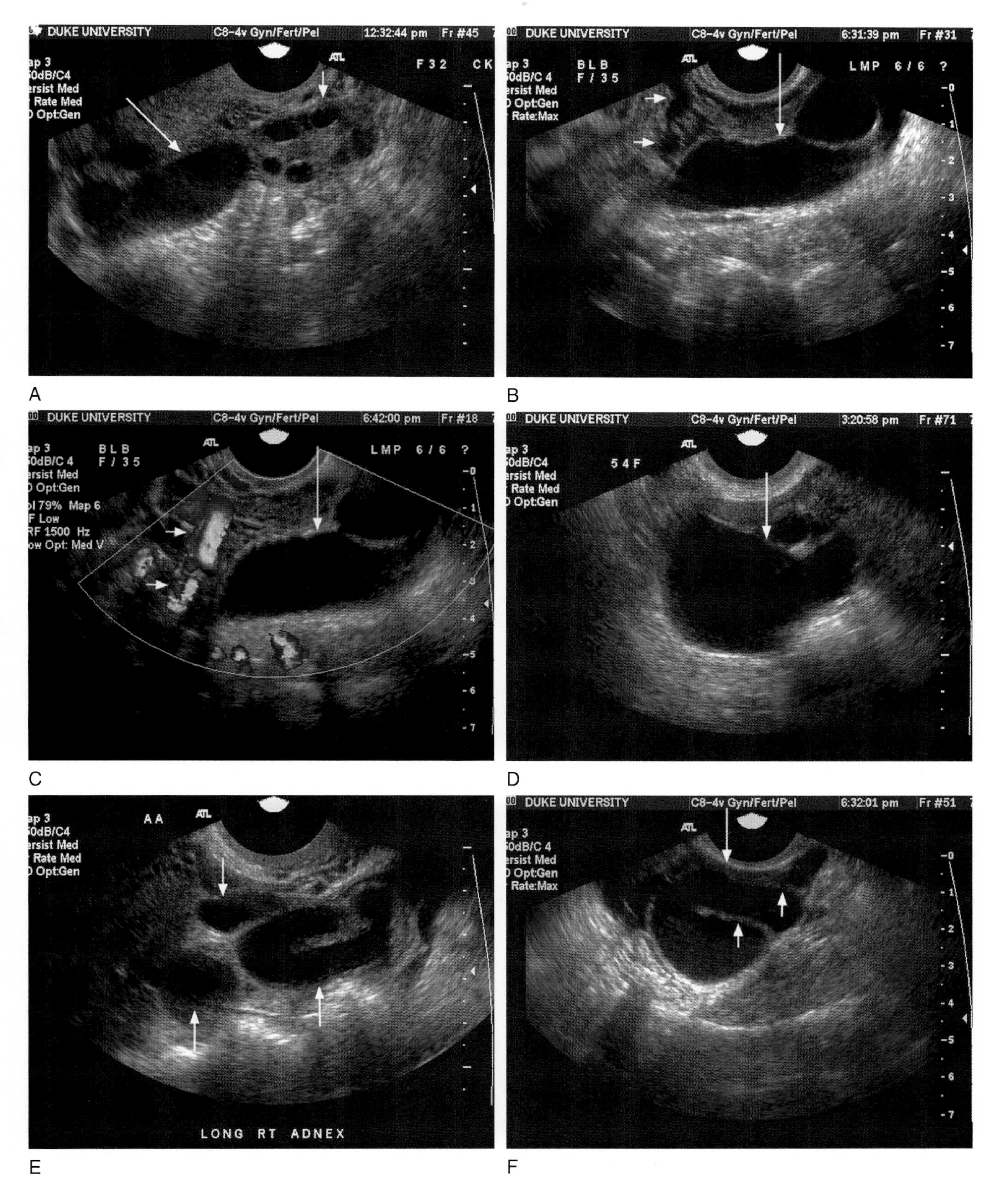

Figure 23-16 Examples of hydrosalpinx. **A,** Axial transvaginal image of left adnexa shows a tubular structure corresponding to hydrosalpinx *(long arrow)* adjacent to left ovary *(short arrow)*. **B,** Longitudinal transvaginal gray-scale scan of left adnexa shows mildly dilated *(short arrows)* and moderately dilated *(long arrow)* tubular structures. **C,** Longitudinal transvaginal color Doppler image of left adnexa of the same patient as in **B** shows the mildly dilated tubular structures *(short arrows)* correspond to adnexal blood vessels whereas the larger tubular structure *(long arrow)* is not vascular, consistent with a hydrosalpinx. **D,** Axial transvaginal scan of right adnexa shows an irregularly shaped cystic area *(arrow)* due to a hydrosalpinx, which was initially thought to be a cystic pelvic mass. **E,** Longitudinal transvaginal image of right adnexa shows several segments *(arrows)* of a tortuous hydrosalpinx. **F,** Axial transvaginal image of a hydrosalpinx *(long arrow)* depicts several prominent mucosal folds *(short arrows)* in the dilated tube.

adnexal blood vessel and no flow in a hydrosalpinx (Fig. 23-16B and C).

Hydrosalpinx has variable presentations from a subtle dilated tubular structure of only several millimeters in diameter to a massive tortuous 5 to 6 cm in diameter cystic area, sometimes mistaken for a cystic mass (Fig. 23-16D). If the hydrosalpinx is tortuous, it may be depicted as two or more tubular components (Fig. 23-16E). If the dilated tube has internal echoes, infrequently with a fluid-debris level, it is likely infected and this is called a pyosalpinx. A pyosalpinx can appear as a complex mass. A TV ultrasound is particularly useful for identifying the tubular nature and folds of the dilated tube, thus avoiding the mistaken diagnosis of a mass (Fig. 23-16F).

When a hydrosalpinx or a pyosalpinx is identified, the likelihood of recurrent infection and ectopic pregnancy increases significantly. TA and TV ultrasound can reveal the presence of pelvic intraperitoneal fluid in the cul-de-sac and either a single or multiple abscesses. Pelvic fluid may frequently have internal echoes, septations, and fluid levels (Fig. 23-17A), a sign that the fluid is not simple but rather may be infected or hemorrhagic. Abscesses are typically hypoechoic masses, often with some internal echogenicity and usually with relatively good through transmission (Fig. 23-17B). Their walls are often ill defined and sometimes thick, and they can be multiloculated or contain irregular pockets of pus (Fig. 23-17C). In the setting of extensive PID, the margins of the ovaries and other pelvic structures can become difficult to distinguish from each other. The echogenic inflammatory material can surround pelvic organs and extends across the midline to the adnexa bilaterally, and pockets of pus can extend into and between pelvic organs (Fig. 23-17D and E).

If the pregnancy test result is positive in a woman with previously treated PID, a careful evaluation of the adnexa is indicated even if a normal intrauterine pregnancy is detected. Primarily because PID is often only partially treated, with fallopian tubes damaged but not destroyed, the incidence of an ectopic pregnancy is significantly increased. The possibility of a heterotopic (a concomitant intrauterine and extrauterine) pregnancy, which in the past had been considered a rare occurrence, is now estimated to be as high as 1 in 4000 pregnancies. Therefore, any adnexal mass except an intraovarian cyst should be considered suggestive of an ectopic pregnancy.

Infrequently, particularly in patients with PID resulting from gonorrhea, a pelvic infection may ascend the right flank, causing a perihepatic inflammation. The pain may mimic liver, gallbladder, and even right renal pain. Perihepatic inflammation can be detected sonographically by scanning along the liver margin and identifying a hypoechoic rim between the liver and the adjacent ribs. This perihepatic inflammation is called the Fitz-Hugh-Curtis syndrome.

OVARIAN TORSION

Ovarian torsion is an unusual but serious problem because it accounts for 3% of gynecologic operative emergencies. Torsion typically involves not only the ovary but frequently also the fallopian tube. It is most common in women during the fertile years and even occurs during pregnancy in 20% of the cases. Torsion may, however, present at any time in female life from childhood to the postmenopausal period. Occasionally, the lead point is an ovarian mass. Once torsion has occurred, there is a 10% increased incidence of torsion occurring in the contralateral adnexa.

Acute severe unilateral pain is typically the presenting symptom in patients with torsion. Intermittent pain may precede the acute pain by weeks. These symptoms can be mimicked by many other pelvic or lower abdominal processes and therefore quite frequently torsion is part of a differential diagnostic list. As a general rule, ovarian torsion is very unlikely when the ovary is normal in size and echo pattern at ultrasound. The torsed ovary is typically enlarged and heterogeneous in appearance, owing to edema, hemorrhage, and/or necrosis (Fig. 23-18A to C). On the other hand, the detection of a complex ovarian mass leads to a range of differential diagnostic possibilities, which includes torsion in the appropriate clinical setting. There is often a lead mass, but in some cases the lead mass is not appreciated because it is mixed in with the necrosis and hemorrhage of the torsed mass. Torsed masses are often large (>4 cm in diameter), vary in their appearance from cystic to solid, and vary in echogenicity from relatively anechoic to markedly hyperechoic.

Sonographically, the differentiation of torsion from other adnexal masses is often not possible unless there is clinical suspicion. Doppler evaluation, particularly color Doppler analysis, appears to have limited value. There may be no detectable Doppler signals in a normal ovary, and asymmetric signals between the two ovaries are often normal during each menstrual cycle. If a mass is detected, its Doppler evaluation may have little diagnostic significance. Documentation of blood flow in an ovary does not exclude torsion (Fig. 23-18D and E). Indeed, Doppler sonography not uncommonly detects arterial and/or venous flow in a torsed ovary. If torsion is intermittent, a "hyperemic" increased diastolic flow during the times when torsion is not present may be seen. Additionally, lack of a detectable Doppler signal within the mass may not be of value because some adnexal masses do not have a detectable Doppler flow.

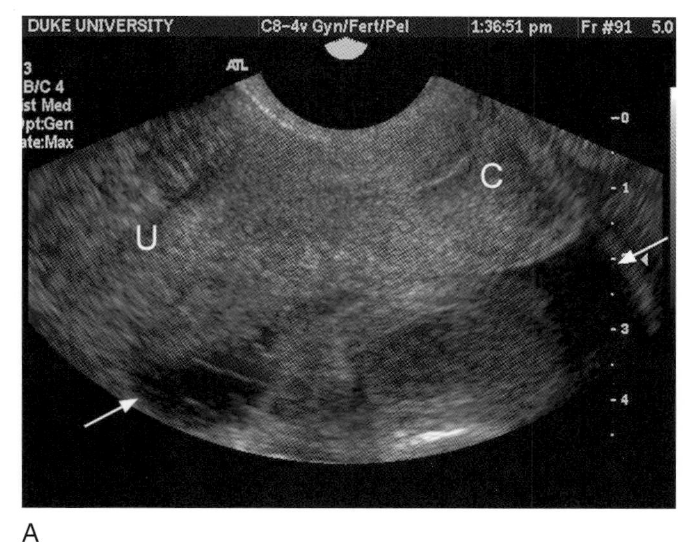

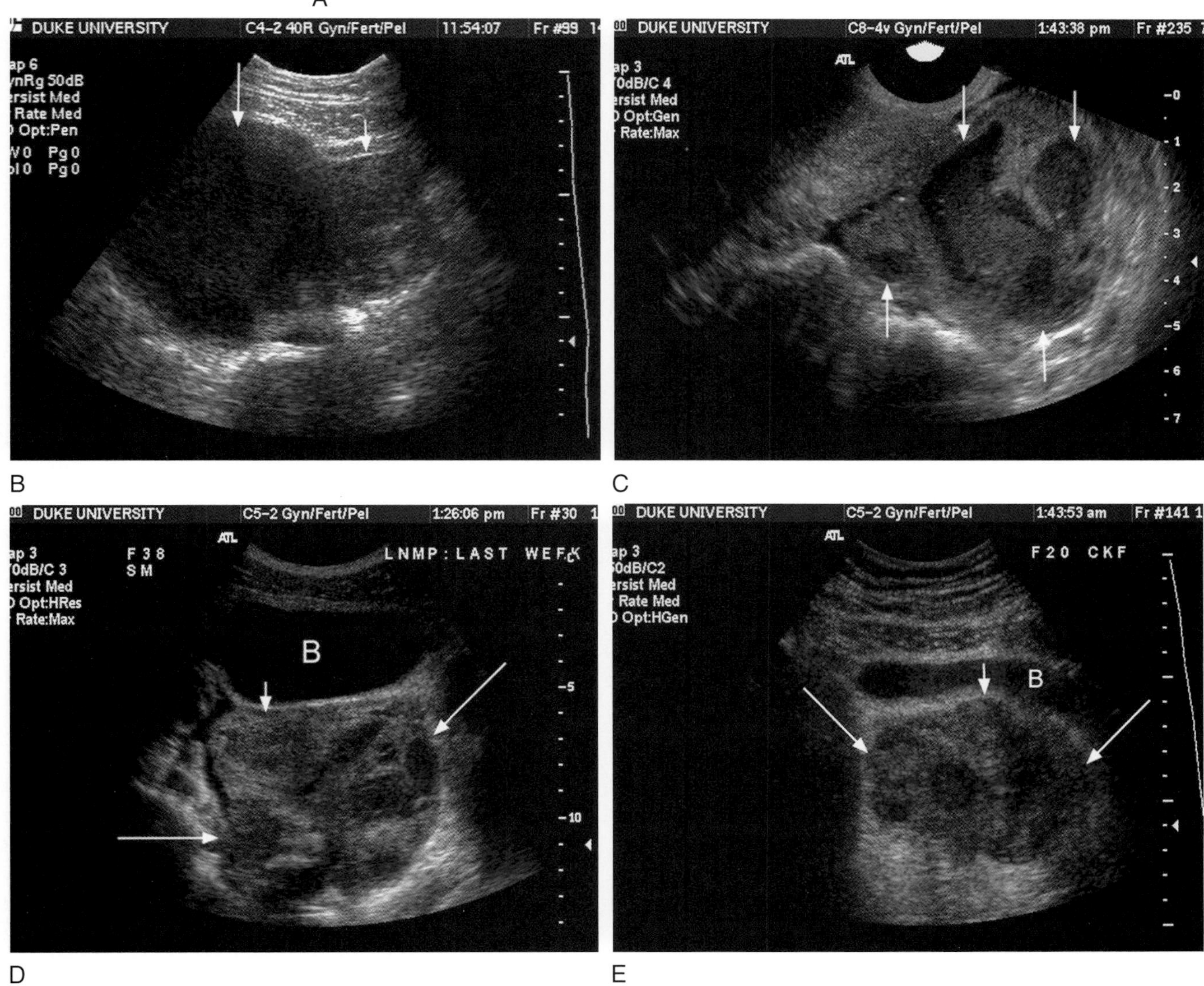

Figure 23-17 Pelvic inflammatory disease (PID). **A,** Infected pelvic fluid. Midline longitudinal transvaginal scan shows complicated fluid collection *(arrows)* with internal echoes and septations posterior to the uterus (U). C, cervix. **B,** Large unilocular pelvic abscess. Transverse transabdominal scan of right pelvis shows a large rounded hypoechoic mass *(long arrow)* with internal echoes due to an abscess in a patient with PID. *Short arrow,* uterus. **C,** Multiple irregular collections of pus. Longitudinal transvaginal scan of left adnexa shows multiple pockets of pus *(arrows)* in ovary and adjacent adnexal tissue. **D** and **E,** Extensive bilateral PID obscuring margins of pelvic organs. Axial transabdominal scans of pelvis in two different patients with severe PID show confluent bilateral adnexal masses with indistinguishable margins *(long arrows)* due to heterogeneous infected material extending throughout the pelvis. *Short arrow,* uterus; B, bladder.

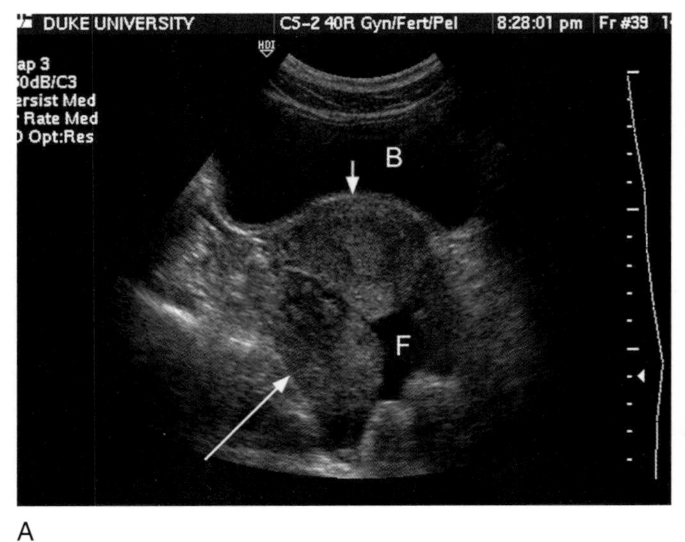

A

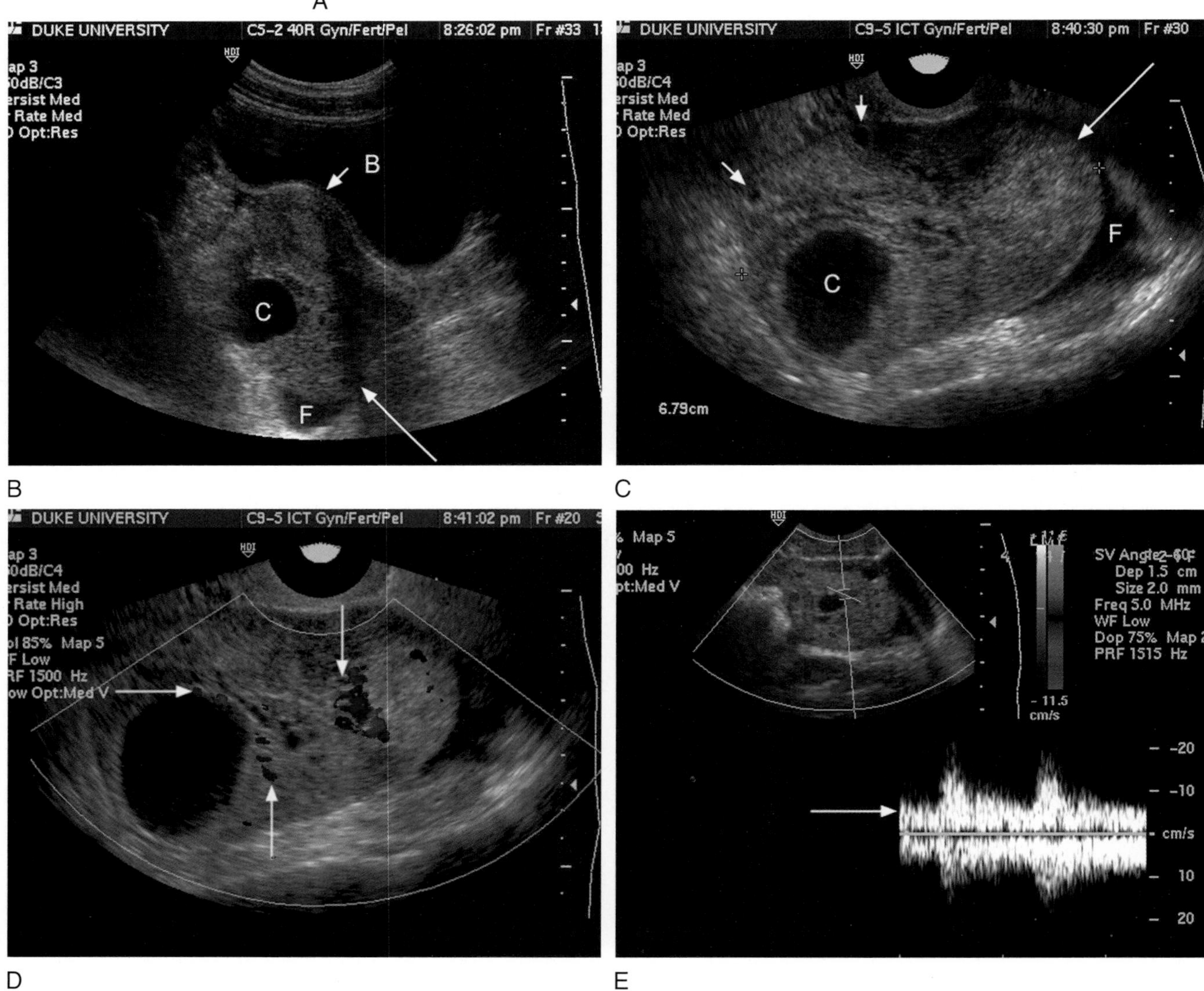

B C D E

Figure 23-18 Ovarian torsion. **A** and **B,** Axial (**A**) and longitudinal (**B**) transabdominal images of pelvis show a heterogeneous right adnexal mass *(long arrow)* corresponding to an enlarged torsed ovary with hemorrhage and necrosis. Short arrow, uterus; F, free fluid; B, bladder; C, corpus luteal cyst. **C,** Longitudinal transvaginal scan of same patient as in **A** and **B** confirms enlargement and abnormal echo pattern of the right ovary *(long arrow),* which contains geographic areas of increased and decreased echogenicity, a corpus luteal cyst (C), and only a few small recognizable follicles *(short arrows).* F, free fluid. **D,** Transvaginal color Doppler image corresponding to the gray-scale image in **C** shows blood flow *(arrows)* in the torsed ovary. **E,** Spectral Doppler evaluation shows arterial flow *(arrow)* but no venous flow in the torsed ovary.

OVARIAN MALIGNANCY

Ovarian cancer is often detected by a combination of physical examination, laboratory, and imaging findings. Because of its availability, an ultrasound examination is almost always the first imaging study used to confirm the suspicion of an adnexal abnormality. Sixty percent of the ovarian malignancies occur in women between 40 and 60 years of age, encompassing both the fertile and postmenopausal periods. The other 40% of cases occur both earlier and later, in women from the early 20s to women into the 90s.

Ovarian malignancy is a "silent" cancer. Because of its relative absence of symptoms early in the disease, ovarian cancer commonly is not detected until advanced, either having spread beyond the capsule but still within the pelvis (stage II) or into the abdomen (stage III). In fact, at the time of initial detection, 50% of women present with stage III spread. The adnexal findings on physical examination are protean, ranging from almost "normal" to slightly enlarged firm irregular ovaries to pelvic masses. In advanced disease, ascites and omental masses may be palpated. The blood chemistry test CA 125 is helpful in some patients but has been disappointing as a screening test because of its lack of ability to detect many cases of ovarian cancer. It has many false-positive and false-negative results, and elevated levels are found in only 50% of patients with stage III ovarian cancer. If a baseline level is known, however, such as in patients who have undergone resection of primary ovarian cancer, then an elevated follow-up level has greater significance.

Ovarian cancer can present as either a complex cystic or a solid mass but is more likely predominantly cystic. As many as 20% are bilateral. Differential diagnosis includes endometriosis, hemorrhagic ovarian cyst, ovarian torsion, PID, and benign ovarian neoplasms (e.g., serous cystadenoma [Fig. 23-19], mucinous cystadenoma

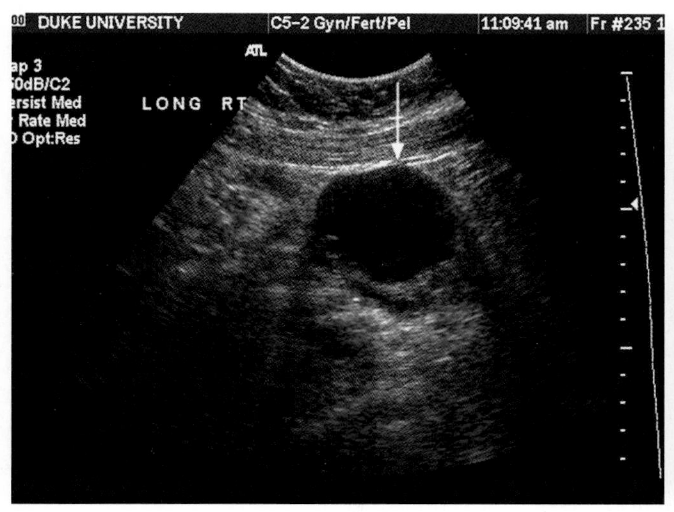

A

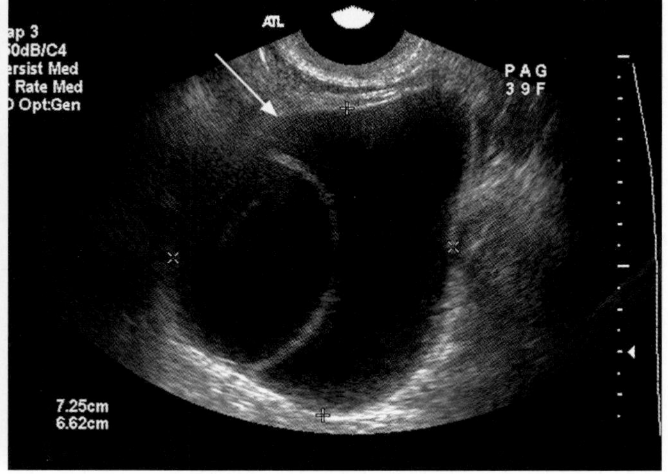

B

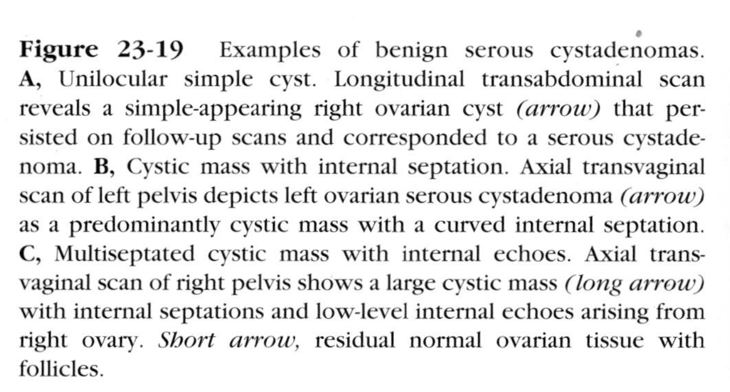

Figure 23-19 Examples of benign serous cystadenomas. **A,** Unilocular simple cyst. Longitudinal transabdominal scan reveals a simple-appearing right ovarian cyst *(arrow)* that persisted on follow-up scans and corresponded to a serous cystadenoma. **B,** Cystic mass with internal septation. Axial transvaginal scan of left pelvis depicts left ovarian serous cystadenoma *(arrow)* as a predominantly cystic mass with a curved internal septation. **C,** Multiseptated cystic mass with internal echoes. Axial transvaginal scan of right pelvis shows a large cystic mass *(long arrow)* with internal septations and low-level internal echoes arising from right ovary. *Short arrow,* residual normal ovarian tissue with follicles.

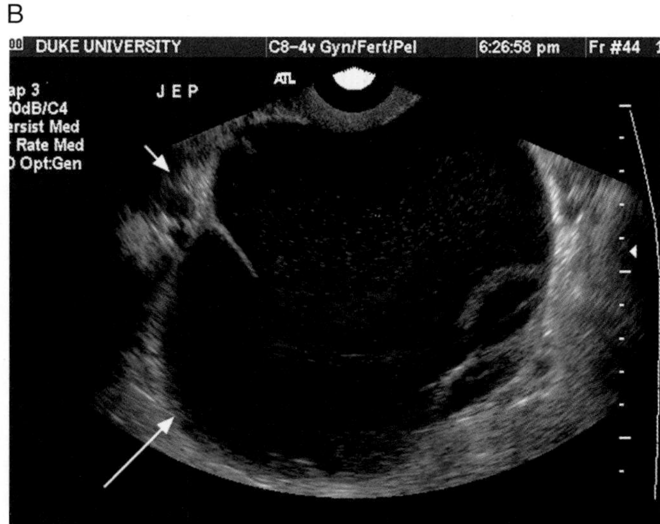

C

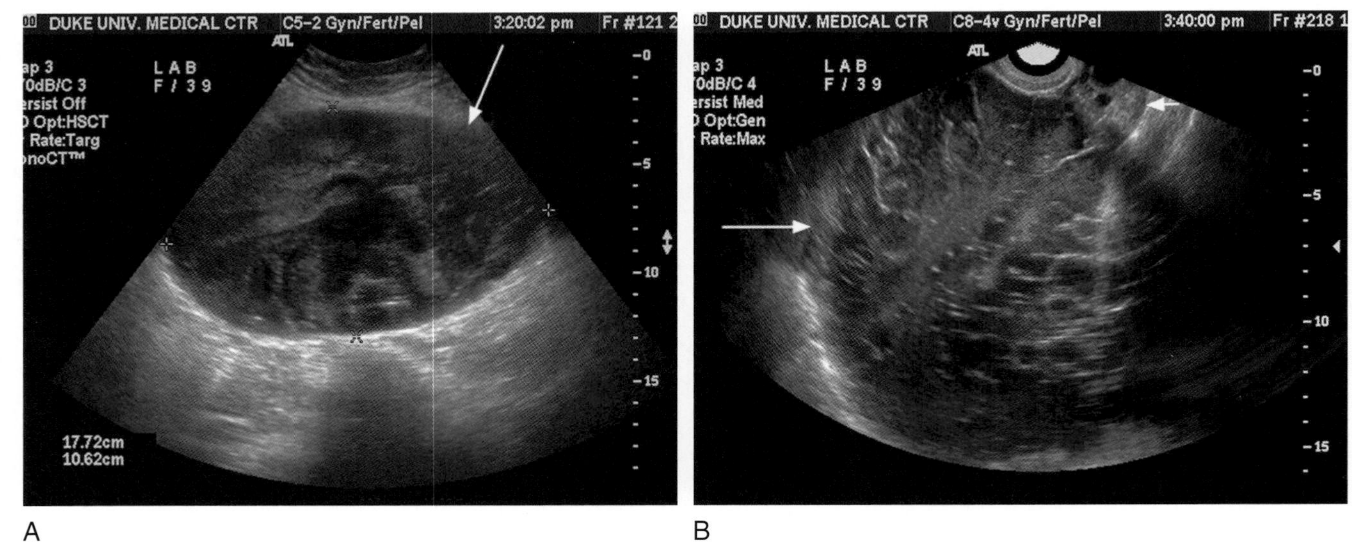

Figure 23-20 Mucinous cystadenoma. **A** and **B,** Axial transabdominal (**A**) and transvaginal (**B**) scans of right ovary show a huge cystic mass *(long arrow)* with internal echoes and numerous septations due to a benign mucinous cystadenoma. *Short arrow,* residual normal ovarian tissue with follicles.

[Fig. 23-20], dermoid [see Fig. 23-14], fibroma, thecoma). An exophytic fibroid or a nongynecologic mass may also appear in the adnexa and resemble an ovarian neoplasm. Unless obvious additional pelvic and abdominal abnormalities exist, such as complex ascites and adenopathy, malignancy cannot be definitively diagnosed before surgery. As a general rule, however, the likelihood of malignancy is increased by the greater the amount of solid tissue in a complex ovarian mass.

Most ovarian cancers are detected as masses. In general, the size of the mass, the age of the patient, and the ultrasound characteristics of the mass relate directly to its potential for being malignant. Masses less than 5 cm in their longest axis are much more likely to be benign; masses larger than 10 cm are much more likely to be malignant; the malignant potential in intermediately sized masses is intermediate. A postmenopausal study on ovarian masses conducted by Rulin and Preston showed that the incidence of malignancy in masses less than 5 cm, 5 to 10 cm, and more than 10 cm in diameter increased from 3% to 11% to 64%, respectively. These incidences might have been lower if premenopausal masses had been included. Increasing age also correlates with an increased incidence of malignancy. In the same postmenopausal study, the incidence of malignancy increased with each decade, from 24% (between the ages 50 and 60 years) to more than 60% (after the age of 80).

Ultrasound characteristics of the mass are also important. Unilocular or thinly septated cysts are more likely to be benign (see Fig. 23-19). Multilocular thickly septated masses and masses with solid nodules are more likely to be malignant (see Table 23-4) (Fig. 23-21). In advanced stages, peritoneal carcinomatosis with malignant ascites and peritoneal implants can be seen (Fig. 23-22).

TA and TV ultrasound by determining ovarian size and echogenicity are also of value in detecting more subtle ovarian abnormalities than can be detected by physical examination. The ovaries are often identified in menstruating women. Their location, size, typical ovoid appearance, and follicles allow for easy detection. Any change in echogenicity and/or volume of more than 20 mL should be considered suspicious. In the postmenopausal period, the ovaries become atrophic, quite frequently do not have follicles, and can be difficult to identify. Only women receiving hormone replacement therapy continue to have normal-sized ovaries. Nevertheless, abnormal ovaries suggestive of malignancy are defined as more than 2 SD above the norm (for the woman's age), as twice the size of the other, or as showing abnormal echogenicity.

The ovaries are more involved with metastatic disease than any other pelvic organ, and these metastases often mimic the appearance of advanced stage II to III primary ovarian cancer. Metastatic cancer can arise from the breast, from the upper gastrointestinal tract, and from other pelvic organs by direct extension or lymphatic spread. Krukenberg tumors are "drop" metastases to the ovaries from the gastrointestinal tract, primarily from the stomach but also from the biliary tract, gallbladder, and pancreas. These masses are typically solid. Cystic metastatic masses appear to result more commonly from

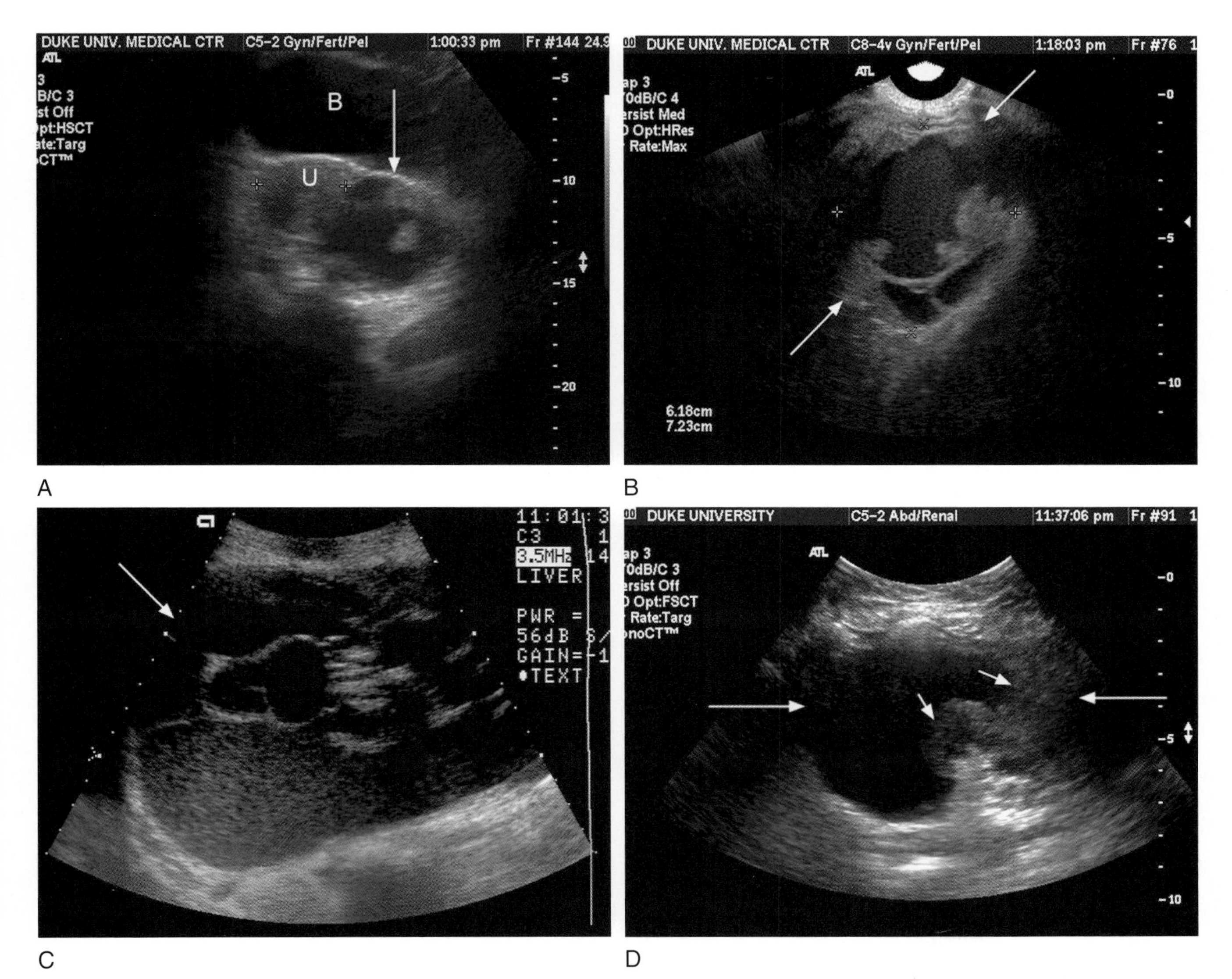

Figure 23-21 Examples of ovarian carcinoma. **A** and **B,** Serous cystadenocarcinoma. Transabdominal (**A**) and transvaginal (**B**) images of complex left ovarian mass *(arrows)* show internal separations and irregular solid components within the mass. U, uterus; B, bladder. **C,** Mucinous cystadenocarcinoma. Longitudinal transabdominal scan of left lower quadrant shows a huge abdominopelvic mass *(arrow)* with internal echoes, septations, and solid components. **D,** Mixed serous cystadenocarcinoma/endometrioid carcinoma. Axial transabdominal scan of right ovary shows complex predominantly cystic mass *(long arrows)* with significant solid components *(short arrows)*. Pathologic evaluation revealed a mixture of serous cystadenocarcinoma and endometrioid carcinoma.

rectosigmoid colon cancers. Regardless of the site of origin, when there are metastases to the ovaries these malignancies are often widespread, with metastasis to the peritoneum (including ascites) and to the mesentery. To further complicate the diagnosis, the incidence of ovarian cancer is greatly increased in women who have had breast and colon cancer. This appears primarily related to genetic mutations in the *BRCA1* and *BRCA2* genes and less commonly in the *MSH2* and *MLH1* genes.

While ultrasound is able to identify masses and subtle changes in ovaries, it is not often able to distinguish benign from malignant lesions. Doppler imaging has been studied to determine if it can detect the neovascularity of malignant masses. Color Doppler analysis is used to survey large areas of tissue and identify areas of flow. Pulsed Doppler imaging is then performed to analyze, if detected, its arterial component. At present, only the solid and complex soft tissue areas of the abnormal ovary or mass have been evaluated. The surrounding soft tissues, their feeding blood vessels, and normal ovaries have not been well studied. When evaluating the soft tissues from the margins of the abnormal ovary or mass, care must be taken so that the sample volume does not obtain flow patterns from adjacent structures.

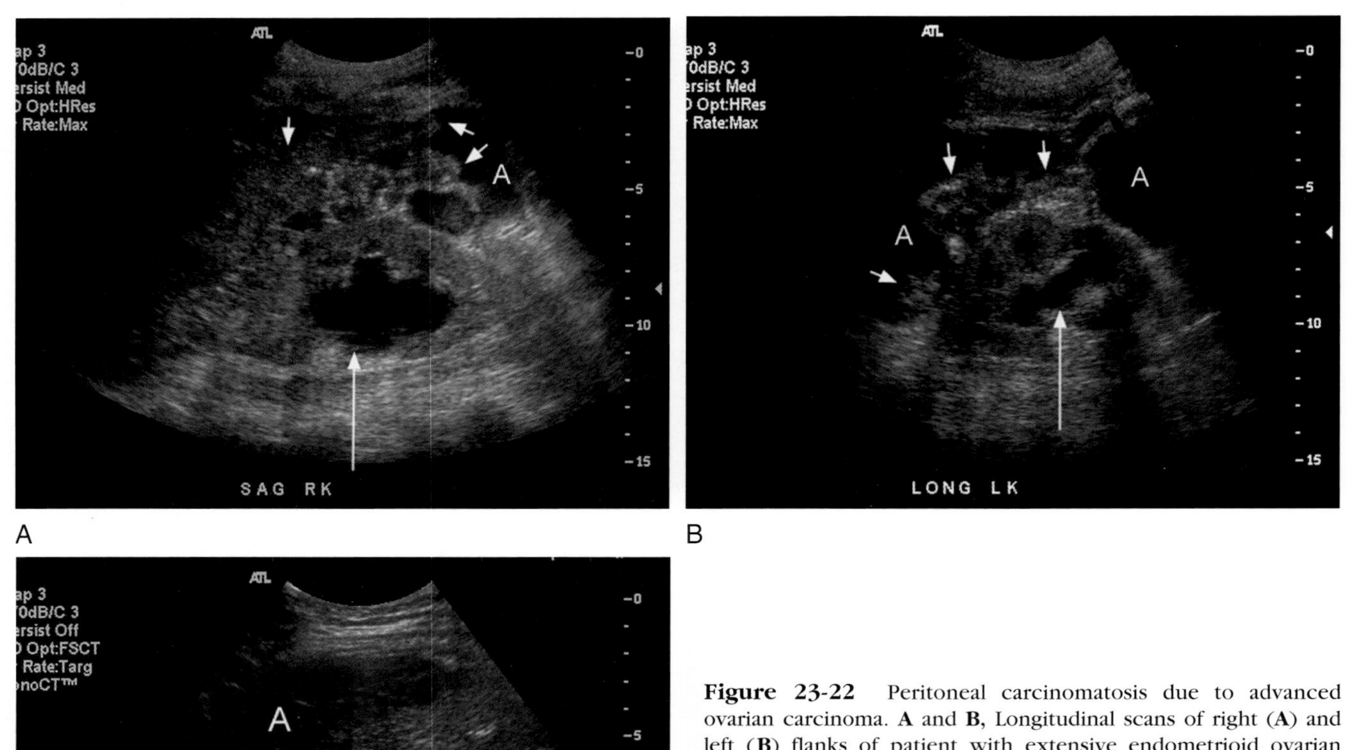

Figure 23-22 Peritoneal carcinomatosis due to advanced ovarian carcinoma. **A** and **B**, Longitudinal scans of right (**A**) and left (**B**) flanks of patient with extensive endometrioid ovarian carcinoma demonstrate malignant ascites (A) containing a large amount of irregular solid tissue *(short arrows)* due to peritoneal implants. There is also bilateral hydronephrosis *(long arrows)* due to ureteral obstruction by pelvic masses. **C**, Axial transabdominal scan of right upper quadrant shows complicated fluid with internal echoes and septations anterior to the liver (L) due to malignant ascites (A).

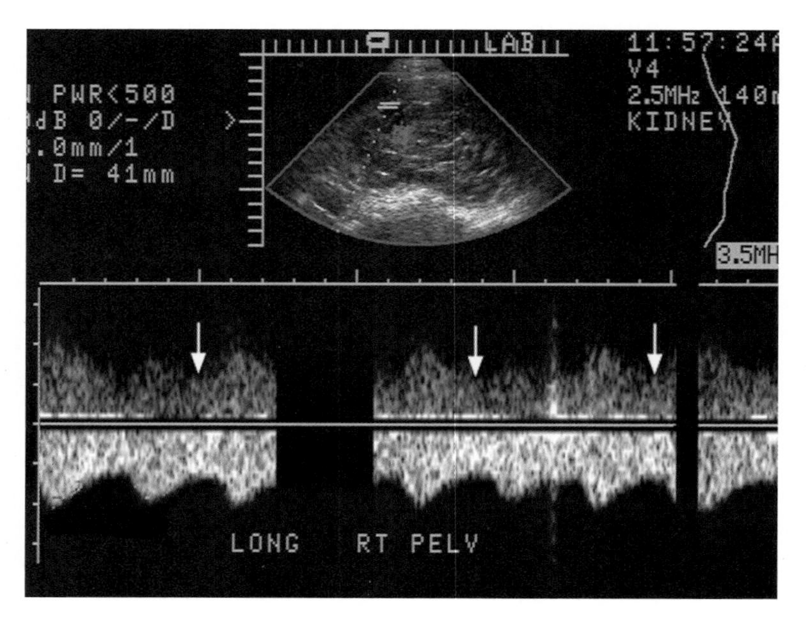

Figure 23-23 Spectral Doppler tracing from ovarian carcinoma. Longitudinal transabdominal scan with spectral Doppler assessment of a right ovarian mucinous cystadenocarcinoma shows a low-resistance waveform with high diastolic flow (*arrows*).

The color Doppler distribution of the small arteries within an ovarian mass may be important. It has been suggested that their presence at the center of an ovarian mass favors malignancy. Two pulsed Doppler indices have also been analyzed, comparing the relative amount of the diastolic to the systolic components of their arterial waveforms. The pulsatility index (PI) is calculated as (peak systolic velocity minus end-diastolic velocity) divided by mean velocity. The resistive index (RI) is the (peak systolic velocity minus the end-diastolic velocity) divided by the peak systolic velocity. Although both indices have different cut-off values, with both, increased diastolic flow suggests neovascularity and the likelihood of malignancy (Fig. 23-23). The cut-off value for the PI is 1.0 and the value for the RI is 0.4, with malignancy considered more likely below and benignity more likely above these values. Other abnormalities may, however, give low indices, thus mimicking cancer. These include inflammatory masses, active endocrine tumors, and trophoblastic disease (ectopic pregnancies). In addition, many index values are borderline, making differentiation impossible.

A mass showing a complete absence of or very little diastolic flow (very elevated RI and PI values) is usually benign. A diastolic notch (in early diastole) may also be a sign of benignity. In theory this notch is caused by arterial rebound and indicates the presence of a normal smooth muscle wall. Neovascular vessels do not have this smooth muscle and should not have this notch. However, this finding is not often noted and its absence has no diagnostic value.

In the fertile years (menstrual and perimenstrual), the PI and RI values vary considerably during each menstrual cycle and this can complicate the pulse Doppler analysis. In the first 7 days, the flow to the ovaries has the greatest resistance with the lowest diastolic flow and the indices are at their highest. Later in each cycle, the diastolic flow increases particularly to the dominant ovary and may lower the indices sufficiently to falsely suggest a malignant process. A Doppler study can be performed at any time during the cycle. If the indices are in the benign range, they do not need repeating. However, if a suspicious mass is present, the indices suggest possible malignancy and are expected to affect management, a repeat study should be performed to confirm the abnormal indices in the first week of another cycle.

Ultrasound screening for ovarian cancer has been recommended by some examiners. However, screening has many problems when it is applied to the ovaries. For screening to be of value, it is necessary to divide women into two distinct groups: those at such low risk that a "safe" interval between studies can be established and those at higher risk who require more immediate attention. This division is not at present possible with ovarian evaluation. At best, only 80% of postmenopausal ovaries can now be identified sonographically. If all ovaries are not identified, all cannot be examined. Equally fundamental, the doubling time of ovarian cancer is not known and without this information the appropriate reexamination interval cannot be established. It has been estimated that to more completely evaluate ovarian cancer, a very large multiyear study would be needed consisting of up to 100,000 women studied for as much as 10 years. Currently no such study has been published. Because of these basic flaws, screening for ovarian cancer is not generally performed.

Key Features

The ovarian position is not constant. While most commonly lateral to the body of the uterus, the ovaries can be displaced to a more superior position by uterine position, by a uterine mass, or by a pregnancy.

The size of the ovary may be expressed as a volume, calculated by the prolated ellipse formula: length × width × anteroposterior dimension × 0.5.

In the fertile (ovulating) women, usually between 14 and 50 years of age, the ovaries are typically ovoid, have a low-level echogenicity, and have a thin hyperechoic rim. With continually developing follicles (functioning cysts), the appearance or each ovary changes throughout each menstrual cycle.

By mid cycle the dominant follicle is usually between 20 and 25 mm in diameter. It may rarely approach 40 mm.

Fertility medications commonly overstimulate the ovaries to produce multiple enlarged follicles, with each ovary occasionally greater than 20 cm in diameter. When the follicles become so numerous that they involve all of the ovarian tissue, the possibility of an early ovarian hyperstimulation syndrome (OHS) must be considered. OHS can become so severe as to cause a marked transudative ascites requiring hospitalization particularly if the woman becomes pregnant.

In the premenstrual years, the ovaries begin to enlarge from early childhood on with acceleration as puberty approaches. Follicles can be seen at any time and are usually 4 to 8 mm in diameter.

In the postmenopausal period, in the absence of hormone replacement therapy, the ovaries steadily shrink. Follicles can, however, still be identified in up to 20% of women.

Both TA and TV techniques are thought to be equal in their ability to identify the site of origin of an abnormality. TV ultrasound is superior, however, in characterizing an abnormality.

TA scanning should be performed in most women undergoing an ultrasound examination for the first time, with a TV examination also performed if needed. Often the TV study may be used exclusively for a subsequent evaluation.

Nonfunctioning cysts (persistent and not under hormonal influence) are usually benign and are of either ovarian or para-ovarian in origin. However, a cystic neoplasm cannot be excluded, and the likelihood of malignancy increases when the mass is more than 5 cm in diameter.

Polycystic ovaries have varied presentation but classically appear rounded with multiple small peripherally placed cysts. These can be clinically related to Stein-Leventhal syndrome, which includes obesity and hirsutism.

The differential diagnosis of complex adnexal cysts includes numerous possibilities. Hemorrhagic cysts, a mimicker of many of these cystic masses, will often resolve or markedly decrease within 4 to 6 weeks. Therefore, unless malignancy is strongly suspected, a follow-up study should be performed.

Cystic teratomas (dermoids) are benign masses of varied size and echogenicity, typically found in young women. The most "classic" patterns are the "tip of the iceberg" sign, the "dermoid plug" sign, the "target" sign, and a lipid-fluid level. A dermoid is also diagnosed if sharp shadowing can be identified and a pelvic radiograph shows a tooth.

Endometriosis is the presence of endometrial glands or stroma in abnormal locations and most commonly has two forms: adenomyosis of the uterus and endometriosis of the adnexa.

In many cases, endometriosis is diagnosed on clinical grounds and is not detectable by ultrasound. When identified, it presents as an adnexal mass or masses (endometriomas) of variable echogenicity, shape, and size.

Ultrasound has limited value during acute pelvic inflammatory disease (PID). In the setting of chronic PID, ultrasound can identify dilated fallopian tubes (hydrosalpinx or pyosalpinx), abscess, and complex intraperitoneal fluid.

Ovarian torsion accounts for 3% of gynecologic emergencies. In the context of acute pain or intermittent cyclic worsening pain, an adnexal mass may be torsed. Doppler imaging at present has only limited value in identifying this condition.

Ovarian cancers are complex cystic or solid masses often presenting with advanced disease and suspected in the following setting: mass or masses larger than 5 cm in long axis often with prominent soft tissue, spread into the abdomen especially with ascites, and in a woman of advanced age.

Metastatic disease to the ovaries can mimic advanced primary ovarian malignancy.

Doppler evaluation of an ovarian mass has been shown to be of limited use. If the arterial waveforms show no diastolic flow (i.e., high resistance), these masses are more likely benign. The possibility of ovarian malignancy increases for masses or abnormal ovaries showing increased diastolic flow (low resistance), but this pattern overlaps other diagnostic considerations, including inflammatory disease.

SUGGESTED READINGS

Albayram F, Hamper UM: Ovarian and adnexal torsion: Spectrum of sonographic findings with pathologic correlation. J Ultrasound Med 20:1083, 2001.

Andolf E, Jørgensen C: A prospective comparison of transabdominal and transvaginal ultrasound with surgical findings in gynecologic disease. J Ultrasound Med 9:71, 1990.

Andolf E, et al: Ultrasound measurement of the ovarian volume. Acta Obstet Gynecol Scand 66:387, 1987.

Baltarowich OH: Female pelvic organ measurements. In Goldberg BB, Kurtz AB (eds): Atlas of Ultrasound Measurements. Chicago, Year Book Medical, 1990.

Baltarowich OK, et al: The spectrum of sonographic findings in hemorrhagic ovarian cysts. AJR Am J Roentgenol 148:901, 1987.

Barloon TJ, et al: Predictive value of normal endovaginal sonography in excluding disease of the female genital organs and adnexa. J Ultrasound Med 13:395, 1994.

Bohm-Velez M, Mendelson E, Bree R, et al: Ovarian cancer screening. American College of Radiology. ACR Appropriateness Criteria. Radiology 215(S):861, 2000.

Bromley B, Goodman H, Benacerraf BR: Comparison between sonographic morphology and Doppler waveform for the diagnosis of ovarian malignancy. Obstet Gynecol 83:434, 1994.

Brown DL, Doubilet PM, Miller FH, et al: Benign and malignant ovarian masses: Selection of the most discriminating gray-scale and Doppler sonographic features. Radiology 208:103, 1998.

Brown DL, et al: Ovarian masses: Can benign and malignant lesions be differentiated with color and pulse Doppler US. Radiology 190:333, 1994.

Cohen HL, Tice HM, Mandel FS: Ovarian volumes measured by US: Bigger than we think. Radiology 177:189, 1990.

Conway C, Zalud I, Dilena M, et al: Simple cyst in the postmenopausal patient: Detection and management. J Ultrasound Med 17:369, 1998.

Fleischer AC: New developments in the sonographic assessment of ovarian, uterine, and breast vascularity. Semin Ultrasound CT MR 1:42, 2001.

Fleischer AC, Stein SM, Cullinan JA, et al: Color Doppler sonography of adnexal torsion. J Ultrasound Med 14:523, 1995.

Fleischer AC, et al: Assessment of ovarian tumor vascularity with transvaginal color Doppler sonography. J Ultrasound Med 10:563, 1991.

Fried AM, Kenney CM, Stigers KB, et al: Benign pelvic masses: Sonographic spectrum. Radiographics 6:321, 1996.

Garel L, Dubois J, Grignon A, et al: US of the pediatric female pelvis: A clinical perspective. Radiographics 6:1393, 2001.

Hamper UM, et al: Transvaginal color Doppler sonography of adnexal masses: Differences in blood flow impedance in benign and malignant lesions. AJR Am J Roentgenol 160:1225, 1993.

Hertzberg BS, Kliewer MA: Sonography of benign cystic teratoma of the ovary: Pitfalls in diagnosis. AJR Am J Roentgenol 167:1127, 1996.

Hertzberg BS, Kliewer MA, Paulson EK: Ovarian cyst rupture causing hemoperitoneum: Imaging features and the potential for misdiagnosis. Abdom Imag 24:304, 1999.

Jain KA: Prospective evaluation of adnexal masses with endovaginal gray-scale and duplex and color Doppler US: Correlation with pathologic findings. Radiology 191:63, 1994.

Jain KA: Sonographic spectrum of hemorrhagic ovarian cysts. J Ultrasound Med 21:879, 2002.

Kim JS, Woo SK, Suh SJ, et al: Sonographic diagnosis of paraovarian cysts: Value of detecting a separate ipsilateral ovary. AJR Am J Roentgenol 164:1441, 1995.

Kurtz AB, Tsimikas JV, Tempany CM, et al: Diagnosis and staging of ovarian cancer: Comparative values of Doppler and conventional US, CT, and MR imaging correlated with surgery and histopathologic analysis: Report of the Radiology Diagnostic Oncology Group. Radiology 212:19, 1999.

Leibman AJ, Kruse B, McSweeney MB: Transvaginal sonography: Comparison with transabdominal sonography in the diagnosis of pelvic masses. AJR Am J Roentgenol 151:98, 1988.

Levine D: Pelvic Doppler. Semin Ultrasound CT MR 20:239, 1999.

Levine D, Feldstein VA, Babcock CJ, et al: Sonography of ovarian masses: Poor sensitivity of resistive index for identifying malignant lesions. AJR Am J Roentgenol 162:1355, 1994.

Levine D, et al: Simple adnexal cysts: The natural history in postmenopausal women. Radiology 184:653,1992.

Lewis V: Polycystic ovary syndrome: A diagnostic challenge. Obstet Gynecol Clin North Am 28:1, 2001.

Patel MD, Feldstein VA, Lipson SD, et al: Cystic teratomas of the ovary: Diagnostic value of sonography. AJR Am J Roentgenol 171:1061, 1998.

Ritchie WGM: Sonographic evaluation of normal and induced ovulation. Radiology 161:1, 1986.

Rosado WM Jr, et al: Adnexal torsion: Diagnosis by using Doppler sonography. AJR Am J Roentgenol 159:1251, 1992.

Salem S, White LM, Lai J: Doppler sonography of adnexal masses: The predictive value of the pulsatility index in benign and malignant disease. AJR Am J Roentgenol 163:1147, 1994.

Sassone AM, et al: Transvaginal sonographic characterization of ovarian disease: Evaluation of a new scoring system to predict ovarian malignancy. Obstet Gynecol 78:70, 1991.

Sheth S, et al: The variable sonographic appearances of ovarian teratomas: Correlation with CT. AJR Am J Roentgenol 151:331, 1988.

Steer CV, et al: Transvaginal colour flow imaging of the uterine arteries during the ovarian and menstrual cycles. Hum Reprod 5:391, 1990.

Taylor KJW, Schwartz PE: Screening for early ovarian cancer. Radiology 192:1, 1994.

Tepper R, Zalel Y, Markov S, et al: Ovarian volume in postmenopausal women: Suggestions to an ovarian size nomogram for menopausal age. Acta Obstet Gynecol Scand 74:208, 1995.

Tessler FN, et al: Endovaginal sonographic diagnosis of dilated fallopian tubes. AJR Am J Roentgenol 153:523, 1989.

Yeh H-C, Futterweit W, Thornton JC: Polycystic ovarian disease: US features in 104 patients. Radiology 163:111, 1987.

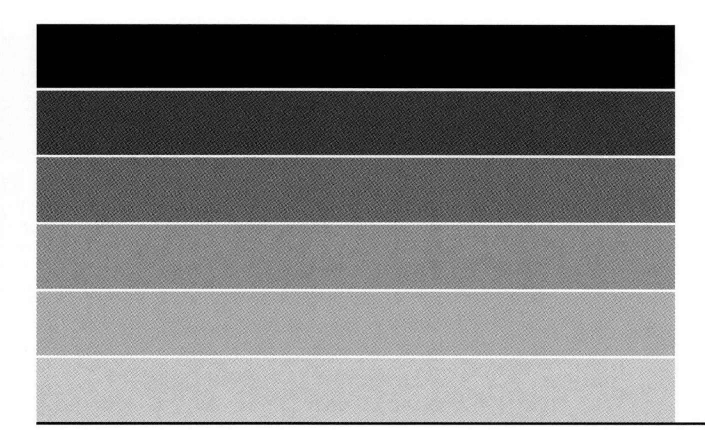

Index

Note: Page numbers followed by the letter f refer to figures, those followed by t refer to tables, and those followed by b refer to boxed material.

B

C

G

M

N